W9-BKF-856

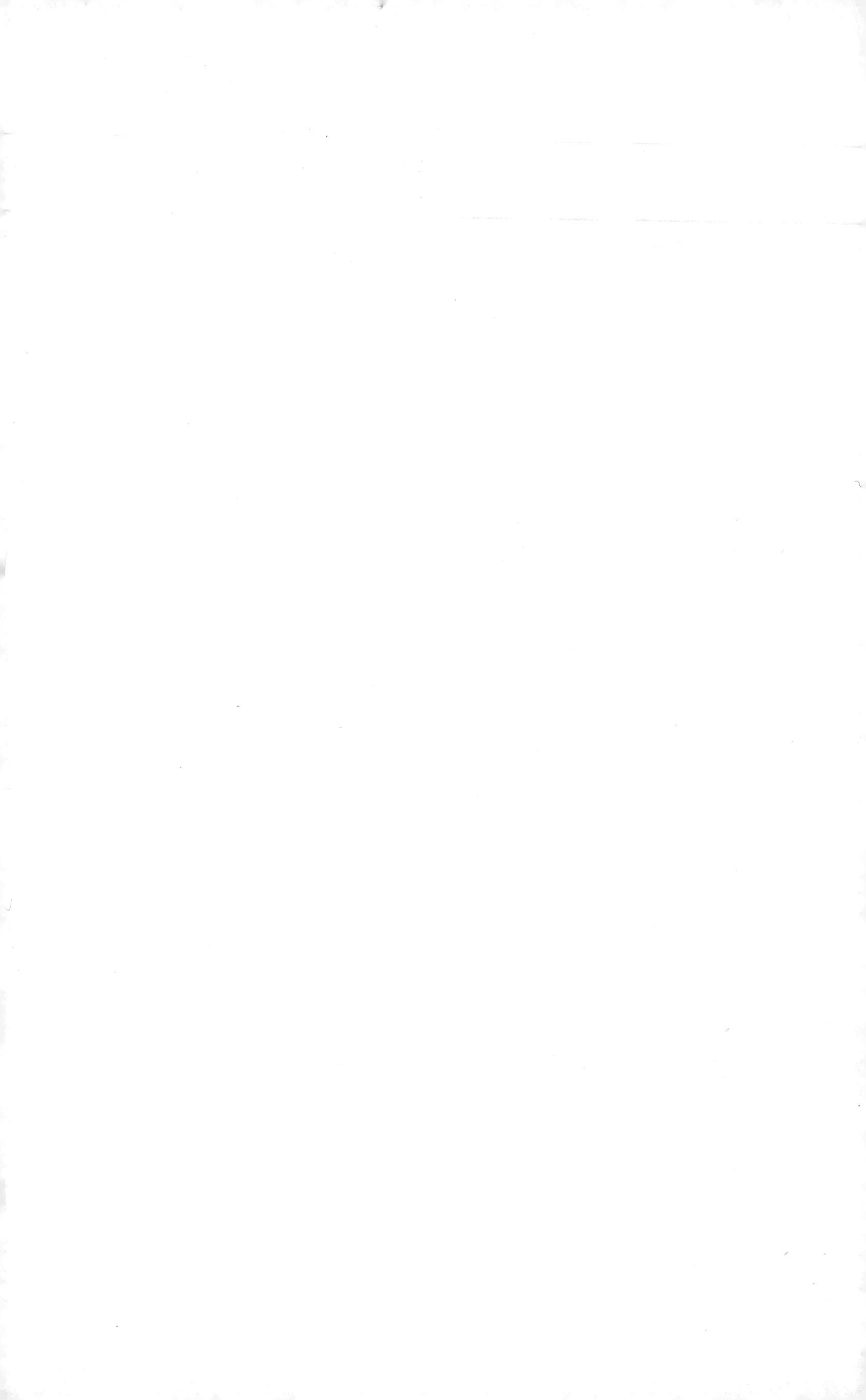

CRC Series in CONTEMPORARY FOOD SCIENCE

Fergus M. Clydesdale, Series Editor
University of Massachusetts, Amherst

Published Titles:

America's Foods Health Messages and Claims: Scientific, Regulatory, and Legal Issues
James E. Tillotson

New Food Product Development: From Concept to Marketplace
Gordon W. Fuller

Food Properties Handbook
Shafiur Rahman

Aseptic Processing and Packaging of Foods: Food Industry Perspectives
Jarius David, V. R. Carlson, and Ralph Graves

The Food Chemistry Laboratory: A Manual for Experimental Foods, Dietetics, and Food Scientists
Connie Weaver

Handbook of Food Spoilage Yeasts
Tibor Deak and Larry R. Beauchat

Food Emulsions: Principles, Practice, and Techniques
David Julian McClements

Getting the Most Out of Your Consultant: A Guide to Selection Through Implementation
Gordon W. Fuller

Antioxidant Status, Diet, Nutrition, and Health
Andreas M. Papas

Forthcoming Titles:

Food Shelf Life Stability
N. A. Michael Eskin and Davis S. Robinson

Bread Staling
Pavinee Chinachoti and Yael Vodovotz

Antioxidant Status, Diet, Nutrition, *and* Health

Edited by

Andreas M. Papas, Ph.D.

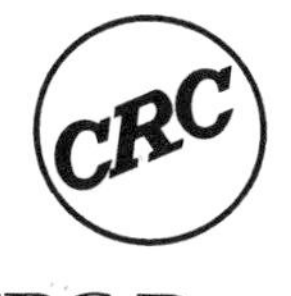

CRC Press
Boca Raton London New York Washington, D.C.

Library of Congress Cataloging-in-Publication Data

Antioxidant status, diet, nutrition and health / editor, Andreas M.
Papas.
p. cm.
Includes index.
ISBN 0-8493-8009-X
1. Antioxidants--Health aspects. 2. Free radicals (Chemistry)-
-Pathophysiology. 3. Nutrition. I. Papas, Andreas M.
RB170.A578 1998
616.07—dc21 98-22208
CIP

This book contains information obtained from authentic and highly regarded sources. Reprinted material is quoted with permission, and sources are indicated. A wide variety of references are listed. Reasonable efforts have been made to publish reliable data and information, but the author and the publisher cannot assume responsibility for the validity of all materials or for the consequences of their use.

Direct all inquiries to CRC Press LLC, 2000 Corporate Blvd., N.W., Boca Raton, Florida 33431.

International Standard Book Number 0-8493-8009-X
Library of Congress Card Number 98-22208
Printed in the United States of America 1 2 3 4 5 6 7 8 9 0
Printed on acid-free paper

Preface

We all know that diet is a major factor affecting human health, and the one single factor that would do much to decrease the incidence of cancer and cardiovascular disease is to encourage consumption of more fruits, grains and vegetables, even in smokers. It is also widely thought that antioxidants in these foods are responsible for some of the beneficial effects, which has led to aggressive marketing of antioxidant "dietary supplements." The evidence is often hard to disentangle from the mass of literature.

This book is an attempt to summarize current knowledge of antioxidant status, diet, nutrition and health. Expert contributors take us effortlessly from the basic chemistry of free radicals and antioxidants through determinations of antioxidant status in humans and how this is affected by specific dietary habits. Each of the major types of antioxidant is carefully reviewed, but the "up-and-coming" agents such as phenolics are not neglected. The effects of antioxidants on a wide range of diseases are considered, including atherosclerosis, skin and colon cancer, eye disorders and neurological diseases. All the chapters carefully and authoritatively balance the evidence and illustrate the difficulties in distinguishing protective effects of diets rich in antioxidants from direct effects of the antioxidants themselves.

This is an excellent book and I recommend it to all who are interested in nutrition, as well as to the whole free radical/antioxidant research community.

Barry Halliwell, D.Sc., Professor
International Antioxidant Research Centre
King's College, University of London

Foreword

Research on the role of antioxidants in human health and disease has advanced from basic metabolic and animal studies to major epidemiological investigations and intervention trials. The vast new knowledge has attracted the interest of the scientific community, but there is also strong public interest for the application of this knowledge in the fields of nutrition, medicine, and public health. To accomplish this, it is necessary to understand the effects of physiological, nutritional and clinical factors on the antioxidant status in humans, and the methods for evaluating it. The ways by which antioxidant compounds affect health status and disease processes need to be better understood. Last, it is essential to bring together the various fields that have contributed to the knowledge concerning antioxidants and their effects and to facilitate the interaction among the scientists who serve these diverse fields. This book represents an important contribution towards these objectives.

This book integrates the basic chemistry of free radicals and antioxidants with practical aspects of diet and nutrition, and evaluates their effects on antioxidant status, health, and disease. Prominent international experts, including biochemists, nutritionists and physicians, contribute to the integration of this very diverse knowledge. The multidisciplinary approach ensures a wide perspective on the status of our knowledge and a balanced discussion of the issues. Thus, it allows physicians and other health professionals to evaluate and apply the emerging knowledge about the role of antioxidants in nutrition, health, and disease.

This book should be useful to a wide range of readers, including students, researchers, physicians and other health professionals who are interested in antioxidants per se, as well as their role in physiological and pathological processes. It covers both theoretical and practical issues and addresses the needs of both the uninitiated and the sophisticated researcher. Antioxidants are likely to be critical in human physiology and pathology, and the reader of this book will be in a favorable position to understand the developments and apply the emerging knowledge in this important field.

Dimitrios Trichopoulos, M.D.
Vincent L. Gregory Professor of Cancer Prevention
Professor of Epidemiology
Harvard School of Public Health

Contributors

Demetrius **Albanes**, M.D., Senior Investigator, Division of Clinical Sciences, National Cancer Institute, 6006 Executive Blvd. Room 321, National Institutes of Health, Bethesda, Maryland 20892-7058 USA

Nathalie **Augè**, Department of Gynecology and Obstetrics, Emory University, Atlanta, Georgia 30322 USA

Angelo **Azzi**, Ph.D., Professor, Institute of Biochemistry and Molecular Biology, University of Bern, Buhlstrasse 28, 3012 Bern, SWITZERLAND

Marvin L. **Bierenbaum**, M.D., Director, Kenneth L. Jordan Research Group, 48 Plymouth Street, Montclair, New Jersey 07042-2625 USA

Jeffrey B. **Blumberg**, Ph.D., Associate Director and Chief, Antioxidants Research Laboratory, USDA Human Nutrition Research Center on Aging, 711 Washington Street, Boston, Massachusetts 02111-1524 USA

Tom W.M. **Boileau**, B.Sc., Division of Nutritional Sciences, University of Illinois, Urbana, Illinois 61801 USA

John W. **Erdman**, Ph.D., Professor and Director, Division of Nutritional Sciences, 451 Bevier Hall University of Illinois, Urbana, Illinois 61801 USA

Angela **Giampaolo**, M.S., 35 High Street #9, Amherst, Massachusetts 01002 USA

Andrew D. **Halpner**, Ph.D., USDA Human Nutrition Research Center on Aging, 711 Washington Street, Boston, Massachusetts 02111-1524 USA

Garry J. **Handelman**, Ph.D., Assistant Professor, USDA Human Nutrition Research Center on Aging, 711 Washington Street, Boston, Massachusetts 0211-1524 USA

Terryl J. **Hartman**, Ph.D., M.P.H., R.D., Senior Staff Fellow, Division of Clinical Sciences, National Cancer Institute, 6006 Executive Blvd. Room 321, National Institutes of Health, Bethesda, Maryland 20892-7058 USA

Charles H. **Hennekens**, M.D., Dr.PH, John Snow Professor of Medicine and Ambulatory Care and Chief, Division of Preventive Medicine Brigham and Women's Hospital, 900 Commonwealth Avenue, Boston, Massachusetts 02215-1204 USA

Suzanne **Hendrich**, Ph.D., Professor, Department of Food Science and Human Nutrition, Iowa State University, 1127 Le Baron Addition, Ames, Iowa 50011-0001 USA

Antonios **Kafatos**, M.D., F.N.C.A. Professor, Director of Preventive Medicine and Nutrition Clinic School of Social Medicine University of Iraklion School of Medicine, P.O. Box 1393, Iraklion, Crete, GREECE

Kim **Kramer-Stickland**, Ph.D., Department of Pharmacology and Toxicology, College of Pharmacy, 1703 Mabel Street, University of Arizona, Tuscon, Arizona 85721 USA

Pagona **Lagiou**, M.D., Athens School of Public Health, 196 Alexandra Avenue, GR115 21 Athens, GREECE

William E. M. **Lands**, Ph.D., Senior Scientific Advisor, NIAAA, NIH, 6000 Executive Blvd., Willco Bldg., Rm 400, Bethesda, Maryland 20892-7003 USA

Sharon **Landvik,** M.S., R.D., Manager VERIS, 5701 Bernard Place Edina, Minnesota 55436 USA

Mark A. **Levine,** M.D., Laboratory of Cell Biology and Kinetics National Institute of Diabetes, Digestive and Kidney Diseases, National Institutes of Health, Bldg. 10, Room 4D5215, Bethesda, Maryland 20892 USA

Daniel **Liebler**, Ph.D., Professor, Department of Pharmacology and Toxicology, College of Pharmacy, 1703 Mabel Street, University of Arizona, Tuscon, Arizona 85721 USA

Hsiao-Kuang **Lin**, M.S., Department of Food Science and Human Nutrition, Ames, Iowa 50011-0001 USA

Maralee **McVean**, Ph.D., Department of Pharmacology and Toxicology, College of Pharmacy, 1703 Mabel Street, University of Arizona, Tuscon, Arizona 85721 USA

Simin N. **Meydani**, Ph.D., Professor of Nutrition, Nutritional Immunology Laboratory USDA Human Nutrition Research Center on Aging, 711 Washington Street, Boston, Massachussetts 02111-1524 USA

Kenneth P. **Mitton**, Ph.D., Ophthalmology Department, Kellogg Eye Center, University of Michigan Medical Center, 1000 Wall Street Ann Arbor, Michigan 48106 USA

Amy C. **Moore**, B.Sc., Division of Nutritional Sciences, University of Illinois, Urbana, Illinois 61801 USA

Patricia A. **Murphy**, Ph.D., Professor, Department of Food Science and Human Nutrition, Iowa State University, 2312 Food Science Bldg., Ames, Iowa 50011 USA

Etsuo **Niki**, Ph.D., Professor, Research Center for Advanced Science and Technology, University of Tokyo, 4-6-1 Komaba, Meguro, Tokyo 153, JAPAN

Noriko **Noguchi**, Ph.D., Research Center for Advanced Science and Technology, University of Tokyo, 4-6-1 Komaba, Meguro, Tokyo 153, JAPAN

Nesrin Kartal **Õzer**, Ph.D., Professor, Department of Biochemistry, Faculty of Medicine, Marmara University, 81326 Haydarpasa, Istanbul, TURKEY

Lester **Packer**, Ph.D., Professor, Department of Molecular and Cell Biology, University of Berkeley, 251 Life Sciences Addition, Berkeley, California 94270-3200 USA

Andreas M. **Papas**, Ph.D., Health and Nutrition, Eastman Chemical Company, PO Box 1974, Kingsport, Tennessee 37662-5230 USA

Sampath **Parthasarathy**, Ph.D., Professor, Emory University School of Medicine, PO Box 21246, Atlanta, Georgia 30322 USA

Robert J. **Pawlosky,** Ph.D., Research Fellow, Laboratory of Membrane Biochemistry and Biophysics, NIAAA National Institutes of Health, 12501 Washington Avenue, Rockville, Maryland 20852 USA

William A. **Pryor**, Ph.D., Director, Biodynamics Institute, Thomas and David Boyd Professor, Louisiana State University, 711 Choppin Hall, Baton Rouge, Louisiana 70803-1800 USA

Steven **Rumsey**, Ph.D., Laboratory of Cell Biology and Kinetics, National Institute of Diabetes, Digestive and Kidney Diseases, National Institutes of Health, Bethesda, Maryland 20892 USA

Norman **Salem**, Ph.D., Chief, Laboratory of Membrane Biochemistry and Biophysics, NIAAA National Institutes of Health, 12501 Washington Avenue, Rockville, Maryland 20852 USA

Nalini **Satanam,** Department of Gynecology and Obstetrics, Emory University, Atlanta, Georgia 30322 USA

Artemis P. **Simopoulos**, M.D., President, The Center for Genetics, Nutrition and Health, 2001 S Street NW, Suite 530, Washington, DC 20009 USA

Ronald J. **Sokol**, M.D., Professor, Department of Pediatric Gastroenterology, University of Colorado School of Medicine, Denver, Colorado 80262 USA

William L. **Stone**, Ph.D., Director, Pediatric Research, Department of Pediatrics, James H. Quillen College of Medicine, East Tennessee State University, Johnson City, Tennessee 37614-0578 USA

Bee-Yen **Tew**, M.S., Department of Food Science and Human Nutrition, Ames, Iowa 50011-0001 USA

John R. **Trevithick**, Ph.D., Professor, Department of Biochemistry, Faculty of Medicine, University of Western Ontario, London, Ontario, CANADA N6A 5C1

Antonia **Trichopoulou**, M.D., Professor, of Nutrition and Biochemistry, Athens School of Public Health, 196 Alexandra Avenue, GR115 21 Athens, GREECE

Gui-Juan **Wang**, M.S., Department of Food Science and Human Nutrition, Ames, Iowa 50011-0001 USA

Huei-Ju **Wang**, Ph.D., Department of Food Science and Human Nutrition, Ames, Iowa 50011-0001 USA

Yaohui **Wang**, Ph.D., Laboratory of Cell Biology and Kinetics, National Institute of Diabetes, Digestive and Kidney Diseases, National Institutes of Health, Bethesda, Maryland 20892 USA

Tom R. **Watkins**, Ph.D., Laboratory Director, Kenneth L. Jordan Heart Foundation and Research Center, 48 Plymouth Street, Montclair, New Jersey 07042-2625 USA

Daywong **Wu**, Ph.D., Nutritional Immunology Laboratory, USDA Human Nutrition Research Center on Aging, 711 Washington Street, Boston, Massachusetts 02111-1524 USA

Xia **Xu**, Ph.D., Department of Food Science and Human Nutrition, Ames Iowa 50011-0001 USA

To Popi and Kostakis

Introduction

This book consists of twenty-seven chapters covering the wide range of topics necessary to achieve its objective of integrating the basic chemistry of free radicals and antioxidants with the effects of diet and physiological stage on antioxidant status in humans in order to understand their impact on nutrition and health. The book is organized in seven parts.

Part 1 focuses on the chemistry of reactive oxygen species and antioxidants, the factors affecting the antioxidant status in humans and the methods for evaluating it.

Part 2 focuses on the role of diet on the antioxidant status. It includes chapters on the evolutionary aspects and genetic variation and the special characteristics of the Mediterranean diet, which has been associated with lower incidence of chronic disease.

Part 3 reviews the major antioxidants present in our diet, including, vitamins A, C, E, carotenoids and antioxidant phytochemicals. It also reviews briefly other major antioxidants including synthetic antioxidants used in foods or as nutritional supplements.

Part 4 focuses on the effects of physiological stage or conditions on antioxidant status. The effects of aging, exercise, prematurity and alcohol consumption are discussed.

Part 5 reviews the proposed mechanisms of action of antioxidants on oxidation of low-density lipoprotein (LDL), immunity, skin carcinomas and colon cancer.

Part 6 focuses on the role of antioxidants in chronic and degenerative diseases. Individual chapters review the role of antioxidants in heart disease, cancer, chronic diseases of the eye, and neurologic diseases.

The final part, Part 7, discusses current issues and emerging research on the role of antioxidants in nutrition and health.

The contributors bring diverse expertise ranging from chemistry, molecular biology, physiology and immunology to nutrition, medicine and public health. They also bring diverse perspectives from their professional experience in academia, government and industry. The high caliber and diversity of the contributors are major assets of this book.

Andreas M. Papas, Ph.D.

Contents

Part 6. Antioxidants and Disease

Part 7. Current Issues and Emerging Research

Epilogue

Index

Part 1

Antioxidant Status in Humans

- Chemistry of Active Oxygen Species and Antioxidants
- Determinants of Antioxidant Status
- Evaluation of Antioxidant Status

1

Chemistry of Active Oxygen Species and Antioxidants

Noriko Noguchi, Ph.D. and Etsuo Niki, Ph.D.
Research Center for Advanced Science and Technology
University of Tokyo, JAPAN

FREE RADICALS AND ACTIVE OXYGEN SPECIES

Introduction

Free radicals are chemical species, which have unpaired electrons. Molecules are composed of atoms and electrons. Electrons are present generally in pairs. However, under certain conditions, molecules have unpaired electrons and as such they are called free radicals. Unpaired electrons usually seek other electrons to become paired. Thus, free radicals are in general reactive and attack other molecules, although some radicals are not reactive but stable enough to have long life. Examples of reactive free radicals are the hydroxyl

0-8493-8009-X/98/$0.00+$.50

($HO^•$) and alkoxyl ($LO^•$) radicals, while the nitric oxide ($^•NO$), vitamin E (tocopheroxyl), and vitamin C (dehydroascorbate) radicals are examples of stable radicals.

Active oxygen species (also known as reactive oxygen species) denote oxygen-containing molecules, which are more active than the triplet oxygen molecule present in air. Superoxide ($O_2^{•-}$), hydrogen peroxide (H_2O_2), hydroxyl radical, and singlet oxygen ($^1O_2$) are accepted as typical active oxygen species, but in broader sense, other species such as alkoxyl radical, peroxyl radical ($LO_2^•$), nitrogen dioxide ($NO_2^•$), lipid hydroperoxide (LOOH), protein hydroperoxide, and hypochlorite (HOCl) are also considered as active oxygen species. Some of them have unpaired electrons and are free radicals, but others are not. Table 1 summarizes the active oxygen species, which are relevant to lipid peroxidation and oxidative stress *in vivo*. Nitric oxide and thiyl radical ($RS^•$), which do not bear unpaired electrons on oxygen are also included.

Table 1
Active Oxygen and Related Species

Radicals		Non-radicals	
$O_2^{•-}$	superoxide	H_2O_2	hydrogen peroxide
$HO^•$	hydroxyl radical	$^1O_2$	singlet oxygen
$HO_2^•$	hydroperoxyl radical	LOOH	lipid hydroperoxide
$L^•$	lipid radical	Fe=O	iron-oxygen complexes
$LO_2^•$	lipid peroxyl radical	HOCl	hypochlorite
$LO^•$	lipid alkoxyl radical		
$NO_2^•$	nitrogen dioxide		
$^•NO$	nitric oxide		
$RS^•$	thiyl radical		
$P^•$	protein radical		

Physiological Functions and Effects

Active oxygen and related species play an important physiological role and, at the same time, they may exert toxic effects as well. The active oxygen species are essential for production of energy, synthesis of biologically essential compounds, and phagocytosis, a critical process of our immune system. They also play a vital role in signal transduction, which is important for cell communication and function. On the other hand, there is now increasing evidence which shows that these active oxygen species may play a causative role in a variety of diseases including heart disease and cancer, and aging. Consequently, the role of antioxidants, which suppress such oxidative damage, has received increased attention. It is important to elucidate the mechanisms and dynamics of the oxidative damage in order to understand its biological significance and develop strategies to prevent it. Both active oxygen species and antioxidants are double-edged swords and the balance of their beneficial and toxic effects is determined by the relative importance of many competing biological reactions.

Formation of Free Radicals and Active Oxygen Species

Free radicals and active oxygen species are formed by various extrinsic and intrinsic sources such as light, heat, and metals. They are formed *in vivo* by various ways at different times and sites as summarized in Table 2.

Reactions of Free Radicals and Active Oxygen Species and Their Reactivities

Free radicals and active oxygen species attack lipids, sugars, proteins, and DNA and induce their oxidation, which may result in oxidative damage such as deterioration of foods, membrane dysfunction, protein modification, enzyme inactivation, and break of DNA strands and modification of its bases. The important reactions of free radicals underlying these events may be classified into the following categories:

1. Hydrogen Atom Transfer Reaction

$$X^\bullet + RH \rightarrow XH + R^\bullet \qquad (1a)$$

$$X^\bullet + RH \rightarrow X^{\bullet -} + RH^{\bullet +} \rightarrow XH + R^\bullet \qquad (1b)$$

2. Addition Reaction

$$X^\bullet + \gt C{=}C\lt \longrightarrow X{-}\overset{|}{\underset{|}{C}}{-}\overset{|}{\underset{|}{C}}{}^\bullet \qquad (2)$$

3. Aromatic Substitution Reaction

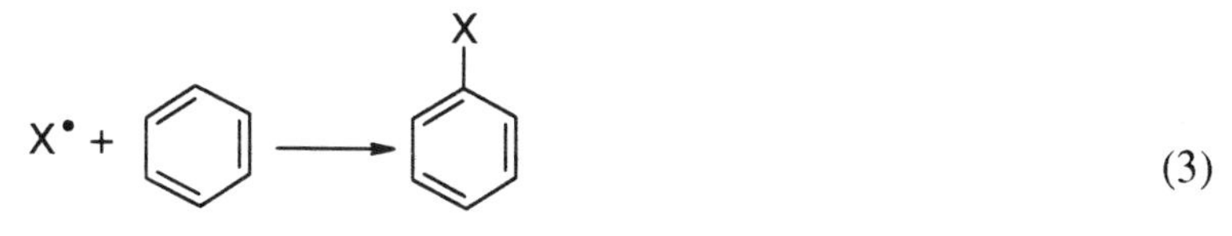

(3)

4. *β*-Scission Reaction

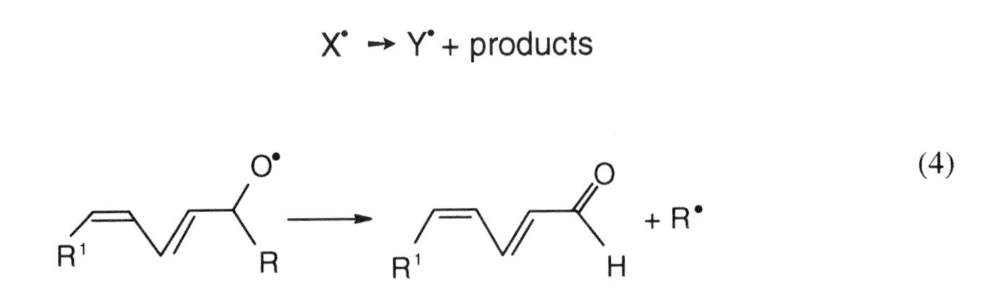

5. Coupling Reactions

$$R^{\bullet} + R^{\bullet} \rightarrow R\text{–}R \tag{5}$$

The hydrogen atom transfer reaction is an important key step in lipid peroxidation, protein modification, and DNA damage. It may proceed by direct hydrogen atom abstraction by free radical (reaction 1a) or by electron transfer reaction followed by proton transfer (reaction 1b). The hydrogen atom abstraction from lipids by peroxyl radicals is the key step in determining the rate and product distribution in lipid peroxidation. They are determined by the reactivities of the attacking radicals as well as those of lipids. Table 3 shows the rate constants for hydrogen atom abstraction from lipids by various free radicals. The reactivities of free radicals toward lipids vary quite extensively by a factor of 10^{10}! The reactivity of the free radical $X^{\bullet}$ can be estimated by the bond dissociation energy of the X–H bond, BDE(X–H). The larger the bond dissociation energy of the X–H bond, the higher the reactivity of $X^{\bullet}$ radical. The bond dissociation energy of HO–H bond is 119 kcal/mol (498 kJ/mol), while that of LOO–H is 88 kcal/mol (368 kJ/mol), and the $HO^{\bullet}$ radical is much more reactive than peroxyl radical in hydrogen atom abstraction.

The bond dissociation energy of the C–H bond being attacked is also important in determining the rate. The bond dissociation energies of the primary, secondary, and tertiary C–H bonds of saturated hydrocarbons are 98, 95, and 92 kcal/mol and those of secondary allylic and bisallylic C–H bonds are 85 and 75 kcal/mol, respectively (Figure 1). The weaker the C–H bond, the faster the hydrogen is abstracted. Hydroxyl radical is so reactive that it is capable of abstracting any type of hydrogen from lipids rapidly, whereas peroxyl radical is much less reactive and it selectively abstracts only reactive hydrogen such as bisallylic hydrogen of polyunsaturated lipids.

Table 2
Production of Active Oxygen Species

Active oxygen species	Formation
Superoxide (Hydoperoxyl radical) $O_2^{\bullet-}$ ($HO_2^{\bullet}$)	Enzymatic and non-enzymatic one electron reduction of oxygen $O_2 + e \rightarrow O_2^{\bullet-} \rightleftarrows HO_2^{\bullet}$ (pK=4.8)
Hydroxyl radical, $HO^{\bullet}$	Radiolysis of water, metal-catalyzed decomposition of hydrogen peroxide, interaction of NO and superoxide $NO + O_2^{\bullet-} \rightarrow ONOO^- \xrightarrow{H^+} HO^{\bullet} + NO_2$
Alkoxyl and peroxyl radicals $LO^{\bullet}$, $LO_2^{\bullet}$	Metal-catalyzed decomposition of hydroperoxides
Hydrogen peroxide, H_2O_2	Dismutation of superoxide, oxidation of sugars
Iron-oxygen complex, Fe=O, etc	Hemoglobin, myoglobin, etc.
Singlet oxygen, $^1O_2$	Photosensitized oxidation, bimolecular interactions between peroxyl radicals, reaction of hypochlorite and hydrogen peroxide
Lipid and protein hydroperoxides	Oxidation of lipids and proteins
Nitrogen dioxide, $NO_2^{\bullet}$	Reaction of peroxyl radical and NO, polluted air and smoking
Nitric oxide, $^{\bullet}NO$	Nitric oxide synthase, nitroso thiol, and polluted air
Thiyl radical, $RS^{\bullet}$	Hydrogen atom transfer from thiols
Protein radical	Hydrogen atom transfer from protein

Table 3
Abstraction of Hydrogen Atom from Lipid by Oxygen Radical

$$X^{\bullet} + LH \xrightarrow{k} XH + L^{\bullet}$$

		-----------------*k*, $M^{-1}s^{-1}$-----------------		
Radical, $X^{\bullet}$	**BDE[a] (X–H) (*k*cal/mol)**	**Saturated**	**Allylic**	**Bis-allylic**
	BDE (L–H)	95	85	75
Hydroxyl, $HO^{\bullet}$	119	10^8	10^9	10^9
Alkoxyl, $LO^{\bullet}$	104	10^5	10^6	10^7
Peroxyl, $LOO^{\bullet}$	88	10^{-2}	1	10^2
Nitrogen dioxide, $NO_2^{\bullet}$	78	0	small	?
Nitric oxide, $^{\bullet}NO$	50	0	0	0

[a] BDE = Bond Dissociation Energy

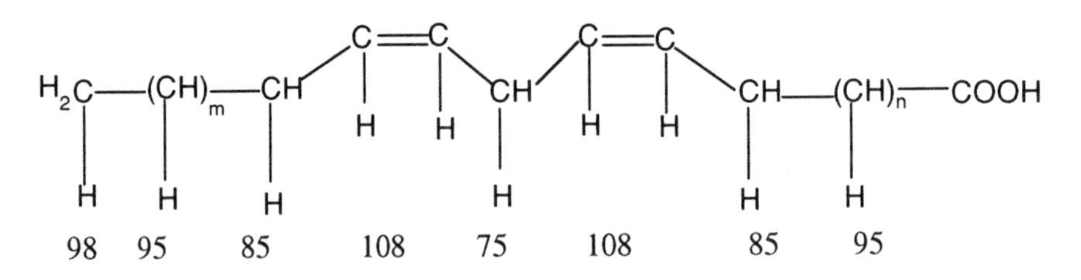

Figure 1. Bond strength of C–H bonds of polyunsaturated fatty acids, kcal/mol.

Lipid Peroxidation

The reactions of free radicals and active oxygen species are considered in this section taking lipid peroxidation as a model reaction. Lipid peroxidation is important in, for example, food deterioration and oxidative modification of low density lipoprotein (LDL) which is now accepted as a key initial event in the progression of atherosclerosis.[1] Lipid peroxidation proceeds by three different pathways: (1) non-enzymatic, free radical-mediated chain reaction, (2) non-enzymatic, non-radical oxidation, and (3) enzymatic reaction. These pathways are discussed below.

1. Non-Enzymatic, Free Radical-Mediated Chain Oxidation

The characteristic of this oxidation is that it proceeds by a chain reaction as illustrated in Figure 2.

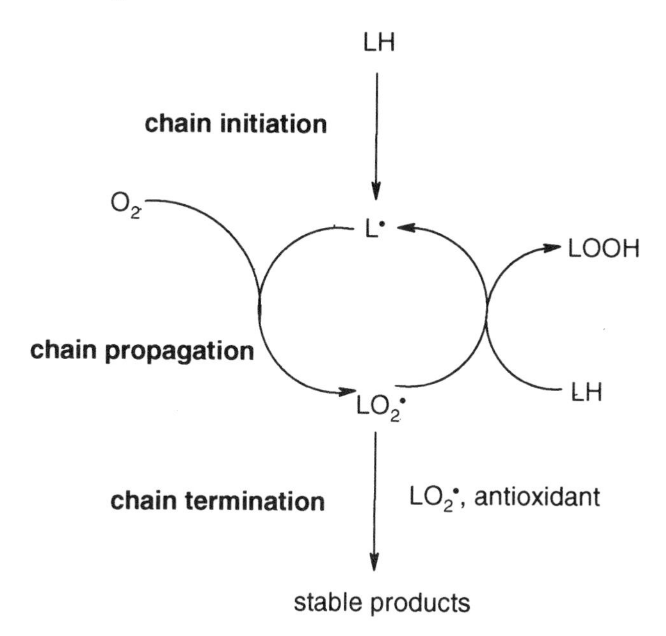

Figure 2. Oxidation of lipids by free radical chain mechanism. LH: lipid; $L^{\bullet}$: carbon-centered lipid radical; LO_2: lipid peroxyl radical; LOOH: lipid hydroperoxide.

It consists of three steps, namely, chain initiation, chain propagation, and chain termination. In the chain initiation step, the free radical is formed and attacks the lipid. The free radical (reaction 6) may be formed by various sources such as light, heat, metal, and some physiological reactions. Foods are stored in the dark and at low temperature to suppress the formation of free radicals. If free radicals are not formed, lipids are stable and not oxidized. However, if radicals are formed, they may attack lipid and generate lipid radicals (reaction 7). The rate and site of this reaction depend on the attacking radical and the lipids. As described above, the hydroxyl radical attacks lipid quite rapidly and randomly, while the peroxyl radical selectively abstracts bisallylic hydrogen. This is true for different classes of lipids such as free fatty acids, phospholipids, triglycerides, and cholesterol esters.[2]

Chain initiation → radical $X^{\bullet}$ (6)

$$X^{\bullet} + LH \text{ (lipid)} \rightarrow XH + L^{\bullet} \text{ (lipid radical)} \quad (7)$$

Chain propagation:

$$L^{\bullet} + O_2 \rightarrow LO_2^{\bullet} \text{ (lipid peroxyl radical)} \quad (8)$$

$$LO_2^{\bullet} + LH \rightarrow LOOH + L^{\bullet} \quad (9)$$

The lipid radical $L^{\bullet}$ reacts with oxygen molecule quite rapidly to give lipid peroxyl radical (reaction 8), although under low oxygen concentration the lipid radical may live longer. The lipid peroxyl radical attacks another lipid molecule and abstracts hydrogen atom to yield lipid hydroperoxide and at the same time another lipid radical (reaction 9), which reacts with oxygen and continues the second oxidation sequence. Thus, the chain is propagated and one molecule of chain-initiating radical may cause the oxidation of many molecules.The number of chain propagations per each chain initiation is called kinetic chain length and shows how long the chain reaction continues. It has been shown that the *in vitro* oxidation of erythrocytes[3] and LDL[4] proceed by a chain reaction, but it is not clearly known how long the chain continues *in vivo*. It is noteworthy that the chain is propagated by lipid peroxyl radical independent of the chain initiating species, whether it is initiated by hydroxyl radical or NO_2, and that polyunsaturated lipids having two or more double bonds are selectively oxidized. The mechanism of lipid peroxidation has been studied extensively and is now well understood[5] (Figure 3). As seen in Figure 4, linoleic acid and its esters are oxidized to give four types of conjugated diene hydroperoxides as primary products, while the oxidation of lipids of higher unsaturation give cyclic peroxides as well as conjugated diene hydroperoxides. Isoprostanes are also known to be formed during the oxidation of arachidonate and accepted as markers of lipid peroxidation.[6]

The chain propagation does not continue forever, but the chain oxidation is terminated when lipid radical or lipid peroxyl radical is scavenged by an antioxidant such as vitamins E and C or when two lipid peroxyl radicals react to give non-radical products such as ketones and alcohols (reaction 10).

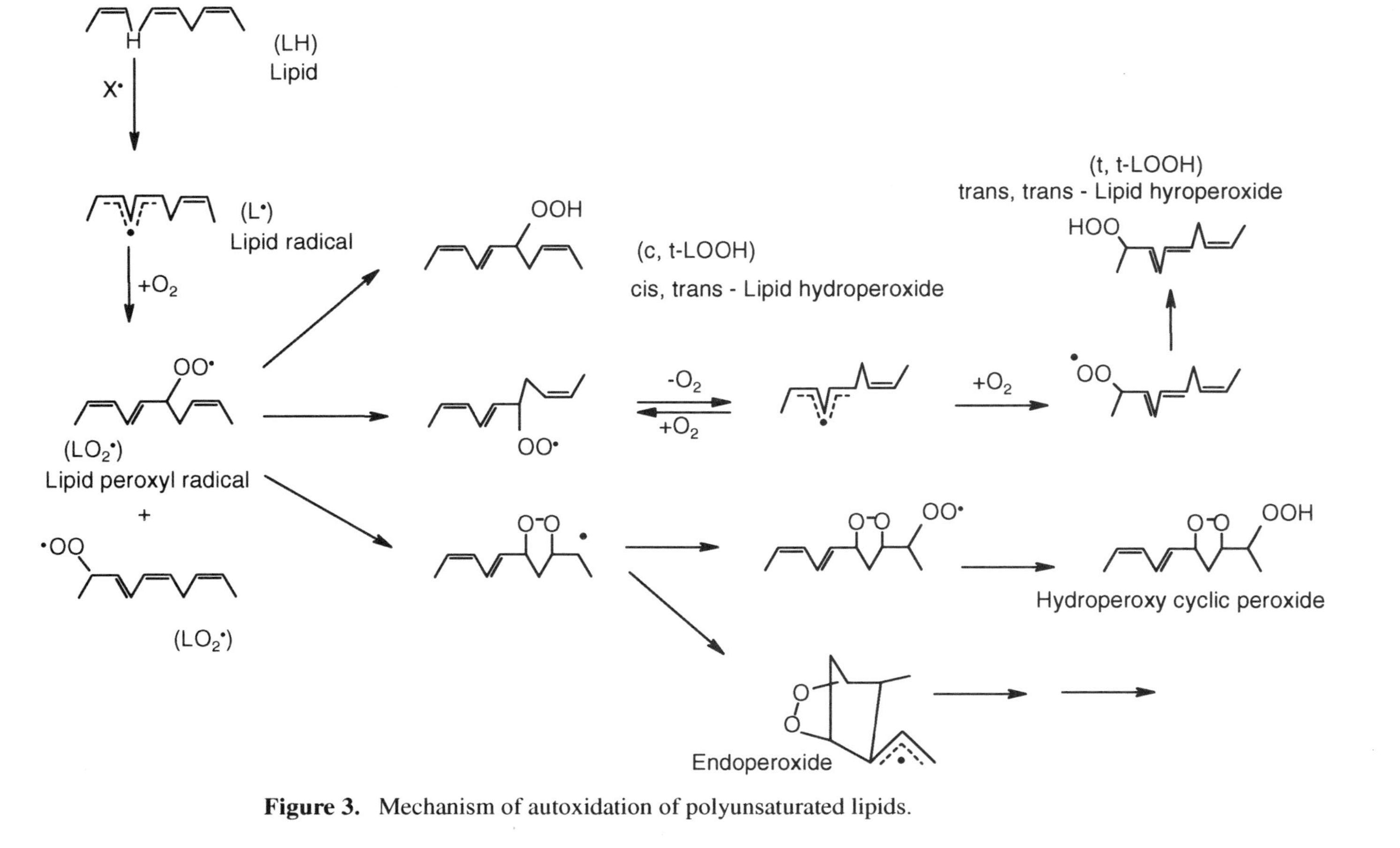

Figure 3. Mechanism of autoxidation of polyunsaturated lipids.

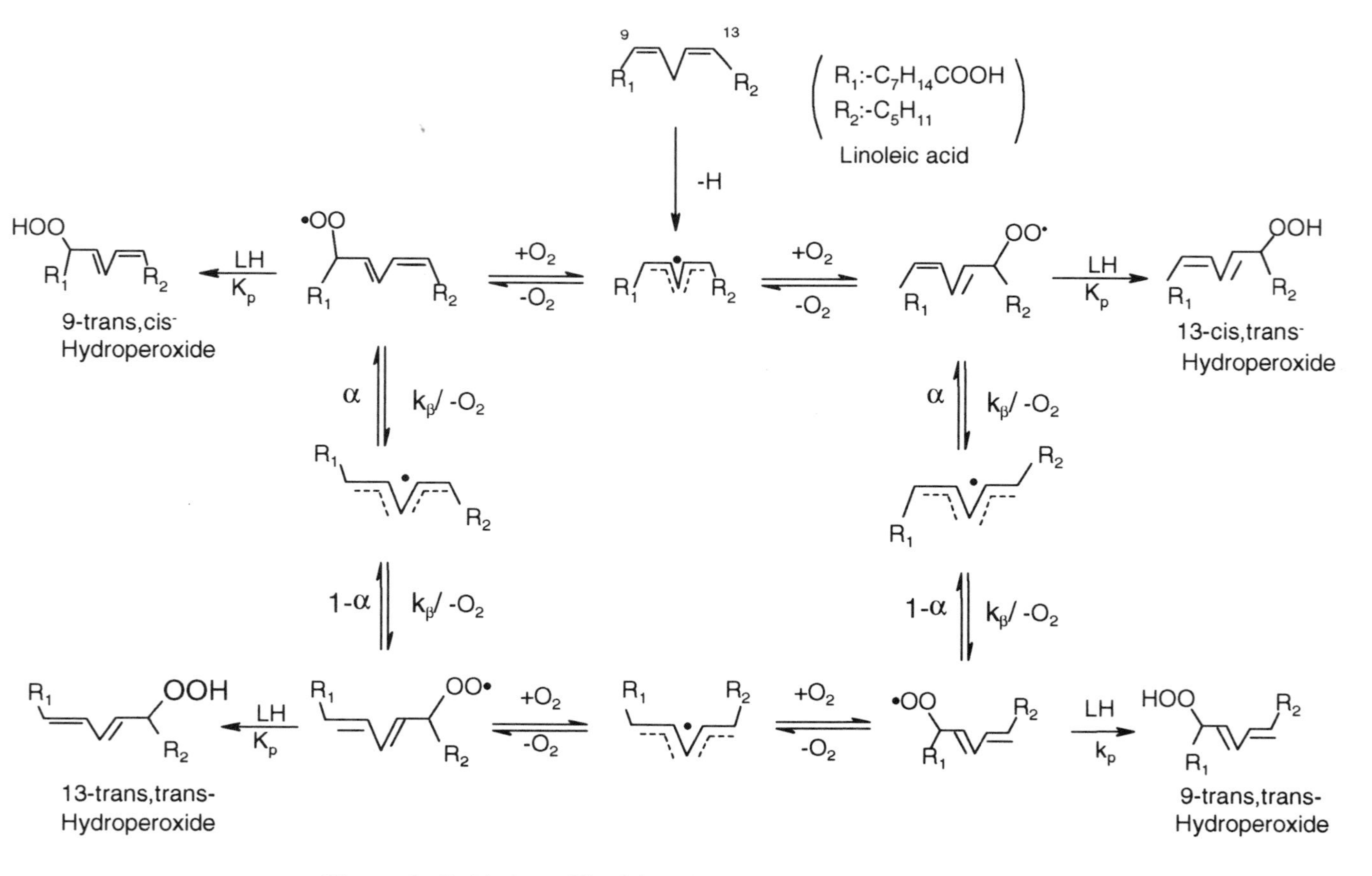

Figure 4. Oxidation of linoleic acid.

Chain termination:

$$2LO_2^{\bullet} \rightarrow \text{ketone} + \text{alcohol} + O_2 \quad (10)$$

2. *Non-Enzymatic, Non-Radical Lipid Peroxidation*

Some active oxygen species oxidize lipids by non-radical mechanisms. A typical example is the oxidation by singlet oxygen, which adds to the double bond rapidly to give hydroperoxide and/or cyclic peroxide instead of abstracting hydrogen from lipids to produce free lipid radical. For example, oleic acid is oxidized by singlet oxygen to give two kinds of hydroperoxides (reaction 11).

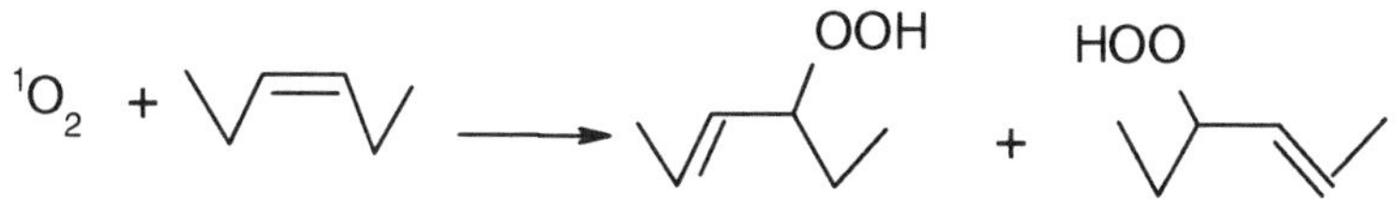

$^1O_2$ + [olefin] ⟶ [allylic hydroperoxide, OOH] + [allylic hydroperoxide, HOO] (11)

It should be noted that, in the oxidation by singlet oxygen, the double bond migrates. Free cholesterol is also oxidized by singlet oxygen to give a specific hydroperoxide.[7] As shown above, free radicals oxidize predominantly polyunsaturated lipids, whereas singlet oxygen oxidizes mono-olefines as well. It may be also noted that, although singlet oxygen oxidizes lipids faster than the peroxyl radical, this oxidation is stoichiometric and one molecule of singlet oxygen oxidizes only one lipid molecule.

3. *Enzymatic Lipid Peroxidation*

Lipids are oxidized by lipoxygenases and cyclooxygenases. The so-called arachidonate cascade is well known and its physiological importance has been well established.[8] Lipoxygenases are non-heme iron containing dioxygenases which oxygenate polyenoic fatty acids containing a 1Z,4Z-pentadiene system to their 1-hydroperoxy-2(E),4(Z)-pentadiene product. In contrast to the non-enzymatic, free radical-mediated lipid peroxidation, the lipoxygenase reaction is in general regiospecific and enantiospecific with respect to the initial hydrogen abstraction and subsequent oxygen insertion. Originally, it was believed that lipoxygenase can oxidize only free polyenoic fatty acids. However, more recent studies indicated that certain plant and mammalian lipoxygenases are capable of specifically oxidizing phospholipids and cholesterol esters in biomembranes and lipoproteins.[9] Thus, a stereospecific pattern of oxidation products in cells and tissues may be regarded as indicator for the *in vivo* action of a lipoxygenase. The detection of stereospecific products of oxidized polyenoic fatty acids in atherosclerotic lesions suggested that 15-lipoxygenases may contribute to lipid peroxidation in the early stages of atherogenesis.

ANTIOXIDANTS

Aerobic organisms are protected from oxidative stress induced by free radicals and active oxygen species by an array of defense systems. As summarized in Table 4, various kinds of antioxidants with different functions play an important role in these defense systems. The preventive antioxidants acting in the first defense line suppress the formation of free radicals and active oxygen species. The radical scavenging antioxidants are responsible in the second defense line and inhibit chain initiation and/or break the chain propagation. The antioxidant enzymes such as phospholipases, proteases, DNA repair enzymes, and transferases act as the third line defense. In addition, the appropriate antioxidant is generated and transferred to the right site at the right time and at the right concentration when the oxidative stress takes place. This adaptation mechanism is also important in the total defense system.

With increasing experimental, clinical, and epidemiological evidence which shows the involvement of free radicals and active oxygen species in a variety of diseases, cancer, and aging, the role of antioxidants has received increasing attention. For example, recent epidemiological studies showed that high intake of vitamin E, a potent radical-scavenging antioxidant, reduces the risk of coronary heart disease and that low levels of vitamin E seem to correlate with an increased incidence of myocardial infarction. Furthermore, probucol, a synthetic radical-scavenging antioxidant, is widely used as a drug in the treatment of hypercholesterolemia and atherosclerosis.

Mechanism of Action of Antioxidants

Inhibition of Lipid Peroxidation

The role and action of antioxidants will be reviewed briefly using lipid peroxidation as an example. Lipid peroxidation can be inhibited by suppressing chain initiation and chain propagation and/or by enhancing chain termination. Metals often play an important role in radical generation. For this reason, proteins such as ferritin and ceruloplasmin, which sequester metal ions are also important antioxidants. Hydroperoxide and hydrogen peroxide are precursors of oxygen radicals and, hence, peroxidases such as glutathione peroxidase (GPX) also act as antioxidants. Superoxide dismutase (SOD) acts as an antioxidant by dismutating superoxide to triplet oxygen and hydrogen peroxide. Various carotenoids may act as quenchers of singlet oxygen.

Table 4
Defense Systems *In Vivo* Against Oxidative Damage

1. Preventive antioxidants: suppress the formation of free radicals

(a) Non-radical decomposition of hydroperoxides and hydrogen peroxide

Catalase	Decomposition of hydrogen peroxide $2H_2O_2 \rightarrow 2H_2O + O_2$
Glutathione peroxidase (cellular)	Decomposition of hydrogen peroxide and free fatty acid hydroperoxides $H_2O_2 + 2GSH \rightarrow 2H_2O + GSSG$ $LOOH + 2GSH \rightarrow LOH + H_2O + GSSG$
Glutathione peroxidase (plasma)	Decomposition of hydrogen peroxide and phospholipid hydroperoxides $PLOOH + 2GSH \rightarrow PLOH + H_2O + GSSG$
Phospholipid hydroperoxide glutathione peroxidase	Decomposition of phospholipid hydroperoxides
Peroxidase	Decomposition of hydrogen peroxide and lipid hydroperoxides $LOOH + AH_2 \rightarrow LOH + H_2O + A$ $H_2O_2 + AH_2 \rightarrow 2H_2O + A$
Glutathione S-transferase	Decomposition of lipid hydroperoxides

(b) Sequestration of metal by chelation

Transferrin, lactoferrin	Sequestration of iron
Haptoglobin	Sequestration of hemoglobin
Hemopexin	Stabilization of heme
Ceruloplasmin, albumin	Sequestration of copper

(c) Quenching of active oxygen species

Superoxide dismutase (SOD)	Disproportionation of superoxide $2O_2^{\bullet -} + 2H^+ \rightarrow H_2O_2 + O_2$
Carotenoids, vitamin E	Quenching singlet oxygen

2. Radical-scavenging antioxidants: scavenge radicals to inhibit chain initiation and break chain propagation

Hydrophilic: Vitamin C, uric acid, bilirubin, albumin
Lipophilic: Vitamin E, ubiquinol, carotenoids, flavonoids

Table 4 (continued)
Defense Systems *In Vivo* Against Oxidative Damage

---

3. Repair and *de novo* enzymes: Repair the damage and reconstitute membranes

Lipase, protease, DNA repair enzymes, transferase

4. Adaptation: Generate appropriate antioxidant enzymes and transfer them to the right site at the right time and in the right concentration

---

The chain propagation can be stopped quite efficiently by eliminating oxygen. Thus, foods are often stored *in vacuo* or under nitrogen. Aerobic organisms, however, need oxygen. The lipid radical reacts with oxygen quite rapidly to give lipid peroxyl radical, which continues the chain propagation reactions. This chain reaction can be terminated by scavenging the chain-carrying lipid peroxyl radical. Vitamins C and E, uric acid, bilirubin, and ubiquinol, a reduced form of coenzyme Q, are important radical-scavenging antioxidants. These antioxidants must scavenge the radical rapidly before it attacks the lipid. Therefore, the more reactive the compound is toward the radical, the more potent it is as an antioxidant. This reactivity is, however, not the only factor that determines the antioxidant potency. It is also determined by many other factors such as the type and location of the radical, site of antioxidant, concentration and mobility of the antioxidant at the microenvironment, fate of antioxidant-derived radical, and interactions with other antioxidants. These factors will be discussed briefly for vitamin E (Figure 5).

Factors Affecting the Function of Antioxidants

Solubility and Location

The site of radical generation and antioxidant localization is important. For example, vitamins C and E have roughly similar reactivities toward oxygen radicals, but their location is quite different. Vitamin C is present in the aqueous phase, while vitamin E is localized in lipophilic compartments such as membranes and lipoproteins. Apparently, vitamin C scavenges aqueous radicals more efficiently than vitamin E, whereas vitamin E is more effective than vitamin C for scavenging radicals within the lipophilic domain. The efficiency of radical scavenging also depends on the attacking radical. As summarized in Table 3, the hydroxyl radical is too reactive for any type of

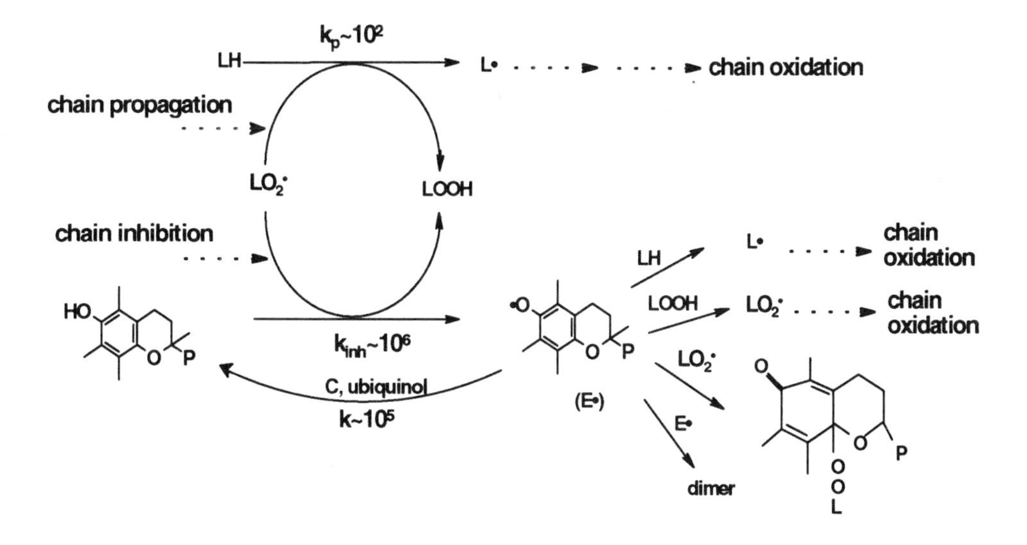

Figure 5. Inhibition of oxidation of lipid by α-tocopherol. LH, lipid; L •, lipid radical; LO_2 •, lipid peroxyl radical; LOOH, lipid hydroperoxide; C, vitamin C; P, phytyl side chain $C_{13}H_{27}$; E •, α-tocopheroxyl radical; k, rate constant in $M^{-1}s^{-1}$.

antioxidant to scavenge it efficiently. For example, vitamin C may scavenge the hydroxyl radical with a rate constant of 10^9 $M^{-1}s^{-1}$. However, the hydroxyl radical reacts with many biological molecules such as lipids, proteins, and sugars with a rate constant of 10^8 $M^{-1}s^{-1}$. Considering the concentration of vitamin C, it is evident that substantially all hydroxyl radicals react with target molecules before vitamin C can scavenge them. It has been suggested that vitamin E is effective for scavenging peroxyl radicals, but not for alkoxyl nor hydroxyl radicals.[10]

The location of lipophilic antioxidants in the membranes or lipoproteins and their mobility are also important factors. For example, it has been shown that the efficacy of radical scavenging by vitamin E decreases as the radical goes deeper into the interior of the membranes and LDL.[11] In contrast, β-carotene, which is about 30 times less reactive than α-tocopherol toward peroxyl radical, scavenges the peroxyl radicals faster than α-tocopherol within the membranes.[12] These results may be explained by a low vertical mobility of α-tocopherol in the membrane.

Antioxidant Radicals and Other Metabolic Products

When antioxidants scavenge radicals, they form antioxidant radicals. For example, when α-tocopherol (vitamin E) scavenges the peroxyl radical, α-tocopheroxyl radical is formed. The fate of this radical derived from the antioxidant is also important in determining the efficacy of antioxidant. The vitamin E radical may scavenge another peroxyl radical to produce an adduct, react with another vitamin E radical to yield a dimer (or disproportionation products), be reduced by reductants such as vitamin C or ubiquinol to regenerate vitamin E, or react with lipid or lipid hydroperoxide to generate lipid or lipid peroxyl radical which may initiate a new chain reaction. The relative importance of these competing reactions is dependent on reaction conditions and it determines the total antioxidant efficacy. The β-carotene radical is resonance stabilized, but it reacts with oxygen to give peroxyl radical which is not stable and it continues the chain oxidation. Thus, the antioxidant potency of β-carotene is higher at lower oxygen concentration. Potent antioxidants form a radical which is stabilized by resonance and steric hindrance.

Interactions of Antioxidants

Another important factor is the interaction between antioxidants. It has been shown that the appropriate combination of two or more antioxidants may result in the synergistic inhibition of lipid peroxidation. The well-known examples are the combination of vitamin C and vitamin E or that of vitamin E and ubiquinol.

Chemical Form and Analogues

There has been some interest and controversy regarding the antioxidant activities of vitamin E compounds. It has been accepted that α-tocopherol has the highest bioactivity in the vitamin E groups, but it has been reported recently that γ-tocopherol may be superior to α-tocopherol under certain conditions.[13,14] Furthermore, it has been also reported that α-tocotrienol may act as a more potent antioxidant than α-tocopherol.[15] The relative antioxidant potency may vary with the conditions and it is important to examine how the antioxidant activities have been assessed, in what kind of medium, and how various factors affect the antioxidant potency. Eventually, these points should be clearly established.

Prooxidant Effects of Antioxidants

It has been known that the antioxidant can act as a prooxidant as well as an antioxidant. For example, it has been observed that α-tocopherol may accelerate lipid peroxidation under certain circumstances especially at high concentrations. The prooxidant action of α-tocopherol in the oxidation of isolated LDL has been discussed extensively by Stocker in terms of phase transfer and chain transfer mechanisms.[16] This effect stems from the abstraction of hydrogen from lipid or lipid hydroperoxide by α-tocopheroxyl radical. The instability of β-carotene peroxyl radical has also been discussed.[12] It is also well known that ascorbic acid promotes oxidation under certain conditions. In fact, the combination of iron and ascorbic acid has been used in the *in vitro* experiment to initiate lipid peroxidation. α-Tocopherol may also act as a prooxidant by reducing metal ions such as Fe(III) or Cu(II), since the reduced forms Fe(II) and Cu(I) react with hydroperoxides to give free radicals faster than Fe(III) and Cu(II), respectively.

However, these prooxidant actions of antioxidants observed *in vitro* may not be important *in vivo*. For example, the prooxidant action of α-tocopherol is diminished by the presence of ascorbic acid[17,18] since ascorbic acid reduces α-tocopheroxyl radical rapidly. Metal ions such as iron and copper are sequestered *in vivo* by proteins such as transferrin and ceruloplasmin, respectively (Table 4), and neither ascorbic acid nor α-tocopherol exerts prooxidant effect with such protein bound metal ions. The relevance of the results of *in vitro* experiments in simplified systems to the *in vivo* situation should be carefully considered.

CONCLUSIONS

Active oxygen and related species play an important physiological role and, at the same time, they may exert toxic effects as well. The active oxygen species are essential for production of energy, synthesis of biologically essential compounds, phagocytosis, and signal transduction. Active oxygen species, however, may play a causative role in a variety of diseases including heart disease and cancer, and aging. Antioxidants, which suppress such oxidative damage play an important role in aerobic organisms. It is important to understand that the total antioxidant potency is determined not simply by a chemical reactivity of the compound toward the radical but also by many other factors described above. This is particularly important and should be considered very seriously when assessing the antioxidant activity of new compounds.

REFERENCES

1. Steinberg D, Parthasarathy S, Garew T, Khoo J, Witztum J. Beyond cholesterol. Modification of low density lipoprotein that increase its atherogenicity. *New England Journal of Medicine,* 320, 915, 1989.

2. Simic MG, Jovanovic SV, Niki E. *Lipid Oxidation in Food.* American Chemical Society, Washington D.C, 1992, 14.
3. Yamamoto Y, Niki E, Eguchi J, Kamiya Y, Shimasaki H. Oxidation of biological membranes and its inhibition. 1. Free radical chain oxidation of erythrocyte ghost by oxygen. *Biochimica et Biophysica Acta,* 819, 29, 1985.
4. Sato K, Niki E, Shimasaki H. Free radical-mediated chain oxidation of low density lipoprotein and its synergistic inhibition by Vitamin E and vitamin C. *Archives of Biochemistry and Biophysics,* 279, 402, 1990.
5. Porter NA, Caldwell SE, Mills KA. Mechanisms of free radical oxidation of unsaturated lipids. *Lipids,* 30, 277, 1995.
6. Morrow JD, Awad JA, Kato T, Takahashi K, Badr KF, Roberts LJ, Burk RF. Formation of novel non-cyclooxygenase-derived prostanoids (F2-isoprostanes) in carbon tetrachloride hepatotoxicity. An animal model of lipid peroxidation. *Journal of Clinical Investigation,* 90, 2502, 1992.
7. Smith L. Cholesterol autoxidation. *Chemistry and Physics of Lipids,* 44, 87, 1987.
8. Yamamoto S. Mammalian lipoxygenases: Molecular structures and functions. *Biochimica et Biophysica Acta,* 1128, 117, 1992.
9. Murray JJ, Brash AR. Rabbit reticulocyte lipoxygenase catalyzes specific 12(S) and 15(S) oxygenation of arachidonoylphosphatidylcholine. *Archives of Biochemistry and Biophysics,* 265, 514, 1988.
10. Niki E, Noguchi N, Tsuchihashi H, Gotoh N. Interaction among vitamin C, vitamin E, and β-carotene. *American Journal of Clinical Nutrition,* 62 (suppl.), 1322S, 1995.
11. Gotoh N, Noguchi N, Tsuchiya J, Morita K, Sakai H, Shimasaki H, Niki E. Inhibition of oxidation of low density lipoprotein by vitamin E and related compounds. *Free Radical Research,* 24, 123, 1996.
12. Tsuchihashi H, Kigoshi M, Iwatsuki M, Niki E. Action of β-carotene as an antioxidant against lipid perioxidation. *Archives of Biochemistry and Biophysics,* 323, 137, 1995.
13. Cooney RV, Franke AA, Harwood PJ, Match Pigott V, Custer LJ, Mordan LJ. α-Tocopherol detoxification of nitrogen dioxide: Superiority to α-tocopherol. *Proceedings of National Academy of Science,* USA, 90, 1771, 1993.
14. Christen S, Woodall AA, Shigenaga MK, Southwell-Keely PT, Duncan MW, Ames BN. α-Tocopherol traps mutagenic electrophiles such as NO_x and complements α-tocopherol: Physiological implications, *Proceedings of National Academy of Science,* USA, 94, 3217, 1997.
15. Packer L. *Nutrition, Lipids, Health, and Disease.* AOCS Press, Champaign, 1995, 8.
16. Waldeck AR, Stocker R. Radical-initiated lipid peroxidation in low density lipoproteins: Insights obtained from kinetic modeling. *Chemical Research of Toxicology,* 8, 954, 1996.
17. Terao J, Matushita S. The peroxidising effect of α-tocopherol on autoxidation of methyl linoleate in bulk phase. *Lipids,* 21, 255, 1986.
18. Takahashi M, Yoshikawa Y, Niki E. Oxidation of lipids. XVII. Crossover, effect of tocopherols in the spontaneous oxidation of methyl linoleate. *Bulletin of Chemical Society of Japan,* 62, 1885, 1989.

2

Determinants of Antioxidant Status in Humans

Andreas M. Papas, Ph.D.
Health and Nutrition
Eastman Chemical Company, Kingsport, Tennessee, USA

INTRODUCTION

Oxidation and production of free radicals and reactive oxygen-containing species (ROS) are an integral part of life and our metabolism.[1] Actually, free radicals and ROS may be produced in our body deliberately to serve important biological functions. For example, activated phagocytes use ROS to kill some strains of invading bacteria and fungi. Superoxide plays a useful role in the regulation of cell growth and intercellular signaling.[2] Free radicals and ROS are useful, however, only when they are produced at the right amount and at the right place and time. Otherwise, they can be very damaging because they are extremely reactive and almost instantly attack molecules, which are very close to them. Free radicals and ROS, therefore, react with

0-8493-8009-X/98/$0.00+$.50

nonradicals and can initiate adverse chain reactions such as lipid peroxidation. They also damage other important molecules including proteins, carbohydrates, and DNA. These reactions were discussed in the previous chapter.

In order to defend against damage from free radicals and ROS, humans and other living organisms developed powerful and complex antioxidant systems.[3] Components of these systems are antioxidants, a diverse group of molecules that protect key biological sites from oxidative damage. They usually act by removing or inactivating chemical intermediates that produce free radicals. Antioxidants are either produced in the body (endogenous) or derived from the diet. They are classified on the basis of several criteria such as solubility in lipid or water; chemical and physical characteristics (proteins, enzymatic and non-enzymatic, or small molecules) etc. It is important to note that individual antioxidants function not in isolation, but as part of systems with significant interdependence and additive or synergistic effects. These systems represent highly specialized strategies developed by various sites in the body for dealing with free radicals and ROS.

Endogenous components of the antioxidant system include:

- glutathione (GSH, also present in foods) and Se-glutathione peroxidase
- Fe-catalase
- NADPH
- ubiquinol-10 (reduced coenzyme Q_{10})
- Mn, Cu, Zn-superoxide dismutase (SOD)
- uric acid
- lipoic acid
- hormones with antioxidant activity (melatonin, DHEA, etc.)
- metal binding proteins including albumin (and albumin bound thiols and bilirubin), Fe and Cu-binding proteins (transferrin, ceruloplasmin) and Fe-complex binding proteins (heptoglobin, hemopexin)

Dietary and exogenous antioxidants include:

- tocopherols and tocotrienols (vitamin E)
- ascorbate (vitamin C)
- vitamin A and carotenoids (β-carotene, lycopene, lutein, etc.)
- Se (and other metals essential for the function of antioxidant enzymes)
- phytochemicals with antioxidant activity
- dietary and other supplements (CoQ_{10}, glutathione, lipoic acid, etc.)
- food antioxidants (BHA, BHT, propyl gallate, TBHQ, rosemary extract)

A large number of phytochemicals in foods have antioxidant activity.[4] Many foods contain natural (tocopherols, rosemary extract, etc.) or synthetic antioxidants (BHA, BHT, propyl gallate, and TBHQ) as additives to inhibit lipid peroxidation.[5] These may also have antioxidant effects in the body.

This chapter will provide a brief overview and discuss the factors that determine the antioxidant status in humans. The major dietary antioxidants and the major factors determining the antioxidant status in humans will be discussed in detail in later chapters.

ANTIOXIDANT STATUS

Antioxidant status is the balance between the antioxidant system and prooxidants in living organisms.[2] This balance is dynamic and, in the human body, is probably tipped slightly in favor of oxidation, which is essential for the production of energy.[1] The body has adapted to this slight imbalance favoring oxidation by developing repair mechanisms, which include several enzymes such as ligases, nucleases, polymerases, proteinases, phospholipases, etc. In addition, gradual and modest increase in oxidation induces production of endogenous antioxidants thus providing a type of feedback regulation mechanism.

A serious imbalance favoring oxidation is defined as oxidative stress. It may result from:

- excessive production of ROS and free radicals and/or
- weakening of the antioxidant system due to lower intake or endogenous production of antioxidants or from increased utilization.

Oxidative stress can cause cell damage and is believed to contribute to aging and the development of chronic disease including heart disease and cancer.[6-14] Thus, prevention of oxidative stress may be important for good health and prevention of disease.

FACTORS AFFECTING ANTIOXIDANT STATUS

The antioxidant status is affected either from increased dietary supply of antioxidants or from endogenous production. It is also affected by the production of free radicals and ROS, which cause increased utilization of antioxidants. Major factors affecting the antioxidant status are summarized in Table 1.

Table 1
Determinants of Antioxidant Status in Humans

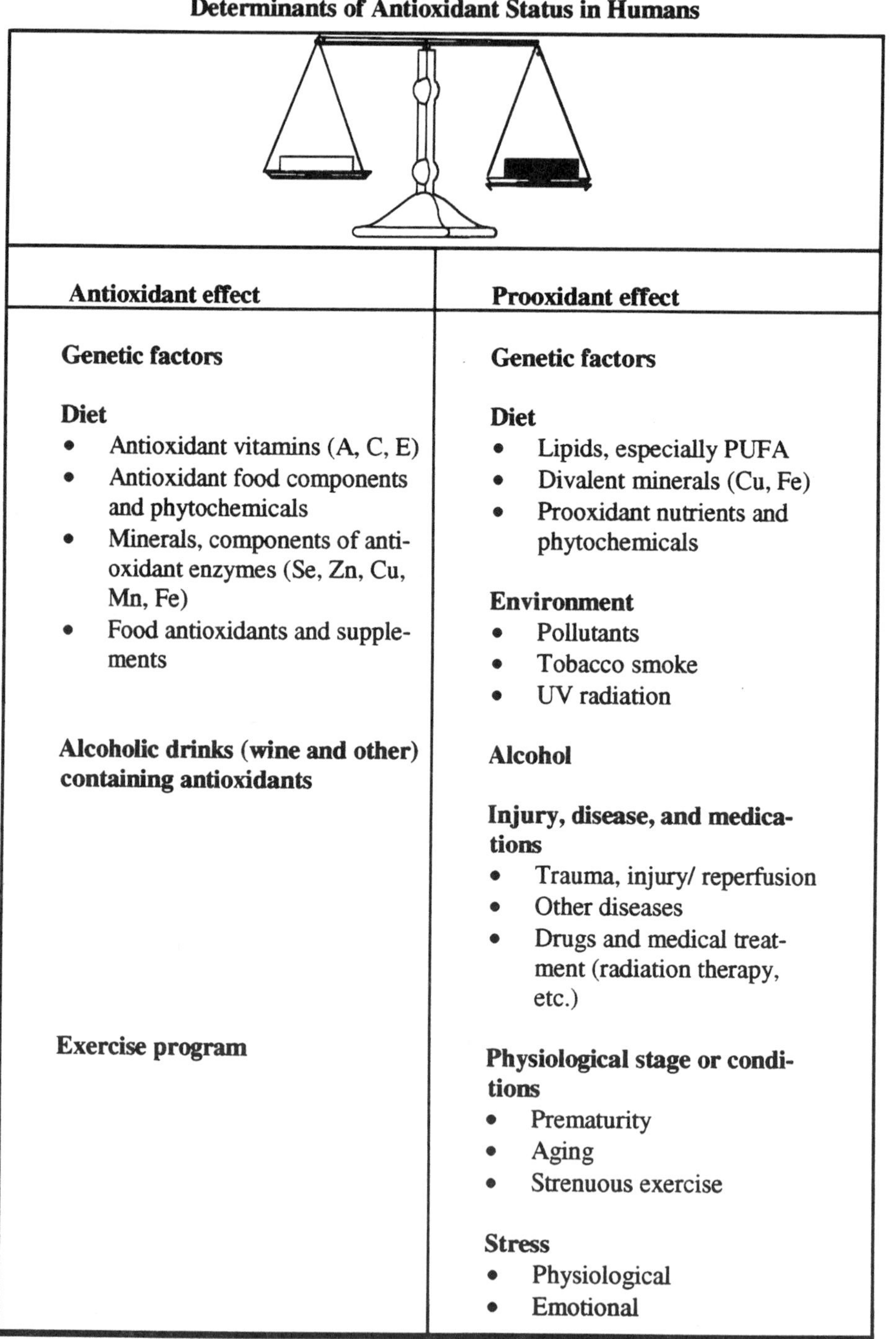

Antioxidant effect	Prooxidant effect
Genetic factors	**Genetic factors**
Diet • Antioxidant vitamins (A, C, E) • Antioxidant food components and phytochemicals • Minerals, components of antioxidant enzymes (Se, Zn, Cu, Mn, Fe) • Food antioxidants and supplements	**Diet** • Lipids, especially PUFA • Divalent minerals (Cu, Fe) • Prooxidant nutrients and phytochemicals
	Environment • Pollutants • Tobacco smoke • UV radiation
Alcoholic drinks (wine and other) containing antioxidants	**Alcohol**
	Injury, disease, and medications • Trauma, injury/ reperfusion • Other diseases • Drugs and medical treatment (radiation therapy, etc.)
Exercise program	**Physiological stage or conditions** • Prematurity • Aging • Strenuous exercise
	Stress • Physiological • Emotional

Diet

More than any other factor, diet can directly affect the antioxidant status in both positive and negative manner. By supplying antioxidants and cofactors of endogenous antioxidants, the antioxidant system can be strengthened. In contrast, some components of the diet such as polyunsaturated fatty acids (PUFA) and divalent metals not bound to proteins, may be easily oxidized or act as prooxidants.[15-17]

Diet affects the antioxidant status in many ways. These include the amount, chemical form, chirality, absorption, bioavailability and biochemical interactions between dietary antioxidants and other factors. Also storage, handling, processing and cooking of food, amount and saturation of lipid material, presence of oxidation promoting metals and food antioxidants are important factors.[18]

Due to its major importance, the role of diet will be discussed in more detail in Chapter 5.

Environment

Air pollutants, tobacco smoke, and exposure to chemicals, ionizing and UV radiation are major environmental factors initiating free radical reactions.

Air Pollutants

The most damaging pollutants are nitrogen dioxide (NO_2) and ozone.[19,20] NO_2 induces the peroxidation of lipids and nitrates aromatic amino acids, whereas ozone particularly damages proteins.

NO_2 is produced primarily from combustion in automobile engines. Ozone is produced mostly from NO_2 by photochemical reactions and from oxygen and gasoline vapors. NO_2 adds to double bonds and abstracts labile hydrogen atoms initiating lipid peroxidation and production of free radicals. It also reacts directly with vitamin C and oxidizes it. Lipids from lungs of rats exposed to NO_2 had lower PUFA and increased oxidation products such as diene hydroperoxides, thiobarbituric acid reactive substances (TBARS), and cholesterol epoxides.[20,21] NO_2 reduced phagocytic activity of alveolar macrophages, changed the metabolism of eicosanoids, and stimulated other inflammatory processes.[22-24]

Ozone, although not a free radical, is a strong oxidant and may lead to free radical production by reacting with PUFA to form ozonides and by inducing autoxidation of lipids. It has also been suggested that the intermediate product of an ozone-olefin reaction, called the Criegee zwiterion, breaks down to hydroperoxide, which can initiate autoxidation, and aldehydes which have been suggested to be signals for inflammation.[20,25] Ozone reacts directly with vitamin E. Vitamin C also may be affected because it is believed to reduce the tocopherol radical. It was also reported that vitamin E was higher in the lungs of animals exposed to ozone probably as defensive response[26] while in skin it was depleted.[27] It has been shown that animals with low vitamin E status were easily injured by chronic ozone exposure and that vitamins E and C were protective.[20] In humans, however, the role of antioxidants in reducing the adverse effects of ozone has not been fully evaluated.

Other environmental pollutants include halogenated hydrocarbons and pesticides. Although many chemicals do not spontaneously generate free radicals, their metabolism by the cytochrome P-450 enzyme system may produce active intermediates causing free radical reactions.[28-30]

Tobacco Smoke

More than 1,000 chemical compounds are found in the gas and tar fractions of tobacco smoke. NO_2, one of the major compounds in the gas phase, has been suggested to react with smoke olefins to form carbon-centered radicals. Alcoxyl radicals were also detected by spin trapping methods.[20,31,32] In addition, tobacco smoke probably increases free radical production indirectly by activating neutrophils, which may cause inflammation. It has been suggested that nitric oxide, the precursor of NO_2, reacts with $O_2^{\bullet -}$ to form peroxynitrite, which inactivates a-1-proteinase. The tar phase contains a semiquinone radical promoting formation of H_2O_2, which along with transition metals, may inhibit the a-1-proteinase, but at a slower rate. This inhibition may be related to increased production of elastase and development of emphysema.[33] Several studies have shown that smokers have lower plasma levels of vitamins E, C, β-carotene, and other antioxidants due to both lower intake and increased metabolic use[34-36] but others observed no effect or even higher levels.[26] Even larger differences in favor of nonsmokers were reported for alveolar fluid.[37]

These findings and supporting epidemiological data provided impetus for evaluating the effect of supplemental antioxidants on the incidence of lung cancer. The alpha-tocopherol beta-carotene study (ATBC or Finnish) and carotene and retinol efficacy trial (CARET), however, failed to show any reduction of lung cancer in male smokers receiving supplemental β-carotene and/or vitamin E (ATBC study) or a combination of β-carotene and vitamin A (CARET study). Actually, incidence of lung cancer appeared to be higher in current smokers receiving β-carotene. No conclusive explanation for these unexpected results is available. The major proposed hypotheses are discussed in several later chapters.

Ionizing Radiation

Sunlight, and especially its ultraviolet (UV) component, initiates free radical reactions within the cells including lipid peroxidation and DNA damage. Artificial sources of light with similar spectrum and other sources of ionizing radiation produce similar effects. Considerable evidence indicates that skin cancer and skin aging are associated with damage from free radical reactions. UV radiation reduces the level of antioxidants in the skin and induces inflammation and other adverse reactions.[38-42] Antioxidants, and particularly dietary or topically applied vitamin E, inhibited lipid peroxidation and immunosuppression and restored thymidine incorporation in mice.[38,43-45] There has been significant progress in understanding the mechanism of vitamin E interaction with UV light.[46] Dr. Liebler and his co-workers review the adverse effects of UV radiation on the skin and the protective role of vitamin E in Chapter 18.

Alcohol

Modest consumption of alcohol appears to cause desirable increase in high-density lipoprotein (HDL) and reduction in platelet aggregation.[47,48] Some alcoholic drinks, especially wine and, to a lesser extent, dark beers, supply phytochemicals (isoflavones, tannins, etc.) having antioxidant properties. Increasing evidence suggests that these compounds, which in wine include quercetin, catechin, epicatechin, and resveratrol, may provide additional benefits to those from a modest amount of alcohol especially by reducing oxidation of LDL.[49] Others, however, found no effect on LDL oxidation.[50] It appears that there are multiple effects of these compounds such as synergistic or sparing effect with other antioxidants, especially vitamin E and coenzyme Q_{10}, and even inhibition of platelet aggregation by resveratrol but with a different mechanism than alcohol.[48,51]

At even modestly high levels, alcohol stimulates LDL oxidation.[52] Excessive consumption damages the liver and increases the risk for chronic disease and especially some forms of cancer. It is now recognized that alcohol causes formation of acetaldehyde, which is toxic to the liver, not only by the main alcohol dehydrogenase mediated reaction, but also by an accessory microsomal pathway that generates oxygen radicals. A third and minor pathway producing acetaldehyde involves catalase located in peroxisomes. As a result, glutathione levels are depressed and some enzymes are inactivated causing production of ethane and pentane, which can be detected in the breath. In addition, iron in the liver is reduced further catalyzing oxidation and production of free radicals.[53] Plasma and liver antioxidants, especially ascorbic acid, tocopherols, and Se are lower in men consuming even modest amounts of alcohol compared to controls, while malondialdehyde and other indicators of oxidative stress were higher.[54-57] In contrast, alcoholic men and women drinking moderately have higher levels of serum β-carotene.[58] Alcohol also activates many xenobiotic compounds, such as carbon tetrachloride, and drugs, such as acetaminophen, to toxic metabolites that often are free radicals. In the digestive and upper respiratory tracts, alcohol appears to increase the activation of procarcinogens by affecting enzymes of the cytochrome P450 system. Finally, alcohol may affect antioxidant status by reducing food intake and by altering metabolism of key nutrients, thereby promoting deficiencies (vitamin A) or toxic interactions with food components. A toxic interaction of alcohol and β-carotene in the liver[58] has received increased attention, and has been suggested as partial explanation for the absence of positive effect of β-carotene and even for the suggestion of an increase in the incidence of lung cancer in smokers in the ATBC study. A large number of smokers in this study were also heavy drinkers.

The effect of alcohol on antioxidant status and health will be discussed in Chapter 15.

Injury and Disease

Oxidative stress is considered a major factor contributing to development of chronic disease. After it develops, however, chronic disease can have a secondary effect on antioxidant status. This effect results from tissue damage and activation of phagocytes. It also has a major indirect effect, because chronic disease reduces appetite and causes physical and emotional stress, which affect the antioxidant status.[2]

Tissue damage is caused by a variety of factors including infection, trauma and burns, ultrasound, X-ray and other radiation, surgery and ischemia, reperfusion, exposure to high oxygen levels, excessive exercise, medications, toxins, etc. Chronic disease such as heart disease, cancer, and others also cause tissue damage and inflammation. In acute injury and infection, production of ROS, free radicals, and mediators of inflammation is a secondary phenomenon, yet possibly very important in causing additional damage.

Tissue injury causes free radical formation by releasing heme proteins and transition metals, primarily Fe, leading to activation of enzymes involved in free radical generating reactions, increased utilization of antioxidants, and disruption of electron transport chains.[59,60] In addition, tissue injury is associated with increased production of mediators such as prostaglandins, leucotrienes, interleukins, interferons, and tumor necrosis factors, which cause inflammation. Peroxynitrite, formed by reaction of superoxide and nitric oxide, appears to be an important tissue-damaging species generated at sites of inflammation.[61] In addition, macrophages, which are activated during inflammation, are major sources of free radicals.

Diseases Affecting the Supply of Dietary Antioxidants

Many disease conditions and drugs depress appetite and thus affect the supply of dietary antioxidants and cofactors of endogenous antioxidants. Other diseases, such as cholestasis, fat malabsorption syndrome, short bowel syndrome, abetalipoproteinemia, and cystic fibrosis impair absorption or transport of vitamin E and other dietary antioxidants leading to serious deficiencies which cause major damage to the nerve and muscle tissues.[62] The mechanisms causing vitamin E deficiency and associated diseases are discussed in a later chapter on antioxidants and neurological disorders.

Other diseases associated with intestinal infections with pathogenic bacteria, fungi, and other pathogens causing inflammation and diarrhea can impair absorption of nutrients. For example, lower blood levels of some vitamins and minerals in AIDS patients[63] may be due in part to impaired absorption.

Injury and Disease Associated with Iron-Catalyzed Radical Reactions

Disease conditions such as sickle-cell anemia, other hemoglobinopathies, iron overload disease, cerebrospinal hemorrhage, and other diseases causing tissue damage and hemolysis, release Fe and other transition metals which catalyze free radical reactions producing peroxy radicals.[2,59,60,64] Similarly, premature babies and even normal-term babies have iron forms capable of catalyzing free radical reactions. Exposure of premature babies to high concentrations of oxygen causes retinopathy, probably due to oxidative damage and deficiency of fat-soluble vitamins primarily vitamin E.[65-67]

Ischemia and Reperfusion

Ischemia forces cells into anaerobic metabolism and causes uncoupling of the electron transport system, release of catecholamines, and production of xanthine oxidase. Reoxygenation catalyzes the breakdown of purines to uric acid concomitant production of $O_2^{\bullet-}$, other radicals and H_2O_2 from the uncoupled electron transport, autoxidation of catecholamines and activation of phagocytes. In addition, hemoglobin released from damaged cells, accelerates production of free radicals. Vitamin E showed considerable promise in reducing damage associated with ischemia and reperfusion.[2,68,69]

Other Diseases, Medical Treatments, and Medications

In addition to reducing appetite, causing diarrhea, or otherwise affecting absorption and utilization of nutrients, other diseases, including infectious diseases, affect the antioxidant status by causing cell damage or by causing inflammation and increased production of phagocytes as described above. Drugs may have direct effects on absorption, transport, and utilization of nutrients.[70]

Radiation treatment causes lipid peroxidation and other free radical reactions similar to those produced by environmental radiation. Drugs and toxins may cause free radical reactions directly or through metabolites produced by the cytochrome P-450 detoxification system.

Physiological Stage, Aging, Exercise, and Other Factors

Premature babies are susceptible to oxidative stress due to immature liver (low bile production), intestinal and lung function, hemolysis, and iron mediated free radical production as discussed above. At the other end of the spectrum, oxidative damage has been suggested as contributing in the aging process.[6] Aging has a secondary effect on antioxidant status because it is associated with higher incidence of inadequate nutrient intake, decline of organ function, weaker immunity, chronic disease, and higher intake of medications.[70,71] Strenuous exercise was reported to produce biochemical reactions similar to acute infection and cell damage and thus it induces similar free radical reactions as evidenced by increased indices of oxidation including breath pentane.[72-75]

It is believed that other factors which cause major emotional and/or physical stress, such as fear, grief, physiological and hormonal changes can affect the antioxidant status either by reducing appetite and/or by causing biochemical reactions in the body which cause production of free radicals.

The factors affecting the antioxidant status in aging and exercise will be discussed in Chapter 13 and for premature and term babies in Chapter 14.

EVALUATION OF ANTIOXIDANT STATUS

There is very strong interest and large potential benefits in accurate and easy-to-use methods for evaluating the antioxidant status in humans. Such methods can be used to assess the status both in health and disease and make diet and other changes to reduce oxidative stress.

Antioxidant status can be evaluated by direct measurements of components of the system such as glutathione, tocopherol, ascorbate and others, or more commonly, indirectly by measuring oxidative stress.[76-79] Because free radicals and ROS are extremely reactive and have very short life, they can be measured directly only by electron spin resonance. In practice, the electron spin trap is used to measure radical spin adducts. Most other methods measure adducts, end-products, or other compounds which are indicators of oxidative damage. These include lipid hydroperoxides, oxidized DNA, TBARS, malondialdehyde, conjugated dienes, oxidized LDL, volatile hydrocarbons, eicosanoids, H_2O_2, and others.

Due to strong preference for non-invasive methods for humans, the focus has been on indicator products present in breath (volatile hydrocarbons, H_2O_2), urine (TBARS, malondialdehyde, eicosanoids) and blood (TBARS, oxidized LDL, H_2O_2, glutathione, and others).

Due to its major importance, the evaluation of antioxidant status is discussed in detail in the next chapter.

ANTIOXIDANT STATUS: WHAT IS OPTIMAL?

Scientists agree that a significant imbalance in the antioxidant status favoring prooxidants is harmful. Would tipping the balance in favor of prooxidants, however, be beneficial? The answer is probably not for several reasons. We derive our energy from oxidation, which requires at least slightly prooxidant conditions.[1,80,81] In addition, it is not practical or even desirable to eliminate production of reactive oxygen species and free radicals because, at least some, are essential components of our body's defense mechanism against invading microorganisms.

We do not know whether it is possible to create, under practical conditions, an imbalance favoring antioxidants. Even if this were possible, it would probably be undesirable because it would cause significant changes in the metabolism with unknown consequences for health. For this reason, the current focus is on preventing or reversing oxidative stress but not in creating an overall environment which completely inhibits oxidation and production of free radicals.

A number of very important issues, some of them controversial, are closely related to the antioxidant status. Because of their importance, they will be discussed in Chapter 27. The nutritional, physiological, and other aspects of antioxidant status are also discussed in several other chapters. These issues are:

- Prooxidant effects of antioxidants
- Optimum dose and safety of antioxidants
- Use of antioxidant nutritional supplements
- Antioxidant status of the digesta

At this time we do not have sufficient knowledge to establish normal or preferred ranges of antioxidant status. Before we are able to do so, we need to find accurate and easy-to-use measures of the antioxidant status oxidative stress. In addition, we need to understand better the benefits and risks of changing the antioxidant status. While this is a very daunting and challenging task, there is significant reason for optimism based on the scope and quality of ongoing research.

There are, however, significant practical applications of the available knowledge to date. For example, consumption of antioxidant rich fruits and vegetables has been increasing. Use of antioxidant vitamins primarily E and C has also increased, even though use of high doses remains controversial. Some laboratories are providing estimates of antioxidant status based on a battery of tests and some health professionals use them to recommend changes in diet, behavior such as smoking, use of nutritional supplements, and other changes. The accuracy and use of these tests are limited now but is likely to increase substantially with the advent of new knowledge.

CONCLUSIONS

The antioxidant status in the human body is dynamic and is affected by many factors including diet, environment, physiological stage, exercise, injury and disease, and others. The antioxidant defense includes a variety of antioxidant systems, which evolved over a very long time. It is very important to consider individual antioxidants as components of systems with major interdependence and interactions.

Ongoing and future research will help establish normal or preferred ranges of antioxidant status and methods for its accurate evaluation. This research will also help resolve major controversies on the optimum intake of antioxidants, prooxidant effects and safety and make possible the development of nutrition and public health recommendations on the use of antioxidants.

REFERENCES

1. Davies KJ. Oxidative stress: the paradox of aerobic life. *Biochem Soc Symp* 1995;61:1-31.
2. Halliwell B. Antioxidants and human disease: a general introduction. *Nutr Rev* 1997;55:S44-9; discussion S49-52.
3. Sies H. Strategies of antioxidant defense. *Eur J Biochem* 1993;215:213-219.
4. Lin RI-S. *Phytochemicals and Antioxidants in Functional Foods*. New York: Chapman and Hall 1995.
5. Papas AM. Oil-soluble antioxidants in foods. *Toxicol Ind Health* 1993;9:123-49.
6. Harman D. Free-radical theory of aging: Increasing the functional life span. *Ann NY Acad Sci* 1994;717:1-15.

7. Parthasarathy S, Rankin SM. Role of oxidized low density lipoprotein in atherogenesis. *Prog Lipid Res* 1992;31:127-43.
8. Cerutti PA, Trump BF. Inflammation and oxidative stress in carcinogenesis. *Cancer Cells* 1991;3:1-7.
9. Baynes JW. Role of oxidative stress in development of complications in diabetes. *Diabetes* 1991;40:405-412.
10. Spector A. Oxidative stress-induced cataract: mechanism of action. *FASEB J* 1995;9:1173-1182.
11. Ebadi M, Srinivasan SK, Baxi MD. Oxidative stress and antioxidant therapy in Parkinson's disease. *Prog Neurobiol* 1996;48:1-19.
12. Brown RK, Kelly FJ. Evidence for increased oxidative damage in patients with cystic fibrosis. *Pediatr Res* 1994;36:487-93.
13. Lyras L, Cairns NJ, Jenner A, Jenner P, Halliwell B. An assessment of oxidative damage to proteins, lipids, and DNA in brain from patients with Alzheimer's disease. *J Neurochem* 1997;68:2061-9.
14. Owen AD, Schapira AH, Jenner P, Marsden CD. Oxidative stress and Parkinson's disease. *Ann NY Acad Sci* 1996;786:217-23.
15. Lynch SM, Frei B. Mechanisms of copper- and iron-dependent oxidative modification of human low density lipoprotein. *J. Lipid Res* 1993;34:1745-1753.
16. Nelson RL. Dietary iron and colorectal cancer risk. *Free Rad Biol Med* 1992;12:161-168.
17. Gower JD. A role for dietary lipids and antioxidants in the activation of carcinogens. *Free Radic Biol Med* 1988;5:95-111.
18. Papas AM. Determinants of antioxidant status in humans. *Lipids* 1996;31:S77-82.
19. Pryor WA. Ozone in all its reactive splendor. *J Lab Clin Med* 1993;122:483-486.
20. Menzel DB. The toxicity of air pollution in experimental animals and humans: the role of oxidative stress. *Toxicol Lett* 1994;72:269-77.
21. O'Neill C, van der Vliet A, Eiserich JP, Last JA, Halliwell B, Cross CE. Oxidative damage by ozone and nitrogen dioxide: synergistic toxicity *in vivo* but no evidence of synergistic oxidative damage in an extracellular fluid. *Biochem Soc Symp* 1995;61:139-52.
22. Erroi A, Pagani P, Sironi M, Salmona M. *In vivo* exposure to NO_2 reduces TNF and IL-6 production by endotoxin- stimulated alveolar macrophages. *Am J Physiol* 1996;271:L132-8.
23. Devalia JL, Bayram H, Rusznak C, *et al.* Mechanisms of pollution-induced airway disease: *in vitro* studies in the upper and lower airways. *Allergy* 1997;52:51UI-97351776.
24. Peden DB. Mechanisms of pollution-induced airway disease: *in vivo* studies. *Allergy* 1997;52:37-44.
25. Pryor WA. Mechanisms of radical formation from reactions of ozone with target molecules in the lung. *Free Rad Biol Med* 1994: 451-456.
26. Elsayed NM, Mustafa MG, Mead JF. Increased Vitamin E content of the lung after ozone exposure: a possible mobilization in response to oxidative stress. *Arch Biochem Biophys* 1990: 263-269.
27. Thiele JJ, Traber MG, Tsang K, Polefka T, Cross C, Packer L. Ozone-exposure depletes vitamin E and induces lipid peroxidation in murine stratum corneum. *J Invest Dermatol* 1997;108:753-757.
28. Cheeseman KH, Albano EF, Tomasi A, Slater TF. Biochemical studies on the metabolic activation of halogenated alkanes. *Environ Health Perspect* 1985;64:85-101.
29. Bagchi D, Bagchi M, Hassoun EA, Stohs SJ. *In vitro* and *in vivo* generation of reactive oxygen species, DNA damage and lactate dehydrogenase leakage by selected pesticides. *Toxicology* 1995;104:129-40.
30. Lodovici M, Casalini C, Briani C, Dolara P. Oxidative liver DNA damage in rats treated with pesticide mixtures. *Toxicology* 1997;117:55-60.

31. Frei B, Forte TM, Ames BN, Cross CE. Gas Phase Oxidants of Cigarette Smoke induce Lipid Peroxidation and Changes in Lipoprotein Properties in Human Blood Plasma. *Biochem J* 1991:277:133-8.
32. Pryor WA, Stone K. Oxidants in cigarette smoke. *Ann NY Acad Sci* 1992:29.
33. Evans MD, Pryor WA. Cigarette smoking, emphysema, and damage to alpha 1-proteinase inhibitor. *Am J Physiol* 1994;266:L593-611.
34. Ross MA, Crosley LK, Brown KM, *et al.* Plasma concentrations of carotenoids and antioxidant vitamins in Scottish males: influences of smoking. *Eur J Clin Nutr* 1995;49:861-5.
35. Driskell JA, Giraud DW, Sun J, Martin HD. Plasma concentrations of carotenoids and tocopherols in male long-term tobacco chewers, smokers and nonusers. *Int J Vitam Nutr Res* 1996;66:203-9.
36. Handelman GJ, Packer L, Cross CE. Destruction of tocopherols, carotenoids, and retinol in human plasma by cigarette smoke. *Am J Clin Nutr* 1996;63:559-65.
37. Wurzel H, Yeh CC, Gairola C, Chow CK. Oxidative damage and antioxidant status in the lungs and bronchoalveolar lavage fluid of rats exposed chronically to cigarette smoke. *J Biochem Toxicol* 1995;10:11-7.
38. Darr D, Combs S, Dunston S, Manning T, Pinnell S. Topical vitamin C protects porcine skin from ultraviolet radiation-induced damage. *Brit J Derm* 1992;127:247-253.
39. Fuchs J, Huflejt ME, Rothfuss LM, Wilson DS, Carcamo G, Packer L. Impairment of enzymic and nonenzymic antioxidants in skin by UVB irradiation. *J Invest Derm* 1989;93:769-773.
40. Grewe M, Trefzer U, Ballhorn A, Gyufko K, Henninger H, Krutmann J. Analysis of the mechanism of ultraviolet (UV) B radiation-induced prostaglandin E2 synthesis by human epidermoid carcinoma cells. *J Invest Dermatol* 1993;101:528-531.
41. Podda M, Traber MG, Weber C, Yan L-J, Packer L. UV-Irradiation Depletes Antioxidants and Causes Oxidative Damage in a Model of Human Skin. *Free Radic Biol Med* 1998;24:55-65.
42. Thiele JJ, Traber MG, Packer L. Depletion of human stratum corneum vitamin E: an early and sensitive *in vivo* marker of UV induced-photo-oxidation. *J Invest Dermatol* 1998;110:756-761.
43. Weber C, Podda M, Rallis M, Traber MG, Packer L. Efficacy of topical application of tocopherols and tocotrienols in protection of murine skin from oxidative damage induced by UV-irradiation. *Free Radic Biol Med* 1997;22:761-769.
44. Jurkiewicz BA, Bissett DL, Buettner GR. Effect of topically applied tocopherol on ultraviolet radiation-mediated free radical damage in skin. *J Invest Derm* 1995;104:484-488.
45. Gensler HL, Magdaleno M. Topical vitamin E inhibition of immunosuppression and tumorigenesis induced irradiation. *Nutr Cancer* 15 1991: 97-106.
46. Kramer KA, Liebler DC. UVB induced photooxidation of vitamin E. *Chem Res Toxicol* 1997;10:219-24.
47. Ganziano MJ, Buring JE, Breslow JL, *et al.* Moderate alcohol intake, increased levels of high-density lipoprotein and its subfractions, and decreased risk of myocardial infarction. *N Engl J Med* 1993: 1829-1834.
48. Pace-Asciak CR, Hahn S, Diamandis EP, Soleas G, Goldberg DM. The red wine phenolics *trans*-resveratrol and quercetin block human platelet aggregation and eicosanoid synthesis: implications for protection against coronary heart disease. *Clin Chim Acta* 1995;235:207-19.
49. Frankel EN, Kanner J, German JB, Parks E, Kinsella JE. Inhibition of oxidation of human low-density lipoprotein by phenolic substances in red wine. *Lancet* 341 1993: 454-457.

50. de Rijke YB, Demacker PN, Assen NA, Sloots LM, Katan MB, Stalenhoef AF. Red wine consumption does not affect oxidizability of low-density lipoproteins in volunteers. *Am J Clin Nutr* 1996;63:329-34.
51. Abu-Amsha R, Croft KD, Puddey IB, Proudfoot JM, Beilin LJ. Phenolic content of various beverages determines the extent of inhibition of human serum and low-density lipoprotein oxidation *in vitro*: identification and mechanism of action of some cinnamic acid derivatives from red wine. *Clin Sci (Colch)* 1996;91:449-58.
52. Croft KD, Puddey IB, Rakic V, Abu-Amsha R, Dimmitt SB, Beilin LJ. Oxidative susceptibility of low-density lipoproteins--influence of regular alcohol use. *Alcohol Clin Exp Res* 1996;20:980-4.
53. Lieber CS. Alcohol and the liver: 1994 update. *Gastroenterology* 1994:1085-1105.
54. Lecomte E, Herbeth B, Pirollet P, *et al.* Effect of alcohol consumption on blood antioxidant nutrients and oxidative stress indicators. *Amer J Clin Nutr* 1994:255-261.
55. Meydani M, Seitz HK, Blumberg JB, Russell RM. Effect of chronic ethanol feeding on hepatic and extrahepatic distribution of vitamin E in rats. *Alcohol Clin Exp Res* 1991;15:771-4.
56. Sadrzadeh SM, Nanji AA, Meydani M. Effect of chronic ethanol feeding on plasma and liver alpha- and gamma-tocopherol levels in normal and vitamin E-deficient rats. Relationship to lipid peroxidation. *Biochem Pharmacol* 1994;47:2005-10.
57. von Herbay A, de Groot H, Hegi U, Stremmel W, Strohmeyer G, Sies H. Low vitamin E content in plasma of patients with alcoholic liver disease, hemochromatosis and Wilson's disease. *J Hepat* 1994;20:41-6.
58. Leo MA, Kim CI, Loe N, Lieber CS. Interaction of ethanol with b-carotene. Delayed clearance and enhanced hepatotoxicity. *Hepatology* 1992;15:883-891.
59. Stohs SJ, Bagchi D. Oxidative mechanisms in the toxicity of metal ions. *Free Radic Biol Med* 1995;18:321-36.
60. Herbert V, Shaw S, Stopler-Kasdan T. Most free-radical injury is iron related: It is promoted by iron, hemin, holoferritin, and vitamin C, and inhibited by desferrioxamine and apoferritin. *Stem Cells* 12 1994: 289-303.
61. Pryor WA, Squadrito GL. The chemistry of peroxynitrite: A product from the reaction of nitric oxide with superoxide. *Am J Physiol* 1995;268:L699-L722.
62. Sokol RJ. Vitamin E deficiency and neurological disorders. In: Packer L, Fuchs J, Eds. *Vitamin E in Health and Disease*. New York, NY: Marcel Dekker, Inc. 1993:815-849.
63. Baum MK, Shor-Posner G, Bonvechi P, *et al.* Influence of HIV infection on vitamin status and requirement. *Ann NY Acad Sci* 1992: 165-173.
64. Young IS, Trouton TG, Torney JJ, McMaster D, Callender ME, Trimble ER. Antioxidant status and lipid peroxidation in hereditary haemochromatosis. *Free Rad Biol Med* 1994: 393-397.
65. Kaempf D, Miki M, Ogihara T, Okamoto R, Konishi K, Mino M. Assessment of vitamin E nutritional status in neonates, infants and children--on the basis of alpha-tocopherol levels in blood components and buccal mucosal cells. *Intl J Vit Nutr Res* 1994;64:185-91.
66. Argao EA, Heubi JE. Fat-soluble vitamin deficiency in infants and children. *Curr Opin Pediatr* 1993;5:562-6.
67. Oski FA, Barness LA. Vitamin E deficiency: a previously unrecognized cause of hemolytic anemia in the premature infant. *J Pediatr* 1967;70:211-20.
68. Murphy ME, Kolvenbach R, Aleksis M, Hansen R, Sies H. Antioxidant depletion in aortic crossclamping ischemia: increase of the plasma alpha-tocopheryl quinone/alpha-tocopherol ratio. *Free Radic Biol Med* 1992;13:95-100.
69. Janero D. Therapeutic Potential of Viamin E Against Myocardial Ischemic-Reperfusion Injury. *Free Radic. Biol. Med.* 1991;10:315-324.

70. Halpner AD, Blumberg JB. Assessment of antioxidant vitamin status in older adults. In: Rosenberg IH, Ed. *Nutritional Assessment of Elderly Populations*: Measure and Function. New York: Raven Press 1995:147-165.
71. Blumberg JB, Suter P. Pharmacology, nutrition, and the elderly: Interactions and implications in geriatric nutrition. In: Chernoff R, Ed. *Geriatric Nutrition*. Rockville, MD.: Aspen Publishers Inc. 1991:337-361.
72. Cannon JG, Meydani SN, Fielding RA, *et al.* Accute phase response in exercise. II. Associations between vitamin E, cytokines, and muscle proteolysis. *Am J Physiol* 1991: R1235-R1240.
73. Packer L. Oxidants, antioxidant nutrients and the athlete. *J Sports Sci* 1997;15:353-63.
74. Papas AM. Vitamin E and exercise: aspects of biokinetics and bioavailability. *World Rev Nutr Diet* 1993;72:165-76.
75. Simon-Schnass IM. Nutrition in high altitude. *J. Nutr* 1992;122: 778-781.
76. Pryor WA. Measurement of oxidative stress status in humans. *Cancer Epidemiol Biomarkers Prev* 1993;2:289-92.
77. Pryor WA, Godber SS. Noninvasive measures of oxidative stress status in humans. *Free Radic Biol Med* 1991;10:177-84.
78. Pryor WA, Godber SS. Oxidative stress status: an introduction. *Free Radic Biol Med* 1991;10:173.
79. Hageman JJ, Bast A, Vermeulen NP. Monitoring of oxidative free radical damage *in vivo*: analytical aspects. *Chem Biol Interact* 1992;82:243-93.
80. Halliwell B. Antioxidants: the basics—what they are and how to evaluate them. *Adv Pharmacol* 1997;38:3-20.
81. Halliwell B. Oxidative stress, nutrition and health. Experimental strategies for optimization of nutritional antioxidant intake in humans. *Free Radic Res* 1996;25:57-74.

3

Evaluation of Antioxidant Status in Humans

Garry J. Handelman, Ph.D.
USDA Human Nutrition Research Center on Aging
Boston, Massachusetts, USA

William A. Pryor, Ph.D.
Biodynamics Institute, Louisiana State University
Baton Rouge, Louisiana, USA

INTRODUCTION

Antioxidant status reflects the balance between the antioxidant defenses and oxidants in living organisms. Impairment of the antioxidant defenses (for example due to inadequate intake of dietary antioxidants) and/or high levels of oxidants (from smog, cigarette smoke, illness, etc.) can lead to oxidative stress. Oxidative stress in humans has been implicated in the pathogenesis of major chronic diseases. Specifically, a role of oxidative stress has been demonstrated for inflammation, ischemia-reperfusion, carcinogenesis and atherosclerosis, and suggested for many other diseases and for aging. For this reason, there has been strong interest in preventing oxidative stress and maintaining an antioxidant status that supports good health. A prerequisite for achieving these objectives is the ability to measure accurately the antioxidant status and oxidant stress in humans.

In this chapter, we review methods for measuring antioxidant status in humans and discuss their advantages and limitations. In the first part we consider the relationship between measurable components and the total physiological system; in the second part, we discuss useful methods for measuring antioxidant nutrient status in humans; and in the third part, we discuss methods for evaluating oxidant stress. Finally, in Appendix 1, we discuss, very briefly, methods for evaluating the antioxidant status that appear promising and may find utility in the future after further development and evaluation.

IMPORTANT CONSIDERATIONS

Direct Versus Indirect Measures

Many biologically important oxidants and radicals are highly reactive and therefore short lived; however, it should be recognized that not all free radicals have high reactivity. Indeed, the lifetimes of reactive oxygen species (ROS) vary from 10^{-9} sec for the hydroxyl radical (HO•) to lifetimes of seconds for peroxyl radicals (ROO•) and even infinitely long lifetimes for semiquinone radicals such as the cigarette tar free radical.[1] However, in general, the direct measurement of free radicals by electron spin resonance is possible only in special circumstances and, at present, does not appear likely to become the basis of clinical tests in humans for oxidative status. The one exception to this is the ascorbate radical, which is a relatively stable semiquinone radical that is seen in almost all human liquid tissue such as blood, semen, etc.[2] Some ROS are relatively stable molecules and not radicals; examples include lipid hydroperoxides and hydrogen peroxide. Nevertheless, it is a general statement that most ROS can only be directly measured with some difficulty, owing either to their short lifetimes or to the lack of suitably sensitive methods to detect the low levels that occur in cells.

Since the oxidants or radicals themselves can be directly observed only in special circumstances, stable products from the reactions of radicals and/or oxidants with their biological target molecules generally are measured. These products are, in a sense, the "footprints" left by the more fleeting ROS themselves. These footprint molecules include oxidatively damaged lipids, proteins, and DNA, which are measured as surrogate markers for ROS.

The levels of antioxidants in animals and cells are dynamic and have many components ranging from antioxidant nutrients and phytochemicals to enzymes, proteins, and others. As with oxidative stress, the methods to measure selected components of these antioxidant systems using the least invasive procedures such as blood sampling, etc. pose challenging research problems.

In this chapter, we will focus on these indirect methods because, as discussed above, they are commonly used and have practical significance. These may be grouped in the following major categories of methods measuring:

1. Antioxidant nutrients, enzymes and other components of the antioxidant system, primarily in the blood but also in some other tissues.
2. Markers of oxidative stress primarily in blood, urine, breath and, to a lesser extent, other tissues.

Balance between Synthesis and Breakdown

The biochemistry of oxidant stress markers includes both synthetic and catabolic steps. For this reason, a level of a marker measured at one time may not be representative of its real value. For example, rapid hepatic degradation and a shorter protein half-life would correspond to a lower steady-state level of damaged circulating proteins (such as protein-bound nitrotyrosine) and underestimate the extent of damage from ROS.

Models of ROS status should integrate both synthetic and degradative processes in the steady-state approximation. The same considerations apply to levels of tissue antioxidant nutrients. For example, very high plasma vitamin E levels in some hyperlipidemias may be attributed incorrectly to increased dietary intake of vitamin E if the elevated level of lipoproteins is not considered.

The Antioxidant System Has Many Components

The antioxidant system is composed of exogenous components derived from the diet and endogenous components. Those obtained from the diet include vitamins such as E and C, minerals such selenium, and other components such as carotenoids and phytochemicals. Those synthesized in the body include the tripeptide glutathione, the iron-binding proteins transferrin and ferritin, and the enzymes catalase and superoxide dismutase. Individual antioxidants do not function in isolation, but as components of this system with many interactions, synergies, and antagonisms. For example, it is believed that vitamin C and glutathione regenerate vitamin E. These interactions of dietary antioxidants extend to their absorption, transport, and tissue uptake. Examples are discussed below. For this reason, single components may not be reliable indicators of antioxidant status.

Localized Versus Systemic Measures

When produced at the proper location and in controlled amounts, ROS perform useful biological functions. For example, lipid peroxides formed during eicosanoid biosynthesis,[3,4] nitrogen oxides generated in the vascular system,[5] and superoxide released by activated phagocytes[6] play important roles in gene expression, cell growth, and communication and immunity.

Oxidative stress and associated damage from excess production of ROS may be localized at cellular sites, tissues, or organs. Thus, the oxidative stress status of some tissues and organs may not be reflected in general systemic measures and may require additional, more site-specific measures.

Markers: Populations Versus Individuals

Epidemiological studies of several markers of antioxidant status, such as the rate of oxidation of low-density lipoprotein (LDL) *in vitro* or the levels of vitamin E and ascorbate in plasma, provided insights into associations of antioxidants and disease and also into the mechanisms of disease. Continued use of these oxidative stress measures for population studies therefore is very likely to be rewarding. However, markers are useful for individuals only if they can be compared to well-established normal ranges, and more work is needed to establish ranges associated with good health and prevention of disease. For this reason, classification of individuals into normal or high-risk groups should be done with extreme care and only on the basis of multiple measures.

MEASUREMENT OF COMPONENTS OF THE ANTIOXIDANT SYSTEM

Antioxidant Nutrients and Phytochemicals

A large number of studies, primarily observational, conducted in the last 50 years (reviewed in Part 6 of this book) find a positive association of elevated blood and tissue antioxidants such as vitamin E, vitamin C, and carotenoids with long-term positive health outcomes. For some antioxidants, beneficial effects have been reported for doses well above the minimal amounts required to saturate biochemical pathways.[7-9] For example, evidence from epidemiological and limited intervention studies suggest that higher vitamin E intakes are associated with less risk of development of atherosclerosis.[10-12] These associations have generated strong interest in using blood and tissue levels of antioxidants as indicators of antioxidant status.

We will discuss the methods that can be used to determine the major antioxidant nutrients and phytochemicals.

Vitamin E

The tocopherol group, known collectively as vitamin E, consists of 4 tocopherols and 4 tocotrienols designated as α, β, γ, and δ (see Chapter 10).

Vitamin E status can be estimated by the measurement of the levels of the tocopherols and tocotrienols in plasma and/or adipose tissue. The major plasma tocopherols, α and γ, are readily measured by high pressure liquid chromatography (HPLC).[13] The National Institutes of Standards and Technology (NIST) provide calibrated plasma samples for an external plasma tocopherol reference.[14] Older methods for vitamin E included gas chromatography (GC) and the ability of the organic extract to reduce ferric ions to ferrous. These and other earlier methods have been rendered obsolete by HPLC methods.

Vitamin E status can also be estimated by HPLC determination of its components in platelets and erythrocytes, but since these bloodstream components are in rapid equilibrium with plasma lipids, a reliable status estimate can be obtained from plasma. Americans that are not currently taking vitamin supplements have plasma α-tocopherol levels in the range of 15-25 μM. For every tenfold increase in dietary α-tocopherol, there is approximately a twofold increase in plasma levels, so that the following approximate relationship is observed (Figure 1),[8] with substantial between-person variation and smaller increase at higher intake levels.

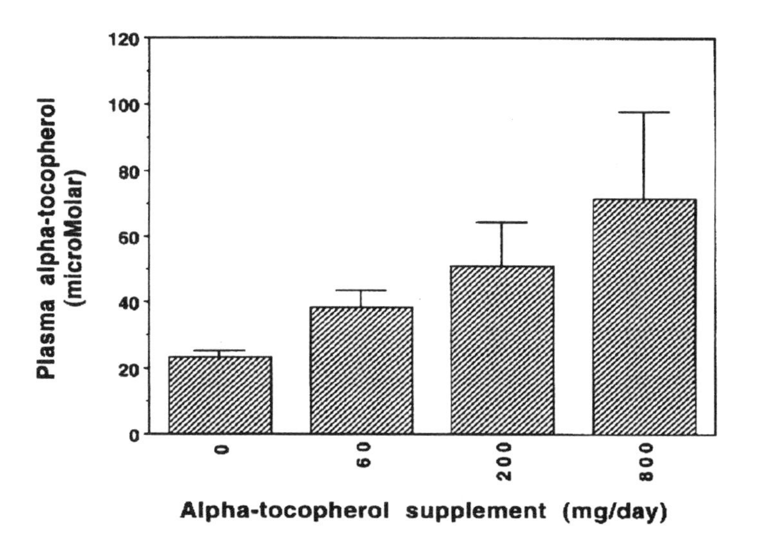

Figure 1. Change in plasma α-tocopherol in healthy elderly subjects receiving 60, 200, and 800 mg dl-α-tocopheryl acetate daily. Reproduced with permission from Reference 8 (Meydani *et al., JAMA* 277:1380-1386, 1997. Copyright 1997, American Medical Association).

Important considerations. In most studies, plasma or adipose α-tocopherol levels are reported as the chief indicator of vitamin E status.

Plasma α-tocopherol levels are typically much higher than plasma γ-tocopherol levels, even though the typical American diet contains more γ-tocopherol than α-tocopherol (see Chapter 10). Commercial supplements consist primarily of α-tocopherol, and high intake of α-tocopherol further depresses γ-tocopherol levels both in plasma[13,15] and in adipose tissue.[16] Part of the interaction between α-tocopherol and γ-tocopherol levels is due to the function of the hepatic α-tocopherol-binding protein, which selectively enriches newly-synthesized lipoproteins with the natural isomer, RRR-α-tocopherol.[17] Measurements of tocopherols in adipose tissue have been preferred as a long-term marker of dietary α-tocopherol supplementation; the α/γ tocopherol ratio in adipose tissue may also be an excellent indicator of α-tocopherol supplement use.[16]

Recent work[18] suggests that γ-tocopherol, but not α-tocopherol, can be nitrated by peroxynitrite at the unsubstituted aromatic carbon atom adjacent to the γ-tocopherol OH group; whether or not this is significant *in vivo* is not clear, but if this reaction were important then γ-tocopherol would possess protective properties that α-tocopherol does not. The tocotrienols and other tocopherols may also have important antioxidant functions (see Chapters 10 and 22). For these reasons, estimates of the vitamin E status based exclusively on α-tocopherol levels may be incomplete or even erroneous.

High doses of fish oil might lead to decreased intestinal absorption of α-tocopherol and depressed plasma values of α-tocopherol.[19] Thus, plasma α-tocopherol might be low even with adequate dietary intake. For interpretation of the plasma α-tocopherol level, it may be appropriate for the investigator to include review of other dietary practices, including consumption of fish oil.

Plasma α-tocopherol levels are influenced by plasma lipids. Independent of any change in dietary intake, a doubling in plasma cholesterol is associated with a very large increase in plasma α-tocopherol. Thus, two people on similar diets may have very different levels of α-tocopherol. For this reason, the use of the α-tocopherol/cholesterol ratio in plasma has been recommended as more appropriate for estimating vitamin E status.

Selenium (Se)

Selenium is a co-factor for the antioxidant enzyme glutathione peroxidase (Se-GSH-Px),[20,21] which has multiple forms.[22,23] Selenium also has a role in the thyroid deiodinase[24] and thioredoxin reductase[25] enzyme systems. Additional proteins that contain Se are likely to be discovered in the future.

Selenium deficiency may be important for human populations in New Zealand, the Keshan region of China, and other areas with low Se content in the soil and a restricted ability to consume foodstuffs grown in other locales.[26,27] The deficiency is clearly demonstrated by low plasma Se-GSH-Px values and low plasma Se levels.[26] The deficiency may be associated with certain forms of heart disease, but it responds readily to a dietary supplement of 100 μg of Se, either as selenite or Se-rich yeast (primarily selenomethionine).

The measurement of Se status is more challenging than other antioxidant nutrients. Plasma Se can be analyzed by graphite-furnace atomic absorption.[28] Erythrocyte Se is a better long-term indicator of Se status, but its analysis is formidable, due to the interference from iron and copper in the hemolysate, and, for this reason, wet-digestion using perchloric and nitric acid is essential for erythrocyte Se analysis.

Se-GSH-Px can be measured in plasma, platelets, and RBC. Few Americans will show any changes in plasma Se-GSH-Px levels following dietary supplementation. The analysis of Se-GSH-Px in platelets may be a reliable indicator of supplementation.[29]

Important considerations. Because many different factors (see Appendix 2) influence the measured level of Se-GSH-Px activity, standardization between different laboratories will be very difficult to achieve. A single laboratory, however, should be able to generate consistent long-term measurements.

Platelet Se-GSH-Px activity saturates when individuals consume an optimal dietary intake of Se, and this relationship can form the basis of a sensitive assay for dietary Se status. If platelet Se-GSH-Px is observed to be relatively low compared to other subjects, a moderate Se dose (100 μg/day for 30 days) can be administered. If the platelet Se-GSH-Px increases following this supplement[29] (see Figure 3), then suboptimal dietary intake is likely and the individual should be advised to increase Se intake. However, if platelet Se-GSH-Px fails to increase following this supplement, other factors may be involved.

Ascorbate (Vitamin C)

The classical role of ascorbate is to maintain transition metals in the reduced form, since the metals are co-factors for biochemical pathways such as proline hydroxylation and steroid biosynthesis.[30] The ability of ascorbate to scavenge aqueous peroxyl radicals[31] has led to the hypothesis that ascorbate is part of the antioxidant defense mechanisms of the vertebrate. In model systems, ascorbate has been shown to reduce the tocopheroxyl radical to tocopherol;[32] this observation has led to the hypothesis that ascorbate serves to maintain vitamin E in the reduced form,[33] thereby enhancing the *in vivo* antioxidant potency of α-tocopherol. However, controlled investigations with guinea pigs[34] and humans[35] have failed to establish that ascorbate recycles α-tocopherol *in vivo*.

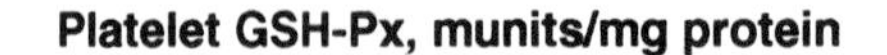

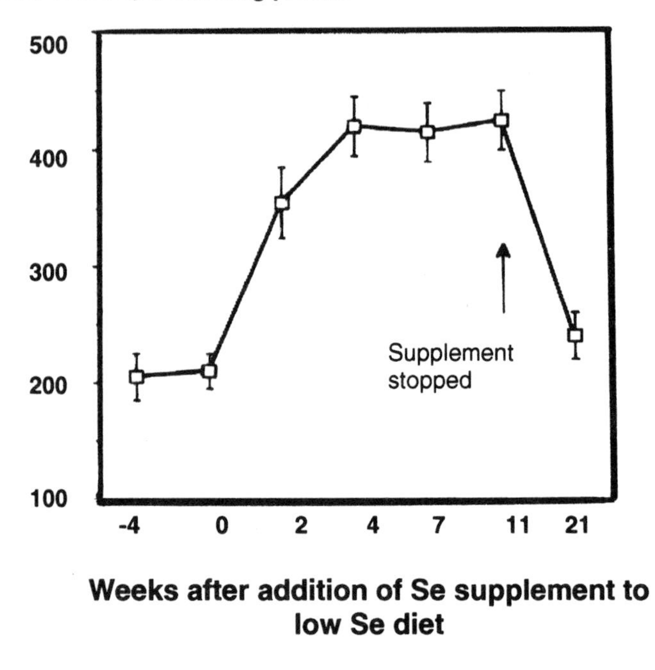

Figure 2. Increase of Se-GSH-Px in human platelets following selenium supplementation of a low selenium diet. Reproduced with permission from Reference 29 (Levander *et al.*, *Am J Clin Nutr* 37:887-897, 1983. Copyright 1983, American Institute of Nutrition).

A validated HPLC method[36] is available for assaying plasma ascorbate. This method requires the use of an electrochemical detector and is more sophisticated than HPLC methods for other antioxidants. Externally standardized plasma samples for calibration have been made available.[36] Ascorbate in plasma degrades to secondary products even if stored at –70 °C if the plasma sample is not stabilized at the time of collection. Metaphosphoric acid has been shown to be satisfactory for this purpose.[36]

Important Considerations. Low levels of ascorbate are prevalent in several populations including cigarette smokers,[37] low-income groups,[38] and elderly confined to nursing facilities.[39] The amount of dietary ascorbate required to achieve plasma saturation is approximately 200 mg/day.[40] Cigarette smoke contains abundant free radicals,[41] and decreased ascorbate levels in smokers may arise from direct attack of smoke constituents on tissue ascorbate[42] and not from reduced intake. Foods rich in ascorbate, as well as dietary supplements, increase plasma ascorbate in smokers to normal levels.[43] Measurement of plasma ascorbate is an important parameter for determining the antioxidant status in smokers.

When studied *in vitro*, ascorbate can also be a prooxidant, because ascorbate can reduce ferric to ferrous ion and promote the Fenton reaction.[44] The role of ascorbate as prooxidant *in vivo* remains controversial.

Carotenoids

HPLC measurements of individual plasma carotenoids are now readily performed in clinical laboratories.[45] Plasma lycopene and β-carotene are the most commonly measured carotenoids and are often used as indicators of carotenoid status, but other carotenoids, such as lutein, astaxanthin, and cryptoxanthin are increasingly used as indices of carotenoid status.

Important Considerations. Effects of dietary supplements can be evaluated in serial measurements. Plasma carotenoid levels reflect a complex interaction between dietary intake, other dietary components, individual gastrointestinal physiology, and lipoprotein turnover. Some dietary carotenoids (primarily β-carotene and α-carotene) have an established role as vitamin A precursors. For this reason, high intakes of preformed vitamin A may influence the plasma levels of these precursors. Other carotenoids such as lutein and zeaxanthin have a role in the human retina.[46,47] For these reasons, measurement of several carotenoids[48] provide a better indicator of carotenoid status than a single one. It is, however, difficult to measure all the known carotenoids, which number in the hundreds and whose importance as biological antioxidants is not yet known.

Several methods have been established to allow the analysis of the complex carotenoid profile found in biological tissues. These methods employ different combinations of HPLC columns and mobile phase gradients.[49,50]

Although carotenoids react rapidly with singlet oxygen and can also efficiently quench other ROS *in vitro*,[51] their role *in vivo* as antioxidants is not fully understood. High-dose supplements of β-carotene may be injurious to cigarette smokers.[52,53] This may be due the smoke-initiated breakdown of β-carotene in the lung to harmful products.[54-56]

Antioxidant Phytochemicals

A large number of phytochemicals have attracted interest for their role in nutrition and health. Many of these phytochemicals affect the antioxidant status directly due to their function as antioxidants, indirectly by chelating prooxidant divalent metals such as Fe and Cu, or by sparing other antioxidants. A group of these phytochemicals, the isoflavones, are discussed in Chapter 11. Blood and tissue levels of some of these compounds may be relevant to the antioxidant status in humans but their role as biological antioxidants is not yet fully understood.

Endogenous Components of the Antioxidant System

Glutathione

The most prevalent water-soluble antioxidant in humans is the tripeptide glutathione (GSH), which serves as a co-factor for the GSH-Px and GSH-S-transferase family of enzymes. GSH also has other roles, including conversion of oxidized ascorbate to reduced ascorbate, amino acid transport, and detoxification. Biosynthesis of GSH requires the sulfur amino acids cysteine and methionine; if these are deficient in the diet, GSH levels in tissue decline. The levels of sulfur amino acid intake can be evaluated by dietary analysis, but plasma levels of GSH are not a simple reflection of dietary intake of sulfur amino acids.[57]

GSH can be measured in plasma, erythrocytes, and lymphocytes. The most reliable measurements employ HPLC methods.[58] There is a colorimetric assay that is satisfactory for GSH levels for RBC and lymphocytes.[59] Normal human levels in RBC and WBC are 2 mmoles/L packed cells. Some of the GSH in tissues is present as oxidized glutathione (GSSG). The HPLC method[58] allows the measurement of both GSH and GSSG in plasma, cells, and tissues.

Important Considerations. During intensive exercise, erythrocyte GSH declines and plasma GSSG increases.[60] The lymphocyte levels of GSH are decreased during diseases with an inflammatory component, such as HIV.[61] The variation of GSH levels in exercise and aging requires further validation. For normal individuals in good health, these GSH measurements are of limited value, since tissue levels do not vary much in response to changes in diet. There have been reports that erythrocyte GSH changes during illness, but levels can both increase and decrease, and systematic study of erythrocyte GSH levels is needed.

Iron-Binding Proteins

The toxic prooxidant effects of iron, which derive in part from the Fenton reaction,[44] are largely prevented by iron-binding proteins, including transferrin, ferritin, and ceruloplasmin. Iron toxicity may occur through excess absorption of dietary iron (hemochromatosis), or through a very rare hereditary lack of transferrin.[62] The hypothesis has been advanced that diets rich in heme-iron may overload tissue stores of iron, with associated increases in degenerative diseases of aging.[63] The bleomycin assay[64,65] detects non-heme iron that is not tightly bound to transferrin or ferritin. The bleomycin assay may be positive in iron overload due to hemochromatosis.[66] Studies in neonates have shown that bleomycin-detectable iron can activate the iron-dependent responsive aconitase.[67]

Important Considerations. After several decades of investigation, the origin of many cases of hemochromatosis has been localized to a gene in the human histocompatibility (HL-A) locus.[68] Since this mutation can be identified by genomic analysis, it may be a useful part of ROS status determination to screen for this common mutation. Several of the oxidative stress markers reviewed here might be elevated in iron overload, and this should be a useful area for further investigations.

MARKERS OF OXIDATIVE STRESS

These markers consist primarily of adducts or end-products of reactions of ROS with lipids, proteins, carbohydrates, DNA, and other molecules. These products, as discussed above, have longer half-lives than ROS and are accessible to measurement. For these reasons, these markers have been used often in the evaluation of the antioxidant status and oxidative stress.

Thiobarbituric Acid Reactive Substances (TBARS)

The TBARS assay, as adapted for plasma by Yagi and co-workers,[69] has been a frequently utilized marker of increased *in vivo* oxidant stress. The TBARS assay forms a colored product (absorption maximum, 532 nm) which can be measured by a simple spectrophotometric assay. Fluorescence and HPLC modifications of the method have been developed.

The primary TBARS chromogen is the reaction product of thiobarbituric acid and malonaldehyde (MDA), which is generated during the analytical procedure from the decomposition of lipid hydroperoxides in the sample.[69] Additional plasma MDA exists covalently bound to amino groups on proteins or phospatidylethanolamine, and is liberated for reaction with thiobarbituric during the analytical procedure.

Several other sources contribute to color development in the TBARS assay.[70] For example, other aldehydes, such as acrolein, can contribute to color development.[71] MDA is also formed as a side reaction during prostaglandin biosynthesis,[72] such that plasma MDA may also be a marker for platelet activation and inflammation. Therefore, high TBARS cannot be assumed to mean high rates of lipid peroxidation *in vivo*.

A recent determination of plasma lipid hydroperoxides with the colorimetic ferrous xylenol orange (FOX) assay (*vide infra*) found that the direct FOX values and the TBARS values did not correlate.[73] This lack of correlation may be due to several factors, including the presence of other preformed MDA and other aldehydes in the plasma sample that contribute to the TBARS values, and variable yield of MDA from decomposition of different chemical species of lipid hydroperoxides.

Important Considerations. MDA, one of the chromogens that contributes to TBARS, could be a promising marker if its level in plasma could be measured directly, without interference from MDA generated during sample preparation. HPLC methods are promising, but may suffer interference from other aldehydes.[74] The use of gas chromatography/mass spectrometry (GC/MS) may provide specific measurement of pre-formed MDA in plasma.[75] It would be useful to apply a chemically defined, validated assay for MDA to animal or human models of oxidative stress, and subsequently to normal humans. An improved MDA assay would carefully differentiate between MDA intrinsic to the sample, and MDA formed from the decomposition of lipid peroxides in the sample during analysis.

Values obtained with the TBARS assay are often accepted as corresponding to plasma levels of lipid hydroperoxides. However, direct measurement of lipid hydroperoxides can be achieved only by HPLC or GC/MS measurement of the hydroperoxides in different lipid classes.

Breath Hydrocarbons

The diverse mixture of products formed during peroxidation of polyunsaturated fatty acids (PUFA), includes pentane present from ω-6 fatty acids such as 18:2ω6 and 20:4ω6, and ethane from ω-3 fatty acids such as 20:5ω3 and 22:6ω3.[76] A portion of these volatile compounds is released into the breath, which can be collected and analyzed by GC. Elevated values of these hydrocarbons in the breath of oxidant-stressed experimental animals was first reported in 1977.[77] The technique of breath analysis has undergone considerable refinement with application to capillary GC to achieve maximum resolution.[78]

The unsaturated branched-chain hydrocarbon isoprene (C_5H_8) is produced as a secondary product of the HMG-CoA-reductase pathway in adult humans, and appears in the breath.[79] Isoprene and pentane may co-elute during GC analysis of breath (Figure 3), and there is usually more isoprene in normal breath than pentane.[80] Because of this interference, pentane values reported in adult humans may not be reliable. However, breath ethane measurement can be carried out with minimal interference.

Important Considerations. This is one of the least invasive assays. The complexity of the analysis, however, has been underestimated, leading to substantial variation in results from different investigations.[81] This widely used assay will benefit from critical efforts at standardization. Breath ethane levels are elevated in smokers,[82] consistent with the increased oxidative stress imposed by smoking.[41] Breath hydrocarbons are higher after strenuous exercise and in some conditions such as diabetes.

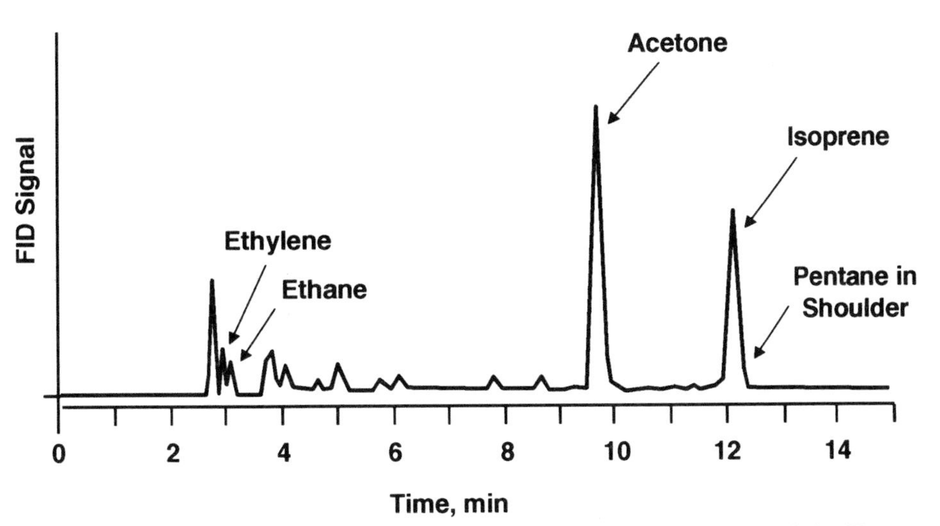

Figure 3. Chromatogram of hydrocarbons in human breath sample (courtesy of Dr. Terence Risby, School of Public Health, Johns Hopkins University, Baltimore, MD). Column, fused silica capillary, 60 M length, 0.53 mm ID, dimethysilicone stationary phase (nonpolar), helium carrier gas. Temperature program: 0-10 min, 25 °C, ramp to 200 °C at 5 °C/min, hold at 200 °C for 5 min. Detection: FID. Polar GC stationary phases are necessary to resolve pentane and isoprene.

Isoprostanes

Pryor *et al.*[72] hypothesized in the 1970s that the radical oxidation of polyunsaturated fatty acids with 3 or more double bonds could undergo a cyclization to give non-enzymatically derived products analogous to prostaglandin H2; when the fatty acid is arachidonic acid, these radical-mediated oxidations would give isoeicosanoids. In recent years, non-enzymatically formed isoprostanes have been identified in animal and human tissues, along with enzymatically formed eicosanoids, and these isoprostanes have proven to be one of the most useful probes of radical/oxidant activity in cells. Some of these stable products of arachidonic acid autoxidation have been identified in tissue lipids during both normal and pathological conditions.

One heterogeneous group of stable isoprostanes have 3 hydroxy groups (Figure 4). Although structurally similar to prostaglandins, isoprostanes have different stereochemistry than the enzymatically controlled eicosanoids and many different stereoisomers may exist. For example, 128 diastereomers of the four regioisomers of the F2 class of isoprostanes gives rise to 512 potentially distinct compounds that are derived from arachidonic acid.[83] The formation of E2 and D2 isoprostanes occurs less frequently than F2 compounds and these compounds are not often detected in plasma. Measurements of both urinary and plasma levels of the isoprostane 8-epi-F2-alpha have been gaining acceptance as a useful index of free radical-mediated injury. Plasma isoprostane levels are elevated in non-insulin-dependent diabetes,[84] and urinary values are increased in scleroderma.[85]

Both physical and immunological methods have been developed to analyze isoprostanes. An immunoassay method for 8-epi-F2-alpha-isoprostane was developed to determine isoprostanes in excretions. This method, similar to other enzyme-linked assays (ELISA), has a high degree of sensitivity but is hampered by cross-reactions with other prostanoids. Several GC/MS methods have been successfully developed to analyze for various isoprostanes. Although analyses by these methods are expensive, the sensitivity and specificity are unrivaled.

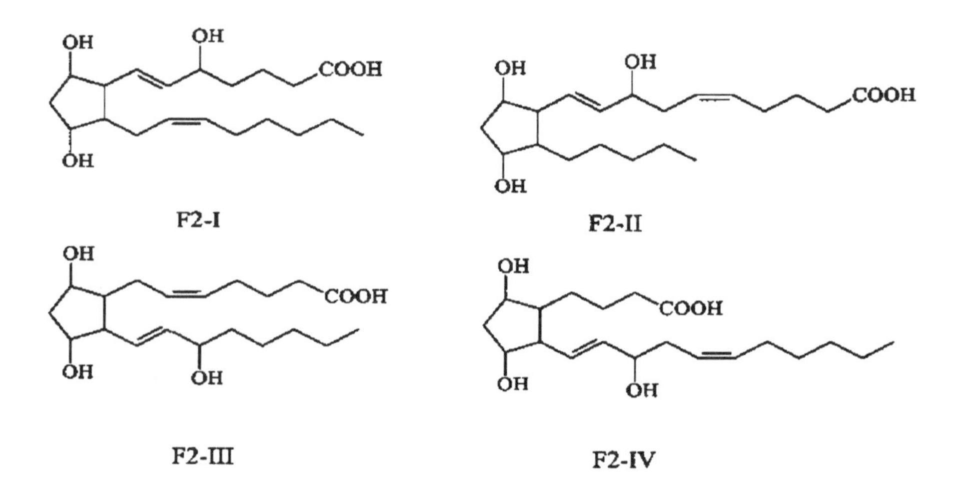

Figure 4. Basic structures of the F-2 isoprostanes. Each compound may exist in many different stereoisomers.

Important Considerations. For measurements of total isoprostanes in plasma, both the GC/MS method and the ELISA kit require extensive sample preparation. The main obstacle to further study is the need to simplify, reduce the cost, and standardize the measurements of isoprostanes.

There is no evidence to date that isosprostanes can be used as markers of oxidative stress in normal individuals, except for smokers, where levels are elevated twofold.[86] Studies of the effects of dietary antioxidants and PUFA intake are needed.

LDL Oxidation *ex vivo*

An accumulating body of research indicates that oxidative damage to LDL enhances atherogenicity. In basic research studies, oxidized LDL has been shown to accelerate several steps in atherogenesis including endothelial damage, monocyte/macrophage recruitment, increased uptake of LDL by foam cells, alteration in vascular tone, induction of growth factors, and formation of autoantibodies. For this reason, the LDL oxidation assay *ex vivo* is widely used as a research tool to evaluate the effect of dietary antioxidants, particularly vitamin E, on the ability of LDL to resist oxidation (discussed in Chapter 16).

The most common LDL oxidation assay involves LDL isolation from blood, challenge with oxidants such as Cu^{2+}, and measurement of the lag-time before oxidation. The detailed protocols for LDL isolation, oxidative challenge, and assessment of damage to LDL vary substantially among different laboratories,[87] and direct comparison of results between different laboratories is usually not possible.

The measurement of LDL susceptibility to oxidation *ex vivo* has been used as a research tool to study the relationship between diet and heart disease. However, no evidence has been presented for its relevance as an indicator for individual vulnerability to development of heart disease.

Important Considerations. The LDL oxidation assay is not standardized between laboratories at this time, so all measurements need to be conducted in a single clinical laboratory.

This assay is useful in evaluating changes in the LDL resistance to oxidation for individuals. For example, improved resistance to *ex vivo* oxidation determined by serial sampling before and after intervention is a promising indicator for cardiovascular health of an individual. Whether single measures can be used to classify people in high or low risk groups remains controversial.

The Ferrous Xylenol Orange (FOX) Assay

The hydroperoxide content of the lipid fraction of plasma can be determined from its ability to oxidize Fe^{2+} to Fe^{3+}. The Fe^{3+} formed is detected as a complex with xylenol orange reagent,[88] which is measured at 560 nm.

$$ROOH + Fe^{2+} \longrightarrow RO\cdot + HO^- + Fe^{3+}$$

$$Fe^{3+} + \text{xylenol orange} \longrightarrow \text{blue chromophore } (\lambda \text{ max} = 560\text{nm})$$

This assay is simple to use and is a candidate for standardization between different laboratories. First the measurement is made with normal plasma. Then the measurement is made in plasma treated with triphenylphosphine to eliminate hydroperoxides. The FOX value is the difference between these two measurements.

Important Considerations. The FOX assay values are 2 to 3-fold higher in subjects with diabetes.[72] Because the nature of the chemical assay is straightforward and simple to use, this assay is an important candidate for epidemiological studies and for the effects of changing diet or behavior in individuals followed over time.

OTHER METHODS

A number of other methods may be used for evaluating antioxidant status in humans. Some of these methods have very specific uses and/or require further development and validation. We briefly summarize some of these methods in Appendix 1.

STANDARDIZATION

Standardization is a useful step in the development of new methods, since it allows investigators separated in space and time to compare results. Measurements of antioxidant nutrient and oxidative stress status may become more common in the future with the increasing use of automated laboratory instruments. While some assays (isoprostanes and Se levels) may remain expensive and labor-intensive, others (vitamin E, ascorbate, carotenoids, and the FOX and Se-GSH-Px assays) might become affordable if they were widely adopted.

For medical diagnosis, clinical tests performed in different laboratories can be used with confidence due to excellent standardization and validation of the methods used. Widely used clinical laboratory tests are standardized through surveys by reference laboratories and by the distribution of quality-control materials to participating laboratories.

Many of the measures of antioxidants and oxidative stress have not yet been subjected to this type of standardization and such standardization may be difficult. For example, the measured enzymatic activity of plasma Se-GSH-Px is a simultaneous function of several parameters (see Appendix 2). Therefore, and in direct contrast to the rigorously standardized plasma cholesterol measurements, usually it is not possible to directly compare Se-GSH-Px values reported from different laboratories, and the nature of the Se-GSH-Px assay makes this a difficult goal to achieve.

Basic Laboratory Requirements for Non-Standardized Methods

The successful application of the non-standardized assays discussed in this review of clinical and research problems depends on the capabilities of the laboratory that will carry out the analyses. The following criteria may be considered:

- Estimate of the range of biological variation based on a broad spectrum of individuals.
- Satisfactory reproducibility – both within and between days for replicate analysis of the same sample.
- Quality control procedures, such as pooled serum aliquots, which insure the accuracy of the results.
- Repeated measurements, especially when evaluating the effect of dietary changes or other interventions.

If these requirements are met, then the clinician or researcher can proceed with optimism, even in the absence of between-laboratory standardization of the analytical methods. Many of these assays can be used to evaluate changes in a single subject after dietary or other interventions even when the variation between subjects is large.

CONCLUSION

The interest in evaluating the antioxidant status in humans will increase further due to accumulating evidence for a role of oxidative stress in health and disease. The methods reviewed in this chapter may be useful in evaluating the antioxidant status of humans. At this time, no single method can provide an accurate estimate of antioxidant status. Therefore, we strongly recommend the use of several methods, each with its own characteristic strengths and limitations. In this way, accurate and useful measures of oxidative stress can be obtained, especially in monitoring changes in a given subject over time. Further development and validation of new methods can be expected to provide significant tools for research in this rapidly developing field.

Acknowlegement

We thank Dr. Paul Jacques for critical review of the manuscript.

APPENDIX 1
PROMISING METHODS FOR EVALUATING ANTIOXIDANT STATUS AND OXIDATIVE STRESS

The following methods may find wide applicability after further development and evaluation.

Changes in Gene Expression

Work in experimental animals indicates changes in tissue gene expression following oxidative stress, but comparable changes have not yet been observed in circulating human lymphocytes. For example, changes in lymphocyte AP-1 or NF-κB would be of interest, but for relevance to healthy humans, these markers need to be followed in freshly isolated human lymphocytes. This is not practical with current technology. Breakthroughs undoubtedly will occur in the near future in this area of ROS research.

Total capacity to trap oxygen radicals

Several assays, such as ORAC[89] and TRAP[90] estimate the total capacity of a plasma or tissue sample to scavenge oxygen radicals. The method is under wide investigation, but its predictive value in human disorders remains to be determined.

Plasma bioflavonoids

HPLC analysis of bioflavonoids has been refined, using electrochemical detection, to allow measurement of low levels of these phenolic compounds. Recent studies have shown that polyphenolics in plasma can be measured after ingestion of bioflavonoid-rich foods,[91,92] but levels are generally in the micromolar range, even directly after consumption of polyphenol-rich foods.

Markers of ROS attack on tyrosine

Tyrosine is readily attacked by several ROS, including peroxynitrite, hypochlorite, and the HO• radical. The products include nitrotyrosine,[93] chlorotyrosine, and meta-OH-tyrosine, both free and protein-bound. Reactive species that cause nitration of tyrosine residues are released by activated neutrophils.[94] Free nitrotyrosine can be measured by HPLC, and nitrotyrosine can be detected in the plasma of individuals with rheumatoid arthritis[95] and with chronic renal failure.[96] Protein-bound nitrotyrosine can also be measured.[97]

Sensitive methods need to be employed to measure the low levels of modified tyrosine likely to be found in the plasma of healthy subjects.

HPLC analysis of plasma lipid hydroperoxides

Several protocols have been established for HPLC measurement of plasma lipid hydroperoxides using chemiluminescence detection,[98,99] and both cholesterol ester hydroperoxides and phospholipid hydroperoxides can be measured. These methods are sensitive and have good chemical specificity, but they require a high level of technical competence to make measurements in biological samples. Calibration with lipid hydroperoxide standards poses special difficulties. Cholesterol ester hydroperoxides in plasma are at the detection limit in healthy subjects, but are higher in subjects with intracranial hemorrhage.[100]

Protein carbonyls

The assay of protein carbonyls, using carbonyl-specific reagents, has achieved wide application.[101] The methods in use provide an estimate of the total protein-bound carbonyl groups, but lack specificity for chemical structure. The carbonyl assay has been effectively employed for studies of *in vitro* oxidative damage to proteins.[102]

Hydroxy-alkenals formed during lipid peroxidation

The peroxidation of lipids *in vivo* generates the toxic by-product 4-hydroxynonenal and other alkenals, which can be measured in biological samples by GC/MS[103,104] and other chromatographic methods. Elevated plasma nonenal levels have been observed concurrent with plasma free-iron during cardiopulmonary bypass.[105]

Markers of DNA damage by ROS

Two major developments have occurred in this promising area:

1. Measurement of the oxidized DNA base, 8-oxo-dG.[106] Most analyses have been carried out by HPLC with electrochemical detection following an elaborate DNA digestion and extraction procedure. An ELISA kit is available commercially that can determine 2-fold changes in the level of 8-oxo-dG; extensive sample preparation is also required for the ELISA kit. Values of 8-oxo-dG were elevated in seminal DNA in subjects with low ascorbate intake.[107] Levels of 8-oxo-dG can be measured in urine, but urinary values may be largely determined by the metabolic rate.[108]
2. The COMET assay for damage to DNA.[109,110] Nicks (fragments of dam-

aged DNA) can be formed in the DNA strand by a variety of agents, including ROS. These nicks can be quantified by DNA electrophoresis, since nicked DNA migrates as a streak on the gel. The great majority of data has been obtained with DNA that was damaged *in vitro* by ROS.[110]

Lipofuscin bound to plasma proteins

Fluorescent substances, called lipofuscin, can be measured in forms that bind to human plasma proteins, including albumin. These fluorophores remain in the aqueous phase following organic solvent extraction of plasma. Their chemical structures have not yet been characterized, but they have been postulated to arise from oxidative stress. This form of lipofuscin increases with age in humans.[111] Plasma protein-bound lipofuscin is elevated in adult respiratory distress syndrome.[112]

Additional ROS markers in breath

Several new assays for direct measurement of ROS in breath have recently been developed. The non-invasive nature of breath sampling may lead to significant use of this methodology in the future.

1. Volatile aldehydes appear in the breath along with ethane and pentane.[113] These aldehydes have been useful in studies of ozonation *in vitro*[114] and *in vivo*.[115] Because of the complexity of the mixture, the analysis of aldehydes in human breath has been technically challenging.
2. Hydrogen peroxide can be measured in human breath samples,[116,117] and is generally elevated in asthma because of chronic inflammation.
3. Nitric oxide can be measured in breath;[118] nitric oxide levels are elevated in asthmatics.

APPENDIX 2 FACTORS AFFECTING THE ASSAY OF GLUTATHIONE PEROXIDASE (Se-GSH-Px)

Measurements of Se-GSH-Px activity obtained in different laboratories are usually not comparable because of the large number of parameters that affect the measured enzymatic rate.

1. The measured activity of Se-GSH-Px increases steadily as GSH concentration in the cuvette increases, and as buffer pH increases, and no plateau can be detected for either variable. Thus, Se-GSH-Px assay values can vary sharply between different laboratories, and even over time for the same laboratory. For good long-term reproducibilty, both GSH con-

centration and buffer pH, along with assay temperature, must be rigorously standardized.[119,120]

2. For RBC measurements, MetHb in the sample generates interference.
3. In tissue homogenates, GSH-S-transferase may contribute to activity, if an organic hydroperoxide is used as substrate.[121]
4. Some antiocoagulants, such as EDTA, can interfere with the activity of Se-GSH-Px,[122] and blood samples collected for Se-GSH-Px assay should be obtained with heparin anticoagulant.

REFERENCES

1. Pryor WA. Oxy-radicals and related species: their formation, lifetimes and reactions. *Annu Rev Physiol* 48:657-667, 1986.
2. Sasaki R, Kurokawa T, Tero-Kubota S. Ascorbate radical and ascorbic acid level in human serum and age. *J Gerontol* 38:1983.
3. Granstrom E. The arachidonic acid cascade. The prostaglandins, thromboxanes and leukotrienes. *Inflammation* 8:S15-S25, 1984.
4. Smith WL. Prostanoid biosynthesis and mechanisms of action. *Am J Physiol* 263:F181-F191, 1992.
5. Moncada S, Higgs A. The L-arginine-nitric oxide pathway. *N Engl J Med* 329:2002-2012, 1993.
6. Rosen GM, Pou S, Ramos CL, *et al.* Free radicals and phagocytic cells. *FASEB J* 9:200-209, 1995.
7. Clark LC, Combs GFJ, Turnbull BW, *et al.* Effects of selenium supplementation for cancer prevention in patients with carcinoma of the skin. A randomized controlled trial. Nutritional Prevention of Cancer Study Group. *JAMA* 276:1957-1963, 1996.
8. Meydani SN, Meydani M, Blumberg JB, *et al.* Vitamin E supplementation and *in vivo* immune response in healthy elderly subjects. A randomized controlled trial. *JAMA* 277:1380-1386, 1997.
9. Stephens NG, Parsons A, Schofield PM, *et al.* Randomised controlled trial of vitamin E in patients with coronary disease: Cambridge Heart Antioxidant Study (CHAOS). *Lancet* 781-786, 1996.
10. Gey KF, Puska P, Jordan P, Moser UK. Inverse correlation between plasma vitamin E and mortality from ischemic heart disease in cross-cultural epidemiology. *Am J Clin Nutr* 53:326S-334S., 1991.
11. Rimm EB, Stampfer MJ, Ascherio A, *et al.* Vitamin E consumption and the risk of coronary heart disease in men. *New Engl J Med* 328:1450-1456, 1993.
12. Stampfer MJ, Hennekens CH, Manson JE, *et al.* Vitamin E consumption and the risk of coronary disease in women. *New Engl J Med* 328:1444-1449, 1993.
13. Handelman GJ, Machlin LJ, Fitch K, *et al.* Oral α-tocopherol supplements decrease plasma γ-tocopherol levels in humans. *J Nutr* 115:807-813, 1985.
14. National Institutes of Standards and Technology. Standard Reference Material #968B. Fat-Soluble Vitamins and Cholesterol in Human Serum. Gaithersburg, MD: 1995.
15. Baker H, Handelman GJ, Short S, *et al.* Comparison of plasma alpha and gamma tocopherol levels following chronic oral administration of either all-rac-α-tocopheryl-acetate or RRR-α-tocopheryl acetate. *Am J Clin Nutr* 43:382-387, 1986.

16. Handelman GJ, Epstein WL, Peerson J, *et al.* Human adipose alpha-tocopherol and gamma-tocopherol kinetics during and after 1 y of alpha-tocopherol supplementation. *Am J Clin Nutr* 59:1025-1032, 1994.
17. Traber MG, Sies H. Vitamin E in humans: demand and delivery. *Annu Rev Nutr* 16:321-347, 1996.
18. Christen S, Woodall AA, Shigenaga MK, *et al.* Gamma-tocopherol traps mutagenic electrophiles such as NO(X) and complements alpha-tocopherol: physiological implications. *Proc Natl Acad Sci USA* 94:3217-3222, 1997.
19. Meydani SN, Shapiro AC, Meydani M, *et al.* Effect of age and dietary fat (fish, corn and coconut oils) on tocopherol status of C57BL/6Nia mice. *Lipids* 22:345-350, 1987.
20. Rotruck JT, Pope AL, Ganther HE, *et al.* Selenium: biochemical role as a component of glutathione peroxidase. *Science* 179:588-590, 1973.
21. Flohe L, Gunzler WA, Schock HH. Glutathione peroxidase: a selenoenzyme. *FEBS Lett* 32:132-134, 1973.
22. Ursini F, Bindoli A. The role of selenium peroxidases in the protection against oxidative damage of membranes. *Chem Phys Lipids* 44:255-276, 1987.
23. Ursini F, Maiorino M, Brigelius-Flohe R, *et al.* Diversity of glutathione peroxidases. *Methods Enzymol* 252:38-53, 1995.
24. Croteau W, Davey JC, Galton VA, St Germain DL. Cloning of the mammalian type II iodothyronine deiodinase. A selenoprotein differentially expressed and regulated in human and rat brain and other tissues. *J Clin Invest* 98:405-417, 1996.
25. Liu SY, Stadtman TC. Heparin-binding properties of selenium-containing thioredoxin reductase from HeLa cells and human lung adenocarcinoma cells. *Proc Natl Acad Sci USA* 94:6138-6141, 1997.
26. Diplock AT. Indexes of selenium status in human populations. *Am J Clin Nutr* 57:256S-258S., 1993.
27. Foster LH, Sumar S. Selenium in health and disease: areview. *Crit Rev Food Sci Nutr* 37:211-228, 1997.
28. Alegria A, Barbera R, Clemente G, *et al.* Selenium and glutathione peroxidase reference values in whole blood and plasma of a reference population living in Valencia, Spain. *J Trace Elem Med Biol* 10:223-228, 1996.
29. Levander OA, Alfthan G, Arvilommi H, *et al.* Bioavailability of selenium to Finnish men as assessed by platelet glutathione peroxidase activity and other blood parameters. *Am J Clin Nutr* 37:887-897, 1983.
30. Levine M, Runsey S, Wang Y, *et al.* Vitamin C. In E. E. Ziegler & L. J. Filer Jr., Eds. *Present Knowledge in Nutrition*. Washington, D.C.: ILSI Press; 1996;pp. 146-159.
31. Frei B, Stocker R, Ames BN. Antioxidant defenses and lipid peroxidation in human plasma. *Proc Natl Acad Sci USA* 85:9748-9752, 1988.
32. Packer JE, Slater TF, Willson RL. Direct observation of a free radical interaction between vitamin E and vitamin C. *Nature* 278:737-738, 1979.
33. Chan AC. Partners in defense, vitamin E and vitamin C. *Can J Physiol Pharmacol* 71:725-731, 1993.
34. Burton GW, Wronska U, Stone L, *et al.* Biokinetics of dietary RRR-alpha-tocopherol in the male guinea pig at three dietary levels of vitamin C and two levels of vitamin E. Evidence that vitamin C does not "spare" vitamin E *in vivo*. *Lipids* 25:199-210, 1990.
35. Jacob RA, Kutnink MA, Csallany AS, *et al.* Vitamin C nutriture has little short-term effect on vitamin E concentrations in healthy women. *J Nutr* 126:2268-2277, 1996.
36. Margolis SA, Duewer DL. Measurement of ascorbic acid in human plasma and serum: stability, intralaboratory repeatability, and interlaboratory reproducibility. *Clin Chem* 42:1257-1262, 1996.

37. Mezzetti A, Lapenna D, Pierdomenico SD, *et al.* Vitamins E, Cand lipid peroxidation in plasma and arterial tissue of smokers and non-smokers. *Atherosclerosis* 112:91-99, 1995.
38. Block G, Sorenson A. vitamin C intake and dietary sources by demographic characteristics. *Nutr Cancer* 10:53-65, 1987.
39. Lowik MR, Hulshof KF, Schneijder P, *et al.* Vitamin C status in elderly women: a comparison between women living in a nursing home and women living independently. *J Am Diet Assoc* 93:167-172, 1993.
40. Levine M, Conry-Cantilena C, Wang Y. Vitamin C pharmacokinetics in healthy volunteers: evidence for a recommended dietary allowance. *Proc Natl Acad Sci USA* 93:3704-3709, 1996.
41. Pryor WA, Stone K. Oxidants in cigarette smoke. Radicals, hydrogen peroxide, peroxynitrate, and peroxynitrite. *Ann NY Acad Sci* 686:12-27, 1993.
42. Cross CE, O'Neill CA, Reznick AZ, *et al.* Cigarette smoke oxidation of human plasma constituents. *Ann NY Acad Sci* 686:72-89, 1993.
43. Abbey M, Noakes M, Nestel PJ. Dietary supplementation with orange and carrot juice in cigarette smokers lowers oxidation products in copper-oxidized low-density lipoproteins. *J Am Diet Assoc* 95:671-675, 1995.
44. Koppenol WH. The centennial of the Fenton reaction. *Free Radic Biol Med* 15:645-651, 1993.
45. Handelman GJ, Shen B, Krinsky NI. High-resolution HPLC analysis of carotenoids in human plasma. *Methods Enzymol* 213:336-346, 1991.
46. Bone RA, Landrum JT, Fernandez L, Tarsis SL. Analysis of the macular pigment by HPLC: retinal distribution and age study. *Invest Opthalmol Vis Sci* 29:843-849, 1988.
47. Handelman GJ, Dratz EA, Reay CC, van Kuijk FJ GM. Carotenoids in the human macula and whole retina. *Invest Ophthalmol Vis Sci* 29:850-855, 1988.
48. Britton G. Structure and properties of carotenoids in relation to function. *FASEB J* 9:1551-1558, 1995.
49. Craft N. Carotenoid reversed-phase high-performance liquid chromatography methods: reference compendium. *Methods Enzymol* 213:185-205, 1992.
50. Stahl W, Sies H. Separation of geometrical isomers of beta-carotene and lycopene. *Methods Enzymol* 234:388-400, 1994.
51. Handelman GJ. Carotenoids as scavengers of active oxygen species. In E. Cadenas and L. Packer, Eds. *Handbook of Antioxidants.* New York: Marcel Dekker; 1995;pp. 259-314.
52. The Alpha-Tocopherol and Beta Carotene Cancer Prevention Study Group. The effect of vitamin E and beta carotene on the incidence of lung cancer and other cancers in male smokers. *N Engl J Med* 330:1029-1035, 1994.
53. Omenn GA, Goodman GE, Thornquist MD, *et al.* The effects of a combination of beta carotene and vitamin A on lung cancer and cardiovascular disease. *New Engl J Med* 334:1150-1155, 1996.
54. Handelman GJ, Packer L, Cross CE. Destruction of tocopherols, carotenoids and retinol human plasma by cigarette smoke. *Am J Clin Nutr* 63:559-565, 1996.
55. Mayne ST, Handelman GJ, Beecher G. Beta-carotene and lung cancer promotion in heavy smokers--a plausible relationship? *J Natl Cancer Inst* 88:1513-1515, 1996.
56. Salgo MG, Cueto R, Winston GW, *et al.* The effects of ß-carotene and its oxidation products on the binding of benzo(a)pyrene to calf thymus DNA. *Free Radic Biol Med* 1998 (in press).
57. Flagg EW, Coate RJ, Eley JW, *et al.* Dietary glutathione intake in humans and the relationship between intake and plasma total glutathione level. *Nutr Cancer* 21:33-46, 1994.
58. Fariss MW, Reed D. High-performance liquid chromatography of thiols and disulfides: dinitrophenol derivatives. *Methods Enzymol* 143:101-109, 1987.

59. Ellman GL. Tissue sulfhydryl groups. *Arch Biochem Biophys* 82:70-77, 1959.
60. Sen CK, Rankinen T, Vaisanen S, Rauramaa R. Oxidative stress after human exercise: effect of N-acetylcysteine supplementation. *J Appl Physiol* 76:2570-2577, 1994.
61. Herzenberg LA, De Rosa SC, Dubs JG, *et al.* Glutathione deficiency is associated with impaired survival in HIV disease. *Proc Natl Acad Sci USA* 94:1967-72, 1997.
62. Hamill RL, Woods JC, Cook BA. Congenital atransferrinemia. A case report and review of the literature. *Am J Clin Pathol* 96:215-218, 1991.
63. Salonen JT, Nyyssonen K, Korpela H, *et al.* High stored iron levels are associated with excess risk of myocardial infarction in eastern Finnish men. *Circulation* 86:803-822, 1992.
64. Gutteridge JM, Rowley DA, Halliwell B. Superoxide-dependent formation of hydroxyl radicals in the presence of iron salts. Detection of 'free' iron in biological systems by using bleomycin-dependent degradation of DNA. *Biochem J* 199:263-265, 1981.
65. Gutteridge JM, Quinlan GJ, Evans TW. Transient iron overload with bleomycin detectable iron in the plasma of patients with adult respiratory distress syndrome. *Thorax* 49:707-710, 1994.
66. Grootveld M, Bell JD, Halliwell B, *et al.* Non-transferrin-bound iron in plasma or serum from patients with idiopathic hemochromatosis. Characterization by high performance liquid chromatography and nuclear magnetic resonance spectroscopy. *J Biol Chem* 264:4417-4422, 1989.
67. Gutteridge JM, Mumby S, Koizumi M, Taniguchi N. "Free" iron in neonatal plasma activates aconitase: evidence for biologically reactive iron. *Biochem Biophys Res Commun* 229:806-809, 1996.
68. Feder JN, Gnirke A, Thomas W, *et al.* A novel MHC class I-like gene is mutated in patients with hereditary haemochromatosis. *Nat Genet* 13:399-408, 1996.
69. Ohkawa H, Ohishi N, Yagi K. Assay for lipid peroxides in animal tissues by thiobarbituric acid reaction. *Anal Biochem* 95:351-358, 1979.
70. Janero DR. Malondialdehyde and thiobarbituric acid-reactivity as diagnostic indices of lipid peroxidation and peroxidative tissue injury. *Free Radic Biol Med* 9:515-540, 1990.
71. Witz G, Lawrie NJ, Zaccaria A, *et al.* The reaction of 2-thiobarbituric acid with biologically active alpha,beta-unsaturated aldehydes. *J Free Radic Bol Med* 2:33-39, 1986.
72. Pryor WA, Stanley JP, Blair E. Autoxidation of polyunsaturated fatty acids. II. A suggested mechanism for the formation of TBA-like material from prostaglandin-like endoperoxides. *Lipids* 11:370-379, 1976.
73. Nourooz-Zadeh J, Tajaddini-Sarmadi J, McCarthy S, *et al.* Elevated levels of authentic plasma hydroperoxides in NIDDM. *Diabetes* 44:1054-1058, 1995.
74. Bailey AL, Wortley G, Southon S. Measurement of aldehydes in low density lipoprotein by high performance liquid chromatography. *Free Radic Biol Med* 23:1078-1085, 1997.
75. Liu J, Yeo HC, Doniger SJ, Ames BN. Assay of aldehydes from lipid peroxidation: gas chromatography-mass spectrometry compared to thiobarbituric acid. *Anal Biochem* 245:161-166, 1997.
76. Dumelin EE, Tappel AL. Hydrocarbon gases produced during *in vitro* peroxidation of polyunsaturated fatty acids and decomposition of preformed hydroperoxides. *Lipids* 12:894-900, 1977.
77. Dillard CJ, Dumelin EE, Tappel AL. Effect of dietary vitamin E on expiration of pentane and ethane by the rat. *Lipids* 12:109-114, 1977.
78. Foster WM, Jiang L, Stetkiewicz PT, Risby TH. Breath isoprene: temporal changes in respiratory output after exposure to ozone. *J Appl Physiol* 80:706-710, 1996.
79. Stone BG, Besse T, Duane WC, *et al.* Effect of regulating cholesterol biosynthesis on breath isoprene excretion in men. *Lipids* 28:705-708, 1993.
80. Kohlmuller D, Kochen W. Is n-pentane really an index of lipid peroxidation in humans and animals? A methodological reevaluation. *Anal Biochem* 268-276, 1993.

81. Springfield JR, Levitt MD. Pitfalls in the use of breath pentane measurements to assess lipid peroxidation. *J Lipid Res* 35:1497-1504, 1994.
82. Habib MP, Clemens NC, Garewall HS. Cigarette smoking and ethane exhalation in humans. *Am. J Resp Crit Care Med* 15:1368-1372, 1995.
83. Morrow JD, Roberts LJ. The isoprostanes: Unique bioactive products of lipid peroxidation. *Prog Lipid Res* 36:1-21, 1997.
84. Gopaul NK, Anggard EE, Mallet AI, *et al.* Plasma 8-epi-PGF2 alpha levels are elevated in individuals with non-insulin dependent diabetes mellitus. *FEBS Lett* 368:225-229, 1995.
85. Stein CM, Tanner SB, Awad JA, *et al.* Evidence of free radical-mediated injury (isoprostane overproduction) in scleroderma. *Arthrit Rheum* 39:1146-1150, 1996.
86. Morrow JD, Frei B, Longmire AW, *et al.* Increase in circulating products of lipid peroxidation (F2-isoprostanes) in smokers. Smoking as a cause of oxidative damage. *N Engl J Med* 332:1198-1203, 1995.
87. Esterbauer H, Gebicki J, Puhl H, Jurgens G. The role of lipid peroxidation and antioxidants in oxidative modification of LDL. *Free Radic Biol Med* 13:341-390, 1992.
88. Nourooz-Zadeh J, Tajaddini-Sarmadi J, Wolff SP. Measurement of plasma hydroperoxide concentrations by the ferrous oxidation-xylenol orange assay in conjunction with triphenylphosphine. *Anal Biochem* 220:403-409, 1994.
89. Cao G, Verdon CP, Wu AH, *et al.* Automated assay of oxygen radical absorbance capacity with the COBAS FARA. *Clin Chem* 41:1738-1744, 1995.
90. Aejmelaeus RT, Holm P, Kaukinen U, *et al.* Age-related changes in the peroxyl radical scavenging capacity of human plasma. *Free Radic Biol Med* 23:69-75, 1997.
91. Hollman PC, van der Gaag M, Mengelers MJ, *et al.* Absorption and disposition kinetics of the dietary antioxidant quercetin in man. *Free Radic Biol Med* 21:703-707, 1996.
92. Unno T, Kondo K, Itakura H, Takeo T. Analysis of (-)-epigallocatechin gallate in human serum obtained after ingesting green tea. *Biosci Biotechnol Biochem* 60:2066-2068, 1996.
93. Beckman JS, Koppenol WH. Nitric oxide, superoxide, and peroxynitrite: the good, the bad, and ugly. *Am J Physiol* 271:C1424-C1437, 1996.
94. Eiserich JP, Hristova M, Cross CE, et al. Formation of nitric oxide-derived inflammatory oxidantd by myeloperoxidase in neutrofils. *Nature* 391:393-397, 1998.
95. Kaur H, Halliwell B. Evidence for nitric oxide-mediated oxidative damage in chronic inflammation. Nitrotyrosine in serum and synovial fluid from rheumatoid patients. *FEBS Lett* 350:9-12, 1994.
96. Fukuyama N, Takebayashi Y, Hida M, *et al.* Clinical evidence of peroxynitrite formation in chronic renal failure patients with septic shock. *Free Radic Biol Med* 22:771-774, 1997.
97. Shigenaga MK, Lee HH, Blount BC, *et al.* Inflammation and NO(X)-induced nitration: assay for 3-nitrotyrosine by HPLC with electrochemical detection. *Proc Natl Acad Sci USA* 94:3211-3216, 1997.
98. Yamamoto Y, Brodsky MH, Baker JC, Ames BN. Detection and characterization of lipid hydroperoxides at picomole levels by high-performance liquid chromatography. *Anal Biochem* 160:7-13, 1987.
99. Miyazawa T. Determination of phospholipid hydroperoxides in human blood plasma by a chemiluminescence-HPLC assay. *Free Radic Biol Med* 7:209-217, 1989.
100. Polidori MC, Frei B, Rordorf G, *et al.* Increased levels of plasma cholesteryl ester hydroperoxides in patients with subarachnoid hemorrhage. *Free Radic Biol Med* 23:762-767, 1997.
101. Stadtman ER. Protein oxidation and aging. *Science* 257:1220-1224, 1992.
102. Levine RL, Garland D, Oliver CN, *et al.* Determination of carbonyl content in oxidatively modified proteins. *Methods Enzymol* 186:464-478, 1990.

103. van Kuijk F, Thomas DW, Stephens RJ, Dratz EA. Occurrence of 4-hydroxyalkenals in rat tissues determined as pentafluorobenzyl oxime derivatives by gas chromatography-mass spectrometry. *Biochem Biophys Res Commun* 139:144-149, 1986.
104. Bruenner BA, Jones AD, German JB. Direct characterization of protein adducts of the lipid peroxidation product 4-hydroxy-2-nonenal using electrospray mass spectrometry. *Chem Res Toxicol* 8:552-559, 1995.
105. Quinlan GJ, Mumby S, Pepper J, Gutteridge JM. Plasma 4-hydroxy-2-nonenal levels during cardiopulmonary bypass, and their relationship to the iron-loading of transferrin. *Biochem Molec Biol Int* 34:1277-1282, 1994.
106. Shigenaga MK, Aboujaoude EN, Chen Q, Ames BN. Assays of oxidative DNA damage biomarkers 8-oxo-2'-deoxyguanosine and 8-oxoguanine in nuclear DNA and biological fluids by high-performance liquid chromatography with electrochemical detection. *Methods Enzymol* 234:16-33, 1994.
107. Fraga CG, Motchnik PA, Shigenaga MK, *et al.* Ascorbic acid protects against endogenous oxidative DNA damage in human sperm. *Proc Natl Acad Sci USA* 88:11003-11006, 1991.
108. Loft S, Astrup A, Buemann B, Poulsen HE. Oxidative DNA damage correlates with oxygen consumption in humans. *FASEB J* 8:534-537, 1994.
109. Duthie SJ, Ma A, Ross MA, Collins AR. Antioxidant supplementation decreases oxidative DNA damage in human lymphocytes. *Cancer Res* 56:1291-1295, 1996.
110. Fairbairn DW, Olive PL, O'Neill KL. The comet assay: a comprehensive review. *Mutat Res* 339:37-59, 1995.
111. Tsuchida M, Miura T, Mizutani K, Aibara K. Fluorescent substances in mouse and human sera as a parameter of *in vivo* lipid peroxidation. *Biochim Biophys Acta* 834:196-204, 1985.
112. Roumen RM, Hendriks T, de Man BM, Goris RJ. Serum lipofuscin as a prognostic indicator of adult respiratory distress syndrome and multiple organ failure. *Br J Surg* 81:1300-1305, 1994.
113. Lin Y, Dueker SR, Jones AD, *et al.* Protocol for collection and HPLC analysis of volatile carbonyl compounds in breath. *Clin Chem* 41:1028-1032, 1995.
114. Cueto R, Squadrito GL, Pryor WA. Quantifying aldehydes and distinguishing aldehydic product profiles from autoxidation and ozonation of unsaturated fatty acids. *Methods Enzymol* 233:174-182, 1994.
115. Pryor WA, Bermudez E, Cueto R, Squadrito GL. Detection of aldehydes in bronchoalveolar lavage of rats exposed to ozone. *Fundam Appl Toxicol* 34:148-156, 1996.
116. Dohlman AW, Black HR, Royall JA. Expired breath hydrogen peroxide is amarker of acute airway inflammation in pediatric patients with asthma. *Am Rev Respir Dis* 148:955-960, 1993.
117. Kietzmann D, Kahl R, Muller M, *et al.* Hydrogen peroxide in expired breath condensate of patients with acute respiratory failure and with ARD. *Intensive Care Med* 19:78-81, 1993.
118. Lundberg JO, Weitzberg E, Lundberg JM, Alving K. Nitric oxide in exhaled air. *Eur Respir J* 9:2671-2680, 1996.
119. Chaudiere J, Tappel AL. Purification and characterization of selenium-glutathione peroxidase from hamster liver. *Arch Biochem Biophys* 226:448-457, 1983.
120. Maddipati KR, Marnett LJ. Characterization of the major hydroperoxide-reducing activity of human plasma. Purification and properties of aselenium-dependent glutathione peroxidase. *J Biol Chem* 262:17398-403, 1987.
121. Burk R. Lipid peroxides as substrates for GSH-S-transferase. *J Biol Chem* 100:1-10, 1980.
122. Hussein KSM, Jones BEV. Effects of different anticoaugulants on determination of erythrocyte glutathione peroxidase. *Acta Vet Scand* 22:472-479, 1981.

Part 2

Effect of Diet on Antioxidant Status

- Genetic Variation and Evolutionary Aspects of Diet
- Diet and Antioxidant Status
- Mediterranean Diet and Antioxidants
- Case Study: The Cretan Experience

4

Genetic Variation and Evolutionary Aspects of Diet

Artemis P. Simopoulos, M.D.
The Center for Genetics, Nutrition and Health, Washington DC, USA

INTRODUCTION

The interaction of genetics and environment, nature, and nurture is the foundation for all health and disease. This concept, based on molecular biology and genetics, was originally defined by Hippocrates. In 480 B.C. Hippocrates stated the concept of positive health as follows:

Positive health requires a knowledge of man's primary constitution (which today we call genetics) and of the powers of various foods, both those natural to them and those resulting from human skill (today's processed food). But eating alone is not enough for health. There must also be exercise, of which the effects must likewise be known. The combination of these two things makes regimen, when proper attention is given to the season of the year, the changes of the winds, the age of the individual and the situation of his home. If there is any deficiency in food or exercise the body will fall sick.

0-8493-8009-X/98/$0.00+$.50

In the last decade it has been shown that genetic factors determine susceptibility to disease and environmental factors determine which genetically susceptible individuals will be affected.[1] Nutrition is an environmental factor of major importance. Whereas major changes have taken place in our diet over the past 10,000 years since the beginning of the Agricultural Revolution, our genes have not changed. The spontaneous mutation rate for nuclear deoxyribonucleic acid (DNA) is estimated at 0.5% per million years. Therefore, over the past 10,000 years there has been time for very little change in our genes, perhaps 0.005%. In fact, our genes today are very similar to the genes of our ancestors during the Paleolithic period 40,000 years ago during the time our genetic profile was established.[2] Genetically speaking, humans today live in a nutritional environment that differs from that for which our genetic constitution was selected.

Studies on the evolutionary aspects of diet indicate that major changes have taken place in the type and amount of essential fatty acids and in the antioxidant content.[2,3] Advances in human biochemical genetics have produced data that suggest considerable biochemical variability within and between human populations. Therefore, the relevance of this genetic information for human nutrition is considerable. Variation in nutritional requirements and the interaction of certain nutrients with genetically determined biochemical and metabolic factors suggest different requirements for individuals. This variation (like sex differences) is inborn and needs to be differentiated from variations caused by the life cycle (growth, pregnancy, and old age). Research is now defining the mechanisms by which genes influence nutrient absorption, metabolism and excretion, taste perception, and degree of satiation; and the mechanisms by which nutrients influence gene expression. Furthermore, advances in molecular and recombinant DNA technology have led to exquisite studies in the field of Genetics and the recognition in a much more specific way, through DNA sequencing, how unique each one of us is, and the extent to which genetic variation occurs in human beings. The importance of the effects of genetic variation has been extensively studied and applied in drug development and evaluation of their metabolism and adverse reactions.[4-8] In the past two decades, physicians, geneticists, and nutritionists began to study the effects of genetic variation and gene-nutrient interactions in the management of chronic diseases.[1,9,10]

Whereas evolutionary maladaptation leads to reproductive restriction (or differential fertility), the rapid changes in our diet, particularly the last 150 years, are potent promoters of chronic diseases such as atherosclerosis, essential hypertension, obesity, diabetes, and many cancers. In addition to diet, sedentary life styles and exposure to noxious substances interact with genetically controlled biochemical processes leading to chronic disease.

This chapter will discuss genetic individuality and polymorphisms; genetic variation and dietary response; gene-nutrient interactions and their role in nutritional requirements and gene expression; and evolutionary aspects of diet with emphasis on the balance of ω-6:ω-3 fatty acids and antioxidants.

GENETIC VARIATION

Genetic Individuality and Polymorphisms

Human populations represent storehouses of genetic variability, greater than appreciated until recently. Advances in genetic studies have pinpointed significant variability in biochemical and immunologic characteristics for individuals that involve many enzymes, proteins, blood groups, human leukocyte antigen (HLA) systems, etc. Human variability has been demonstrated by use of linkage, other family studies, somatic cell genetic hybridization studies, and molecular genetic studies. Molecular genetics indicate that more extensive variability occurs at the DNA level.

Common alleles (variants at a single locus) or polymorphisms form the basis of human diversity, including the ability to handle environmental challenge. In humans and practically all organisms examined, 30% of loci have polymorphic variants (defined as two or more alleles with frequency of at least 1% or more) in the population. An average individual is heterozygous at about 10% of the loci. Alleles that confer selective advantage in the heterozygous state are likely to have increased in prevalence because positive selection affects the number of variants. Changes in nutritional environment will affect heritability of the variant phenotypes that are dependent, to a lesser or greater degree, on the nutrient environment for their expression.[11]

Individuality is determined by genes - (both major genes and modifiers), constitutional factors (age, sex, developmental stage, parental factors) and environmental factors (time, geography, climate, socioeconomic status, occupation, education, and diet). All sorts of interactions among these three sources of variation are possible.

Genes do not provide an unalterable blueprint but merely a set of options, each more or less conditional, and to be taken up according to what is being experienced as well as what has been experienced. Thus, gene-environment (nutrient) interaction must be described in the context of development and in a dynamic, dialectical mode[12,13] (Figure 1).

The importance of advances in molecular biology and their application to genetic diseases has revolutionized our concepts and has provided the impetus to use the new techniques to identify those specifically at risk for chronic degenerative diseases. Thus, by the use of the tools of molecular genetics, which combine classical family genetic studies with the newest in recombinant DNA techniques, it is now possible to develop diagnostic tests for specific inherited diseases. These studies were first used for the diagnosis of single gene defects. It is now possible to use this approach to detect an individual's susceptibility to diseases caused by multiple factors. Research advances have developed data pertaining to the diagnosis of genetic predisposition to four major multifactorial polygenic diseases: atherosclerosis, hypertension, diabetes, and cancer.

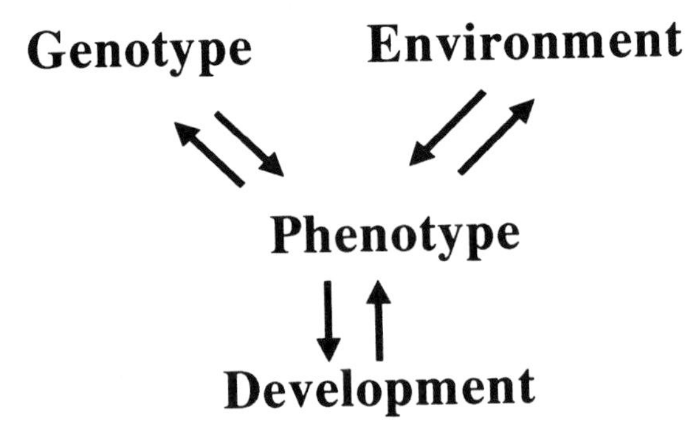

Figure 1. Relationships among genes, environment, and development are dynamic.

Genetic Variation and Dietary Response

Genetics deal with variation. A fundamental aspect of the genetics approach to disease is an appreciation of human variation: its nature and extent, its origin and maintenance, its distribution in families and populations, its interaction with environment, and its consequences for normal development and homeostasis.[14]

In the U.S. and other countries, general dietary guidelines have been issued for the prevention of chronic diseases. The effects of genetic variation on dietary response have not been considered, despite such evidence in the response to dietary cholesterol, dietary sodium, or dietary calcium intake.

Genetic Variation and Dietary Cholesterol

It has been known for at least 20 years that the response of plasma cholesterol concentration to cholesterol feeding is heterogeneous, although the mechanisms only recently are being understood.[15-22]

In certain situations, the response to diet appears to be determined by the genetic variant of apolipoprotein as, for example, in the case with apolipoprotein E (Apo E). Apo E4 is associated with hypercholesterolemia, whereas the variant form of Apo E2 is associated with the development of type III hyperlipoproteinemia and the accumulation of chylomicron and very-low-density lipoprotein (VLDL) remnants in the plasma.[23] Only one person in 50 with Apo E2 variant develops hypertriglyceridemia. Since triglyceride removal is genetically determined, an increase in intake of energy, trans fatty acids or carbohydrate (particularly in women) leads to hypertriglyceridemia. Obesity, diabetes, and hypothyroidism facilitate Apo E2 variant gene expression.[23]

Additional studies show that women of the Apo 3/2 phenotype stand to benefit the least from a high polyunsaturate:saturate (P:S) diet because of reduction in the more "protective" high density lipoprotein (HDL) cholesterol, whereas men of the Apo 4/3 phenotype showed the greatest improvement in the LDL:HDL ratio. Therefore, a general recommendation to increase the polyunsaturated fatty acid (PUFA) content of the diet to decrease plasma cholesterol level and the risk for coronary artery disease is not appropriate for women with Apo 3/2 phenotype.[24]

Oat bran has been shown to decrease serum cholesterol levels in some studies but not in others. Recently, it was shown that only subjects with Apo E3/3 phenotype had a hypocholesterolemic response to oat bran at 4 weeks, but no change was noted in individuals with Apo E4/4 or 4/3 type.[25] Thus, specific genetic information is needed to define the optimal diet for an individual. General recommendations are not appropriate for disease prevention and treatment.

The variant Apo A-IV-1/2 decreases the response of the plasma cholesterol concentration to dietary cholesterol.[26] In the United States, about one person in seven is heterozygote. In other words, 13% of the population carries the Apo A-IV-1/2 allele. The homozygote state is Apo IV-1/1. Increasing dietary cholesterol from 200 mg/day to 1100 mg/day by the addition of four eggs/day increased total cholesterol 22 mg/dl in the Apo IV-1/1 group and only 6 mg/dl in the Apo IV-1/2 group. The mean plasma LDL cholesterol increased by 19 in the Apo IV-1/1 group and only 1 mg/dl in the Apo A-IV-1/2 group. Neither group had any changes in the plasma triglycerides or HDL cholesterol concentration. These results clearly show the genetic effects of the response to dietary cholesterol.

Genetic Variation and Dietary Sodium

Adducin is a protein found in the renal tubule. A polymorphism has been described (Gly 460 Trp) that is associated with changes in blood pressure that may help identify patients who will benefit from sodium restriction or depletion. Hypertensive patients with a 460 Trp allele had a greater decrease in mean arterial blood pressure to both acute and chronic sodium depletion than those homozygous for the wild type mutation.[27]

Genetic Variation and Dietary Calcium

There are important interactions among the vitamin D receptor (VDR) genotype, calcium absorption, and dietary calcium levels. VDR genotypes were significantly associated with bone density only among those premenopausal women with low dietary calcium intakes.[28] Older postmenopausal women with the BB genotype had lower values for calcium absorption than those with the bb genotype, while eating a low-calcium diet, but not while eating a high-calcium diet, suggesting that the women with the BB genotype could not adapt to a low calcium intake.[29] The current RDA for calcium is 800-1200 mg/day, whereas estimated intake during the Paleolithic period was 1580 mg/day. At the level of RDA of 800 mg, a significant proportion of the population with the BB genotype will not be absorbing adequate amounts of calcium.

Gene-Nutrient Interactions

Major advances have occurred over the past 15 years in both the field of Genetics and Nutrition.[1,9,10,30-33] Nutritional health depends on the interaction between the environmental factors affecting dietary intake and the genetically controlled aspects of digestion in the form of proteins such as receptors, carriers, enzymes, and hormones as shown in Figure 2.

Nutritional Requirements

The interaction of certain nutrients with genetically determined biochemical and metabolic factors suggest different requirements for individuals, i.e., familial hypercholesterolemia, familial hypertriglyceridemia, and familial combined hyperlipidemia.[34,35] The healthy individual lives in a 'nutritional window' between the lower and upper thresholds with regard to his intake of each dietary component. An illustration of the 'nutritional window' concept is provided by the healthy adult, in whom one criterion of health is constancy of the body composition.[36] His protein intake can vary from about 50 g to at least 150 g/day without apparent ill effect and without any progressive change in body nitrogen content. His sodium chloride intake can vary from 0.10 g/day to at least 20 g/day, without any progressive change in body sodium chloride content. The constancy of the body content of nitrogen or of sodium chloride in the face of marked changes of intake reflects the ability of the healthy adult to regulate the entry or exit of these nutrients into or out of the body. Such regulatory adjustments are adequate as long as the dietary intakes are above the minimum daily requirement and below the maximal tolerance; if these dietary thresholds are violated, the capacity of the regulatory mechanisms to defend body composition will be exceeded and illness will result.

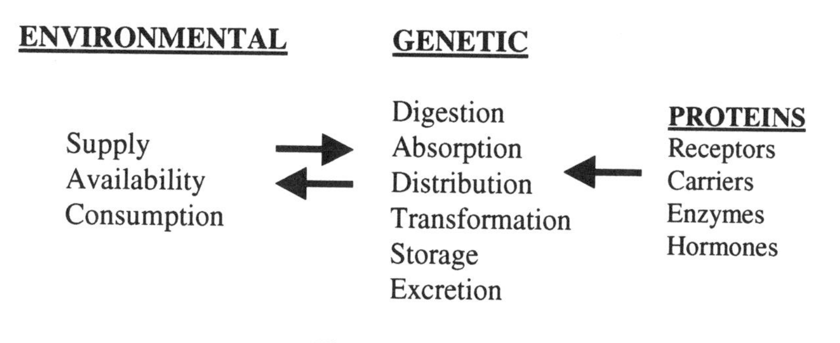

Figure 2. Nutritional health

Nutritional thresholds are defined as being a value between the minimum requirement and the maximum tolerance. The minimum requirement is the smallest amount of a nutrient that the individual must consume in order to promote optimal growth and to prevent illness associated with deficiency. The maximum tolerance for a nutrient is the largest amount that an individual can consume or be administered without an adverse effect. Only the essential nutrients have a lower threshold while all dietary components theoretically have an upper threshold.

These nutritional thresholds are influenced by a number of factors. A threshold for one nutrient is influenced by the intake of another nutrient; by genetically programmed life cycle events (e.g., pregnancy, lactation, infancy, old age); by environment (heat or cold stress); by the level of physical activity, and by altered inherited metabolic characteristics. For many of the threshold-determining mechanisms, genetic variability is now recognized. As a result, individuals and families may differ in a nutritional threshold. The adverse effects of violating these genetically altered thresholds include the single gene defects seen in the pediatric age groups, e.g., in amino acid and carbohydrate metabolic defects and in young adulthood and middle age, e.g., salt-sensitive hypertension, familial hyperlipidemia, and type II diabetes mellitus.[1]

The adverse health outcomes of nutrient consumption below the requirement or above the tolerance can be prompt or delayed. The prompt outcomes of growth arrest, weight loss, and neurologic, skeletal, or hematologic disorders make up the monovalent deficiency syndromes (such as scurvy, beriberi, rickets, or kwashiorkor) which were the focus of clinical nutritionists during the first half of the 20th century. Only in the last 30 years have we realized the delayed effects of inadequate or excessive intake of a nutrient,[17,18] such as: fluoride versus dental caries; calcium versus osteoporosis; calories versus obesity and diabetes; salt-sensitive hypertension; familial hyperlipidemia; ω-3 fatty acids and coronary heart disease, diabetes and arthritis; vitamin E and coronary heart disease[37] and possibly vitamin E and osteoporosis;[38] and vitamin A versus head and neck cancer. In other words, the definition of a nutritional threshold must be based on the prevention of delayed as well as prompt adverse health effects.[36]

The importance of genetic variation in establishing dietary reference values is demonstrated by the study of Molloy *et al.*[39] These investigators studied two groups of healthy women (242 pregnant and 318 non-pregnant). They identified the thermolabile variant of 5,10-methylenetetrahydrofolate reductase (C677T) genotype and measured red-cell folate concentrations. The C677T genotype causes mild hyperhomocysteinemia and is positively associated with the development of vascular disease and the risk of neural-tube defects. Red-cell folate is a reliable marker for tissue folate. The study showed that the red-cell folate was significantly lower in women with C677T as was the plasma folate. In this study, 8.3% of the pregnant and 12.9% of the non-pregnant women were positive for C677T. About 5-15% of the general population is homozygous for C677T indicating that a substantial minority of people in the general population may have increased folate needs. Currently the dietary reference values for folate, as for other nutrients, are targeted to the general and supposedly normal population, not people with special needs, such as those with genetic or metabolic abnormalities or diseases.[39] The Molloy study clearly shows that a substantial minority of the population is at a disadvantage because of current recommendations for folate intake, and the reference-value system should take this into account.

The Role of Nutrients in Gene Expression

There has been an increase in the use of concepts evolved from molecular biology in the study of food components and essential nutrients as factors in the control of gene expression.[31] In terms of chronic diseases, particularly relevant are the effects of dietary cholesterol and fatty acids on gene expression. Dietary cholesterol exerts a profound inhibitory effect on the transcription of the gene for HMG-CoA reductase.[40] Dietary PUFA suppress the hepatic mRNA production of fatty acid synthase for lipoproteinemia in adult and weanling rats. This ability to suppress the abundance of mRNAs for lipogenic proteins is dependent on the degree of fatty acid unsaturation. Eicosapentaenoic acid (EPA) and docosahexaenoic acid (DHA) in the form of fish oils are thus more effective than arachidonic acid (AA).[41] Dietary ω-3 fatty acids reduce levels of mRNA for platelet-derived growth factor[42] (PDGF) and for IL-1β indicating regulation at the transcriptional level.[43] This area of research is expanding very rapidly[44] (Tables 1 and 2).

Table 1
Effects of PUFA on Several Genes Encoding Enzyme Proteins Involved in Lipogenesis, Glycolysis, and Glucose Transport

	Hepatic Cells		Mature Adipocytes	
Fatty Acid	Lipogenesis[a]	Glycolysis[b]	Glut 4[51]	Glut 1[51]
Linoleic acid	↓	*		
Linolenic acid	↓	↓		
Arachidonic acid	↓	↓	↓	↑
Eicosapentanoic acid	↓	↓	↓	↑
Docosahexanoic acid	↓↓	↓		

[a] FAS Ref. 41,45-47; S14 Ref. 41,45-47; SCDI Ref. 48; SCDII Ref. 49, ACC Ref. 47; ME Ref. 47.
[b] G6PD Ref. 50; GK Ref. 50; PK.
* LA does not suppress PK but suppresses GK and G6P
↓ = suppress or decrease; ↑ = induce or increase.

EVOLUTIONARY ASPECTS OF DIET

The foods commonly available to pre-agricultural humans (lean meat, fish, green leafy vegetables, fruits, nuts, berries, and honey) shaped modern human's genetic nutritional requirements. Cereals did not become part of our food supply only very recently - 10,000 years ago - with the advent of the Agricultural Revolution. Up to that time, humans were non-cereal eating hunter-gatherers since the emergence of Homo erectus 1.7 million years ago. During this very long period, humans ate an enormous variety of wild plants, whereas today about 17% of plant species provide 90% of the world's food supply, with the greatest percentage contributed by cereal grains.[55]

Table 2
Effects of PUFA on Several Genes of Enzyme Proteins

Fatty Acid	Cell growth and early gene expression[a]	Adhesion molecules[b]	Inflam-mation[c]	β-oxi-dation[d]	Growth factors[e]
Linoleic				↑	
Linolenic				↑	
Arachidonic	↑	↑	↑	↑	↑
Eicosa-pentanoic	↓	*	↓	↑	↓
Docosa-hexanoic	↓	↓	↓	↑↑	↓

[a] c-fos,Egr-1, Ref. 52.
[b] VCAM1, mRNA, Ref. 53. Monounsaturates also suppress VCAM1 mRNA, but to a lesser degree than DHA, and induce acyl-CoA oxidase mRNA.
[c] IL-1b mRNA, Ref. 54.
[d] acyl-coA oxidase mRNA, Ref. 47. Comment on footnote b also applies.
[e] PDFG mRNA, Ref. 42.
* EPA has no effect by itself but enhances the effect of DHA
↓ = suppress or decrease ↑ = induce or increase

Three cereals, namely, wheat, maize, and rice together account for 75% of the world's grain production. The nutritional implications of such high grain consumption upon human health are enormous. There is no evolutionary precedent in our species for grass seed consumption.[2] Therefore, we had little time (<500 generations) since the beginning of the Agricultural Revolution to adapt to a food type which now represents humanity's major source of both calories and protein. Cereal grains are high in carbohydrates and ω-6 fatty acids, but low in ω-3 fatty acids and in antioxidants. Recent studies show that low fat/high carbohydrate diets increase insulin resistance and hyperinsulinemia, conditions that increase the risk for coronary heart disease, diabetes, and obesity.[56-58]

A number of anthropological, nutritional, and genetic studies indicate that human's overall diet, including energy intake and energy expenditure, has changed over the past 10,000 years with major changes occurring during the past 150 years in the type and amount of fat[2,59-61] (Table 3, Figure 3).

Table 3
Characteristics of Hunter-Gatherer and Western Lifestyles and Diet

Characteristic	Hunter-Gatherer	Western
Physical activity	high	low
Diet		
Energy density	low	high
Energy intake	moderate	high
Protein	high	low-moderate
Animal	high	low-moderate
Vegetable	very low	low-moderate
Carbohydrate	low-moderate (slowly absorbed)	moderate (rapidly absorbed)
Fiber	high	low
Fat	low	high
Vegetable	very low	moderate to high
Animal	low and as PUFA	high, saturated
ω-6/ω-3 ratio	low (2.4)	high(12)
Linolenic and linoleic	low (3.3 g/day)	high (12.3 g/day)
Long chain ω-6 and ω-3	high (2.3 g/day)	low (0.2 g/day)
Vitamins, mg/d	**Paleolithic period**	**Current U.S. intake**
Riboflavin	6.49	1.34-2.08
Folate	0.357	0.149-0.205
Thiamin	3.91	1.08-1.75
Ascorbate	604	77-109
Carotene	5.56	2.05-2.57
(Retinol equivalent)	(927)	-
Vitamin A	17.2	7.02-8.48
(Retinol equivalent)	(2870)	(1170-429)
Vitamin E	32.8	7-10

Eaton and Konner[2] have estimated higher intakes for protein, calcium, potassium, and ascorbic acid and lower sodium intakes for the diet of the late Paleolithic period than the current U.S. and western diet. Most of our food is calorically concentrated in comparison with wild game and the uncultivated fruits and vegetables of the Paleolithic diet. The Paleolithic man consumed fewer calories and drank water, whereas today most drinks to quench thirst contain calories. Today industrialized societies are characterized by (1) an increase in energy intake and decrease in energy expenditure; (2) an increase in saturated fat, ω-6 fatty acids and trans fatty acids, and a decrease in ω-3 fatty acid intake; (3) a decrease in complex carbohydrates and fiber; (4) an increase in cereal grains and a decrease in fruits and vegetables; and (5) a decrease in protein, antioxidants, and calcium intake.[2]

The various roles of (1) essential fatty acids, including their influence on gene expression, and (2) antioxidants have been recognized as important factors in growth and development and in chronic diseases. The functions of essential fatty acids (EFA) and antioxidants are intertwined.[62] Therefore, the dietary changes that have occurred in EFA and selected antioxidants through evolution will be discussed.

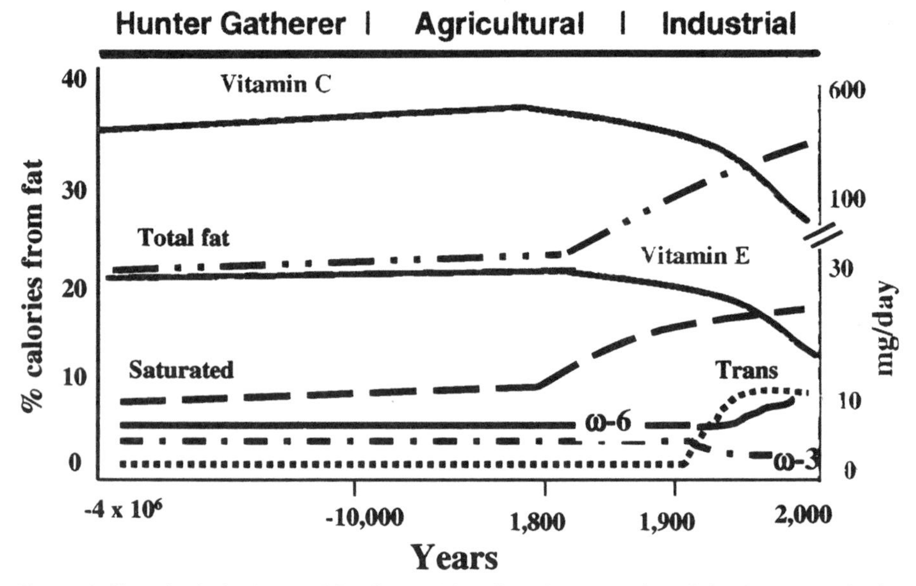

Figure 3. Hypothetical scheme of fat, fatty acid (ω-3, ω-6, trans and total) intake (as % of calories from fat) and intake of vitamins E and C (mg/day). Data were extrapolated from cross-sectional analyses of contemporary hunter-gatherer populations and from longitudinal observations and their putative changes during the preceding 100 years. Intake of vitamins E and C are from Ref. 2 and 77.

Essential Fatty Acids and the ω-6/ω-3 Balance

Large-Scale Production of Vegetable Oils

The increased consumption of ω-6 fatty acids in the last 100 years is due to the development of technology at the turn of the century that marked the beginning of the modern vegetable-oil industry and to modern agriculture with emphasis on grain feeds for domestic livestock (grains are rich in ω-6 fatty acids). The invention of the continuous screw press, named Expeller® by V. D. Anderson, and the steam-vacuum deodorization process by D. Wesson made possible the industrial production of cottonseed oil and other vegetable oils for cooking.[63] Solvent extraction of oilseeds came into increased use after World War I as the large-scale production of vegetable oils became more efficient and more economical. Subsequently, hydrogenation was applied to oils to solidify them.[64] The partial selective hydrogenation of soybean oil reduced the alpha-linolenic acid (LNA) content of the oil while leaving a high concentration of linoleic acid (LA). LNA content was reduced because LNA in soybean oil caused many organoleptic problems. It is now well known that the hydrogenation process and particularly the formation of trans fatty acids has led to increases in serum cholesterol concentrations, whereas LA in its regular state in oil is associated with a reduced serum cholesterol concentration.[65] Since the 1950s, research on the effects of ω-6 PUFAs in lowering serum cholesterol concentrations has dominated research support on the role of PUFAs in lipid metabolism. Although a number of investigators contributed extensively, the paper by Ahrens *et al.*[66] in 1954 and subsequent work by Keys *et al.*[67] firmly established ω-6 fatty acids as the important fatty acids in the field of cardiovascular disease. The availability of methods for production of vegetable oils and their use in lowering serum cholesterol concentration led to an increase in both the fat content of the diet and the greater increase in vegetable oils rich in ω-6 fatty acids.

Agribusiness and Modern Agriculture

Agribusiness contributed further to the decrease in ω-3 fatty acids in animal carcasses. Wild animals and birds who feed on wild plants are very lean, with a carcass fat content of only 3.9% and contain about five times more PUFAs per gram than is found in domestic livestock.[68-70] Most important, 4% of the fat of wild animals contains EPA. Domestic beef contains very small or undetectable amounts of LNA because cattle are fed grains rich in ω-6 fatty acids and poor in ω-3 fatty acids[71] whereas deer that forage on ferns and mosses contain more ω-3 fatty acids (LNA) in their meat.

Modern agriculture with its emphasis on production has decreased the ω-3 fatty acid content in many foods such as green leafy vegetables, animal meats, eggs, and even fish.[72-75] Foods from edible wild plants contain a good balance of ω-6 and ω-3 fatty acids. Table 4 shows purslane and compares it to spinach, red leaf lettuce, buttercrunch lettuce, and mustard greens. Purslane has 8 times more alpha-linolenic acid than the cultivated plants. Farmed fish generally contain less ω-3 and more ω-6 than their counterparts in the wild.[73]

As can be seen from Table 5 comparing the fatty acid composition of egg yolk from free-ranging chicken and the standard U.S. Department of Agriculture (USDA) egg, the former has an ω-6/ω-3 ratio of 1.3 whereas the USDA egg has an ω-6/ω-3 ratio of 19.4.[74] By enriching the chicken feed with fishmeal or flax, this ratio decreased to 6.6 and 1.6 respectively.[74]

Table 4
Fatty Acid Content of Plants[a]

Fatty Acid	Purslane	Spinach	Red Leaf Lettuce	Buttercrunch Lettuce	Mustard
	mg/g of wet weight				
14:0	0.16	0.03	0.03	0.01	0.02
16:0	0.81	0.16	0.10.	0.07	0.13
18:0	0.20	0.01	0.01	0.02	0.02
18:1ω9	0.43	0.04	0.01	0.03	0.01
18:2ω6	0.89	0.14	0.12	0.10	0.12
18:3ω3	4.05	0.89	0.31	0.26	0.48
20:5ω3	0.01	0.00	0.00	0.00	0.00
22:6ω3	0.00	0.00	0.002	0.001	0.001
Other	1.95	0.43	0.12	0.11	0.32
Total	8.50	1.70	0.702	0.60	1.101

[a] Adapted from Simopoulos AP, Salem Jr, N, Ref. 72.

Imbalance of ω-6/ω-3

It is evident that food technology and agribusiness provided the economic stimulus that dominated the changes in the food supply. From per capita quantities of foods available for consumption in the U.S. national food supply in 1985, the amount of EPA is reported to be about 50 and the amount of DHA is 80 mg/capita/day. The two main sources are fish and poultry.[75]

It has been estimated that the present western diet is 'deficient' in ω-3 fatty acids with a ratio of ω-6/ω-3 of 20 to 25:1, instead of 1:1 as is the case with wild animals and, presumably, human beings.[71-76] Before the 1940s, cod-liver oil was given to children as a source of vitamins A and D with the usual dose being a teaspoonful. Once these vitamins were synthesized, consumption of cod-liver oil was drastically decreased. Thus an absolute and relative

Table 5
Fatty Acid Levels in Chicken Egg Yolks[a,b,c]

Fatty Acid	Greek Egg	Supermarket Egg	Fishmeal Egg	Flax Egg
Monounsaturates	142.8	115.4	108.9	99.1
Saturates	100.7	80.7	92.9	86.9
ω-6				
18:2ω6	16.0	26.1	67.8	42.4
18:3ω6	-	0.3	0.3	0.2
20:2ω6	0.2	0.4	0.6	0.4
20:3ω6	0.5	0.5	0.5	0.4
20:4ω6	5.4	5.0	4.4	2.6
22:4ω6	0.7	0.4	0.3	-
22:5ω6	0.3	1.2	0.2	-
Total ω-6	23.1	33.9	74.1	46.0
ω-3				
18:3ω3	6.9	0.5	4.1	21.3
20:3ω3	0.2	-	0.1	0.4
20:5ω3	1.2	-	0.2	0.5
22:5ω3	2.8	0.1	0.4	0.7
22:6ω3	6.6	1.1	6.5	5.1
Total ω-3	17.7	1.7	11.3	28.0
Polyunsaturate saturate ratio	0.4	0.4	0.9	0.9
Monounsaturate saturate ratio	1.4	1.4	1.2	1.1
ω6/ω3 ratio	1.3	19.9	6.6	1.6

[a] Modified from Simopoulos AP, Salem Jr N, Ref. 74.

[b] The eggs were hard-boiled, and their fatty acid composition and lipid content were assessed as described in Ref. 74.

[c] Greek eggs, free-ranging chickens; supermarket eggs, standard US Department of Agriculture eggs found in US supermarkets; fish meal eggs, main source of fatty acids provided by fish meal and whole soybeans; flax eggs, main source of fatty acids provided by flax flour.

change of ω-6/ω-3 in the food supply of Western societies occurred over the last 100 years[59] (Figure 3). A balance existed between ω-6 and ω-3 for millions of years during the long evolutionary history of the genus Homo, and genetic changes occurred partly in response to these dietary influences.[2] However, rapid dietary changes over short periods of time as have occurred over the past 100-150 years is a totally new phenomenon in human evolution.

A balance between the ω-6 and ω-3 fatty acids is a more physiologic state in terms of prostaglandin and leukotriene metabolism and interleukin-1 (IL-1) production.[3] The current recommendation to substitute vegetable oils (ω-6) for saturated fats leads to increases in IL-1, prostaglandins of the 2 series and leukotrienes of the 4 series, which are proinflammatory, prothrombotic, and vasoconstrictive; it is not consistent with human evolution; and may lead to maladaptation in those genetically predisposed.[3]

Antioxidants

Dietary Evolution and Antioxidant Intake

Just as the ω-3 fatty acids were depleted from the food supply and led to an imbalance in the ω-6 and ω-3 ratio, the antioxidant intake has also decreased. Our ancestors ate meat, fish, and fresh fruits and vegetables whereas today most of the vegetables eaten are cooked and are limited in number. Prior to the Agricultural Revolution, humans typically used many species of wild plants for food, mostly green leafy vegetables. In addition, they consumed roots, beans, nuts, tubers, and fruit. These foods are rich sources of antioxidants.

It is very difficult to estimate the antioxidant intake during the Paleolithic period and before. There are strong indications, however, that it was higher during the Paleolithic period and earlier. These indications are based on anthropological studies of present day hunters and gatherers,[78] findings of archeological excavations, and comparative data on the antioxidant content of wild and cultivated plants used as major food sources. The major evolutionary changes in the diet summarized in Table 3 include a decline in the intake of vitamins A, C, E and β-carotene. The estimated intakes[2,77] of the antioxidant vitamins E and C are shown in Figure 3.

Antioxidant Content of Wild Plants Used as Food

Wild plants are rich in antioxidant vitamins E and C and other important antioxidants such as glutathione and carotenoids. The study of wild plants such as purslane provides information about the antioxidant intake of our ancestors. Purslane seeds found in caves date back to 16,400 years ago. This finding is of particular interest in terms of human evolution.

We studied the fatty acid composition and antioxidant content of purslane (Table 6).[79] It is particularly rich in α-tocopherol and glutathione. The role of α-tocopherol as a major fat-soluble antioxidant is discussed extensively in other chapters. Glutathione is also a major component of the antioxidant system and has been suggested to play a role in the prevention and treatment of chronic diseases.[80-82] Purslane contains higher levels of vitamin C but lower levels of β-carotene in comparison to spinach.[83]

Table 6
Comparison of α-Tocopherol, Ascorbic Acid, and β-Carotene in Purslane and Spinach Leaves

	α-Tocopherol	Ascorbic Acid	β-Carotene
	.... mg/100 g fresh weight[a]		
Chamber-grown purslane[b]	12.2 ± 0.4	26.6 ± 0.8	1.9 ± 0.08
Spinach	1.8 ± 0.09	21.7 ± 0.5	3.3± 0.5
	.... mg/100 g dry weight[a]		
Chamber-grown purslane	230 ± 9	506 ± 17	38.2 ± 2.4
Spinach	36 ± 4	430 ± 15	63.5 ± 5.7

[a] Data represent mean value from four analyses each with three replicates per species/type.[79]
[b] Purslane is rich in glutathione and alpha-linolenic acid (14.8 and 400 mg/100g wet weight, respectively).

Purslane is one of the 8 most common plants dispersed on planet Earth and has been part of the diet of both humans and animals. Purslane was part of the diet of hunter-gatherers in the Pacific Northwest section of the U.S. The large native population encountered in the years 1790-1850 was non-agricultural and obtained their food by foraging and harvesting natural localized species of plants and animals. Norton *et al.* studied the vegetable food products of foraging economies of the Pacific Northwest and found them to be valuable sources of calcium, magnesium, iron, zinc, and ascorbic acid.[78] Norton states:

These members of the Lily, Purslane, Barberry, Currant, Rose, Parsley, Heath, Honeysuckle, Sunflower and Water-Plantain families are among those regularly collected by these foraging groups whose economic strategies were keyed to the use of multiple resources and the storage of large quantities of processed foods. Stored vegetable food along with dried fish provided ample and nutritious diets during seasonal periods of resource non-productivity... Analyses show that these native foods are superior to cultigens in necessary fiber, minerals and vitamins making substantial contributions to pre-contact diets.

A wide variety of foods were used to meet nutritional needs. Vegetable foods were systematically gathered and processed in quantity. The native preparation and preservation techniques were important factors in retaining nutrients and in maintaining a balanced diet during seasons of low productivity. Of the 1,300 known food plants, fewer than 20 are currently providing most of our food needs, making humans heavily dependent on a few crops to provide food, yet plants have influenced the evolution of human beings. Paleolithic humans ate a greater variety of wild plants and fruits that were richer in vitamins and minerals than today's limited cultivated varieties. Table 7 shows the levels of vitamins C and E in wild plants and Table 8 shows the vitamin C content in some of the wild fruits in the diet of Australian aborigines.[84] A number of these plants are rich sources of vitamins E and C. In addition, plants supply a wide variety of phytochemicals many of which have strong antioxidant activity.

Table 7
Vitamin E and C Content of Different Plant Species[a]

Plant Species	Ascorbic Acid	α-Tocopherol
	mg/100 g dry weight	
Morning glory	2 ± 1	10 ± 3
Lamb's quarter	58 ± 18	12 ± 3
Alfalfa	143 ± 12	10 ± 1
Pigweed	504 ± 24	10 ± 1
Buckwheat	53 ± 27	28 ± 2
Mustard	469 ± 24	50 ± 9
Sicklepod	861 ± 73	60 ± 6
Velvetleaf	92 ± 7	50 ± 4
Jimson weed	114 ± 29	83 ± 16

[a] Values represent the mean ± SE of 6 plants of each species (Ref. 83).

Evolution and Oxidative Stress

There is little information on the comparative stress of modern and ancient humans. Some modern environmental factors are known to increase oxidative stress. The modern diet for example, is rich in animal fat, which

Table 8
Vitamin C (Ascorbate) Content of Selected Fruits

Taxonomic Name	Common Name	Ascorbic Acid mg/100 g raw
Buchanania obovata	Green Plum	53
Santalum Lanceolatum	Bush Plum	54
Solanum chippendalei	Bush Tomato	59
Antidesma bunis	Wild Cherry	69
Microcitrus australasica var.sanguinus	Finger Lime	82
Capparis umbonata		89
Morinda citrifolia	Great Morinda Cheese Fruit	90
Capparis mitchellii	Wild Orange	98
Ximenia citrifolia	Sea Lemon	108
Morinida americana		123
Terminalia aff. latipes	Wild Olives	146
Cynanchum pedunculatum		174
Minusops elengi	Tanjong Tree	223
Anacardium occidentale	Cashew Fruit	265
Phyllanthus emblica		316
Rosa cania	Rose Hips	468
Ficus opposita	Sandpaper Fig	918
Terminalia latipes		1800
Terminalia carpentariae		1995
Terminalia ferdinandiana	Billy Goat Plum	5320

contains lower levels of fat-soluble antioxidants such as tocopherols than vegetable oils. In addition, the vegetable oils used in modern diets supply more ω-6 and less ω-3 than evolutionary and other diets. Oil seeds and nuts are good sources of tocopherols and other antioxidants. The modern oil refining processes, however, remove the larger part of the tocopherols and other antioxidants.

As discussed earlier, ω-6 fatty acids induce inflammation, which increases oxidative stress. Phagocytes, for example, produce large amounts of free radicals. Saturated fatty acids, which are common in animal fats, appear to be atherogenic, a condition which involves phagocytes and inflammatory responses. In contrast, ω-3 fatty acids are antiinflammatory. Thus the change in the ratio ω-6:ω-3 may have contributed to conditions of oxidative stress. Other major evolutionary changes in diet discussed earlier, such as higher intake of carbohydrates and especially refined sugars, produce hormonal and other metabolic changes and seem to contribute to development of chronic diseases such as diabetes and heart disease. It is believed that oxidative stress plays a major role in the pathogenesis of these diseases.

Environmental factors such as air pollutants, UV radiation, and others increase oxidative stress but their comparative impact on modern and ancient humans is not clearly understood.

CONCLUSIONS

Genetic variation is an important consideration in establishing dietary reference values for nutrients. For this reason, general dietary recommendations are not appropriate for the prevention or management of chronic diseases and are not applicable to different populations.

Humans evolved on a diet that was very different from current Western diets. It was lower in total fat, saturated fat, trans fatty acids, and ω-6 fatty acids while it was higher in ω-3 fatty acids, protein, ascorbic acid, and probably other antioxidants such as α-tocopherol and glutathione. These dietary changes came about as a result of the Agricultural Revolution which occurred about 10,000 years ago, and for the past 50 years by agribusiness, food technology, and the economic factors that provided the stimulus for the expansion of processed foods. The latter brought about rapid changes more in the form of cultural evolution. Cultural evolution may completely suppress natural selection. In so doing, it may increase the incidence of chronic disease, and unveil a number of diseases that did not exist before, or were very rare.[85,86]

Eaton has presented some very good arguments for the need to consider the dietary intake of the Paleolithic period in making dietary recommendations and in setting dietary reference values.[2,77] Significant evidence suggests that the ratio of ω-6:ω-3 should be reduced to 4:1 or lower, and intake of ascorbic acid, vitamin E, and folate should be increased.

Genetic research should enhance the understanding of mechanisms involved in the development of chronic diseases, which may eventually lead to improved management of cancer and cardiovascular diseases. It will be a special challenge to bridge the divide between molecular biology and public health.

REFERENCES

1. Simopoulos AP, Childs B, Eds. Genetic Variation and Nutrition, Vol. 63, *World Rev Nutr Diet*, Basel, 1990.
2. Eaton SB, Konner M. Paleolithic nutrition. A consideration of its nature and current implications. *New Engl J Med*, 312, 283, 1985.
3. Simopoulos AP. Omega-3 fatty acids in health and disease and in growth and development. *Am J Clin Nutr*, 54, 438, 1991.
4. Gonzalez FJ, Skoda RC, Kimura S, *et al.*, Characterization of the common genetic defect in humans deficient in debrisoquine metabolism, *Nature*, 331, 442, 1988.
5. Price Evans D.A, in *Ethnic Differences in Reactions to Drugs and Xenobiotics*, Kalow W, Goedde HW, Agarwal DP, Eds. Liss, New York, 1986, 491.
6. Price Evans DA, Harmer D, Downham DY, *et al.*, The genetic control of sparteine and debrisoquine in metabolism in man with new methods of analyzing bimodal distributions, *J Med Genet*, 20, 321, 1983.
7. Idle JR, Poor metabolizers of debrisoquine reveal their true colours, *Lancet* ii, 1097, 1989.
8. Wolf CR, Moss JE, Miles JS, Gough AC, Spurr NK, Detection of debrisoquine hydroxylation phenotypes, *Lancet*, 336, 1452, 1990.
9. Simopoulos AP, Herbert V, Jacobson B, *The Healing Diet*, Macmillan, New York, 1995.
10. Goldbourt U, de Faire U, Berg K, *Genetic Factors in Coronary Heart Disease*, Kluwer, Dordrecht, 1994.
11. Scriver CR Nutrient-gene interactions: the gene is not the disease and vice versa. *Am J Clin Nutr*, 48, 1505, 1988.
12. Childs B. Genetic variation and nutrition. *Am J Clin Nutr*, 48, 1500, 1988.
13. Lewontin RC. Gene, organism and environment, in *Evolution from Molecules to Man*, Bendall DS, Ed. Cambridge University Press, Cambridge, 1983.
14. Bowman JE, Murray RF. *Genetic Variation and Disorders in Peoples of African Origin*. The Johns Hopkins University Press, Baltimore, 1990.
15. Simopoulos AP, Nestel P, Eds. Genetic Variation and Dietary Response, Vol. 80, *World Rev Nutr Diet*, 1997.
16. Simopoulos AP. Diet and gene interactions. *Food Technology*, 51(3), 66, 1997.
17. Simopoulos AP. Part 1. Genetic variation and nutrition. Populations differences due to single gene defects and population differences in multifactorial diseases due to polygenic effects. *Nutr Today*, 30(4), 157, 1995.
18. Simopoulos AP. Part 2. Genetic variation and nutrition. Genetic variation, nutrition and chronic diseases. *Nutr Today*, 30(5), 194, 1995.
19. Beynen AC, Katan MB, Van Zutphen LFM. Hypo- and hyperresponders: individual differences in the response of serum cholesterol concentration to changes in diet. *Adv Lipid Res*, 22, 115, 1987.
20. Miettinen TA, Kensaniemi YA. Cholesterol absorption: regulation of cholesterol synthesis and elimination and within-population variations of serum cholesterol levels. *Am J Clin Nutr*, 49, 629, 1989.
21. Nestel PJ, Poyser A. Changes in cholesterol synthesis and excretion when cholesterol intake is increased. *Metabolism*, 25, 1591, 1976.
22. Glatz JF, Turner PR, Katan MD, Stalenhoef AF, Lewis B. Hypo- and hyperresponse of serum cholesterol level and low density lipoprotein production and degradation to dietary cholesterol in man. *Ann NY Acad Sci*, 676, 163, 1993.
23. Mahley RW, Weisgraber KH, Innerarity TL, Rall SC. Genetic defects in lipoprotein metabolism. Elevation of atherogenic lipoproteins caused by impaired catabolism. *JAMA*, 265, 78, 1991.

24. Cobb MM, Teitlebaum H, Risch N, Jekel J, Ostfeld A. Influence of dietary fat, apolipoprotein E phenotype, se xon plasma lipoprotein levels, Circulation, 86, 849, 1992.
25. Uusitupa MIJ, Ruuskanen E, Makinen E, *et al.* A controlled study on the effect of beta-glucan-rich oat bran on serum lipids in hypercholesterolemic subjects: relation to apolipoprotein E phenotype. *J Am College Nutr*, 11, 651, 1992.
26. McCombs RJ, Marcadis DE, Ellis J, Weinberg RB. Attenuated hypercholesterolemic response to a high-cholesterol diet in subjects heterozygous for the apolipoprotein A-IV-2 allele. *N Engl J Med*, 331, 706, 1994.
27. Cusi D, Barlassina C, Azzani T, *et al.* Polymorphisms of alpha-adducin and salt sensitivity in patients with essential hypertension. *Lancet*, 349, 1353, 1997.
28. Salamone LM, Glynn NW, Black DM, *et al.* Determinants of premenopausal bone mineral density: the interplay of genetic and lifestyle factors. *J Bone Miner Res*, 11, 1557, 1996.
29. Dawson-Hughes B, Harris SS, Finneran S. Calcium absorption on high and low calcium intakes in relation to vitamin D receptor genotype. *J Clin Endocr Metab*, 80, 3657,1995.
30. Velazquez A, Bourges H, Eds. *Genetic Factors in Nutrition*, Acad. Press, Orlando, 1984.
31. Rucker R,, Tinker D. The role of nutrition in gene expression: a fertile field for the application of molecular biology. *J Nutr*, 116, 177, 1986.
32. Castro CE, Towle HC. Nutrient-genome interaction. Fed. Proc, 45, 2392, 1986.
33. Berdanier CD, Hargrove JL, Eds. *Nutrition and Gene Expression*, CRC Press, Boca Raton, 1993.
34. Goldstein JL. Genetics and cardiovascular disease, in *Heart Disease: A Textbook of Cardiovascular Medicine,* 2nd ed, Vol. 2, WB Saunders, Philadelphia, 1984, 1606.
35. Simopoulos AP. *Nutrition policies for the prevention of atherosclerosis in industrialized societies, in Diet and Life Style. New Technology*, Moyal, MF, Ed, John Libby, Paris, 1988, 373.
36. Rudman D, Williams PJ. Pathophysiologic principles of nutrition, in *Pathophysiology: The Biomedical Principles of Disease*, Smith LH, Ed, W. B. Saunders, Philadelphia, 1985.
37. Losonczy KG, Harris TB, Havlik RJ. Vitamin E and vitamin C supplement use and risk of all-cause and coronary heart disease mortality in older persons: the Established Populations for Epidemiologic Studies of the Elderly. *Am J Clin Nutr,* 64, 190, 1996.
38. Watkins BA, Seifert MF, Allen KGD. Importance of dietary fat in modulating PGE2 responses and influence of vitamin E on bone morphometry, in Nutrition and Fitness: Metabolic and Behavioral Aspects in Health and Disease, Vol. 82, Simopoulos AP, Pavlou KN, Eds, *World Rev Nutr Diet*, 1997.
39. Molloy AM, Daly S, Mills JL, *et al.* Thermolabile variant of 5,10-methylenetetrahydrofolate reductase associated with low red-cell folates: implications for folate intake recommendations. *Lancet,* 349, 1591, 1997.
40. Osborn TF, Goldstein JL, Brown MS. 5'-End of HMG-CoA reductase gene contains sequences responsible for cholesterol-mediated inhibition of transcription. *Cell* 42, 203, 1985.
41. Clarke SD, Jump DB. Regulation of hepatic gene expression by dietary fats: a unique role for polyunsaturated fatty acids, in *Nutrition and Gene Expression*, Berdanier CD, Hargrove JL, Eds, CRC Press, Boca Raton, 1993.
42. Kaminski WE, Jendraschak C, Kiefl R, von Schacky C. Dietary omega-3 fatty acids lower levels of platelet-derived growth factor mRNA in human mononuclear cells. *Blood* 81(7) 1871, 1993.
43. Urakaze M, Sugiyama E, Xu L, Auron P, Yeh E, Robinson D. Dietary marine lipids suppress IL-1B mRNA levels in lipopolysaccharide stimulated monocytes. *Clin Res*, 23, 1991.

44. Simopoulos AP. The role of fatty acids in gene expression: health implications. *Ann Nutr Metab,* 40, 303, 1996.
45. Clarke SD, Romsos DR, Leveille GA. Differential effects of dietary methylesters of long chain saturated and polyunsaturated fatty acids on rat liver and adipose tissue lipogenesis. *J Nutr* 107, 1170, 1977.
46. Clarke SD, Armstrong MK, Jump DB. Nutritional control of rat liver fatty acid synthase and S14 mRNA abundance. *J Nutr*, 120, 218, 1990.
47. Clarke SD, Jump DB. Polyunsaturated fatty acid regulation of hepatic gene transcription. *Lipids*, 31, 7, 1996.
48. Ntambi JM. Dietary regulation of stearoyl-CoA desaturase I gene expression in mouse liver. *J Biol Chem*, 267, 10925, 1991.
49. DeWillie JW, Farmer SJ. Linoleic acid controls neonatal tissue-specific stearoyl-CoA desaturase mRNA levels. *Biochim Biophys Acta*, 1170, 291, 1993.
50. Jump DB, Clarke SD, Thelen A, Liimatta N. Coordinate regulation of glycolytic and lipogenic gene expression by polyunsaturated fatty acids. *J Lipid Res*, 35, 1076, 1994.
51. Tebbey PW, McGowan KM, Stephens JM, Buttke TM, Pekata PH. Arachidonic acid down-regulates the insulin-dependent glucose transporter gene (Glut 4) in 3T3-L1 adipocytes by inhibiting transcription and enhancing mRNA turnover. *J Biol Chem*, 269, 639, 1994.
52. Sellmayer A, Danesch U, Weber P.C. Effects of different polyunsaturated fatty acids on growth-related early gene expression and cell growth. *Lipids*, 31(suppl), S37, 1996.
53. De Caterina R, Libby P. Control of endothelial leukocyte adhesion molecules by fatty acids. *Lipids*, 31(suppl), S57, 1996.
54. Robinson DR, Urakaze M, Huang R, *et al.* Dietary marine lipids suppress the continuous expression of interleukin-1B gene transcription. *Lipids*, 31(suppl), S23, 1996.
55. Simopoulos AP, Ed. *Plants in Human Nutrition. World Rev Nutr Diet*, Vol. 77, Karger, Basel, 1995.
56. Fanaian M, Szilasi J, Storlien L, Calvert GD. The effect of modified fat diet on insulin resistance and metabolic parameters in type II diabetes. *Diabetologia*, 39(suppl 1), A7, 1996.
57. Simopoulos AP. Is insulin resistance influenced by dietary linoleic acid and trans fatty acids?, *Free Rad Biol & Med*, 17(4), 367, 1994.
58. Simopoulos AP. Fatty acid composition of skeletal muscle membrane phospholipids, insulin resistance and obesity. *Nutr Today*, 2, 12, 1994.
59. Leaf A, Weber P.C. A new era for science in nutrition. *Am J Clin Nutr*, 45, 1048, 1987.
60. Simopoulos AP. Dietary risk factors for hypertension. *Comp Ther*, 18(10), 26, 1992.
61. Simopoulos AP. The Mediterranean diet: Greek column rather than an Egyptian pyramid. *Nutrition Today*, 30(2), 54, 1995.
62. Karlsson J *Antioxidants and Exercise*. Human Kinetics Publishers, Champaign, IL, 1997.
63. Kirshenbauer HG. *Fats and Oils*, 2nd Ed., Reinhold Publishing, New York, 1960.
64. Emken EA. Nutrition and biochemistry of trans and positional fatty acid isomers in hydrogenated oils. *Annu Rev Nutr*, 4, 229, 1984.
65. Troisi R, Willett WC, Weiss ST. Trans-fatty acid intake in relation to serum lipid concentrations in adult men, *Am J Clin Nutr*, 56, 1019, 1992.
66. Ahrens EH, Blankenhorn DH, Tsaltas TT. Effect on human serum lipids of substituting plant for animal fat in the diet. *Proc Soc Exp Biol Med*, 86, 872, 1954.
67. Keys A, Anderson JT, Grande F. Serum cholesterol response to dietary fat. *Lancet*, 1, 787, 1957.
68. Ledger HP. Body composition as a basis for a comparative study of some East African mammals. *Symp Zool Soc London*, 21, 289, 1968.

69. Crawford MA. Fatty acid ratios in free-living and domestic animals. *Lancet*, 1, 1329, 1968.
70. Wo CKW, Draper HH. Vitamin E status of Alaskan Eskimos. *Am J Clin Nutr*, 28, 808, 1975.
71. Crawford MA, Gale MM, Woodford MH. Linoleic acid and linolenic acid elongation products in muscle tissue of Syncerus caffer and other ruminant species. *Biochem J*, 115, 25, 1969.
72. Simopoulos AP, Salem NJr, Purslane: a terrestrial source of omega-3 fatty acids. N. Engl. *J Med*, 315, 833, 1986.
73. van Vliet T, Katan MB. Lower ratio of n-3 to n-6 fatty acids in cultured than in wild fish. *Am J Clin Nutr*, 51, 1, 1990.
74. Simopoulos AP, Salem NJr. Egg yolk as a source of long-chain polyunsaturated fatty acids in infant feeding. *Am J Clin Nutr* 55, 411, 1992.
75. Raper NR, Cronin FJ, Exler J Omega-3 fatty acid content of the US food supply. *J Am College Nutr*, 11(3), 304, 1992.
76. Hunter JE. Omega-3 fatty acids from vegetable oils in Dietary ω-3 and ω-6 Fatty Acids: *Biological Effects and Nutritional Essentiality*, Series A: Life Sciences, Vol. 171, Galli, C, and Simopoulos, AP, Eds, Plenum Press, New York, 1989, 43.
77. Eaton SB, Eaton SB III, Konner MJ, Shostak, M. An evolutionary perspective enhances understanding of human nutritional requirements. *J Nutr*, 126, 1732, 1996.
78. Norton HH, Hunn, ES, Martinsen CS, Keely, P.B. Vegetable food products of the foraging economies of the Pacific Northwest. *Ecol Food & Nutr*, 14, 219, 1984.
79. Simopoulos AP, Norman HA, Gillaspy JE, Duke, JA. Common purslane: a source of omega-3 fatty acids and antioxidants. *J Am College Nutr*, 11(4), 374, 1992.
80. Oleinick NL, Xue L, Friedman LR, Donahue LL, Biaglow, JE. Inhibition of radiation-induced DNA-protein cross-link repair by glutathione depletion with l-buthionine sulfoximine. *NCI Monogr*, 6, 225, 1988.
81. Fuchs JA. Glutaredoxin, in Glutathione. *Chemical, Biochemical and Medical Aspects*, Dolphin, D, Avramovic, O, Pulson, R, Eds, Wiley, New York, 1989, 551.
82. Buhl R, Holroyd KJ, Mastrangeli A, Cantin AM, Jaffee HA, *et al.* Systemic glutathione deficiency in symptom-free HIV-seropositive individuals. *Lancet*, ii, 1294, 1989.
83. Simopoulos AP, Norman, HA, Gillaspy, JE. Purslane in human nutrition and its potential for world agriculture, in Plants in Human Nutrition, Simopoulos, AP, Ed, *World Rev Nutr Diet*, Vol. 77, Karger, Basel, 1995, 47.
84. Miller JB, James KW, Maggiore PMA. *Tables of Composition of Australian Aboriginal Foods*. Aboriginal Studies Press, Canberra, 1993.
85. Simopoulos AP, Ed. Metabolic Consequences of Changing Dietary Patterns. *World Rev Nutr Diet*, Vol. 79, Karger, Basel, Switzerland, 1996.
86. Wahlqvist ML, Lo CS, Myers, KA. Food variety is associated with less macrovascular disease in those with type II diabetes and their healthy controls. *J Am Coll Nutr*, 8, 515, 1989.

5

Diet and Antioxidant Status

Andreas M. Papas, Ph.D.
Health and Nutrition
Eastman Chemical Company, Kingsport, Tennessee, USA

INTRODUCTION

The link of diet and chronic disease is very well documented. Poor diet combined with lack of exercise is the second leading cause of death in the United States, accounting for over 300,000 deaths every year.[1] Heart disease, the leading cause of death in the United States and many industrialized countries, is greatly influenced by diet, especially by the amount and type of fat. As much as one third of all cancers are related to our diet.

Nutritionists, dietitians, and health professionals disagree on many issues related to nutrition and disease. They are, however, practically unanimous in their recommendation of diets rich in fruits and vegetables for good health and for reducing the risk of heart disease and some cancers. Many epidemiological and limited clinical studies provided the basis for this recommendation.[2,3] Particularly prominent were studies that documented a striking lower

0-8493-8009-X/98/$0.00+$.50

incidence of heart disease and cancer in the Mediterranean countries than in North Europe and North America (Figure 1). The Mediterranean diet, which is rich in fruits and vegetables and low in saturated fats,[4,5] appeared to account for most of the difference (see Chapter 6). Other studies documented diet related differences in chronic disease in the people of North America and Europe as compared with people of Japan and some other Asian countries. This lower incidence of disease has been attributed, in large part, to higher consumption of soy and fish[6-9] and lower consumption of meat and saturated fat.[10]

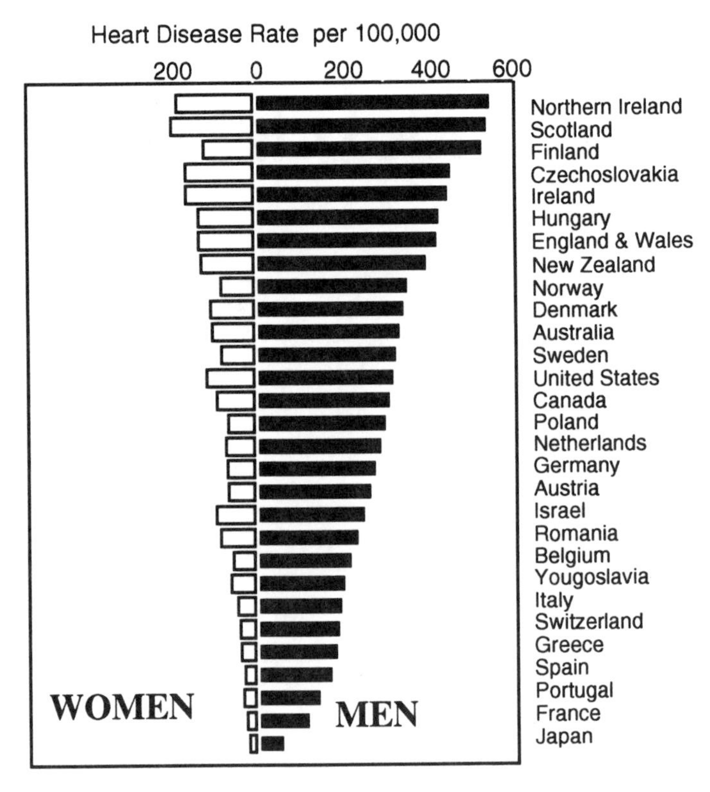

Figure 1. Country differences in the incidence of heart disease. Diet is believed to be among the major factors accounting for these differences. Data from the World Health Organization.

The beneficial effects of fruits and vegetables and the Mediterranean diet are very likely due to many of their components such as fiber, micronutrients, and others. Antioxidants, which are among their major components, have been proposed, but not confirmed yet, as the principle active agents for reducing the risk of chronic disease.[11] For soy, the suggested beneficial agents include isoflavones such as daidzein and genistein.[6] These are phenolic compounds with several biological functions including antioxidant activity (see Chapter 11).

Diet has a profound effect on antioxidant status and ranks among the top factors under our control. Unlike other factors such as smoking, stress, and disease, that have only a prooxidant effect, diet, depending on its components, can have antioxidant or prooxidant effects.

This chapter will discuss the major dietary factors affecting antioxidant status. The term diet in this chapter will include natural foods and drinks, additives and nutritional supplements.

DIETARY FACTORS AFFECTING THE ANTIOXIDANT STATUS

The overall effect of the diet, whether antioxidant or prooxidant, is determined by its components and related factors including:

- Antioxidant and prooxidant nutrient and nonnutrient components
- Absorption and bioavailability
- Food processing and storage
- Food additives and nutritional supplements
- Chemical, chiral form and formulation of additives and supplements.

Some of the above factors such as the major dietary antioxidants (vitamins E and C, carotenoids, flavonoids and other phytochemicals, alcohol) are discussed in separate chapters. This chapter will focus on the remaining factors.

DIETARY ANTIOXIDANTS AND PROOXIDANTS

Dietary Antioxidants

Our diet contains antioxidants recognized as essential nutrients and others, which have antioxidant activity even though they are not essential nutrients.

Nutrient Antioxidants

Nutrient antioxidants in the diet include:

- Vitamin E (tocopherols and tocotrienols)

- Vitamin C or ascorbic acid
- Vitamin A and its non-nutrient precursor β-carotene
- Nutrients essential for normal function of endogenous antioxidant systems. For example, the minerals Cu, Mn, Zn, Se, Fe and the vitamin riboflavin are important cofactors of antioxidant enzyme systems.

Non-nutrient Antioxidants

The diet also contains enzymes, peptides, proteins and other compounds similar to those present in our body. Glutathione, coenzyme Q_{10}, catalases, superoxide dismutases (SOD), albumins, and others are good examples. From these, small peptides, like glutathione may escape hydrolysis and can be absorbed intact. Larger proteins, however, such as catalases, SOD, and albumins are denatured and hydrolyzed in the digestive system and, thus, little, if any, is absorbed in the active form.

Finally, a large number of phytochemicals, not recognized as essential nutrients, apparently play an important antioxidant role in the body. Practically all diets contain at least some phytochemicals. Fruits, vegetables, and herbs are particularly rich sources.[12] Many phytochemicals are now studied extensively for their potential role in reducing the risk and even preventing and treating some diseases.[13] Major classes of phytochemicals with potential for antioxidant activity are listed in Table 1.

Table 1
Major Classes of Phytochemicals with Antioxidant Activity

Class of Phytochemicals	Example Compounds
Carotenoids	lycopene, lutein, astaxanthin
Bioflavonoids	genistein, diadzein, quercetin
Phytosterols	sitosterol, stigmasterol, oryzanol
Tannins	catechins and other polyphenol compounds
Chlorophylls	chlorophyll A and chlorophyllin
Terpenoids	limonin and limonene
Allylic compounds	diallyl sulfide and disulfide
Indoles	indole-3-carbinol.

Dietary Components that may Function as Prooxidants

Dietary components, which can be easily oxidized or can promote oxidation, have a major impact on the antioxidant status. The following have major practical significance.

Polyunsaturated Fatty Acids (PUFA)

Our diets contain significant amounts of lipids such as triglycerides, phospholipids, cholesterol, and others. Lipids are susceptible to attack by free radicals and their oxidation can be very damaging because, as discussed in Chapter 1, it proceeds as a chain reaction. Lipids containing PUFA are particularly prone to attack by free radicals. In recent decades, consumption of PUFA-rich vegetable oils has been increasing because saturated fats have been associated with higher risk of heart disease and cancer.[10] The ω-3 PUFA (α-linolenic, eicosapentaenoic, and docohexaenoic), believed to be the beneficial agents in fish,[14] are now added to infant formula and some foods in some countries. They are also available in many countries including the United States as nutritional supplements. In the absence of appropriate antioxidants, PUFA form free radicals and can have a significant prooxidant effect leading to significant depletion of vitamin E and increased oxidation products.[15-18] It is important to note, however, that PUFA-rich vegetable oils are also good sources of tocopherols and/or tocotrienols and other fat-soluble phytochemicals that have antioxidant function.

Transition Metals

Iron (Fe) and copper (Cu) are considered as transition metals because they have variable oxidation numbers, i.e., Fe^{2+} or Fe^{3+} and Cu^{+} or Cu^{2+}. Because they can accept or donate electrons, they are major promoters of free radical reactions. The reaction of Fe^{2+} salts with H_2O_2, known as the Fenton reaction, yields Fe^{3+} and the extremely reactive hydroxyl radical ($HO^{\bullet}$). Fe^{3+} and Cu^{2+} can be reduced to Fe^{2+} and Cu^{+}, respectively, by ascorbate (vitamin C). Iron also hydrolyzes lipid hydroperoxides to alcoxy and hydroxy radicals. These radicals are major initiators of lipid peroxidation.

Transition metals may act as prooxidants in the food, especially in stored fats and oils,[19] in the digestive tract,[20-22] and, after absorption, in our tissues.[23-25] Their practical importance, however, is generally higher in foods and the digestive tract, because absorbed Fe and Cu is almost completely bound to proteins and enzymes. For example, hemoglobin contains 55-60% of all body iron, followed by ferritin/hemosiderin with 30%, myoglobin with 10%, and transferrin with 0.1%. Fe and Cu bound to proteins and enzymes are shielded from surrounding media and do not act as prooxidants. Actually, caeruloplasmin, the major protein containing Cu, inhibits lipid peroxidation.

Absorbed Fe is carried by transferrin, a glycoprotein with high affinity for Fe^{3+}. Excess binding capacity (70-80%) of transferrin assures that concentration of free Fe^{3+} in blood is maintained at extremely low levels (less than 10^{-12} M). Inside the cell, Fe concentration is also very low and is regulated by the expression of the transferrin receptor and ferritin. Oxidative stress causes release of Fe primarily from ferritin. Superoxide and nitric oxide probably mediate this release. Iron is also released from hemoglobin and other proteins and enzymes when red blood cells are hemolyzed or tissue is injured. In people suffering from the hereditary diseases, idiopathic hemochromatosis and thalassemia (hemoglobin is defective) excess unbound Fe catalyzes oxidation and production of free radicals.[24-26]

Feces have high levels of bile pigments (such as bilirubin, biliverdin), which can chelate iron in a form capable of supporting the superoxide driven Fenton reactions. In our diet, heme iron, available primarily in animal products and especially red meat, is better absorbed at rates of 10-35%. Most of our dietary Fe, however, is derived from plants in the insoluble non-heme Fe^{3+} form and commonly complexes with oxalates or phenolic compounds. In order to be absorbed, it requires reduction to the more soluble Fe^{2+} ion. This is achieved by the action of the stomach hydrochloric acid, which aids solubilization of Fe^{3+} and thus allows reducing agents, such as vitamin C, to reduce it to the Fe^{2+} form. Thus, vitamin C and other organic acids such as lactic and citric, enhance the absorption of Fe (non-heme Fe is absorbed at rates ranging from 2-20%).

This effect is highly desirable when dietary Fe is low and has low bioavailability (non-heme form) especially for menstruating women and children, who have high nutritional requirements. If, however, the amount of dietary Fe is high, the effect of vitamin C and other reducing agents may be harmful because it may lead to excessive Fe absorption. There is serious concern that in people suffering from idiopathic hemochromatosis, thalassemia, or other conditions causing iron overload, vitamin C may have a prooxidant effect by further increasing absorption, but may also cause ferritin to release Fe^2.[2,25] The role of vitamin C, however, as a prooxidant even in conditions of iron overload, remains highly controversial. Specifically it is suggested that, at high serum levels, reduced ascorbic acid drives through the pores of the ferritin protein shell to the inside surface, where it converts the Fe^2 to catalytic Fe^3, which then leaks out of the pores and generates free radicals.[27] In addition, it was suggested that high levels of vitamin C inhibit the antioxidant activities of caeruloplasmin and, specifically, the conversion of Fe^2 to Fe^3. Other researchers, however, reported results showing that is unlikely; however, oral supplementation with vitamin C can raise plasma levels sufficiently to inhibit caeruloplasmin.[28] They also dispute the prooxidant effect of vitamin C *in vivo*, even in conditions of Fe overload.[29]

While this discussion focused on Fe, the same considerations apply to Cu and other transition metals. Because Cu levels in our body and diet are much lower than Fe, its practical significance as prooxidant may be lower even though Cu is more reactive. The adult male body contains about 4.5 g Fe and only about 75 mg Cu. The daily Fe RDA for adults is 10-15 mg and only 1.5-3.0 mg for Cu. It is estimated that 1 mg of Fe is absorbed daily. A large part of dietary iron is not absorbed and is concentrated in feces at a level calculated to be 10-fold greater than in most tissues.

We proposed that the antioxidant status of the digesta has a direct effect on the production of free radicals and possibly the development of colon cancer.[20] The amount of Fe and its ionic form are important considerations. In addition to vitamin C, flavonoids and superoxide ions reduce Fe^{3+} thus increasing the lipid peroxidation and other harmful reactions. Other phytochemicals, such as tannins, bind metals including Fe and reduce their absorption. Vitamin C appears to counteract the inhibition of phenolic compounds.[30]

Phytochemicals

Many phytochemicals have antioxidant properties,[12,31] which are discussed in several other chapters. Phytochemicals may also have prooxidant effects. For example, phenolic flavonoids, which have been shown to have lipid antioxidant properties can also form hydroxyl radicals either by autoxidation or when complexed with metals such as Cu or Fe.[31]

Some phytochemicals affect the antioxidant status directly, others indirectly, and some may have both direct and indirect effects. For example, phytates, tannins, and other phenolic compounds, may have a direct antioxidant effect by scavenging free radicals. They also bind metals such as Fe, Cu, Zn, Mn and reduce their absorption.[32] It has been suggested that the effect of phenolic compounds in Fe absorption depends on their content of iron-binding galloyl groups, whereas the phenolic catechol groups seem to be of minor importance.[33] If such binding causes a deficiency of these essential antioxidant enzyme cofactors the net effect would be prooxidant. If, however, there is sufficient amount for optimal enzymatic activity, binding of the Fe and Cu will prevent them from acting as prooxidants.

FOOD PROCESSING

Storage, handling, processing, and cooking of food can result in oxidative damage. The degree of damage and the resulting oxidation products depend on a variety of factors including temperature, exposure to light and air, amount and saturation of lipid material, presence of oxidation promoting metals, and other factors.[19,23] Peroxides and prooxidants in processed foods affect antioxidant status.

Processing has a major effect on absorption and bioavailability. Carotenoids provide excellent examples. Absorption of lycopene from fresh tomatoes and β-carotene from fresh carrots is significantly lower than from tomato juice or cooked carrots and carrot juice. Heat processing of tomato and carrot juice further increases bioavailability.[34-37] Processing to produce juice and heating breaks the carotenoid protein complexes. In addition, heating causes isomerization such as conversion of *cis* to *trans* β-carotene, which as discussed below, may affect bioavailability. Excessive heating may decrease absorption and bioavailability by promoting oxidation or formation of complexes of antioxidants with carbohydrates and proteins.

ABSORPTION

Absorption and bioavailability determine whether dietary antioxidants and prooxidants have a direct effect in the blood and other tissues in addition to their effects in the digestive tract. From the many factors affecting absorption and bioavailability of antioxidants, the following have major significance.

Dietary Fat

Antioxidant fat-soluble vitamins and phytochemicals are absorbed as micelles. For example, bile emulsifies the tocopherols incorporating them into micelles along with other fat-soluble compounds, thereby facilitating absorption. Lipases are required to hydrolyze esterified antioxidants such as vitamins A and E. Dietary fat stimulates the secretion of bile and lipases and has direct effect on the absorption of fat-soluble antioxidants (see example of beta-carotene). When dietary fat is replaced by non-lipid fat replacers such as Olestra[R], which do not stimulate production of lipases and bile, absorption of fat soluble antioxidants is reduced. It is for this reason that Olestra[R] is fortified with some fat-soluble nutrients and phytochemicals.[38,39]

Physiological conditions or diseases, which reduce the secretion of bile or production of lipases, have a direct effect on absorption.[40] Examples include alcoholic hepatitis, which damages liver function; cholestasis, a genetic disease, which impairs bile secretion; and cystic fibrosis, a genetic disorder which impairs the function of the pancreas and production of lipases (discussed in Chapter 25).

Even though excess dietary fat is a major public health issue, there are small segments of the population where very low dietary fat impairs absorption of major antioxidants but also of some prooxidants.

Interactions between Dietary Antioxidants and Nutrients

Some of the well-known interactions of minerals affect the antioxidant status. For example, high calcium levels in the diet reduce the absorption of other minerals such as Fe, Cu, manganese, zinc, and selenium. The net effect of impaired absorption on the antioxidant status of the blood and other tissues may be harmful if it leads to deficiency for normal enzyme and other physiological functions; their effect, however, may be neutral or positive if they prevent excessive absorption. Their effect on the antioxidant status of the digesta is different. When absorption is reduced, these minerals remain in the gut and their effect depends on the degree and type of binding to other compounds.

Physiological Conditions, Disease, and Drugs

The absorption of some nutrient and non-nutrient antioxidants in babies, especially premature babies, and the elderly are discussed in other chapters. Disease conditions, especially those causing inflammation of the gut or significantly change its microflora, may impair the absorption of nutrients. Of particular current interest is the malabsorption occurring in advanced stages of AIDS primarily due to colonization of the gut by pathogenic fungi and diarrhea.[41] Many AIDS patients develop steatorrhea, a condition associated with serious fat malabsorption including fat-soluble antioxidants.[42] Some drugs have a direct effect on absorption of nutrients including antioxidants.[43,44] Others, especially antibiotics, have direct effect on microflora and thus may affect absorption.

Intestinal Microflora

Intestinal microflora is concentrated primarily in the lower gut; their number increases by six orders of magnitude between the ileum and the colon. The abundance of gut microflora is illustrated by the fact that they constitute about 40-55% of the dry weight of feces.[45] Significant interactions of the microflora with components of the diet and with gastric secretions directly affect absorption and the antioxidant status.

Major examples of such effects include the hydrolysis by intestinal microflora of the non-absorbable glucoside forms of lignans, flavonoids and other phytochemicals to their absorbable aglucone form.[46,47] For example, the isoflavones diadzein and genistein are absorbed in their aglucone form after they are hydrolyzed with the aid of gut microflora.

Carbohydrates, proteins, and lipids can be modified by gut microflora with direct effects on absorption. Cellulose, a major component of the fiber in our diet, not digestible by mammalian enzymes, is partially hydrolyzed and metabolized by bacteria to short chain fatty acids including butyric, propionic, and acetic which are readily absorbed even from the lower gut. Butyric acid and, to a lesser extent, propionic, have been associated with lower risk of colon cancer.[48,49] Other carbohydrates such as starch and sugars can be fermented by gut bacteria to short chain fatty acids. Proteins are also partially hydrolyzed to fatty acids and ammonia. PUFA are partially hydrogenated by anaerobic gut bacteria. Because easily digestible food components such as starch, sugars, proteins, and lipids are largely digested and absorbed before they reach the lower gut, the effect of microflora is rather minimal.

The respiratory activity of bacteria in the gut produces superoxide radicals ($O_2^{\bullet -}$) that, in the presence of chelated Fe, generate hydroxyl radicals. These radicals cause lipid peroxidation and other reactions, which modify nutrients and other dietary components and non-dietary compounds such as drugs.[22,50,51]

BIOAVAILABILITY

Bioavailability is discussed separately from absorption in order to emphasize their respective importance in understanding the role of dietary components on antioxidant status. The following example of tocopherols and tocotrienols, all compounds of the vitamin E family, discussed in detail in an earlier chapter, illustrates this point. α-Tocopherol and γ-tocopherol are equally well absorbed. However, α-tocopherol is preferentially secreted by the liver into the blood lipoproteins. The naturally occurring RRR stereoisomer and the synthetic all-rac-α-tocopherol are also equally well absorbed, yet levels of α-tocopherol in the blood and tissues increase significantly more with RRR than all-rac. A tocopherol binding protein is responsible for incorporating preferentially α-tocopherol over γ and other tocopherols into nascent VLDL entering the blood. The same mechanism has been proposed for the preference of RRR over all-rac-α-tocopherol.[52] It has been suggested that tocopherols and particularly non-α-tocopherol and all-rac-α-tocopherol are secreted into the intestine via bile. Tocotrienols appear in the blood and tissues at significantly lower levels than tocopherols even when ingested at equivalent or higher amounts.[53] It is unlikely that significantly lower absorption accounts for this difference suggesting other mechanisms are involved.

Other examples abound: *cis* β-carotene appears in blood and tissues at significantly lower concentrations than the corresponding *trans* form even when ingested at equivalent or higher amounts. Using labeled compounds, Dr. Parker and his associates showed that, after absorption, the *cis* form β-carotene is converted to the *trans* form.[36] This conversion increases the apparent bioavailability of the *trans* form at the expense of the *cis* form.[54] Other compounds may be rapidly modified after absorption to compounds that have similar or opposite antioxidant effects. It is thus apparent that understanding absorption and bioavailability is essential for evaluating the effects of the diet on antioxidant status.[53]

FOOD ADDITIVES, FORTIFIED FOODS, AND NUTRITIONAL SUPPLEMENTS

Some of our foods contain food additives that have a direct and/or indirect effect on the antioxidant status. The following are examples with practical significance.

Food Antioxidants

Synthetic and natural food antioxidants are used routinely in some foods especially those containing oils and fats. Lipids in foods and particularly those containing PUFA are easily oxidized in a chain reaction. Natural tocopherols, the synthetic α-tocopherol, and other phenolic antioxidants such as BHA (butylated hydroxyanisole), BHT (butylated hydroxytoluene), PG (propyl gallate), TBHQ (tertiary butylhydroquinone) are effective chain-breaking antioxidants.[19] Rosemary extract is also used as an antioxidant.

Water-soluble antioxidants such ascorbic and citric acids are also used extensively. Ascorbic acid is a synergist for tocopherols because it regenerates oxidized tocopherols.[55,56] Some compounds have an indirect antioxidant effect. Citric acid, lecithin, and others bind prooxidant metals such as Fe and Cu or (lecithin and melanoidins) decompose hydroperoxides to stable products.

The effect of food antioxidants is not restricted in the food. Natural antioxidants such as tocopherols and antioxidant phytochemicals have a major impact on the antioxidant status in the whole digestive tract. They are also absorbed, at least in part, and have an antioxidant effect in our body. Synthetic antioxidants and their metabolites are also absorbed and may have some tissue effects. For example, it was reported that BHA is largely absorbed (70-100%) and excreted in the urine as the glucuronide conjugate of BHA or TBHQ. The strong scrutiny of synthetic antioxidants, and particularly BHA and BHT, for their potential toxic effects at very high levels,[19] overshadowed several reports of beneficial effects directly related to their antioxidant function.[57-60] Food antioxidants may have contributed to the dramatic decrease in stomach cancer during the last 60 years.

Fortified Foods

Antioxidant vitamins and other antioxidants have been routinely added to foods. The traditional fortification of foods like cereals, milk, and flour with vitamins and minerals is now expanding to many new products. Fortification is expanded and includes antioxidant phytochemicals such as carotenoids, flavonoids, and others. Examples of such products are drinks fortified with carotenoids, vitamins, and minerals; orange juice fortified with vitamins C, E, and calcium; snack bars fortified with a variety of vitamins, minerals, and phytochemicals; margarines fortified with β-carotene and sterols. Of course, fortification provides both antioxidants and prooxidants such as Fe and Cu and some phytochemicals can act as prooxidants under certain conditions.[31]

Nutritional Supplements

National surveys indicate that 40-50% of Americans take vitamin supplements mostly in the form of tablets and capsules.[61] New formats such as drinks and snack bars, which blur the differences from fortified foods, are also becoming popular. A smaller percentage regularly takes supplements of individual vitamins such as E (10%), C (17%), or groups of nutrients such as B vitamin complex (6%), mixture of antioxidant vitamins plus selenium, ω-3 fatty acids, etc. In addition, consumption of herbs, herb extracts, and phytochemicals is increasing rapidly. Japan has been leading the way in the use of nutritional supplements and with new product formats such as drinks, teas, and herbal extracts. These products are widely available including in vending machines. Europeans and people in developing countries have been using herbs and their extracts extensively but their use of tablets and capsules has been significantly lower than in the United States and Japan.

Intake of antioxidant nutrients from nutritional supplements is usually in excess of the RDAs. For example, the most popular doses of vitamin E are 400 and 200 and 800 IU (RDA is 10-15 IU and USRDA 30 IU) and of vitamin C, 500, 1,000, and 250 mg (RDA is 60 mg).

Chemical, Chiral Form and Formulation

Chemical and Chiral Form

In the past, the role of chirality and chemical form on antioxidant activity received little attention. It has now come to the forefront as a result of major studies. Vitamin E provides an excellent example. The differences of various chemical forms of vitamin and particularly α and γ tocopherols were discussed briefly above and will be discussed in detail in a later chapter. Also, the major differences between the naturally occurring RRR stereoisomer and the synthetic racemic mixture of α -tocopherol which approaches the ratio of 2:1 for blood and some tissues shows the dramatic effect of chirality.[52,62,63] Other examples of β-carotene and lycopene were mentioned above and will also be discussed in later chapters. Even simple changes in chemical form can have major impact on physical characteristics, stability, and antioxidant effect. For example, the palmitate ester of ascorbic acid has some solubility in oil while ascorbic acid and sodium ascorbate are insoluble. The acetate ester of α-tocopherol is yellow oil while the succinate ester is white solid. Both esters are extremely stable in storage while the free tocopherol is easily oxidized when exposed to air, heat, and especially in the presence of oxidizing agents such as Fe and Cu. In our body, these esters function as antioxidants only after hydrolysis and release of the free tocopherol. Thus the tocopheryl esters do not function as antioxidants in food, the oral cavity, the esophagus, the stomach and the duodenum because their active hydroxyl group is blocked. Esters must by hydrolyzed by pancreatic lipases prior to absorption of the α-tocopherol, a major consideration for people with cystic fibrosis, premature infants, and the elderly.

Formulation

Formulation can dramatically change absorption and bioavailability of antioxidants. Carotenoids provide excellent examples. Less than 10% of β-carotene in raw carrots is absorbed. Absorption is higher in cooked carrots and carrot juice.[36,37] Commercial β-carotene, in viscous oil form, is absorbed at approximately 10-20%. In contrast, absorption of β-carotene microencapsulated with gelatin, is significantly higher.[64]

The effect of formulation on solubility and other physical characteristics can be dramatic. Microencapsulated β-carotene is a white solid completely dispersible in water while extracted β-carotene is very viscous oil. The importance of chemical form and formulation is illustrated in the following example. In the major ATBC intervention study on the role of α-tocopherol and β-carotene in lung cancer in smokers, the daily dose of β-carotene was 20 mg of microencapsulated synthetic form with estimated absorption exceeding 90%. The estimated average daily intake of β-carotene is 3.0 mg; thus the dose used would be 6.7 times the daily intake. If we, however, factor the approximate absorption of 10% from food sources and 90% from the supplement, then the effective dose is 18 mg (20mg x 90%) versus 0.30 mg from the food (3.0 mg x 10%). Thus the effective dose was 60 times higher.

Unfortunately, in many clinical studies the chemical and chiral forms and formulation are not considered, thus creating major difficulty in the interpretation of the results.

ANTIOXIDANT FUNCTION IN FOODS, *IN VITRO* AND IN HUMANS: A NEW LOOK

The relative ability of compounds to prevent oxidation in foods or *in vitro* systems is often extrapolated to their antioxidant function in the tissue. Such extrapolations are usually inaccurate and not very meaningful. Tocotrienols were reported to prevent oxidation of low-density lipoproteins (LDL) *in vitro* at least equal to or several-fold better than α-tocopherol.[65,66] α-Tocopherol, however, is by far the most abundant antioxidant in LDL and is the principal antioxidant for LDL[67] and in cell membranes. Similarly, on the basis of their function as food antioxidants and from some *in vitro* systems, β, γ, and δ tocopherols and synthetic compounds such as trolox, BHA, BHT, TBHQ, and propyl gallate are effective chain-breaking antioxidants, yet their role in humans for preventing LDL oxidation is very low compared to α-tocopherol. These apparent contradictions may be due to several reasons. For example, α-tocopherol is preferentially secreted into the lipoproteins over the other tocopherols and tocotrienols. Furthermore, while natural phenolic and synthetic antioxidants share the same active group they lack the phytyl chain, which provides tocopherols their unique ability to be positioned in the cell membrane.

Because antioxidants act as components of a complex system, comparisons based on single test or criterion are not very meaningful. Although γ-tocopherol may play a lesser role than α-tocopherol in preventing lipid oxidation in LDL, it may play a more important role in neutralizing nitrogen radicals. The major sites of its action may also be different.[20] Glutathione, coenzyme Q_{10}, and vitamin C have additive, synergistic effects or regenerate tocopherols.[23,55,56] In addition, unique physical and chemical properties such as solubility, enzymatic activity, and others allow individual antioxidants to perform specialized functions. The water-soluble vitamin C plays a critical role in the cytoplasm while the lipophilic vitamin E is an important antioxidant in membranes but both are essential components of the antioxidant system. Coenzyme Q_{10} is a critical component of the electron transfer system in the mitochondria, the basic process for generating energy in the cell. In the absence of vitamin E in the mitochondrial membrane or vitamin C in the cytoplasm this process would not function efficiently.

CONCLUSION

The diet is one of the leading factors under our control affecting the antioxidant status. The effect of the diet must be considered in its totality and should include the digestive system. For this reason, our view of absorption and bioavailability of food components must be expanded to include their effect in the digestive and urinary systems. These considerations are particularly important when using advance techniques of food processing and nutrient formulation, which change dramatically their absorption and bioavailability characteristics. Similarly they must be considered in the design of clinical trials evaluating the health effects of foods, nutrients, and phytochemicals. Major changes in the diet can have diverse and even opposing effects on the antioxidant status. Lower fat in the diet or fat substitutes reduce the amount of fatty acids, especially PUFA available for oxidation. Very low fat diets, however, reduce the absorption of fat-soluble nutrients and phytochemicals including many antioxidants.

REFERENCES

1. McGinnis JM, Foege WH. Actual causes of death in the United States. JAMA 1993;270:2207-12.
2. Block G, Patterson B, Subar A. Fruit, vegetables, and cancer prevention: a review of the epidemiological evidence. Nutr Cancer 1992;18:1-29.
3. Gillman MW, Cupples A, Cagnon D, *et al.* Protective effect of fruits and vegetables on development of stroke in men. JAMA 1995;273: 1114-1117.

4. Trichopoulou A, Toupadaki N, Tzonou A, *et al.* The macronutrient composition of the Greek diet: estimates derived from six case-control studies. Eur J Clin Nutr 1993;47:549-58.
5. Willett WC, Sacks F, Trichopoulou A, *et al.* Mediterranean diet pyramid: a cultural model for healthy eating. Am J Clin Nutr 1995;61:1402S-1406S.
6. Adlercreutz CH, Goldin BR, Gorbach SL, *et al.* Soybean phytoestrogen intake and cancer risk. J Nutr 1995;125:757S-770S.
7. Anderson JW, Johnstone BM, Cook-Newell ME. Meta-analysis of the effects of soy protein intake on serum lipids. N Engl J Med 1995;333:276-82.
8. Messina M. Modern applications for an ancient bean: soybeans and the prevention and treatment of chronic disease. J Nutr 1995;125:567S-569S.
9. Daviglus ML, Stamler J, Orencia AJ, *et al.* Fish consumption and the 30-year risk of fatal myocardial infarction. N Engl J Med 1997;336:1046-53.
10. Weisburger JH. Dietary fat and risk of chronic disease: mechanistic insights from experimental studies. J Am Diet Assoc 1997;97:S16-23.
11. Block G. The data support a role for antioxidants in reducing cancer risk. Nutr Rev 1992;50:207-13.
12. Lin RI-S. Phytochemicals and antioxidants. In: Goldberg Ie, Ed. in *Functional Foods*. New York: Chapman and Hall, 1995:393-441.
13. Steele VE, Moon RC, Lubet RA, *et al.* Preclinical efficacy evaluation of potential chemopreventive agents in animal carcinogenesis models: methods and results from the NCI Chemoprevention Drug Development Program. J Cell Biochem Suppl 1994;20:32-54.
14. Simopoulos AP. Omega-3 fatty acids in health and disease and in growth and development. Am J Clin Nutr 1991;54:438-63.
15. Brown JE, Wahle KW. Effect of fish-oil and vitamin E supplementation on lipid peroxidation and whole-blood aggregation in man. Clin Chim Acta 1990;193:147-56.
16. Meydani M, Natiello F, Goldin B, *et al.* Effect of long-term fish oil supplementation on vitamin E status and lipid peroxidation in women. J Nutr 1991;121:484-91.
17. Meydani SN. Effect of (n-3) polyunsaturated fatty acids on cytokine production and their biologic function. Nutrition 1996;12:S8-14.
18. Wander RC, Du SH, Ketchum SO, Rowe KE. Alpha-tocopherol influences *in vivo* indices of lipid peroxidation in postmenopausal women given fish oil. J Nutr 1996;126:643-52.
19. Papas AM. Oil-soluble antioxidants in foods. Toxicol Ind Health 1993;9:123-49.
20. Stone WL, Papas AM. Tocopherols and the etiology of colon cancer. J Natl Cancer Inst 1997;89:1006-14.
21. Nelson RL. Dietary iron and colorectal cancer risk. Free Rad Biol and Med 1992;12:161-168.
22. Chadwick RW, George SE, Claxton LD. Role of gastrointestinal mucosa and microflora in the bioactivation of dietary and environmental mutagens or carcinogens. Drug Metabolism Rev 1992;24:425-492.
23. Halliwell B, Murcia MA, Chirico S, Aruoma O. Free radicals and antioxidants in food and *in vivo*: What they do and how they work. Crit. Rev. Food Sci. Nutr 1995;35: 7-20.
24. Lynch SM, Frei B. Mechanisms of copper- and iron-dependent oxidative modification of human low density lipoprotein. J. Lipid Res. 1993;34:1745-1753.
25. Herbert V, Shaw SJ, E., Stopler-Kasdan T. Most free-radical injury is iron related: It is promoted by iron, hemin, holoferritin, and vitamin C, and inhibited by desferrioxamine and apoferritin. Stem Cells 12, 1994: 289-303.
26. Stohs SJ, Bagchi D. Oxidative mechanisms in the toxicity of metal ions. Free Radic Biol Med 1995;18:321-36.

27. Herbert V, Shaw S, Jayatilleke E. Vitamin C-driven free radical generation from iron [published errata appear in J Nutr 1996 Jun;126(6):1746 and 1996 Jul;126(7):1902]. J Nutr 1996;126:1213S-20S.
28. Berger TM, Polidori MC, Dabbagh A, *et al.* Antioxidant activity of vitamin C in iron-overloaded human plasma. J Biol Chem 1997;272:15656-60.
29. Gutteridge JM. Plasma ascorbate levels and inhibition of the antioxidant activity of caeruloplasmin. Clin Sci (Colch) 1991;81:413-7.
30. Siegenberg D, Baynes RD, Bothwell TH, *et al.* Ascorbic acid prevents the dose-dependent inhibitory effects of polyphenols and phytates on nonheme-iron absorption. Am J Clin Nutr 1991;53:537-41.
31. Cao G, Sofic E, Prior RL. Antioxidant and prooxidant behavior of flavonoids: structure-activity relationships. Free Radic Biol Med 1997;22:749-60.
32. Tuntawiroon M, Sritongkul N, Brune M, *et al.* Dose-dependent inhibitory effect of phenolic compounds in foods on nonheme-iron absorption in men. Am J Clin Nutr 1991;53:554-7.
33. Brune M, Rossander L, Hallberg L. Iron absorption and phenolic compounds: importance of different phenolic structures. Eur J Clin Nutr 1989;43:547-57.
34. Stahl W, Sies H. Uptake of lycopene and its geometrical isomers is greater from heat-processed than from unprocessed tomato juice in humans. J Nutr 1992;122:2161-6.
35. Gartner C, Stahl W, Sies H. Lycopene is more bioavailable from tomato paste than from fresh tomatoes. Am J Clin Nutr 1997;66:116-22.
36. Parker RS. Absorption, metabolism, and transport of carotenoids. FASEB J 1996;10:542-51.
37. Erdman JW, Jr., Bierer TL, Gugger ET. Absorption and transport of carotenoids. Ann N Y Acad Sci 1993;691:76-85.
38. Schlagheck TG, Kesler JM, Jones MB, *et al.* Olestra's effect on vitamins D and E in humans can be offset by increasing dietary levels of these vitamins. J Nutr 1997;127:1666S-85S.
39. Cooper DA, Webb DR, Peters JC. Evaluation of the potential for olestra to affect the availability of dietary phytochemicals. J Nutr 1997;127:1699S-709S.
40. Sokol RJ. Vitamin E deficiency and neurological disorders. In: Packer L, Fuchs J, Eds. *Vitamin E in Health and Disease.* New York, NY: Marcel Dekker, Inc., 1993:815-849.
41. Koch J, Garcia-Shelton YL, Neal EA, Chan MF, Weaver KE, Cello JP. Steatorrhea: a common manifestation in patients with HIV/AIDS. Nutrition 1996;12:507-10.
42. Lambl BB, Federman M, Pleskow D, Wanke CA. Malabsorption and wasting in AIDS patients with microsporidia and pathogen-negative diarrhea. Aids 1996;10:739-44.
43. Blumberg JB, Suter P. Pharmacology, nutrition, and the elderly: Interactions and implications in geriatric nutrition. In: Chernoff R, Ed. *Geriatric Nutrition.* Rockville, MD.: Aspen Publishers Inc., 1991:337-361.
44. Halpner AD, Blumberg JB. Assessment of antioxidant vitamin status in older adults. In: Rosenberg IH, Ed. *Nutritional Assessment of Elderly Populations: Measure and Function.* New York: Raven Press, 1995:147-165.
45. Stephen AM, Cummings JH. The microbial contribution to human faecal mass. J Med Microbiol 1980;13:45-56.
46. Xu X, Harris KS, Wang HJ, Murphy PA, Hendrich S. Bioavailability of soybean isoflavones depends upon gut microflora in women. J Nutr 1995;125:2307-15.
47. Borriello SP, Setchell KD, Axelson M, Lawson AM. Production and metabolism of lignans by the human faecal flora. J Appl Bacteriol 1985;58:37-43.
48. Velazquez OC, Lederer HM, Rombeau JL. Butyrate and the colonocyte. Implications for neoplasia. Dig Dis Sci 1996;41:727-39.

49. Gamet L, Daviaud D, Denis-Pouxviel C, Remesy C, Murat JC. Effects of short-chain fatty acids on growth and differentiation of the human colon-cancer cell line HT29. Int J Cancer 1992;52:286-9.
50. Blakeborough MH, Owen RW, Bilton RF. Free radical generating mechanisms in the colon: their role in the induction and promotion of colorectal cancer? Free Radic Res Commun 1989;6:359-367.
51. Van Tassell RL, Kingston DGI, Wilkins TD. Metabolism of dietary genotoxins by the human colonic microflora; the fecapentaenes and heterocyclic amines. Mutation Res. 1990;238:209-221.
52. Kayden HJ, Traber MG. Absorption, lipoprotein transport and regulation of plasma concentrations of vitamin E in humans. J. Lipid Res. 1993;34:343-358.
53. Hayes KC, Pronczuk A, Liang JS. Differences in the plasma transport and tissue concentrations of tocopherols and tocotrienols: observations in humans and hamsters. Proc Soc Exp Biol Med 1993;202:353-9.
54. Stahl W, Schwarz W, von Laar J, Sies H. All-*trans* beta-carotene preferentially accumulates in human chylomicrons and very low density lipoproteins compared with the 9-*cis* geometrical isomer. J Nutr 1995;125:2128-33.
55. Niki E, Tsuchiya J, Tanimura R, Kamiya Y. The regeneration of vitamin E from alpha-chromanoxyl radical by glutathione and vitamin C. Chem. Lett. 1982;6:789-792.
56. Packer JE, Slater TF, Willson RL. Direct observation of a free radical interaction between vitamin E and vitamin C. Nature 1979;278:737-738.
57. Black HS, Mathews-Roth MM. Protective role of butylated hydroxytoluene and certain carotenoids in photocarcinogenesis. Photochem Photobiol 1991;53:707-16.
58. Slaga TJ. Inhibition of the induction of cancer by antioxidants. Adv Exp Med Biol 1995;369:167-74.
59. Williams GM, Iatropoulos MJ. Inhibition of the hepatocarcinogenicity of aflatoxin B1 in rats by low levels of the phenolic antioxidants butylated hydroxyanisole and butylated hydroxytoluene. Cancer Lett 1996;104:49-53.
60. Arroyo PL, Hatch Pigott V, Mower HF, Cooney RV. Mutagenicity of nitric oxide and its inhibition by antioxidants. Mutat Res 1992;281:193-202.
61. Dickinson A. Optimal nutrition for good health: the benefits of nutritional supplements. Washington, DC: Council for Responsible Nutrition, 1998.
62. Burton GW, Traber MG, Acuff RV, *et al.* Human plasma and tissue alpha-tocopherol concentrations in response to supplementation with dueterated natural and synthetic vitamin E. Am J Clin Nutr 1998;67:669-84.
63. Acuff RV, Thedford SS, Hidiroglou NN, Papas AM, Odom TA, Jr. Relative bioavailability of RRR- and all-rac-alpha-tocopheryl acetate in humans: studies using deuterated compounds. Am J Clin Nutr 1994;60:397-402.
64. Gaziano JM, Johnson EJ, Russell RM, *et al.* Discrimination in absorption or transport of beta-carotene isomers after oral supplementation with either all-*trans*- or 9-*cis*-beta-carotene. Am J Clin Nutr 1995;61:1248-52.
65. Kamal-Eldin A, Appelqvist LA. The chemistry and antioxidant properties of tocopherols and tocotrienols. Lipids 1996;31:671-701.
66. Serbinova EA, Kagan VE, Han D, Packer L. D-alpha tocotrienol is a more powerful membrane antioxidant than d-alpha tocopherol. In: Davies KJA, Ed. *Oxidative Damage And Repair: Chemical, Biological And Medical Aspects*. Oxford, England, UK: Pergamon Press, 1991:77-81.
67. Esterbauer H, Gebicki J, Puhl H, Jurgens G. The role of lipid peroxidation and antioxidants in oxidative modification of LDL. Free Rad. Biol. Med. 1992;13:341-390.

6

Mediterranean Diet: Are Antioxidants Central to Its Benefits?

Antonia Trichopoulou, M.D. and Pagona Lagiou, M.D.
Department of Nutrition and Biochemistry
National School of Public Health, Athens, GREECE

Andreas M. Papas, Ph.D.
Health and Nutrition
Eastman Chemical Company, Kingsport, Tennessee, USA

THE MEDITERRANEAN DIET

The dietary patterns that prevail in the Mediterranean have many common characteristics, most of which stem from the fact that olive oil occupies a central position in all of them. Olive oil has several beneficial properties, but it also allows the consumption of large quantities of vegetables and leg-

0-8493-8009-X/98/$0.00+$.50

umes in the form of salads and cooked foods. Other essential components of the Mediterranean diet are wheat and grapes, and their various derivative products. Total lipids may be high, but in all instances the ratio of monounsaturated fatty acids to saturated fatty acids is much higher than in other places of the world, including northern Europe and North America. We will concentrate on the Greek variant of the Mediterranean diet, because most studies that pointed to the beneficial effects of the Mediterranean diet have been undertaken in Greece, and because of the nationality of the authors.[1,2]

The traditional Mediterranean diet, and in particular the Greek version of it, may be thought of as having 8 components[3-6] summarized in Table 1.

Table 1
Major Components of the Mediterranean Diet[a]

1. High monounsaturated-to-saturated fat ratio
2. Moderate ethanol consumption
3. High consumption of legumes
4. High consumption of cereals (including bread)
5. High consumption of fruits
6. High consumption of vegetables
7. Low consumption of meat and meat products
8. Moderate consumption of milk and dairy products

[a] For more details see References 3-6.

MEDITERRANEAN DIET AND HEALTH

Epidemiological and Other Evidence

Mortality statistics have provided the earliest evidence that something unusual has been favorably affecting the health of the Mediterranean populations. Even though health care for many of these populations has been inferior to that available to people in northern Europe and North America, and the prevalence of smoking has been unusually high,[7] death rates in the Mediterranean region have been, and still are, generally lower than those prevailing in the economically more developed countries of northern Europe and North

America, particularly among men. Cause-specific mortality statistics indicate that the health advantage of the Mediterranean populations is mainly accounted for by lower mortality rates from coronary heart disease, as well as from cancers of the large bowel, breast (Table 2), endometrium, ovary, and prostate.

The classic international study launched by Keys in the '50s reported follow-up findings that were focused primarily on the role of diet in the occurrence of coronary heart disease (CHD). Although it was clear that Mediterranean populations had lower incidence not only of CHD, but also of other important causes of morbidity and mortality, the lasting conclusion was that Mediterraneans were privileged by having low rates of coronary heart disease simply because they consumed diets with low saturated fat content.[2] The argument of several scientists from Mediterranean countries, that the diet of their region is more than a low saturated fat diet and has implications for diseases other than CHD, was not appreciated by the wider scientific community.[1]

Table 2
Standardized[a] Mortality Rates in 10 DAFNE Countries and the USA, Circa 1990 *(per 100,000 person-years)*

Country	Coronary Heart Disease (CHD)	Colon Cancer	Breast Cancer	Stomach Cancer
Greece	**95**	**10**	**21**	**11**
Spain	**73**	**17**	**24**	**16**
Belgium	103	26	37	13
Germany	149	28	33	16
Hungary	240	36	32	24
Ireland	238	27	37	13
Luxembourg	108	25	39	10
Norway	187	26	27	12
Poland	121	19	23	21
UK	215	26	40	13
USA	180	22	32	5

[a] Standardized to the European population of 1991.
Source: Health for All, WHO Regional Office for Europe 1992.

Mechanistic Considerations

Biochemical, clinical, and epidemiological studies during the last two decades have provided strong indications concerning the mechanisms underlying the health benefits of the Mediterranean diet. It has been established that moderate drinking of alcoholic beverages reduces the risk of coronary heart disease, probably by increasing levels of serum high-density lipoprotein (HDL) cholesterol.[8] Moreover, it has now been established that monounsaturated lipids, including olive oil, increase HDL cholesterol more than polyunsaturated lipids and substantially more than carbohydrates.[9,10]

In addition, recently accumulated evidence on the deleterious role of plasma homocysteine levels on CHD risk provides a plausible explanation for the inverse association between consumption of vegetables on the one hand, and CHD and peripheral arterial disease on the other,[11,12] because homocysteine levels are reduced by folic acid found mainly in vegetables. Last, there is overwhelming evidence that consumption of vegetables and fruits reduces the risk of most forms of cancer, although the responsible compounds or processes have not been established.[13]

ARE ANTIOXIDANT PROCESSES CENTRAL IN THE MEDITERRANEAN DIET?

Two of the most prominent characteristics of the Mediterranean diet are the high, on the average, consumption of olive oil, vegetables, and fruits (Table 3), as well as the high variability of this consumption. The latter is due to the fact that part of the Mediterranean population remains loyal to the traditional diet, while another part has adopted westernized food consumption patterns. Both these population characteristics are expected to facilitate the documentation, if any, of empirical associations between olive oil, vegetables, and fruits on the one hand, and chronic diseases on the other. For example, due to the partial adoption of westernized diet, the low incidence of cardiovascular disease in Greece increased substantially in the last 40 years while the higher rate in North America and Western Europe declined (Figure 1). These significant trends may be due in part to changes in the diet. The association of changes in the diet from the traditional Mediterranean to a more western type diet and increased incidence of CHD was studied in the island of Crete and will be discussed in the next chapter.

Table 3
Availability of Selected Food Groups in 10 DAFNE[a] Countries Circa 1990 (and the USA)[b], *(g/person/day)*

Country	Fruits	Vegetables	Meat	Added Lipids
Greece	**341**	**252**	**175**	**82**
Spain	**307**	**178**	**178**	**59**
Belgium	198	162	168	44
Germany	202	143	140	39
Hungary	159	201	190	53
Ireland	104	129	138	42
Luxembourg	234	181	186	57
Norway	174	103	129	35
Poland	100	202	187	59
UK	133	157	138	32
USA	162	194	181	74[c]

[a] DAFNE I and II projects of the European Commission, except for USA.
[b] U.S. Department of Agriculture, Agricultural Research Service, 1997.
[c] Total fat intake.

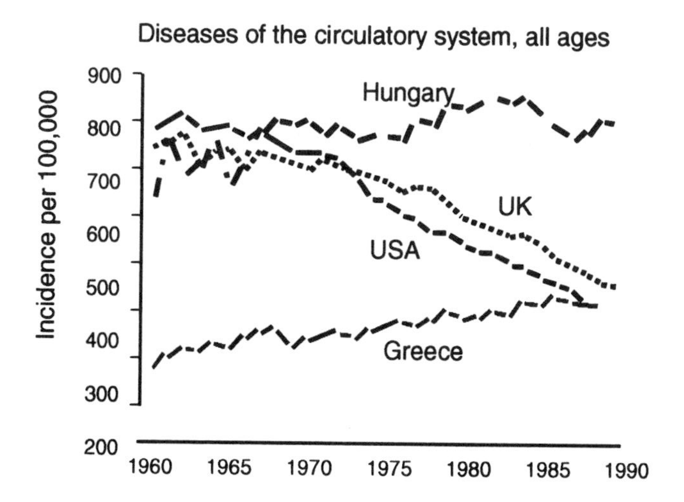

Figure 1. Changes in the incidence of cardiovascular disease in Greece, USA, UK, and Hungary. Source: Health for All, WHO Regional Office for Europe, 1992.

Fruits and Vegetables

Some of the earliest studies, demonstrating an inverse association between vegetables and fruits and various forms of cancer, have been reported from Mediterranean countries and particularly from Greece, where the consumption of vegetables has been and remains exceptionally high. A few years later, Trichopoulos and his colleagues found that individuals consuming high quantities of lemons, oranges, and raw salad-type vegetables as well as whole-grain bread, were less likely to be affected by cancer of the stomach.[15]

Perhaps more important, an early study from Greece[16] was the first to point out that consumption of vegetables, as a group, and, within that group, of cucumber, lettuce, and carrot was inversely associated with breast cancer risk. This inverse association was later confirmed by several authors and it was also noticed in a more comprehensive investigation in Greece.[17] Other epidemiological studies of cancer in the Greek population have also documented an apparent protective effect of vegetables and/or fruits. An effect of fruits was more evident with respect to lung cancer,[18] whereas crude fiber, mostly from vegetables, was the discriminatory protective agent in studies of pancreatic cancer[19] and ovarian cancer.[20] Last, vegetables and fruits were the only food groups inversely related to cancer of the endometrium[21] and to adenocarcinoma of the esophagus,[22] although these associations were not always significant.[21] It is noteworhty, however, that, in most of these studies, associations with particular vitamins or micronutrients, including β-carotene and vitamin C, were generally weaker than those with vegetables and fruits as a whole, an observation suggesting that other, or additional factors were operating. Studies in Greece were not unique in documenting an apparent protective effect from high intake of vegetables and fruits. In fact, such associations represent the main thrust of nutritional epidemiology of cancer.[13] Greek studies, however, have been unusual in their consistent documentation of a protective effect of vegetables and fruits against a wide spectrum of human malignancies.

Studies in Greece have also provided evidence that high intake of vegetables and fruits, reflected in high intake of total carbohydrates and crude fiber, may play a dominant beneficial role against the occurrence of atherosclerosis, as manifested in peripheral arterial occlusive disease[23] and CHD.[24] These findings have received support from the results of other extensive and sophisticated investigations.[25,26] An inverse association between vegetable intake and atherosclerosis could be explained in terms of the homocysteine hypothesis,[11,12] but it is also compatible with a generalized beneficial effect of a diet rich in antioxidant substances.

Olive Oil

The antioxidant hypothesis may also be relevant to the recent evidence indicating that intake of olive oil may be inversely related to the occurrence of breast cancer and perhaps other malignancies. Studies in Spain, Greece, and Italy, recently reviewed,[27] converge in suggesting that consumption of olive oil conveys protection against breast cancer, whereas studies in Greece indicate that this protection may also cover cancers of the ovary[20] and the endometrium.[21]

Olive oil is probably the only vegetable oil obtained from whole fruit. Palm oil is also extracted from the fruit but only the mesocarp is used. Other major vegetable oils are extracted from seed and contain very little or no carotenoids and flavonoids. As compared to other vegetable oils such as soy and palm, olive oil has a peculiar fatty acid composition[23,28] characterized by high levels of monounsaturated fatty acids and low levels of polyunsaturated and saturated fatty acids (Table 4). Phenolic compounds (up to 800mg/kg oil) can predict olive oil stability to oxidation, and hydroxytyrosol, in particular, appears to be critical to the oil's resistance to rancidity.[29,30] Extra virgin olive oil is particularly rich in phenols.[28]

Table 4
Composition of Olive, Soy and Palm Oils

Component	Olive Oil[a]	Soy Oil[b]	Palm Oil[b]
Fatty acid, % (mol/mol) of methyl esters			
Oleic	56.0-83.0	23.3	39.3
Palmitic	7.5-20.0	10.6	44.4
Linoleic	3.5-20.0	53.7	10.0
Stearic	0.5-3.5	4.0	4.1
Palmitoleic	0.3-3.5	0.1	0.2
Linolenic	0.0-1.5	7.6	0.3
Myristic	0.0-0.05	0.1	1.0
Other compounds, mg/kg			
Tocols[c]	126	890	800-1175
Phytosterols	2,210	2,500	1,000[d]

[a] From References 23 and 28.
[b] USDA Nutrient Database for Standard Reference, Release 11-1 (August 1997).
[c] Tocols is the sum of tocopherols and tocotrienols.
[d] Unpublished data.

The antioxidant activity of olive oil has been clearly established *in vitro* and it is likely that the responsible compounds also block oxidation of low density lipoprotein (LDL) cholesterol, the pre-eminent risk factor for atherosclerosis. The exact mechanism of action has not been established, but compounds in olive oil are believed to act as free radical scavengers that may play a role in forfeiting some early steps in the carcinogenic process.[31,32]

It is important to note that the tocopherol plus tocotrienol content of olive oil is significantly lower than in soy and palm oil. Its high content of phytochemical antioxidants such as flavonoids and polyphenols, particularly hydroxytyrosol, may account for its strong antioxidant and other biological effects. It is important to note that consumption of added lipids in Greece is higher than the total fat intake in the United States (Table 3), yet the incidence of heart disease and some cancers is higher in the United States (Table 2), suggesting that these differences are not due to the amount of fat consumed but rather the type of fat and other components of the diet. Studies reviewed in this chapter strongly suggest that olive oil may account for a large number of these differences.

ANTIOXIDANTS IN THE GREEK DIET

The Greek version of the Mediterranean diet is dominated by the consumption of olive oil and by high consumption of vegetables and fruits. Antioxidants represent a common element in these foods and an antioxidant action provides a plausible explanation for the apparent benefits. The potential benefits of olive oil were discussed above.

Vegetables and fruits are the richest source of antioxidant vitamins, including vitamins C, E and β-carotene, which are frequently invoked for the explanation of the well-documented inverse associations of vegetables and fruits with several forms of cancer.[33-35] It is also possible that antioxidants may play a key role in reducing the establishment and progression of atherosclerosis and, therefore, the occurrence of CHD.[36,37] Vegetables and fruits, however, also contain a large number of other non-nutritive compounds, which appear to have pronounced biologic activity and beneficial potential. Pre-eminent among these are flavonoids, and in particular flavonols and flavones[38] (Table 5), and for both of these groups, there is evidence that can affect, in a beneficial way, the occurrence of cancer and CHD.[39,40] Thus, antioxidants are likely mediators, at least in part, of the benefit derived from consumption of vegetables and fruits, and, inferentially, the Mediterranean diet.

Table 5
Flavonol Content Of Greens in The Greek Island of Crete
(mg per 100g of green)

Plant	Myri-cetin	Querce-tin	Lute-olin	Kaemp-ferol	Apige-nine	Isorham-netin
Lapatho	5.73	86.2	<0.02	10.31	<0.05	<0.03
Stafilinakas	0.44	1.08	34.07	0.23	12.59	<0.06
Koutsounada	1.13	26.29	0.2	2.34	0.09	1.08
Tsohos	3.62	15.95	6.48	3.84	3.78	0.71
Agrioprasso	<0.03	10.37	0.35	12.48	<0.07	8.5
Caucalis	1.56	29.28	0.61	2.89	<0.08	5.08
Maratho	19.81	46.81	0.06	6.54	<0.07	9.29

Source: Trichopoulou A, Vassilopoulou E, Kromhout D, Hollman P. Study of traditional green foods (unpublished data).

This is not to imply that the Mediterranean diet could be equated to an antioxidant process – indeed, as previously indicated, selected antioxidant vitamins, including β-carotene and vitamin C, do not adequately explain the apparent protective effect of vegetables and fruits against various forms of cancer, or different manifestations of atherosclerosis. Nevertheless, a reductionist approach may be necessary if the beneficial effects of the Mediterranean diet were to be transplanted into populations with different lifestyles than those prevailing in the Mediterranean basin.

High consumption of legumes probably is the third most important component of the Mediterranean diet, but the mode of action of these foods is poorly understood and there is little evidence that antioxidants play a role in it. Like soy, the legumes consumed in the Mediterranean, which include beans, lentils, chick peas, and fava beans are good sources of tocopherols. In contrast to soy, however, these legumes contain little isoflavones such as daidzin and genistin. It appears, however, that frequent consumption of legume seeds and derivatives is associated with reduced levels of LDL cholesterol in the blood.[41] The mechanisms causing these effects have not been identified. Dry legumes are usually prepared with leafy vegetables such as those in Table 5, onions and herbs, which may provide flavonoids and other antioxidants.

It is also possible, although not yet established, that some of the beneficial effect of moderate wine consumption may be due to antioxidant substances, particularly catechin, which is found in higher concentrations in red rather than white wine.[42,43]

CONCLUSION

The health benefits of the Mediterranean diet are probably associated with its major components including high intake of olive oil, fruits, vegetables, cereals, and legumes and moderate consumption of alcoholic drinks. Olive oil, fruits, vegetables, grains, legumes, and wine are good sources of major antioxidants. While there is no direct evidence that these antioxidants are central to the benefits of the Mediterranean diet, indirect evidence from epidemiological data and the increasing understanding of their mechanisms of action suggest that antioxidants may play a major role. Ongoing research will help elucidate the role of antioxidants in the significant benefits of the traditional Mediterranean diet.

REFERENCES

1. Trichopoulou A, Lagiou P. Healthy traditional Mediterranean diet - An expression of culture, history and lifestyle. Nutrition Reviews 1998;55:383-9.
2. Keys A. *Seven countries: a multivariate analysis of death and coronary heart disease.* Cambridge: Harvard University Press, 1980.
3. Helsing E, Trichopoulou A, Eds. The Mediterranean diet and food culture: a symposium. Eur J Clin Nutr 1989;43(suppl 2):1-92.
4. Trichopoulou A, Katsouyanni K, Gnardellis Ch. The traditional Greek diet. Eur J Clin Nutr 1993;47(suppl):76-81.
5. Trichopoulou A, Kouris-Blazos A, Vassilakou T, Gnardellis Ch, Polychronopoulos E, Venizelos M, Lagiou P, Walhqvist ML, Trichopoulos D. Diet and survival of elderly Greeks: a link to the past. Am J Clin Nutr 1995;61 (suppl):1346S-50S.
6. Trichopoulou A, Kouris-Blazos A, Walhqvist ML, Gnardellis Ch, Lagiou P, Polychronopoulos E, Vassilakou T, Lipworth L, Trichopoulos D. Diet and overall survival in elderly people. BMJ 1995;311:1457-60.
7. World Health Organization. Tobacco or health: A global status report. Geneva, WHO, 1997.
8. Rimm EB, Giovannucci EL, Willett WC, Colditz GA, Ascherio A, Rosner B, et al. Prospective study of alcohol consumption and risk of coronary disease in men. Lancet 1991;331:464-8.

9. Mattson FH, Grundy SM. Comparison of effects of dietary saturated, monounsaturated, and polyunsaturated fatty acids on plasma lipids and lipoproteins in man. J Lipid Res 1985;26:194-202.
10. Mensink RP, Katan MB. Effect of monounsaturated fatty acids versus complex carbohydrates on high-density lipoproteins in healthy men and women. Lancet 1987;I:122-5.
11. Stampfer MJ, Malinow MR, Willett WC, et al. A prospective study of plasma homocyst(e)ine and risk of myocardial infarction in US physicians. JAMA 1992;268:877-81.
12. Nygard O, Nordrehhaug JE, Refsum H, Ueland PM, Farstad M, Vollset SE. Plasma homocysteine levels and mortality in patients with coronary artery disease. N Engl J Med 1997;337:230-6.
13. Willett WC, Trichopoulos D. Nutrition and cancer: A summary of the evidence. Cancer Causes and Control 1996;7:178-80.
14. Manousos O, Day NE, Trichopoulos D, Gerovassilis F, Tzonou A. Diet and colorectal cancer: a case-control study in Greece. Int J Cancer 1983;32:1-5.
15. Trichopoulos D, Ouranos G, Day NE, Tzonou A, Manousos O, Papadimitriou Ch, Trichopoulos A. Diet and cancer of the stomach: a case-control study in Greece. Int J Cancer 1985:36:291-7.
16. Katsouyanni K, Trichopoulos D, Boyle P, Xirouchaki E, Trichopoulou A, Lisseos B, Vasilaros S, MacMahon B. Diet and breast cancer: a case-control study in Greece. Int J Cancer 1986;38:815-20.
17. Trichopoulou A, Katsouyanni K, Stuver S, Tzala L, Gnardellis Ch, Rimm E, Trichopoulos D. Consumption of olive oil and specific food groups in relation to breast cancer risk in Greece. J Natl Cancer Inst 1995;87:110-6.
18. Kalandidi A, Katsouyanni K, Voropoulou N, Bastas G, Saracci R, Trichopoulos D. Passive smoking and diet in the etiology of lung cancer among non-smokers. Cancer Causes and Control 1990;1:15-21.
19. Kalapothaki V, Tzonou A, Hsieh C-c, Karakatsani A, Trichopoulou A, Toupadaki N, Trichopoulos D. Nutrient intake and cancer of the pancreas: a case-control study in Athens, Greece. Cancer Causes and Control 1993;4:383-9.
20. Tzonou A, Hsieh C-c, Polychronopoulou A, Kaprinis G, Toupadaki N, Trichopoulou A, Karakatsani A, Trichopoulos D. Diet and ovarian cancer: a case-control study in Greece. Int J Cancer 1993;55:411-4.
21. Tzonou A, Lipworth L, Kalandidi A, Trichopoulou A, Gamatsi I, Hsieh C-c, Notara V, Trichopoulos D. Dietary factors and the risk of endometrial cancer: a case-control study in Greece. Brit J Cancer 1996;73:1284-90.
22. Tzonou A, Lipworth L, Garidou A, Signorello L, Lagiou P, Hsieh C-c, Trichopoulos D. Diet and risk of esophageal cancer by histologic type in a low-risk population. Int J Cancer 1996;68:300-4.
23. Katsouyanni K, Skalidis Y, Petridou E, Polychronopoulou-Trichopoulou A, Willett W, Trichopoulos D. Diet and peripheral arterial occlusive disease:the role of poly-, mono- and saturated fatty acids. Am J Epidemiol 1991;133:24-31.
24. Tzonou A, Kalandidi A, Trichopoulou A, Hsieh C-c, Toupadaki N, Willett W, Trichopoulos D. Diet and coronary heart disease: a case-control study in Athens, Greece. Epidemiology 1993;4:511-6.
25. Gramenzi A, Gentile A, Fasoli M, Negri E, Parazzini F, La Vecchia C. Association between certain foods and risk of acute myocardial infarction in women. BMJ 1990;300:771-3.
26. Rimm EB, Ascherio A, Giovannucci E, Spiegelman D, Stampfer MJ, Willett WC. Vegetable, fruit, and cereal fiber intake and risk of coronary heart disease among men. JAMA 1996;275:447-451.

27. Lipworth L, Martinez ME, Angeli J, Hsieh C-c, Trichopoulos D. Olive oil and human cancer: an assessment of the evidence. Preventive Medicine 1997;26:181-90.
28. Visioli F, Galli C. Natural antioxidants and prevention of coronary heart disease: the potential role of olive oil and its minor constituents. Nutr Metab Cardiovasc Dis 1995;5:306-14.
29. Chimi H, Rahmani H, Cillard J, Cillard P. Autooxydation des huiles d' olive: role des composes phenoliques. Rev Franc Corps Gras 1990;11/12:363-7.
30. Montedoro GF, Servili M, Baldioli M, Miniati E. Simple and hydrolyzable phenolic compounds in virgin olive oil. 1. Their extraction, separation and quantitative and semiquantitative evaluation by HPLC. J Agric Food Chem 1992;40:1571-6.
31. Visioli F, Bellomo G, Montedoro GF, Galli C. Low density lipoprotein oxidation is inhibited *in vitro* by olive oil constituents. Atherosclerosis 1995;117:25-32.
32. Afanas'ev IB, Dorozhko AI, Brodskii AV, Kostyuk VA, Potapovitch AI. Chelating and free radical scavenging mechanisms of inhibitory action of rutin and quercetin in lipid peroxidation. Biochem Pharmacol 1989;38:1763-9.
33. Steinmetz KA, Potter JD. Vegetables, fruits, and cancer. I. Epidemiology. Cancer Causes and Control 1991;2:325-57.
34. Steinmetz KA, Potter JD. Vegetables, fruits, and cancer. II. Mechanisms. Cancer Causes and Control 1991;2:427-42.
35. Block G, Patterson B, Subar A. Fruit, vegetables, and cancer prevention: A review of the epidemiological evidence. Nutr Cancer 1992;17:1-29.
36. Wiztum JL, Steinberg D. Role of oxidised low-density lipoprotein in atherogenesis. J Clin Invest 1991;88:1785-92.
37. Gey KF, Moser UK, Jordan P, et al. Increased risk of cardiovascular disease at suboptimal plasma concentrations of essential antioxidants: an epidemiological update with special attention to carotene and vitamin C. Am J Clin Nutr Suppl 1993;57:787-97.
38. Hertog MGL, Hollman PCH, Katan MB. Content of potentially anticarcinogenic flavonoids of 28 vegetables and 9 fruits commonly consumed in the Netherlands. J Agricult Food Chem 1992;40:2379-83.
39. Hertog MGL, Feskens EJM, Hollman PCH, Katan MB, Kromhout D. Dietary flavonoids and cancer risk in The Zutphen Elderly Study. Nutr Cancer 1994;22:175-84.
40. Hertog MGL, Feskens EJM, Hollman PCH, Katan MB, Kromhout D. Dietary antioxidant flavonoids and risk of coronary heart disease. The Zutphen Elderly Study. The Lancet 1993;342:1007-11.
41. Kingman SM. The influence of legume seeds on human plasma lipid concentrations. Nutrition Research Reviews 1991;4:97-123.
42. Fuhrman B, Lavy A, Aviram M. Consumption of red wine with meals reduces the susceptibility of human plasma and low-density lipoprotein to lipid peroxidation. Am J Clin Nutr 1995;61:549-54.
43. Carbonneau MA, Leger CL, Monnier L, Bonnet C, Michel F, Fouret G, Dedieu F, Descomps B. Supplementation with wine phenolic compounds increases the antioxidant capacity of plasma and vitamin E of low-density lipoprotein without changing the lipoprotein Cu^{2+}-oxidizability: Possible explanation by phenolic location. Eur J Clin Nutr 1997;51:682-90.

7

Diet, Antioxidants, and Health – Case Study: The Cretan Experience

Anthony G. Kafatos, M.D., F.A.C.N.
University of Crete School of Medicine, Iraklion, Crete, GREECE.

INTRODUCTION

The Mediterranean diet is well known internationally from the results of the Seven Countries Study[1] in which the population of Crete was found to have the lowest coronary heart disease (CHD) mortality rate compared to the other populations of the study. This low CHD mortality in Crete has been attributed to the high olive oil, vegetable, and fruit consumption. The olive oil consumption was approximately 100 g per person per day (one third of the total daily energy intake).[2] According to recent research, high olive oil consumption is believed not only to decrease low density lipoprotein (LDL) cholesterol levels in the blood, but also to prevent LDL-oxidation owing to the antioxidant substances in olive oil such as tocopherols, polyphenols, squalenes and others.[3] In addition, olive oil does not lower high density lipo-

0-8493-8009-X/98/$0.00+$.50

protein (HDL) cholesterol levels as do other vegetable oils rich in polyunsaturated fatty acids.[4] The latter are sensitive to oxidation and are a major source of lipid peroxides and oxidative modification of lipoproteins, which is considered to be the first step in the development of arterial intima lipid deposition and foam cell formation. On the other hand, monounsaturated fatty acids such as olive oil have been reported to protect lipoproteins from oxidation.

OXIDIZED LDL CHOLESTEROL HYPOTHESIS

The low mortality rates and longevity of the population of Crete in comparison to other countries has proved consistent in the periodic follow-up studies of the original cohorts of the Seven Countries Study.[5] In addition, it has recently been shown[6] that men from the Mediterranean, having the same total cholesterol levels with men of the same age from Northern Europe and the United States, have two to three times lower risk of dying from coronary heart disease. As shown in Figure 1, at cholesterol level of about 210 mg/dl coronary heart disease mortality varied from 4 to 5% in Japan and Mediterranean Southern Europe to 10% in Inland Southern Europe, 12% in the USA and 15% in Northern Europe.[6] Men in the lowest cholesterol quartile in Northern Europe (mean cholesterol 190 mg/dl) had almost a two-fold higher risk of dying from CHD compared to the highest cholesterol quartile of men from Mediterranean Southern Europe (mean cholesterol 250 mg/dl). Statistical adjustment for age, smoking, and blood pressure indicates that these differences in risk could not be attributed to these factors.

These significant recent findings from the Seven Countries Study suggest that it may not be possible to reduce CHD mortality in the USA and Northern Europe by focusing on decreasing total serum cholesterol levels. The only hypothesis that seems to explain these paradoxical findings is the role of oxidized LDL (ox-LDL), which is the most atherogenic cholesterol. The level, therefore, of total serum cholesterol in the blood may not be as important a determinant of the atherosclerotic process as the levels of ox-LDL cholesterol.

The amount of ox-LDL in the blood seems to be related to oxidative stress such as smoking and the lack of protective antioxidant substances such as carotenoids, tocopherols, polyphenols, flavonoids, ascorbate, and some trace elements. Another important determinant of the susceptibility of LDL to oxidation is its fatty acid composition. A predominance of polyunsaturated fatty acids from seed oils increases the susceptibility to oxidation while monounsaturated fatty acids are resistant to the oxidation process.

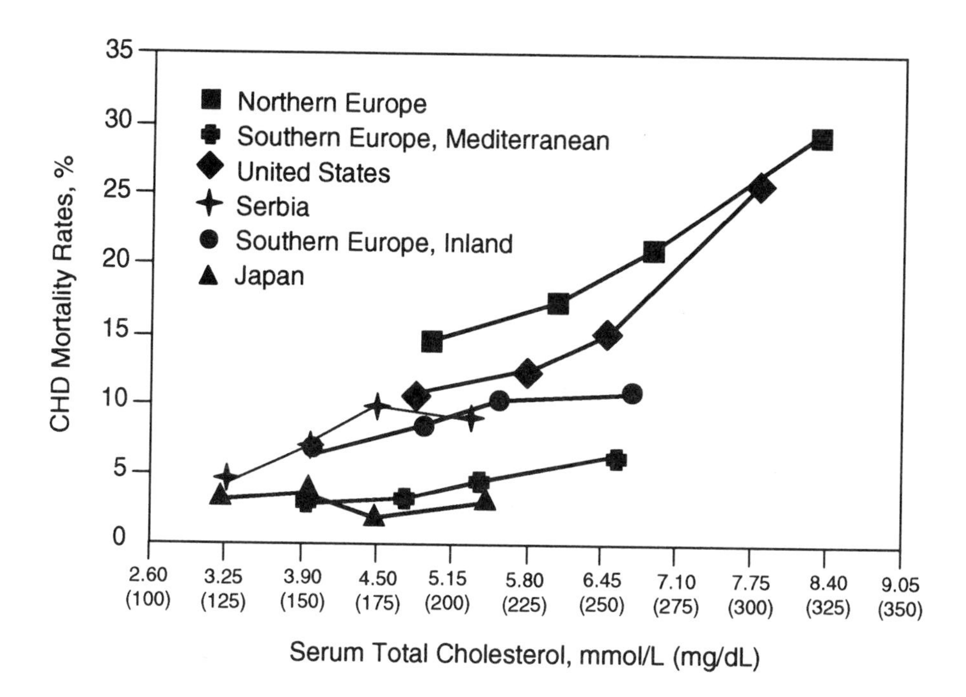

Figure 1. Twenty five-year coronary heart disease (CHD) mortality rates per baseline cholesterol quartile, adjusted for age, cigarette smoking, and systolic blood pressure. From Verschuren *et al.*, Serum total cholesterol and long-term coronary heart disease mortality in different cultures. *JAMA* 1995: 274: 131-136 (Copyright 1995, American Medical Association, with permission).

DIETARY CHANGES AND ANTIOXIDANT STATUS

Over the last 30 years there has been a large increase in saturated fatty acids intake from 8% of total energy in 1960 to 12% in 1991, with a parallel reduction in monounsaturated fatty acids.[7] Cheese intake, providing the most atherogenic fatty acid lauric and myristic, has increased by 396% since 1960 (Figure 2). As a result of these dietary changes in the Greek population, there has been a 40% increase in total cholesterol over the same period. CHD morbidity and mortality rates have been continuously increasing in Greece for the last 35 years as compared to some other developed countries.

In a recent comparative metabolic experiment with high-risk target groups (the first degree relatives of myocardial infarction patients) in Crete, Ireland, and the UK, the serum lipoproteins in the Mediterranean populations were shown to be rich in monounsaturated fatty acids coming from olive oil.[7]

The antioxidant capacity is, however, influenced by the level of antioxidant substances in the diet. The Mediterranean diet, and more specifically the Cretan diet, has been known since the early 1960s to contain more fruits, vegetables, and fish, and less meat and dairy products compared to diets in Northern Europe and the USA.[8] As a result, as shown in Table 1, there was a significant difference in serum levels of α-tocopherol between the populations at high risk of myocardial infarction in Crete and in Northern Europe, while carotenoids and retinol levels were not significantly different. These differences could possibly be attributed to the high tocopherol and fat soluble polyphenol intake by the population of Crete, both present in high quantities in virgin olive oil. Data from these experiments also reflect the recent general trend of reduced consumption of vegetables and fruits among younger generations of Greeks, as shown in Figure 2. Comparisons between the food intake of Cretan men in the 1960s with those of comparable age in 1988[9] indicate that there has been a 6% reduction in total vegetable and fruit intake over the last 30 years.

Table 1
Serum Levels of Antioxidant Vitamins in Men, First Degree Relatives of Subjects with Premature Ischaemic Heart Disease From Northern Europe and Crete[a, b]

Antioxidant	Ireland N=12	United Kingdom N=13	Crete, N=25	
			Initial	Two months
β-Carotene, μM	0.68±0.59	0.58±0.18	0.50±0.29	0.52±0.27
Lycopene, μM	0.48±0.37	0.57±0.42	0.30±0.26	0.55±0.54
Tocopherol, μM	17.44±2.73	16.92±3.26*	24.26±8.16*	20.44±5.11
Retinol, μM	3.04±0.9	3.09±0.67	2.6±0.7	3.00±0.87

[a] Unpublished data, University of Crete School of Medicine.
[b] Values are mean ± SD; * P<0.01.

A recent chemical analysis of the diet of Cretans in comparison with the diets of the other Seven Countries Study populations gave interesting results.[10,11] The intake of antioxidant vitamins and other substances with antioxidant activities were among the highest in the populations of Crete and Corfu (Table 2). These data on nutrient intake support the recent experimental data[7] of significantly higher serum levels of α-tocopherol in the Greek populations.

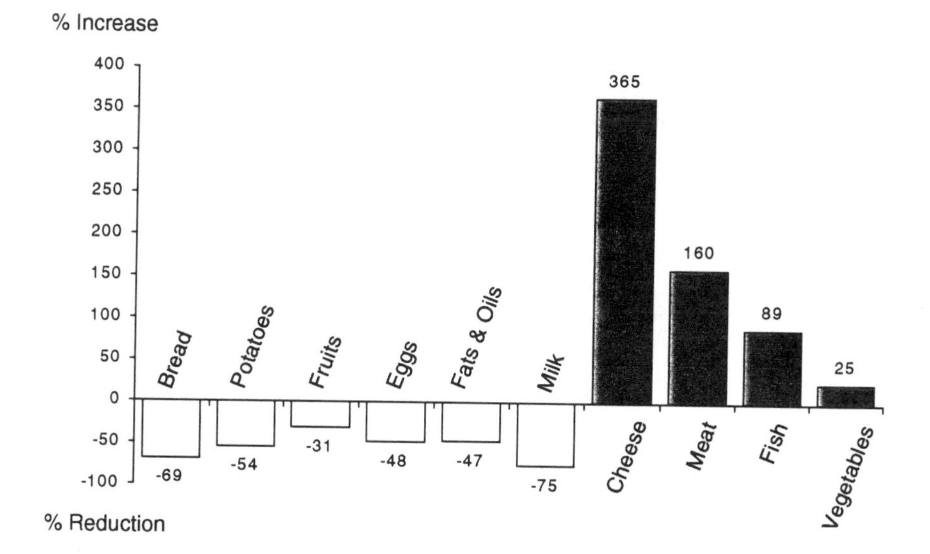

Figure 2. Change in food consumption of Cretan men aged 40-60 years from 1960 to 1988.

Table 2
Average Daily Antioxidant Intake of the 16 Cohorts of the Seven Countries Study (II)

Cohort	β-Carotene	Vitamin C	α-Tocopherol
Croatia - Dalmatia	4.2	60	15.9
Croatia - Slavonia	3.4	41	15.2
Serbia - Velica Krsna	0.6	17	7.8
Serbia - Zrenjanin	2.1	112	12.1
Serbia - Belgrade	1.7	70	18.3
Greece - Corfu	2.1	125	31.2
Greece - Crete	1.8	136	21.4
Italy - Rome	2.6	53	14.3
Italy - Crevalcore	1.2	50	15.7
Italy - Montegiorgio	2.8	44	13.2
The Netherlands - Zutphen	2.9	110	8.6
Finland - West	2.1	65	9.1
Finland - East	1.4	80	9.6
USA - Railroad	2.5	142	6.8
Japan - Tamushimaru	1.8	39	4.7
Japan - Ushibuka	1.4	45	6.3

From Ocké *et al.*, Average intake of antioxidant (pro) vitamins and subsequent cancer mortality in the 16 cohorts of the Seven Countries study. *Int. J. Cancer* 1995: 61: 480-484 (with permission).

HEALTH IMPLICATIONS

α-Tocopherol, as a fat-soluble vitamin, may exert higher antioxidant activity for the LDL-cholesterol as compared to ascorbic acid, flavonoids, and quercetin, which are mainly water-soluble substances. Although flavonoid and quercetin intake is the highest in Japan, CHD and cancer mortality rates are not the lowest (Table 3). The same holds true for saturated fat intake which was lower in the Japanese population compared to the population of Crete, although the CHD mortality rate was lower in Crete.[10] The antioxidant flavonoids intake is related to lower CHD mortality in the populations of the Seven Countries Study. The saturated fatty acid intake is, however, the major determinant of the differences of CHD among the Seven Countries populations, explaining 73% of the total variance. The flavonoid intake explains independently another 8% of the total variance of CHD disease.[10]

Other water soluble antioxidants such as ascorbic acid have been shown to have a strong inverse relationship to the 25-year stomach cancer mortality of the 16 cohorts of the Seven Countries Study (Figure 3), but not to mortality from lung and colon cancer. The intake of carotenoids and α-tocopherol was not associated with these types of cancer.

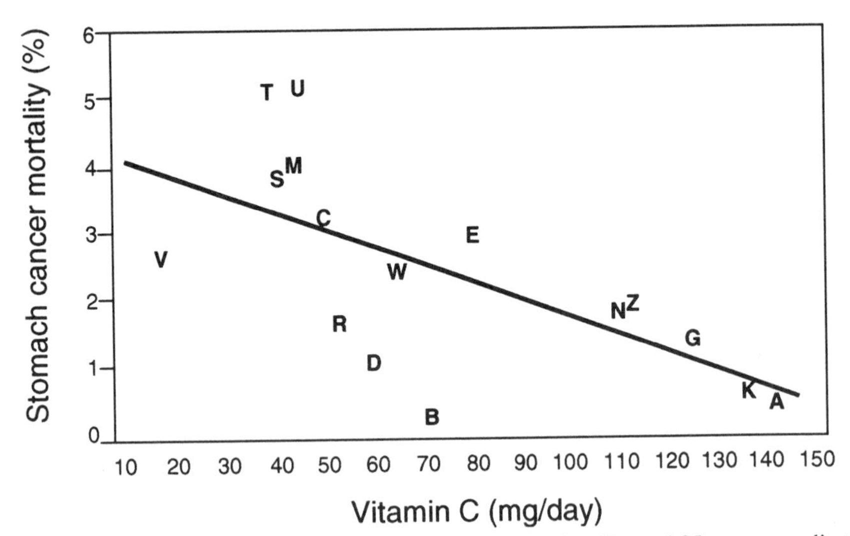

Figure 3. Univariate associations between vitamin C intake at baseline and 25-year age-adjusted mortality from stomach cancer in the Seven Country Study. A U.S. railroad, B Belgrade, C Crevalcore, D Dalmatia, E East Finland, G Corfu, K Crete, M Montegiorgio, N Zuphen, R Rome railroad, S Slavonia, T Tanushimaru, U Ushibuka, V Velika Krsna, W West Finland, Z Zrenjanin. From Ocké *et al.*, Average intake of antioxidant (pro) vitamins and subsequent cancer mortality in the 16 cohorts of the Seven Countries study. *Int. J. Cancer* 1995: 61: 480-484 (with permission).

Table 3
Average Risk Factor Levels at Baseline and Age-Adjusted Mortality From Several Causes After 25 Years of Follow-up in 16 Cohort Groups of the Seven Countries Study[10]

Cohort	N	Intake of			Smoking	Age-Adjusted 25-Year Mortality, %					
		Flavonoids mg/d	Quercetin mg/d	SFA[a] g/d	%	CHD[b]	Cancer	Lung Cancer	Colorectal Cancer	Stomach Cancer	All Causes
West Finland	860	2.6	2.6	73.0	57	19.2	12.3	4.4	0.9	2.3	50.3
Velika Krsna, Serbia	511	9.0	9.0	52.0	49	12.2	10.3	1.6	1.7	2.6	50.0
East Finland	817	9.6	9.6	88.6	69	28.8	12.7	7.3	0.1	2.9	59.7
US railroad	2571	12.9	11.0	55.3	59	20.2	11.4	3.3	2.0	0.5	45.1
Zrenjanin, Serbia	516	13.0	13.1	55.0	63	17.7	13.1	2.1	1.4	1.8	57.9
Belgrade, Serbia	536	13.3	7.7	57.3	44	11.8	8.4	2.1	0.6	0.2	29.5
Corfu, Greece	529	15.6	14.1	28.0	64	9.5	10.9	2.8	0.4	1.3	40.4
Crete, Greece	686	15.7	15.0	21.8	57	4.6	8.8	2.0	0.9	0.5	31.4
Rome railroad, Italy	768	23.1	17.2	46.9	65	13.2	12.2	3.3	1.4	1.6	39.7
Crevalcore, Italy	993	23.3	18.3	54.1	63	13.4	17.0	3.0	1.6	3.2	49.8
Zutphen, The Netherl.	878	33.1	13.1	60.9	75	19.7	17.8	7.2	2.0	1.7	48.0
Montegiorgio, Italy	719	33.9	26.8	31.4	59	11.5	12.2	1.0	1.1	4.0	46.2
Dalmatia, Croatia	671	40.2	21.0	67.0	58	8.1	10.0	3.5	0.5	1.0	43.3
Slavonia, Croatia	696	58.2	38.2	64.4	60	14.2	10.8	1.8	1.1	3.8	51.0
Tanushimaru, Japan	508	60.8	27.2	10.1	71	4.5	13.1	1.0	1.6	5.1	39.4
Ushibuka, Japan	502	68.2	34.6	14.0	78	6.3	18.1	2.6	1.0	5.1	51.5

[a] SFA: Saturated Fatty Acids
[b] CHD: Coronary Heart Disease
From: Hertog *et al.*, Flavonoid intake and long-term risk of coronary heart disease and cancer in the Seven Countries study. *Arch. Intern. Med.* 1995: 155: 381-386. (Copyright 1995, American Medical Association, with permission).

The high dietary intake of ascorbic acid by the population of Crete has been confirmed in other recent studies.[9,12] The plasma levels, however, of ascorbic acid in the Eurogast Study were not significantly associated with gastric cancer.[13] In this study the population of Crete had the highest plasma ascorbic acid levels.

The differences in the CHD and cancer mortality among the Seven Countries cohorts can also be partly attributed to other factors such as genetic (apolipoprotein E), cultural, and geographic which may play a role in explaining differences in absolute risk. Even lung cancer mortality is not the highest in the population of Crete although Crete, and Greece more generally, has the highest rates of smoking in the world. The high olive oil, fruit, and vegetable intake may protect Cretans from the heavy smoking habits. Despite the recent decline in fruit and vegetable consumption, particularly among younger generations of Greeks,[9] fruit and vegetable intake (excluding potatoes) at approximately 600 g per day in Greece is still the highest compared with other European Union populations.

Post-prandial lipemia has been shown recently to explain differences in the atherogenic and thrombogenic profile between Northern Europeans (UK and Ireland) and Cretans. This is attributed to the habitual high olive oil intake favoring a faster clearance of chylomicrons and chylomicron remnants from the circulation.[7] In addition to faster post-prandial clearance of chylomicrons from the blood of Cretans in comparison to Northern Europeans, the high antioxidant content of olive oil protects the lipoproteins from oxidative damage.[14]

CONCLUSION

The Cretan cohort of the Seven Countries Study, examined prospectively for the last 38 years, has provided valuable morbidity and mortality data which has been evaluated in relation to the diet of the population. This relationship supports the widely accepted concept that the diet of Crete is mainly responsible for the relative health and longevity of the population in comparison with 16 other populations.

In recent years there has been a great deal of interest in developing food-based dietary guidelines. Typical 24-hour meal schedules, derived from Keys and Christakis' dietary records of men in Crete in the early 1960s, have been analyzed by use of the USDA food data base, modified by the Department of Preventive Medicine and Nutrition at the University of Crete.[1,2,15] The fatty acid composition of 105 Greek foods providing 95% of the fat in the diet were analyzed by the European Union supported TRANSFAIR study in 1997.

As can be seen from Table 4, the antioxidant vitamin intake of a middle-aged Cretan farmer exceeds the RDA.

Table 4
Traditional Diet of Crete, early 1960s

Breakfast /Snack	Lunch	Dinner
Goat milk, 200 ml Ground wheat, 50 g 1 pear **Snack 10:00AM** Home made cheese, 40 g Dried whole wheat bread	Salted cod with potatoes, 100 g and tomatoes, 30 g Salad greens, 100 g, Carrots 40 g, 6 olives and olive oil, 20 g Whole wheat bread, 50 g 1 glass red wine, 120 ml 1 apple	Broad beans, 250 g and olive oil, 30 g Radish, 100 g and olive oil, 15 g Whole wheat bread, 60 g 1 glass red wine, 120 ml 2 oranges

Nutrient	Amount	% of Energy	% of RDA
Protein, g	98		155.4
Total fat, g	114	35.9	
Carbohydrate, g	337	47.2	
Dietary fiber, g	45.5		
Calories, kcal	2860		124.3
Calcium, mg	1279		162.2
Iron, mg	23		228.0
Magnesium, mg	412		117.7
Phosphorus, mg			203.6
Potassium, mg	5460		
Sodium, mg	2978		
Vitamin A, mg RE	1878		187.8
Ascorbic acid, mg	256		426.8
α-Tocopherol, mg	7.8		78
Vitamin B1, mg	1.7		141.1
Vitamin B2, mg	1.3		91.2
Vitamin B6, mg	1.8		176.7
Cholesterol, mg	135		
Saturated fatty acids, g	25	8.0	
Monounsaturated fatty acids, g	67.1	21.1	
Polyunsaturated fatty acids, g	11	3.4	
Total *trans* unsaturated, g	0.8	0.3	
C 12:0 + C 14:0 + C 16:0, g	17	5.5	
ω-6, g	9.0	2.8	
ω-3, g	0.6	0.2	

The daily meals included simple foods produced at home. Meat was eaten once a week while dietary products were used in small quantities. Home-made whole-wheat bread, olive oil, olives, and legumes were the main sources of energy. An abundant variety of wild and cultivated vegetables, fruits, and nuts were necessary daily complements to the main meals.

Some of the main elements of the Cretan diet of the early 1960s have been used by developed nations in setting goals for dietary changes in their own populations. Such elements, which characterized the Cretan diet in the 1960s, include: 8% of total energy from saturated fats; fiber intake exceeding 30 g/day, and over 600 g/day of fruit and vegetables, excluding potato intake. Unfortunately, contemporary Greeks have been adopting westernized dietary patterns. The results are reflected in the increasing CHD mortality rates in Greece over the last 35 years, which serve as a potent argument in urging the resumption of traditional dietary patterns.

REFERENCES

1. Keys, A. (Ed) Coronary heart disease in Seven Countries. Circulation 1970, 41 Suppl. 1, I-211.
2. Keys, A.(Ed). *Seven Countries: A multivariate analysis of death and coronary heart disease.* Cambridge MA/London: Harvard University Press, 1980.
3. Halliwell, B. Free radicals and antioxidants: A personal view. Nutrition Review 1994, 52: 253-265.
4. Mensink, R.P., Katan, M.B. Effects of a diet enriched with monounsaturated or polyunsaturated fatty acids on levels of low-density and high-density lipoprotein cholesterol in healthy women and men. N. Eng. J. Med. 1989: 321: 436-441.
5. Menotti, A., Keys A., Aravanis, C., *et al.* Seven Countries Study. First 20-year mortality data in 12 cohorts of six countries. Ann. Med. 1989: 21: 175-9.
6. Verschuren, M., Jacobs, D.R., Bloemberg B. P. M., Kromhout D, Menotti, A. Aravanis, C., Blackburn, H., Buzina, R., Dontas, A., Fidanza, F., Karvonen M.J. Nedeljkovic S., Nissinen, A., Toshima H. Serum total cholesterol and long-term coronary heart disease mortality in different cultures. JAMA 1995: 274: 131-136.
7. Kafatos, A., Mamalakis G., Williams C. M., Gibney M., Roche H., Zampelas A. Effect of monounsaturated fatty acids enriched diet on serum lipids and on non-esterified phospholipid fatty acids in men with familial history of coronary artery disease. Third International Conference, Dietary Assessment Methods The Netherlands May 6-9, 1998.
8. Kromhout, D., Keys, A. Aravanis, C. *et al.*, Food Consumption Patterns in the 1960s in Seven Countries. Am. J. Clin. Nutr. 1989: 49: 889-94.
9. Kafatos, A.G., Kouroumalis I. *et al.*, Coronary-heart disease risk-factor status of the Cretan urban population in the 1980's. Am. J. Clin. Nutr. 1991: 54: 591-8.
10. Hertog M., Kromhout, D. Aravanis C., Blackburn H., Buzina R., Fidanza F., Giampaoli S., Jansen A., Menotti A., Nedeljkovic S., Pekkarinen M., Simic B.S., Toshima H., Feskens E., Hollman P., Katan M.B. Flavonoid intake and long-term risk of coronary heart disease and cancer in the Seven Countries Study. Arch. Intern. Med. 1995: 155: 381-386.

11. Ocké, M.C., Kromhout, D. Menotti A., Aravanis C., Blackburn H., Buzina R., Fidanza F., Jansen A., Nedeljkovic S., Nissinen A., Pekkarinen M. Average intake of antioxidant (pro) vitamins and subsequent cancer mortality in the 16 cohorts of the Seven Countries Study. Int. J. Cancer 1995: 61: 480-484.
12. Kafatos A.G., Diakatou A., Labadarios D., Kounali D., Apostolaki J., Vlachonikolis J., Mamalakis G., Megremis S. Nutritional status of the elderly in Anogia, Crete, Greece. J. Am. College Nutr. 1993: 12: 685-692.
13. Webb P.M., Bates C., Pall D., Forman D and the Eurogast Study group: Gastric cancer, gastritis and plasma vitamin C: results from an International correlation and cross-sectional study. Int. J. Cancer 1997: 73: 684-689.
14. Hassapidou M., Manoukas A. Tocopherol and tocotrienol composition of raw table olive fruit. J. Sci. Food Agric. 1993: 61: 277-280.
15. Christakis G., Sevringhaus E. L., Maldonado Z., *et al.*. Crete: A study in metabolic epidemiology of coronary heart disease. Am. J. Cardiol. 1965: 15: 320-332.

Part 3

Major Dietary and Other Antioxidants

- Carotenoids and Vitamin A
- Vitamin C
- Vitamin E: Tocopherols and Tocotrienols
- Isoflavones
- Other Antioxidants

8

Carotenoids and Vitamin A

Thomas W.M. Boileau, B.Sc., Amy C. Moore, B.Sc.
and John W. Erdman, Jr., Ph.D.
Division of Nutritional Sciences, University of Illinois
Champaign-Urbana, Illinois, USA

CHEMISTRY, OCCURRENCE, ABSORPTION, AND TRANSPORT

Major Classes of Carotenoids

Carotenoids are a group of over 600 naturally occurring plant pigments that provide the yellow, orange, and red colors seen in many fruits and vegetables.[1,2] β-Carotene, the most well-known carotenoid, can be converted within the intestinal mucosal cell to two identical molecules of retinal, or vitamin A (VA), by the enzyme β-carotene 15,15'-dioxygenase.[3,4] Most carotenoids are devoid of VA, activity. For example, lycopene, the carotenoid responsible for giving tomatoes their red color, cannot be converted to VA. The

0-8493-8009-X/98/$0.00+$.50

fact that few of the carotenoids found in human serum and tissues are converted to VA has sparked interest in the health benefits of carotenoids aside from their role as VA precursors.

To date, 34 dietary carotenoids have been found in human serum.[5] Not all carotenoids found in foods are efficiently absorbed by humans. Capsanthin, the red color in paprika, is not typically found in human serum or tissues. Carotenoids found in human serum and tissues have in common two major structural features (see Figure 1). The first is a system of 9 conjugated double bonds. This characteristic of the molecules is responsible for absorbing visible light to give carotenoids their characteristic color. The second major structural feature is the end group. Pro-VA active carotenoids have at least one unsubstituted β-ionone ring at the end of their conjugated double bond chain. Non- pro-VA carotenoids may have substituted (oxygenated) β-ionone rings, as seen in lutein; no ring structure at all, as is the case with lycopene; or altered double bond structures.

Carotenoids can be classified into two major groups based on structure. Xanthophylls are oxygenated carotenoids containing carboxyl and/or hydroxyl group(s) as end group substituents. Lutein is the major xanthophyll found in human serum, but zeaxanthin and cryptoxanthin are also present. β-cryptoxanthin is a pro-VA xanthophyll. Carotenoids not containing oxygen molecules are classified as hydrocarbon carotenoids or carotenes. The major pro-VA carotenoids, β-carotene and α-carotene, as well as lycopene are found in this group.[2]

Geometric isomers of the above carotenoids may have distinct biological roles. Most naturally occurring carotenoids are found in the linear or *all-trans* configuration. Exposure to light and/or heat may facilitate the *trans* to *cis* isomerization of one or more double bonds.[6] Many *cis*-isomers of carotenoids are found in human serum and tissues. They differ in structure from *trans* isomers in that they have a *cis* bond or "kink" introduced in the double bond chain (see Figure 1). β-Carotene is found predominately in human serum in the *all-trans* form while three major *cis*-isomers (9-,13-, and 15-*cis*) are found to varying degrees in tissues.[7] Human serum contains 13- and 15-*cis* β-carotene, but very low 9-*cis* β-carotene. 9-*cis*-β-Carotene may be found only in small amounts in serum to limit the quantities available for conversion to 9-*cis*-retinoic acid, a potent hormone.[8,9] Lycopene, on the other hand, is found in human tissues and serum mainly in *cis*-configurations. As many as 18 geometrical isomers of lycopene are seen in human prostate tissue and over 50% of lycopene isomers in serum are in the *cis*-configuration.[7,10] The differences seen between isomers present in food and isomers present in human serum and tissues may be accounted for by selective absorption or *in vivo* isomerization of the given carotenoid.[11,12]

ABSORPTION AND TRANSPORT

Absorption

The intestinal absorption of dietary carotenoids is facilitated by the formation of bile acid micelles. The hydrocarbon structure of the carotenoids prevents them from being water soluble and, like other non-polar lipids, are solubilized within the gastrointestinal tract when micelles are formed. Micellar solubilization facilitates the diffusion of lipids across the unstirred water layer.[13,14] The presence of fat in the small intestine stimulates the secretion of bile from the gall bladder and improves the absorption of carotenoids by increasing the size and stability of micelles thus allowing more carotenoids to be solubilized. Dietary fat has previously been shown to significantly improve the serum response to dietary crystalline β-carotene.[15,16] The uptake of β-carotene by the enterocyte is believed to occur by passive diffusion. This has been demonstrated *in vivo* in the rat intestinal perfusion model.[17] Uptake by the villus-associated enterocytes alone, however, is not sufficient for absorption. Once inside the enterocyte, carotenoids must also be incorporated into chylomicrons and released into the lymphatics. Carotenoids possessing vitamin A activity may either be absorbed intact or cleaved to form vitamin A prior to secretion into the lymph. Carotenoid cleavage is accomplished either by the intestinal mucosal enzyme β-carotene 15, 15'-dioxygenase (EC 1.13.11.21)[18] or by non-central cleavage mechanisms.[19] The rate of conversion of a highly bioavailable source of β-carotene to retinol in man has been shown to be between 60 and 75%[20] but likely varies with vitamin A status. Remaining carotenoids may then be incorporated into chylomicrons and secreted into the lymphatics. Carotenoids that are taken up by the mucosal cells but not incorporated into chylomicrons are sloughed off when the enterocytes turn over, and spill their contents into the lumen of the gastrointestinal tract. Portal transport of carotenoids is minimal due to the lipophilic nature of their structures.

Transport

The carotenoids are transported in the serum exclusively by lipoproteins.[21] It is thought that β-carotene and other hydrocarbon carotenoids reside in the hydrophobic core of the particles, while the more polar xanthophylls reside closer to the surface.[21] The carotenoid content of the individual lipoprotein classes is not homogeneous. In the fasted state, the hydrocarbon carotenoids such as β-carotene, α-carotene, and lycopene are carried predominantly by LDL with the remaining being carried by HDL and, to a lesser extent, VLDL.[22] In one study, the percentage of these carotenoids carried by LDL ranged from 77.9 (± 24.5) to 87.4 (± 10.5).[23] In contrast, the more polar xanthophylls such as lutein and zeaxanthin are found predominantly in HDL.[21,24,25]

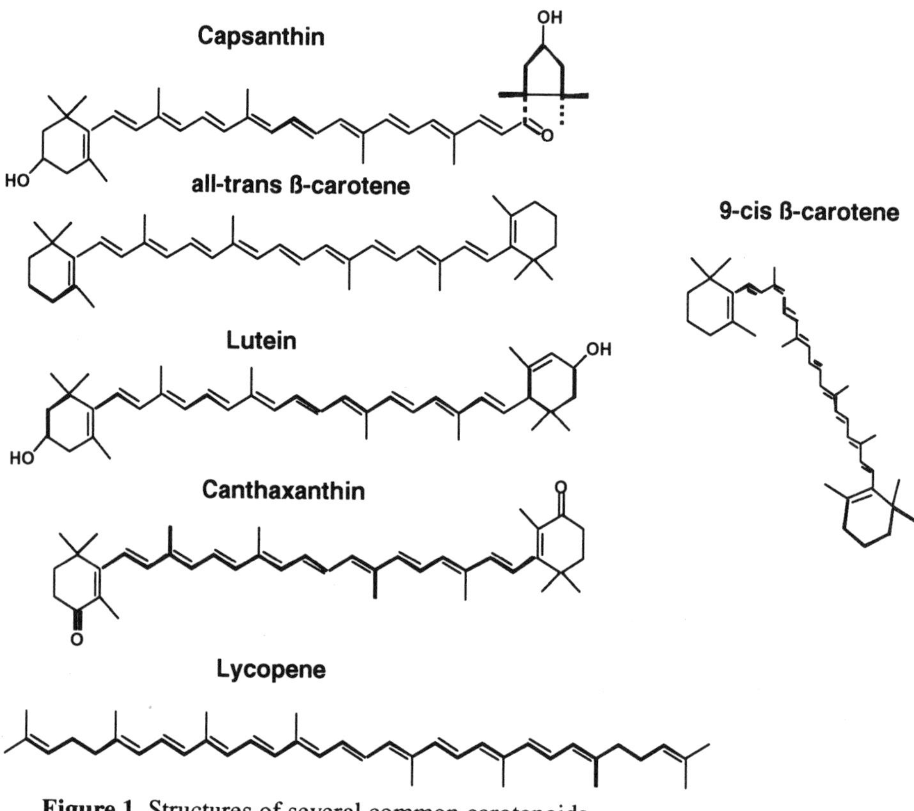

Figure 1. Structures of several common carotenoids.

Blood and Tissue Concentrations

At present, 34 carotenoids have been identified in human serum and breast milk.[5] Of these, 13 are geometrical isomers of their *all-trans* parent structures and 8 are metabolites. This is in contrast to the up to 50 carotenoids that have been identified in the U.S. diet.[5] The most prevalent carotenoids in human serum include β-carotene, lycopene, and lutein.[26] These are also the most prevalent in the diet. *cis*-Isomers of lycopene are commonly found in the serum and in fact have been shown to constitute more than 50%

of the total serum lycopene.[7] In contrast, *cis*-isomers of β-carotene are considerably less common in serum. In addition to these, α-carotene, zeaxanthin, and cryptoxanthin are also major serum carotenoids.[27] The concentrations of the various carotenoids in human serum and tissues are highly variable and likely dependent on a number of factors (Table 1).

Table 1
Concentrations of Selected Carotenoids in Human Serum and Tissues[a]

Carotenoid	Serum (μmol/L)	Liver (μmol/g)	Kidney (μmol/g)	Lung (μmol/g)
Lycopene	0.13-0.82	0.20-17.2	0.093-2.4	0.1-1.0
β-carotene	0.09-0.91	0.39-19.4	0.093-2.8	0.1-1.6
Lutein	0.16-0.72	0.10-3.0	0.037-2.1	0.1-2.3
β-cryptoxanthin	0.05-0.38	0.037-20.0	0.019-3.9	0.1-2.5
α-carotene	0.02-0.22	0.075-10.8	0.037-1.5	0.1-1.0

[a] Data from Schmitz *et al.*[33] and Kaplan *et al.*[34] for tissues and NHANES III[30] for serum.

For many years investigators have studied human serum responses to doses of carotenoids from both synthetic sources and food sources. By measuring the change from baseline of serum carotenoids following a single dose or ingestion of a test meal, investigators are able to estimate absorption. Data from such studies are complicated by a very large inter-subject variability and the existence of non-responders. For example, one investigator reported that only 4 out of 11 subjects had a plasma response to a single oral 120 mg dose of β-carotene.[22] A number of explanations for the existence of non-responders have been proposed including inefficient uptake and/or absorption and extremely efficient conversion to vitamin A.[21] The serum appearance of carotenoids after a single dose is relatively slow, with peak concentrations being reached between 24 and 48 hours.[28] This reflects the lag time between initial transport to the liver and subsequent repackaging of carotenoids into lipoprotein particles. The earliest post-prandial serum appearance of carotenoids is in the chylomicron fraction. One investigator has proposed using this triglyceride-rich lipoprotein fraction when quantitating carotenoid absorption.[29] This would provide a more direct measure of absorption since total serum carotenoid content is not an exclusive measure of newly absorbed carotenoids.

Unpublished data from NHANES III demonstrate the variability of normal serum carotenoid concentrations. The following ranges have been reported: lycopene 0.13-0.82 μmol/L, lutein+zeaxanthin 0.16-0.72 μmol/L, β-carotene 0.09-0.91 μmol/L, β-cryptoxanthin 0.05-0.38 μmol/L, and α-carotene 0.02-0.22 μmol/L.[30] This variability is attributed to a variety of lifestyle and physiological factors. In a recent population-based study, Brady *et al.* reported that lower serum concentrations of β-carotene, α-carotene, β-cryptoxanthin, lutein+zeaxanthin, but not lycopene were generally associated with male gender, smoking, younger age, lower HDL cholesterol, greater ethanol consumption, and higher body mass index.[31] Several of these factors were similarly related to reduced dietary intake suggesting that carotenoid intake itself may be influenced by these factors. Lipid-lowering drugs have also been shown to dramatically decrease serum carotenoids.[32] In a double-blind, randomized trial, treatment with cholestyramine (lipid-lowering resin) for 4 months and probucol (antioxidant and lipid-lowering drug) for 2 months resulted in a 65% reduction in serum β-carotene and 51% reduction in lycopene. The reductions were attributed to reduced intestinal absorption of lipids by cholestyramine and reduced lipoprotein particle number and size by probucol.

The delivery of carotenoids to extra-hepatic tissue is accomplished through the interaction of lipoprotein particles with receptors and degradation of lipoproteins by extra-hepatic enzymes such as lipoprotein lipase. Carotenoids are present in a number of human tissues including adipose, liver, kidney, and adrenal.[33] Adipose tissue and liver appear quantitatively to be the main storage sites.[27] However, based on a wet tissue weight basis, the liver, adrenal gland, and testes contain the highest per gram concentrations.[7] Similar to what is reported in serum, β-carotene, lycopene, and lutein are the main tissue carotenoids, although α-carotene, zeaxanthin, and cryptoxanthin are also detected.[27,33,34] In contrast to serum profiles, 9-*cis* β-carotene is consistently present in storage tissues.[7,10] In both serum and tissue storage, lycopene *cis*-isomers constitute greater than 50% of the total lycopene present.[7,10]

Interactions of Carotenoids

Various factors are known to impact the intestinal absorption of carotenoids including food matrix effects, dietary fiber, fat level, and various other physiological factors.[35,36] Interactions during the absorptive process has been an emerging area of research interest. The observation that not all dietary carotenoids have been identified in serum and the recent widespread use of β-carotene supplements have prompted investigators to study these interactions.

Interactions with Other Carotenoids

An interaction between β-carotene and lutein was reported in a study evaluating the impact of chronic β-carotene supplementation on the plasma concentrations of other carotenoids.[37] In this study, recipients of commercial β-carotene beadlets in either 12 mg or 30 mg capsules for 6 weeks had significantly lower plasma lutein than subjects obtaining β-carotene and lutein from food sources. In addition, plasma β-carotene was higher in the subjects receiving β-carotene beadlets demonstrating the superior bioavailability of this source. Interactions between β-carotene and lutein have also been described by other investigators. When subjects were given purified crystalline β-carotene and crystalline lutein in a combined dose, β-carotene significantly reduced the serum area under the curve (AUC) value (a measure of total absorption) for lutein.[38] Lutein in a combined dose with β-carotene significantly enhanced β-carotene AUC in subjects whose AUC for β-carotene (when dosed alone) was lowest.

The carotenoid profile of Betatene™, (0.5% lutein, 0.75% zeaxanthin, 3.6% α-carotene, 70.3% *trans* β-carotene, and 22.7% *cis* β-carotene) a natural carotenoid source extracted from algae, was shown to be vastly different from the carotenoid profile of human chylomicrons following Betatene™ ingestion.[39] In this study, the investigators reported a 14-fold higher concentration of lutein relative to β-carotene in the chylomicron fraction when compared to the composition of Betatene™ ingested by the subjects. The proportion of α-carotene in chylomicrons was equivalent to that in the Betatene™ while the β-carotene content of the chylomicrons was lower. This suggests that either lutein and α-carotene are more bioavailable than β-carotene from this source, or that β-carotene is being efficiently converted to vitamin A.

Interactions between β-carotene and canthaxanthin in humans have also been reported.[40] In this study, the carotenoids were administered either separately or in combined doses with a meal as water-dispersible beadlets in water. The combined dose resulted in a significantly lower serum response to canthaxanthin when compared to dosing with canthaxanthin alone. In contrast, the serum response to β-carotene was not reduced by a combined dose when compared to dosing with β-carotene alone. A similar study carried out in the ferret model demonstrated a reduction in β-carotene bioavailability when β-carotene and canthaxanthin as water-dispersible beadlets were given in a combined dose.[41] In the rat, significant interactions have been reported between lycopene and canthaxanthin.[42] In this study, rats that were fed a diet supplemented with lycopene as tomato paste and canthaxanthin as water-dispersible beadlets had a decreased serum concentration as well as decreased liver levels of canthaxanthin when they were fed the highest level of tomato paste (90 mg/kg diet). The reciprocal relationship was also present since feeding canthaxanthin dramatically reduced liver lycopene. No lycopene was detected in the plasma of any of the rats regardless of dietary treatment. Interaction data such as this, however, is complicated by the use of purified sources of carotenoids and food sources of carotenoids in the same study. The superior bioavailability of water-soluble beadlets and other purified sources becomes apparent when they are compared to food sources of the same carotenoids.

Effect of 9-cis β-Carotene Supplementation on all-trans β-Carotene

Numerous human studies have consistently demonstrated a blunted serum response to the ingestion of 9-*cis* β-carotene in comparison to *all-trans* β-carotene.[12,39,43-46] These studies seem to suggest that *all-trans* β-carotene is preferentially absorbed over its 9-*cis* isomer. One explanation may be that 9-*cis* β-carotene isomerizes to *all-trans* β-carotene during the absorptive process. This has been demonstrated *in vivo* in humans using stable isotopes of *all-trans* or 9-*cis* β-carotene.[47] Another explanation is that dietary 9-*cis* β-carotene undergoes enzymatic conversion to 9-*cis* retinoic acid. This conversion has been demonstrated *in vivo* in the ferret[8] and also in human intestinal mucosa *in vitro*.[48] 9-*cis* retinoic acid has been shown to be a high affinity ligand for the retinoid X receptor.[49]

Does β-Carotene Supplementation Affect Blood α-Tocopherol?

The effects of long term β-carotene supplementation on serum vitamin E concentrations has been addressed by a number of investigators and is currently equivocal. In one study, a 40% decrease in plasma α-tocopherol was reported after 9 months of daily β-carotene supplementation.[50] In this study, 45 normal subjects were assigned to either 15, 30, 45, or 60 mg β-carotene per day. The reported reduction in α-tocopherol was seen in all supplementation groups and without an effect of dose. In contrast to these findings, when 505 patients from a clinical trial (antioxidant vitamin prevention of colonic polyp recurrence) were administered 25 mg β-carotene per day for 9 months, no change in serum vitamin E occurred.[51] No effect of β-carotene supplementation on serum vitamin E has been reported in normal, well-nourished adults.[52] In that study, 30 mg of β-carotene was administered daily for 16 weeks. The majority of studies support no negative impact of supplemental β-carotene on vitamin E.

CAROTENOIDS IN FOODS

The ability to estimate a person's carotenoid intake is limited by the accuracy of the available food composition data. Prior to 1993, food composition tables contained information for total carotenoid content rather than for individual carotenoids.[53,54] The estimation process improved dramatically in 1993 when the USDA and the NCI developed a food composition database for 120 foods that contained values for 5 commonly occurring carotenoids: β-carotene, α-carotene, lutein, lycopene, and β-cryptoxanthin.[54] This data was then used to compile a database containing values of these carotenoids for 2,458 fruits, vegetables, and multicomponent foods.[55] The second database was then used to evaluate the main food contributors of carotenoids for 1,102 women aged 19-50 in the U.S. According to the data, carrots constitute the primary source of both β-carotene (25%) and α-carotene (51%) in the diets of the women surveyed. Cantaloupe, broccoli, and soups containing carrots and tomatoes ranked second, third, and fourth, respectively. Orange juice and raw oranges were the primary dietary sources of β-cryptoxanthin. The primary sources of lutein and zeaxanthin were spinach, collard, mustard, or turnip greens, and broccoli. Tomatoes, tomato-based sauces, and catsup were the primary sources of lycopene. Tomatoes and most tomato products do contain appreciable β-carotene, but the predominant carotenoid is lycopene.[56] For example, tomato sauce contains about 0.45 mg of β-carotene and 17.98 mg of lycopene per 100 g of sauce. Cooked, canned, or frozen carrots contain on average 9.8 mg of β-carotene and 3.7 mg α-carotene per 100 grams.[54] Table 2 summarizes the major carotenoid content of selected foods.

Table 2
Content of Carotenoids in Various Foods[a]

Carotenoid	Broccoli	Cantaloupe	Carrot	Spinach	Tomato	Water-melon
	μg/100g					
Lutein & Zeaxanthin	1800			10200	100	
β-Caroteme	1300	3000	7900	4100	520	230
Lycopene					3100	4100
α-Carotene		35	3600			

[a] Data from Mangels *et al.*[54] Values are expressed as medians.

Factors Affecting Bioavailability of Food Carotenoids

Bioavailability of carotenoids from foods, concentrated extracts or synthetic products is quite variable (Figure 2). The following factors affect absorption and bioavailability.

a. Food Processing

The bioavailability of carotenoids from whole foods can be quite variable. Plant carotenoids can be bound in carotenoproteins or may be associated with the plant matrix.[36] The hypothesis that cooking may improve the bioavailability of these carotenoids has been tested. The bioavailability of lycopene from tomato juice, for example, is vastly improved by heat treatment.[11] When subjects consumed tomato juice equivalent to a single lycopene dose of 2.5 μmol/kg body weight that had been heated at 100 °C for 1 hour with oil, they experienced a serum lycopene peak at 24-48 hours. In contrast, the equivalent doses that were not heat treated did not result in an increase in serum lycopene. Steaming has also been shown to increase the amount of extractable carotenoids in spinach and carrots.[57] In one study, 10 g each of spinach and carrots were steamed for 3 min at 100°C and subsequently analyzed for their content of both α-carotene and β-carotene. Steamed carrots contained 139% of the α-carotene contained in the raw carrots and the steamed spinach 132% of the β-carotene of the raw spinach. In addition, a feeding study done in the preruminant calf demonstrated a slight enhancement of the bioavailability of β-carotene from steamed carrots versus raw carrots.[58]

b. Storage

The stability of carotenoids during cold storage and thermal processing has been evaluated in a number of carotenoid-rich foods. Following harvest, foods are subjected to handling and storage. The ability of light to degrade carotenoids has been evaluated during the cold storage of spinach and carrots.[59] Exposure of spinach to light during 8 days of cold storage resulted in a 60% loss of violaxanthin (an epoxy carotenoid), a 22% loss of lutein, a 41% loss of *all-trans* β-carotene, and a 48% loss of 9-*cis* β-carotene. In contrast, dark, cold storage for 8 days resulted in no losses of either violaxanthin or lutein and only 18% and 10% losses of *trans* and 9-*cis* β-carotene, respectively. This study reported no appreciable loss of carotenoids during either light or dark cold storage of carrots. The dense and compact structure of carrots likely explains the attenuated loss of carotenoids from carrots during storage. On the other hand, spinach leaves contain considerably greater surface area thus allowing a greater degree of exposure of carotenoids to light.

In contrast to steaming, more prolonged exposure to high temperatures (boiling) can negatively impact the carotenoid content of vegetables. An extreme example is the thermal processing of mango.[60] The carotenoid profile of both the raw and frozen mango consists of a variety of xanthophylls and hydrocarbon carotenoids. The carotenoid profile of samples of canned mango demonstrated complete degradation of xanthophylls leaving β-carotene as the predominant carotenoid.

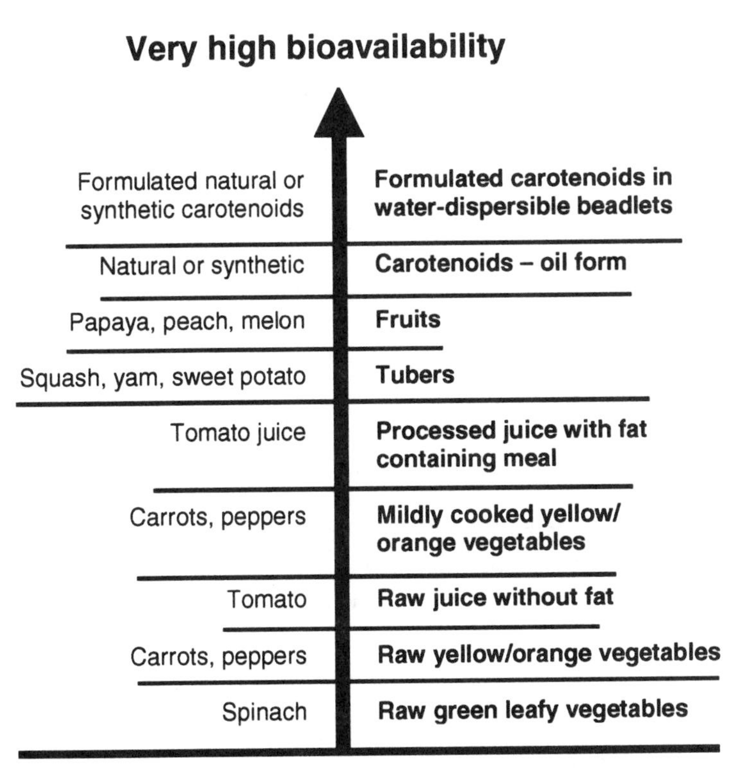

Figure 2. Effect of food matrix and processing on bioavailability of carotenoids.

c. Cooking

Cooking has also been shown to cause a differential rate of carotenoid loss in green, leafy vegetables.[61] Microwave cooking of brussel sprouts and kale for 6 minutes in a small amount of water produced a loss of 19-57% of the xanthophylls and 15% loss of the hydrocarbon carotenoids. Xanthophylls comprised 80-90% of the total carotenoids in the raw form of both of these vegetables.

The effects of microwave cooking and boiling on the carotenoid content of green beans has also been evaluated.[62] Lutein, α-carotene, and β-carotene remained stable after both microwave cooking (4 minutes) and boiling (9 minutes). However, considerable violaxanthin was lost after both cooking methods. When the green beans were boiled for 1 hour, the epoxy carotenoids including violaxanthin were completely destroyed while lutein, α-carotene, and β-carotene continued to remain stable. The canning process to preserve foods also involves extensive thermal processing and results in the formation of *cis*-isomers.[63] For example, canned carrots contain 73% *all-trans* β-carotene, 19% 13-*cis* β-carotene, and 8% 9-*cis* β-carotene while fresh carrots contain 100 % of the β-carotene in the *all-trans* configuration.

Although cooking at high temperatures can reduce the amount of carotenoids in foods, cooking may exert a greater impact on other nutrients in foods. In one study it was shown that cooking spinach in an open pan for 30 minutes reduced the vitamin C content by 90% while the β-carotene content was reduced by only 50%.[64]

It is important to keep in mind that the net effect of mild cooking such as steaming may be to increase the amount of carotenoid that is available for absorption. This process denatures proteins, which releases more carotenoids from the food matrix than are destroyed by the mild heat. In this case, the net effect is positive. In contrast, cooking at higher temperatures for longer periods of time (boiling) destroys a much higher percentage of the carotenoids in foods and is detrimental.

CAROTENOIDS AND HUMAN HEALTH

Much of the current research on the carotenoids focuses on their role as precursors to VA. Carotenoids are the primary source of VA for most people living in developing countries. Of the carotenoids, β-carotene has the highest VA value. Carotenoids such as α-carotene and β-cryptoxanthin have half of the VA value as β-carotene. As previously mentioned, research on the bioavailability of β-carotene and other pro-VA carotenoids from various food sources, the mechanisms by which carotenoids are converted to VA, and development of physiologically relevant animal models to study carotenoid and

VA metabolism are at the forefront of pro-VA carotenoid research.[65-67]

Retinoids are well known for their ability to induce cellular differentiation, reducing the ability of many cell types to proliferate. Conversion of carotenoids to retinoids, then, is one mechanism by which carotenoids may protect from various cancers and other diseases. However, conversion of carotenoids to VA is only one of numerous protective roles carotenoids are thought to play in biological systems. Some proposed mechanisms by which β-carotene and other carotenoids may decrease risk for the development of cancers include their ability to quench singlet oxygen and other reactive species,[68-76] upregulate gap junction communication between cells,[71,77-80] increase immune system efficiency,[81-84] and induce detoxifying enzymes.[85-88]

Carotenoids have also been implicated in protection from cardiovascular disease,[76,89] macular degeneration,[90-92] and have been used in the treatment of certain photosensitivity disorders.[93] At this time, however, the role of carotenoids in preventing LDL oxidation and modulating activities of detoxifying enzymes seems to be equivocal.[94-96]

Lycopene, a non-pro-VA carotenoid, has recently been epidemiologically correlated with decreased risk of prostate cancer,[97] and is the predominant carotenoid in human prostate tissue.[10] Lycopene is the most potent biological quencher of singlet oxygen,[69,70] and is able to stimulate gap junctional communication *in vitro*.[98] *In vivo* formation of oxidation products of lycopene may modulate some of lycopene's protective functions.[5,26]

Other nonpro-VA carotenoids are thought to have distinct roles in biological systems. Lutein and zeaxanthin have been the subject of much interest because of their role in the retina and macular pigment.[90,99] Canthaxanthin has been shown to be one of the most effective carotenoids at inducing gap junctions,[80] and has also been used with β-carotene in the treatment of photosensitivity disorders.[93] Astaxanthin has been studied for a possible role in enhancing immune function.[100-103] However, astaxanthin is not abundant in foods and to date has not been identified in human serum.

MOLECULAR MECHANISMS OF CAROTENOIDS

Carotenoids as Quenchers of Reactive Species

The human body is constantly under insult by a variety of reactive species that are able to modify DNA, proteins, and lipids, resulting in increased incidence of certain diseases. Reactive oxygen species, which include hydrogen peroxide, superoxide anion, and singlet oxygen as well as nitrogen oxides are endogenously produced daily by aerobic metabolism and by the cells of the immune system. Reactive compounds entering the body from exogenous sources such as cigarette smoke or the diet may also act deleteriously within the body.[104] The reactions of carotenoids with and inactivation of these reactive compounds has been proposed as a mechanism by which carotenoids may protect cells from damage and hence decrease risk for cancer and cardiovascular disease.

Carotenoids are the most potent biological quenchers of singlet oxygen.[70] Singlet oxygen is produced when a light-excited photosensitizer passes its energy on to molecular oxygen.[105] The reaction of β-carotene with singlet oxygen was first shown in 1968 by Foote *et al.*[68] The efficiency with which carotenoids can quench singlet oxygen is related to their chemical structures. Because singlet oxygen quenching is directly related to polyene chain length, lycopene appears to be the most efficient carotenoid at quenching singlet oxygen.[69] Its isolated double bonds, open chain, and lack of oxygen substituents apparently increase its activity.[70] Other carotenoids such as neurosporene have a greater ability to quench singlet oxygen, but they are not found in human serum or tissues in large quantities.[69] Astaxanthin, β-carotene, and lycopene but not canthaxanthin have been shown to protect from singlet oxygen-induced membrane damage to human lymphoid cells.[106] Carotenoids interact with singlet oxygen either via a physical quenching mechanism, in which the excited energy from singlet oxygen is transferred to the carotenoid and then dissipated to the surroundings as heat, or chemical quenching, in which the carotenoid is destroyed in the process by addition of oxygen to its double bond system.[74]

The action of carotenoids as chain-breaking antioxidants has also been investigated.[72,107] Free radicals generated within the body can react with polyunsaturated fatty acids to cause a chain reaction which can destroy many lipid molecules in a short period of time. For a molecule to be a good chain-breaking antioxidant, it must be able to form a stable radical by donating a hydrogen to the damaging unstable radical. α-Tocopherol, the best chain-breaking antioxidant, can donate its phenolic hydrogen to a lipid radical while in the process forming a stable carbon-centered radical. The reaction of β-carotene with a lipid radical results in the formation of a carbon-centered β-carotene radical intermediate. This intermediate structure has two possible fates; it can act as a prooxidant by reacting with molecular oxygen or it can react with another lipid radical to form stable products. In environments with high oxygen partial pressures such as in lung tissue, β-carotene may act via the first mechanism, while in other tissues with lower oxygen pressures, it more likely acts as an antioxidant to terminate lipid oxidation.[72,74,107]

Martin *et al.* have recently shown both β-carotene and the oxygenated carotenoid lutein to protect HepG2 cells against oxidative damage induced by *tert*-butylhydroperoxide (TBHP).[108] Overnight incubation of cells with β-carotene or lutein in the presence of the oxidant TBHP resulted in protection of cells from lipid peroxidation and membrane damage as measured by decreased cellular release of lactate dehydrogenase as compared to untreated controls.

Carotenoid *cis*-isomers may play a role in radical chain-reaction termination. 9-*cis*-β-Carotene has been shown *in vivo* and *in vitro* to be a better free radical scavenger than the *all-trans* form.[73,109]

Carotenoids and Macular Degeneration

Age-related macular degeneration is the leading cause of irreversible blindness in people over the age of 65. It is a result of blue-light-mediated free radical damage to the retina.[110] The macular region of the eye has a distinct yellow coloration because of the presence of two carotenoids, lutein and zeaxanthin. These two carotenoids are found within the entire retina and macula and are thought to protect this area from light-mediated damage via an antioxidant mechanism. Zeaxanthin is found mainly in the macular region, while lutein is found throughout the retina.[90] Epidemiological studies have indicated a relationship between intake of vegetables containing lutein and zeaxanthin and decreased risk for macular degeneration.[91,92]

Carotenoids and the Immune Response

Dietary patterns have long been thought to influence the activity of the immune system, but not until recently have studies shown the mechanisms by which nutrients, including carotenoids, modulate the immune response. It is important to remember, though, that *in vivo* studies conducted with pro-VA carotenoids may yield results that are attributed to the conversion of carotenoids to VA or retinoids, not the effects of the intact carotenoid.

A recent study by Hughes *et al.* provides information on the mechanisms by which β-carotene may enable immune cells to act more efficiently.[83] In this study, subjects were supplemented for 26 days with either 15 mg β-carotene or placebo. Subjects receiving the β-carotene treatment had an increase in expression of adhesion molecules by monocytes, an increase in *ex vivo* secretion of tumor necrosis factor-α, and an increased percentage of monocytes expressing MHC II, a cell surface molecule responsible for presenting antigen to T-helper cells.

A series of studies by Jyonouchi *et al.* have focused on the carotenoid astaxanthin and its *in vitro* and *in vivo* effects on several parameters of the immune response.[100-103,111] In these studies, astaxanthin has been shown to be more effective than β-carotene in enhancing T cell-dependent immune responses. The effects seen, therefore, are not thought to be mediated via a conversion to retinoids since astaxanthin does not possess VA activity.

Other aspects of the immune response that carotenoids are thought to modulate include increasing natural killer cell activity in the elderly,[112,113] increasing lymphocyte response to mitogens,[114,115] protection of immune cells from their own bactericidal production of reactive species,[116] and increasing total white blood cells and CD4/CD8 ratios in HIV infected humans.[117]

Modulation of Gap Junctions

Non-transformed cells communicate via either hormonal signals or gap junctional communication. Cell-cell communication is essential for tissue homeostasis. Alterations in the way in which cells communicate may lead to uncontrolled cell growth and ultimately to cancer. Most gap junctions are comprised of a six sub-unit protein termed connexin. These proteins form pores in cellular membranes and allow the transfer of molecules between adjacent cells. Molecules that flow through gap junctions are small (less than 1000 daltons in weight) and may be charged or uncharged. Signaling molecules such as cAMP, calcium, and inositol triphosphate have been shown to move from cell to cell via gap junctions and are important in the maintenance of controlled, uniform growth of cells.[118]

Carotenoids have been implicated in increasing cell-cell communication via up-regulation of gap-junctions, specifically by increasing connexin-43 expression. Zhang *et al.* were the first to investigate the potential ability of carotenoids to increase cell-cell communication.[80] This group had previously shown that carotenoids inhibit neoplastic transformation *in vitro*[119] and hypothesized that carotenoids inhibited transformation by increasing cell-cell communication. In this study they utilized a mouse embryo fibroblast cell line (C3H/10T1/2) to investigate the ability of six carotenoids (lycopene, α- and β-carotene, canthaxanthin, lutein, and methyl bixin) to increase cell-cell transfer of a fluorescent dye. Carotenoids were introduced into cell media via tetrahydrofuran (THF) as a vehicle. Cells treated with β-carotene, canthaxanthin, and lutein increased intercellular dye transfer at concentrations of 10^{-5} M over a 28-day period. Lycopene increased only intercellular transfer for 14 days post-treatment. To investigate whether the increase in cellular communication seen was due to the conversion of carotenoids to retinoids, this group looked at expression of connexin-43 in the same cell culture model.[98] They found that treatment with 10^{-5} M β-carotene, canthaxanthin, or lycopene increased expression of connexin-43 mRNA and protein. Treatment with canthaxanthin, however, did not upregulate the gene encoding the retinoic acid receptor-β (RAR-β). Since the RAR-β gene is known to respond only to retinoids, these findings suggest that carotenoids do not act via conversion to retinoids to increase connexin-43 expression.

Hanusch *et al.* have shed more light on the mechanism by which carotenoids, namely canthaxanthin, enhance gap junctional communication.[79] This group isolated decomposition products of canthaxanthin and tested their ability to stimulate expression of connexin-43 mRNA *in vitro*. Two oxidative decomposition products, *all-trans* and 13-*cis*-4-oxoretinoic acid were shown to increase connexin-43 mRNA expression at 10^{-6} M. Canthaxanthin itself was also shown to be active, but at higher concentrations (10^{-5} M). This finding is of particular interest because of the recent finding that 4-oxoretinol as well as 4-oxoretinoic acid are both ligands for RAR-β.[120,121]

Stahl *et al.* have further investigated the ability of other natural and synthetic carotenoids to induce gap junctional communication.[71] They found that carotenoids with six-membered rings are efficient at inducing gap-junctional communication, while synthetic carotenoids with only five-membered rings are not as effective. The addition of oxygen atoms to the ring structure appears to have little effect on gap junctional induction.

It is important to consider, though, that carotenoids are relatively unstable under the cell culture conditions of light and heat. Carotenoids are also insoluble in water, so delivery of carotenoids to cell culture systems is difficult. Williams *et al.* have shown that the most physiological vehicle to deliver carotenoids to cell culture is lipoproteins.[122] High amounts of carotenoid degradation were seen during typical cell culture incubations when THF, liposomes, or water dispersible beadlets, but not carotenoid-rich lipoprotein, were used as delivery vehicles to cells in culture. Ninety-five percent of the β-carotene remained in the media after a 72-hour incubation when lipoproteins were used as the delivery method while only 37 percent remained when THF was used. Since cells take up only a small percentage of the initial carotenoid from the media, carotenoid degradation to various metabolites, not the intact carotenoid, may modulate some of the protective functions seen in cell culture studies.

Carotenoids and Cardiovascular Disease

Because carotenoids are primarily transported in low-density lipoprotein (LDL) in serum and because they have been shown to be good quenchers of reactive species, their role in the prevention of LDL oxidation and hence reducing risk of cardiovascular disease has been investigated. Several epidemiological studies support a role for β-carotene in the prevention of heart disease. These studies will be reviewed elsewhere in this book.

In vitro models of LDL oxidation have produced equivocal results. Jialal *et al.* have shown β-carotene at 2 μM to inhibit both cell-free copper induced LDL oxidation and uptake of modified LDL by a human macrophage cell line.[89] Using laser Doppler electrophoresis, Packer *et al.* have shown β-carotene to protect LDL from oxidation. In both of these studies, β-carotene was incorporated into LDL *in vitro*.[76]

Conversely, Reaven *et al.*,[96] Princen *et al.*,[95] and Gaziano *et al.*,[94] have shown β-carotene to be ineffective at preventing LDL oxidation *in vitro* after *in vivo* supplementation of human subjects with β-carotene. In all studies, supplementation raised serum and LDL β-carotene concentrations.

A recent study by Fuhrman *et al.* has suggested that β-carotene and lycopene may be able to act independently of their antioxidant properties to lower LDL cholesterol and upregulate LDL receptor activity.[123] In this study, 10 μM β-carotene or lycopene inhibited cholesterol synthesis from ^{3}H-acetate, but not from ^{14}C-mevalonate in a macrophage cell line. Since carotenoids are synthesized in plants via the HMG-CoA pathway, the authors suggest that carotenoids may act via a feedback mechanism to inhibit HMG-CoA reductase in humans. An *in vivo* trial conducted in this same study resulted in a 14% decrease in plasma LDL-cholesterol with supplementation of 60 mg/d lycopene for 3 months in 6 males.

Modulation of Xenobiotic Metabolizing Enzymes

Dietary factors have been shown to modulate expression and/or activity of xenobiotic metabolizing enzymes. Phase I xenobiotic metabolizing enzymes act to add a polar group onto many foreign substances. In many cases phase I enzymes activate a procarcinogen into a carcinogen. Phase II enzymes further act on xenobiotics to make them unreactive and more easily excreted. Ideally then, increasing activity of phase II enzymes without increasing activity of phase I enzymes would allow for efficient clearance of xenobiotics from the body and less risk of damage by the potential carcinogens.

The evidence for a role of carotenoids in modulating activities of phase I and phase II enzymes is uncertain at this time. Gradelet *et al.* have shown canthaxanthin, astaxanthin, and β-Apo-8'-carotenal to be inducers of both phase I and phase II enzymes in the liver of the male rat.[86,87] *Trans* and *cis*-β-carotene, lutein, and lycopene had little if any effect on the activities of rat liver xenobiotic metabolizing enzymes. In mice, Astorg *et al.* have recently shown that canthaxanthin increased phase I CYP-1A activity while β-carotene, astaxanthin, and β-apo-8'-carotenal had no effect.[85] Astaxanthin and canthaxanthin increased phase II NAD(P)H:quinone reductase (QR) activity. Wang *et al.* have shown β-carotene, but not lycopene, to induce QR in human colon cancer cells. This effect is thought to be mediated by retinoids rather than by β-carotene itself. No effect was seen by any treatment on glutathione-s-transferase, another phase II enzyme.[88] In a study designed to investigate lifestyle and nutritional correlates of phase I CYP1A2 activity in humans, Le Marchand *et al.* have found that in both healthy and colorectal cancer patients plasma lutein was negatively correlated with activity, while plasma lycopene was positively correlated with CYP1A2 activity. More research on the mechanisms by which carotenoids may modulate detoxifying enzymes is needed.[124]

RECOMMENDATIONS

The typical intake of β-carotene in the U.S. is 3.0 mg/d. Total carotenoid intakes have been shown to be 5-7 mg/d.[125] As with all dietary substances, more is not necessarily better. Data from recent intervention studies have failed to demonstrate a protective effect of β-carotene supplementation at 20 mg/d,[126] or 30 mg/d β-carotene taken with 25,000 IU VA on lung cancer incidence in smokers.[127] On the other hand, β-carotene intakes of greater than 4.0 mg/d are associated with reduced risk of chronic diseases in most epidemiological studies.[128] In these studies the carotenoids ingested were from whole foods, not from supplements.

It has been postulated that up to 70% of all cancers are related to dietary intake.[129] The American Cancer Society currently recommends the consumption of five servings of fruits and/or vegetables per day to lower the risk of cancer. Eating "five a day" would provide at least 5.0 mg/d β-carotene. These recommendations are based on the concept that whole foods provide many chemoprotective compounds such as carotenoids and vitamin C as well as other potentially protective compounds not found in supplements. A synergy may also exist between protective compounds found in whole foods. For example, the role of vitamin C in the recycling of vitamin E is well known.[130] Some compounds found in whole foods may act only in a protective manner when other compounds are ingested with them. They may not be protective when ingested alone in supplemental form. Thus, the consumption of a diet high in carotenoids (from foods) appears to protect against many cancers and other chronic diseases. This protective effect, however, may not be attributed to carotenoids alone, but to the combination of nutrients found in these whole foods.

REFERENCES

1. Olson JA, Krinsky NI. Introduction: the colorful, fascinating world of the carotenoids: important physiological modulators. FASEB Journal 1995;9:1547-1550.
2. Britton G. Structure and properties of carotenoids in relation to function. FASEB Journal 1995;9:1551-1558.
3. Olson JA. The conversion of radioactive β-carotene into vitamin A by rat small intestine *in vivo*. Journal of Biological Chemistry 1961;236:349-356.
4. Olson JA. Provitamin A function of carotenoids: the conversion of β-carotene into vitamin A. Journal of Nutrition 1989;119:105-108.
5. Khachik F, Spangler CJ, Cecil J, Smith J. Identification, quantification, and relative concentrations of carotenoids and their metabolites in human milk and serum. Analytical Chemistry 1997;69:1873-1881.
6. Rock CL, Swendseid ME. Plasma β-carotene response in humans after meals supplemented with dietary pectin. American Journal of Clinical Nutrition 1992;55:96-99.
7. Stahl W, Schwarz W, Sundquist AR, Sies H. *Cis-trans* isomers of lycopene and β-carotene in human serum and tissues. Archives of Biochemistry and Biophysics 1992;294:173-177.
8. Hebuterne X, Wang X-D, Johnson E, Krinsky NI, Russell RM. Intestinal absorption and metabolism of 9-*cis* β-carotene *in vivo*: biosynthesis of 9-*cis* retinoic acid. Journal of Lipid Research 1995;36:1264-1273.
9. Nagao A, Olson JA. Enzymatic formation of 9-*cis*, 13-*cis*, and *all-trans* retinals from isomers of β-carotene. FASEB Journal 1994;8:968-973.
10. Clinton SK, Emenhiser C, Schwartz SJ, Bostwick DG, Williams AW, Moore BJ, John W. Erdman J. *cis-trans* lycopene isomers, carotenoids, and retinol in the human prostate. Cancer Epidemiology, Biomarkers & Prevention 1996;5:823-833.
11. Stahl W, Sies H. Uptake of lycopene and its geometrical isomers is greater from heat-processed than from unprocessed tomato juice in humans. Journal of Nutrition 1992;122:2161-2166.
12. Gaziano JM, Johnson EJ, Russell RM, Manson JE, Stampfer MJ, Ridker PM, *et al.* Discrimination in absorption or transport of β-carotene isomers after oral supplementation with either *all*-trans or 9-*cis* β-carotene. American Journal of Clinical Nutrition 1995;61(1995):1248-1252.
13. Hollander D. Intestinal absorption of vitamins A, E, D, and K. The Journal of Laboratory and Clinical Medicine 1981;97:449-462.
14. Simmonds WJ. The role of micellar solubilization in lipid absorption. Australian Journal of Experimental Biology and Medical Sciences 1972;50:403-421.
15. Dimitrov NV, Meyer C, Ullrey DE, Chenoweth W, Michelakis A, Malone W, Boone C, Fink G. Bioavailability of β-carotene in humans. American Journal of Clinical Nutrition 1988;48:298-304.
16. Prince MR, Frisoli JK. Beta-carotene accumulation in serum and skin. American Journal of Clinical Nutrition 1993;57:175-181.
17. Hollander D, Muralidhara KS. Vitamin A intestinal absorption *in vivo*: influence of luminal factors on transport. American Journal of Physiology 1977;232:E471-E477.
18. Van Vliet T, Van Schaik F, Van Den Berg H. Beta-carotene metabolism: the enzymatic cleavage to retinal. Voeding 1992;53:186-190.
19. Wang XD, Krinsky NI, Tang G, Russell RM. Retinoic acid can be produced from exentric cleavage of β-carotene in human intestinal mucosa. Archives Chemistry, Biochemistry and Biophysics 1992;293:298-304.

20. Blomstrand R, Werner B. Studies on the intestinal absoprtion of radioactive β-carotene and vitamin A in man. Scandinavian Journal of Clinical Laboratory Investigation 1967;19:339-345.
21. Parker RS. Absorption, metabolism, and transport of carotenoids. FASEB Journal 1996;10:542-551.
22. Johnson EJ, Russell RM. Distribution of orally administered β-carotene among lipoproteins in healthy men. American Journal of Clinical Nutrition 1992;56:128-135.
23. Ziouzenkova O, Winklhofer-Roob BM, Puhl H, Roob JM, Esterbauer H. Lack of correlation between the alpha tocopherol content of plasma and LDL, but high correlations for gamma tocopherol and carotenoids. Journal of Lipid Research 1996;37:1936-1946.
24. Clevidence BA, Bieri JG. Association of carotenoids with human plasma lipoproteins. In: Abelson J, Simon MI, editors. *Methods in Enzymology*. Volume 214. San Diego: Academic Press, Inc.; 1993. 33-46.
25. Reddy PP, Clevidence BA, Berlin E, Taylor PR, Bieri JG, Smith JC. Plasma carotenoid content and vitamin E profile of lipoprotein fractions of men fed a controlled typical U.S. diet. FASEB J. 1989;3:A955.
26. Khachik F, Beecher GR, J. Cecil Smith J. Lutein, lycopene, and their oxidative metabolites in chemoprevention of cancer. Journal of Cellular Biochemistry 1995;22(supplement):236-246.
27. Parker RS. Carotenoids in human blood and tissues. Journal of Nutrition 1989;119:101-104.
28. Bowen PE, Mobarhan S, J. Cecil Smith J. Carotenoid absorption in humans. Methods in Enzymology 1993;214:3-17.
29. Van Vliet T, Schreurs WH, Van Den Berg H. Intestinal β-carotene absorption and cleavage in men: response of β-carotene and retinyl esters in the triglyceride-rich lipoprotein fraction after a single oral dose of β-carotene. American Journal of Clinical 1995;62:110-116.
30. NCHS. Unpublished NHANES III data 1996. Washington, D.C.
31. Brady WE, Mares-Perlman JA, Bowen P, Stacewicz-Sapuntzakis M. Human serum carotenoid concentrations are related to physiologic and lifestyle factors. Journal of Nutrition 1996;126:129-137.
32. Elinder LS, Hadell K, Johansson J, Holme JM, Olsson AG, Walldius G. Probucol treatment decreases serum concentrations of diet-derived antioxidants. Arteriosclerosis, Thrombosis and Vascular Biology 1995;15:1057-1063.
33. Schmitz HH, Poor CL, Wellman RB, Erdman JW, Jr. Concentrations of selected carotenoids and vitamin A in human liver, kidney and lung tissue. Journal of Nutrition 1991;121:1613-1621.
34. Kaplan LA, Lau JM, Stein EA. Carotenoid composition, concentrations and relationships in various human organs. Clinical Physiology and Biochemistry 1990;8:1-10.
35. Parker RS. Bioavailability of carotenoids. European Journal of Clinical Nutrition 1997;51(Suppl. 1):S86-S90.
36. Erdman JW, Jr., Bierer TL, Gugger ET. Absorption and transport of carotenoids. Annals of the New York Academy of Sciences 1993;691(Carotenoids in Human Health):76-85.
37. Micozzi MS, Brown ED, Edwards BK, Bieri JG, Taylor PR, Khachik F, Beecher GR, J. Cecil Smith J. Plasma carotenoid response to chronic intake of selected foods β-carotene supplements in men. American Journal of Clinical Nutrition 1992;55:1120-1125.
38. Kostic D, White WS, Olson JA. Intestinal absorption, serum clearance, and interactions between lutein and β-carotene when administered to human adults in separate and combined oral doses. American Journal of Clinical Nutrition 1995;62:604-610.

39. Gärtner C, Stahl W, Sies H. Preferential increase in chylomicron levels of the xanthophylls lutein and zeaxanthin compared to β-carotene in the human. International Journal of Vitamin Research 1996;66:119-125.
40. White WS, Stacewicz-Sapuntzakis M, Erdman JW, Bowen PE. Pharmacokinetics of β-carotene and canthaxanthin after ingestion of individual and combined doses by human subjects. Journal of the American College of Nutrition 1994;13:665-671.
41. White WS, Peck KM, Bierer TL, Gugger ET, Erdman JW. Interactions of oral β-carotene and canthaxanthin in ferrets. Journal of Nutrition 1993;123:1405-1413.
42. Brown ED, Blakely SR, Babu U, Grundel E, Mitchell GV. Vegetable concentrates interact with canthaxanthin to affect carotenoid bioavailability and superoxide dismutase activity but not immune response in rats. Nutrition Research 1997;17:989-998.
43. Ben-Amotz A, Levy Y. Bioavailability of a natural isomer mixture compared with synthetic *all-trans* β-carotene. American Journal of Clinical Nutrition 1996;63:729-734.
44. Stahl W, Schwarz W, Laar Jv, Sies H. *All*-trans β-carotene preferentially accumulates in human chylomicrons and very low density lipoproteins compared with the 9-*cis* geometrical isomer. Journal of Nutrition 1995;125:2128-2133.
45. Tamai H, Morinobu T, Murata T, Manago M, Mino M. 9-*cis*-β-carotene in human plasma and blood cells after ingestion of β-carotene. Lipids 1995;30:493-498.
46. Stahl W, Schwarz W, Sies H. Human serum concentrations of *all-trans* β-carotene and alpha-carotene but not 9-*cis* β-carotene increase upon ingestion of a natural isomer mixture obtained from *Dunaliella salina* (Betatene). Journal of Nutrition 1993;123:847-851.
47. You C-S, Parker RS, Goodman KJ, Swanson JE, Corso TN. Evidence of *cis-trans* isomerization of 9-*cis*-β-carotene during absorption in humans. American Journal of Clinical Nutrition 1996;64:177-183.
48. Wang X-D. Review: absorption and metabolism of β-carotene. Journal of the American College of Nutrition 1994;13:314-325.
49. Heyman RA, Mangelsdorf DJ, Dyck JA, Stein RB, Eichele G, Evans RM, Thaller C. 9-*cis* retinoic acid is a high affinity ligand for the retinoid X receptor. Cell 1992;68:397-406.
50. Xu MJ, Plezia PM, Alberts DS, Emerson SS, Peng YM, Sayers SM, Liu Y, Ritenbaugh C, Gensler HL. Reduction in plasma or skin alpha-tocopherol concentrations with long-term oral administration of beta-carotene in humans and mice. Journal of the National Cancer Institute 1992;84:1559-1565.
51. Nierenberg DW, Stukel TA, Mott LA, Greenberg ER. Steady-state serum concentration of alpha tocopherol not altered by supplementation with oral beta carotene. Journal of the National Cancer Institute 1994;86:117-120.
52. Willett WC, Stampfer MJ, Underwood BA, Taylor JO, Hennekens CH. Vitamins A, E, and carotene: effects of supplementation on their plasma levels. American Journal of Clinical Nutrition 1983;38:559-566.
53. Rodriguez-Amaya DB. Critical review of provitamin A determination in plant foods. Journal of Micronutrient Analysis 1989;5:191-225.
54. Mangels AR, Holden JM, Beecher GR, Forman MR, Lanza E. Carotenoid content of fruits and vegetables: an evaluation of analytic data. Journal of the American Dietetic Association 1993;93:284-296.
55. Chug-Ahuja JK, Holden JM, Forman MR, Mangels AR, Beecher GR, Lanza E. The development and application of a carotenoid database for fruits, vegetables, and selected multicomponent foods. Journal of the American Dietetic Association 1993;93:318-323.
56. Tonucci LH, Holden JM, Beecher GR, Khachik F, Davis CS, Mulokozi G. Carotenoid content of thermally processed tomato-based food products. Journal of Agriculture and Food Chemistry 1995;43:579-586.

57. Dietz JM, Kantha SS, Erdman JW. Reversed phase HPLC analysis of α-carotene and β-carotene from selected raw and cooked vegetables. Plant Foods for Human Nutrition 1988;38:333-341.
58. Poor CL, Bierer TL, Merchen NR, George C. Fahey J, Erdman JW. The accumulation of alpha and beta-carotene in serum and tissue of preruminant calves fed raw and steamed carrots. Journal of Nutrition 1993;123:1296-1304.
59. Kopas-Lane LM, Warthesen JJ. Carotenoid photostability in raw spinach and carrots during cold storage. Journal of Food Science 1995;60:773-776.
60. Cano MP, Ancos Bd. Carotenoid and carotenoid ester composition in mango fruit as influenced by processing method. Journal of Agricultural and Food Chemistry 1994;42:2737-2742.
61. Micozzi MS, Beecher GR, Taylor PR, Khachik F. Carotenoid analysis of selected raw and cooked foods associated with a lower risk for cancer. Journal of the National Cancer Institute 1990;82:282-285.
62. Khachik F, Beecher GR, Goli MB, Lusby WR. Separation, identification, and quantification of carotenoids in fruits, vegetables and human plasma by high performance liquid chromatography. Pure & Applied Chemistry 1991;63:71-80.
63. Chandler LA, Schwartz SJ. HPLC separation of *cis-trans* carotene isomers in fresh and processed fruits and vegetables. Journal of Food Science 1987;52:669-672.
64. Yadav SK, Sehgal S. Effect of home processing on ascorbic acid and β-carotene content of spinach (*Spinacia oleracia*) and amaranth (*Amaranthus tricolor*) leaves. Plant Foods for Human Nutrition 1995;47:125-131.
65. de Pee S, West CE, Muhilal, Karyadi D, Hautvast GAJ. Lack of improvement in vitamin A status with increased consumption of dark-green leafy vegetables. Lancet 1995;346:75-81.
66. Wolf G. The enzymatic cleavage of β-carotene: still controversial. Nutrition Reviews 1995;53:134-137.
67. Solomons NW. Plant sources of Vitamin A and human nutrition: renewed strategies. Nutrition Reviews 1996;54:89-91.
68. Foote CS, Chang YC, Denny RW. Chemistry of singlet oxygen. X. Carotenoid quenching parallels biological protection. Journal of the American Chemical Society 1970;92:5216-5218.
69. Hirayama O, Nakamura K, Hamada S, Kobayasi Y. Singlet oxygen quenching ability of naturally occuring carotenoids. Lipids 1994;29:149-150.
70. Di Mascio P, Kaiser S, Sies H. Lycopene as the most efficient biological carotenoid singlet oxygen quencher. Archives of Biochemistry and Biophysics 1989;274:532-538.
71. Stahl W, Nicolai S, Briviba K, Hanusch M, *et al.* Biological activities of natural and synthetic carotenoids: induction of gap junctional communication and singlet oxygen quenching. Carcinogenesis 1997;18:89-92.
72. Burton GW, Ingold KU. β-Carotene: an unusual type of lipid antioxidant. Science 1984;224:569-573.
73. Levin G, Yeshurun M, Mokady S. *In vivo* antiperoxidative effect of 9-*cis* β-carotene compared with that of the *all-trans* isomer. Nutrition and Cancer 1997;27:293-297.
74. Liebler DC. Antioxidant reactions of carotenoids. Annals of the New York Academy of Sciences 1993;691:20-31.
75. Olson JA. Vitamin A and carotenoids as antioxidants in a physiological context. Journal of Nutrition Science Vitaminology 1993;39:s57-s65.
76. Packer L. Antioxidant action of carotenoids *in vitro* and *in vivo* and protection against oxidation of human low-density lipoproteins. Annals of The New York Academy of Sciences 1993;691:48-60.

77. Bertram J. Cancer prevention by carotenoids: mechanistic studies in cultured cells. Annals of The New York Academy of Sciences 1993;691:177-191.
78. Bertram JS, Bortkiewicz H. Dietary carotenoids inhibit neoplastic transformation and modulate gene expression in mouse and human cells. American Journal of Clinical Nutrition 1995;62(suppl):1327s-1336s.
79. Hanusch M, Stahl W, Schulz WA, Sies H. Induction of gap junctional communication by 4-oxoretinoic acid generated from its precursor canthaxanthin. Archives of Biochemistry and Biophysics 1995;317:423-428.
80. Zhang L-X, Cooney RV, Bertram JS. Carotenoids enhance gap junctional communication and inhibit lipid peroxidation in C3H/10T1/2 cells: relationship to their cancer chemopreventive action. Carcinogenesis 1991;12:2109-2114.
81. Bendich A. Carotenoids and the immune response. Journal of Nutrition 1989;119:112-115.
82. Bendich A. Biological functions of dietary carotenoids. Annals of the New York Academy of the Sciences 1993;691:61-67.
83. Hughes DA, Wright AJA, Finglas PM, Peerless ACJ, Bailey AL, Astley SB, Pinder AC, Southon S. The effect of β-carotene supplementation on the immune function of blood monocytes from healthy male nonsmokers. Journal of Laboratory and Clinical Medicine 1997;129:309-317.
84. Baker KR, Meydani M. β-Carotene as an antioxidant in immunity and cancer. Journal of Optimal Nutrition 1994;3:39-50.
85. Astorg P, Gradelet S, Leclerc J, Siess MH. Effects of provitamin A or non-provitamin A carotenoids on liver xenobiotic-metabolizing enzymes in mice. Nutrition and Cancer 1997;27:245-249.
86. Gradelet S, Leclerc J, Siess M-H, Astorg PO. β-Apo-carotenal, but not β-carotene, is a strong inducer of liver cytochromes p4501A1 and 1A2 in rat. Xenobiotica 1996;26:909-919.
87. Gradelet S, Astorg PO, Leclerc J, Chevalier J, Vernevaut MF, Siess M-H. Effects of canthaxanthin, astaxanthin, lycopene and lutein on liver xenobiotic-metabolizing enzymes in the rat. Xenobiotica 1996;26:49-63.
88. Wang W, Higuchi CM. Induction of NAD(P)H:quinone reductase by vitamins A, E, and C in Colo205 colon cancer cells. Cancer Letters 1995;98:63-69.
89. Jialal I, Norkus EP, Cristol L, Grundy SM. β-Carotene inhibits the oxidative modification of low-density lipoprotein. Biochimica et Biophysica Acta. 1991;1086:134-138.
90. Handelman GJ, Dratz EA, Reay CC, van Kuijk JG. Carotenoids in the human macula and whole retina. Investigative Opthamology and Visual Science 1988;29:850-855.
91. Seddon JM, Ajani UA, Sperduto RD, Hiller R, *et al.* Dietary carotenoids, vitamins A, C, and E, and advanced age-related macular degeneration. JAMA 1994; 272:1413-1420.
92. Snodderly DM. Evidence for protection against age-related macular degeneration by carotenoids and antioxidant vitamins. American Journal of Clinical Nutrition 1995;62(suppl):1448s-1461s.
93. Mathews-Roth MM. Carotenoids in erythropoietic protoporphyria and other photosensitivity diseases. Annals of the New York Academy of Sciences 1993;691:127-138.
94. Gaziano JM, Hatta A, Flynn M, Johnson EJ, Krinsky NI, Ridker PM, Hennekens CH, Frei B. Supplementaion with β-carotene *in vivo* and *in vitro* does not inhibit low density lipoprotein oxidation. Atherosclerosis 1995;112:187-195.
95. Princen HMG, Poppel Gv, Vogelezang C, Buytenhek R, Kok FJ. Supplementation with Vitamin E but not β-carotene *in vivo* protects low density lipoprotein from lipid peroxidation *in vitro*: effect of cigarette smoking. Arteriosclerosis and Thrombosis 1992;12:554-562.

96. Reaven PD, Khouw A, Beltz WF, Parthasarathy S, witztum JL. Effect of dietary antioxidant combinations in humans; protection of LDL by vitamin E but not β-carotene. Arterioscelrosis and Thrombosis 1993;13:590-600.
97. Giovannucci E, Ascherio A, Rimm EB, Stampfer MJ, Colditz GA, Willet WC. Intake of carotenoids and retinol in relation to prostate cancer risk. Journal of the National Cancer Institute 1995;87:1767-1776.
98. Zhang L-X, Cooney RV, Bertram JS. Carotenoids up-regulate connexin 43 expression independent of their provitamin A or antioxidant properties. Cancer Research 1992;52:5707-5712.
99. Schalch W. Carotenoids in the retina: a review of their possible role in preventing or limiting damage caused by light and oxygen. Free Radicals and Aging 1992:280-298.
100. Jyonouchi H, Hill RJ, Tomita Y, Good RA. Studies of immunomodulating actions of carotenoids: I. Effects of β-carotene and astaxanthin on murine lymphocyte functions and cell surface marker expression in *in vitro* culture system. Nutrition and Cancer 1991;16:93-105.
101. Jyonouchi H, Zang L, Gross M, Tomita Y. Immunomodulating actions of carotenoids: enhancement of *in vivo* and *in vitro* antibody production to T-dependent antigens. Nutrition and Cancer 1994;21:47-58.
102. Jyonouchi H, Sun S, Gross M. Effect of carotenoids on *in vitro* immunoglobin production by human peripheral blood mononuclear cells: astaxanthin, a carotenoid without vitamin A activity, enhances *in vitro* response to a T-dependent stimulant antigen. Nutrition and Cancer 1995;23:171-183.
103. Jyonouchi H, Sun S, Tomita Y, Gross MD. Astaxanthin, a carotenoid without vitamin A activity, augments antibody responses in cultures including T-helper cell clones and suboptimal doses of antigen. Journal of Nutrition 1995;125:2483-2492.
104. Ames BN, Shigenaga MK, Hagen TM. Oxidants, antioxidants, and the degenerative diseases of aging. Proceedings of the National Academy of Science 1993;90:7915-7922.
105. Krinsky NI. The biological properties of carotenoids. Pure and Applied Chemistry 1994;66:1003-1010.
106. Tinkler JH, Bohm F, Schalch W, Truscott TG. Dietary carotenoids protect human cells from damage. Journal of Photochemistry and Photobiology B: Biology 1994;26:283-285.
107. Burton GW. Antioxidant actions of carotenoids. Journal of Nutrition 1989;119:109-111.
108. Martin KR, Failla ML, Smith JC, Jr. β-Carotene and lutein protect HepG2 human liver cells against oxidant-induced damage. Journal of Nutrition 1996;126:2098-2106.
109. Levin G, Mokady S. Antioxidant activity 9-*cis* compared to *all-trans* β-carotene *in vitro*. Free Radicals in Biology and Medicine 1994;17:77-82.
110. Gerster H. Review: antioxidant protection of the ageing macula. Age and Ageing 1991;20:60-69.
111. Jyonouchi H, Sun S, Mizokami M, Gross MD. Effects of various carotenoids on cloned effector-stage T-helper cell activity. Nutrition and Cancer 1996;26:313-324.
112. Santos MS, Meydani SN, Leka L, Wu D, *et al.* Natural killer cell activity in elderly men is enhanced by β-carotene supplementation. American Journal of Clinical Nutrition 1996;64:772-777.
113. Prabhala RH, Garewal HS, Meyskens FL, Watson RR. Immunomodulation in humans by β-carotene and vitamin A. Nutrition Research 1990;10:1473-1786.
114. Bendich A, Shapiro SS. Effect of β-carotene and canthaxanthin on the immune responses of the rat. Journal of Nutrition 1986;116:2254-2262.
115. Kramer TR, Burri BJ. Modulated mitogenic proliferative responsiveness of lymphocytes in whole-blood cultures after a low-carotene diet and mixed-carotenoid supplementation in women. American Journal of Clinical Nutrition 1997;65:871-875.

116. Anderson R, Theron AJ. Physiological potential of ascorbate, β-carotene and α-tocopherol individually in combination in the prevention of tissue damage, carcinogenesis and immune dysfunction mediated by phagocyte-derived reactive oxidants. World Review of Nutrition and Diet 1990;62:27-58.
117. Coodley G, Nelson H, Loveless MO, Folk C. β-Carotene in HIV infection. Journal of Acquired Immune Deficiency Syndromes 1993;6:272-276.
118. Yamasaki H. Gap junctional intercellular communication and carcinogenesis. Carcinogenesis 1990;11:1051-1058.
119. Bertram JS, Pung A, Churley M, Kappock TJ, Wilkins LR, Conney RV. Diverse carotenoids protect against chemically induced neoplastic transformation. Carcinogenesis 1991(671-678).
120. Pijnappel W, Hendriks H, Folkers G, *et al.* The retinoid ligand 4-oxo-retinoic acid is a highly active modulator of positional specification. Nature 1993;366:340-344.
121. Achkar C, Derguini F, Blumberg B, *et al.* 4-oxoretinol, a new natural ligand and transactivator of the retinoic acid receptors. Proceedings of the National Academy of Sciences 1996;93:4879-84.
122. Williams AW, Boileau TWM, Clinton SK, Erdman JW, Jr. β-Carotene-enriched bovine serum - a physiological vehicle to deliver carotenoids to prostate cancer cells in culture. FASEB J. 1996;10(abstract):A241.
123. Fuhrman B, Elis A, Aviram M. Hypocholesterolemic effect of lycopene and β-carotene is related to suppression of cholesterol synthesis and augmentation of LDL receptor activity in macrophages. Biochemical and Biophysical Research Communications 1997;233:658-662.
124. Marchand LL, Franke AA, Custer L, Wilkens LR, Cooney RV. Lifestyle and nutritional correlates of cytochrome CYP1A2 activity; inverse association with plasma lutein and alpha-tocopherol. Pharmacogenetics 1997;7:11-19.
125. Nebeling LC, Forman MR, Graubard BI, Snyder RA. The impact of lifestyle characteristics on carotenoid intake in the United States: the 1987 national health interview survey. American Journal of Public Health 1997;87:268-271.
126. The ATBC Group. The effect of vitamin E and beta carotene on the incidence of lung cancer and other cancers in male smokers. The New England Journal of Medicine 1994;330:1029-1035.
127. Omenn G, Goodman G, Thornquist M, Balmes J, Cullen M, *et al.* Effects of a combination of beta carotene and vitamin A on lung cancer and cardiovascular disease. The New England Journal of Medicine 1996;334:1150-1155.
128. CARIG. Beta-carotene and the carotenoids: beyond the intervention trials. Nutrition Reviews 1996;54:185-188.
129. Steinmetz KA, Potter JD. Vegetables, fruit, and cancer prevention: A review. Journal of the American Dietetic Association 1996;96:1027-1039.
130. Groff JL, Gropper SS. *Advanced Nutrition and Human Metabolism.* St. Paul, MN: West Publication Company; 1995.

9

Vitamin C

Steven C. Rumsey, Yaohui Wang, and Mark Levine

National Institute of Diabetes and Digestive and Kidney Diseases
National Institutes of Health, Bethesda, Maryland, USA

INTRODUCTION

Vitamin C (ascorbic acid) is a required nutrient for humans. Most animals are capable of synthesizing ascorbic acid with the exception of humans, non-human primates, Indian fruit bats, bulbuls, guinea pigs, and some fish.[1] Humans and non-human primates lack the enzyme gulonolactone oxidase which catalyzes the last step in the endogenous synthesis of ascorbic acid from glucose.[2]

Lack of ascorbate in the diet leads to the deficiency disease scurvy. Scurvy is characterized by small areas of bleeding under the skin, coiled hairs, bleeding gums, hyperkeratosis, joint pain, shortness of breath, and lethargy.[3-5] Fatigue is an important early symptom in vitamin C deficiency. It was mentioned in James Lind's classic work on scurvy in sailors more than 200 years ago[6] and was noted to be the first symptom of deficiency in a recent study at the National Institutes of Health.[7] Overt ascorbate deficiency can still be found in the United States in people with cancer cachexia, poor intake, malabsorption, alcoholism, or chemical dependency.[8] Because a substantial fraction of the population ingests <1 fruit or vegetable daily,[9-11] subclinical vitamin C deficiency may be much more common than overt deficiency. The current recommendation of ascorbate intake given by the Food and Nutrition Board of the National Academy of Sciences, last updated in 1989, is 60 mg/day.[12] This recommendation was arrived at by estimating, based on available data at the time, the amount of ascorbate required to maintain body stores and to avoid deficiency for up to a month of total absence of vitamin C in the diet. Recent data, however, suggest that the data upon which these recommendations are based may be flawed,[7] and that recommended intake should be higher than 60 mg/day. These issues will be discussed more fully below. In addition, evidence exists that specific populations may have increased requirements. Consequently, the recommended intake for pregnant women is 70 mg/day, for lactating women 95 mg/day, and for smokers is 100 mg/day.[12]

The basis of the Food and Nutrition Board recommendation regarding vitamin C was to prevent deficiency disease. Little consideration was given to amounts of ascorbic acid intake that may be appropriate for optimal health.[13] This is primarily due to the inherent difficulty of achieving a satisfactory definition of optimal health, especially based on biochemical criteria. However, because of scientific advances and the decreased prevalence of overt deficiency diseases in recent years, investigators in the field of nutrition have become increasingly focused on disease prevention and have begun to define ways to scientifically examine the elusive concept of optimal health.[14]

Various investigators have postulated a role of ascorbic acid in the prevention of cancer, heart disease, and in the augmentation of immune function such as in the prevention of the common cold.[15,16] A scientific consensus concerning the efficacy of ascorbate in preventing chronic diseases or immune function has still not been reached despite many years of study and despite the fact that ascorbic acid is the most-consumed vitamin supplement in the United States. The reasons for this discrepancy are based in part on assay methodologies and on the state of scientific knowledge. At the biochemical level, there were limitations in the ability to accurately measure cellular vitamin C content prior to 1980, and little was known about the mechanisms which govern vitamin C transport across cell membranes. Lack of knowledge of these factors greatly hampered the ability to examine optimal levels of ascorbate *in vitro*. At the clinical level, well controlled pharmacologic studies using state-of-the-art measurement techniques have only recently been performed in normal men (see discussion below).

Accurate measurement of vitamin C is crucial for study of both its biochemistry and its pharmacokinetic properties. Assays should be sensitive, specific, reproducible, and free of interference from other biological compounds. Many older studies of vitamin C relied upon assays which did not meet these criteria, and therefore results of these studies must be evaluated in light of the possibility for measurement error. Assay methods for ascorbic acid and dehydroascorbic acid have been reviewed extensively elsewhere and will not be discussed here.[17]

In order to evaluate *in vitro* and *in vivo* data, plan new studies, and arrive at scientific consensus, the role of ascorbic acid in biological systems must be well understood. Consideration of *in vivo* functions and requirements of vitamin C must include two factors: first, its biochemical properties, including the ability of vitamin C to act both as an antioxidant and as an enzyme cofactor; second, its pharmacokinetics. The latter includes intestinal absorption, serum concentration, cellular distribution, utilization, and excretion. This chapter will provide an overview of the current data concerning the state of knowledge in these areas, and will discuss how this knowledge may contribute towards achieving a recommendation for vitamin C intake.

BIOCHEMISTRY

Chemical Reactions

Vitamin C (ascorbic acid) is a six carbon weak acid with a pK of 4.2. It is reversibly oxidized with the loss of one electron to form the free radical, semidehydroascorbic acid[18] (Figure 1). Compared to other free radical species, semidehydroascorbic acid is relatively stable with a rate constant of decay of approximately 10^{-5} M^{-1} sec^{-1}.[19] Further oxidation of semidehydroascorbic acid results in dehydroascorbic acid which probably exists *in vivo* in multiple forms.[18] Dehydroascorbic acid can be reduced back to ascorbic acid via the same intermediate radical. Alternatively, the ring structure of dehydroascorbic acid can irreversibly hydrolyze to yield diketogulonic acid. The latter may be metabolized further to form oxalate, threonate, xylose, xylonic acid, and lynxonic acid.[20] Dehydroascorbic acid is unstable in aqueous solution, with a half-life at 37°C of approximately 6-20 min, as a function of concentration.[21]

Ascorbic acid is an outstanding antioxidant and reducing agent. In chemical terms this signifies that ascorbic acid easily loses electrons. The overall values for the standard redox potential of the DHA/AA couple are approximately +0.06 to 0.1 volts.[20,22] In physiologic terms this means that ascorbic acid provides electrons for enzymes, for chemical compounds that are oxidants, or for other electron acceptors. In addition to its redox potential, other properties of ascorbic acid make it an excellent electron donor in biological systems. First, its intermediate free radical, semidehydroascorbic acid, is relatively non-reactive, especially with oxygen.[23] Second, the ascorbic acid oxidation product dehydroascorbic acid is efficiently reduced by cells back to ascorbic acid, which then becomes available for reuse[17,24] (see discussion below).

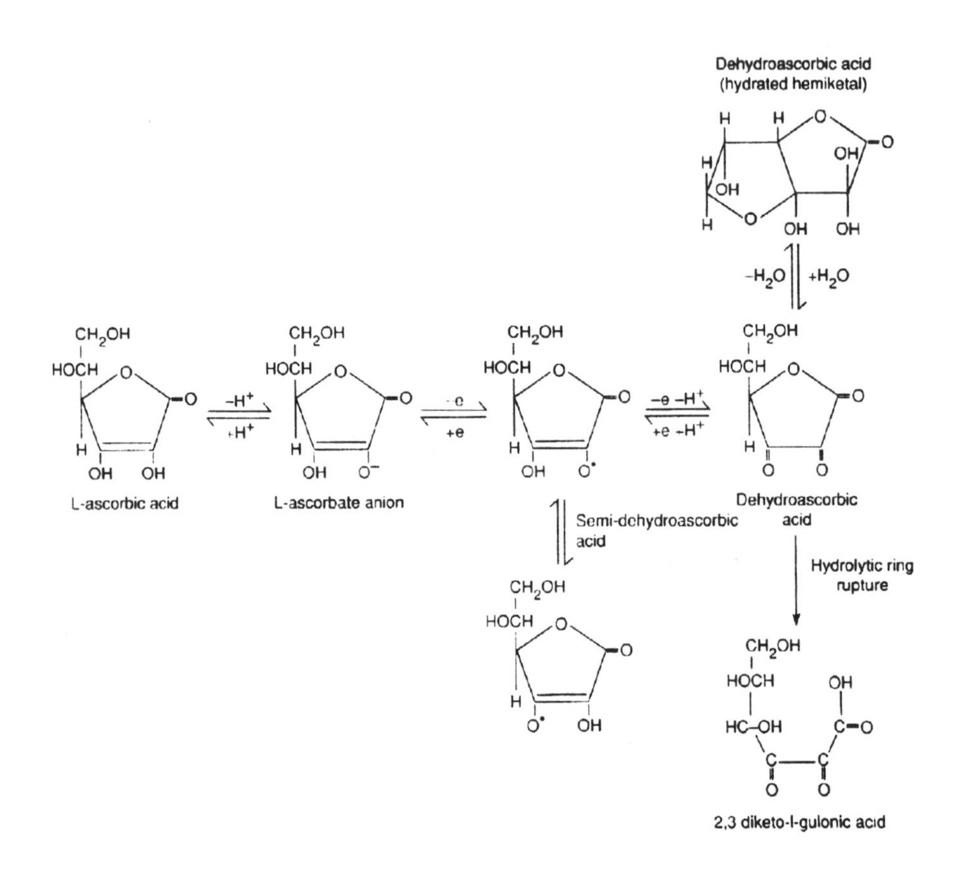

Figure 1. Ascorbic acid and its oxidation products. Dehydroascorbic acid exists in more than one form, and only two are shown here for simplicity. The hydrated hemiketal is proposed to be the favored form in aqueous solutions.[18] It is unknown which form is found in biological systems. Semidehydroascorbic acid might also have other configurations which are omitted here.[20,158] Formation of 2,3,-diketogulonic acid by hydrolytic ring rupture is probably irreversible. (From Washko *et al.*, 1992.)[159]

Ascorbate is an electron donor (reducing agent) for chemical reactions that occur either inside or outside cells. Ascorbate reduces superoxide, hydroxyl radical, hypochlorous acid, and other reactive oxidant species, which can be present both intracellularly and extracellularly. All of these oxidant products can be produced in great quantities by specialized immune cells such as neutrophils and macrophages in response to bacterial infection.[25] Some oxidant products may be slowly released within cells as a normal byproduct of cellular mitochondrial metabolism, as in the case of superoxide. Because oxidants might affect DNA transcription or could damage DNA, proteins, or membrane structures, ascorbate might have a central role in cellular oxidant defense.[26,27] Ascorbate within cells is also utilized as an electron donor as part of the interaction between iron and ferritin.[28] Outside of cells ascorbate may act in conjunction with tocopherols (vitamin E), present in lipid membranes, to quench free radicals and prevent lipid peroxidation.[29] In this manner, ascorbate may help prevent the oxidation of low density lipoprotein (LDL),[30] which is thought to be a major initiating event in the genesis of atherosclerosis. In summary, because of its electrochemical and physiological properties, vitamin C may play a major role in protecting cells and cell components against free radicals and oxidant damage.

Enzymatic Reactions

Ascorbate is a co-factor or co-substrate for 8 isolated enzymes (Table 1).

Table 1
Biochemistry of Ascorbic Acid

ENZYMATIC REACTIONS
Proline hydroxylase (EC 1.14.11.2)
Procollagen-proline 2-oxoglutarate-3-dioxygenase (EC 1.14.11.7)
Lysine hydroxylase (EC 1.14.11.4)
Gamma-butyrobetaine 2-oxoglutarate 4-dioxygenase (EC 1.14.11.1)
Trimethyllysine-2-oxoglutarate dioxygenase (EC 1.14.11.8)
Dopamine beta-monooxygenase (EC 1.14.17.1)
Peptidyl glycine alpha-amidating monooxygenase (EC 1.14.17.3)
4-Hydroxylphenylpyruvate dioxygenase (EC 1.13.11.27)
CHEMICAL REACTIONS
Intracellular reactions
Quenching of reactive oxidants
Iron-ferritin interaction
Extracellular reactions
Quenching of reactive oxidants
Electron transfer to oxidized tocopherol
Prevention of LDL oxidation
Iron absorption in the gastrointestinal tract

Three enzymes require ascorbate for proline or lysine hydroxylation in collagen biosynthesis: proline hydroxylase, procollagen-proline 2-oxoglutarate-3-dioxygenase, and lysine hydroxylase.[31-33] The enzymes gamma-butyrobetaine 2-oxoglutarate 4-dioxygenase and trimethyllysine-2-oxoglutarate dioxygenase require ascorbate in the biosynthetic pathway for carnitine. Carnitine is crucial for ATP synthesis via fatty acid oxidation in mitochondria.[34,35] Dopamine beta-monooxygenase and peptidyl-glycine alpha monooxygenase are necessary for hormone synthesis. Each contains an active site copper moiety and requires ascorbate for maximal activity. The former enzyme catalyzes the synthesis of norepinephrine from dopamine.[36,37] The latter enzyme mediates amidation at the carboxy-terminus of peptide hormones, thereby conferring stability to hormones such as thyrotropin-releasing hormone, ACTH, vasopressin, oxytocin, and cholecystokinin.[38,39] Ascorbate is also required for enzymatic metabolism of tyrosine by 4-hydroxylphenylpyruvate dioxygenase.[40] For each of the above enzymes, the role of ascorbate with purified enzymes *in vitro* has been characterized.

PHARMACOKINETICS

The pharmacokinetics of vitamin C are defined by its intestinal absorption, plasma concentration, cellular distribution, utilization, and excretion. To have a firm foundation for dietary recommendations it is necessary to have knowledge of vitamin C biology in all of these areas. We will review the current state of knowledge in these areas and then provide a rationale for dietary recommendations of vitamin C based on the available data.

Recently, new pharmacokinetic data about vitamin C were published, based on 7 men who were in-patients for 4-6 months at the National Institutes of Health (NIH).[7] Vitamin C ingestion from foods was <5 mg daily. Ascorbate was measured by HPLC with coulometric electrochemical detection. When subjects achieved plasma concentrations of <10 μM ascorbate, each of 7 ascorbate repletion doses from 30 to 2500 mg daily were administered in succession. For each dose each volunteer reached a steady-state plasma value before the next dose was administered. This study represents the most complete in-patient study of vitamin C to date, and will be discussed in detail below as it relates to each pharmacokinetic parameter.

Intake and Bioavailability

To provide vitamin C to tissues, humans must ingest the vitamin and absorb it in the gastrointestinal tract. Ascorbic acid in the reduced form constitutes the majority (80-90%) of this vitamin in food.[41] Studies utilizing sections of human ileum[42] determined that ascorbic acid is absorbed in the human intestine by a Na^+-dependent active transport system. Absorption is greatest in the proximal intestine.[43]

It is not known whether there are individual differences in ascorbic acid absorption. In addition, the possibility exists that vitamin C intestinal transport is regulated. In guinea pigs, for example, prior feeding of large doses of ascorbic acid decreased transport across isolated intestinal mucosa.[44] However, to date there are no direct data showing regulation of intestinal ascorbic acid transport mechanisms in humans.

Little information is available on the intestinal absorption of dehydroascorbic acid in humans. In isolated guinea pig intestinal mucosa, dehydroascorbic acid absorption is a Na^+-independent, saturating process.[45] The majority of dehydroascorbic acid is immediately reduced upon crossing the serosal membrane and is present intracellularly as ascorbic acid.[46] Although dehydroascorbic acid can prevent scurvy in humans,[47,48] some studies suggest that absorption is less than that of ascorbic acid.[49] It is not known whether the composition of ingested food or its antioxidant content affects dehydroascorbic acid reduction to ascorbic acid or hydrolysis to diketogulonic acid prior to absorption.

It is unclear which form physically crosses intestinal membranes: ascorbic acid or dehydroascorbic acid or both. The data imply that both species are transported but by separate mechanisms. Direct experiments to validate this concept remain to be performed.

Absorption is clinically determined using the pharmacokinetic principles of bioavailability. True bioavailability is defined as the increase in the amount of a substance in plasma after an oral dose compared with the increase in plasma after the same dose is given intravenously.[50] Prior to administration of an oral dose, baseline plasma values are obtained. Once the dose is given, plasma values rise and then return to baseline. When the data are displayed, there is an area under the curve and above baseline represented by the oral dose: this area is AUC_{po}. When values return to baseline, the same dose is given intravenously. After an intravenous bolus, plasma values usually rise much faster because the gastrointestinal system is bypassed. Plasma values then return to baseline. When the data are displayed, the area under the curve and above baseline represents the increment from the intravenous dose, and is called AUC_{iv}. True bioavailability is defined pharmacologically as AUC_{po}/AUC_{iv}, and is often displayed as a percent, with 100% bioavailability representing complete absorption. Studies of true bioavailability are difficult to perform because subjects must be at steady-state for the tested dose, the substance must be administered intravenously, and many samples must be analyzed for each tested dose. Ideally, several different doses should be studied and true bioavailability calculated for each.

Until recently, true bioavailability of ascorbate was unknown. Because of the above mentioned difficulties most investigators have estimated ascorbate bioavailability indirectly. In some studies instead of measuring plasma ascorbate concentrations, oral absorption of ascorbate was compared to urine excretion.[51-54] Other studies determined relative bioavailability by comparing absorption of one form of vitamin C (i.e., in foods) to another form (i.e., in a supplement).[55-58] With both methods, because subjects are often not at steady state, pharmacokinetic parameters such as absorption, utilization, and excretion may vary from individual to individual and from hour to hour. While these data may be useful to provide comparative results concerning vitamin C absorption in one individual, they cannot be used to make conclusions about true bioavailability.

The first data to provide detailed information about true bioavailability were part of NIH in-patient study of vitamin C.[7] After attaining steady-state status for a given ascorbic acid dose, subjects were given pure ascorbic acid solutions either by mouth or intravenously. The data obtained from one subject for bioavailability of 200 mg or 1250 mg ascorbic acid are shown in Figure 2.

Based on data for the seven subjects and using a five-compartment pharmacokinetic model, ascorbate bioavailability at steady-state was calculated to be 90% for ≤200 mg, 73% for 500 mg, and 49% for 1250 mg.[59]

The above data for true bioavailability of vitamin C were based on vitamin C administration alone, with the vitamin given either in the fasting state or at least 90 minutes before meals. There are no data for true bioavailability of vitamin C administered with foods or with compounds found in foods. Studies which have examined relative bioavailability have found little difference in absorption between pure ascorbic acid and ascorbic acid in foods[58,60-62] with the exception of one study which showed ascorbic acid relative bioavailability was increased by 35% when the vitamin was accompanied with a citrus extract.[63] One must keep in mind, however, that the majority of these studies were performed using imprecise assays, and further study into this area is warranted.

The true bioavailability of dehydroascorbic acid is unknown. As mentioned above, dehydroascorbic acid has been shown to be antiscorbutic,[47-49] but to a lesser extent than ascorbic acid. However, because intravenous dehydroascorbic acid may be toxic, at least at high doses,[64] studies of true bioavailability have not been performed.

Plasma Concentrations

Until recently, steady-state plasma ascorbate concentrations as a function of consumed dose were unknown.[7] Previous investigations of vitamin C metabolism were not adequately designed to address this issue or were hampered by assays which were not specific. The basis of the current RDA of vitamin C for adults are the in-patient ascorbic acid metabolism studies performed on male prisoner volunteers in Iowa.[12,65-67] Prisoner subjects were given ≤66.5 mg of ascorbate daily, except for one who received 130.5 mg daily. Not enough doses were given to determine a dose-concentration relationship, and samples were analyzed by the imprecise dinitrophenylhydrazine assay technique. The investigators themselves realized that this colorometric assay produced falsely elevated results, especially at the lowest ascorbate doses.[68] Other in-patient studies were limited because only one dose was given above 60 mg daily or because only 3 vitamin C doses were given and samples were measured by an imprecise technique.[69]

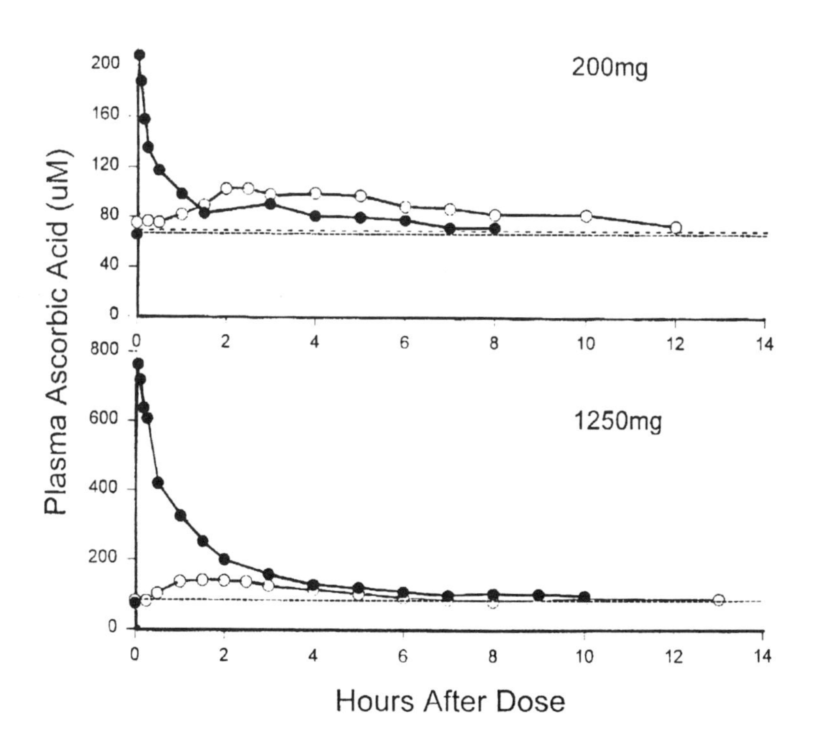

Figure 2. Ascorbic acid bioavailability in plasma. As part of the recent NIH in-patient study,[7] the bioavailability of ascorbic acid was measured. The curves represent data from one subject. Ascorbic acid (200 mg or 1250 mg) was administered orally (o) and the same dose was administered 24 hours later intravenously (•). Blood samples were obtained at the times indicated and plasma ascorbic acid was measured. Baseline ascorbic acid concentration is indicated by the dashed line. (From Levine *et al.*, 1996.)[7]

The relationship between ascorbate dose and serum concentration has also been examined using out-patient studies.[51,70-72] Out-patient studies have the strong disadvantage of not being able to control the essential parameters of dietary ascorbate and ascorbate ingestion. These studies are predominantly based on dietary recall surveys, which can result in both misleading information and underreporting, especially over narrow dose ranges.[73] Nonetheless, similar to previous in-patient studies, out-patient studies have also used insufficiently narrow dose ranges or non-specific assay techniques.

In the recent NIH study, patients were given vitamin C doses ranging from 30 to 2500 mg daily. Measurement of plasma vitamin C showed that there was a sigmoid relationship between ascorbate dose and steady-state plasma concentration (Figure 3). The plasma concentration produced by the present RDA (60 mg/day) was on the bottom third of the steep portion of the curve; the 200 mg dose was beyond the steep portion of the curve and produced >80% plasma saturation. Plasma ascorbate completely saturated at the 1000 mg daily dose.

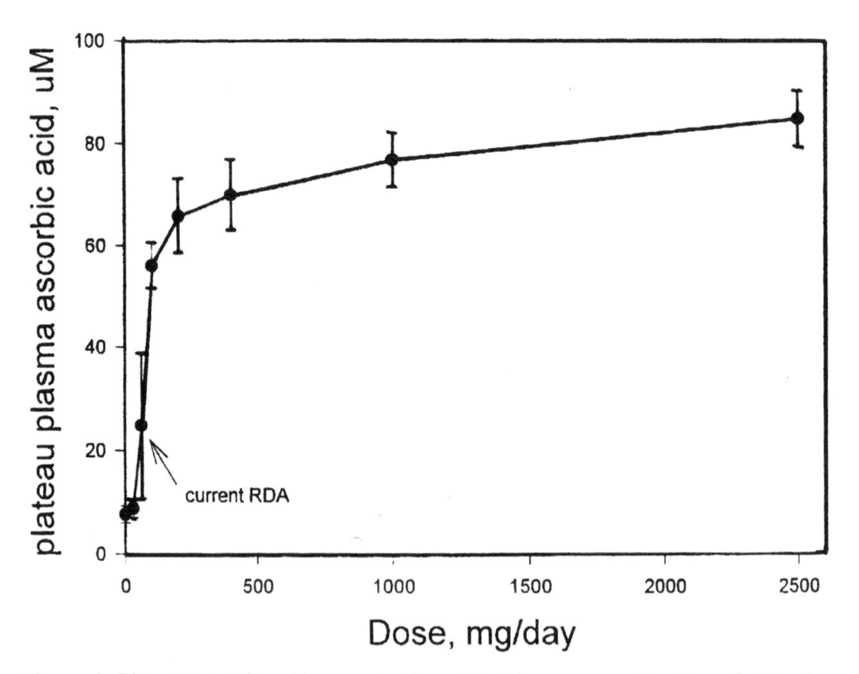

Figure 3. Plasma ascorbic acid concentrations (μM) in men as a function of daily dose. Seven healthy volunteers were hospitalized for 4-6 months and consumed a diet containing <5mg vitamin C daily.[160] Steady-state plasma and tissue concentrations were determined at 7 vitamin C daily doses from 30-2500 mg.[7] All data represent morning fasting samples. Values are means of plateau ascorbic acid from seven men at all doses. The plasma ascorbic acid concentration achieved with intake equivalent to the current RDA (60 mg/day) is indicated by the arrow. (From Levine *et al.*, 1996.)[7]

Dehydroascorbic acid is probably not present in blood under normal circumstances. Limitations of assay methodology hamper efforts to accurately measure low amounts of dehydroascorbic acid in plasma. Measurement of dehydroascorbic acid by prior reduction to ascorbic acid using HPLC with electrochemical detection has yielded concentrations of dehydroascorbic acid <1-2% of plasma ascorbic acid.[74] A fluorescent-based post-column derivatization HPLC assay gave a higher value of 7.6%[75] and some investigators have postulated that in diabetes, plasma dehydroascorbic acid may be elevated even further.[76] However, the latter results may well be the result of assay artifact due to increased oxidation of plasma ascorbic acid during sample processing.

Cellular Distribution

Because it is water soluble, vitamin C is available to all tissues of the body by means of the circulation. Uptake and accumulation of ascorbic acid in tissues is a function of plasma concentration, transport across cellular membranes, and mechanisms which maintain ascorbate intracellularly. Vitamin C content of human tissues varies over a wide range. Tissues with the greatest quantity of vitamin C include adrenal and pituitary glands with 30-50 mg/100g tissue, followed by liver, spleen, eye lens, pancreas, kidney, and brain with between 10 and 30mg/100g.[77]

Dehydroascorbic acid, on the other hand, is not found in appreciable levels in tissues.[17,78,79] Dehydroascorbic acid is avidly taken up by cells, but is immediately reduced intracellularly to ascorbic acid (see discussion below).

Steady-State Concentrations in Cells and Tissues

Unlike other cells, circulating cells can be relatively easily obtained. It has therefore been possible to examine the concentrations of vitamin C in these cells and the relationship between vitamin C intake and cell content in humans. Similar to plasma data, however, until very recently there have been no well controlled studies in humans examining the relationship between cell vitamin C content and dietary intake over a wide range. Previous studies examining the relationship between vitamin C intake and intracellular ascorbate were compromised by few doses.[69,80] A recent study provided new information about ascorbate in seminal fluid but similarly was hampered by a narrow dose range, with only 1 dose above 60 mg daily.[81]

The recent NIH volunteer study examined the vitamin C content of neutrophils, monocytes, and lymphocytes at each dose from 30 mg to 2500 mg daily.[7] The intracellular concentration of ascorbate in all cell types saturated at the 100 mg daily dose, which was less than the dose at which plasma ascorbate began to show saturation (Figure 4). At 100 mg daily, intracellular vitamin C concentrations were 1-4 mM, at least 14-fold higher than plasma. The corresponding plasma concentration at this dose was 55-60 μM.

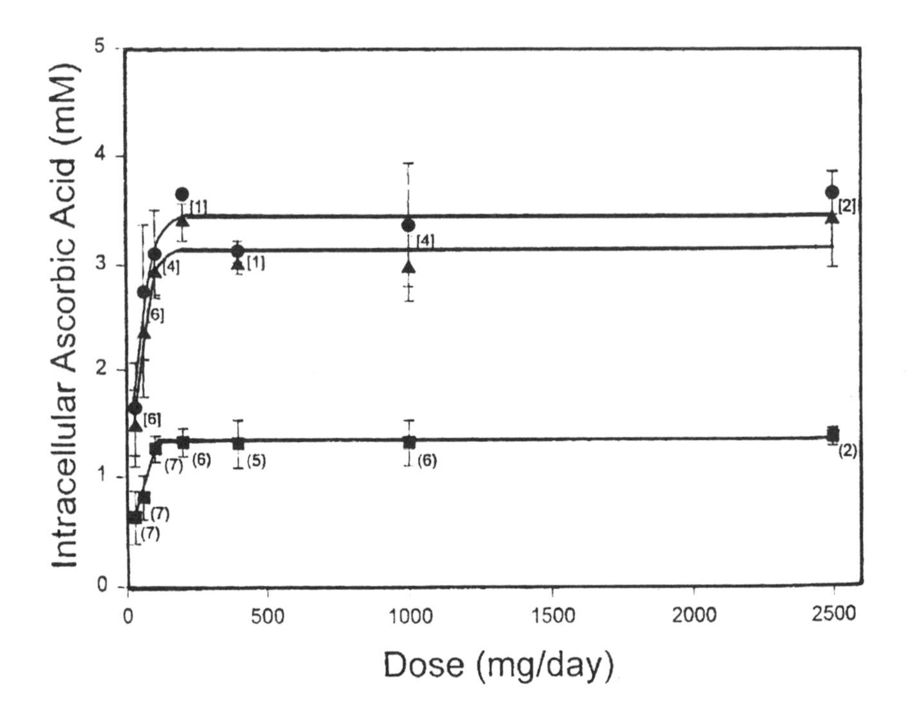

Figure 4. Intracellular ascorbic acid concentration (mM) in circulating immune cells as a function of dose. When NIH in-patient volunteers reached plateau for each dose of ascorbic acid, neutrophils (■), monocytes (▲), and lymphocytes (•) were isolated and intracellular ascorbic acid was measured. Numbers in parentheses at each dose indicate the number of volunteers from whom cells were obtained. (From Levine *et al.*, 1996.)[7]

Biological Transport of Ascorbic Acid and Dehydroascorbic Acid

The extent to which vitamin C accumulates in tissues is a function of external vitamin C concentration and net transport across the cell membrane. Both ascorbic acid and dehydroascorbic acid are transported across cell membranes. Ascorbic acid transport exhibits saturable kinetics and in most cases is Na^+-dependent.[79,82-86] Ascorbic acid transport has been specifically shown to require metabolic energy.[42,85-88] The apparent transport affinity (K_M) of ascorbic acid in human tissue is in the range of 5-20μM with V_{MAX} of uptake saturating at approximately 50-100μM.[82,83,85,86] The protein responsible for ascorbic acid transport has not been isolated.

Transport of dehydroascorbic acid is Na^+-independent,[17,79,89] and does not require metabolic energy. The generally proposed mechanism is one of cellular trapping. Upon cell entry, dehydroascorbic acid is immediately reduced to ascorbic acid, which produces an effective gradient of dehydroascorbic acid across the membrane.[17,90] The apparent K_M for dehydroascorbic acid transport is generally much higher than that of ascorbic acid and ranges from 0.75 to 3.7mM.[91-94]

For many years *in vitro* data suggested that dehydroascorbic acid may be transported by the same transporter as glucose.[89,91,95,96] Seven glucose transporter isoforms (GLUT 1-5, SGLT1, and SGLT2) have been characterized,[97-99] which vary in substrate affinity and tissue distribution. Recent experiments utilizing *Xenopus laevis* oocytes to express individual glucose transporter isoforms demonstrated that GLUT1[94,100] and GLUT3[94] act as dehydroascorbic acid transport proteins with an affinity similar to or lower than that for glucose (1-2mM). The insulin sensitive glucose transport protein, GLUT4, also mediates the transport of dehydroascorbic acid but at a lower rate compared to glucose. The kinetics of dehydroascorbic acid transport via GLUT4 have not yet been defined. None of the glucose transporter isoforms transport ascorbic acid.[94] GLUT1 is constitutively expressed in most cells, GLUT3 is localized to neuronal tissue, testes, and platelets, and GLUT4 is found predominantly in muscle, adipose, heart, and brain.[101,102] It is not known whether other proteins exist that mediate the transport of dehydroascorbic acid into cells. Because glucose transport proteins are ubiquitous and show a high affinity for dehydroascorbic acid, they are likely to be the primary proteins responsible for cellular dehydroascorbic acid uptake.

The mechanisms of cellular accumulation of ascorbic acid have been controversial for many years. Some investigators contended that all ascorbic acid transport was due to conversion of ascorbic acid to dehydroascorbic acid with subsequent transport of only dehydroascorbic acid.[100,103,104] Because of the ease of interconversion between ascorbic acid and dehydroascorbic acid under some redox conditions, the nature of the substrate present *in vitro* is not always straightforward, and care must be taken when interpreting experimental data. However, based on extensive data, ascorbic acid and dehydroascorbic acid transport are different with respect to Na^+ and energy dependence, rate constants, effect of reducing agents, transport via expressed glucose transporters, and tissue specificity. In addition, recent experiments performed in human neutrophils using ascorbic acid analogs conclusively demonstrated separate ascorbic acid and dehydroascorbic acid transport activities.[79] Based on these data, therefore, it is very unlikely that ascorbic acid transport occurs exclusively by oxidation to dehydroascorbic acid.

The *in vivo* contribution of ascorbic acid and/or dehydroascorbic acid toward cellular ascorbic acid accumulation remains an open issue. The rate of dehydroascorbic acid uptake appears to be much greater than that of ascorbic acid for most tissues studied. When both ascorbic and dehydroascorbic acid transport were measured in myeloid cell lines, 15 to 30-fold more dehydroascorbic acid was transported compared to ascorbic acid.[79] However, net transport is dependant on substrate availability. Normal plasma concentrations of ascorbic acid (20-100μM) are consistent with ascorbic acid transporter affinity and saturation. By contrast, dehydroascorbic acid is either not detectable or measured in very low concentrations (<1-2μM) in the circulation.[74]

Intracellular Dehydroascorbic Acid Reduction

It has been known for many years that in most tissues examined intracellular dehydroascorbic acid is immediately reduced to ascorbic acid.[105] Intracellular reduction is mediated by two major pathways: chemical reduction by glutathione[106] and enzymatic reduction.[24,107] The role of these two processes *in vivo* is probably tissue specific and remains to be resolved.[106-108]

Isolated proteins which have been shown to have dehydroascorbic acid reducing activity include glutaredoxin from neutrophils,[24] pig liver, bovine thymus and human placenta,[109] bovine protein disulfide isomerase,[107,109] 3-α-hydroxysteroid dehydrogenase,[110] and an as yet unidentified protein of MW 31,000 isolated from rat liver.[111] Although glutaredoxin is responsible for most of dehydroascorbic acid reduction in human neutrophils, the relative role of these other proteins in tissues is not known. The tissue distribution in humans of glutaredoxin and other dehydroascorbic acid reducing protein activities and their regulation under normal and oxidative stress conditions remain to be examined.

As mentioned above, it is likely that the intracellular reduction of dehydroascorbic acid to ascorbic acid is the driving force for dehydroascorbic acid transport across cell membranes. The result is an outside to inside dehydroascorbic acid gradient, favoring entry. It is unknown whether differences in cellular dehydroascorbic acid reducing capacity may regulate cellular ascorbic acid accumulation. Because ascorbic acid appears to exit cells at comparatively slow rates,[79,90] high intracellular concentrations of ascorbic acid can be maintained. Separate ascorbic acid transport activity probably also helps to maintain high internal concentrations.

Ascorbic Acid Recycling

The most comprehensive model of ascorbic acid accumulation consistent with available data is ascorbic acid recycling. In this model, transport of both dehydroascorbic acid and ascorbic acid occurs, but is dependent on substrate availability. Under normal conditions ascorbic acid accounts for the majority of ascorbic acid accumulation, because it is the dominant and perhaps only substrate in plasma.[74] However, when ascorbic acid is oxidized, dehydroascorbic acid may transiently form. This could be particularly relevant in the extracellular space, where local oxidant concentration may be higher. With increased availability of dehydroascorbic acid, this substrate is preferentially transported (≥10-

fold faster than ascorbic acid), followed by immediate intracellular reduction.

Ascorbic acid recycling has been experimentally demonstrated in neutrophils.[17] In resting cells, ascorbic acid is transported constitutively as ascorbic acid, and internal ascorbic acid can be maintained at mM concentrations. When neutrophils are activated by contact with bacteria, reactive oxygen species are produced and extracellular ascorbic acid is oxidized to dehydroascorbic acid. Dehydroascorbic acid is then rapidly transported across the cell membrane and immediately reduced intracellularly to ascorbic acid (Figure 5).

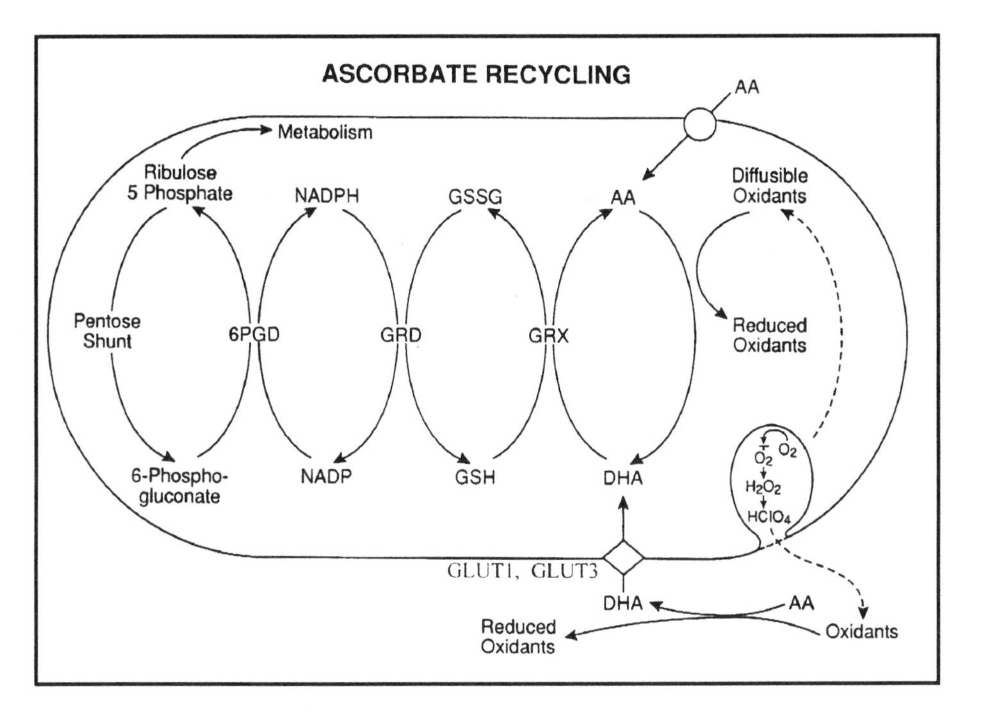

Figure 5. A model of dehydroascorbic acid and ascorbate transport and recycling in human neutrophils. Constitutive ascorbate transport (open circle) likely maintains mM concentrations of ascorbate inside neutrophils.[82] With activation, neutrophils secrete reactive oxygen species which oxidize extracellular ascorbate to dehydroascorbic acid, resulting in rapid uptake of dehydroascorbic acid (open diamond) and immediate intracellular reduction to ascorbate.[17] In neutrophils, glutaredoxin is responsible for the majority of intracellular reduction.[24] As a result of this internalization pathway, as much as 10-fold higher internal concentrations of the vitamin are achieved compared to activity of the ascorbate transporter alone.[17,79] The proposed mechanism of reduction could require glutathione, NADPH, and the enzymes shown.[24] Dehydroascorbic acid entry may be mediated by the glucose transporter isoforms GLUT1 and GLUT3.[94] Abbreviations: AA, ascorbate; DHA, dehydroascorbic acid; GRX, glutaredoxin; GSH, reduced glutathione; GSSG, oxidized glutathione; 6-PGD, 6-phosphogluconate dehydrogenase; GRD, glutathione reductase.

In this manner as much as 10 to 20-fold increases in intracellular ascorbic acid concentration can be rapidly achieved.[17,79,112] Ascorbic acid transport also occurs but at a much slower rate. The results imply that dehydroascorbic acid formation and transport could occur during bacterial infection or inflammation.[112]

Rapid dehydroascorbic acid uptake and intracellular reduction may be a protective mechanism for cells. The resulting sudden increase in intracellular ascorbic acid accumulation may blunt oxidative stress. Bacteria do not possess mechanisms to efficiently transport either ascorbic acid or dehydroascorbic acid, and do not accumulate ascorbic acid.[112] Thus, recycling may confer a specific benefit to neutrophils during a bacterial challenge. If ascorbic acid recycling can be demonstrated *in vivo*, the next challenges would be to determine the functional consequences of recycling and its regulation *in vivo*. Whether this mechanism is important in the function of immune cells and in protection against environmental oxidants has yet to be determined.

The lack of dehydroascorbic acid in plasma is consistent with the mechanisms of intracellular dehydroascorbic acid reduction and ascorbic acid recycling. Because of the high expression of glucose transport proteins on erythrocytes, newly formed dehydroascorbic acid would likely be rapidly removed from the circulation. Some investigators suggested that erythrocytes contain the highest fraction of vitamin C among blood cells because of their abundance.[113] However, determination of erythrocyte vitamin C is problematic because of the presence of very large quantities of highly reactive heme-iron, which can easily oxidize vitamin C during sample preparation or storage prior to measurement. As yet, satisfactory analysis of erythrocyte vitamin C content has not been achieved.

In summary, both ascorbic acid and dehydroascorbic acid may be important for transport *in vivo*. Substrate availability probably plays a key role in which species are transported at a particular time. Because of its relatively high plasma concentration, low transporter affinity, and ubiquitous presence extracellularly, ascorbic acid is the form likely utilized by cells for constitutive ascorbic acid uptake. By contrast, dehydroascorbic acid concentration would be dependent on acute oxidation of ascorbic acid, and dehydroascorbic acid uptake would then be induced by substrate formation and limited by substrate availability.

Excretion

Ascorbic acid is filtered at the glomerulus of all species studied and is reabsorbed at the proximal tubule by an active transport process.[114,115] In humans the upper range of ascorbic acid concentration in blood is limited by tubular reabsorption.[116] Maximal tubule reabsorption rates have been determined in men and women of different ages and found to be relatively constant between groups at about 1.5 mg/100 ml glomerular filtrate.[114,117] As in the intestine, ascorbic acid transport in the kidney tubule is Na^+-dependent.[118,119] Tubule reabsorption presumably is related to the tubule concentration of ascorbate. It is unknown whether ascorbic acid reabsorption can be regulated by other mechanisms, and it is not clear whether there is also active secretion of ascorbic acid into renal tubules.

In contrast to ascorbic acid, dehydroascorbic acid transport in isolated kidney tubules is Na^+-independent, insensitive to transmembrane electrical potential difference, and is not concentrated against a gradient.[120] *In vitro*, transported dehydroascorbic acid is rapidly reduced to ascorbic acid in isolated tubules from rat and guinea pig,[121] and transport of ascorbic acid and dehydroascorbic acid at the renal basolateral membrane appear to be Na^+-independent processes of comparable rate.[121] No evidence is available on the renal excretion or reuptake of dehydroascorbic acid *in vivo* because no measurable amounts can be found in plasma. Measurement of dehydroascorbic acid in urine is fraught with similar methodological difficulties as is plasma. Most likely, dehydroascorbic acid is present only at very low quantities or not at all in urine. Greater quantities are probably a result of experimental artifact.[122]

Early clinical studies implied that ascorbic acid was excreted in urine of volunteers who were at steady-state for a 60 mg daily dose.[65] This information is part of the basis for the current recommended dietary allowance of ascorbic acid at 60 mg daily.[12] However, the actual data were not published in the scientific literature. The findings can also be questioned because the assay for ascorbic acid was subject to false-positive interference, especially at low ascorbic acid concentrations.[123] Using a sensitive electrochemical HPLC assay to measure ascorbic acid, the recent NIH study showed that ascorbic acid appeared in urine only at doses greater or equal to 100 mg/day,[7] which corresponded to an average plasma concentration of 57 μM. At higher doses, ≥500 mg/day, virtually all of the absorbed vitamin was excreted in urine.

Adverse Effects

Vitamin C is remarkably non-toxic. Because of its pharmacokinetics, described above, vitamin C does not accumulate to toxic levels in healthy humans. Excessive amounts of ingested vitamin C are both poorly absorbed and almost completely excreted in the urine. Metabolic byproducts of ascorbic acid such as urate and oxalate may be increased as a result of high vitamin C intake but data are conflicting.

Increased urate secretion was reported when some subjects received a large dose of ascorbate intravenously[124] or orally,[125] although these findings were contradicted by others.[126] The conflicting findings may be due to lack of steady-state for vitamin C, differences in plasma concentrations, or the duration of vitamin administration. In the NIH volunteer study, uric acid excretion was increased at the 1 gram dose of vitamin C compared to lower doses.[7] There were fewer subjects whose urine was available for measurement at the 1 gram dose, and it is possible that the observed increased uric acid excretion was transient and would not persist if these doses were administered for longer periods.

The data concerning enhanced oxalate secretion with high vitamin C ingestion are also contradictory for several reasons.[127-129] Substantial confusion has been due to the difficulty in measuring oxalate accurately. In oxalate assays commonly used more than 10 years ago, ascorbate produced falsely elevated measurement of oxalate.[130] We believe that the best explanation of the data is that subsets of patients may have enhanced oxalate excretion from ascorbate. In particular, patients with hyperoxalemia who form oxalate stones may have enhanced oxalate excretion associated with ascorbate ingestion $\geq$1000 mg, and for these patients megadoses of ascorbate could be harmful.[129] Because hyperoxalemia may be clinically ocult in the general population, safe doses of vitamin C are $<$1000 mg daily.

Although vitamin C is non-toxic for normal individuals, there are additional special considerations. Vitamin C will enhance iron absorption by maintaining iron in its reduced form.[131] In cases of iron overload, such as in patients with thalassemia major, hemochromatosis, and sideroblastic anemia, increased vitamin C intake may be harmful. For individuals who are heterozygous for hemochromatosis available data show no adverse affects of increased vitamin C intake.[7,132] Some health-care practitioners administer ascorbate intravenously in doses of many grams. In patients with glucose-6-phosphate dehydrogenase deficiency, hemolysis occurred after ascorbate was administered intravenously[133,134] and after a 6-gram single oral dose.[135]

Many harmful effects have been mistakenly attributed to vitamin C ingestion, especially at doses above 1 gram. These misconceptions include hyperglycemia, rebound scurvy, infertility, mutagenesis, and destruction of vitamin B12. It is erroneous to conclude that gram doses of vitamin C produce these effects. In addition, it has been proposed that excess ascorbic acid may accelerate oxidant damage in the presence of free cations, especially iron.[136] However, this hypothesis is based on *in vitro* experiments with excessive concentrations of free cations. *In vivo*, cations are very efficiently sequestered and generally are not freely available.

In situ Kinetics and Recommended Intake

The goal of *in situ* kinetics is to study vitamin function directly in organelles, cells, tissues, or animals, including humans. Although more complex than *in vitro* experiments, *in situ* studies are essential for the determination of recommended intake. Vitamin function in living tissue is a consequence of local vitamin concentration and competing reactions and may be different from that found with isolated reactions or proteins.[74,137] *In situ* kinetics have both biochemical and clinical components (Table 2).[138] The biochemical component concerns how vitamin concentration affects vitamin biochemical or molecular function *in situ*. The clinical component entails how these effective *in situ* vitamin concentrations are achieved in people.

Biochemical Component

The goal of the biochemical component of *in situ* kinetics is to describe the kinetics of vitamin-dependent reactions directly in organelles, cells, or tissues. Once kinetics have been determined, optimal vitamin ingestion would be the amount that produced maximal function, or V_{MAX}, of different reactions, but with no adverse consequences.[14] The reaction should have potential benefit for the organism. There must be a sensitive and specific means to measure the vitamin, and to adjust its concentration in the tissue over a wide range. It must also be possible to specifically measure the vitamin-mediated reaction. As described above, vitamin C participates in 8 known enzymatic reactions as well as in non-enzymatic oxidant quenching reactions (Table 2).

Table 2
***In situ* Kinetics**

BIOCHEMICAL COMPONENT
Vitamin biochemical and molecular function in relation to vitamin concentration

- Assay for vitamin
- Ability to have different vitamin concentrations *in situ*: transport, depletion, repletion
- Distribution of vitamin *in situ*
- Assay for vitamin function
- Determination of vitamin function *in vitro* and *in situ*
- Localization of vitamin function *in situ* and relationship to vitamin distribution
- Specificity of vitamin function *in vitro* and *in situ*
- Vitamin function in relation to different vitamin concentrations *in situ*

CLINICAL COMPONENT
Achieving effective vitamin concentrations in people

- Availability of the vitamin in the diet
- Steady-state vitamin concentration in plasma as a function of dose
- Steady-state vitamin concentration in tissues as a function of dose
- Vitamin bioavailability
- Vitamin excretion
- Vitamin safety and adverse effects
- Beneficial effects in relation to dose: direct effects and epidemiologic observations

In situ kinetics of vitamin C have been described for norepinephrine biosynthesis and ascorbate transmembrane electron transfer in animal tissue, but are not known for other reactions.[74,137] Inhibition of LDL oxidation as a function of vitamin C concentration has been described, but not in a true *in situ* system.[30] Other reactions for which maximal enzyme activity may be beneficial include proline and lysine hydroxylation for wound healing, oxidant quenching both intracellularly and extracellularly, carnitine biosynthesis for ATP generation, and hormone biosynthesis. A fundamental component for understanding *in situ* kinetics for different reactions is vitamin C transport. As described earlier, apparent K_M for ascorbic acid transport in human cells is 5-20μM, with transport V_{MAX} occuring at external concentrations of 50-100μM.

Clinical Component

The goals of the clinical component of *in situ* kinetics are to determine the manner in which vitamin concentrations are achieved in humans and the effect of these concentrations on clinical parameters. The clinical component has seven parts (Table 2). Initially the vitamin should be available in the food supply. Vitamin C can easily be obtained by eating fruits and vegetables, with five servings daily providing roughly 200 mg.[139,140] Despite its potential availability, less than 28% of Americans consume five serving of fruit or vegetable daily and up to a third of the population consumes less than 60 mg of vitamin C daily.[9,141-143]

The relationship between intake and steady-state vitamin concentrations in plasma and tissues must be determined. As described above, until recently these data were not available for vitamin C. The recent NIH in-patient study provided this data for 7 normal men. Plasma concentration reached a plateau at approximately 200 mg daily, with plasma concentrations of 65μM. Further supplementation up to 1000 mg/day increased plasma concentrations only slightly to 80μM. Cellular concentration of ascorbic acid measured in neutrophils, monocytes, and lymphocytes saturated earlier at an ingested dose of 100 mg/day. Intracellular concentration accumulated to mM concentrations.[7]

Bioavailability and urine excretion were also examined in the NIH study. At doses of up to 200 mg/day vitamin C was almost completely absorbed in the intestine, but with higher doses absorption declined markedly.[7,59] Urinary excretion followed a converse pattern. Up until 100 mg/day no ascorbic acid was excreted in the urine. By contrast, at doses ≥500 mg/day virtually all of the absorbed vitamin C was excreted unchanged in urine.[7]

Other important components of *in situ* kinetics are vitamin toxicity, which were discussed above, and considerations derived from epidemiological studies.

The effects of vitamin C on various chronic diseases such as cancer, coronary heart disease, stroke, cataract, and overall survival are controversial.[144-154] Potential reasons for the discrepancies include: first, that ingestion is often calculated using food-recall surveys, which are often inaccurate;[73] and second, in many of these studies tissue and plasma concentrations of vitamin C were unknown. Based on what is now known about the pharmacokinetics of vitamin C intake it is quite possible that vitamin C ingestion in many subjects was above the steep portion of the dose-concentration curve. In other words, vitamin C concentrations in plasma and tissues would be close to saturation at the initiation of the study and thus little change would occur with supplementation.

The best data correlating vitamin C with beneficial clinical outcome comes from data regarding its intake as a component of fruits and vegetables. High fruit and vegetable intake is associated with lower risk for heart disease and cancer, particularly gastrointestinal cancers.[144] However, it is unknown which factors in fruits and vegetables are protective. The benefit may be due to complex interactions between vitamin C and other components of these foods, or independent of vitamin C altogether. Epidemiologic studies have an important role in determining vitamin recommendations, but should not be used alone.[155] Limitations of epidemiologic studies should be recognized, and the steep dose-concentration curve in the range of 30-100 mg daily for ascorbate should be accounted for.

CONCLUSIONS

The principles of *in situ* kinetics described have been used to recommend vitamin C ingestion of 200 mg daily.[7,108,138,156] This amount of vitamin C is easily obtained by eating five daily servings of fruits and vegetables.[140] Ingestion of vitamin C in foods is clearly preferably to supplementation because of the association of fruits and vegetables with lowered risk of various chronic diseases.[144] Vitamin doses of 500 mg and higher are incompletely absorbed in normal men, and of that which is absorbed, virtually all is excreted in the urine.[7] Such doses may be beneficial if there are advantages to having unabsorbed vitamin C in the gastrointestinal tract or in the urine. However, no data are available concerning these issues. Although doses less than or equal to 200 mg/day appear to be completely absorbed, the influence of food composition on vitamin C bioavailability is not well understood, and more information is needed. If food substantially alters absorption of vitamin C, then 200 mg would be a minimal estimate for recommended ingestion.

Vitamin C pharmacokinetics may be affected by parameters not yet mentioned, including gender, age, or differing metabolic states such as stress or disease. Evidence exists suggesting that smokers might have an increased requirement for vitamin C.[157] These data are far from complete, but remain the basis for the increased RDA of 100 mg/day for smokers. Other conditions such as sepsis or renal insufficiency might also profoundly affect vitamin C pharmacokinetics by increasing vitamin C utilization or excretion, respectively. Specific studies examining these issues have not yet been performed.

Although direct data concerning the relationship between vitamin C concentration and function *in situ* are lacking for most of the reactions in which the vitamin participates, recommendations for vitamin C ingestion are still necessary. To make recommendations for optimal vitamin C consumption, both biological and clinical components should be considered. Data from epidemiological studies can be used synergistically with pharmacokinetic and functional studies to provide an improved perspective which none can provide alone. Recommendations can be divided categorically. For example, 60 mg daily could be considered the required dose to prevent subtle symptoms of deficiency, whereas 200 mg daily may be a better dose for optimal function. Based on current available data a safe upper limit is likely <1000 mg daily.[7] Patients with specific diseases, i.e., renal failure or iron overload, may require individualized intake recommendations.

REFERENCES

1. Chatterjee M and Ghosh, JJ. An experimental study on the evaluation of amino-aciduria in premature (low birth weight) babies, *J Indian Med Assoc* 61:69-73 1973.
2. Nishikimi M, Fukuyama R, Minoshima S, Shimizu N, and Yagi K. Cloning and chromosomal mapping of the human nonfunctional gene for L-gulono-gamma-lactone oxidase, the enzyme for L-ascorbic acid biosynthesis missing in man, *J Biol Chem* 269:13685-13688 1994.
3. Hodges, JR and Hotston, RT. Suppression of adrenocorticotrophic activity in the ascorbic acid deficient guinea-pig, *Br J Pharmacol* 42:595-602 1971.
4. Baker, EM, Hodges, RE, Hood, J, Sauberlich, HE, March, SC, and Canham, JE. Metabolism of 14C- and 3H-labeled L-ascorbic acid in human scurvy, *Am J Clin Nutr* 24:444-454 1971.
5. Kinsman, RA and Hood, J. Some behavioral effects of ascorbic acid deficiency, *Am J Clin Nutr* 24:455-464 1971.
6. Lind, *A Treatise on the Scurvy*, A. Millar, London, (1753).
7. Levine, M, Conry-Cantilena, C, Wang, Y, Welch, RW, Washko, PW, Dhariwal, KR, Park, JB, Lazarev, A, Graumlich, J, King, J, and Cantilena, LR. Vitamin C pharmacokinetics in healthy volunteers: evidence for a Recommended Dietary Allowance, *Proc Natl Acad Sci USA* 93:3704-3709 1996.
8. Massachusetts General Hospital, Case records of the Massachusetts General Hospital. Case 39-1955. A 72 year old man with exertional dyspnea, fatigue, and extensive ecchymoses and purpuric lesions, *N Engl J Med* 333:1695-1702 1995.
9. Life Sciences Research Office, Third Report on Nutrition Monitoring in the United States, U. S. Government Printing Office, Washington, DC. (1995).
10. Simon, JA, Schreiber, GB, Crawford, PB, Frederick, MM, and Sabry, ZI. Dietary vitamin C and serum lipids in black and white girls, *Epidemiology* 4:537-542 1993.

11. Basch, CE, Syber, P, and Shea, S. 5-a-day: dietary behavior and the fruit and vegetable intake of Latino children, *Am J Public Health* 84:814-818 1994.
12. Food and Nutrition Board (USRC), Recommended Dietary Allowances, National Academy Press, Washington, DC. (1989).
13. Levine, M. New concepts in the biology and biochemistry of ascorbic acid, *N Engl J Med* 314:892-902 1986.
14. Levine, M, Dhariwal, KR, Washko, PW, Butler, JD, Welch, RW, Wang, YH, and Bergsten, P. Ascorbic acid and *in situ* kinetics: a new approach to vitamin requirements, *Am J Clin Nutr* 54:1157S-1162S 1991.
15. Pauling, L. Vitamin C the common cold and the flu, WH Freeman and Co. San Francisco, (1976).
16. Hemila, H. Vitamin C and plasma cholesterol, *Crit Rev Food Sci Nutr* 32:33-57 1992.
17. Washko, PW, Wang, Y, and Levine, M. Ascorbic acid recycling in human neutrophils, *J Biol Chem* 268:15531-15535 1993.
18. Tolbert and Ward JB. Dehydroascorbic Acid, in: *Ascorbic Acid: Chemistry, Metabolism, and Uses,* PA. Seib *et al.*, American Chemical Society, Washington, DC. pp. 101-123 (1982).
19. Bielski, BH, Richter, HW, and Chan, PC. Some properties of the ascorbate free radical, *Ann N Y Acad Sci* 258:231-7:231-237 1975.
20. Lewin, *Vitamin C: Its Molecular Biology and Medical Potential*, Academic Press, London, (1976).
21. Penney, JR and Zilva, SS. Chemical behavior of dehydro-l-ascorbic acid *in vitro* and *in vivo*, *Biochem J* 37:403-417 1943.
22. Buettner, GR and Moseley, PL. EPR spin trapping of free radicals produced by bleomycin and ascorbate, *Free Radic Res Commun* 19 Suppl 1:S89-93:S89-93 1993.
23. Buettner, GR. The pecking order of free radicals and antioxidants: lipid peroxidation, alpha-tocopherol, and ascorbate, *Arch Biochem Biophys* 300:535-543 1993.
24. Park, JB and Levine, M. Purification, cloning, and expression of dehydroascorbic acid reduction activity from human neutrophils: identification as glutaredoxin, *Biochem J* 315:931-938 1996.
25. DeChatelet, LR. Oxidative bactericidal mechanisms of polymorphonuclear leukocytes, *J Infect Dis* 131:295-303 1975.
26. Frei, B, England, L, and Ames, BN. Ascorbate is an outstanding antioxidant in human blood plasma, *Proc Natl Acad Sci U S A* 86:6377-6381 1989.
27. Halliwell, B. Free radicals and antioxidants: a personal view, *Nutr Rev* 52:253-265 1994.
28. Hoffman, KE, Yanelli, K, and Bridges, KR. Ascorbic acid and iron metabolism: alterations in lysosomal function, *Am J Clin Nutr* 54:1188S-1192S 1991.
29. Niki, E, Noguchi, N, Tsuchihashi, G, and Gotoh, N. Interaction among vitamin C, vitamin E and β-carotene, *Am J Clin Nutr* 62:1322S-1326S 1995.
30. Jialal, I, Vega, GL, and Grundy, SM. Physiologic levels of ascorbate inhibit the oxidative modification of low density lipoprotein, *Atherosclerosis* 82:185-191 1990.
31. Peterkokshy, B and Udenfriend, S. Enzymatic hydroxylation of proline microsomal polypeptide leading to formation of collagen, *Proc Natl Acad Sci U S A* 53:335-342 1965.
32. Puistola, U, Turpeenniemi-Hujanen, TM, Myllyla, R, and Kivirikko, KI. Studies on the lysylhydroxylase reaction. II. Inhibition kinetics and the reaction mechanism, *Biochim Biophys Acta* 611:51-60 1980.
33. Kivirikko, KO, Myllyla, R, and Pihlajaniemi, T. Protein hydroxylation: prolyl 4-hydroxylase, an enzyme with four cosubstrates and a multifunctional subunit, *FASEB J* 3:1609-1617 1989.
34. Lindblad, B, Lindstedt, G, Lindstedt, S, and Rundgren, M. Purification and some properties of human 4-hydroxyphenylpyruvate dioxygenase (I), *J Biol Chem* 252:5073-5084 1977.

35. Dunn, WA, Rettura, G, Seifter, E, and Englard, S. Carnitine biosynthesis from gamma-butyrobetaine and from exogenous protein-bound 6-N-trimethyl-L-lysine by the perfused guinea pig liver. Effect of ascorbate deficiency on the *in situ* activity of gamma-butyrobetaine hydroxylase, *J Biol Chem* 259:10764-10770 1984.
36. Friedman, S and Kaufman, S. 3,4-dihydroxyphenylethylamine beta-hydroxylase. Physical properties, copper content, and role of copper in the catalytic activity, *J Biol Chem* 240:4763-4773 1965.
37. Levine, M. Ascorbic acid specifically enhances dopamine beta-monooxygenase activity in resting and stimulated chromaffin cells, *J Biol Chem* 261:7347-7356 1986.
38. Wand, GS, Ney, RL, Baylin, S, Eipper, B, and Mains, RE. Characterization of a peptide alpha-amidation activity in human plasma and tissues, *Metabolism* 34:1044-1052 1985.
39. Eipper, BA and Mains, RE. The role of ascorbate in the biosynthesis of neuroendocrine peptides, *Am J Clin Nutr* 54:1153S-1156S 1991.
40. La Du, BN and Zannoni, VG. The role of ascorbic acid in tyrosine metabolism, *Ann N Y Acad Sci* 92:175-191 1961.
41. Vanderslice, JT and Higgs, DJ. Vitamin C content of foods: sample variability, *Am J Clin Nutr* 54:1323S-1327S 1991.
42. Stevenson, NR. Active transport of L-ascorbic acid in the human ileum, *Gastroenterology* 67:952-956 1974.
43. Stewart, JS and Booth, CC. Ascorbic acid absorption in malabsorption, *Clin Sci* 27:15-22 1964.
44. Karasov, WH, Darken, BW, and Bottum, MC. Dietary regulation of intestinal ascorbate uptake in guinea pigs, *Am J Physiol* 260:G108-G118 1991.
45. Bianchi, J and Rose, RC. Dehydroascorbic acid and cell membranes: possible disruptive effects, *Toxicology* 40:75-82 1986.
46. Rose, RC. Transport of ascorbic acid and other water-soluble vitamins, *Biochim Biophys Acta* 947:335-366 1988.
47. Todhunter, EN, McMillan, T, and Ehmke, A. Utilization of dehydroascorbic acid by human subjects, *J Nutr* 42:297-308 1950.
48. Linkswiler, H. The effect of the ingestion of ascorbic acid and dehydroascorbic acid upon the blood levels of these two components in human subjects, *J Nutr* 63:43-54 1957.
49. Sabry, JH, Fisher, KH, and Dodds, ML. Human utilization of dehydroascorbic acid, *J Nutr* 68:457-466 1958.
50. Gibaldi and D. Perrier, *Pharmacokinetics*, Marcel Dekker, New York & Basel, (1982).
51. Kallner, A, Hartmann, D, and Hornig, D. On the absorption of ascorbic acid in man, *Int J Vitam Nutr Res* 47:383-388 1977.
52. Yung, S, Mayersohn, M, and Robinson, JB. Ascorbic acid absorption in humans: a comparison among several dosage forms, *J Pharm Sci* 71:282-285 1982.
53. Mayersohn, M. Ascorbic acid absorption in man--pharmacokinetic implications, *Eur J Pharmacol* 19:140-142 1972.
54. Melethil, SL, Mason, WE, and Chiang, C-J. Dose dependent absorption and excretion of vitamin C in humans, *Int J Pharm* 31:83-89 1986.
55. Richards, TW, Cheraskin, E, and Ringsdorf, WM, Jr. Effect of sustained release versus regular multivitamin supplement upon vitamin C state, *Int Z Vitaminforsch* 39:407-415 1969.
56. Zetler, G, Seidel, G, Siegers, CP, and Ivens, H. Pharmacokinetics of ascorbic acid in man, *Eur J Clin Pharmacol* 10:273-282 1976.
57. Piotrovskij, VK, Kallay, Z, Gajdos, M, Gerykova, M, and Trnovec, T. The use of a nonlinear absorption model in the study of ascorbic acid bioavailability in man, *Biopharm Drug Dispos* 14:429-442 1993.

58. Mangels, AR, Block, G, Frey, CM, Patterson, BH, Taylor, PR, Norkus, EP, and Levander, OA. The bioavailability to humans of ascorbic acid from oranges, orange juice and cooked broccoli is similar to that of synthetic ascorbic acid, *J Nutr* 123:1054-1061 1993.
59. Graumlich, JF, Ludden, TM, Conry-Cantilena, C, Cantilena, LR, Jr, Wang, Y, and Levine, M. Pharmacokinetic model of ascorbic acid in healthy male volunteers during depletion and repletion, *Pharmaceutical Research* 14:1133-1139 1997.
60. Clayton, MM and Folsom, MT. A method for the study of the availability for human nutrition of the vitamin C in foods, with an application to the study of the potato, *J Home Econ* 32:390-395 1940.
61. Todhunter, EN and Fatzer, AS. A comparison of the utilization by college women of equivalent amounts of ascorbic acid (vitamin C) in red raspberries and in crystalline form, *J Nutr* 19:121-130 1940.
62. Hartzler, ER. The availability of ascorbic acid in papayas and guavas, *J Nutr* 30:355-365 1945.
63. Vinson, JA and Bose, P. Comparative bioavailability to humans of ascorbic acid alone or in a citrus extract, *Am J Clin Nutr* 48:601-604 1988.
64. Patterson, JW. The diabetogenic effect of dehydroascorbic and dehydroisoascorbic acids, *J Biol Chem* 183:81-88 1950.
65. Baker, EM, Hodges, RE, Hood, J, Sauberlich, HE, and March, SC. Metabolism of ascorbic-1-14C acid in experimental human scurvy, *Am J Clin Nutr* 22:549-558 1969.
66. Hodges, RE, Baker, EM, Hood, J, Sauberlich, HE, and March, SC. Experimental scurvy in man, *Am J Clin Nutr* 22:535-548 1969.
67. Hodges, RE, Hood, J, Canham, JE, Sauberlich, HE, and Baker, EM. Clinical manifestations of ascorbic acid deficiency in man, *Am J Clin Nutr* 24:432-443 1971.
68. Hodges, RE. What's new about scurvy? *Am J Clin Nutr* 24:383-384 1971.
69. Jacob, RA, Pianalto, FS, and Agee, RE. Cellular ascorbate depletion in healthy men, *J Nutr* 122:1111-1118 1992.
70. Kallner, A, Hartmann, D, and Hornig, D. Steady-state turnover and body pool of ascorbic acid in man, *Am J Clin Nutr* 32:530-539 1979.
71. VanderJagt, DJ, Garry, PJ, and Bhagavan, HN. Ascorbic acid intake and plasma levels in healthy elderly people, *Am J Clin Nutr* 46:290-294 1987.
72. Garry, PJ, Goodwin, JS, Hunt, WC, and Gilbert, BA. Nutritional status in a healthy elderly population: vitamin C, *Am J Clin Nutr* 36:332-339 1982.
73. Hegsted, DM. Defining a nutritious diet: need for new dietary standards, *J Am Coll Nutr* 11:241-245 1992.
74. Dhariwal, KR, Hartzell, WO, and Levine, M. Ascorbic acid and dehydroascorbic acid measurements in human plasma and serum, *Am J Clin Nutr* 54:712-716 1991.
75. Koshiishi, I and Imanari, T. Measurement of ascorbate and dehydroascorbate contents in biological fluids, *Anal Chem* 69:216-220 1997.
76. Cox, BD and Whichelow, MJ. The measurement of dehydroascorbic acid and diketogulonic acid in normal and diabetic plasma, *Biochem Med* 12:183-193 1975.
77. Hornig, D. Distribution of ascorbic acid, metabolites and analogues in man and animals, *Ann N Y Acad Sci* 258:103-118 1975.
78. Damron, CM, Monier, MM, and Roe, JH. Metabolism of L-ascorbic acid, dehydro L-ascorbic acid and diketo-L-gulonic acid in the guinea pig, *J Biol Chem* 195:599-606 1952.
79. Welch, RW, Wang, Y, Crossman, A, Jr, Park, JB, Kirk, KL, and Levine, M. Accumulation of vitamin C (ascorbate) and its oxidized metabolite dehydroascorbic acid occurs by separate mechanisms, *J Biol Chem* 270:12584-12592 1995.

80. Jacob, RA, Omaye, ST, Skala, JH, Leggott, PJ, Rothman, DL, and Murray, PA. Experimental vitamin C depletion and supplementation in young men. Nutrient interactions and dental health effects, *Ann N Y Acad Sci* 498:333-346 1987.
81. Fraga, CG, Motchnik, PA, Shigenaga, MK, Helbock, HJ, Jacob, RA, and Ames, BN. Ascorbic acid protects against endogenous oxidative DNA damage in human sperm, *Proc Natl Acad Sci U S A* 88:11003-11006 1991.
82. Washko, PW, Rotrosen, D, and Levine, M. Ascorbic acid transport and accumulation in human neutrophils, *J Biol Chem* 264:18996-19002 1989.
83. Dixon, SJ and Wilson, JX. Adaptive regulation of ascorbate transport in osteoblastic cells, *J Bone Miner Res* 7:675-681 1992.
84. Lam, KW, Yu, HS, Glickman, RD, and Lin, T. Sodium-dependent ascorbic and dehydroascorbic acid uptake by SV-40-transformed retinal pigment epithelial cells, *Ophthalmic Res* 25:100-107 1993.
85. Welch, RW, Bergsten, P, Butler, JD, and Levine, M. Ascorbic acid accumulation and transport in human fibroblasts, *Biochem J* 294:505-510 1993.
86. Bergsten, P, Yu, R, Kehrl, J, and Levine, M. Ascorbic acid transport and distribution in human B lymphocytes, *Arch Biochem Biophys* 317:208-214 1995.
87. Wright, JR, Castranova, V, Colby, HD, and Miles, PR. Ascorbate uptake by isolated rat lung cells, *J Appl Physiol* 51:1477-1483 1981.
88. Castranova, V, Wright, JR, Colby, HD, and Miles, PR. Ascorbate uptake by isolated rat alveolar macrophages and type II cells, *J Appl Physiol* 54:208-214 1983.
89. Ingermann, RL, Stankova, L, and Bigley, RH. Role of monosaccharide transporter in vitamin C uptake by placental membrane vesicles, *Am J Physiol* 250:C637-C641 1986.
90. Hughes, RE and Maton, SC. The passage of vitamin C across the erythrocyte membrane, *Br J Haematol* 14:247-253 1968.
91. Bigley, R, Wirth, M, Layman, D, Riddle, M, and Stankova, L. Interaction between glucose and dehydroascorbate transport in human neutrophils and fibroblasts, *Diabetes* 32:545-548 1983.
92. Stahl, RL, Farber, CM, Liebes, LF, and Silber, R. Relationship of dehydroascorbic acid transport to cell lineage in lymphocytes from normal subjects and patients with chronic lymphocytic leukemia, *Cancer Res* 45:6507-6512 1985.
93. Vera, JC, Rivas, CI, Zhang, RH, Farber, CM, and Golde, DW. Human HL-60 myeloid leukemia cells transport dehydroascorbic acid via the glucose transporters and accumulate reduced ascorbic acid, *Blood* 84:1628-1634 1994.
94. Rumsey, SC, Kwon, O, Xu, GW, Burant, CF, Simpson, I, and Levine, M. Glucose transporter isoforms GLUT1 and GLUT3 transport dehydroascorbic acid, *J Biol Chem* 272:18982-18989 1997.
95. Mann, GV and Newton, P. The membrane transport of ascorbic acid, *Ann N Y Acad Sci* 258:243-252 1975.
96. Mooradian, AD. Effect of ascorbate and dehydroascorbate on tissue uptake of glucose, *Diabetes* 36:1001-1004 1987.
97. Keller, K and Mueckler, M. Different mammalian facilitative glucose transporters expressed in Xenopus oocytes, *Biomed Biochim Acta* 49:1201-1203 1990.
98. Hediger, MA, Coady, MJ, Ikeda, TS, and Wright, EM. Expression cloning and cDNA sequencing of the Na+/glucose co-transporter, *Nature* 330:379-381 1987.
99. Kanai, Y, Lee, WS, You, G, Brown, D, and Hediger, MA. The human kidney low affinity Na+/glucose cotransporter SGLT2. Delineation of the major renal reabsorptive mechanism for D-glucose, *J Clin Invest* 93:397-404 1994.
100. Vera, JC, Rivas, CI, Fischbarg, J, and Golde, DW. Mammalian facilitative hexose transporters mediate the transport of dehydroascorbic acid, *Nature* 364:79-82 1993.

101. Haber, RS, Weinstein, SP, O'Boyle, E, and Morgello, S. Tissue distribution of the human GLUT3 glucose transporter, *Endocrinology* 132:2538-2543 1993.
102. Maher, F, Vannucci, SJ, and Simpson, IA. Glucose transporter proteins in brain, *FASEB J* 8:1003-1011 1994.
103. Hendry, JM, Easson, LH, and Owen, JA. The uptake and reduction of dehydroascorbic acid by human leukocytes, *Clin Chim Acta* 9:498-499 1964.
104. Bigley, RH and Stankova, L. Uptake and reduction of oxidized and reduced ascorbate by human leukocytes, *J Exp Med* 139:1084-1092 1974.
105. Borsook, H, Davenport, HW, Jeffreys, CEP, and Warner, RC. The oxidation of ascorbic acid and its reduction *in vitro* and *in vivo*, *J Biol Chem* 117:237-279 1936.
106. Winkler, BS, Orselli, SM, and Rex, TS. The redox couple between glutathione and ascorbic acid: a chemical and physiological perspective, *Free Radic Biol Med* 17:333-349 1994.
107. Wells, WW and Xu, DP. Dehydroascorbate reduction, *J Bioenerg Biomembr* 26:369-377 1994.
108. Levine, SC. Rumsey, Y. Wang, JK. Park, O, W. Xu, and N. Amano, Vitamin C, in: *Present Knowledge in Nutrition*, LJ. Filer *et al.,* International Life Sciences Institute, Washington, DC. pp. 146-159 (1996).
109. Wells, WW, Xu, DP, Yang, Y, and Rocque, PA. Mammalian thioltransferase (Glutaredoxin) and protein disulfide isomerase have dehydroascorbate reductase activity, *J Biol Chem* 265:15361-15364 1990.
110. Del Bello, B, Maellaro, E, Sugherini, L, Santucci, A, Comporti, M, and Casini, AF. Purification of NADPH-dependent dehydroascorbate reductase from rat liver and its identification with 3 alpha-hydroxysteroid dehydrogenase, *Biochem J* 304:385-390 1994.
111. Maellaro, E, Del Bello, B, Sugherini, L, Santucci, A, Comporti, M, and Casini, AF. Purification and characterization of glutathione-dependent dehydroascorbate reductase from rat liver, *Biochem J* 301:471-476 1994.
112. Wang, Y, Russo, TA, Kwon, O, Chanock, S, Rumsey, SC, and Levine, M. Ascorbate recycling in human neutrophils: Induction by bacteria, *Proc Natl Acad Sci USA* 94:13816-13819 1997.
113. Evans, RM, Currie, L, and Campbell, A. The distribution of ascorbic acid between various cellular components of blood, in normal individuals, and its relation to the plasma concentration, *Br J Nutr* 47:473-482 1982.
114. Ralli, EP, Friedman, GJ, and Rubin, SH. The mechanism of the excretion of vitamin C by the human kidney, *J Clin Invest* 17:765-770 1938.
115. Bowers-Komro, DM and McCormick, DB. Characterization of ascorbic acid uptake by isolated rat kidney cells, *J Nutr* 121:57-64 1991.
116. Friedman, GJ, Sherry, S, and Ralli, E. The mechanism of excretion of vitamin C by the human kidney at low and normal plasma levels of ascorbic acid, *J Clin Invest* 19:685-689 1940.
117. Oreopoulos, DG, Lindeman, RD, VanderJagt, DJ, Tzamaloukas, AH, Bhagavan, HN, and Garry, PJ. Renal excretion of ascorbic acid: effect of age and sex, *J Am Coll Nutr* 12:537-542 1993.
118. Toggenburger, G, Hausermann, M, Mutsch, B, Genoni, G, Kessler, M, Weber, F, Hornig, D, O'Neill, B, and Semenza, G. Na+-dependent, potential-sensitive L-ascorbate transport across brush border membrane vesicles from kidney cortex, *Biochim Biophys Acta* 646:433-443 1981.
119. Rose, RC. Ascorbic acid transport in mammalian kidney, *Am J Physiol* 250:F627-F632 1986.
120. Bianchi, J and Rose, RC. Transport of L-ascorbic acid and dehydro-L-ascorbic acid across renal cortical basolateral membrane vesicles, *Biochim Biophys Acta* 820:265-273 1985.
121. Rose, RC, Choi, JL, and Koch, MJ. Intestinal transport and metabolism of oxidized ascorbic acid (dehydroascorbic acid), *Am J Physiol* 254:G824-G828 1988.

122. Wang, YH, Dhariwal, KR, and Levine, M. Ascorbic acid bioavailability in humans. Ascorbic acid in plasma, serum, and urine, *Ann N Y Acad Sci* 669:383-386 1992.
123. Washko, P and Levine, M. Inhibition of ascorbic acid transport in human neutrophils by glucose, *J Biol Chem* 267:23568-23574 1992.
124. Stein, HB, Hasan, A, and Fox, IH. Ascorbic acid-induced uricosuria. A consequence of megavitamin therapy, *Ann Intern Med* 84:385-388 1976.
125. Sutton, JL, Basu, TK, and Dickerson, JW. Effect of large doses of ascorbic acid in man on some nitrogenous components of urine, *Hum Nutr Appl Nutr* 37:136-140 1983.
126. Mitch, WE, Johnson, MW, Kirshenbaum, JM, and Lopez, RE. Effect of large oral doses of ascorbic acid on uric acid excretion by normal subjects, *Clin Pharmacol Ther* 29:318-321 1981.
127. Wandzilak, TR, D'Andre, SD, Davis, PA, and Williams, HE. Effect of high dose vitamin C on urinary oxalate levels, *J Urol* 151:834-837 1994.
128. Tinchieri, A, Mandressi, A, Luongo, P, Longo, G, and Pisani, E. The influence of diet on urinary risk factors for stones in healthy subjects and idiopathic renal calcium stone formers, *Br J Urol* 67:230-236 1991.
129. Urivetzky, M, Kessaris, D, and Smith, AD. Ascorbic acid overdosing: a risk factor for calcium oxalate nephrolithiasis, *J Urol* 147:1215-1218 1992.
130. Li, MG and Madappally, MM. Rapid enzymatic determination of urinary oxalate, *Clin Chem* 35:2330-2333 1989.
131. Hallberg, L, Brune, M, and Rossander-Hulthen, L. Is there a physiological role of vitamin C in iron absorption? *Ann N Y Acad Sci* 498:324-32:324-332 1987.
132. Cook, JD and Monsen, ER. Vitamin C, the common cold, and iron absorption, *Am J Clin Nutr* 30:235-241 1977.
133. Campbell, GD, Jr, Steinberg, MH, and Bower, JD. Letter: Ascorbic acid-induced hemolysis in G-6-PD deficiency, *Ann Intern Med* 82:810 1975.
134. Mehta, JB, Singhal, SB, and Mehta, BC. Ascorbic-acid-induced haemolysis in G-6-PD deficiency [letter], *Lancet* 336:944 1990.
135. Rees, DC, Kelsey, H, and Richards, JD. Acute haemolysis induced by high dose ascorbic acid in glucose-6-phosphate dehydrogenase deficiency, *BMJ* 306:841-842 1993.
136. Herbert, V, Shaw, S, Jayatilleke, E, and Stopler-Kasdan, T. Most free-radical injury is iron-related: it is promoted by iron, hemin, holoferritin and vitamin C, and inhibited by desferoxamine and apoferritin, *Stem Cells (Dayt)* 12:289-303 1994.
137. Dhariwal, KR, Washko, P, Hartzell, WO, and Levine, M. Ascorbic acid within chromaffin granules. *In situ* kinetics of norepinephrine biosynthesis, *J Biol Chem* 264:15404-15409 1989.
138. Levine, M, Rumsey, SC, Wang, Y, Park, J, Kwon, O, and Amano, N. *In situ* kinetics: an approach to recommended intake of vitamin C, *Methods Enzymol* 281:425-437 1997.
139. Haytowitz, D. Information from USDA's Nutrient Data Book, *J Nutr* 125:1952-1955 1995.
140. Lachance, P and Langseth, L. The RDA concept: time for a change? *Nutr Rev* 52:266-270 1994.
141. Koplan, JP, Annest, JL, Layde, PM, and Rubin, GL. Nutrient intake and supplementation in the United States (NHANES II), *Am J Public Health* 76:287-290 1986.
142. Patterson, BH, Block, G, Rosenberger, WF, Pee, D, and Kahle, LL. Fruit and vegetables in the American diet: data from the NHANES II survey, *Am J Public Health* 80:1443-1449 1990.
143. Murphy, SP, Rose, D, Hudes, M, and Viteri, FE. Demographic and economic factors associated with dietary quality for adults in the 1987-88 Nationwide Food Consumption Survey, *J Am Diet Assoc* 92:1352-1357 1992.
144. Byers, R and Guerrieri, N. Epidemiologic evidence for vitamin C and vitamin E in cancer prevention, *Am J Clin Nutr* 62 (suppl):1385S-1392S 1995.

145. Blot, WJ, Li, J-Y, Taylor, PR, *et al.* Nutrition intervention trials in Linxian, China: supplementation with specific vitamin/mineral combinations, cancer incidence, and disease-specific mortality in the general population, *J Natl Cancer Instit* 85:1483-1492 1993.
146. Enstrom, JE, Kanim, LE, and Breslow, L. The relationship between vitamin C intake, general health practices, and mortality in Alameda County, California, *Am J Public Health* 76:1124-1130 1986.
147. Gey, KF, Moser, UK, Jordan, P, Stahelin, HB, Eichholzer, M, and Ludin, E. Increased risk of cardiovascular disease at suboptimal plasma concentrations of essential antioxidants: an epidemiological update with special attention to carotene and vitamin C, *Am J Clin Nutr* 57:787S-797S 1993.
148. Greenberg, ER, Baron, JA, Tosteson, TD, Freeman, DH, Jr, Beck, GJ, Bond, JH, Colacchio, TA, Coller, JA, Frankl, HD, and Haile, RW. A clinical trial of antioxidant vitamins to prevent colorectal adenoma. Polyp Prevention Study Group, *N Engl J Med* 331:141-147 1994.
149. Jacques, PF, Chylack, LT, Jr, McGandy, RB, and Hartz, SC. Antioxidant status in persons with and without senile cataract, *Arch Ophthalmol* 106:337-340 1988.
150. Riemersma, RA, Wood, DA, Macintyre, CC, Elton, RA, Gey, KF, and Oliver, MF. Risk of angina pectoris and plasma concentrations of vitamins A, C, and E and carotene, *Lancet* 337:1-5 1991.
151. Rimm, EB, Stampfer, MJ, Ascherio, A, Giovannucci, E, Colditz, GA, and Willett, WC. Vitamin E consumption and the risk of coronary heart disease in men, *N Engl J Med* 328:1450-1456 1993.
152. Seddon, JM, Ajani, UA, Sperduto, RD, Hiller, R, Blair, N, Burton, TC, Farber, MD, Gragoudas, ES, Haller, J, and Miller, DT. Dietary carotenoids, vitamins A, C, and E, and advanced age-related macular degeneration. Eye Disease Case-Control Study Group, *JAMA* 272:1413-1420 1994.
153. Robertson, JM, Donner, AP, and Trevithick, JR. A possible role for vitamins C and E in cataract prevention, *Am J Clin Nutr* 53:346S-351S 1991.
154. Vitale, S, West, S, Hallfrisch, J, Alston, C, Wang, F, Moorman, C, Muller, D, Singh, V, and Taylor, HR. Plasma antioxidants and risk of cortical and nuclear cataract, *Epidemiology* 4:195-203 1993.
155. Block, F, Kunkel, M, and Sontag, KH. Posttreatment with EPC-K1, an inhibitor of lipid peroxidation and of phospholipase A2 activity, reduces functional deficits after global ischemia in rats, *Brain Res Bull* 36:257-260 1995.
156. Levine, M, Rumsey, S, and Wang, Y. Principles involved in formulating recommendations for vitamin C intake: a paradigm for water-soluble vitamins, *Methods Enzymol* 279:43-54 1997.
157. Kallner, AB, Hartmann, D, and Hornig, DH. On the requirements of ascorbic acid in man: steady-state turnover and body pool in smokers, *Am J Clin Nutr* 34:1347-1355 1981.
158. Bielski, Chemistry of ascorbic acid radicals, in: *Ascorbic Acid: Chemistry, Metabolism, and Uses*, PA. Seib *et al.,* American Chemical Society, Washington, DC. pp. 81-100 (1982).
159. Washko, PW, Welch, RW, Dhariwal, KR, Wang, Y, and Levine, M. Ascorbic acid and dehydroascorbic acid analyses in biological samples, *Anal Biochem* 204:1-14 1992.
160. King, J, Wang, Y, Welch, RW, Dhariwal, KR, Conry-Cantilena, C, and Levine, M. Use of a new vitamin C-deficient diet in a depletion/repletion clinical trial, *Am J Clin Nutr* 65:1434-1440 1997.

10

Vitamin E: Tocopherols and Tocotrienols

Andreas M. Papas, Ph.D.
Health and Nutrition
Eastman Chemical Company, Kingsport, Tennessee, USA

INTRODUCTION

Vitamin E was discovered by Evans and Bishop in 1922 in the course of research on the relationship of nutrition and fertility.[1] Female rats, fed a vitamin E deficient diet for several months, suffered loss of fertility through resorption of the fetus, which was prevented by supplementing their diet with small amounts of fresh lettuce, wheat germ, or dried alfalfa leaves. Originally, the term vitamin E described a lipid extract from plants, which was essential to maintain fertility.[2] Later, 8 compounds exhibiting vitamin E activity were isolated, four tocopherols and four tocotrienols (Figure 1). The tocopherols

0-8493-8009-X/98/$0.00+$.50

were isolated and characterized first in the late '30s; tocotrienols were characterized approximately 25 years later.[3]

α-Tocopherol has become synonymous with vitamin E and has been the main focus of research because it is the predominant form in human and animal tissues. In addition, it is by far the most bioactive form based on the rat fetal resorption test, which is the classical assay for vitamin E activity.[4] The other tocopherols and tocotrienols, however, have important and unique antioxidant and other biological effects in nutrition and health and are now receiving increased attention.[5-7]

Vitamin E is one of the most important lipid soluble antioxidants.[8] This chapter will review its chemistry, absorption, transport, metabolism, and biological function with emphasis on the role of tocopherols and tocotrienols as biological antioxidants. Their role in health and disease will be discussed in several other chapters of this book.

CHEMICAL FORMS AND POTENCY

Tocopherols consist of a chroman ring and a long, saturated phytyl chain. The four tocopherols, designated as α, β, γ, and δ, differ only in the number and position of the methyl groups on the chroman ring. Tocotrienols, also designated as α, β, γ, and δ, have identical chroman rings to the corresponding tocopherols, but their side chain is unsaturated with double bonds in the 3', 7', and 11' positions (Figure 1).

The natural tocopherols all have three asymmetric carbons at the 2, 4', and 8' positions. Biosynthesis of tocopherols in nature yields only the RRR stereoisomer. For example, α-tocopherol derived from natural sources is 2R,4'R,8'R-α-tocopherol. In contrast, tocopherols produced by chemical synthesis, by condensing isophytol with tri-, di-, or monomethyl hydroquinone, are equimolar racemic mixtures (all-rac) of 8 stereoisomers (Figure 2).

The National Research Council (NRC)[11] recommended that, for dietary purposes, vitamin E activity be expressed as d-α-tocopherol equivalents (α-TE; 1.0 mg RRR-α-tocopherol = 1.0 α-TE). *All-rac*-α-tocopherol was assigned a value of 0.74 α-TE (for 1.0 mg). Biopotency of the esterified forms is computed from the RRR or *all-rac*-α-tocopherol content (Table 1). For mixed tocopherols the NRC proposed the following biopotencies in α-TE: β–tocopherol 0.5, γ-tocopherol 0.1, α-tocotrienol 0.3. The biopotency of RRR α-tocopherol and its esters over the corresponding *all-rac* forms is 36%

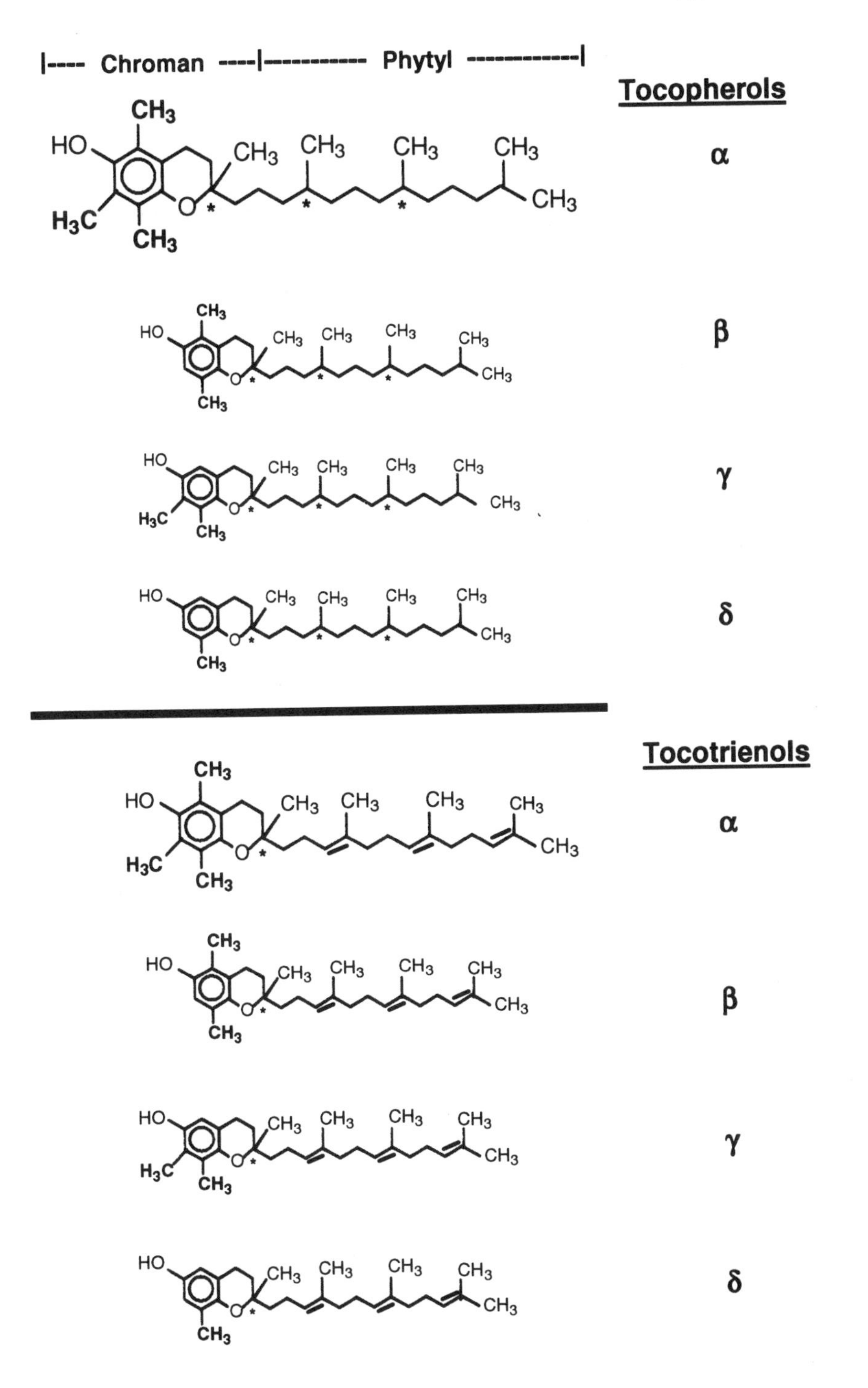

Figure 1. Structure of tocopherols and tocotrienols. Tocopherols and tocotrienols have the same chroman ring but the phytyl tail of tocotrienols contains three double bonds.

higher whether expressed in IU, USP E Units, or α-TE. Commercial products are usually labeled in IU with only limited labeling in α-TE. Vitamin E activity in commercial products is computed only from its α-tocopherol content; no IU or α-TE is included from other tocopherols or tocotrienols. These biopotencies were applied to humans without species adjustments. Recent research, discussed below, indicates that these biopotencies significantly underestimate the advantage of RRR-rac-α-tocopheryl acetate and other RRR forms over the corresponding *all-rac* forms.[12-15]

Table 1
Potencies of Tocopherols and Tocotrienols in International Units (IU) or α-Tocopherol Equivalents (α-TE) [a,b]

	IU/mg	α-TE/mg
α-Tocopherol		
Naturally occurring d- or RRR-α-tocopherol and its esters		
d-α-tocopherol	1.49	**1.0**
d-α-tocopheryl acetate	1.36	0.91
d-α-tocopheryl succinate	1.21	0.81
d-α-tocopheryl polyethylene glycol 1000 succinate (TPGS)	0.39	0.26
Synthetic dl- or *all-rac*-α-tocopherol and its ester		
dl-α-tocopherol	1.10	0.74
dl-α-tocopheryl acetate	**1.0**	0.67
dl-α-tocopheryl succinate	0.89	0.60
Other tocols (only for diets containing natural form:		
d-β-tocopherol	0	0.50
d-γ-tocopherol	0	0.10
d-δ-tocopherol	0	0
d-α-tocotrienol	0	0.30
d-β-tocotrienol	0	0
d-γ-tocotrienol	0	0
d-δ-tocotrienol	0	0

[a] United States Pharmacopeia/National Formulary (Reference 10) the International Formulatory and the International Union of Pure and Applied Chemistry.
[b] National Research Council (Reference 11).

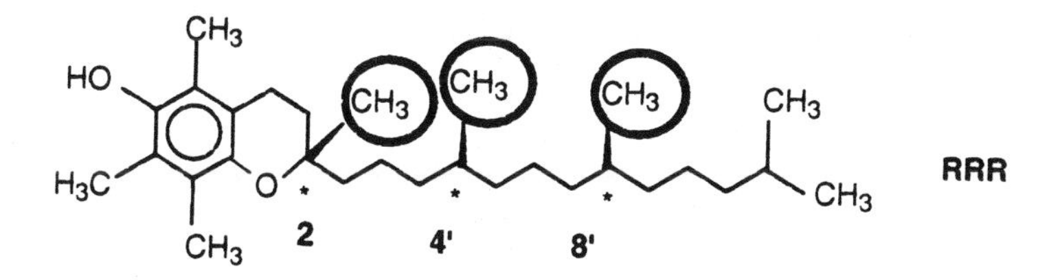

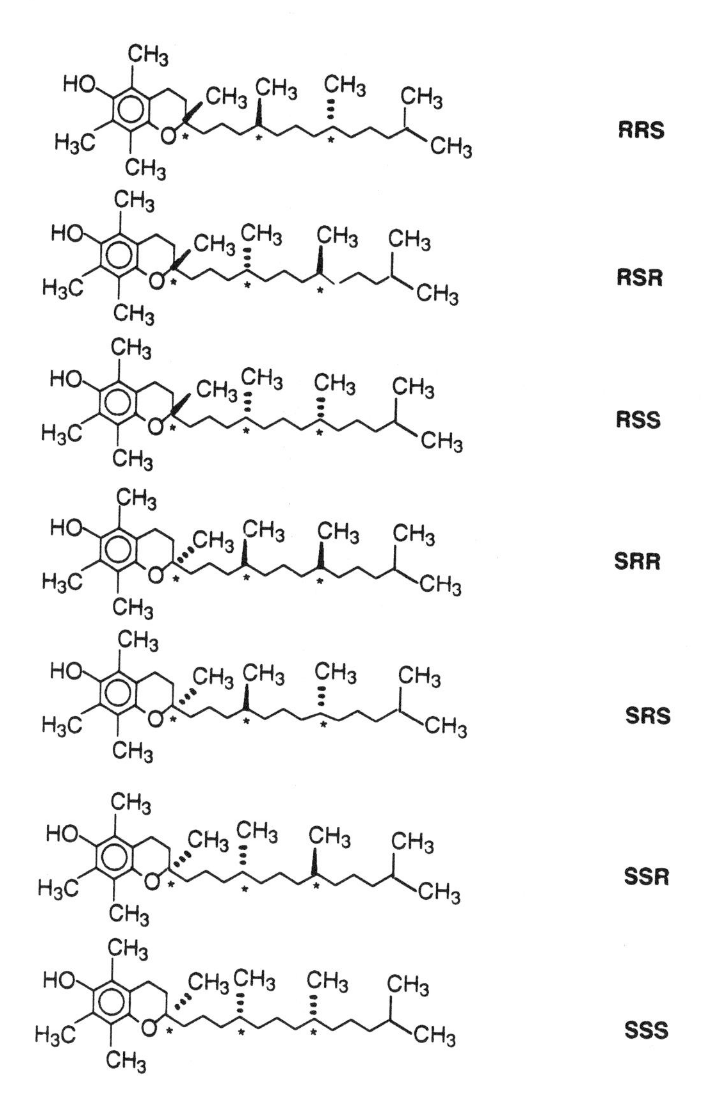

Figure 2. The eight stereoisomers of synthetic *all-rac*-α–tocopherol which result from the random positioning of the methyl groups on the 2, 4', and 8' asymmetric carbons indicated by *. Tocopherols derived from natural sources contain only the RRR stereoisomer.

ABSORPTION, TRANSPORT, AND BIOAVAILABILITY

Absorption and Transport

Vitamin E is absorbed in the same path as other nonpolar lipids such as triglycerides and cholesterol.[12] Bile, produced by the liver, emulsifies the tocopherols incorporating them into micelles along with other fat-soluble compounds, thereby facilitating absorption. Esters of α-tocopherol, such as acetate and succinate, are hydrolyzed by lipases, produced by the pancreas, and are absorbed as free α-tocopherol. Dietary fat, which promotes production of lipases and bile, is essential for absorption of vitamin E. TPGS, a water-soluble form of vitamin E, forms its own micelles and can be absorbed without the aid of lipases or bile salts.[16,17]

Tocopherols are absorbed from the small intestine and secreted into lymph in chylomicrons produced in the intestinal wall (Figure 3). Lipoprotein lipases catabolize chylomicrons rapidly and a small amount of tocopherol may be transferred from chylomicron remnants to other lipoproteins or tissues. During this process, apolipoprotein E binds to chylomicron remnants. Because the liver has specific apolipoprotein E receptors, it retains and clears the majority of the chylomicron remnants. Tocopherols in the remnants are secreted into very low-density lipoproteins (VLDL) and circulated through the plasma. VLDL is hydrolyzed by lipoprotein lipase to low density lipoproteins (LDL), which carry the largest part of plasma tocopherols and appears to exchange them readily with high-density lipoproteins (HDL). Tocopherols in HDL may be readily transferred back to chylomicron remnants as they pass through circulation returning plasma tocopherol to the liver.

Tissue uptake of tocopherols varies widely and is not well understood. Tocopherols may be delivered to tissues during hydrolysis of chylomicrons and VLDL. It is believed, however, that tocopherols are largely transferred from LDL to tissues by the action of LDL receptors on the surface of tissue cells as well as by the direct transfer of tocopherol across membranes from areas of high concentration to areas of low concentration. This transfer may occur from lipoproteins to tissues or from tissues to lipoproteins. Tocopherol uptake by tissues has been described as either rapid (plasma, red blood cells, spleen, and liver) or slow (heart, testes, muscle, brain, and spinal cord).[18,19]

Absorption of tocotrienols appears similar to tocopherols. Their transport and tissue uptake, however, appear to differ from α-tocopherol. Tocotrienols disappear from plasma with chylomicron clearance and are deposited, in conjunction with triglycerides, in the adipose tissue.[20]

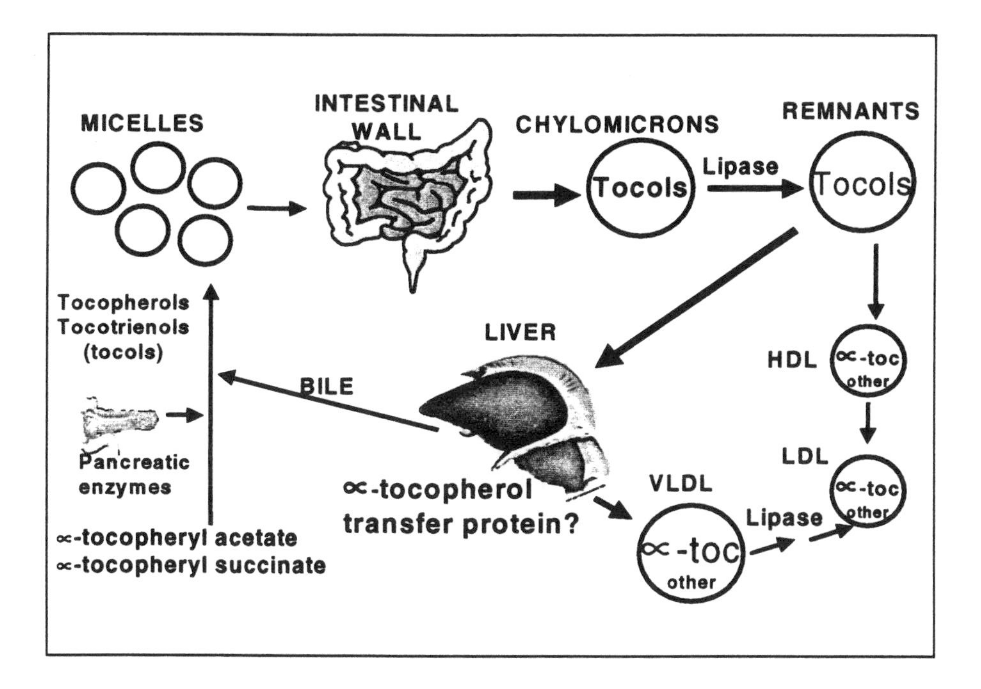

Figure 3. Absorption and transport of tocopherols as proposed in Reference 11. The absorption and transport of tocotrienols is not fully understood.

Biodiscrimination of Tocopherols and Tocotrienols

Our plasma and tissues contain at least 2-3 times more α than γ-tocopherol even though the typical American diet contains more γ than α-tocopherol.[21] Concentration of tocotrienols in plasma and tissues is low even when consumed in comparable amounts with α-tocopherol.[22,23] Similarly, others and we showed that RRR-α-tocopheryl acetate increased blood levels more than an equimolar amount of *all-rac*-α-tocopheryl acetate.[13-15] It appears that biodiscrimination, which takes place largely in the liver, causes these differences.[12] Research in the mechanisms involved was greatly facilitated by the synthesis of tocopherols labeled with deuterium.[24] Researchers supplied these tocopherols to humans and animals individually or in mixtures and studied their absorption, transport, and tissue uptake with significant accuracy because their label made it possible to differentiate them from food and endogenous tocopherols.[12,13,15,18,19,22,25] α-Tocopherol and γ-tocopherol are apparently equally well absorbed. However, α-tocopherol is preferentially secreted into nascent VLDL. Similarly, RRR and the SRR stereoisomer are equally well absorbed, yet the RRR causes higher levels of α-tocopherol in the blood and tissues (Figure 4).

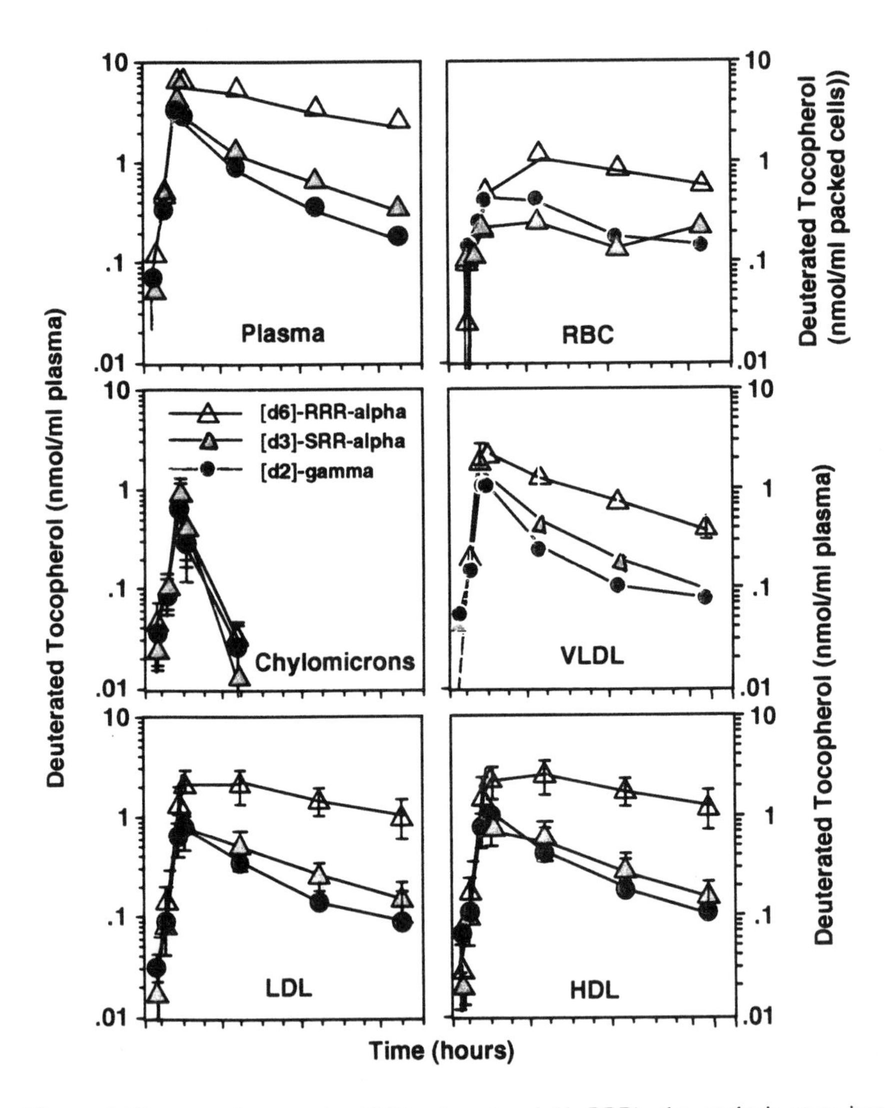

Figure 4. The naturally occurring RRR-α-tocopherol (d_6-RRR), the synthetic stereoisomer SRR-α-tocopherol (d_3-SRR), and RRR-γ-tocopherol (d_2-gamma) appear in similar concentrations in the chylomicrons but RRR-α-tocopherol is preferentially secreted in VLDL and other lipoproteins. (From Traber *et al. J Lipid Res* 1992;33;1171-82 with permission.)

It was proposed that a tocopherol binding protein is responsible for incorporating preferentially RRR-α-tocopherol into nascent VLDL.[12,25,26] This protein has been identified and characterized in the rat, rabbit, and recently humans.[27-33] This protein has greater affinity for RRR-α-tocopherol than other tocopherols. It has been suggested, but not yet confirmed, that the tocopherol binding protein is responsible for the biodiscrimination in favor of the naturally occurring RRR over the synthetic *all-rac*-α-tocopherol.[12] Supporting this hypothesis is evidence from humans and animals, indicating similar absorption for both forms but lower blood and tissue level with the *all-rac* form. Also, in patients with familial isolated vitamin E deficiency, who lack or have defective tocopherol transfer protein, this biodiscrimination is absent or very weak.[34]

Natural vs. Synthetic α-tocopherol (RRR vs. *all-rac*)

The relative biopotencies of RRR and *all-rac*-α-tocopherol were determined by the rat fetal resorption test. Extrapolating from the rat to humans assumes equivalent biodiscrimination. Strong evidence from studies using deuterium labeled tocopherols points to significant differences. Our work in healthy subjects showed a relative bioavailabilty for RRR and *all-rac*-α-tocopheryl acetate, measured as the ratio of the respective α-tocopherol areas under the blood concentration curve, was close to 2:1 (Figure 5); this is significantly higher than the accepted biopotency ratio of 1.36:1.[13] Other researchers confirmed this ratio.[13-15] Furthermore, researchers measured the relative concentration in tissues obtained from humans during elective surgery or from terminally ill patients immediately after their death. Ratios of RRR and *all-rac*-α-tocopherol in various tissues varied, but they were mostly higher than 1.36. Ratios in the liver were lower probably reflecting the ratio prior to the effect of biodiscrimination.[14]

Regulation of Blood and Tissue Levels and Metabolism

The mechanisms for regulating blood and tissue levels of vitamin E and its metabolic fate are not well understood. The tocopherol binding protein probably plays a major role because its affinity for individual tocopherols is reflected in blood and tissue concentrations. Patients lacking this protein have very low concentrations of α-tocopherol.[34] In normal subjects, large doses of α-tocopherol increase blood levels 2 to 4-fold but further increase is rather small even with very large doses.[35] In contrast, infusions of lipid emulsions rich in γ-tocopherol, which bypass temporarily the normal absorption

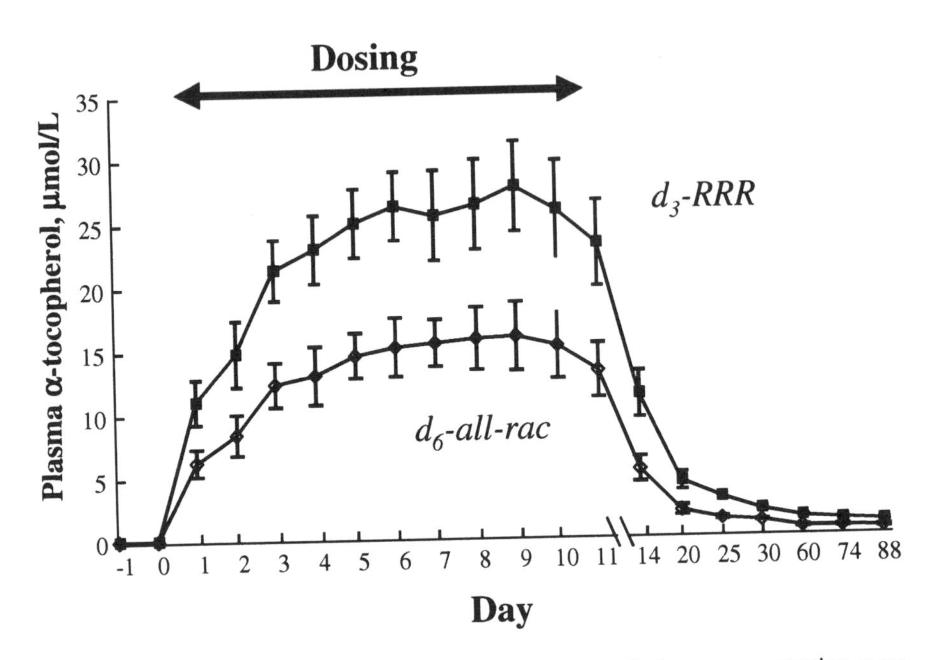

Figure 5. The naturally occurring RRR-α-tocopherol increased plasma concentration more than the synthetic *all-rac*-α-tocopherol (d_6-all-rac) in humans. Both forms were supplied in the same capsule as deuterium labeled acetate esters (150 mg each/day) to 6 people, (From Ref. 13 with permission.)

and transport route, increase its concentration in blood 10-fold but only during the infusion. Within 24 hours, concentrations of γ-tocopherol return to baseline, significantly below the levels of α-tocopherol.[26]

Unlike other fat-soluble vitamins, vitamin E is not stored in the liver and this may account for its low toxicity.[36] Tissue levels increase with dosage but the limited evidence available suggests that it does not accumulate in very large amounts.[14] What then is its metabolic fate? We and others hypothesized that larger proportions of non-α-tocopherols are excreted via the bile in the digesta. We were unable, however, to confirm this hypothesis.

There is only limited information on tissue and fecal levels of tocopherols and tocotrienols in humans. Recent data from elective surgery and terminally ill subjects indicate large variation in their tocopherol content; adipose tissue had the highest. Levels of γ-tocopherol in adipose, muscle, and skin tissues were higher than would be expected from their relative concentration in blood and comprised over 30% or more of total tocopherols.[14] Tocotrienols also seem to accumulate in the skin and adipose tissue. It was suggested that these compounds are delivered by chylomicrons during clearance and before the chylomicron remnants are taken by the liver.[20]

Very little information is available on the catabolism of different tocopherols in tissues. γ-Tocopherol disappears from rat red blood cells, liver, spleen, heart, kidney, testes, and muscle more rapidly than α-tocopherol. Similarly γ-tocopherol disappears from cultured human endothelial cells more rapidly than α-tocopherol.[37] The mechanisms involved and their metabolic products are not well understood. Two metabolic products of α-tocopherol, called the Simon metabolites, have been isolated and characterized in the urine of rabbits, humans, and rats. These are 2-(3-hydroxy-3-methyl-)-3,5,6-trimethyl-1,4-benzoquinone and its γ-lactone.[38] Two other tocopherol metabolites were isolated recently from human urine. The first, 2,5,7,8-tetramethyl-2(2'carboxyethyl)-6-hydroxychroman, a metabolite of α-tocopherol, has been suggested as an indicator of vitamin E supply.[39] The second, 2,7,8-trimethyl-2-(β-carboxyethyl)-6-hydroxychroman is believed to be a metabolite of γ-tocopherol.[40] This metabolite, named LLU-α, is probably part of the natriuretic system, which controls extracellular fluids. It is believed that oxidized tocopherols (quinones) and other metabolic products are secreted in the bile but information on their structure and relative abundance is very limited.

TOCOPHEROLS AND TOCOTRIENOLS AS ANTIOXIDANTS

Antioxidant Functions

A major antioxidant function of vitamin E in humans, studied mostly with α-tocopherol, is the inhibition of lipid peroxidation described in Chapter 1. Lipid peroxidation is particularly common in cell and organelle membranes, lipoproteins, the adipose tissue, brain, and other tissues where PUFA are abundant.

α-Tocopherol is present in membranes in the approximate ratio of 1 molecule to 1000 lipid molecules. Its phytyl tail gives it the unique ability to position itself in the membrane bilayer with the active chroman ring close to the surface.[41] This allows not only for efficient function as lipid antioxidant but also enables it to regenerate itself from its oxidized form by interacting with other antioxidants. An intriguing synergy with vitamin C, which results in the regeneration of the tocopheryl radical, was demonstrated conclusively *in vitro*[42] but its importance *in vivo* remains controversial. Nevertheless, synergy with other antioxidants, especially water soluble ones, is a particularly important feature of the antioxidant system.

Vitamin E also plays a critical role in preventing lipid oxidation in lipoproteins. α-Tocopherol is the main vitamin E form responsible for this effect in LDL because it is the most abundant[43] and the best scavenger of peroxyl radicals. Chylomicrons, however, may carry other tocopherols and tocotrienols in similar or even higher concentration than α-tocopherol, depending on the diet, and they may also play an important role as lipid antioxidants. They may also function as important lipid antioxidants in adipose tissue and the liver. Some *in vitro* studies suggested that tocotrienols are significantly more effective than tocopherols in inhibiting LDL oxidation;[44] in contrast, studies with plasma obtained from rats fed tocotrienol rich diets indicate approximately similar inhibition by α-tocotrienol and α-tocopherol; γ-tocopherol and γ-tocotrienol had similar effect but lower than the α forms.[45] It is difficult to extrapolate these findings directly to humans because the dynamic environment is different. In addition, the liver biodiscrimination reviewed above causes preferential enrichment of LDL with α-tocopherol thus explaining, in large part, its major importance.

In addition to peroxy radicals, tocopherols and tocotrienols trap singlet oxygen,[46] and other reactive species and free radicals. The antioxidant effect of vitamin E on nitrogen reactive species has been receiving increasing attention.[5,6,46] In biological systems, nitrogen dioxide (NO_2) is produced from the reaction of nitrogen oxide (NO) with oxygen. α-Tocopherol reacts with NO_2 to yield a nitrosating agent but this does not occur with γ-tocopherol. In contrast, γ-tocopherol reduces NO_2 to NO or reacts with it without generating a nitrosating species.[47] The unique ability of γ-tocopherol, probably due to the number and positioning of the methyl groups on the chroman ring, may be particularly important in carcinogenesis,[48] arthritis, and neurologic diseases because nitrosating agents can deaminate DNA bases causing mutations or interfere with important physiological and immune functions. γ-Tocotrienol may also play an important role in preventing the harmful effects of NO_2 (see Chapter 22).

Antioxidant Activity, Vitamin E Activity (Biopotency) and Bioavailability – A Unified Concept?

Early *in vitro* studies showed a clear superiority of α-tocopherol for trapping peroxyl radicals followed by β, γ, and δ. Their relative reactivities with lipid peroxyl radicals were 100/60/25/27[49] and seemed to account in large part for their relative vitamin E activity (100/50/15/0). However, later studies showed that their relative reactivities in trapping singlet oxygen were100/100/76/34 for α/β/γ/δ[46] while γ-tocopherol was reported to be superior to α-tocopherol for quenching nitrogen dioxide and peroxynitrite radicals.[5,6] From the four tocotrienols only α and γ-tocotrienols have measurable, but very low vitamin E activity. Yet, as discussed above, tocotrienols are strong antioxidants *in vitro* and in some systems are stronger or similar antioxidants as tocopherols.[44,45] Further undermining a direct relationship is the lower vitamin E activity of various stereoisomers of *all-rac*-α-tocopherol even though their *in vitro* antioxidant activity is similar.

The biodiscrimination mechanism in the liver explains in part these contradictions. Since all tocopherols (and tocotrienols?) are apparently absorbed in a similar manner, yet secreted in the blood at significantly different rates, biodiscrimination may account, in large part, for their differences in biopotency. Thus the lower biopotency of γ-tocopherol may be due, in large part, to the lower amount secreted into VLDL and entering blood and taken up by the tissues. The same may be true for other tocopherols and tocotrienols. Bioavailability for individual tocopherols and tocotrienols may be affected by the others present. Specifically, high intake of α-tocopherol depresses the levels of γ-tocopherol in blood and adipose tissue.[23]

It is apparent that antioxidant properties of tocopherols and tocotrienols have no direct relationship to their vitamin E activity (and biopotency). The emerging new information on the roles and sites of action of various tocopherols and tocotrienols[5-7,45,50,51] indicates that their vitamin E activity does not predict their role as biological antioxidants. We believe that this information underscores the need to take a fresh look at the function of all tocopherols and tocotrienols as biological antioxidants.

Tocopherols and Tocotrienols as Antioxidants – Practical Considerations

The active site of both tocopherols and tocotrienols is the 6-hydroxyl group on their chroman ring. When esterified, their 6-hydroxyl group is blocked. For this reason, tocopherols and tocotrienols can be used as food antioxidants only in their free, unesterified form.[52] The esters are, however, more stable than free tocopherols when exposed to oxidizing agents such as air, light, metals, and others and are used commercially to fortify foods or as nutritional supplements. In our digestive system, esters are hydrolyzed by lipases and are absorbed in the free tocopherol form. Tocopherols and tocotrienols in human blood and tissues are in their free, unesterified form.

RRR-α-tocopherol and RRR-α-tocopheryl acetate are equally bioavailable in healthy humans. RRR-α-tocopheryl succinate appears to have lower bioavailability in short-term but not in long-term studies.[53,54] This is probably due to slower hydrolysis in the gut and not to liver biodiscrimination since all forms are absorbed as α-tocopherol.

Tocopherols and tocotrienols applied on the skin function as antioxidants both on the surface and after they penetrate into the skin; in contrast, tocopherol esters function as antioxidants after they penetrate the skin and are hydrolyzed to the free tocopherol form.[55] This explains why α-tocopherol was effective in reducing carcinogenesis in preventing carcinogenesis in mice from ultraviolet radiation while its acetate and succinate esters were ineffective or even had a negative effect.[56]

BEYOND ANTIOXIDANT FUNCTION: OTHER BIOLOGICAL EFFECTS OF VITAMIN E

Tocopherols and tocotrienols and their metabolites appear to have significant and sometimes quite different metabolic effects, which may be independent or only partially related to their function as antioxidants. The following are major examples of such effects:

- Signal transduction. α-Tocopherol is a stronger inhibitor of Protein Kinase C (PKC), an important isoenzyme in signal transductions, than β, γ, and δ-tocopherols and α-tocotrienol.[57,58] The mechanisms involved and the biological significance of these phenomena are discussed by Drs. Őzer and Azzi in Chapter 20.
- Platelet adhesion. This is the initial event in a cascade, which converts the soluble fibrinogen to insoluble fibrin and causes blood to clot. Platelet adhesion and aggregation are absolutely essential for prevention of hemorrhaging to death. Adhesion, however, of platelets to atherosclerotic lesions accelerates the formation of plaque and heart disease. α-Tocopherol and its quinone form, reduce the rate of adhesion of platelets in a dose-dependent manner.[59,60] An antioxidant effect cannot explain the activity of the quinone. Vitamin E compounds appear to modulate the function of phospholipase A_2 and lipoxygenases and production of prostacyclin, a major metabolite of arachidonic acid.
- Post-transcriptional suppression of 3-hydroxy-3-methylglutaryl-coenzyme A (HMG-CoA) reductase. This enzyme is important for the synthesis of cholesterol. Tocotrienols appear to inhibit its activity *in vitro* and animal models.[61]
- Control of extracellular fluids. LLU-α, a proposed metabolite of γ-tocopherol, may inhibit the 70 pS K^+ channel in the apical membrane in the kidney. LLU-α is considered an endogenous natriuretic factor.[40]

- Inhibition of modification of brain and lymphocyte band 3 proteins. These proteins transport anions and CO_2, regulate acid-base balance, and link the plasma membrane to cytoskeleton. Their oxidation generates senescent cell antigen (SCA) which binds on aging cells and provides the signal for apoptosis, the process by which cells die. Vitamin E, fed to rats as d-α-tocopheryl acetate, reduced the age-related decline of anion transport in lymphocytes and reduced production of SCA.[62] It is possible that these protective effects were due exclusively to its antioxidant protection of band 3 proteins, as the authors of this study suggested. Because modification of proteins often involves enzymatic hydrolysis, non-antioxidant effects cannot be ruled out.
- Whether completely or partially independent of their antioxidant function, the above effects of tocopherols and tocotrienols have profound indirect impact on the overall antioxidant status. For example, inhibition of lipoxygenase, PKC, IL-1β, and NFκB reduces production of free radicals. Similarly, disturbances of the cell respiration and acid-base balance are major metabolic changes affecting antioxidant status.

VITAMIN E IN HEALTH AND DISEASE

Vitamin E Deficiency

The observation made in the early 1920s that a nutritional factor, later identified as vitamin E, was required for prevention of fetal resorption in rats was the first association of vitamin E and health. Later, it was found that it was required for normal fertility in male animals. Eventually deficiency of vitamin E was associated with a large number of pathological conditions:[2,63]

- Encephalomalacia, first studied in chicks
- Muscular dystrophy, first studied in rabbits and guinea pigs
- Hemolysis in humans and animals leading to anemia (common in premature babies)
- Neurologic abnormalities including areflexia and ataxia
- Muscle and other tissue damage
- Clinical symptoms of deficiency develop very slowly but they are mostly irreversible. In addition to malnutrition, malabsorption, impaired transport system and secretion of α-tocopherol in nascent VLDL in the liver, cause clinical deficiency often associated with major neurological and other health problems.

Malabsorption and Impaired Transport System

The same conditions which impair absorption of fat cause malabsorption of vitamin E because they follow a similar path. Such conditions are associated with diet, genetic diseases, infectious diseases, and others.

Very low fat or fat-free diets provide insufficient stimulation for production of bile in the liver, which is required for the formation of micelles and absorption of vitamin E. Some fat substitutes like Olestra reduce absorption of fat-soluble vitamins including vitamin E and, for this reason, it is fortified.[64] Dietary factors, like excessive alcohol consumption and infections of the liver, can cause hepatitis and thus impair liver function. Hepatitis can reduce production of bile and impair secretion of α-tocopherol in the VLDL.

Some physiological conditions and infectious diseases can affect absorption. Premature babies absorb lipids, including vitamin E rather inefficiently. In the elderly, absorption of nutrients is modified with some nutrients being absorbed at higher rates and others at lower rates. Diseases, which cause inflammation of the gut, changes in its microflora, and diarrhea reduce absorption. For example, in advanced stages of AIDS, fungi that colonize the intestinal wall causing serious diarrhea impair absorption. Short bowel syndrome, a disease associated with major inflammation of the gut, reduces absorption of vitamin E and other nutrients. These conditions are discussed in later chapters.

The following neurodegenerative diseases associated with malabsorption and impaired transport of vitamin E are discussed in Chapter 25.

- Cholestasis, a rare liver disease which causes insufficient production of bile and is associated with very serious neurologic disorders.
- Cystic fibrosis, a pancreatic disease that reduces production of enzymes including lipases, impairs formation of micelles.
- Abetalipoproteinemia, a rare defect in the secretion of chylomicrons by the intestinal wall and VLDL by the liver also associated with serious neurologic disorders.
- Familial Isolated Vitamin E Deficiency (FIVE) syndrome, an extremely rare disease. It has been suggested that a defective or absent a-tocopherol transfer protein in the liver causes this disease.

The water-soluble vitamin E TPGS is absorbed by patients whose malabsorption is due to insufficient production of bile and pancreatic enzymes, factors that prevent sufficient formation of micelles.[16] This is due to its ability to form its own micelles. In addition, it appears to be improving the vitamin E status of patients suffering from short bowel syndrome.[65]

Beyond Deficiency: Health Benefits of Vitamin E

The focus of research on the health benefits of vitamin E shifted in the last decade from deficiency to prevention of disease. Major epidemiological studies and limited, mostly short-term, intervention studies, suggested that vitamin E, studied mostly as α-tocopherol, reduced the risk of heart disease, some cancers, cataracts, some complications of diabetes, and slowed progression of some neurological and other diseases. In addition, it has been suggested that it reduces muscle damage from strenuous exercise. These benefits did not appear to result from correction of deficiency, as we understand it today. In contrast, in many cases, these effects appear associated with intakes 1-30 times the recommended dietary allowance (RDA).[66-69] The following mechanisms have been proposed as being responsible for the health benefits of vitamin E and will be discussed in later chapters of this book.

- Protection of cells from oxidative damage.
- Protection of LDL from oxidation (Chapter 16).
- Enhancement of the immune system (Chapters 13 and 17).
- Reduction of oxidative damage of specialized tissues such as the eye lens, nerve tissue, blood vessels, cartilage, and others (Chapter 24).
- Reduction of cholesterol synthesis by inhibition of the enzyme HMG-CoA reductase (Chapter 22).
- Enhancement of the antioxidant status of the digesta (Chapter 19).
- Mechanisms not related to their function as antioxidants (Chapter 20).

OPTIMUM DOSE AND SAFETY

There is considerable controversy as to the optimum dose for vitamin E. The USDA RDA is 30 IU and the NRC RDI is even lower.[10,11,70,71] It is generally assumed that the vitamin E requirement is for α-tocopherol and there is no official RDA for other tocopherols and tocotrienols.

It is estimated that intake from our diet is less than 15 IU/day.[72] Multivitamin supplements and fortified foods claiming to supply the RDA contain 30 IU per tablet, capsule, or serving. It is estimated that over 10% of Americans and a smaller percentage of the population, primarily in industrialized countries, take supplements of vitamin E alone or with other nutrients, primarily antioxidants. The most common supplemental doses are 400, 800, 100, and 200 IU.

Arguments against supplementation over the RDA include:

- There is no conclusive evidence from clinical intervention studies that higher levels are helpful for prevention of disease.[73]
- At high levels, vitamin E may act as prooxidant instead of antioxidant.
- Long-term intake of high levels of vitamin E may be toxic.

Arguments in favor of supplementation over the RDA include:

- The old concept of preventing deficiency is not applicable to maintaining good health and preventing disease. The requirements may be significantly different.
- Dose response studies measuring resistance of LDL oxidation or immune responses indicate that intake in excess of 200 IU is necessary for best response.[69]
- Epidemiological data and limited clinical intervention studies indicate that levels in excess of 100 IU are needed for prevention of disease.[66,67]
- Anthropological studies suggest that in ancient times, humans getting their diet from nature, consumed significantly more vitamin E than available in modern diets.[74]

Unlike other fat-soluble vitamins, toxicity of vitamin E is very low probably because it is not stored in the liver. Side effects have been rare, mostly gastrointestinal, with doses of over 1200 IU/day.[36] In a major study patients in early stages of Parkinson's disease received 2,000 IU/day *all-rac*-α-tocopheryl acetate for 2 years without significant side effects.[75] Two major ongoing clinical studies evaluate 300 and 400 IU RRR-α-tocopheryl acetate. In one, the Women's Health Study, 20,000 women will receive 600 IU RRR-α-tocopheryl acetate every other day for over 6 years thus providing information for prolonged use. It is unlikely that adverse effects will be observed because consumers have been taking such or higher levels without major reports of side effects.

Large doses may exacerbate blood coagulation in persons with vitamin K deficiency or those taking anticoagulant drugs. Toxicity of vitamin E has been studied primarily with α-tocopherol and little is known about the toxicity of other tocopherols and tocotrienols. It is very likely that toxicity of the other tocopherols is low because they have been used as nutritional supplements and food antioxidants for decades without any significant reports of toxicity.

CONCLUSION

Vitamin E is a major fat-soluble antioxidant and has significant antioxidant functions especially in cell membranes and lipoproteins. Epidemiological and limited intervention studies suggest that vitamin E may help reduce the risk of cardiovascular disease, some cancers, and other chronic diseases. A number of major intervention clinical trials are now in progress for further evaluation of the health effects of vitamin E. While α-tocopherol has been the focus of most research in the past, other tocopherols and tocotrienols are now receiving increased attention. Early results suggest that they may have antioxidant and other functions different from α-tocopherol.

REFERENCES

1. Evans HM, Bishop KS. On the existence of a hitherto unrecognized dietary factor essential for reproduction. *Science* 1922;56:650-651.
2. Mason KE. The first two decades of vitamin E. *Fed Proc* 1977;36:1906-10.
3. Pennock JF, Hemming FW, Kerr JD. A reassessment of tocopherol in chemistry. *Biochem Biophys Res Commun* 1964;17:542-8.
4. Desai DI. Assay methods. In: Machlin LJ, Ed. *Vitamin E: A Comprehensive Treatise.* New York, NY: Marcel Dekker, Inc., 1980.
5. Cooney RV, Franke AA, Harwood PJ, *et al.* Gamma-tocopherol detoxification of nitrogen dioxide: superiority to alpha-tocopherol. *Proc Natl Acad Sci U S A* 1993;90:1771-1775.
6. Christen S, Woodall AA, Shigenaga MK, *et al.* Gamma-tocopherol traps mutagenic electrophiles such as NO(X) and complements alpha-tocopherol: physiological implications. *Proc Natl Acad Sci U S A* 1997;94:3217-22.
7. Stone WL, Papas AM. Tocopherols and the etiology of colon cancer. *J Natl Cancer Inst* 1997;89:1006-14.
8. Burton GW, Joyce A, Ingold KU. First proof that vitamin E is major lipid-soluble, chain-breaking antioxidant in human blood plasma. *Lancet* 1982;8292 ii:327.
9. Anonymous. Nomenclature policy: genetic descriptors and trivial names for vitamins and related compounds. *J Nutr* 1987;117:7-14.
10. Anonymous. The United States Pharmacopeia 23/The National Formulary 18. The United States Pharmacopeial Convention, Inc. Rockville, MD, 1995.
11. NRC. *Recommended Dietary Allowances.* 10 ed. Washington, DC: National Academy Press, 1989.
12. Kayden HJ, Traber MG. Absorption, lipoprotein transport and regulation of plasma concentrations of vitamin E in humans. *J Lipid Res* 1993;34:343-358.
13. Acuff RV, Thedford SS, Hidiroglou NN, Papas AM, Odom TA, Jr. Relative bioavailability of RRR- and *all-rac*-alpha-tocopheryl acetate in humans: studies using deuterated compounds. *Am J Clin Nutr* 1994;60:397-402.
14. Burton GW, Traber MG, Acuff RV, *et al.* Human plasma and tissue alpha-tocopherol concentrations in response to supplementation with deuterated natural and synthetic vitamin E. *Am J Clin Nutr* 1998;67:669-84.

15. Kiyose C, Muramatsu R, Kameyama Y, Ueda T, Igarashi O. Biodiscrimination of alpha-tocopherol stereoisomers in humans after oral administration. *Am J Clin Nutr* 1997;65:785-9.
16. Sokol RJ, Heubi JE, Butler-Simon N, *et al.* Treatment of vitamin E deficiency during chronic childhood cholestasis with oral d-α-tocopheryl polyethylene glycol 1000 succinate (TPGS). I. Intestinal absorption, efficacy and safety. *Gastroenterology* 1987;93:975-985.
17. Traber MG, Kayden HJ, Green JB, Green MH. Absorption of water miscible forms of vitamin E in a patient with cholestasis and in rats. *Am J Clin Nutr* 1986;44:914-923.
18. Burton GW, Ingold KU. Biokinetics of vitamin E using deuterated tocopherols. In: Packer L, Fuchs J, Eds. *Vitamin E in Health and Disease.* New York, NY: Marcel Dekker, 1993:329-344.
19. Ingold KU, Burton GW, Foster DO, *et al.* Biokinetics of and discrimination between dietary RRR- and SRR-alpha-tocopherols in the male rat. *Lipids* 1987;22:163-172.
20. Hayes KC, Pronczuk A, Liang JS. Differences in the plasma transport and tissue concentrations of tocopherols and tocotrienols: observations in humans and hamsters. *Proc Soc Exp Biol Med* 1993;202:353-9.
21. Bieri JG, Evarts RP. Tocopherols and fatty acids in American diets. *J Am Diet Assoc* 1973;62:147-151.
22. Traber MG, Kayden HJ. Preferential incorporation of alpha-tocopherol vs gamma-tocopherol in human lipoproteins. *Am J Clin Nutr* 1989;49:517-526.
23. Handelman GJ, Epstein WL, Peerson J, Spiegelman D, Machlin LJ. Human adipose α-tocopherol and γ-tocopherol kinetics during and after 1 y of α-tocopherol supplementation. *Am J Clin Nutr* 1994;59:1025-1032.
24. Burton GW, Ingold KU, Cheeseman KH, Slater TF. Application of deuterated alpha-tocopherols to the biokinetics and bioavailability of vitamin E. *Free Radic Res Commun* 1990;11:99-107.
25. Traber MG, Burton GW, Ingold KU, Kayden HJ. *RRR*- and *SRR*-α-tocopherols are secreted without discrimination in human chylomicrons, but *RRR*-α-tocopherol is preferentially secreted in very low density lipoproteins. *J Lipid Res* 1990;31:675-685.
26. Traber MG. Regulation of human plasma vitamin E. In: Sies H, Ed. *Antioxidants in Disease Mechanisms and Therapeutic Strategies.* San Diego: Academic Press, 1996:49-63.
27. Dutta Roy AK, Leishman DJ, Gordon MJ, Campbell FM, Duthie GG. Identification of a low molecular mass (14.2 kDa) alpha-tocopherol-binding protein in the cytosol of rat liver and heart. *Biochem Biophys Res Commun* 1993;196:1108-12.
28. Gordon MJ, Campbell FM, Dutta-Roy AK. α–Tocopherol-binding protein in the cytosol of the human placenta. *Biochem Soc Trans* 1996;24:202S.
29. Kuhlenkamp J, Ronk M, Yusin M, Stolz A, Kaplowitz N. Identification and purification of a human liver cytosolic tocopherol binding protein. *Prot Exp Purific* 1993;4:382-389.
30. Leishman DJ, Duthie G, Dutta Roy AK. Identification of a vitamin E-binding protein in rat heart cytosol. *Biochem Soc Trans* 1992;20:339s.
31. Sato Y, Arai H, Miyata A, *et al.* Primary structure of alpha-tocopherol transfer protein from rat liver. Homology with cellular retinaldehyde-binding protein. *J Biol Chem* 1993;268:17705-10.
32. Tozuka M, Fidge N. Purification and characterization of two high density lipoprotein binding proteins from rat and human liver. *Biochem J.* 1989;261:239-244.
33. Yoshida H, Yusin M, Ren I, *et al.* Identification, purification, and immunochemical characterization of a tocopherol-binding protein in rat liver cytosol. *J Lipid Res* 1992;33:343-350.
34. Traber MG, Sokol RJ, Kohlschutter A, *et al.* Impaired discrimination between stereoisomers of alpha-tocopherol in patients with familial isolated vitamin E deficiency. *J Lipid Res* 1993;34:201-10.

35. Dimitrov MV, Meyer C, Gilliland D, Ruppenthal M, *et al.* Plasma tocopherol concentrations in response to supplemental vitamin E. *Am J Clin Nutr* 1991;53:723-729.
36. Kappus H, Diplock A. Tolerance and safety of vitamin E: a toxicological position report. *Free Rad Biol Med* 1992;13:55-74.
37. Tran K, Chan AC. Comparative uptake of alpha- and gamma-tocopherol by human endothelial cells. *Lipids* 1992;27:38-41.
38. Dutton PJ, Hughes LA, Foster DO, Burton GW, Ingold KU. Simon metabolites of alpha-tocopherol are not formed via a rate-controlling scission of the 3'C-H bond. *Free Radic Biol Med* 1990;9:435-9.
39. Schultz M, Leist M, Petrzika M, Gassmann B, Brigelius-Flohé R. A novel urinary metabolite of α-tocopherol, 2,5,7,8-tetramethyl-2(2'carboxyethyl)-6-hydroxy chroman (α-CEHC) as an indicator of an adequate vitamin E supply? *Am J Clin Nutr* 1995;62 (suppl):1527S-1534S.
40. Wechter WJ, Kantoci D, Murray ED, Jr, *et al.* A new endogenous natriuretic factor: LLU-alpha. *Proc Natl Acad Sci U S A* 1996;93:6002-7.
41. Kagan VE, Serbinova EA, Bakalova RA, *et al.* Mechanisms of stabilization of biomembranes by alpha-tocopherol. The role of the hydrocarbon chain in the inhibition of lipid peroxidation. *Biochem Pharmacol* 1990;40:2403-13.
42. Niki E, Tsuchiya J, Tanimura R, Kamiya Y. The regeneration of vitamin E from alpha-chromanoxyl radical by glutathione and vitamin C. *Chem Lett.* 1982;6:789-792.
43. Esterbauer H, Dieber-Rotheneder M, Striegl G, Waey G. Role of vitamin E in preventing the oxidation of low density lipoprotein. *Am J Clin Nutr* 1991;53:314S-321S.
44. Serbinova EA, Tsuchiya M, Goth S, Kagan VE, Packer L. Antioxidant action of α-tocopherol and α-tocotrienol in membranes. In: Packer L, Fuchs J, Eds. *Vitamin E in Health and Disease.* New York, NY: Marcel Dekker, Inc., 1993:235-243.
45. Suarna C, Food RL, Dean RT, Stocker R. Comparative antioxidant activity of tocotrienols and other natural lipid-soluble antioxidants in a homogeneous system, and in rat and human lipoproteins. *Biochim Biophys Acta* 1993;1166:163-170.
46. Kaiser S, Di-Mascio P, Murphy ME, Sies H. Physical and chemical scavenging of singlet molecular oxygen by tocopherols. *Arch Biochem Biophys* 1990;277:101-8.
47. Cooney RV, Harwood PJ, Franke AA, *et al.* Products of gamma-tocopherol reaction with NO2 and their formation in rat insulinoma (RINm5F) cells. *Free Radic Biol Med* 1995;19:259-269.
48. Arroyo PL, Hatch Pigott V, Mower HF, Cooney RV. Mutagenicity of nitric oxide and its inhibition by antioxidants. *Mutat Res* 1992;281:193-202.
49. Burton GW, Ingold KU. Autoxidation of biological molecules. I. The antioxidant activity of vitamin E and related chain-breaking phenolic antioxidants *in vitro. J Amer Chem Soc* 1981;103:6472-6477.
50. Tomeo AC, Geller M, Watkins TR, Gapor A, Bierenbaum ML. Antioxidant effects of tocotrienols in patients with hyperlipidemia and carotid stenosis. *Lipids* 1995;30:1179-83.
51. Kamal-Eldin A, Appelqvist LA. The chemistry and antioxidant properties of tocopherols and tocotrienols. *Lipids* 1996;31:671-701.
52. Papas AM. Oil-soluble antioxidants in foods. *Toxicol Ind Health* 1993;9:123-49.
53. Papas AM. Vitamin E and exercise: aspects of biokinetics and bioavailability. *World Rev Nutr Diet* 1993;72:165-76.
54. Cheeseman KH, Holley AE, Kelly FJ, Wasil M, Hughes L, Burton G. Biokinetics in humans of RRR-alpha-tocopherol: the free phenol, acetate ester, and succinate ester forms of vitamin E. *Free Radical Biol Med* 1995;19:591-598.
55. Norkus EP, Bryce GF, Bhagavan HN. Uptake and bioconversion of alpha-tocopheryl acetate to alpha-tocopherol in skin of hairless mice. *Photochem Photobiol* 1993;57:613-5.

56. Gensler HL, Aickin M, Peng YM, Xu M. Importance of the form of topical vitamin E for prevention of photocarcinogenesis. *Nutr Cancer* 1996;26:183-91.
57. Clement S, Tasinato A, Boscoboinik D, Azzi A. The effect of alpha-tocopherol on the synthesis, phosphorylation and activity of protein kinase C in smooth muscle cells after phorbol-12-myristate-13-acetate down-regulation. *Eur J Biochem* 1997;246:745-9.
58. Tasinato A, Boscoboinik D, Bartoli GM, Maroni P, Azzi A. d-alpha-tocopherol inhibition of vascular smooth muscle cell proliferation occurs at physiological concentrations, correlates with protein kinase C inhibition, and is independent of its antioxidant properties. *Proc Natl Acad Sci U S A* 1995;92:12190-4.
59. Dowd P, Zheng ZB. On the mechanism of the anticlotting action of vitamin E quinone. *Proc Natl Acad Sci U S A* 1995;92:8171-5.
60. Richardson PD, Steiner M. Adhesion of human platelets inhibited by vitamin E. In: Packer L, Fuchs J, Eds. *Vitamin E in Health and Disease*. New York, NY: Marcel Dekker, Inc., 1993:297-311.
61. Parker RA, Pearce BC, Clark RW, Gordon DA, Wright JJ. Tocotrienols regulate cholesterol production in mammalian cells by post-transcriptional suppression of 3-hydroxy-3-methylglutaryl-coenzyme A reductase. *J Biol Chem* 1993;268:11230-8.
62. Poulin JE, Cover C, Gustafson MR, Kay MB. Vitamin E prevents oxidative modification of brain and lymphocyte band 3 proteins during aging. *Proc Natl Acad Sci U S A* 1996;93:5600-3.
63. Sokol RJ. Vitamin E and neurologic function in man. *Free Rad Biol Med* 1988;6:189-207.
64. Schlagheck TG, Kesler JM, Jones MB, *et al.* Olestra's effect on vitamins D and E in humans can be offset by increasing dietary levels of these vitamins. *J Nutr* 1997;127:1666S-85S.
65. Traber MG, Schiano TD, Steephen AC, Kayden HJ, Shike M. Efficacy of water soluble vitamin E in the treatment of vitamin E malabsorption in the short bowel syndrome. *Am J Clin Nutr* 1994;59:1270-1274.
66. Rimm EB, Stampher MJ, Ascherio A, Giovannuci E, Colditz MB, Willet WC. Vitamin E consumption and the risk of coronary disease in men. N Engl J Med, 1993: 1450-1456.
67. Stampher MJ, Hennekens CJ, Manson JE, *et al.* Vitamin E consumption and the risk of coronary disease in women. N Engl J Med, 1993: 1444-1449.
68. Meydani SN, Meydani M, Blumberg JB, *et al.* Vitamin E supplementation and *in vivo* immune response in healthy elderly subjects. A randomized controlled trial. *JAMA* 1997;277:1380-6.
69. Jialal I, Fuller CJ, Huet BA. The effect of α-tocopherol supplementation on LDL oxidation. A dose-response study. *Arterioscler Thromb Vasc Biol* 1995;15:190-198.
70. Nesaretnam K, Guthrie N, Chambers AF, Carroll KK. Effect of tocotrienols on the growth of a human breast cancer cell line in culture. *Lipids* 1995;30:1139-43.
71. Catignani GL, Bieri JG. Rat liver α-tocopherol binding protein. *Biochim Biophys Acta* 1977;497:349-357.
72. Murphy SP, Subar AF, Block G. Vitamin E intakes and sources in the United States. *Am J Clin Nutr* 1990;52:361-7.
73. Hennekens CH, Gaziano JM, Manson JE, Buring JE. Antioxidant vitamin-cardiovascular disease hypothesis is still promising, but still unproven: the need for randomized trials. *Am J Clin Nutr* 1995;62:1377S-1380S.
74. Eaton SB, Eaton SB, 3rd, Konner MJ, Shostak M. An evolutionary perspective enhances understanding of human nutritional requirements. *J Nutr* 1996;126:1732-40.
75. Group. Effects of tocopherol and deprenyl on the progression of disability in early Parkinson's disease. The Parkinson Study Group. *N Engl J Med* 1993;328:176-83.

11

Isoflavone Metabolism and Bioavailability

Suzanne Hendrich, Ph.D., Gui-Juan Wang, M.S., Hsiao-Kuang Lin, M.S., Xia Xu, Ph.D., Bee-Yen Tew, M.S., Huei-Ju Wang, Ph.D., and Patricia A. Murphy, Ph.D.
Food Science and Human Nutrition, Iowa State University, Ames, Iowa, USA

INTRODUCTION

Flavonoids and Isoflavones: Biological Effects

Flavonoids are widely dispersed in the human food supply in fruits and vegetables (Table 1), and several of these compounds have anticarcinogenic effects (reviewed elsewhere).[1,2] Isoflavones are structural isomers of the flavonoid and, given those structural similarities (Figure 1), these two classes of compounds would likely be metabolized in relatively similar manners, and therefore, also may have similar health effects. Isoflavones and flavonoids share some general biological effects, including anticarcinogenic,[3,4] tyrosine kinase,[5,6] and aromatase-inhibiting[7,8] abilities. The potency of various members of these chemical classes with respect to these general effects can vary by at least an order of magnitude. For example, the isoflavone biochanin A

0-8493-8009-X/98/$0.00+$.50

Table 1
Flavonoids (~ 2000 in nature), Structurally Related to Flavone (2-phenylbenzopyrone)

Group	Name / *IUPAC Name*	Food Source
Flavone	Tangeretin *3',4',5,6,7,8-hexamethoxy-flavone*	Tangerine rind & juice
	Apigenin *4',5,7-trihydroxy-flavone*	Grapefruit rind & juice Flower petals-petunias
Flavanol	Quercetin *3',4',3,5,7-pentahydroxy-flavanol*	All green leaves, onions, stone fruits (cherries, plums, etc.) grapes, strawberries
Flavanone	Naringenin *3',5,7-trihydroxy-flavanone*	Citrus peels & juices
	Hesperitin *3',5,7-trihydroxy-4'-methoxy-flavanone*	Grapefruit peel and juices
Isoflavone	Genistein *4',5,7-trihydroxy-isoflavone*	Soybeans
	Daidzein *4',7-dihydroxy-isoflavone*	Soybeans, kudzu
Catechin	Epicatechin *3',4',3,5,7-flavanpentol*	Tea leaves

inhibits aromatase-inhibited human preadipocyte aromatase in amounts of 100 μmol, whereas chrysin, a flavonoid, was effective at 5 μmol in the same assay system.[8] This review focuses on the isoflavones, but it is reasonable to deduce that the same general trends for bioavailability and metabolism will hold true for many flavonoids. The isoflavones are a more limited structural group than are the flavonoids, insofar as one considers the major isoflavones presently known in the human diet. The fewer different compounds in a class, the more readily they can be studied and compared. Thus, isoflavones may give us insights into the greater class of flavonoid food components.

Isoflavones are found in soy beans in amounts of 1-3 mg/g[9] and in soy foods in amounts of 0.025 to 3 mg/g.[10] The isoflavones are found primarily as glycosides, genistin, daidzin, and glycetin, which may also be malonated and acetylated.[9] The aglycone forms, genistein, daidzein, and glycetein, are also

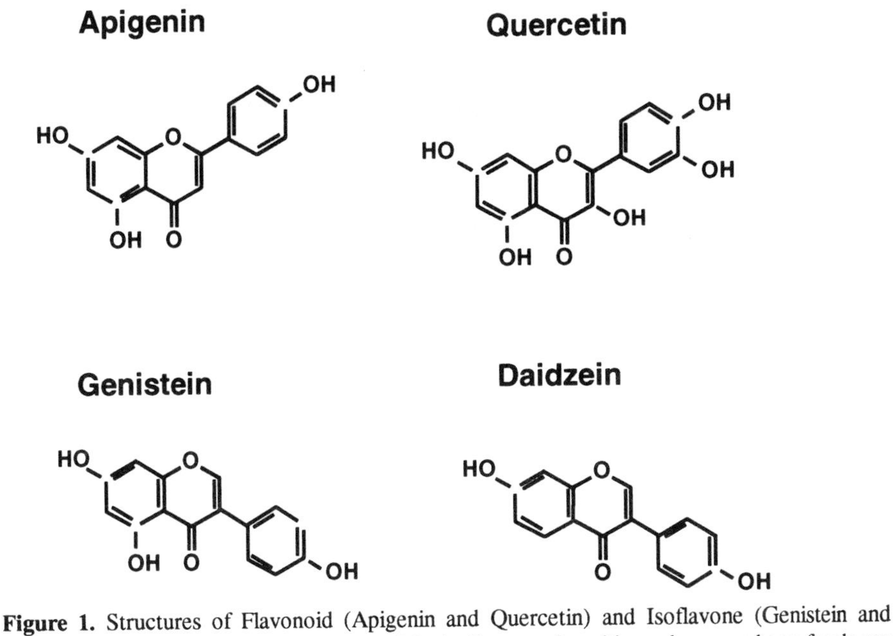

Figure 1. Structures of Flavonoid (Apigenin and Quercetin) and Isoflavone (Genistein and Daidzein) aglycones. The glucone forms of the isoflavones found in soybeans and soy foods are 7-O-glucosides which may also occur as 6"-O-acetyl- or -malonyl-glucosides.

present in foods, especially if fermentation has been used during processing, as for miso.[10] Soybeans generally contain slightly more genistein than daidzein (both predominantly as glycosides), with glycetein and its glycosides representing less than 10% of total isoflavones, but daidzein and glycetein glycosides are the major isoflavones in soy germ. Only trace amounts of isoflavones are found in other legumes, making soybeans a unique source of these potentially beneficial food components. Isoflavones are antioxidants *in vitro* and *in vivo*.[11,12] Their weak estrogenicity may be related to both toxic and potentially beneficial effects.[13] Isoflavones are tyrosine kinase[6] and DNA topoisomerase II inhibitors.[14] They also inhibit angiogenesis in an *in vitro* model.[15] Any or all of these functions might account for the anticarcinogenic effects of isoflavones. Isoflavone extracts made from toasted, defatted soy flakes in amounts of 1 mmol total isoflavone per kg of diet are anticarcinogens at the stage of promotion in rat hepatocarcinogenesis models.[4,16] The anticarcinogenic ability of purified isoflavones remains to be proven, although the present evidence supports this claim, at least in some model systems. For example, genistein administered in the perinatal is strongly protective against rat mammary carcinogenesis.[17] The major mechanisms of action of isoflavones *in vivo* remain to be ascertained.

Isoflavones: Significance of Bioavailability and Metabolism

The ability of isoflavones to exert their anticarcinogenic and other possible health effects depends upon their bioavailability, defined in a nutritional sense as the relative ability of these compounds to reach their sites of action in biologically active forms. Bioavailability of dietary compounds depends upon their structure, dose (amount in foods), time course of dosing (meal frequency), and characteristics of their food matrices. In many cases, interactions of the compounds with gut microflora may also be significant in determining the compounds' biological effects.

ISOFLAVONE METABOLISM

Biotransformation of Isoflavones

Biotransformation Reactions

The phenolic structure of isoflavones seems to be a major determinant of their availability because such hydroxyls are readily metabolized to glucuronide conjugates by reactions catalyzed by UDP-glucuronosyltransferases (UGTs) involving UDP-glucuronic acid (UDPGA) as the cosubstrate. Isoflavone glucuronides are excreted rapidly in bile[18] and urine.[19] The hydroxyl groups of phenolic compounds can also be transformed by sulfotransferase (STs) with the cosubstrate phosphoadenosylphosphosulfate (PAPS).[20] The relative extent of transformation of phenolics to glucuronide versus sulfate conjugates is species and gender dependent. For example, feline biotransformation lacks UGTs, whereas swine and brachymorphic mice lack ST20. Males have greater ST activity than females and, therefore, sulfate conjugates will be present to a greater extent in males than in females,[21] although this remains to be confirmed in humans. But the predominant metabolite of genistein and daidzein (the major soybean isoflavones and the major isoflavones in the human diet, in general) in men and women are glucuronides of both isoflavones, and probably, specifically the 7-O-glucuronides. Zhang[19] showed that the major isoflavone metabolites in human urine after consumption of soy milk had the same retention times as did 7-O-glucuronides of daidzein and genistein synthesized using rat hepatic microsomal UGT. The isoflavone glucuronides formed by rat liver microsomes were confirmed to be 7-O-glucuronides by the absence of bathochromic shifts when these metabolites were dissolved in methanol/sodium acetate, and mass spectroscopy. It seems likely that human UGTs would form the same glucuronides as formed in rats. The daidzein and genistein glucuronides made up more than 90% of total isoflavones found in both plasma and urine samples in humans.

Biliary Excretion

Biliary excretion is likely the main limiting factor with respect to the dose percentage of isoflavones that is systemically available, meaning the proportion of the total dose that reaches the general circulation. This systemic availability is reflected in the total amount of isoflavones excreted in the urine. Although some portion of the isoflavones reaching the general circulation may be excreted by the bile, the biliary portion of isoflavone excretion cannot be readily measured in humans. The first-pass effect, meaning the fraction of ingested isoflavones entering hepatic portal circulation from the intestine that is immediately passed back out into the intestine by biliary excretion,[22] may be considerable[18] based on the observation that 75% of a dose of ^{14}C-genistein was recovered from bile within 4 h after duodenal infusion of rats. The biliary isoflavone metabolite of genistein was the 7-O-glucuronide. Given the glucuronidase activity of gut microflora, significant enterohepatic recirculation of isoflavones is theoretically possible. But the recovery of isoflavones from feces is usually nearly nil,[23-25] and recovery of a total of less than 50% of ingested isoflavones in urine[23-27] suggests that biliary excretion of isoflavones is followed by their breakdown, catalyzed by gut microorganisms.[24]

Biotransformation Sites

Most tissues in most animals have biotransformation capacity. The Phase II biotransformation of phenolics by UGTs and STs is thought to occur mainly in the intestine and liver. When portal blood was collected from rats infused intestinally with ^{14}C-genistein, the genistein was found predominantly in its glucuronidated form.[18] Thus, the intestinal mucosa was the major site of biotransformation in rats. This would seem likely to occur in humans as well. The implication of this finding is either that isoflavone glucuronides are responsible for the observed health effects of isoflavones, or that mechanisms exist for deconjugation of isoflavones near the cell surface or within cells. The deconjugation of isoflavone glucuronides is improbable, although granulocytes possess glucuronidase activity.[28] If such deconjugation occurs it would be a minor reaction, because generally less than 10% of total isoflavones in blood plasma is found as isoflavone aglycones. Given the range of isoflavone concentrations found in circulation after isoflavone-containing meals of 1-10 µmol/L, the circulating isoflavone aglycone concentrations would be only 0.1-1 µmol/L, and only mechanisms operating at such low isoflavone concentrations could be considered to be physiologically relevant.

Roles of the Gut in Metabolism of Flavonoids and Isoflavonoids

Deconjugation and Biotransformation

Isoflavones in the human diet exist largely as glycosides. Such compounds seem to be virtually unabsorbable by the intestine as they have never been reported to be found in human blood or urine, using HPLC conditions that would be able to detect such compounds.[23] Intestinal glucosidases are needed to permit absorption of isoflavones as aglycones (Figure 2). There are no reports describing deconjugation of isoflavones or related compounds by mammalian β-glucosidases. Flavonoids seem to be poor substrates for mammalian glucosidases,[29] but gut microfloral β-glucosidases may readily act to deconjugate isoflavone glucosides permitting passive absorption of seemingly as much as 75% of the dose of isoflavones as aglycones.[18]

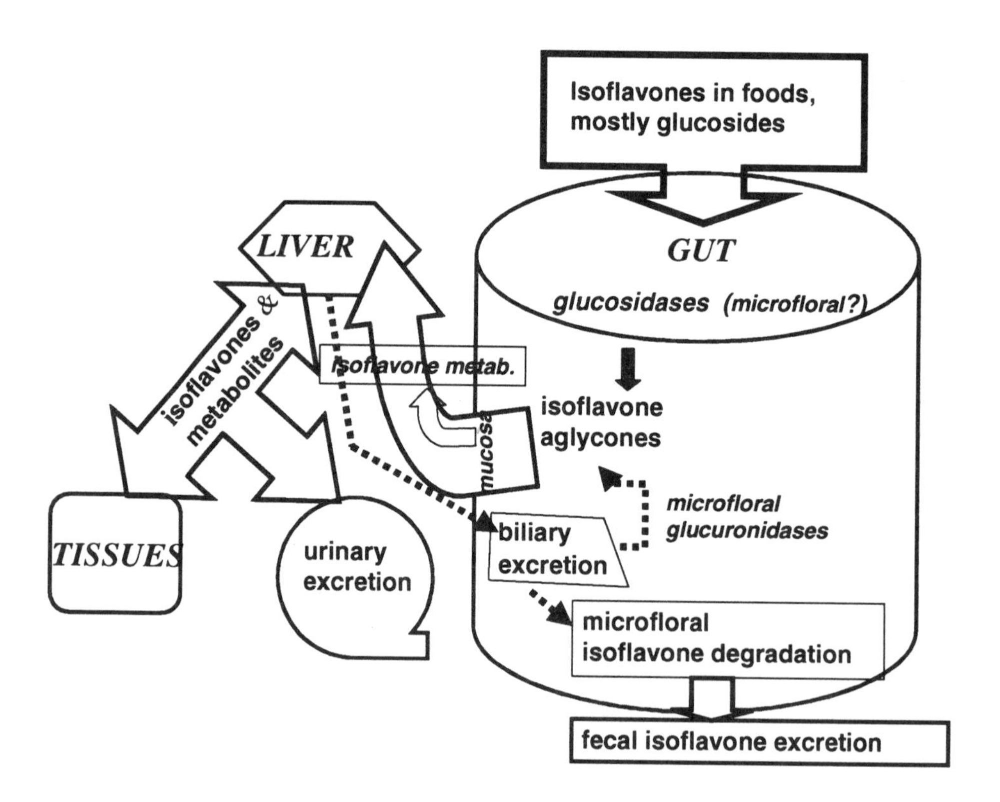

Figure 2. Isoflavones: routes of metabolism and excretion, and influence of gut microflora.

Gut microflora further biotransform isoflavones after their post-biliary reentry into the gut, first deconjugating isoflavone glucuronides and then forming O-desmethylangolensin[30] and equol[31] from daidzein. Equol formation seemingly results from gut microfloral adaptation to the presence of dietary isoflavones, because equol has never been found in studies of the bioavailability of single meals containing isoflavones, and studies of repeated isoflavone feeding show equol excretion only after several days of soy feeding.[32,33] Not all individuals possess the ability to form equol, presumably due to the lack of unidentified species of microoorganisms that catalyze the conversion of daidzein to equol. Approximately only one-third[32] to two-thirds[33] of human subjects are equol formers. Equol has estrogenic activity,[34] and the variability in formation of equol may contribute to variation in biological effects of soy consumption.

Degradation

Because human fecal recovery of isoflavones after soy feeding is usually only a few percent of the ingested dose, and urinary recovery of total isoflavones is usually only between 10-50% of ingested dose,[23-25,27] the fate of a large proportion of ingested isoflavones is uncertain. The degradation of isoflavones by gut microflora was demonstrated *in vitro*.[24] The flavonoid C-ring can be broken by human gut microflora,[35] and it is reasonable to assume that the isoflavonoid C-ring would also be susceptible to such degradation. Interindividual variation in human gut microfloral ability to degrade isoflavones seems to be linked with the extent of urinary excretion of these compounds, as well as to plasma levels. Approximately 25% of women fed soy milk[24] had tenfold greater fecal isoflavone excretion than did the rest of the women studied. The greater fecal isoflavone excretion was associated with threefold greater urinary isoflavone excretion, twofold greater plasma isoflavone concentrations at 24 h after soy milk feeding, and greater and longer retention especially of genistein in the body.[24] Degradation of isoflavones and flavonoids to monophenolic compounds may be of particular interest, because some monophenolics have antiproliferative effects, e.g., methyl *p*-hydroxyphenyllactate which can inhibit growth of MCF-7 cells *in vitro*.[36] Specific monophenolic degradation products of isoflavones have not yet been identified. Under some conditions, dihydrodaidzein and dihydrogenistein may also be formed by intestinal microflora, but this microbial ability seems to vary greatly among individuals.[37] The dihydroisoflavones are probably intermediate or side products in isoflavone degradation by gut microorganisms, because they were produced in media containing fiftyfold more dilute fecal samples than used in similar media in a study showing apparently complete breakdown of isoflavones by human fecal microflora.[38] Dihydroisoflavones were only rarely found in human urine.[37] The relative ratio of gut microorganisms to isoflavones passing through the gut is likely to be far greater than under the conditions used to produce dihydroisoflavones *in vitro*.[37] Dihydroisoflavones are probably not physiologically important isoflavone metabolites. But, in general, biotransformation and degradation of isoflavones by gut microflora are likely to be important influences on the biological effects and interindividual variation in effects of isoflavones because the gut microflora clearly affect isoflavone bioavailability.

BIOAVAILABILITY OF ISOFLAVONES

Quantitation of Bioavailability

Blood Plasma Kinetics

Classical pharmacokinetic studies of drugs or toxicants quantify bioavailability as the total amount of a substance found in the blood or blood plasma during the administration and complete disposition of the substance. Measurement of the substance in repeated blood samples, coupled with measurement or estimation of blood or blood plasma volume are used to estimate the area under the curve or AUC, the total amount of the substance in the blood or blood plasma over its time of administration and disposition.[39] Estimation of plasma volume may be based upon the percentage of body weight composed of the blood, which varies by species and some physiological states, e.g., pregnancy. The percentage of body weight (bwt) composed of blood minus the blood volume multiplied by the percentage of blood composed of red blood cells (easily determined by obtaining the hematocrit) is the plasma volume as percentage of body weight:

Plasma volume (% bwt) = Blood volume (% bwt) – Blood volume (Hematocrit (%/100%)).

The AUC is thought to reflect the amount of a substance that is available to its sites of action in tissues, and is considered to be the best measurement of a substance's bioavailability. If a peak plasma concentration of a substance is known and repeated subsequent plasma concentrations are known, the plasma half-life of the substance, i.e., the time for peak plasma concentration to be reduced by half, can be estimated. This is also a useful measurement of bioavailability, although at present, there are no reports of AUC values or plasma half-lives for isoflavones in humans. Human urinary excretion half-lives for soy isoflavones during one month of feeding 12 ounces of soy milk at each of 3 meals per day to healthy men (21-35 y of age) were estimated by Lu *et al.*[40] to be approximately 3-4 h for daidzein, 4-5 h for genistein, and 5-10 h for equol after two single doses of 36 ounces of soy milk given at 2-wk intervals. Plasma isoflavone half-lives would probably be similar. In hooded Wistar male rats, 10 weeks of age, the pharmacokinetics of a single dose of 20 mg genistein/kg bwt and of an amount of soy extract containing mostly genistin and daidzin equivalent to 20 mg genistein/kg bwt showed an apparent peak plasma concentration of 11 μmol/L for genistein and about 5 μmol/L for genistein from soy extract.[26] A crude estimate of plasma genistein disappearance half-life based upon this study would be about 6 h for purified genistein and about 18 h for genistein from soy extract. Rat urinary excretion half-life was approximately 8 h for genistein and 12 h for genistein from soy extract.

Excretion and Balance Studies

Because the measurement of plasma kinetics requires frequent blood sampling, usually with aid of an indwelling catheter, such studies are heroic and relatively uncommon. Less invasive methods may also provide insight into bioavailability. Such methods are routinely used in assessment of nutrient bioavailability, where nutrient balance, the difference between dietary intake and overall excretion (by all routes) of a nutrient may be used to estimate some nutrient requirements.[41] For example, when the intake of a nutrient is equal to its total excretion including the excretion of its metabolites or metabolic products over a day or over a period of several days, that intake is thought to meet an adult's requirement for maintenance:

$$\text{Nutrient Balance} = \text{Nutrient intake} - \text{Nutrient output (excretion)}$$

Total urinary and fecal excretion from apparently healthy adult individuals has been used to estimate requirements of some nutrients, e.g., iron.[42] During growth, nutrients are accumulated to some extent in the body, and nutrient balance would need to be greater than zero to permit such accumulation. The approach to measuring bioavailability of comparing intake and output has yielded insight into the utilization of non-nutrients of potential health significance, such as the soy isoflavones. Urinary excretion reflects the amount of a substance that has been absorbed by the intestinal mucosa and entered the general circulation. Fecal excretion reflects the amount of a substance ultimately not absorbed by the gut mucosa and not metabolized by gut microorganisms. One key limitation of the balance approach is that it is not generally possible to distinguish fecal products of biliary excretion from unabsorbed fecal products of a substance. Thus the balance method may underestimate the total absorption of a substance, but the portion of a substance that is passed through the liver and rapidly excreted through the bile back into the intestine (the "first-pass" portion) would probably have little effect on tissues other than liver and intestine and, therefore, be of only minor systemic significance. Whatever biliary metabolites of a substance are reabsorbed by the intestine and reach the general circulation would be reflected in urinary excretion. Measuring fecal excretion of substances is a crucial aspect of understanding the availability of a substance to the body because the fecal excretion products reflect the proportion of the substance that is apparently unabsorbed. Gut microfloral metabolism may be complex and fecal metabolites difficult to measure, but they may be important to determining the whole picture of bioavailability, and gut microfloral metabolism is certainly an important aspect of isoflavone metabolism and bioavailability.

Animal Studies of Isoflavone Bioavailability and Metabolism

Isoflavone Metabolism and Disposition

Few studies of isoflavone bioavailability in animal models have been performed. A study of genistein pharmacokinetics in mice showed that about 12% of oral genistein was excreted in urine, and genistein was rapidly cleared from the blood.[43] In rats, 18-20% of a single dose of either purified genistein or genistein and its glycone from soy extract was recovered over 48 h, with about 20% of genistein from either source recovered in feces as well.[26] Sfakianos *et al.*[18] showed ready absorption of a dose of genistein infused duodenally into adult female Sprague-Dawley rats, 75% of which was rapidly excreted into bile in the form of genistein-7-O-glucuronide. The glucuronide was also the predominant form of genistein in portal blood, suggesting that this form of genistein could be the major genistein metabolite in the general circulation after a small dose of genistein (about 1 μmol/kg bwt). This dose would be within the range of human exposures (e.g., a dose of 30 mg isoflavones/d would be about 125 μmoles/50 kg or 2.5 μmol/kg bwt). Yasuda *et al.*[44] showed that daidzein and daidzin were converted to glucuronide, sulfate, and sulfate/glucuronide metabolites in rats with daidzein sulfate recovered only in bile and not urine, but that all three of these metabolites were recovered in urine. Daidzein and genistein glucuronides predominated in humans.[19,45]

Disposition of genistein and daidzein was compared with apigenin, the flavonoid isomer of genistein, in female Sprague-Dawley rats.[46] Twenty-four weanling rats, weighing an average of 71 g (Harlan, Indianapolis, IN) were housed in individual metabolic cages designed to permit the separate collection of urine from feces. The experimental protocol was reviewed and approved by the Iowa State University (ISU) Animal Care Committee. Purified genistein, daidzein, and apigenin were fed *ad libitum* at 1 mmole/kg diet for 4 days to groups of six rats. The diet was based on AIN-76 diet but contained 40% of energy as fat from beef tallow and corn oil, substituting for sucrose and cornstarch. Rats were fed at 24-hour intervals and the urine and feces were collected at 4:00 p.m. each day. Blood plasma was obtained on day 4 at 10 a.m. (18 h after food was given) when the rats were killed.

The excretion of genistein, daidzein, and apigenin in urine and feces and plasma concentrations of these compounds were analyzed by reverse-phase high performance liquid chromatography (HPLC).[10,23,47] Purified daidzein (4′, 7-dihydroxyisoflavone, 98%) was purchased from ICN Biochemical, Inc. (Costa Mesa, CA). Genistein (98%) (4′, 5, 7-trihydroxyisoflavone), apigenin (95%) (4′, 5, 7-trihydroxyflavone), and β-glucuronidase/sulfatase (type H2 from Helix pomatia) were obtained from Sigma Chemical Co., (St. Louis, MO). Equol was a generous gift from Dr. Adlercreutz (Helsinki, Finland). Extrelut® QE columns were purchased from EM Separations (Gibbstown, NJ). Sep-Pak C18 cartridges were obtained from Millipore (Marlborough, MA). Syringe filters (13 mm) were purchased from Alltech Associates, Inc. (Deerland, IL) and Milli-Q system from (Millipore Co., Bedford, MA).

One mL urine sample was mixed with 3.75 mL, sodium acetate (200 mM, pH 5.5) and 25 μl fl-glucuronidase/sulfatase to deconjugate these metabolites and produce free parent compound. After incubation for 16 hours at 37°C, 10 mM sodium phosphate buffer (pH 7.0) was added, and the solution was passed through an Extrelut QE column. The column was washed 3 times with 10 mL ethyl acetate (HPLC grade). The effluent was collected in a 100 mL round bottom flask, and dried on a rotary evaporator (Buchler Instruments, Fortlee, NJ). The dried residues were redissolved in ethyl acetate, dried under nitrogen, dissolved in 5 mL 80% methanol in water, and filtered through a Sep-Pak C18 cartridge. The cartridges were washed with 2 mL distilled water, and the eluent recovered in 2 mL of 80% methanol (100% methanol was used for apigenin) was collected for filtration through a 13 mm syringe filter. This filtrate was used for HPLC analysis. Fecal samples were freeze dried on a freeze-dryer (Virtis, Gardiner, NY) and ground to powder by mortar and pestle. A 0.25 g fecal sample was weighed and mixed with 5 mL acetonitrile (ethyl acetate was used in apigenin sample), and 1 mL 0.1 M HCl in 20 mL glass vials. The sample vials were put on a wrist-action shaker (Burrel Co. Pittsburgh, PA) and shaken for 6 hours to extract the desired compounds. After shaking, the mixture was filtered through Whatman No. 1 filter paper, the filtrates dried under nitrogen, and the dried residue dissolved in 5 mL 80% methanol and acidified with 100 μL 1 M HCl. Plasma samples were prepared and HPLC analyses of isoflavones was performed as described.[23] The mobile phase used to analyze apigenin samples was an isocratic mixture, 35% B/A+B (B = 0.1% acetic acid in HPLC grade acetonitrile, A = 0.1% acetic acid in HPLC-grade water). Statistical analysis was performed by ANOVA. The analysis of variance provided the pooled estimates of error used in the comparisons. Significant differences between treatments and times were determined by calculation of the least significant difference (LSD).[48]

No significant differences in food intakes or body weights were observed. The recovery of compounds was about 76.3% ± 8.2%, although the recovery of genistein was moderately lower (65.2% ± 5.6%) than for the other compounds. The modified extraction method for apigenin samples produced a recovery of 92.8% ± 12.7% in urine, 72.8% ± 15.9% in feces, and 75.5% ± 15.6% in plasma. Plasma samples did not contain detectable apigenin. However, genistein and daidzein were found at 0.97 and 0.81 μmole/L, respectively. There was no significant difference between the plasma concentration of genistein and daidzein. Urinary excretion of daidzein did not differ between days 2 and 3 suggesting that excretion of daidzein had reached a steady state, but excretion of equol increased significantly with each day, as did excretion of genistein. Excretion of genistein and daidzein were similar to each other on days 2 and 3, and equol excretion was greater than either daidzein or genistein on day 3. Apigenin excretion was less than the excretion of the isoflavones, and apigenin excretion did not vary with day (Table 2).

Table 2
Urinary Excretion Of Genistein, Daidzein, and Apigenin as a Percentage of Daily Intake of the Compounds in Weanling Female Rats

Treatment	Day 1	Day 2	Day 3
Daidzein	11.9	9.8	11.1
Equol	3.7	10.2	19.6
Genistein	3.2	9.5	11.7
Apigenin	2.2	1.2	1.3

Statistically significant differences occurred among the treatment means, LSD (P = .05) = 4.6, and among the day means, LSD (P = .05) = 1.6.

Daily excretion of daidzein in feces was significantly higher than genistein, and genistein excretion was significantly greater than apigenin. Fecal excretion of daidzein significantly increased from day one to day two, whereas fecal excretion of apigenin significantly increased from day two to day three. The fecal excretion of genistein increased each day over three days (Table 3).

Table 3
Fecal Excretion Of Genistein, Daidzein, and Apigenin as a Percentage of Daily Intake of the Compounds in Weanling Female Rats

Treatment	Day 1	Day 2	Day 3
Genistein	0.5	2.2	4.5
Daidzein	8.1	12.4	13.6
Apigenin	4.1	5.1	6.7

Statistically significant differences occurred among the treatment means, LSD(P = .05) = 2.3, and among the day means, LSD (P = .05) = 1.6.

These data suggest about twofold greater availability of daidzein than of genistein in rats, when daidzein and its metabolite, equol, are combined. Because genistein's urinary excretion increased from day 1 to day 2, this compound may be retained in the body for a longer time than daidzein. Gut microfloral adaptation to the presence of daidzein, reflected in increasing amounts of urinary equol, was also an important aspect of isoflavone bioavailability. The relatively small percentages of isoflavones and apigenin recovered in feces suggests gut microfloral degradation of these compounds, with some adaptation, lessening degradation somewhat and achieving a steady state by day 3 for daidzein, but not for genistein or apigenin. The greater degradation of genistein and apigenin than of daidzein by gut microflora reflect the specificity of this degradation process favoring compounds possessing 5-hydroxyl groups, which are more susceptible to C-ring cleavage.[49] Bioavailability differences after the first day are not representative of the overall picture of bioavailability primarily because of the gut microbial adaptation causing equol production.

Structure/Activity Relationships

Aglycones versus Glucosides. Farmakalidis *et al.*[13] showed that daidzin and genistin had the same estrogenicity in mice as did their respective aglycones, when fed in equivalent molar doses. This suggested that the glycosides were cleaved to aglycones by gut microfloral β-glycosidases before absorption.

The glycosides had much less antioxidant activity than did the aglycones.[11] It seems reasonable that, in general, the glycosides would have less biological activity than the aglycones, even if the glycosides were absorbed, because their greater hydrophilicity and molecular weight would impair their availability to likely sites of action, such as cytosolic estrogen receptors. But, it seems that the glycosides are probably not absorbed. Studies comparing isoflavone aglycones and glycones showed nearly identical total urinary excretion of both compounds, 5% of daidzein or daidzin[44] and 20% of genistein or a soy extract containing predominantly genistin.[26] Neither study reported urinary excretion of isoflavone glycones. Because the isoflavone glycone seems to be metabolized nearly identically to the aglycone, conversion to the aglycone, which is likely catalyzed by gut microflora, before absorption seems extremely likely, and any absorption of glycone isoflavones would be unusual and minimal. Although isoflavone aglycones may be absorbed somewhat more rapidly than are isoflavones from dietary sources containing mostly glycones,[26] the biological activity and ultimate fate of glycones and aglycones do not seem to differ appreciably.

Daidzein, Genistein, and Apigenin. From our study described above, it is clear that the soy isoflavones daidzein and genistein are more bioavailable than is the flavonoid genistein analog apigenin. Apigenin was seemingly less well absorbed than genistein, and just as susceptible as genistein to apparent gut microfloral degradation. The lack of apigenin in plasma suggested more rapid clearance than for genistein and daidzein. The differences between the flavonoid apigenin and the isoflavone genistein in urinary excretion, reflecting systemic bioavailability, are significant but not readily explained. The differences between daidzein and genistein in bioavailability may be partly due to genistein's greater hydrophobicity, which would partly explain genistein's apparently longer retention in the body compared with daidzein. But this is probably less important than are the differences in gut microfloral metabolism between these two compounds that are partly due to their structural differences (the absence of the 5-hydroxyl from daidzein), although in another study, only 6% of daidzein and 20% of genistein from soy extract were recovered in feces after a single dose given to male Wistar rats.[26] Because the isoflavones given in the study of King *et al.*[26] were predominantly in glycone form, this may have protected genistein from microfloral degradation, at least in this strain of rats. The fortuitous conversion of daidzein to equol by gut microflora increases the contribution of dietary daidzein at least with respect to the potential phytoestrogenic effects of the isoflavones.

Human Studies of Isoflavone Bioavailability and Metabolism

Influences of Dose and Time

Dose/Response Measurements. A series of human feeding studies has been performed to assess the influence of isoflavone dose on isoflavone excretion and plasma concentrations and reviewed elsewhere.[50] To briefly summarize those results, urinary excretion of daidzein was generally more than twofold greater than that of genistein, although the doses of daidzein and genistein were nearly equal.[23,24,27,50] Isoflavone dose was linearly related to plasma and urinary isoflavone levels.[23,24,50] The more frequently soybean isoflavone doses were given, the more prolonged was isoflavone retention in the body, as would be expected.[23,24] Moderate gender differences in isoflavone bioavailability seem to occur, at least in young adults, with males showing greater urinary isoflavone excretion than females when fed the same isoflavone dose (mg/kg bwt).[50]

Duration of Exposure. When comparing short-term single dose studies[23,24] with a week-long feeding,[50] 9-day feeding,[32] or with a month of feeding[40] of soybean isoflavones, the same trends emerge of twofold more or greater availability of daidzein than of genistein, and of incomplete bioavailability of the isoflavones (5-50% of the ingested dose excreted in urine). The production of equol observed in the longer studies in some subjects[32,40] is the major effect of a longer duration of isoflavone dosing.

Dietary and Gut Microfloral Influences

Soy Food Type. Soybean isoflavone structure is related to the bioavailability of these compounds, in that daidzein is more available than is genistein, but the relative amounts of various glycones versus aglycones in different foods may have little effect on isoflavone bioavailability. Isoflavones in most soy foods are largely glycosides, which seemingly need to be cleaved by gut microfloral β-glycosidases before the isoflavone aglycones can be absorbed.[29] The presence of malonyl or acetyl side chains on the glycosides may also be insignificant to isoflavone absorption from soy foods, because when women were fed the same amounts of isoflavones from tofu (relatively high in glycones and acetyl glycones) versus texturized vegetable protein (TVP, relatively high malonyl glycone content), urinary and plasma isoflavones did not differ with soy food.[27] When isoflavone bioavailability from single meals of tofu, soybeans, TVP, and tempeh was compared in women, no significant differences were found between the soy foods in terms of percentage of isoflavone dose excreted in urine. About 38-51% of ingested daidzein and 9-16%

of genistein was excreted in urine regardless of soy food type.[51] In another study comparing urinary excretion of tempeh versus soybean pieces during 9 days of feeding in men, 10% of tempeh isoflavones, but only 5% of isoflavones from soybean pieces were excreted.[32] The difference between these two studies remains to be understood, but the evidence combined from animals and humans overall at this time suggests little difference between glycone and aglycone isoflavone absorption because the glycone is converted readily to the aglycone before absorption.

Dietary Interactions. Few studies have examined the influence of dietary components on isoflavone bioavailability. When an *ad libitum* background diet was compared with a diet provided by the investigators (basic foods diet) and a self-selected diet consumed at the same time as the basic foods diets, women showed no difference in isoflavone bioavailability when fed soy milk at each of three meals on a single day.[51] When a diet high in wheat fiber (40 g) was fed to women consuming a single soy food meal (TVP versus tofu), significantly lower plasma genistein at 24 h after feeding but not at 6 h after feeding, and lower total urinary genistein excretion (by 20%) were found, compared with a diet containing only 15 g dietary fiber.[27] Thus, limited data suggest little effect on isoflavone bioavailability of background diet and variation in dietary fiber.

Gut Microfloral Isoflavone Metabolism. The consistently low recovery of isoflavones from feces[23,24,27,32] and urinary recovery of only 10-50% of ingested isoflavones suggests significant gut microbial degradation of these compounds. Flavonoids and isoflavonoids may be degraded by strains of *Clostridium, Butyrivibrio,* and *Eubacterium* found in the guts of rats, cattle, and humans.[52-54] The half-lives of disappearance of isoflavones in an *in vitro* anaerobic incubation of a suspension of human feces in brain/heart infusion (BHI) media were 7.5 and 3.3 h for daidzein and genistein, respectively.[24] Genistein may be more susceptible to C-ring cleavage by virtue of its 5-OH group, a moiety absent from daidzein.[49]

Some individuals have much greater fecal isoflavone excretion, experience more prolonged and greater isoflavone bioavailability, and more equal availability of genistein and daidzein, in contrast with the majority of subjects.[24] This suggests that the presence or absence of certain gut microfloral species may be an important determinant of isoflavone bioavailability.

Gut microfloral metabolism of isoflavones *in vitro* has been studied in 15-20 healthy subjects, who were not soy food consumers, over a ten-month period.[50] Three distinct fecal excretor phenotypes were identified. Low degraders had fecal daidzein degradation constant (k) = 0.012 (n = 5). For moderate degraders, k for daidzein was 0.055 (n = 10) and for high degraders, k for daidzein = 0.299 (n = 5). When observed 300 days later, low (n = 5) and moderate (n = 4) phenotypes had similar daidzein degradation rate constants of 0.053 and 0.073, respectively, differing significantly from the daidzein degradation rate constant of the high excretor phenotype (n = 5), k = 0.326. At day 0, genistein degradation rate constants were 0.023, 0.163, and 0.299 for low, moderate and high excretor phenotypes, respectively, each phenotype significantly different from the other groups ($p < 0.05$). At day 300, genistein degradation rate constants still differed significantly among the three phenotypes, k = 0.049 (Low), 0.233 (Moderate) and 0.400 (High). These data suggest relatively stable human gut microfloral differences in ability to degrade isoflavones, which might influence the biological effects of isoflavones, contributing significantly to interindividual variability in such effects. Eliminating one major source of variability in biological effects might be important to establishing the health consequences of consumption of isoflavones, flavonoids, and related compounds.

CONCLUSIONS

Isoflavone bioavailability depends upon the phenolic nature of these compounds, which determines their major metabolic products, the glucuronide and sulfate conjugates. The future study of the effects of these metabolites will be crucial to determining the health effects of isoflavones. Gut microflora also exert profound effects on isoflavone availability, with microfloral breakdown of these compounds limiting their reabsorption and systemic availability and microfloral metabolism contributing an additional isoflavonoid, equol, to the overall effects of ingested isoflavones. The presence of varying glycosidic and aglycone forms of isoflavones in soy foods probably has little impact on the bioavailability of these compounds, which is linearly related to their dose over a broad dose range, as observed in humans. Isoflavone metabolism and bioavailability may be seen as modeling what is likely to occur with many structurally related phenolic compounds (Figure 2), with glucosides being metabolized to aglycones by gut microflora before their absorption, rapid intestinal mucosal, and hepatic biotransformation to predominantly glucuronide metabolites, subsequent biliary excretion and either enterohepatic recirculation or gut microfloral breakdown occurring before ultimate urinary and fecal excretion. Understanding the metabolism and bioavailability of these compounds is crucial to an appreciation of their potential as health protectants.

REFERENCES

1. Attaway J., Citrus juice flavonoids with anticarcinogenic and antitumor properties, in *Food Phytochemicals for Cancer Prevention I*,.Huang, M.-T., Osawa, T., Ho, C.-T., and Rosen, R. T., Eds, American Chemical Society, Washington, DC, 1994, 240.
2. Formica, J. V. and Regelson, W., Review of the biology of quercetin and related bioflavonoids, *Fd. Chem. Toxicol.*, 33, 1061, 1995.
3. Verma, A. K., Johnson, J. A., Gould, M. N., and Tanner, M. A. Inhibition of 7,12-dimethylbenzo(a)anthracene and N-nitrosomethyl urea induced rat mammary cancer by dietary flavonol quercetin. *Cancer Res.*, 48, 5754, 1988.
4. Lee, K.-W., Wang, H.-J., Murphy, P. A., and Hendrich, S., Soybean isoflavone extract suppresses early but not late promotion of hepatocarcinbogenesis by phenobarbital in female rat liver, *Nutr. Cancer*, 24, 267, 1995.
5. Levy, J., Teurstein, I., and Marbach, M. Tyrosine protein kinase activity in the DMBA induced rat mammary tumour: inhibition of quercetin, *Biochem. Biophys. Res. Comm.* 123, 1227, 1984.
6. Akiyama, T., Ishida, J., Nakagawa, S., Ogaware, H., Watanabe, S., Itoh, N., Shibuya, M., and Fukami, Y., Genistein, a specific inhibitor of tyrosine-specific protein kinases. *J. Biol. Chem.*, 262, 5592, 1987.
7. Adlercreutz, H., Bannwart, C., Wahala, K., Makela, T., Brunow, G., Hase, T., Arosemena, P. J., and Kellis, J. T., Inhibition of human aromatase by mammalian lignans and isoflavonoid phytoestrogens. *J. Steroid Biochem. Molec. Biol.*, 44, 147, 1993.
8. Wang, C. Makela, T., Hase, T., Adlercreutz, H., and Kurzer, M. S., Lignans and flavonoids inhibit aromatase enzyme in human preadipocytes. *J. Steroid Biochem. Molec. Biol.*, 50, 205, 1994.
9. Wang, H.-J. and Murphy, P.A., Isoflavone composition of American and Japanese soybeans in Iowa: effects of variety, crop year, and location. *J. Agric. Food Chem.*, 42, 1674, 1994.
10. Wang, H.-J. and Murphy, P.A., Isoflavone content in commercial soybean foods. *J. Agric. Food Chem.*, 42, 1666, 1994.
11. Naim, M., Gestetner, B., Bondi, A., and Birk, Y., Antioxidant and antihemolytic activities of soybean isoflavones. *J. Agric. Food Chem.*, 24, 1174, 1976.
12. Wei, H., Wei, L., Frenkel, K., Bowen, R., and Barnes, S., Inhibition of tumor-promoter induced hydrogen peroxide formation by genistein *in vitro* and *in vivo*. *Nutr. Cancer,* 20, 1, 1993.
13. Farmakalidis, E., Hathcock, J. N., and Murphy, P.A., Oestrogenic potency of genistein and daidzein in mice, *Food Chem. Toxicol.*, 23, 841, 1985.
14. Okura, A., Arakawa, H., Oka, H., Yoshinari, T., and Monden, Y., Effects of genistein on topisomerase activity on the growth of [val. 12] H3-ras transformed NIH 3T3 cells. *Biochem. Biophys. Res. Comm.*, 157, 183, 1988.
15. Fotsis, T., Pepper, M., Adlercreutz, H., Flerischmann, G., Hase, T., Montesano, R., and Schweigerer, L., Genistein, a dietary-derived inhibitor of *in vitro* angiogenesis. *Proc. Natl. Acad. Sci. U.S.A.*, 90, 1690, 1993.
16. Hendrich, S., Lu, Z., Wang, H.-J., Hopmans, E. C., and Murphy, P. A., Soy isoflavone extract suppresses fumonisin B_1-promoted rat hepatocarcinogenesis. *Amer. J . Clin. Nutr. (suppl.), in press.*
17. Lamartiniere, C. A., Moore, J., Brown, M., Thompson, R., Hardin, M. J., and Barnes, S. Genistein suppresses mammary cancer in rats. *Carcinogenesis,* 16, 2833, 1995.
18. Sfakianos J., Coward, L., Kirk, M., and Barnes, S., Intestinal uptake and biliary excretion of the isoflavone genistein in rats. *J. Nutr.*, 127, 1260, 1997.

19. Zhang, Y., *Daidzein and genistein glucuronides: synthesis, estrogen receptor binding and effect on human natural killer cell activity.* M.S. Thesis, Iowa State University Library, Ames, IA 50011, 1997, 22.
20. Sipes, I. G. and Gandolfi, A. J., Biotransformation of toxicants, in *Casarett and Doullís Toxicology, The Basic Science of Poisons*, Klaassen, C. D., Amdur, M. O., and Doull, J., Eds., Macmillan Publ. Co., New York, NY, 64, 1986.
21. Runge-Morris, M. A., Regulation of expression of the rodent cytosolic sulfotransferases. *FASEB J.*, 11, 109, 1997.
22. Welling, P. G. First-pass metabolism, enterohepatic circulation and physicochemical factors affected absorption, in *Pharmacokinetics; Processes and Mathematics*, Welling, P. G., Ed., American Chemical Society, Washington, D.C., 1986, 35.
23. Xu, X., Wang, H.J., Murphy, P.A., Cook, L., and Hendrich, S., Daidzein is a more bioavailable soymilk isoflavone than is genistein in adult women. *J. Nutr.*, 124, 825, 1994.
24. Xu, X., Harris, K., Wang, H.J., Murphy, P.A., and Hendrich, S., Bioavailability of soybean isoflavones depends upon gut microflora in women. *J. Nutr.* 125, 2307, 1995.
25. Xu, X., Wang, H.-J., Murphy, P. A., Cook, L. R., and Hendrich, S., Disposition of a single dose of soy milk isoflavones in adult females, in *Natural Protectants Against Natural Toxicants*, Bidlack, W. R. and Omaye, S. T., Eds., Technomic Publishing Co., Inc., Lancaster, PA, 1995, 51.
26. King, R. A., Broadbent, J. L., and Head, R. J., Absorption and excretion of the soy isoflavone genistein in rats. *J. Nutr.* 126, 176, 1996.
27. Tew, B.-Y., Xu, X., Wang, H.-J., Murphy, P.A., and Hendrich, S., A diet high in wheat fiber decreases the bioavailability of soybean isoflavones in a single meal fed to women. *J. Nutr.*, 126, 871, 1996.
28. Marshall, T., Shult, P., and Busse, W., Release of lysosomal enzyme beta-glucuronidase from isolated human eosinophils. *J. Allergy Clin. Immunol.*, 82, 550, 1988.
29. Brown, J. P., Hydrolysis of glycosides and esters. in *Role of the Gut Flora in Toxicity and Cancer,* Rowland, I. R., Ed., Academic Press Inc., San Diego, CA, 1988, 109.
30. Bannwart, C., Adlercreutz, H., Fotsis, T., Wahala, K., Hase, T., and Brunow, G., Identification of O-desmethylangolensin, a metabolite of daidzein, and of matairesinol, one likely precursor of the animal lignan enterolactone, in human urine. *Finn. Chem. Lett.*, 4, 120, 1984.
31. Axelson, M., Sjovall, J., Gustafsson, B. E., and Setchell, K. D. R., Soya, a dietary source of the non-steroidal oestrogen equol in man and animals. *J. Endocr.*, 102, 49, 1984.
32. Hutchins, A. M., Slavin, J. L., and Lampe, J. W., Urinary isoflavonoid phytoestrogen and lignan excretion after consumption of fermented and unfermented soy products. *J. Am. Diet. Assoc.* 95, 545, 1995.
33. Setchell, K. D. R., Borrielolo, S. P., Hulme, P., Kirk, D. N., and Axelson, M., Nonsteroidal estrogens of dietary origin: possible roles in hormone-dependent disease. *Am. J. Clin. Nutr.*, 40, 569, 1984.
34. Tang, B. Y, and Adams, N. R., The effect of equol on oestrogen receptors and on synthesis of DNA and protein in the immature rat uterus. *J. Endocr.,* 85, 291, 1980.
35. Winter, J., Moore, L. H., Dowell, V. R. Jr., and Bokkenheuser, V. D., C-ring cleavage of flavonoids by human intestinal bacteria. *Appl. Environ. Microbiol.*, 55, 1203, 1989.
36. Markaverich, B. M., Gregory, R. R., Alejandro, M. A., Clark, J. H., Johnson, G. A., and Middleditch, B. S., Methyl p-hydroxyphenyllactate--an inhibitor of cell growth and proliferation and an endogenous ligand for nuclear type-II binding sites. *J. Biol. Chem.*, 263, 7203, 1988.
37. Chang, Y.-C. and Nair, M. G., Metabolism of daidzein and genistein by intestinal bacteria. *J. Nat. Prod.*, 58, 1892, 1995.

38. Wang, G.-J., *Human gut microfloral metabolism of soybean isoflavones.* M.S. Thesis, Iowa State University Library, Ames. IA 50011, 1997, 21.
39. Klaassen, C. D., Distribution, excretion, and absorption of toxicants, in *Casarett and Doullís Toxicology, The Basic Science of Poisons*, Klaassen, C. D., Amdur, M. O., and Doull, J., Eds., Macmillan Publ. Co., New York, NY, 33, 1986.
40. Lu, L. J., Grady, J. J., Marshall, M. V., and Ramanujam, V. M., Altered time course of urinary daidzein and genistein excretion during chronic soya diet in healthy male subjects. *Nutr. Cancer* 24, 311, 1995.
41. Reeds, P. J. and Beckett, P. R., Protein and amino acids, in *Present Knowledge in Nutrition, 7th edition*, Ziegler, E. E., and Filer, L. J., ILSI Press, Washington, D.C., 67, 1996.
42. Yip, R. and Dallman, P., Iron, in *Present Knowledge in Nutrition, 7th edition*, Ziegler, E. E., and Filer, L. J., ILSI Press, Washington, D.C., 277, 1996.
43. Supko, J. G. and Malspeis, L., Plasma pharmacokinetics of genistein in mice. *Int. J. Oncol.* 7, 847, 1995.
44. Yasuda, T., Kano, Y., Saito, K.-I., and Ohsawa, K., Urinary and biliary metabolites of daidzin and daidzein. *Biol. Pharm. Bull.*, 17, 1369, 1994.
45. Adlercreutz, H., Fotsis, T., Lampe, J., Wahala, K., Makela, T., Brunow, G., and Hase, T., Quantitative determination of lignans and isoflavonoids in plasma of omnivorous and vegetarian women by isotope dilution gas chromatography-mass spectrometry. *Scand. J. Clin. Lab. Invest.* 53 (suppl. 215), 5, 1993.
46. Lin, H.-K., *Genistein, daidzein, and apigenin bioavailability and effects on glutathione peroxidase activity*, M.S. Thesis, Iowa State University Library, Ames, IA, 50011, 1994.
47. Lundh, T. J., Pettersson, H., and Kiessling, K. H. Liquid chromatographic determination of the estrogens daidzein, formononetin, coumestrol, and equol in bovine blood plasma and urine. *J. Assoc. Offic. Anal. Chem.* 71, 938, 1988.
48. Cochran, W. G. and Cox, G. M. *Experimental design, 2nd edition.* Wiley Publications in Statistics, New York, NY, 75, 1957.
49. Griffiths, L. A. and Smith, G. E., Metabolism of apigenin and related compounds in the rat. *Biochem. J.*, 128, 901, 1972.
50. Hendrich, S., Wang, G.-J., Xu, X., Tew, B.-Y., Wang, H.-J., and Murphy, P.A., Human Bioavailability of Soy Bean Isoflavones: Influences of Diet, Dose, Time and Gut Microflora, in *Functional Foods, ACS Monograph,* Shibamoto, T., Ed., ACS Books, Washington, DC, in press.
51. Xu, X., Wang, H.-J., Murphy, P.A., Hendrich, S. Neither diet selection nor type of soy food affect isoflavone bioavailability in women. *J. Nutr.*, submitted.
52. Cheng, K.-J., Jones, G. A., Simpson, F. J., and Bryant, M. P., Isolation and identification of rumen bacteria capable of anaerobic rutin degradation, *Can. J. Microbiol.,* 15, 1365, 1969.
53. Krishnamurty, H. G., Cheng, K.-J., Jones, G. A., Simpson, F. J., and Aatkin, J. E. Identification of products produced by the anaerobic degradation of rutin and related flavonoids by *Butyrivibrio* sp. C_3, *Can. J. Microbiol.*, 16, 759, 1970.
54. Winter, J., Popoff, M. R., Grimont, P., and Bokkenheuser, V. D. *Clostridium orbiscindens* sp. nov., a human intestinal bacterium capable of cleaving the flavonoid C-ring. *Intl. J. System. Bacteriol.,* 41, 355, 1991.

12

Other Antioxidants

Andreas M. Papas, Ph.D.
Health and Nutrition
Eastman Chemical Company, Kingsport, Tennessee, USA

INTRODUCTION

In addition to the major classes of antioxidants reviewed in Chapters 8 to 11, a large number of compounds in our food and our body have antioxidant activity. For some of these compounds, we have a good understanding of their antioxidant function and, to a lesser extent, their role in nutrition and health. For many others, our knowledge is very limited. This chapter will review briefly some of these antioxidants.

0-8493-8009-X/98/$0.00+$.50

COENZYME Q

Chemistry and Occurrence

Coenzyme Q (CoQ, Figure 1), also known as ubiquinone, was first isolated from beef heart and chemically characterized in 1957 by Frederick Crane. Four years later, Peter D. Mitchell elucidated its function and won the Nobel Prize for chemistry in 1978 for this work.[1] The structure of CoQ consists of a quinone ring attached to an isoprene side chain. CoQ is fat-soluble but becomes amphiphilic in the process of translocating electrons and protons. The number of isoprene units in the side chain varies with each species of animal or plant. Human CoQ has 10 isoprene units and is designated as CoQ_{10}.

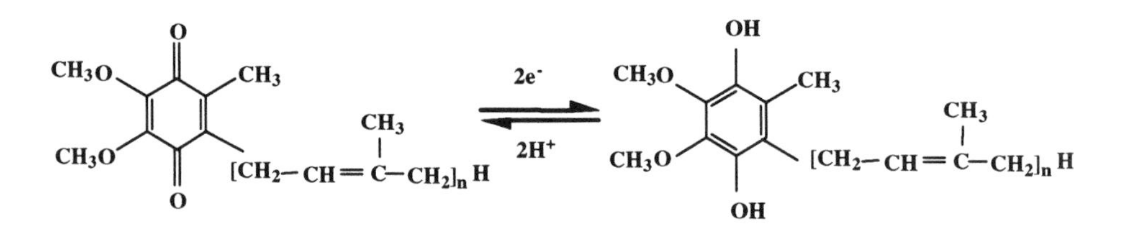

Figure 1. Oxidized and reduced forms of coenzyme Q. In humans, the number of isoprene units (n) is 10 and is known as CoQ_{10}.

CoQ is found naturally in the tissues of animals and plants. In humans, it is fairly abundant in the heart, liver, kidney, and pancreas. Although concentrated in the mitochondria, Golgi apparatus, and lysosomes of cells, it is also present in all plasma membranes including low-density lipoprotein (LDL).[2-4] The major sources of CoQ in our diet are meats, fish, and vegetable oils. Wheat germ, rice bran, soy and some other beans are fairly good sources. With the exception of spinach and broccoli, vegetables are generally low in CoQ. Estimated average daily intake is about 3-5 mg/day.[5]

Although dietary CoQ contributes significantly to the pool of CoQ_{10} in humans,[6,7] the major part is synthesized, primarily in the liver.[8-10] The quinone ring is synthesized from the amino acids tyrosine and phenylalanine, and the polyprenyl side chain is synthesized from acetyl-CoA.

CoQ as Antioxidant and Prooxidant

The two major known functions of CoQ are bioenergetic and antioxidant. CoQ plays a vital role in the production of energy from oxidation of glucose in the mitochondria coupling, the transfer and translocation of electrons, and translocation of protons through the osmotic barrier of the mitochondrial christae membrane. As a donor of electrons, CoQ also has antioxidant properties.[11] These two major functions may be related because free radicals are produced in the mitochondria during the process of respiration.

Two mechanisms of antioxidant action have been proposed. In the first, the reduced ubiquinol form of CoQ, functions independently as chain-breaking antioxidant and reduces peroxyl (ROO*) and alcoxyl radicals.[12]

$$CoQH + ROO^* \rightarrow Q^* + ROOH$$

The second is a redox interaction with the vitamin E radical (TO*) regenerating vitamin E in the same manner as suggested for vitamin C.[13-15]

$$CoQH + TO^* \rightarrow Q^* + ROOH$$

Because CoQ scavenges free radicals *in vitro* less efficiently than vitamin E, it has been suggested that its role in regenerating vitamin E is more important *in vivo*. It appears that CoQ, due to its unique positioning in the membranes, is able to export the radical reaction to the aqueous phase. This may be very important in protecting membrane lipids and LDL. Recently, Stocker and his co-workers[16] showed that α-tocopherol can function *in vitro*, as prooxidant for LDL in the absence of other antioxidants such as ascorbic acid and CoQ_{10}. The same researchers showed in the same *in vitro* system that ascorbic acid and coenzyme Q_{10} prevented the prooxidant effect of α-tocopherol.[17,18] They proposed that small amphiphilic antioxidants are particularly efficient because they can shuttle free radicals out from the lipophilic LDL.[19] This suggests that CoQ, as a component of a complex antioxidant system, may amplify the effect of vitamin E.

CoQ and specifically its intermediate ubisemiquinone, can undergo autoxidation during the redox cycling by electron transport producing superoxide radicals. This reaction requires protons, which are not readily available in the phospholipid membranes because the lipophilic polyisoprenyl side chain resides specifically in the lipid bilayer. When, however, the integrity of the membranes or the redox cycling are disturbed, due to disease, genetic defects, or aging, protons become available and autoxidation can and probably does occur.[12,14] Aging in particular is associated with increase in membrane permeability, which allows protons to oxidize ubisemiquinones.

Nutritional Issues

Because CoQ is not considered an essential nutrient, there is no established recommended dietary allowance (RDA). It is rather poorly absorbed[6,20,21] especially with low-fat or fat-free diets. Supplementation increases the blood and liver concentration but enrichment of other tissues is very slow.[21] Blood levels are lower in people with some chronic diseases including heart disease,[22] cancer,[23] AIDS,[24] and the elderly. It is also low in people with some genetic diseases such as neurologic diseases and myopathies.[25,26] Commercial supplements are available as oxidized CoQ_{10}. It appears that after oral supplementation, CoQ appears mainly in its reduced, antioxidant form in the body. Doses taken as supplements range considerably. Common doses used as supplements are 10-30 mg/day. Therapeutic dosages for serious diseases range from 200-400 mg daily.

CoQ in Health and Disease

Aging

The age-related decline in CoQ, in conjunction with the free radical hypothesis for aging, suggest a potential role for CoQ in maintaining the efficiency of cellular energy production.[27] The potential role of CoQ in age-related brain degenerative diseases is discussed below.

Exercise

Heavy exercise causes increased production of free radicals because it increases energy consumption and oxidation to produce ATP. In addition, hyperthermia may cause uncoupling of the respiratory chain thus producing free radicals. Athletes, as opposed to sedentary individuals, have lower levels of serum CoQ_{10} and higher levels of muscle and heart CoQ_{10}. Several studies suggest that CoQ increases the volume of oxygen uptake and reduces free radical production which may increase energy output and lengthen the time to reach exhaustion.[12,28]

Heart Disease

CoQ_{10} is concentrated in the myocardium and has been suggested as essential for normal heart function. Heart disease has been the main focus for the therapeutic effects of CoQ. A number of clinical studies indicated that CoQ improved heart function and exercise capacity,[29,30] but others showed no benefit. CoQ may protect against heart damage from adriamycin, a common and powerful cytotoxic chemotherapy drug. In addition, CoQ probably plays a role in reducing the risk of heart disease because, as discussed above, it may work with vitamin E to inhibit oxidation of LDL.[17-19] In a recent study with smokers, CoQ_{10} did not increase resistance of LDL and VLDL to copper induced oxidation.[20]

Muscular Dystrophy and Mitochondrial Myopathies

Muscular dystrophy is a group of closely related syndromes characterized by an abnormality in muscle structure that gives rise to the death of the muscle fibers and to abnormal muscle regeneration. Some myopathies are associated with abnormal activities of mitochondrial enzymes.[31] Muscular dystrophy and other myopathies are usually associated with heart disease. The use of CoQ supplementation has been tried in a large number of these syndromes. Results from two double-blind trials were reported recently.[32] In the first, twelve patients, ranging from 7-69 years of age, having diseases including the Duchenne, Becker, the limb-girdle dystrophies, myotonic dystrophy, Charcot-Marie-Tooth disease, and the Welander disease were treated for three months with 100 mg daily of CoQ_{10} and a matching placebo. The second double-blind trial was similar with fifteen patients having the same categories of disease. CoQ appeared to improve physical performance of these patients.

Periodontal Disease

CoQ level is dramatically lower in diseased gingiva. This apparent deficiency provided the impetus for studies to determine the effects of CoQ_{10}, supplied orally or by topical application, on the progression of periodontal disease. Oral administration and especially topical application of CoQ_{10} appeared to reduce gingival inflammation and periodontal pocket-depth in at least some studies.[33]

Immune Function

CoQ appears to stimulate the immune system in both normal and deficient people. Acquired Immune Deficiency Syndrome (AIDS) is associated with significantly depressed CoQ_{10} levels. Human Immunodefficiency Virus (HIV)-positive persons without symptoms have normal levels that decline as they progress to AIDS Related Complex (ARC), and further decline as they develop AIDS. These results stimulated interest in the role of CoQ_{10} in people with AIDS. A pilot study suggested that CoQ_{10} delayed the progression of ARC to AIDS.[24]

Brain Function and Degenerative Brain Diseases

It has been proposed recently that the development of degenerative brain diseases such as Alzheimer's, Parkinson's, and Huntington's may be linked to mithochondrial defects and in particular of the cytochrome oxidase system.[34,35] As a result, oxidation of glucose in the mitochondria to produce energy is disrupted, causing a major increase in the production of free radicals. Thus these diseases may be characterized as "diseases of the bioenergetics." Preliminary studies suggest that supplemental CoQ_{10} or vitamin E may help delay the progress of these diseases.[36,37] There is also strong interest in determining whether CoQ improves brain function in healthy people.

URIC ACID

Chemistry and Occurrence

Uric acid (Figure 2) is produced in our body from the oxidation of xanthine and hypoxanthine by the enzymes xanthine oxidase and dehydrogenase. Unlike other animal species, humans and other higher primates lack the enzyme urate oxidase, which converts urate to allantoin, which is further metabolized to urea and glycoxalate.[38]

Uric acid concentration in our body fluids of 0.2-.0.4 mM is higher than ascorbate another major water-soluble antioxidant.[39,40] At the physiological pH of many bodily fluids, which is higher than 7, uric acid is present as urate. Because of its limited solubility in water at high concentrations, uric acid crystallizes causing gout. Diets rich in purines such as anchovies, sardines, sweetbreads, kidney, or liver increase the concentration of uric acid. The diet, however, accounts for approximately half of the uric acid produced in the body, with the other half produced from endogenous purines.[38]

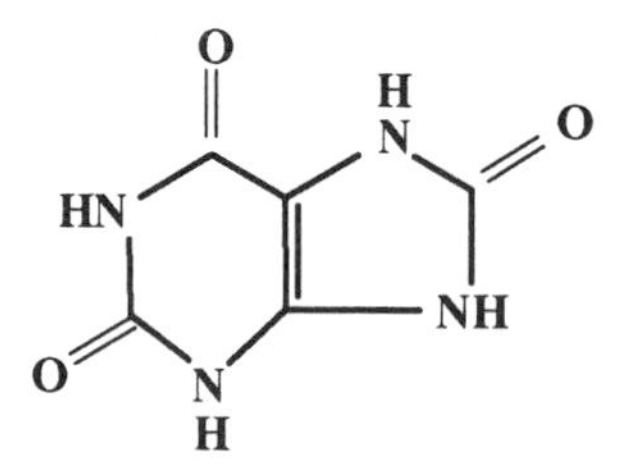

Figure 2. Uric acid.

Antioxidant Function

Uric acid has several antioxidant functions *in vitro*. It binds strong prooxidant transition metals such as Fe and Cu thus preventing their reaction with H_2O_2 to produce hydroxyl radical. In blood, uric acid appears to stabilize ascorbate probably due to binding of Fe and Cu.[41] It also reacts with a variety of reactive oxygen species such as ozone, nitrogen dioxide, peroxynitrite, singlet oxygen, hypochlorous acid, and the OH* radical. It inhibits peroxidation of lipids probably indirectly by binding Fe and Cu. Due to its abundance and its role in stabilizing vitamin C, which regenerates vitamin E, urate is considered a major component of the antioxidant system in humans. Reaction of urate with OH* forms a urate radical, which *in vitro* inactivates enzymes.[42] Ascorbate regenerates the urate radical. Allantoin is the major oxidation product of urate. The ratio of allantoin to urate is used as a measure of oxidative stress in aqueous compartments.

Uric Acid in Health and Disease

Because high blood urate is associated with gout and appears to correlate with increased risk of cardiovascular disease,[43,44] there has been very limited research on its role in reducing the risk of chronic disease. In addition, urate is not an essential nutrient and is produced in our body thus there is no established RDA for it or its precursors. Although pollutants reduce lung concentrations of urate and oxidative stress increases its breakdown, there are no established disease conditions associated with its deficiency. There is, however, significant evidence that urate is an important component of the human antioxidant system.

GLUTATHIONE (GSH)

Chemistry and Occurrence

GSH is a tri-peptide, composed of cysteine, glutamic acid, and glycine (Figure 3). Its active group is the thiol (-SH) of cysteine. Oxidized glutathione (GSSG) consists of two GSH molecules joined by their –SH groups into a disulfide bridge. GSH and associated enzymes, such as GSH peroxidase, are found in tissues of virtually all plants and animals. In humans, the highest levels are found in the liver, lenses of the eyes, pancreas, spleen, and kidneys.[45-47] GSH is the most abundant non-protein thiol in the cells. GSH, unlike vitamins, can be synthesized intracellularly through several enzymatic steps. As a metabolically important compound, tissue concentrations of GSH are highly regulated, and it is therefore difficult to see depletion or excess of GSH in the body.

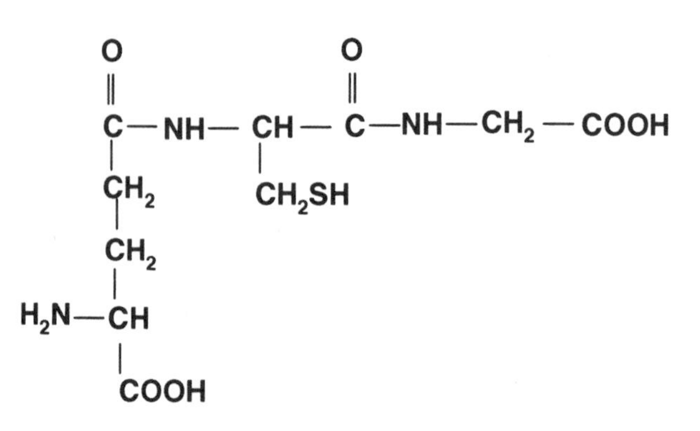

Figure 3. Clutathione (GSH) is composed of the amino acids cysteine, glutamic acid, and glycine.

Antioxidant Function

GSH functions as antioxidant in several ways primarily as a component of an enzyme system containing GSH oxidase and reductase. The GSH peroxidase contains Se and removes H_2O_2 by oxidizing GSH. H_2O_2 is produced in the cytosol by superoxide dismutase (Cu, Zn-SOD) and in the mitochondria by Mn-SOD:

$$2GSH + H_2O_2 \rightarrow GSSG + 2H_2O$$

The GSH reductase, which contains flavin adenine dinucleotide, a derivative of riboflavin, reduces GSSG

$$GSSG + NADPH + H^+ \rightarrow NADP^+ + 2GSH$$

These reactions are probably very important in the proposed regeneration of the tocopheryl radical because GSH can reduce the ascorbyl radical.[46] The ratio of oxidized to reduced GSH has been used as a measure of oxidative stress in premature infants.

GSH also functions as antioxidant independent of the enzymes. For example, it donates hydrogen to repair damaged DNA. For this reason, GSH and other thiol compounds may be important for protecting against damage from radiation and helping to reduce the side effects of chemotherapy and X-rays.

GSH is also a component of a detoxification system, separate from the cytochrome P450, which metabolizes toxic compounds to inactive or less harmful products. The enzyme glutathione transferase catalyzes the binding of these compounds to glutathione.

Glutathione in Nutrition and Health

GSH is not classified as an essential nutrient and, therefore, there is no established RDA. Good food sources are broccoli and green leafy vegetables such as parsley and spinach. Dietary GSH is only partially absorbed because, as a tri-peptide, it is hydrolyzed in part by peptidases and absorption of intact GSH is rather poor. GSH is also available as a nutritional supplement. The diet, however, is a very important factor for the GSH status because it supplies essential cofactors (such as Se, Mn, and Zn) and the sulfur-containing amino acids. In addition, if it contains alcohol, heavy metals and food toxicants, it may cause blood and liver reduction of GSH.[48,49]

The role of GSH in health and disease is twofold. In addition to its antioxidant functions described above, it plays an important role in the detoxification of compounds such as alcohol, pesticides, drugs, and others.[49,50] Its role in immunity and aging is discussed in Chapters 13 and 17.

HIV infection is associated with low levels of GSH in blood.[51] Based on *in vitro* studies showing that low GSH levels promote both HIV expression and impair T cell function, Herzenberg and his associates suggested a link between GSH depletion and HIV disease progression.[52] The same researchers reported data suggesting that low GSH levels predict poor survival in otherwise indistinguishable HIV-infected subjects. Specifically, GSH deficiency in CD4 T cells from such subjects is associated with markedly decreased survival 2-3 years after baseline data collection. Oral administration of the GSH prodrug N-acetylcysteine replenishes GSH in these subjects.

FOOD ANTIOXIDANTS

Chemistry

Synthetic and natural food antioxidants are used routinely in many foods especially those containing oils and fats. Natural tocopherols, the synthetic α-tocopherol, and other phenolic antioxidants such as BHA (butylated hydroxyanisole), BHT (butylated hydroxytoluene), PG (propyl gallate), and TBHQ (tertiary butylhydroquinone) are effective chain-breaking antioxidants and the most commonly used commercially (Figure 4 and Table 1). Water-soluble antioxidants such ascorbic and citric acids are also used extensively. Approved food antioxidants, use levels, and related information were reviewed earlier.[53] The role of antioxidant status in humans was discussed in Chapter 5.

Antioxidant Function

Tocopherols, BHA, BHT, PG, and TBHQ function as chain-breaking antioxidants as described in Chapter 1 by reacting with the peroxyl radical (RCOO*):

$$AH + RCOO^* \rightarrow RCOOH + A^*$$

Other food antioxidants bind prooxidant metals such as Cu and Fe (citric acid, lecithin) or regenerate antioxidants (ascorbic acid) or scavenge free radicals.

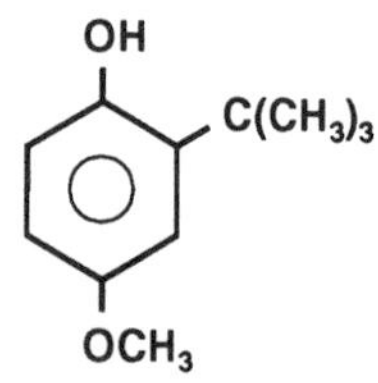

3-tertiary-butyl-4-hydroxyanisole

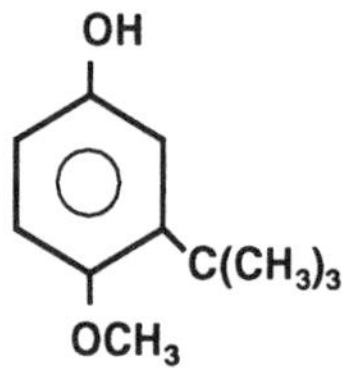

2-tertiary-butyl-4-hydroxyanisole

BHA

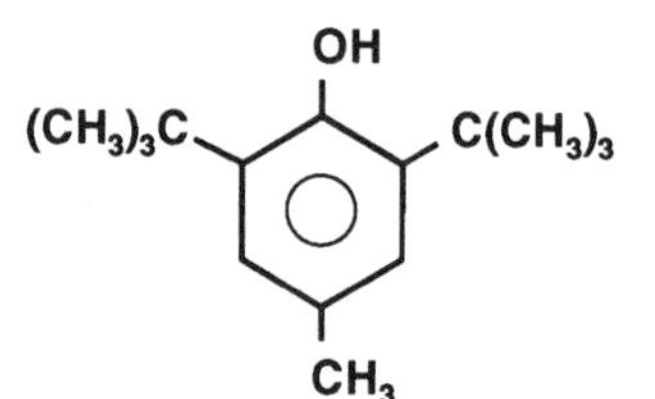

2,6-ditertiary-butyl-4-methyl phenol

BHT

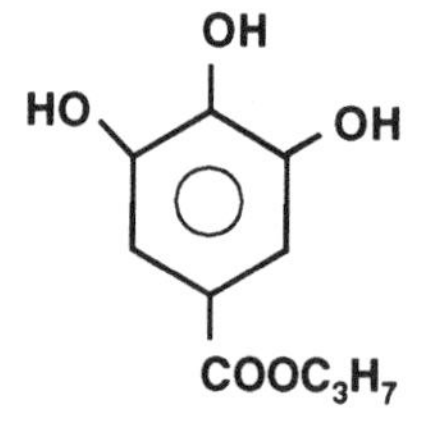

n-propyl ester of 3,4,5-tri-hydroxybenzoic acid

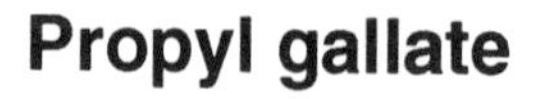

Propyl gallate

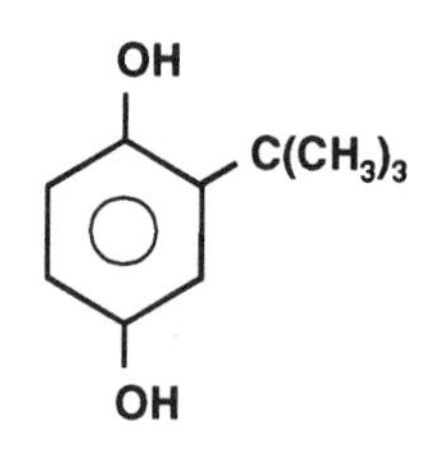

tertiary-butyl-hydroquinone

TBHQ

Figure 4. Structure of the synthetic food antioxidants, BHA, BHT, Propyl Gallate, and TBHQ. They are all phenolic compounds.

Table 1
Major Commercial Food Antioxidants[a]

	United States	Europe[b]	Canada	Japan
Antioxidant	FDA Food Additive Regulation	Food and Drugs Regulation	Food and Drugs Act and Regulation	Ministry of Health
			Table 11, part iv	
BHA	21CRF182.3169	E320	Item b1	Approved
BHT	21CFR182.3173	E321	Item b2	Approved
Propyl gallate	21CFR184.1660	E310	Item p1	Approved
TBHQ	21CFR172.185	Not approved	Not approved	Not approved
Tocopherols	21CFR182.3890	E306	Item t2	Approved

[a] These are the major fat-soluble antioxidants used in foods to protect lipid oxidation. Use of other fat-soluble antioxidants is limited. Most countries approved use of these antioxidants. TBHQ was approved only recently in Europe and Canada.

Food Antioxidants in Health and Disease

The role of tocopherols and tocotrienols in nutrition and health is discussed in several other chapters.

For BHA, BHT, TBHQ, and PG, their indirect benefits to health from inhibition of lipid oxidation in foods are well documented. Research, however, on additional direct health benefits from ingestion of these antioxidants was overshadowed by the controversy about their toxic effects at very high levels. There are considerable indications for a role in reducing the risk of some forms of cancer. BHA and BHT inhibit the carcinogenic effects of afflatoxin.[58,59] There is also evidence that BHT inhibits photocarcinogenesis in animal models and protects against UV-B-induced erythema and UV-B induction of ornithine decarboxylase. BHA, but not PG, reduced the incidence of aberrant crypts on rat colon, a predictor of colon cancer.[55-57,61,62]

Unfortunately, the potential benefits of these antioxidants have not been evaluated in major intervention clinical studies. It is, however, interesting to contemplate whether they had a role in the dramatic reduction of stomach cancer in the last 50 years. This decrease is even more remarkable considering that the incidence of other cancers changed very little and, for lung cancer, it increased substantially. The primary reason was probably the advent of refrigeration that made possible increased consumption of fresh fruits and vegetables and reduced consumption of preserved foods especially those producing nitrosamines. Another major development was the discovery and practical use of food antioxidants that reduced lipid peroxides in our diets.

ALPHA-LIPOIC ACID

Alpha-lipoic acid (thioctic acid) is a naturally occurring metabolite (Figure 5) and has been used, primarily in Germany, for treatment of diabetes and neurologic diseases. As a small molecule, it can be absorbed from the diet. Recently, it received attention as a biological antioxidant.[63,64] Lipoate or its reduced form, dihydrolipoate, reacts with reactive oxygen species such as superoxide radicals, hydroxyl radicals, hypochlorous acid, peroxyl radicals, and singlet oxygen. It was suggested that it interacts with vitamin C and glutathione, which may in turn recycle vitamin E. In addition to its antioxidant activities, dihydrolipoate may exert prooxidant actions through reduction of iron.

Landvic and Packer discuss the function of alpha-lipoic acid as a biological antioxidant and its role in health and disease in Chapter 26.

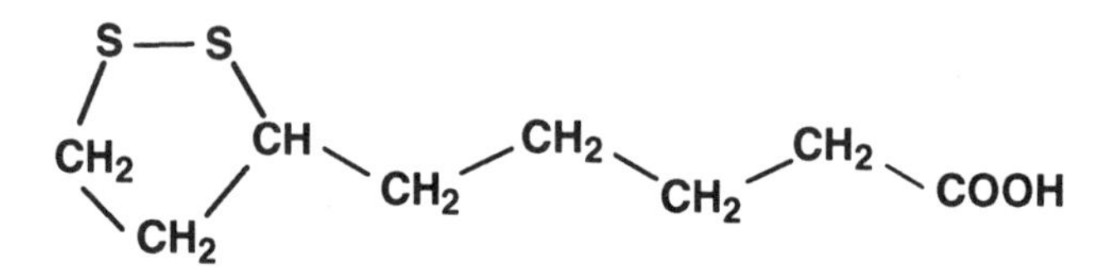

Figure 5. Lipoic acid.

MELATONIN

Chemistry and Occurrence

Melatonin, N-acetyl-5-methoxytryptamine, is a mammalian hormone produced by the metabolism of serotonin (5-hydroxytryptamine) which is derived from tryptophan (Figure 6). It is synthesized primarily in the pineal gland (a pea-sized organ situated in the center of the brain) and, to a lesser extent, in the retina, the gastrointestinal tract, and several other tissues. Melatonin production is higher during darkness and plays an important role in the daily (circadian) and annual (circannual) biological rhythms, such as sleep and hormone patterns. Production of melatonin and blood and tissue levels decline with age. Animal and human studies demonstrated that administration of melatonin can shift their biological rhythms. Depending on the time of administration, melatonin advances or delays the timing of biological rhythms as a result of interaction with the body's internal body clock, which is situated within an area of mammalian hypothalamus.

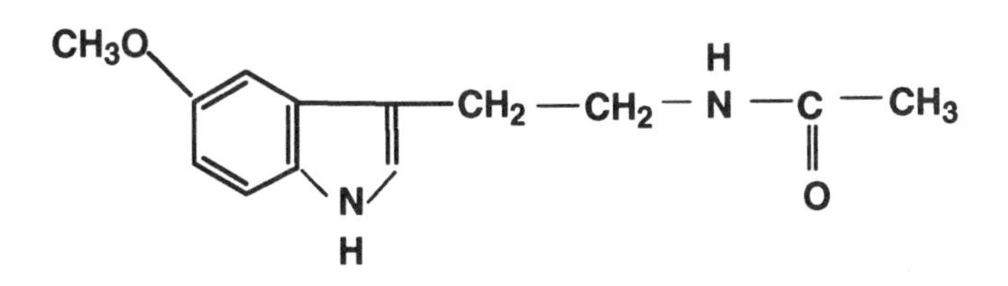

Figure 6. Melatonin.

Antioxidant Function

The antioxidant effects of melatonin have been studied during the last 8 years by Dr. Reiter's group[65,66] at the University of Texas and others. It was reported that melatonin has direct antioxidant effects *in vitro* such as scavenging hydroxyl radicals and reducing peroxidation of neural membranes induced by thiobarbituric acid. *In vivo*, high doses of melatonin reduced paraquat-induced lipid peroxidation in lungs prevented formation of DNA adducts induced by carcinogens, and increased brain glutathione synthesis in rats.[67-69]

The importance of melatonin as an antioxidant in normal physiological conditions is unclear. Melatonin is a weak direct antioxidant but this does not prevent a special role in the brain or indirect antioxidant effects by enhancing endogenous antioxidant enzymes.[70]

Safety

While short-term use of low doses of melatonin appears safe, there is no information on its long-term side effects or interactions with drugs or other antioxidants. Controlled trials of melatonin have been limited to acute studies using healthy individuals aged 20-60. In view of the large number of individuals reportedly taking melatonin, several scientific and health organizations in the United States and Europe raised concerns about the unsupervised long-term use of this hormone. There is also significant controversy as to the appropriate dose level.

Melatonin in Nutrition and Health

Our diet supplies little if any melatonin. The amino acid tryptophan, a precursor of serotonin increases endogenous production of serotonin. Thus diets rich in tryptophan may affect indirectly the production of melatonin. Tryptophan is contained in all proteins and was available as a nutritional supplement. A few years ago, the FDA banned tryptophan as a nutritional supplement following several deaths, later found to be associated with a contaminant.

Melatonin is used to overcome disruptions in the circadian rhythm such as disruption of sleep due to travel and changes in time zones and for treatment of insomnia. It has been also proposed that melatonin may have a large number of health benefits many attributed, at least in part, to its antioxidant function.[65] These proposed benefits include delaying aging and reducing the risk of associated neurodegenerative diseases such as Alzheimer's, reducing the risk of heart disease and damage from ionizing radiation, and treating AIDS patients.[65-69,71] These proposals were based primarily on short-term studies *in vitro* and animals. For example, the proposed effect on aging was based on the surgical exchange of pineal glands from young and old rats that showed dramatic changes in their physiology and appearance.[72] Such promising results, however, need to be evaluated in long-term intervention trials in humans before we fully understand the role and safety of melatonin.[73]

Overall the practical importance of melatonin as antioxidant and its role in health especially in reducing the risk of disease remain unclear and require further study.

CONCLUSION

These antioxidants, whether supplied in the diet, produced in our body, or merely used as food antioxidants play an important role, directly or indirectly, on the antioxidant status in humans. Their role in nutrition and health is discussed further in later chapters.

REFERENCES

1. Crane FL, Hatefi Y, Lester RL, Widmer C. Isolation of a quinone from beef heart mitochondria. 1957. *Biochim Biophys Acta* 1989;1000:362-3.
2. Åberg F, Appelkvist EL, Dallner G, Ernster L. Distribution and redox state of ubiquinones in rat and human tissues. *Arch Biochem Biophys* 1992;295:230-234.
3. Johansen K, Theorell H, Karlsson J, Diamant B, Folkers K. Coenzyme Q_{10}, alpha-tocopherol and free cholesterol in HDL and LDL fractions. *Ann Med* 1991;23:649-656.
4. Lang JK, Gohil K, Packer L. Simultaneous determination of tocopherols, ubiquinols, and ubiquinones in blood, plasma, tissue homogenates, and subcellular fractions. *Anal Biochem* 1986;157:106-16.
5. Weber C, Bysted A, Hllmer G. The coenzyme Q_{10} content of the average Danish diet. *Int J Vitam Nutr Res* 1997;67:123-9.
6. Weber C, Bysted A, Holmer G. Coenzyme Q_{10} in the diet--daily intake and relative bioavailability. *Mol Aspects Med* 1997;18:s251-4.
7. Mohr D, Bowry VW, Stocker R. Dietary supplementation with coenzyme Q_{10} results in increased levels of ubiquinol-10 within circulating lipoproteins and increased resistance of human low-density lipoprotein to the initiation of lipid peroxidation. *Biochim Biophy Acta* 1992;1126:247-254.
8. Olson RE, Rudney H. Biosynthesis of ubiquinone. *Vitam Horm* 1983;40:1-43.
9. Kagan VE, Serbinova EA, Maguire JJ, Shvedova AA, Packer L. On the path from ubiquinone to ubiquinol chain breaking lipid peroxyl radical scavenging or vitamin E radical recycling? In: Davies KJA, Ed. *Oxidative Damage And Repair: Chemical, Biological and Medical Aspects.* Oxford, England, UK: Pergamon Press, 1991:121-125.
10. Mukai K, Morimoto H, Kikuchi S, Nagaoka S. Kinetic study of free-radical-scavenging action of biological hydroquinones (reduced forms of ubiquinone, vitamin K and tocopherol quinone) in solution. *Biochim Biophys Acta* 1993;1157:313-7.
11. Niki E. Chemistry and biochemistry of vitamin E and coenzyme Q as antioxidants. In: Corongiu F, Banni S, Dessi MA, Rice-Evans C, Eds. *Free Radicals and Antioxidants in Nutrition.* London: The Richelieu Press Ltd., 1993:13-25.
12. Beyer RE. An analysis of the role of coenzyme Q in free radical generation and as an antioxidant. *Biochem Cell Biol* 1992;70:390-403.
13. Kagan VE, Serbinova E, Khwaja S, Catudioc J, Maguire JJ, Packer L. *Ubiquinones and vitamin E: Partners or competitors in antioxidation. Active oxygens, lipid peroxides, and antioxidants.* Tokyo: Japan Science Press /CRC Press, 1993:237-245.
14. Maggio B, Diplock AT, Lucy JA. Interactions of tocopherols and ubiquinones with monolayers of phospholipids. *Biochem. J.* 1977;161:111-121.
15. Kagan V, Serbinova E, Packer L. Antioxidant effects of ubiquinones in microsomes and mitochondria are mediated by tocopherol recycling. *Biochem Biophys Res Commun* 1990;169:851-7.
16. Bowry VW, Ingold KU, Stocker R. Vitamin E in human low-density lipoprotein. When and how this antioxidant becomes a pro-oxidant. *Biochem. J.* 1992;288:341-344.
17. Thomas SR, Neuzil J, Stocker R. Cosupplementation with coenzyme Q prevents the pro-oxidant effect of alpha-tocopherol and increases the resistance of LDL to transition metal-dependent oxidation initiation. *Arterio Thromb Vasc Biol* 1996;16:687-696.
18. Ingold KU, Bowry VW, Stocker R, Walling C. Autoxidation of lipids and antioxidation by alpha-tocopherol and ubiquinol in homogeneous solution and in aqueous dispersions of lipids: unrecognized consequences of lipid particle size as exemplified by oxidation of human low density lipoprotein. *Proc Natl Acad Sci U S A* 1993;90:45-9.
19. Thomas SR, Neuzil J, Stocker R. Inhibition of LDL oxidation by ubiquinol-10. A protective mechanism for coenzyme Q in atherogenesis? *Mol Aspects Med* 1997;18:s85-103.

20. Kaikkonen J, Nyyssonen K, Porkkala-Sarataho E, *et al.* Effect of oral coenzyme Q_{10} supplementation on the oxidation resistance of human VLDL+LDL fraction: absorption and antioxidative properties of oil and granule-based preparations. *Free Radic Biol Med* 1997;22:1195-202.
21. Zhang Y, Turunen M, Appelkvist EL. Restricted uptake of dietary coenzyme Q is in contrast to the unrestricted uptake of alpha-tocopherol into rat organs and cells. *J Nutr* 1996;126:2089-97.
22. Folkers K. Heart failure is a dominant deficiency of coenzyme Q_{10} and challenges for future clinical research on CoQ10. *Clin Investig* 1993;71:S51-4.
23. Folkers K, Osterborg A, Nylander M, Morita M, Mellstedt H. Activities of vitamin Q_{10} in animal models and a serious deficiency in patients with cancer. *Biochem Biophys Res Commun* 1997;234:296-299.
24. Folkers K, Langsjoen P, Nara Y, *et al.* Biochemical deficiencies of coenzyme Q_{10} in HIV-infection and exploratory treatment. *Biochem Biophys Res Commun* 1988;153:888-96.
25. Sobreira C, Hirano M, Shanske S, *et al.* Mitochondrial encephalomyopathy with coenzyme Q_{10} deficiency. *Neurology* 1997;48:1238-43.
26. Imagawa M, Naruse S, Tsuji S, Fujioka A, Yamaguchi H. Coenzyme Q10, iron, and vitamin B6 in genetically-confirmed Alzheimer's. *Lancet* 1992;340:671.
27. Sugiyama S, Yamada K, Ozawa T. Preservation of mitochondrial respiratory function by coenzyme Q_{10} in aged rat skeletal muscle. *Biochem Mol Biol Int* 1995;37:1111-20.
28. Shimomura Y, Suzuki M, Sugiyama S, Hanaki Y, Ozawa T. Protective effect of coenzyme Q_{10} on exercise-induced muscular injury. *Biochem Biophys Res Commun* 1991;176:349-55.
29. Mortensen SA. Perspectives on therapy of cardiovascular diseases with coenzyme Q_{10} (ubiquinone). *Clin Investig* 1993;71:S116-23.
30. Morisco C, Trimarco B, Condorelli M. Effect of coenzyme Q_{10} therapy in patients with congestive heart failure: a long-term multicenter randomized study. *Clin Investig* 1993;71:S134-6.
31. Disdier P, Harle JR, Figarella Branger D, Cherif AA, Desnuelle C. Ptosis and asthenia manifesting a mitochondrial myopathy. *Rev Med Interne* 1992;13:381-3.
32. Folkers K, Simonsen R. Two successful double-blind trials with coenzyme Q_{10} (vitamin Q_{10}) on muscular dystrophies and neurogenic atrophies. *Biochim Biophys Acta* 1995;1271:281-6.
33. Folkers K. A critique of 25 years of research which culminated in the successful therapy of periodontal disease with coenzyme Q_{10}. *J Dent Health* 1992;42:258-63.
34. Davis RE, Miller S, Herrnstadt C, *et al.* Mutations in mitochondrial cytochrome c oxidase genes segregate with late-onset Alzheimer disease. *Proc Natl Acad Sci USA* 1997;94:4526-31.
35. Linnane AW, Degli E-M, Generowicz M, Luff AR, Nagley P. The universality of bioenergetic disease and amelioration with redox. *Biochim-Biophys-Acta.* 1995;1271:191-4.
36. Koroshetz WJ, Jenkins BG, Rosen BR, Beal MF. Energy metabolism defects in Huntington's disease and effects of coenzyme Q_{10}. *Ann Neurol* 1997;41:160-5.
37. Sano M, Ernesto C, Thomas RG, *et al.* A controlled trial of selegiline, alpha-tocopherol, or both as treatment for Alzheimer's disease. The Alzheimer's Disease Cooperative Study. *N Engl J Med* 1997;336:1216-22.
38. Becker BF. Towards the physiological function of uric acid. *Free Radic Biol Med* 1993;14:615-31.
39. Wayner DD, Burton GW, Ingold KU, Barclay LR, Locke SJ. The relative contributions of vitamin E, urate, ascorbate and proteins to the total peroxyl radical-trapping antioxidant activity of human blood plasma. *Biochim Biophys Acta* 1987;924:408-19.

40. Motchnik PA, Frei B, Ames BN. Measurement of antioxidants in human blood plasma. In: Packer L, Ed. *Meth. Enzymol.* San Diego, CA: Academic Press, Inc, 1994:269-279.
41. Sevanian A, Davies KJ, Hochstein P. Serum urate as an antioxidant for ascorbic acid. *Am J Clin Nutr* 1991;54:1129S-1134S.
42. Halliwell B. Uric acid: An example of antioxidant evaluation. In: Cadenas CaP, L, Ed. *Handbook of Antioxidants.* New York: Marcell Dekker, Inc, 1997.
43. Iribarren C, Sharp DS, Curb JD, Yano K. High uric acid: a metabolic marker of coronary heart disease among alcohol abstainers. *J Clin Epidemiol* 1996;49:673-8.
44. Persky VW, Dyer AR, Idris-Soven E, *et al.* Uric acid: a risk factor for coronary heart disease? *Circulation* 1979;59:969-77.
45. Meister A. Metabolism and function of glutathione. In: Dolphin D, Poulson R, Avrannovic O, Eds. *Glutathione.* New York: Wiley-Intrasciences Pulication, John Wiley & Sons, Inc., 1989:367-474.
46. Meister A. Glutathione-ascorbic acid antioxidant system in animals. *J. Biol. Chem.* 1994;269:9397-9400.
47. Meister A. Glutathione biosynthesis and its inhibition. *Meth. Enz.* 1995;252:26-30.
48. Dröge W, Schulze-Osthoff K, Mihm S, *et al.* Functions of glutathione and glutathione disulfide in immunology and immunopathology. *FASEB J.* 1994;8:1131-8.
49. Stohs SJ, Bagchi D. Oxidative mechanisms in the toxicity of metal ions. *Free Radic Biol Med* 1995;18:321-36.
50. Lieber CS. Role of oxidative stress and antioxidant therapy in alcoholic and nonalcoholic liver diseases. *Adv Pharmacol* 1997;38:601-28.
51. Look MP, Rockstroh JK, Rao GS, *et al.* Serum selenium, plasma glutathione (GSH) and erythrocyte glutathione peroxidase (GSH-Px)-levels in asymptomatic versus symptomatic human immunodeficiency virus-1 (HIV-1)-infection. *Eur J Clin Nutr* 1997;51:266-72.
52. Herzenberg LA, De Rosa SC, Dubs JG, *et al.* Glutathione deficiency is associated with impaired survival in HIV disease. *Proc Natl Acad Sci U S A* 1997;94:1967-72.
53. Papas AM. Oil-soluble antioxidants in foods. *Toxicol Ind Health* 1993;9:123-49.
54. Ito N, Fukushima S, Tsuda H. Carcinogenicity and modification of the carcinogenic response by BHA, BHT, and other antioxidants. *Crit Rev Toxicol* 1985;15:109-50.
55. Black HS, Mathews-Roth MM. Protective role of butylated hydroxytoluene and certain carotenoids in photocarcinogenesis. *Photochem Photobiol* 1991;53:707-16.
56. Ikezaki S, Nishikawa A, Enami T, *et al.* Inhibitory effects of the dietary antioxidants butylated hydroxyanisole and butylated hydroxytoluene on bronchioloalveolar cell proliferation during the bleomycin-induced pulmonary fibrosing process in hamsters. *Food Chem Toxicol* 1996;34:327-35.
57. Slaga TJ. Inhibition of the induction of cancer by antioxidants. *Adv Exp Med Biol* 1995;369:167-74.
58. Soni KB, Lahiri M, Chackradeo P, Bhide SV, Kuttan R. Protective effect of food additives on aflatoxin-induced mutagenicity and hepatocarcinogenicity. *Cancer Lett* 1997;115:129-33.
59. Williams GM, Iatropoulos MJ. Inhibition of the hepatocarcinogenicity of aflatoxin B1 in rats by low levels of the phenolic antioxidants butylated hydroxyanisole and butylated hydroxytoluene. *Cancer Lett* 1996;104:49-53.
60. Iverson F. Phenolic antioxidants: Health Protection Branch studies on butylated hydroxyanisole. *Cancer Lett* 1995;93:49-54.
61. Hendricks JD, Arbogast DN, Pereira CB, Bailey GS. Long-term, high-dose dietary exposure of rainbow trout to butylated hydroxyanisole is non-carcinogenic. *Cancer Lett* 1994;78:189-93.
62. Stich HF. The beneficial and hazardous effects of simple phenolic compounds. *Mutat Res* 1991;259:307-24.

63. Scott BC, Aruoma OI, Evans PJ, *et al.* Lipoic and dihydrolipoic acids as antioxidants. A critical evaluation. *Free Radic Res* 1994;20:119-33.
64. Packer L, Witt EH, Tritschler HJ. Alpha-lipoic acid as a biological antioxidant. *Free Radic Biol Med* 1995;19:227-50.
65. Reiter RJ. Antioxidant actions of melatonin. *Adv Pharmacol* 1997;38:103-17.
66. Marshall KA, Reiter RJ, Poeggeler B, Aruoma OI, Halliwell B. Evaluation of the antioxidant activity of melatonin *in vitro*. *Free Radic Biol Med* 1996;21:307-15.
67. Garcia JJ, Reiter RJ, Guerrero JM, *et al.* Melatonin prevents changes in microsomal membrane fluidity during induced lipid peroxidation. *FEBS Lett* 1997;408:297-300.
68. Vijayalaxmi, Reiter RJ, Herman TS, Meltz ML. Melatonin reduces gamma radiation-induced primary DNA damage in human blood lymphocytes.*Mutat Res* 1998;397:203-8.
69. Bettahi I, Pozo D, Osuna C, Reiter RJ, Acuna-Castroviejo D, Guerrero JM. Melatonin reduces nitric oxide synthase activity in rat hypothalamus. *J Pineal Res* 1996;20:205-10.
70. Halliwell B. How to characterize an antioxidant: an update. *Biochem Soc Symp* 1995;61:73-101.
71. Pappolla MA, Sos M, Omar RA, *et al.* Melatonin prevents death of neuroblastoma cells exposed to the Alzheimer amyloid peptide. *J Neurosci* 1997;17:1683-90.
72. Lesnikov VA, Pierpaoli W. Pineal cross-transplantation (old-to-young and vice versa) as evidence for an endogenous "aging clock". *Ann N Y Acad Sci* 1994;719:456-60.
73. Kendler BS. Melatonin: media hype or therapeutic breakthrough? *Nurse Pract* 1997;22:66-7, 71-2, 77.

Part 4

Physiological Stage and Antioxidant Status

- Aging and Exercise
- Premature Infants
- Alcoholism

13

Antioxidant Status and Function: Relationships to Aging and Exercise

Jeffrey B. Blumberg, Ph.D. and Andrew D. Halpner, Ph.D.
USDA Human Nutrition Research Center on Aging, Tufts University
Boston, Massachusetts, USA

INTRODUCTION

Substantial experimental evidence indicates a role for oxygen free radicals in the aging process and in the development of chronic diseases common among the elderly. Comparisons between mammalian species reveal a strong correlation between life span, metabolic generation of free radicals, and tissue concentrations of specific antioxidants including α-tocopherol, carotenoids, uric acid, and superoxide dismutase (SOD).[1] Experimental, clinical, and epidemiological studies are converging to reveal a reduced risk of age-related conditions like atherosclerosis, cataract, cancer, and other chronic diseases in groups with high antioxidant vitamin status.[2,3] Diets characterized by high intakes of fruits and vegetables, particularly those rich in antioxidant nutrients, are similarly associated with a lower prevalence of these conditions.

A better understanding of the complex relationships between antioxidants and aging within the context of the free radical theory of aging should be promoted by looking at several facets of this interaction. First, it is important to understand how antioxidant status changes with aging in people, particularly for considerations of revising dietary requirements and proffering recommendations for food fortification and supplementation. Second, the only established model demonstrating a direct relationship between nutrition and aging is that of caloric restriction. Investigations of the impact of caloric restriction on antioxidant defenses are helping to elucidate the mechanisms which underlie the extension of both the health and life span induced by this intervention in animal models. Third, exercise presents an apparent paradox – an activity, which increases the production of reactive oxygen species (ROS) but also provides many health benefits. Studies exploring the role of supplemental antioxidants in physical activity and the biological responses balancing ROS generation and antioxidant protection, particularly in older people, may suggest practical approaches to optimizing recommendations for dietary intake and exercise.

FREE RADICAL THEORY OF AGING

The free radical theory of aging proposed by Harman[4] hypothesizes that the degenerative changes associated with aging might be produced by the accumulation of deleterious side reactions of free radicals generated during cellular metabolism. Oxygen free radicals, particularly superoxide, hydroxyl, and peroxyl radicals, are the most common radicals generated during metabolism and could contribute to aging via several mechanisms. Oxyradicals can also be generated *in vivo* by environmental exposure to prooxidant toxicants like cigarette smoke and smog. Oxyradical-induced DNA cross-links could lead to somatic mutations and loss of essential enzyme expression. Oxidation of sensitive sulfhydryl groups could cause cellular damage to mitotic and cytoplasmic microtubules. Membrane lipid peroxidation could destroy the integrity of subcellular organelles. Macro-molecular cross-links of connective tissue could impede nutrient diffusion and impair tissue viability. While cellular antioxidants effectively quench many reactive oxygen ROS and damage that does occur is usually repaired rapidly, only a small fraction of unrepaired lesions allowed by inadequate antioxidant defenses could contribute to aging and the pathogenesis of chronic diseases. Although supporting evidence keeps the free radical theory of aging both reasonable and attractive, several basic predictions are not observed, particularly the fact that supplementary antioxidants do not lengthen the maximum life span of mammals appreciably. However, rigorous experimental testing of this approach with a full complement of antioxdants has not been conducted.

Pryor[5] has suggested that the free radical hypothesis of aging be reproposed with free radicals considered as involved in the etiology and development of chronic diseases that are most life-limiting, i.e., with radicals implicated in processes that shorten life below the maximum life span possible even if dampening radical reactions cannot lengthen maximum life span. Indeed, free radicals appear to play an important role in the initiation and/or promotion of Alzheimers disease, atherosclerosis, cancer, cataract, Parkinsonism, rheumatoid arthritis, and other chronic diseases common among older adults. Nonetheless, it is important to recognize that tissue injury and many diseases may themselves generate ROS such that oxidant formation is an epiphenomenon that makes little contribution to the progression of the condition. However, increasing antioxidant defenses may prove to be a useful intervention, if not necessarily to slowing the rate of the aging process, for reducing the associated risk of chronic disease.

ANTIOXIDANT STATUS AND INTAKE IN OLDER ADULTS

Assessment of antioxidant nutriture in older adults is complicated by the absence of appropriate and validated age-adjusted standards. Most surveys indicate that antioxidant nutrient intake in non-institutionalized elderly populations are within acceptable ranges of the U.S. Recommended Dietary Allowance and clinical measures of status. Table 1 indicates the ranges found from many investigations of intake and status of vitamins C and E and ß-carotene as well as iron, the mineral cofactor for catalase, selenium, the cofactor for glutathione peroxidase (GSHPx), and zinc, a cofactor for SOD.[6-8] Assessments of copper and manganese, also cofactors for SOD, in elderly populations are not available.

Vitamin E

Vitamin E Status

Serum tocopherol levels increase with age, at least into the seventh decade, in association with its carrier β-lipoprotein and in relation to liver stores of vitamin E.[9] Normal plasma levels of vitamin E in the United States is 23 mol/L with a range of 12-31 mol/L.[10,11] In comparison, vitamin E deficiency, characterized by functional deficits in the muscular, vascular, immune, hematopoietic and nervous systems, is generally associated with plasma levels <12 mol/L and/or intakes <3 α-TE/d.

Table 1
Antioxidant and Other Nutrients in Free Living Older Adults

Antioxidant or Nutrient	Intake		Status	
	1989 RDA	Mean Intake % RDA	Marginal Plasma Concentration	% Below Marg. Concentration
Vitamin C	60 mg - M	95–213	11.4 µM	< 5
	60 mg - F	106–220		
Vitamin E	10 mg - M	83–92	11.6 µM	0 – 3
	8 mg - F	83–89		
Carotenoids	N/A	11 µmol/d[a]	-	-
Iron	10 mg - M	140	45 µg/L[c]	25
	10 mg - F	107		
Selenium	70 µg - M	99	0.6 µM	3 – 4
	55 µg - F	89		
Zinc	15 mg - M	39 – 107[b]	10.8 µM	0 – 18
	12 mg - F			

M = male, F = female. [a] ß-carotene equivalents. [b] M and F combined. [c] Serum ferritin.

Meydani and Blumberg[12] examined the Boston Nutritional Status Survey and reported mean plasma vitamin E decreased from 32 to 21 mol/L in men aged 60–90+ y. A similar pattern was observed in the women with plasma vitamin E falling from 32 to 26 mol/L over this 30+ y span. Institutionalized elderly in this survey presented median plasma vitamin E levels 23% lower than the free-living subjects. Ascherio *et al.*[13] analyzed plasma vitamin E in middle-aged and older American men and women and reported mean α-tocopherol levels of 27 and 26 mol/L, respectively. Campbell *et al.*[14] analyzed the plasma of healthy British adults and elderly and institutionalized elderly and found mean α-tocopherol levels of 24, 26, and 19 mol/L, respectively; a significant age-associated increase in plasma vitamin E concentration was noted to age 60 in the healthy group followed by a decrease after age 80 (but not when vitamin E was expressed in terms of plasma LDL-cholesterol). In contrast, Herbeth *et al.*[15] reported significantly higher plasma levels of vitamin E in older French men and women as 32 and 35 mol/L, respectively. Vandewoude and Vandewoude[16] reported plasma vitamin E concentrations of 31 and 21 mol/L in healthy older adults 60–79 y and 80–94 y, respectively, in Belgium; these values were noted to be significantly lower than those determined in younger adults. None of these studies suggests that older adults are at risk for vitamin E deficiency when a criteria of <12 mol/L (or erythrocyte hemolysis) is employed.

Vitamin E is transported in plasma mainly in the high density lipoprotein and low density lipoprotein fractions and is highly correlated with plasma cholesterol levels. Thus, although only rarely done, vitamin E status is best described in relation to plasma lipids. This relationship is particularly important with regard to considerations of older populations where changes in mean plasma lipid concentrations may be the result of survival selection.

Platelet tocopherol has been suggested as a useful measure of vitamin E status as it is highly correlated with the vitamin E content of other tissues. Vericel *et al.*[17] observed low platelet vitamin E levels in elderly as compared to young adults even though plasma vitamin E in both groups was within ranges accepted as normal. Since α-tocopherol turnover in adipose tissue is very slow, this measure could provide a tool for evaluating long-term intake of vitamin E; however, the required biopsy procedure presents difficulties in collecting samples and no such data appear available in elderly subjects.

Vitamin E Intake

The second U.S. National Health and Nutrition Examination Survey (NHANES II) contains dietary data collected via 24-hour recalls from people aged 19-74 y. Although this method is not appropriate for the assessment of nutrient intakes by individuals, it is useful in establishing rankings between groups. Murphy *et al.*[18] analyzed NHANES II and reported mean vitamin E intake in men and women at 9.6 and 7.0 mg/d, respectively; median intakes were 7.3 and 5.4 mg/d, respectively. Intakes declined steadily with age such that the >65 y men and women were consuming a significantly lower mean of 8.3 and 6.6 mg/d and median of 6.0 and 4.9 mg/d, respectively. Ascherio *et al.*[13] estimated mean vitamin E intakes of 9.2 and 7.1 mg/d in men (mean = 55.7 y) and women (mean = 52.7 y), respectively, from a food frequency questionnaire. Herbeth *et al.* (1989) reported mean vitamin E intakes of 15.3 and 14.4 mg/d in men and women, respectively, from a 7 d diet record.

In considering dietary vitamin E intake, it is important to recognize that the food tables on which these analyses are based do not estimate well the actual vitamin E intake. It has always been appreciated that food processing and storage destroy some of the tocopherol content of most foods. After adjusting for age, body mass index, plasma cholesterol, and triglycerides, Ascherio *et al.*[13] found $r = 0.51$ and 0.41 in men and women, respectively, between plasma α-tocopherol and vitamin E intake as estimated by a food frequency questionnaire. However, this correlation was reduced to $r = 0.11$ and 0.12 in men and women, respectively, when subjects using vitamin E supplements were removed from the calculations. Herbeth *et al.*[15] reported a significant correlation between recorded dietary intake and measured plasma levels of vitamin E in older adults but did not differentiate between supplement users and nonusers in their calculations. Romieu *et al.*[19] found plasma α-tocopherol was poorly correlated ($r = 0.20$) with vitamin E consumption when adjusted for energy intake.

β-Carotene

β-Carotene Status

Johnson and Russell[20] analyzed data from the Boston Nutritional Status Survey and reported mean total carotenoid levels in plasma of 2.4 and 2.5 mol/L in men and women, respectively. Ascherio *et al.*[13] reported mean plasma β-carotene levels of 0.46 and 0.58 mol/L in men and women, respectively. Järvinen *et al.*[21] found the plasma levels of β-carotene in Finnish adults was 0.16 and 0.23 mol/L in men and women, respectively. Ito *et al.*[22] examined β-carotene concentration in the plasma of healthy males and females and reported mean values of 0.34 and 0.63 mol/L, respectively; concentrations remained constant in men 20–69 y but increased in women through 49 y. Results of the Dietary and Nutritional Survey of British Adults showed that serum α-carotene levels increased slightly from young to middle age, β-cryptoxanthin varied little across the life span, lycopene levels decreased sharply after 25–34 y, and β-carotene levels increased significantly with age; values in women were always higher than in men.[23] Serum β-carotene appears to better reflect recent dietary intakes, thus surveys covering long periods of time may not detect significant relationships with functional parameters. For example, Järvinen *et al.*[21] noted confounding results may occur if β-carotene is measured in the plasma of non-fasted subjects.

β-Carotene Intake

Ascherio *et al.*[13] reported mean intakes of carotene at 11.32 and 11.37 mol/d (β-carotene equivalents) in men and women, respectively. While they found only weak correlations between the intake of preformed vitamin A and plasma retinol, a significant relationship between estimated intake of β-carotene (from food frequency questionnaires) and plasma β-carotene was noted with $r = 0.24$ and 0.27 in men and women, respectively; after adjustment for plasma lipids, age, body mass index, and alcohol intake, the correlations increased to $r = 0.30$ and 0.34, respectively. These observations are supported by Järvinen *et al.*[21] who analyzed the relationship between mean β-carotene intake calculated from quantitative dietary history inventories (1.59 and 2.06 mg/d in men and women, respectively) and plasma levels of carotene. They noted $r = 0.35$ and, after adjusting for age and geographical region, $r = 0.38$ in women; these correlations were not statistically significant in men. Romieu *et al.*[19] calculated a correlation of $r = 0.40$ between β-carotene intake and plasma levels.

Vitamin C

Vitamin C Status in Humans

Vitamin C is an effective antioxidant but its essentiality is also based upon its function as a cosubstrate in hydroxylation reactions. Dietary intakes <10 mg/d vitamin C and/or plasma levels <11 mol/L lead to a weakening of collagenous structures, widespread capillary hemorrhaging, and joint pain (scurvy). Generous consumption of dietary ascorbate appears important to the maintenance of immune responsiveness and cholesterol metabolism and is associated with a reduced risk of cataract, cancer, and hypertension and other cardiovascular diseases.

Taylor[24] calculated mean plasma ascorbic acid for the older men and women in the Boston Nutritional Status Survey at 61 and 72 mol/L, respectively; small declines in plasma vitamin C were associated with increased age. Institutionalized elderly maintained plasma ascorbate levels 10–15% lower than free-living groups. Itoh *et al.*[25] observed mean plasma ascorbate in an older Japanese population not consuming vitamin C supplements at 52 and 63 mol/L in men and women, respectively; mean levels were significantly lower in smokers (46 mol/L) than in nonsmokers (56 mol/L). Bates *et al.*[26] reported mean plasma ascorbic acid levels of 15 and 21 mol/L for free-living elderly British men and women, respectively. Heseker *et al.*[27] reported plasma vitamin C levels decreased from 66 to 60 mol/L in German men after 65 y compared to those 55–64 y; older women had significantly higher levels (82 mol/L) and showed no decline with age. Garry *et al.*[28] recruited a population of older Americans and assessed their plasma vitamin C annually over a 5-y period; during this time they reported a range of 51–59 and 62–68 mol/L in men and women, respectively. Newton *et al.*[29] reported significantly lower plasma vitamin C values for female geriatric patients in British hospitals at 10–13 mol/L.

Plasma and leukocyte ascorbate concentrations have been used to assess vitamin C status. While plasma levels of vitamin C are considered indicative of recent dietary intake, concentration in leukocytes appear to reflect tissue stores. Generally, leukocyte ascorbate levels have been reported to decline with age and be lower in older men than older women. Vanderjagt *et al.*[30] reported ascorbic acid concentrations in mononuclear cells of 11–14 and 12–18 nmol/mg protein in elderly men and women, respectively, who consumed 30–150 mg/d vitamin C during 3-wk test periods; increasing vitamin C intakes to 280 mg/d significantly increased mononuclear cell concentrations to 23 and 29 nmol/mg protein, respectively. Elevations in total ascorbate over this range of intake were noted to be due primarily to cellular increases in dehydroascorbic acid. Vanderjagt *et al.*[30] also noted that mononuclear cell aturation levels of ascorbate were not achieved with the intakes tested in their study. Bui *et al.*[31] has employed ascorbic acid concentrations in bronchoalveolar lavage fluid and alveolar macrophages of young men to assess vitamin C status, particularly in smokers, but similar data are not available in older adults.

Vitamin C Intake

Taylor[24] reported the elderly men and women in The Boston Nutritional Status Survey had median dietary vitamin C intakes of 128 and 132 mg/d. The 3-d diet records collected by Itoh *et al.*[25] revealed dietary vitamin C intakes of 145 and 151 mg/d in men and women, respectively; mean intake was significantly lower among smokers than nonsmokers at 126 and 158 mg/d, respectively. Koplan *et al.*[32] found the older adults surveyed in NHANES II reported mean vitamin C intakes of 63 and 64 mg/d in men and women, respectively. Bates *et al.*[26] asked elderly men and women to keep a daily qualitative diet record for 12 mo and reported mean vitamin C intakes of 34 and 36 mg/d, respectively. Garry *et al.*[28] reported mean vitamin C intakes of 127-140 and 124-162 mg/d in the older men and women, respectively, surveyed over a 5-y period. Newton *et al.*[29] documented two groups of institutionalized geriatric patients with mean vitamin C intakes of 14-26 mg/d.

Actual intakes of vitamin C may be considerably lower than the calculated amount in the food ingested, largely because of its destruction by heat and oxygen and its loss in cooking water. Bates *et al.*[26] correlated intakes with serum concentration at $r = 0.22$ and $r = 0.62$ when 12-wk and 7 d diet records were employed prior to the blood draw. Itoh *et al.*[25] reported these correlations from their survey at $r = 0.319$ and $r = 0.297$ in men and women, respectively; when the correlations are computed using the reciprocal of both vitamin C intake and plasma level, they increase to $r = 0.618$ and 0.515, respectively. Sinha *et al.*[33] reported a correlation of $r = 0.43$ between calculated vitamin C intake and plasma levels in middle-aged men. They observed that larger vitamin C intakes were associated with increased plasma ascorbic acid concentrations in a two-phase linear-curvilinear relationship; those subjects not taking supplements accounted for the linear portion of the curve and those taking supplements contributed to the plateau of the curve. Sinha *et al.*[33] concluded that plasma ascorbic acid is an acceptable marker for dietary vitamin C intake except when individuals consume supplements of this nutrient.

Flavonoids

Over 4000 different types of flavonoids have been described to date and total daily intake in the United States has been estimated to be around 1 g, although this is probably an overestimation.[34-36] There are no recent estimations of total flavonoid intake, although Hertog *et al.*[37] calculated the intake of five principal flavonols and flavones at 23 mg/d. Although epidemiologic studies have indicated an inverse association between the intake of selected flavonoids and cancer, coronary heart disease, and stroke among older adults,[38-40] nutrient databases remain inadequate to provide references for age-related intake of this class of antioxidant compounds. Population based references on blood levels of flavonoids is similarly unavailable.

AGING AND ANTIOXIDANTS IN ANIMAL MODELS

Theories of aging are generally based on the principle of either developmentally programmed aging or damage-accumulation aging, both reference mechanisms involving the generation of ROS. For example, for programmed aging, Cutler[1] proposed longevity-determining genes of longer-lived species control the expression of SOD and uric acid metabolism. SOD activity of different mammals is well correlated with the metabolic rate multiplied by the maximum lifespan of the species. On the other hand, Harman[4] originally proposed that normal aging results from random deleterious damage to tissues by free radicals produced and accumulated during normal aerobic metabolism. Targets of ROS are now being characterized and quantified. For example, Ames *et al.*[41] calculated that DNA in rat cells may receive ~100,000 oxidative hits per day with concentrations of 8 hydroxydeoxyguanosine, an indicator of DNA oxidative damage, rising several-fold with age. There is also an age-related two- to three-fold increase in the concentration of oxidatively damaged proteins, reflected by the presence of ~10% of protein molecules with carbonyl modifications and loss of protein -SH groups.[42] Increases with age in lipid peroxidation reactions are indicated by such measures as alkane hydrocarbon exhalation.[43] Further, the ratio of redox couples such as glutathione (GSH):oxidized GSH (GSSG), $NADPH:NADP^+$, and $NADH:NAD^+$ tend to shift toward more prooxidant values during aging.[44]

ROS in Mitochondria

Investigations into the relationship between antioxidants and aging have largely focused on how oxidative processes change with age. Mitochondria, key organelles in aerobic metabolism and a major source of ROS, have served not only as a useful model but perhaps a central functional point as mitochondrial dysfunction may be a principal underlying event in aging.[45] Mitochondrial DNA, which does not contain histones, appears to be particularly sensitive to oxidative modification. The accumulation of mitochondrial DNA mutations may lead to decreased gene expression, a decline in oxidative phosphorylation, inefficient electron transport, and increased oxidant flux.[46] Ames *et al.*[41] have shown that mitochondrial DNA damage is greater in old than in young rats and significantly greater as well than in nuclear DNA. Increased oxidative damage in mitochondria with age may result from increased oxidant generation and/or decreased antioxidant defenses.

Nohl and Hegner[47] were among the first to demonstrate, in mitochondria isolated from rat hearts, an age-associated increase in the generation of ROS. More recently, Sohal *et al.*[48,49] have confirmed this observation in noting a two-fold greater production of oxidants in mitochondria by old mice and gerbils than by young animals. Hagen *et al.*,[50] probing isolated hepatocytes with rhodamine 123, also found significant increases in oxidant generation in old versus young rats. In contrast, Hansford *et al.*[51] attempted to maintain physiological concentrations of substrate during mitochondrial experiments and failed to detect age-related increases in mitochondrial hydrogen peroxide production. Sohal *et al.*[52] also examined this phenomenon by separating 12-d old fruit flies into behaviorally older crawlers and younger fliers and found mitochondrial hydrogen peroxide was twice as high in the crawlers compared with the fliers, a potential reflection of their greater phenotypic age.

Antioxidant Enzymes

While the increase in ROS and oxidized target molecules with age appears relatively similar across species, such consistency is absent in the response of the antioxidant enzymes. Antioxidant enzymes have been reported to increase, decrease, or not change with age; this inconsistency is due, in part, to differences in the tested species, age, gender, and diet.[53] Further complicating this situation is the difficulty in interpreting apparent changes in antioxidant enzyme activity with age as either a normative response to redox events or a response to and index of oxidative stress status.

Sohal *et al.*[49] reported increases in SOD in most tissues of old relative to young gerbils but no differences in GSHPx. In contrast, Mo *et al.*[54] reported significant decreases in SOD activity in the brain of old compared to young mice but no changes in GSHPx activity. Azhar *et al.*[55] also found significant decreases in Cu/Zn- and Mn-SOD activity in adrenal homogenates from old versus young rats but reported a two-fold decrease in GSHPx activity and no change in catalase in old rats. Lüpez-Torres *et al.*[56] found no difference between the activity of SOD, catalase or GSH reductase in the skin of young and old mice although GSHPx activity was reduced. Similarly, Lüpez-Torres *et al.*[57] found liver SOD and catalase, activity unchanged in young and old frogs. Tissue specific differences may account for some of the apparent discrepancies in antioxidant enzyme changes with age. For example, in rats Ji *et al.*[58] observed decreases in cytosolic SOD and GSHPx with age in heart but increases in skeletal muscle. Several but not all laboratories have reported age-related decreases in catalase mRNA,[55,59] GSHPx mRNA,[53] and Cu/Zn- and Mn-SOD mRNA[59,60] in mouse liver although no change was noted in enzyme activity; calorie restriction generally has no effect on either mRNA levels or enzyme activity in this mouse tissue.[53]

Low Molecular Weight Antioxidants

Similar to antioxidant enzyme activity, consistent patterns with age in low molecular weight antioxidants are also absent.[61] Hazelton and Lang[62] reported that tissue GSH is 20-33% lower in old than mid-aged mice. Christon *et al.*[63] reported a significant decrease in GSH in liver cytosol from old compared to young rats while oxidized GSH (GSSG) levels remained unchanged in both groups. In old mice with decreased brain SOD activity, Mo *et al.*[54] observed an association with increased GSSG as well as lipid peroxidation. In contrast, Lüpez-Torres *et al.*[56] reported no difference in GSH, GSSG:GSH or ascorbate in old versus young frog liver or kidney, although GSSG:GSH, was increased in mid-age. Similarly, Lüpez-Torres *et al.*[57] reported a significant increase in GSSG and decrease in GSSG:GSH in the dermis of old mice but found no difference between young and old mice with regard to ascorbate, dehydroascorbate, GSH, GSSG, uric acid, α-tocopherol, or ubiquinol 9 in the epidermis. In rat adrenals, Azhar *et al.*[55] reported significant losses with age of ascorbate and GSH with concomitant increases in GSSG. α-Tocopherol concentrations in the adrenal and liver were significantly greater in old rats, apparently a result of age-related increases in fat droplets in these tissues; little change was noted in the cell membrane content of α-tocopherol in these tissues. Meydani *et al.*[64] reported age-related decreases in the content of α-tocopherol in rat cerebellum and brain stem.

CALORIC RESTRICTION, ANTIOXIDANTS, AND AGING

Caloric Restriction

The only manipulation that has consistently been shown to affect maximal life span in animal models is caloric restriction.[61] Postulated mechanisms of action underlying the efficacy of caloric restriction in extending the life span are numerous and include reduction in body temperature, altered gene expression, and neuroendocrine changes. However, the free radical hypothesis of aging has been invoked to explain the effects of caloric restriction through alterations in metabolic rate and associated changes in the cellular balance between oxidative stresses and antioxidant defenses. Studies do indicate the greater production of ROS associated with aging can be blunted by caloric restriction.[65]

Chipalkatti *et al.*[66] and Rao *et al.*[67] have both reported significant associations between caloric restriction and reduced accumulations of lipofuscin and malondialdehyde, established indices of lipid peroxidation reactions. Rao *et al.*[67] also noted greater activities of SOD and catalase in restricted old rats relative to *ad libitum* fed controls, although age alone had no effect on enzyme activity. Parallel increases in mRNA levels for SOD and catalase were also found, suggesting caloric restriction affects not only enzyme activity but also the expression of the enzymes. In contrast, Luhtala *et al.*[68] observed an increase in the activity of skeletal muscle catalase and GSHPx in old compared to young rats. Calorically restricting these rats blunted the increase in catalase activity and abolished the age-related increase in GSHPx. Rojas *et al.*[69] reported no changes with caloric restriction in mice of liver SOD, catalase, GSHPx, GSH reductase, GSH, or uric acid although ascorbate levels were lower than in controls. However, the time at which caloric restriction is introduced appears to be a critical factor affecting the outcome of many parameters[70] and the intervention by Rojas *et al.*[69] was less than 8 wk in duration.

In caloric-restricted mice, Sohal *et al.*[48] found, in association with the extension of average life span, a reduction in the age-associated increase in the carbonyl content of protein. Moreover, age-associated increases in the mitochondrial generation of hydrogen peroxide and superoxide in heart, brain, and kidney were significantly lower in restricted relative to *ad libitum* fed animals. Despite the increase in the accumulation and/or rate of oxidant stress with age and the slowing of this process by caloric restriction, no change in SOD, catalase, or GSHPx activity was observed. Lee and Devi[71] reported that restricting caloric intake rendered rats more resistant to gastric injury by ethanol compared with *ad libitum* controls. The protection was attributed to a higher GSH concentration in the gastric mucosa of the restricted animals.

Antioxidant Interventions

Another approach to test whether free radical reactions contribute to or cause aging is to intervene directly by feeding antioxidants and examining changes in life span or functional capacity of body systems where age-related changes have been demonstrated. To date, unequivocal interpretation of existing data from survival studies is not possible. It is critical in longevity studies to separate effects due to prevention of disease from those due to modification of the basic aging process. Life span extension requires the longest-lived survivors to pass beyond the maximum limit reported for the species under optimal conditions. Extending the mean life span (MLS) of the population can be attributed to prevention or curing of disease rather than altering the basic aging rate.

Harman[72-74] attempted to prolong life span by supplementing the natural antioxidant protective mechanisms with chronic dietary administration of 2-mercaptoethanol, cysteine HCl, 2-mercaptoethylamine, butylated hydroxytoluene, hydroxylamine, or 2,2-diaminodiethyl disulfide HCl. These compounds did extend the MLS of most, but not all, of the several mouse strains tested. This squaring of the mortality curve may be related to the delay of chronic diseases, especially cancer. Similarly, Clapp *et al.*[75] found that butylated hydroxytoluene increased MLS in mice, but Kohn[76] found no such effect when care was taken to ensure that the control animals lived as long as possible. Comfort *et al.*[77] have extended the MLS and maximum life span of mice with ethoxyquin treatment. Injection of cysteine or thiazolidine carboxylic acid has been reported to increase the life spans of mice and guinea pigs but not rats.[78] Lönnrot *et al.*[79] fed rats ubiquinone (coenzyme Q), a cellular antioxidant which appears to decrease with age, but failed to alter lifespan, lipopigment accumulation, or plasma α-tocopherol levels. Miquel *et al.*[80] found that N-acetylcysteine treatment of mice prevented the age-associated decline in the activity of enzymes associated with oxidative phosphorylation but did not report longevity.

Even the successful antioxidant feeding experiments described above do not show a dramatic effect on the life span of the animals tested. In trying to reconcile this data with the free radical theory of aging, it must be recognized that most of the synthetic antioxidants were developed for industrial uses such as stabilizing rubber or petroleum products and their absorption, distribution, metabolism, and excretion are markedly different from those of the dietary antioxidants.[81] Tissue levels of the synthetic antioxidants in these studies were not measured in most experiments even though they are known to be poorly absorbed and quickly eliminated. Moreover, many of the reports indicate moderate to significant weight loss in the treated animals and thus the results may be confounded by an effect of caloric restriction. Well-controlled life span animal experiments employing a combination of several dietary antioxidants have not yet been performed although several investigators have examined the effect of vitamin E.

Vitamin E has been administered to mice,[82-85] rats,[86,87] fruit flies,[88] rotifers,[89] nematodes,[90] human cell cultures,[91-93] and fungi[94] in an attempt to extend their longevity. Most of these studies show a reduction in lipofuscin accumulation but the majority demonstrated only small increases in MLS or survival time and no increase in maximum life span (except with fruit flies and nematodes).

Using a different approach, Orr and Sohal[95] reported that transgenic fruit flies overexpressing Cu-Zn SOD and catalase exhibited a marked extension in life span and retardation of the loss of physical performance; the protein carbonyl content was found to be significantly lower in the transgenic flies compared to controls.

EXERCISE AND ANTIOXIDANTS DURING AGING

Although there are many documented benefits to health from physical activity, exercise is also associated with increases in whole body oxygen consumption and oxygen flux in muscle and production of superoxide.[96] These changes appear to play a key role in altering the membrane fatty acid composition, permeability and leakage of enzymes, and chemotactic factors, all of which elicit metabolic events that lead to muscle fiber degradation and the subsequent repair processes. Strenuous and exhaustive exercise as well as unaccustomed exercise induce oxidative damage and result in muscle injury.[97,98] The benefits and risks of exercise in older adults and to the aging process itself have not been thoroughly studied although there are indications that exercise has a significant impact on the antioxidant defense network and affects the requirement for dietary antioxidants.[99] Table 2 compares the general metabolic, body composition, and oxidative stress characteristics associ ated with aging and exercise. The impact of exercise on most measures of oxidative stress is strongly dependent upon the parameters of the physical activity, i.e., duration, intensity, and type.

Table 2

Characteristics Associated with Aging and Exercise

Characteristic	Aging	Exercise
Metabolic		
Acute phase reactions	↓	↑
Basal metabolic rate	↓	↑/-
Calcium balance	↓	↑
Glucose tolerance	↓	↑
Insulin responsiveness	↓/-	--
LDL cholesterol	↑	↓
Muscle glycogen	↓	↑
Body Composition		
Bone mass	↓	↑/-
Fat mass	↑	↓
Lean body mass	↓	↑
Total body water	↓	↑/-
Oxidative Stress		
GSH oxidation	↑	↑
Lipid peroxidation	↑	↑/-
Muscle membrane damage[a]	↑/-	↑
Nucleic acid oxidation	↑	↑/-
Protein carbonylation	↑	↑/-

↑ = increase, ↓ = decrease, - = no change.
[a] Muscle enzyme leakage reflected by increased serum activity of creatine kinase and lactate dehydrogenase.

Animal Models

Davies *et al.*[100] reported that rats fed a vitamin E deficient diet and then exercised to exhaustion doubled their production of free radicals (measured by electron spin resonance) in liver and muscle and presented with a significantly lower level of endurance than those fed a vitamin E sufficient diet.

Kanter *et al.*[101] found swimming exercise in mice induced significant increases in the activity of GSHPx, SOD, and catalase in blood. Alessio *et al.*[102] also reported significant increases in the activity of catalase and SOD in liver following acute exercise bouts in trained rats compared to trained controls without acute exercise. Interestingly, the exercise-induced increase in the activity of antioxidant enzymes may be attenuated by age.

Reznick *et al.*[103] exercised young and old mice and found an increase in heart muscle SOD in the young animals but a decrease in the old ones. Zerba *et al.*[104] have observed that muscle from senescent mice is more susceptible to injury and is damaged more severely by lengthening contractions than muscle from young and adult mice; further, a lower maximum isotonic force was noted in the older animals. Pretreatment of old mice with polyethylene glycol-SOD provided immediate protection against injury, indicating that during the lengthening contraction, in addition to mechanical stress, oxidative damage contributes to the initial injury. Although the activity of antioxidant enzymes in muscle may increase with age, the ability of these enzymes to protect against oxidative injury may be inadequate to meet demands under conditions of oxidative stress.[105] Thus, the influence of age on antioxidant enzyme activities may have an impact on antioxidant nutrient requirements.

Quintanilha *et al.*[106] investigated the effect of endurance training on vitamin E status of rats. While α-tocopherol concentrations in liver were not affected by exercise in rats fed a vitamin E sufficient diet, those fed a vitamin E deficient diet and exercised did show marked reductions. Aikawa *et al.*[107]examined α-tocopherol levels in muscle and liver from exercised and sedentary rats fed either a vitamin E sufficient or deficient diet. Rats receiving the sufficient diet and exercise had significantly less muscle α-tocopherol than sedentary controls. Exercise also decreased liver α-tocopherol in rats receiving the deficient diet. In contrast, Gohil *et al.*[108] found endurance training in rats increased the ubiquinol content of adipose tissue and red quadriceps muscle but did not affect α-tocopherol status. Nonetheless, as mitochondria in muscle proliferate during endurance training, the effective concentration of vitamin E may be diminished. Like Davies *et al.*,[100] Gohil *et al.*[109] found rats maintained on a vitamin E deficient diet had a significantly lower endurance capacity when exercised to exhaustion; supplementing the vitamin E deficient diet with vitamin C did not affect the endurance capacity. Novelli *et al.*[110] treated mice with either vitamin E or free radical spin traps and found these compounds effectively increased endurance capacity.

Human Studies

Vitamin E has long been postulated to benefit physical performance in man based largely on findings from tocopherol-deficient animals, e.g., increased urinary excretion of creatine and phosphate, increased oxidation of polyunsaturated fatty acids, decreased ATP production, and increased levels of lactate and pyruvate, leading to a form of muscular dystrophy.[111] While most studies on vitamin E in sports have failed to demonstrate significant ergogenic effects, clinical trials have shown α-tocopherol supplementation reduces exercise-induced lipid peroxidation.[112,113] Simon-Schnazz and Pabst[114] found that vitamin E supplementation prevents the loss in anaerobic threshold seen in mountain climbers at high altitudes. Sumida *et al.*[115] reported that vitamin E supplementation lowered the increases in serum markers of cell membrane damage (malondialdehyde, β-glucuronidase, mitochondrial glutamic-oxaloacetic transaminase) seen after exhaustive exercise on a bicycle ergometer. While these data have been derived from young adults, Meydani *et al.*[116] have indicated that vitamin E may provide particular protection against exercise-induced oxidative injury in older adults. The potential for antioxidant protection against free radical pathology generated during exercise, while promising but not unequivocally proven, has led some investigators to recommend vitamin E supplements for athletes.[117,118]

The increased production of reactive oxygen species associated with exercise has given rise to the hypothesis that in addition to vitamin E other antioxidant nutrients may also play a protective role, if not necessarily an ergogenic one, during strenuous physical activity. Although most studies of vitamin C supplementation show little or no beneficial action, under certain conditions of dose and duration Bramich *et al.*[119] found that ascorbic acid increased muscle strength and reduced VO_2max. High dose combinations of vitamins C and E and β-carotene have been found effective in reducing measures of lipid peroxidation such as serum malondialdehyde and exhaled pentane.[120] Dragan *et al.*[121] supplemented with selenium in a crossover study to Romanian elite swimmers and reported the treatment lowered levels of serum lipid peroxides and increased concentrations of serum GSH. With the exception of vitamin E, the use of antioxidant nutrients singly or in combination has not been tested in older adults engaged in exercise programs.

The overall antioxidant defense system of older adults to cope with the oxidative stress produced by exercise appears to be lower than that of young individuals.[122] Ultrastructural examination of muscle biopsy reveals significantly greater amounts of muscle damage in older men performing high intensity eccentric exercise compared to the damage seen in young men performing the exercise at a similar intensity.[123] Old skeletal muscle appears to be more susceptible to eccentric exercise-induced injury in part because older men are typically less active and fit.[124] Skeletal muscle in older individuals may also contain muscle fibers that are more susceptible to injury.[125] This intrinsic damage seen in older subjects may also be due to the accumulation of oxidized forms of proteins.[105]

As noted, rates of lipid peroxidation as well as antioxidant enzyme activities in skeletal muscle increase with advancing age.[105] However, the age-related accumulation of oxidized proteins in muscle suggests there is a relatively greater increase in pro-oxidant reactions than in antioxidant defenses. This imbalance may contribute to the reduced ability of the elderly to mount an acute phase response to muscle damage. Cannon *et al.*[126] observed greatly attenuated neutrophil and plasma creatine kinase responses in untrained older men when compared to young men following downhill running; vitamin E supplementation significantly increased the post-exercise rise in circulating neutrophils and creatine kinase activity in the older subjects to levels comparable to those of the younger men. At the time of peak concentrations in the plasma, creatine kinase was significantly correlated with superoxide release from neutrophils. The association of this circulating skeletal muscle enzyme with neutrophil mobilization and function supports the concept that neutrophils are involved in the delayed increase in muscle membrane permeability after damaging exercise. Further, increases in superoxide and cytokine production by circulating neutrophils was attenuated when subjects were supplemented with vitamin E.[126,127] These data indicate that vitamin E supplementation may affect the rate of repair of skeletal muscle following muscle damage and that these effects may be more pronounced in older subjects. The alterations observed in fatty acid composition, vitamin E, and lipid conjugated dienes in muscle and in urinary lipid peroxides after the eccentric exercise were consistent with the concept that vitamin E provides protection against exercise-induced oxidative injury.[116] A variety of potential mechanisms of action of vitamin E and other antioxidant nutrients have been proposed with regard to their ability to modulate immune responses during exercise.[128]

CONCLUSION

Free radical-induced oxidative damage has been implicated in the pathogenesis of a number of diseases common among the elderly and in the etiology of the aging process itself. Findings from clinical trials and epidemiologic studies strongly suggest antioxidant nutrient consumption and status are inversely related to loss of function with aging and risk of chronic disease. Preliminary work suggests the need to include in our focus the potential impact of plant polyphenolic and other phytochemical antioxidants as well as vitamins C and E and β-carotene. There is still relatively little direct human data on the relationship of oxidative stress status to antioxidant nutrient intake, aging, and disease risk. Research data suggest oxidative stress status increases with age and in a variety of chronic diseases. If measures of oxidative stress status are incorporated into new studies, it should become possible to test the biological basis of the observed relationship between antioxidant nutrients and aging as well as chronic disease. However, as the targets for free radical injury are numerous and each may be associated with different functional endpoints in aging and disease, any assessment of oxidative stress will have to include several measures. It may also prove important to assess the effects of antioxidant nutrients which are not directly related to their antioxidant mechanisms. These measures could then become tools useful in assessing nutritional and health status and in developing nutrient requirements based on health promotion and disease prevention and a goal of successful aging.

REFERENCES

1. Cutler, R. G. Antioxidants and aging, *Am. J. Clin. Nutr.*, 53, 373S, 1991.
2. Slater, T. F. and Block, G., Eds. Antioxidant Vitamins and ß-carotene in Disease Prevention, *Am. J. Clin. Nutr.*, 53, 1991.
3. Krinsky, N. I. and Sies, H., Eds. Antioxidant vitamins and β-carotene in disease prevention. *Am. J. Clin. Nutr.*, 62, 1995.
4. Harmon, D. Aging: a theory based on free radical and radiation chemistry, *J. Gerontol.*, 2, 298, 1956.
5. Pryor, W. A. The free-radical theory of aging revisited: a critique and a suggested disease-specific theory, in *Modern Biological Theories of Aging*, Warner, H. R., Butler, R. N., and Sprott, R. L., Eds., Raven Press, New York, 1987, 89.
6. Russell, R. M. and Suter, P. M. Vitamin requirements of elderly people: An update, *Am. J. Clin. Nutr.*, 58, 4, 1993.
7. Wood, R. J., Suter, P. M., and Russell, R. M. Mineral requirements of elderly people. *Am. J. Clin. Nutr.*, 62. 493. 1005.
8. Halpner, A. D. and Blumberg, J. G. Assessment of antioxidant vitamin status in older adults, in *Nutritional Assessment of Elderly Populations*, Rosenberg, I. H., Ed., Raven Press, New York, 1995, 147.
9. Blumberg, J. B. Vitamin E requirements during aging, in *Clinical and Nutritional Aspects of Vitamin E*, Hayaishi, O. and Mino, M., Eds., Elsevier Science B.V., Amsterdam, 1987, 53.
10. Farrell, P. M. Deficiency states, pharmacological effects, and nutrient requirements, in *Vitamin E - A Comprehensive Treatise*, Vol. 1, Machlin, L. J., Ed., Marcel Dekker, New York, 1980, 520.
11. Horwitt, M. K. Interpretation of human requirements for vitamin E. In *Vitamin E - A Comprehensive Treatise*, Vol. 1., Machlin, L. J., Ed., Marcel Dekker, New York, 1980, 621.
12. Meydani, M. and Blumberg, J. B. Vitamin E, in *Nutrition in the Elderly - The Boston Nutritional Status Survey*, Hartz, S. C., Russell, R. M., and Rosenberg, I. H., Eds., Smith-Gordon Nishimura, London, 1992, 103.

13. Ascherio, A., Stampfer, M. J., Colditz, G. A., Rimm, E. B., Litin, L., and Willett, W. C. Correlations of vitamin A and E intakes with the plasma concentrations of carotenoids and tocopherols among American men and women, *J. Nutr.*, 1122, 1792, 1992.
14. Campbell, D., Bunker, V. W., Thomas, A. J., and Clayton, B. E. Selenium and vitamin E status of healthy and institutionalized elderly subjects: analysis of plasma, erythrocytes and platelets, *Br. J. Nutr.*, 62, 221, 1989.
15. Herbeth, B., Chavance, M., Musse, N., Mejean, L., and Vernhes, G. Dietary intake and their determinants of blood vitamins in an elderly population. *Eur. J. Clin. Nutr.*, 43, 175, 1989.
16. Vandewoude, M. F. and Vandewoude, M. G. Vitamin E status in a normal population: the influence of age, *J. Am. Coll. Nutr.*, 6, 307, 1987.
17. Vericel, E., Croset, M., Sedivy, P., Courpron, P., Dechavanne, M., and Lagarde, M. Platelets and aging. I. Aggregation, arachidonate metabolism and antioxidant status, *Thromb Res.*, 49, 331, 1988.
18. Murphy, S. P., Subar, A. F., and Block, G. Vitamin E intakes and sources in the United States, *Am. J. Clin. Nutr.*, 52, 361, 1990
19. Romieu, I., Stamfer, M. J., Stryker, W. S., Hernandez, M., Kaplan, L., Sober, A., Rosner, B., and Willett, W. C. Food predictors of plasma beta-carotene and alpha-tocopherol: validation of a food frequency questionnaire, *Am. J. Epidemiol.*, 131, 864, 1990.
20. Johnson, E. J. and Russell, R. Vitamin A, in *Nutrition in the Elderly - The Boston Nutritional Status Survey*, Hartz, S. C., Russell, R. M., and Rosenberg, I. H., Eds., Smith-Gordon Nishimura, London, 1192, 87.
21. Järvinen, R., Knekt, P., Seppnen, R., Heinonen, M., and Aaran, A. K. Dietary determinants of serum beta-carotene and serum retinol, *Eur. J. Clin. Nutr.*, 47, 31, 1993.
22. Ito, Y., Ochiai, J., Sasaki, R., Suzuki, S., Kusuhara, Y., Morimitsu, Y., Otani, M., and Aoki, K. Serum concentrations of carotenoids, retinol, and α-tocopherol in healthy persons determined by high-performance liquid chromatography. *Clin. Chim. Acta.*, 194, 131, 1990.
23. Gregory, J., Foster, K., Tyler, H., and Wiseman, M. The dietary and nutritional survey of British adults, Office of Population Censuses and Surveys, London, HMSO, 1990.
24. Taylor, A. Vitamin C, in *Nutrition in the Elderly - The Boston Nutritional Status Survey*, Hartz, S. C., Russell, R. M., and Rosenberg, I. H., Eds., Smith-Gordon Nishimura, London, 1992, 147.
25. Itoh, R., Yamada, K., Oka, J., Echizen, H., and Murakami, K. Sex as a factor in levels of serum ascorbic acid in a healthy elderly population, *Int. J. Vitam. Nutr. Res.*, 59, 365, 1989.
26. Bates, C. J., Rutishauser, I. H. E., Black, A. E., Paul, A. A., Mandal, A. R., and Patnaik, B. K. Long-term vitamin status and dietary intake of healthy elderly subjects. 2. Vitamin C, *Br. J. Nutr.*, 42, 4356, 1977.
27 Heseker, H., Schneider, R., Moch, K.J., Kohlmeier, M., and Kübler, W. VERA Schriftenreihe, Band IV. Vitaminversorgung Erwachsener in der Bundesrepublik Deutschland. Wissen-schaftlicher Fachverlag Dr. Fleck, Niederkleen.
28. Garry, P. J., Vanderjagt, D. J., and Hunt, W. C. Ascorbic acid intakes and plasma levels in healthy elderly, *Ann. N.Y. Acad. Sci.*, 498, 90, 1987.
29. Newton, H. M. V., Schorah, C. J., Habibzadeh, N., Morgan, D. B., and Hullin, R. P. The cause and correction of low blood vitamin C concentrations in the elderly, *Am. J. Clin. Nutr.*, 42, 656, 1985.
30. Vanderjagt, J. D., Garry, P., and Bhagavan, H. N. Ascorbate and dehydroascorbate distribution in mononuclear cells of healthy elderly people, *Am. J. Clin. Nutr.*, 49, 511, 1989.

31. Bui, M. H., Sauty, A., Collet, F., and Levenberger, P. Dietary vitamin C and concentrations in the body fluids and cells of male smokers and nonsmokers, *J. Nutr.*, 122, 312, 1992.
32 Koplan, J. P., Annest, J. L., Layde, P. M., and Rubin, G. L. Nutrient intake and supplementation in the United States (NHANES II), *Am. J. Public Health*, 76, 287, 1986.
33. Sinha, R., Block, G., and Taylor, P. R. Determinants of plasma ascorbic acid in a healthy male population. *Cancer Epidemiol. Biomarkers Prevent.*, 1, 297, 1992.
34. Khnau, J. The flavonoids: a class of semi-essential food components: Their role in human nutrition, *World Rev. Nutr. Diet*, 24, 117, 1976.
35. Markham, K. R. Flavones, flavonols and their glycosides, *Meth. Plant Biochem.*, 1, 197, 1989.
36. Hertog, M. G. L. and Katan, M. B. Quercetin in foods, cardiovascular disease, and cancer, in *Flavonoids in Health and Disease,* Rice-Evans, C. A. and Packer, L., Eds., Marcel Dekker. New York, 1997, 447.
37. Hertog, M. G. L., Hollman, P. C. H., Katan, M. B., and Kromhout, D. Intake of potentially anticarcinogenic flavonoids and their determinants in adults in The Netherlands, *Nutr. Cancer*, 20, 9, 1993.
38. Hertog, M. G. L., Feskens, E. J. M., Hollman, P. C. H., Katan, M. B., and Kromhout, D. Dietary antioxidant flavonoids and risk of coronary heart disease. The Zutphen Elderly Study, *Lancet,* 342, 1007, 1993.
39. Hertog, M. G. L., Kromhout, D., Aravanis, C., Blackburn, H., Buzine, A., Fidanza, F., Giampaoli, S., Janson, A., Menotti, A., Nedeljkovc, S., Pekkarinen, M., Simic, B. S., Toshima, H., Feskens, E. J. M., Hollman, P. C. H., and Katan, M. B. Flavonoid intake and long-term risk of coronary heart disease and cancer in the Seven Countries Study, *Arch. Intern. Med.,* 155, 381, 1995.
40. Keli, S. O., Hertog, M. G. L., Feskens, E. J. M., and Kromhout, D. Flavonoids, antioxidant vitamins and risk of stroke, The Zutphen Study, *Arch. Intern. Med.*, 154, 637, 1996.
41. Ames, B. N., Shigenaga, M. K., and Hagen, T. M. Oxidants, antioxidants, and the degenerative diseases of aging, *Proc. Natl. Acad. Sci.,* U.S.A., 90, 7915, 1993.
42. Stadtman, E. R. Protein oxidation and aging, [Review] Sciences, 257, 1220, 1992.
43. Sagai, M. and Ichinose, T. Age-related changes in lipid peroxidation as measured by ethane, ethylene, butane and pentane in respired gases of rats, *Life Sciences*, 37, 731, 1980.
44. Noy, N., Schwartz, H., and Gafni, A. Age-related changes in the redox status of rat muscle cells and their role in enzyme-aging, *Mech. Ageing Dev.,* 29, 63, 1985.
45. Shigenaga, M., Hagen, T. M., and Ames, B. N., Oxidative damage and mitochondrial decay in aging, *Proc. Natl. Acad. Sci. U.S.A.*, 91, 10771, 1994.
46. Wallace, D. C. Mitochondrial genetics: a paradigm for aging and degenerative diseases, *Science*, 256, 628, 1992.
47. Nohl, H. and Hegner, D., Do mitochondria produce oxygen radicals *in vivo*? *Eur. J. Biochem.*, 82, 563, 1978.
48. Sohal, R. S., Ku, H., Agarwal, S., Forester, M. J., and Lal, H. Oxidative damage, mitochondrial oxidant generation and antioxidant defenses during aging and in response to food restriction in the mouse, *Mech. Ageing Dev.*, 74, 121, 1994.
49. Sohal, R. S., Agarwal, S., and Sohal, B. H. Oxidative stress and aging in the Mongolian gerbil (*Meriones unguiculatus*), *Mech. Ageing Dev.*, 81, 15, 1995.
50. Hagen, T. M., Yowe, D., Bartholomew, J. C., Wehr, C. M., Do, K. L., Park, J., and Ames, B. N. Mitochondrial decay in hepatocytes from old rats: Membrane potential declines, heterogeneity and oxidants increase, *Proc. Natl. Acad. Sci.,* U.S.A., 94, 3064, 1997.

51. Hansford, R. G., Hogue, B. A., and Mildaziene, V. Dependence of H_2O_2 formation by rat mitochondria on substrate availability and donor age, *J. Bioenerg. Biomembr.*, 29, 89, 1997.
52. Sohal, R. S. Hydrogen peroxide production by mitochondria may be a biomarker of aging, *Mech. Ageing Dev.*, 60, 189, 1991.
53. Mura, C. V., Gong, X., Taylor, A., Villalobos-Molina, R., and Scrofano, M. M. Effects of calorie restriction and aging on the expression of antioxidant enzymes and ubiquitin in the liver of Emory mice, *Mech. Ageing Dev.*, 115, 29, 1996.
54. Mo., J. Q., Hom, D. G., and Anderson, J. K. Decreases in protective enzymes correlates with increased oxidative damage in the aging mouse brain, *Mech. Ageing Dev.*, 81, 73, 1995.
55. Azhar, S., Cao, L., and Reaven, E. Alteration of the adrenal antioxidant defense system during aging in rats, *J. Clin. Invest.*, 96, 1414, 1995.
56. Lüpez-Torres, M., Prez-Campo, R., Rojas, C., Cadenas, S., and Barja, G. Simultaneous induction of SOD, glutathione reductase, GSH, and ascorbate in liver and kidney correlates with survival during aging, *Free Radic. Bio. Med.*, 15, 133, 1993.
57. Lüpez-Torres, M., Shindo, Y., and Packer, L. Effect of age on antioxidants and molecular markers of oxidative damage in murine epidermis and dermis, *J. Invest. Dermatol.*, 102, 476, 1994.
58. Ji, L. L., Dillon, D., and Wu, E. Myocardial aging: antioxidant enzyme systems and related biochemical properties, *Am. J. Physiol.*, 261, R386, 1991.
59. Mote, P. L., Grizzle, J. M., Walford, R. L., and Spindler, S. R. Age-related down regulation of hepatic cytochrome P_1-450, P_3-450, catalase and CuZnSOD RNA, *Mech. Ageing Dev.*, 53, 101, 1990.
60. Mote, P. L., Grizzle, J. M., Walford, R. L., and Spindler, S. R. Influence of age and calorie restriction on expression of hepatic genes for xenobiotic and oxygen metabolizing enzymes in the mouse, *J. Gerontol.*, 46, B95, 1991.
61. Sohal, R. S. and Weindruch, R. Oxidative stress, caloric restriction, and aging, *Science*, 273, 59, 1996.
62. Hazelton, G. and Lang, C., Glutathione contents of tissues in the aging mouse, *Biochem. J.*, 188, 25, 1980.
63. Christon, R., Haloui, R. B., and Durand, G. Dietary polyunsaturated fatty acids and aging modulate glutathione-related antioxidants in rat liver, *J. Nutr.*, 125, 3062, 1995.
64. Meydani, M., Macauley, J. B., and Blumberg, J. B. Influence of dietary vitamin E, selenium and age on regional distribution of α-tocopherol in rat brain, *Lipids*, 21, 786, 1986.
65. Choi, J. and Yu, B. P. Brain synaptosomal aging: Free radicals and membrane fluidity, *Free Radic. Biol. Med.*, 18, 133, 1995.
66. Chipalkatti, S., De, A. K., and Aiyar, A. S. Effect of diet restriction on some biochemical parameters related to aging in mice, *J. Nutr.*, 113, 994, 1983.
67. Rao, G., Xia, E., Nadakavukaren, J., and Richardson, A. Effect of dietary restriction on the age-dependent changes in the expression of antioxidant enzymes in rat liver, *J. Nutr.*, 120, 602, 1990.
68. Luhtala, T. A., Roecker, E. B., Pugh, T., Feuers, R. J., and Weindruch, R. Dietary restriction attenuates age-related increases in rat skeletal muscle antioxidant enzyme activities, *J. Gerontol.*, 49, B231, 1994.
69. Rojas, C., Cadenas, S., Perez-Campo, R., Lüpez-Torres, M., Pamplona, R., Prat, J., and Barja, G. Relationship between lipid peroxidation, fatty acid composition, and ascorbic acid in the liver during carbohydrate and caloric restriction in mice, *Arch, Biochem. Biophys.*, 306, 59, 1993.
70. Yu, B. P. Aging and oxidative stress: Modulation by dietary restriction, *Free Radic. Biol. Med.*, 21, 651, 1996.

71. Lee, M. and Devi, B. G. Effects of dietary restriction on experimental gastric mucosal injury in Fischer 344 rats, *Mech. Ageing Dev.*, 89, 11, 1996.
72. Harman D. Prolongation of the normal life span by radiation protection chemicals, *J. Gerontol.*, 12, 257, 1957.
73. Harman, D. Prolongation of the normal lifespan and inhibition of spontaneous cancer by antioxidants, *J. Gerontol.*, 16, 247, 1961.
74. Harman, D. Free radical theory of aging: effect of free radical reaction inhibitors on the mortality rate of male LAF mice, *J. Gerontol.*, 23, 476, 1968.
75. Clapp, N. K., Satterfield, L. C., and Bowles, N. D. Effects of antioxidant butylated hydroxytoluene (BHT) on mortality in BALB/c mice, *J. Gerontol.*, 34, 497, 1979.
76. Kohn, R. R. Effect of antioxidants on life-span of C57BL mice, *J. Gerontol.*, 26, 378, 1971.
77. Comfort, A., Youhotsky-Gore, I., and Pathmanathan, K. Effect of ethoxyquin on the longevity of C3H mice, *Nature (London)*, 229, 254, 1971.
78. Oeriu, S. and Vochitu, E. The effect of the administration of compounds which contain sulfhydryl groups on the survival rates of mice, rats, and guinea pigs, *J. Gerontol.*, 20, 417, 1965.
79. Lönnrot, K., Mets-Ketel, T., and Alho, H. The role of coenzyme Q-10 in aging: A follow-up study on life-long oral supplementation Q-10 in rats, *Gerontology,* 41, suppl 2, 109, 1995.
80. Miquel, J., Ferrándiz, M. L., De Juan, E., Sevila, I., and MartÌnez, M. N-Acetylcysteine protects against age-related decline of oxidative phosphorylation in liver mitochondria, *Eur. J. Pharmacol.*, 292, 333, 1995.
81. Witting, L. A. Vitamin E and lipid antioxidants in free-radical initiated reactions, in *Free Radicals in Biology,* Pryor, W. A., Ed., Academic Press, New York, 1980, 295.
82. Tappel, A. L., Fletcher, B., and Deamer, D. Effect of antioxidants and nutrients on lipid peroxidation fluorescent products and aging parameters in the mouse, *J. Gerontol.*, 28, 415, 1973.
83. Ledvina, M. and Hodanova, M. The effect of simultaneous administration of tocopherol and sunflower oil on the life-span of female mice, *Exp. Gerontol.* 1980;15:67-71.
84. Blackett, A. D. and Hall, D. A. The action of vitamin E on the aging of connective tissues in the mouse, *Mech. Ageing Dev.*, 14, 305, 1980.
85. Blackett, A. D. and Hall, D. A. Vitamin E--its significance in mouse aging, *Age Ageing*, 10, 191, 1981.
86. Berg, B.N. Study of vitamin E supplements in relation to muscular dystrophy and other diseases in aging rats, *J. Gerontol.*, 14, 174, 1959.
87. Porta, E. A., Joun, N. S., and Nitta, R. T. Effects of the type of dietary fat at two levels of vitamin E in Wistar male rats during development and aging. I. Lifespan, serum biochemical parameters and pathological changes, *Mech. Ageing Dev.*, 13, 1, 1980.
88. Miguel, J., Binnard, R. and Howard, W. H. *Gerontologist*, 3, 37, 1973.
89. Enesco, H. E., and Verdone-Smith, C. alpha-tocopherol increases lifespan in the rotifer Philodina, *Exp. Gerontol.*, 15, 335, 1980.
90. Epstein, J.and Gershon, D. *Mech. Ageing Dev.*, 6, 257, 1970.
91. Packer, L. and Smith, J. R. Extension of the lifespan of cultured normal human diploid cells by vitamin E, *Proc. Natl. Acad. Sci. U.S.A.*, 71, 4763, 1974.
92. Packer, L. and Smith, J. R. Extension of the lifespan of cultured normal human diploid cells by vitamin E: a reevaluation, *Proc. Natl. Acad. Sci. U.S.A.*, 74, 1640, 1977.
93. Sakagami, H. and Yamada, M. Failure of vitamin E to extend the life span of a human diploid cell line in culture, *Cell Struct. Funct.*, 2, 219, 1977.
94. Munkres, K. D. and Minssen, M. Aging of Neurospora crassa. I. Evidence for the free radical theory of aging from studies of a natural-death mutant, *Mech. Ageing Dev.*, 5, 79, 1976.

95. Orr, W. C. and Sohal, R. S. Extension of life-span by overexpression of superoxide dismutase and catalase in *Drosphila melanogaster, Science*, 263, 1128, 1994.
96. Witt, E. H., Reznick, A. Z., Viguie, C. A., Starke-Reed, P., and Packer, L. Exercise, oxidative damage and effects of antioxidant manipulation, *J. Nutr.*, 122, 766, 1992.
97. Evans, W. J. and Cannon, J. G. The metabolic effects of exercise-induced muscle damage, in *Exerc. Sport Sci. Rev.*, Holloszy, J. O., Ed., Williams and Wilkins, Baltimore, 1991, 99.
98. Packer, L. Vitamin E, physical exercise and tissue damage in animals, *Med. Biol.*, 62, 105, 1984.
99. Blumberg, J. B. and Meydani, M. The relationship between nutrition and exercise in older adults, in *Perspectives in Exercise Science and Sports Medicine,* Vol. 8, Gisolfi, C. V., Nadel, E. R., and Lamb, D. R., Eds., Cooper Publishing Group, Carmel, 1995, 353.
100. Davies, K. J. A., Quintanilha, A. T., Brooks, G. A., and Packer, L. Free radicals and tissue damage produced by exercise, *Biochem. Biophys. Res. Com.*, 107, 1198, 1982.
101. Kanter, M. M., Hamlin, R. L., Unverferth, D. V., Davis, H. W., and Merola, A. J. Effect of exercise training on antioxidant enzymes and cardiotoxicity of doxorubicin, *J. Appl. Physiol.*, 59, 1298, 1985.
102. Alessio, H. M. and Goldfarb, A. H. Lipid peroxidation and scavenger enzymes during exercise: adaptive response to training, *J. Appl. Physiol.*, 64, 1333, 1988.
103. Reznick, A. Z., Steinhagen-Thiessen, E., and Gershon, D. The effect of exercise on enzyme activities in cardiac muscles of mice of various ages, *Biochem. Med.*, 28, 347, 1982.
104. Zerba, E., Komorowski, T. E., and Faulkner, J. A. Free radical injury to skeletal muscles of young, adult, and old mice, *Am. J. Physiol.*, 158, C429, 1990.
105. Oliver, C. N., Ahn, B., Moerman, E. J., Goldstein, S., and Stadtman, E. Age-related changes in oxidized proteins, *J. Biol. Chem.*, 262, 5488, 1987.
106. Quintanilha, A. T. Effects of physical exercise and/or vitamin E on tissue oxidative metabolism, *Biochem. Soc. Trans.*, 12, 403, 1984.
107. Aikawa, K. M., Quintanilha, A. T., de Lumen, B. O., Brooks, G. A., and Packer, L. Exercise endurance-training alters vitamin E tissue levels and red-blood-cell hemolysis in rodents, *Biosci. Rep.*, 4, 253, 1984.
108. Gohil, K., Rothfuss, L., Lang, J., and Packer, L. Effect of exercise training on tissue vitamin E and ubiquinone content, *J. Appl. Physiol.*, 63, 1638, 1987.
109. Gohil, K., Packer, L., de Lumen, B., Brooks, G. A., and Terblanche, S. E. Vitamin E deficiency and vitamin C supplements: exercise and mitochondrial oxidation, *J. Appl. Physiol.*, 60, 1986, 1991.
110. Novelli, G. P., Bracciotti, G., and Falsini, S. Spin-trappers and vitamin E prolong endurance to muscle fatigue in mice, *Free Radic. Biol. Med.*, 8, 9, 1990.
111. Shephard, R. J. Vitamin E and athletic performance, *J. Sports Med.*, 23, 461, 1983.
112. Dillard, C. J., Litov, R. E., Savin, W. M., Dumelin, E. E., and Tappel, A. L. Effects of exercise, vitamin E and ozone on pulmonary function and lipid peroxidation, *J. Appl. Physiol.*, 45, 927, 1978.
113. Goldfarb, A. H., Todd, M. K., Boyer, B. T., Alessio, H. M., and Cutler, R. G. Effect of vitamin E on lipid peroxidation at 80% VO_2max, *Med. Sci. Sports Exer.*, 21, S16, 1989.
114. Simon-Schnazz, I. and Pabst, H. Influence of vitamin E on physical performance, *Int. J. Vitam. Nutr. Res.*, 58, 49, 1988.
115. Sumida, S., Tanaka, K., Kitao, H., and Nakadomo, F. Exercise-induced lipid peroxidation and leakage of enzyme before and after vitamin E supplementation, *Int. J. Biochem.*, 21, 835, 1989.

116. Meydani, M., Evans, W. J., Handleman, G., Biddle, L., Fielding, R. A., Meydani, S. N., Burrill, J., Fiatarone, M. A., Blumberg, J. B., and Cannon, J. G. Protective effect of vitamin E on exercised induced oxidative damage in young and older adults, *Am. J. Physiol.*, 264, R992, 1993.
117. Packer, L., Reznick, A. Z., Simon-Schnass, I., and Landvik, S. V. Significance of vitamin E for the athlete, in *Vitamin E in Health and Disease*, Packer, L. and Fuchs, J., Eds., Marcel Dekker, Inc., New York, 1993, 465.
118. Shephard, R. J. Athletic performance and urban air pollution, *Can. Med. Assoc. J.*, 131, 105, 1984.
119. Bramich, K. and McNaughton, L. The effects of two levels of ascorbic acid on muscular endurance, muscular strength and on VO_2max, *Int. Clin. Nutr. Rev.*, 7, 5, 1987.
120. Singh, V. N. A current perspective on nutrition and exercise, *J. Nutr.*, 122, 760, 1992.
121. Dragan I., Dinu, V., Mohora, M., and Cristea, E. Studies regarding the antioxidant effects of selenium on top swimmers, *Rev. Roum. Physiol.*, 27, 15, 1990.
122. Meredith, C. N., Frontera, W. R., Fusher, E. C., Hughes, V. A., Herland, J. C., Edwards, J., and Evans, W. J. Peripheral effects of endurance training in young and old subjects, *J. Appl. Physiol.* 66, 2844, 1989a.
123. Manfredi, T. G., Fielding, R. A., O'Reilly, K. P., Meredith, C. N., Lee, H. Y., and Evans, W.J. Serum creating kinase activity and exercise-induced muscle damage in older men, *Med. Sci. Sports Exerc.*, 23, 1028, 1991.
124. Meredith, C. N., Zackin, M. J., Frontera, W. R., and Evans, W. J. Dietary protein requirements and body protein metabolism in endurance-trained men, *J. Appl. Physiol.*, 66, 2850, 1989b.
125. Armstrong, R. B., Ogilvie, R. W., and Schwane, J. A. Eccentric exercise-induced injury to rat skeletal muscle, *J. Appl. Physiol.*, 54: 80, 1983.
126. Cannon, J. G., Orencole, S. F., Fielding, R. A., Meydani, M., Meydani, S. N., Fiatarone, M. A., Blumberg, J. B., and Evans, W. J. The acute phase response in exercise. I: The interaction of age and vitamin E on neutrophils and muscle enzyme release, *Am. J. Physiol.*, 1990, 259, R1214.
127. Cannon, J. G., Meydani, S. N., Fielding, R. A., Fiatarone, M. A., Meydani, M., Farhangmehr, M., Orencole, S. F., Blumberg, J. B., and Evans, W. J. Acute phase response in exercise. II. Associations between vitamin E, cytokines, and muscle proteolysis, *Am. J. Physiol.*, 260, R1235, 1991.
128. Cannon, J. G. and Blumberg, J. B. Acute phase immune responses in exercise, in *Exercise and Oxygen Toxicity*, Sen, C. K., Packer, L., and Hänninen O., Eds., Elsevier Science Publishers B. V., Amsterdam, 1994, 447.

14

Oxidative Stress and Antioxidants in Premature Infants

William L. Stone, Ph.D.
Professor and Director of Pediatric Research, Department of Pediatrics, East Tennessee State University, Johnson City, Tennessee, USA

SCOPE AND SIGNIFICANCE

Oxidative stress is a physiological condition in which prooxidant factors outweigh antioxidant defenses.[1] Premature infants are born more than six weeks early or before 37 weeks of gestation. They can be further characterized on the basis of their birth weights with low birth weight (LBW) infants weighing between 1501 g and 2500 g, very low birth weight (VLBW) infants weighing between 1001 g and 1500 g, and extremely low weight (ELBW) infants weighing less than 1000 g. About 4.5 million premature infants are born world wide each year and many suffer from diseases that have a well-documented oxidative stress component such as respiratory distress syndrome, intraventricular hemorrhage, persistent ductus arteriosus, and retinopathy of prematurity.[2-4]

0-8493-8009-X/98/$0.00+$.50

Premature birth and low birth weight are significant public health problems in the United States and account for about 75% of all infant deaths occurring soon after birth. The additional cost for low birth weight in the United States is at least $3.5 to 4 billion.[5] In general, the health problems of premature infants increase dramatically with decreasing birth weight and gestational age. Infants born between 23 and 25 weeks of gestation have only a 40% survival rate and half the surviving infants who are less than 750 g have moderate to severe disabilities such as blindness. Despite fairly aggressive clinical efforts, the incidence of preterm births has not decreased in recent years. Moreover, efforts to decrease preterm labor, which is a leading cause of premature births, are limited by our minimal understanding of the physiological events that trigger normal term births.

This chapter will discuss: (1) the *in vivo* and *ex vivo* evidence for oxidative stress in premature infants; (2) the factors and mechanisms contributing to this oxidative stress; and (3) the use of antioxidants to treat or prevent oxidative stress-related diseases in premature infants. Where appropriate, gaps in our current understanding will be identified.

OXIDATIVE STRESS IN PREMATURE INFANTS

Limitations of Research with Premature Infants

Blood Sampling

Research studying the potential role of antioxidants in preventing free radical pathology in premature infants has enormous health related significance and is just beginning to receive its just attention and focus. There are, however, a number of major limitations in this area of research which do not occur with normal term infants. Oxidative stress is often accessed by measuring levels of antioxidants and/or levels of oxidation products in plasma and red blood cells. Premature infants often suffer from an anemia that is likely due to increased red blood cell hemolysis (see below) and/or erythropoietin deficiency. Institutional Review Boards, which monitor all research involving human subjects, are increasingly reluctant (and justifiably so) to permit blood samples to be obtained from premature infants for research purposes only.

Most future research on blood samples from premature infants will be limited to the small volume of packed red blood cells and plasma contained within the microhematocrit tubes used to monitor anemia and the need for blood transfusions. Hematocrits are measured as part of the routine clinical management of premature infants and the hematocrit tubes are normally discarded. Moreover, the fact that premature infants often receive blood transfusions (with blood obtained from adults) also complicates the ability to access oxidative stress from these samples.

Other Markers

A potentially useful and highly sensitive photochemiluminescent technique for measuring the nonenzymatic antioxidant capacity in plasma has been recently described by Popov *et al.*[6] High pressure liquid chromatography with coulometric electrochemical detection (HPLC-EC) is an extremely valuable technique and has been used to measure ubiquinol-10, ubiquinone-10, carotenoids, and tocopherols in the very small volume (10 µl) of plasma contained in a hematocrit tube. We are currently using HPLC-EC to measure tocopherols and tocopheryl quinones in plasma from premature infants and require only a10 µl aliquot of plasma.

Although not suitable for large-scale studies and technically difficult, the measurement of pentane and ethane in expired air as an index of *in vivo* lipid peroxidation is an important noninvasive technique that holds much promise. Urine samples can be readily obtained from premature infants and can be assayed for both antioxidant metabolites and for biomarkers of oxidative stress. Moreover, urine samples are useful for large-scale clinical studies. Premature infants receiving ventilation and surfactant therapy routinely receive endotracheal tube lavage and suctioning. The lung lavage fluid obtained from this suctioning can also be a valuable source of material in which to evaluate oxidative stress.

FACTORS AND MECHANISMS OF OXIDATIVE STRESS IN PREMATURE INFANTS

Table 1 provides a summary of the possible factors and mechanisms implicated in producing oxidative stress in premature infants. Each item listed in Table 1 will be discussed below.

Prematurity

Prematurity itself can be considered a disease with an oxidative stress component. Newborn infants are faced with an abrupt change to a relatively hyperoxic extrauterine environment where alveoli pO2 levels are five times higher than during intrauterine development.[4] Full-term infants show evidence of oxidative stress. For example, Jain *et al.*[7] found elevated levels of the vitamin E oxidation product, tocopheryl quinone, in newborns compared to the levels found in their mothers. Oxidative stress in premature infants is, however, even more extreme since they have lower levels of antioxidant defenses and are often treated with high levels of oxygen for respiratory distress syndrome (RDS). RDS and its complications are the major cause of mortality and morbidity in premature infants. RDS in premature infants is primarily caused by a deficiency of pulmonary surfactant which is essential for preventing the collapse of lung alveoli at the end of respiration. In order to maintain normal arterial oxygen levels, infants with RDS are provided with surfactant and ventilation therapy using high levels of oxygen. The use of oxygen therapy is not, however, without side effects and it contributes to oxidative stress and the development of chronic lung disease (bronchopulmonary dysplasia) in about 20% of the surviving infants.

Table 1

Possible Factors and Mechanisms for Oxidative Stress in Premature Infants

- **Prematurity**
- **Cigarette smoking during pregnancy**
- **Hyperoxia therapy for respiratory distress syndrome**
  - ⇒ **superoxide radicals**
  - ⇒ **hydroxyl radicals**
  - ⇒ **peroxynitrite**
- **Lack of adequate antioxidant defense systems**
  - ⇒ **deficiency of antioxidant enzymes**
  - ⇒ **vitamin E deficiency**

Cigarette Smoking

Cigarette smoking during pregnancy is a major risk factor for low birth weight[8] and is associated with a retardation of intrauterine growth.[9] It has been estimated that smoking during pregnancy may be responsible for 20 to 30% of the incidence of low birth weight.[8] Smoking has also been identified as a major oxidative stress factor and free radical induced damage may be an underlying cause of many smoking related diseases.[10,11] Cigarette smoke contains very high levels of free radicals that can initiate lipid peroxidation reactions.[12] Work by Jendryczko *et al.*[13] has shown that school age children whose parents smoke have increased indices of free radical mediated peroxidation compared with children whose parents did not smoke. If passive smoking is sufficient to cause oxidative stress in children, it is reasonable to suspect that smoking during pregnancy would be an even greater source of oxidative stress to the developing fetus. Nevertheless, the possible molecular mechanisms whereby oxidative stress, induced by maternal smoking, contributes to premature birth are not well understood. This is a research area that clearly deserves more emphasis.

Hyperoxia Increases Oxygen Radical Production in Lung Tissues

Work done in animal models and tissue culture indicates that hyperoxia increases the formation of reactive oxygen species in lung tissues and that reactive oxygen species derived from superoxide radicals are likely to be responsible for the oxidative damage.[14,15] Kelly and Lubec[16] recently examined hyperoxic injury to the lungs of premature guinea pigs to determine the specific reactive oxygen species responsible for oxidative damage. Hydroxyl radicals are known to attack phenylalanine generating o-tyrosine. These investigators found increased levels of o-tyrosine in the lung tissues of preterm guinea pigs treated with 85% O2 compared to levels observed under normoxia. It was concluded that hydroxyl radicals play a key role in hyperoxic lung injury.

When premature infants suffer from respiratory distress, they experience a hypoxia that is treated with hyperoxia. During hypoxia it is well established that hypoxanthine accumulates in tissues and plasma. In a key publication by Saugstad *et al.*[17] it was suggested that the hypoxic-hyperoxic insult experienced by some premature infants could activate the production of superoxide radicals by the hypoxanthine/xanthine oxidase system. These investigators used an animal model to demonstrate that the combination of hypoxanthine and high levels of oxygen causes more lung damage than high oxygen alone. Preterm infants who develop bronchopulmonary dysplasia have a significantly higher level of plasma hypoxanthine than preterm infants who do not develop this disease.[18] Further support for the involvement of the hypoxanthine/xanthine oxidase system in the morbidity of premature infants has been provided by a recent clinical study.[19] In this study, plasma levels of xanthine, oxidase activity, and plasma lipid hydroperoxides were found to be significantly higher (at 4 hr after birth) in premature infants with a poor clinical outcome compared with a control group of premature infants. This work is especially significant because it suggests that serial measurements of plasma xanthine oxidase and plasma lipid hydroperoxides can identify those premature infants at risk for major clinical problems and provide a means of monitoring potential therapeutic interventions with antioxidants. LeClair and Stone have described a microplate method that is well suited for measuring plasma lipid hydroperoxides in a clinical setting.[20]

The increased generation of superoxide radicals in premature infants must be evaluated in the context of nitric oxide production. Nitric oxide, by itself, appears to act as an antioxidant capable of inhibiting lipid peroxidation.[21] However, nitric oxide rapidly reacts with superoxide oxide radicals[22] to form peroxynitrite which is a powerful oxidant:

$$O_2^- + NO \rightarrow ONOO^- \quad (1)$$

Only very limited information is currently available on the production of nitric oxide in premature infants. Urinary levels of nitrite/nitrate were found to be higher in premature infants compared with term infants one week old.[23] These data suggest that nitric oxide production is activated in premature infants but it is not clear whether this is beneficial or not. If the increased level of nitric oxide production is accompanied by an even greater increase in superoxide production, the consequences may not be beneficial. The resulting decreased level of nitric oxide (see reaction 1) could cause a vasoconstriction. Moreover, peroxynitrite can initiate lipid peroxidation and increased formation of F2-isoprostanes which is a potent vasoconstrictor. Nitric oxide inhalation by infants with respiratory distress syndrome has been found to increase systemic arterial blood oxygen tension.[24] These data suggest that despite an increased production of nitric oxide by premature infants the degradation (perhaps by formation of peroxynitrite) of this vasodilator is rapid and inhalation therapy might be useful in promoting oxygen delivery to tissue and relieving pulmonary hypertension.

Lack of Adequate Antioxidant Defense Systems

Deficiencies of Antioxidant Enzymes

The premature infant is not simply a small term infant but is also developmentally delayed and has deficiencies in a number of chemical and enzymatic antioxidant mechanisms. Bazowska and Jendryczko[25] have recently examined the levels of antioxidant enzymes in the lung tissue of neonates who died of respiratory distress syndrome (premature infants) or from inherited heart abnormalities (term infants). The ages in the study population ranged from 31 weeks of gestation to 3 months post term. The lung levels of superoxide dismutase, catalase, and glutathione peroxidase (all key antioxidant enzymes) decreased with decreasing gestational age. Moreover, those infants who died of respiratory distress syndrome had significantly lower lung levels of all three antioxidant enzymes. These data certainly support the notion that oxidative stress in premature infants is, in part, due to a deficiency of key antioxidant enzymes.

Aliakbar *et al.*[26] have used an enzyme-linked immunosorbent method to measure the levels of erythrocyte superoxide dismutase in adults, neonates, and fetuses. These investigators found that erythrocyte superoxide dismutase levels in adults were significantly higher than in neonates who, in turn, had significantly higher levels than found in the erythrocytes of fetuses. Superoxide dismutase levels are known to be sensitive to oxygen levels, i.e., low oxygen pressure reduces and high oxygen pressure increases the levels of this enzyme. Since fetuses experience an oxygen tension much lower (by a factor of 5) than neonates, it is not surprising that erythrocyte superoxide dismutase levels are lowest in fetuses and that adult levels would be achieved only after replacement of the fetal erythrocytes.

Glutathione peroxidase is a seleno-enzyme that detoxifies hydrogen peroxide and lipid hydroperoxides. Reduced glutathione is a substrate for glutathione peroxidase and, as mentioned above, recent studies by Jain *et al.*[27] indicate that premature infants have a glutathione deficiency that increases with the degree of prematurity. Glutathione synthesis requires cysteine which in adults is made from methionine (via homocysteine and cystathionine) using the hepatic cystathionase enzyme. Premature infants have, however, very low levels of this enzyme which may account for the low glutathione levels found in premature infants and suggests that cysteine should be considered an essential amino acid for premature infants.[28]

Deficiency of Vitamin E

Vitamin E is the major lipid soluble antioxidant and it plays a major role in protecting biological membrane and lipoproteins from oxidative damage. The ability of premature infants to resist oxidative stress may be limited by low vitamin E levels in their plasma and erythrocytes. Vitamin E deficiency in premature infants is associated with hemolytic anemia, bilirubinemia, intraventricular hemorrhage, and retinopathy of prematurity. Many investigators have observed low levels of hemoglobin and low hematocrits in VLBW and LBW infants despite frequent transfusions and vigorous efforts to prevent iatrogenic blood loss. Neonatal red blood cells are known to have a shorter life-span than adult red blood cells.[29] Numerous investigators have provided evidence for the role of vitamin E in the hemolytic anemia of VLBW and LBW infants.[30-32] Diets with high iron levels and/or a high polyunsaturated fatty acid (PUFA) content contribute to this vitamin E responsive anemia. It is difficult, however, to ascribe all of the anemia in these infants to a hemolytic process since erythropoietin unresponsiveness (or deficiency) may also contribute. Recent work by Shahal *et al.*[33] has shown that red blood cells from newborns are more sensitive to *in vitro* oxidative stress than adult red blood cells. The exact mechanism for the enhanced susceptibility of neonatal red blood cells to oxidation is not known. Shahal *et al.*[33] point out that most of the intracellular hemoglobin (Hb) in neonatal red blood cells is Hb F which has a stronger tendency to denature and oxidize than HbA. Denatured and oxidized Hb is a potent catalyst for lipid peroxidation. Neonatal red blood cells may, therefore, require a better antioxidant defense system than adult red blood cells because of their intrinsic susceptibility to oxidative stress.

Most preterm LBW infants have a true deficiency of vitamin E at birth that requires early treatment.[34] The biochemical basis for low serum vitamin E levels in LBW and VLBW infants is not yet fully understood. Gestational age, however, is a key factor in determining the intestinal absorption of vitamin E. Infants with a low gestational age (and low birth weight) were least able to absorb vitamin E in the form of α-tocopheryl acetate (*all-rac* or RRR form not specified) despite being given very high doses (e.g., 100 IU). Kelly *et al.*[36] also found that premature infants had low plasma α-tocopherol levels at birth that did not increase after one week despite adequate intake (chemical and stereochemical form not specified). In contrast, term infants with a similar vitamin E intake had a dramatic increase in plasma α-tocopherol over the first week of life. It is not clear, however, what physiologic processes are being impaired by a low gestational age. Some possibilities are:

1. Poor intestinal absorption due to low levels of bile acids
2. Impaired secretion of tocopherol containing VLDL from the liver
3. Poor intestinal esterase activity causing an inability to convert the α-tocopheryl acetate to the free alcohol (necessary for absorption)
4. Low levels of plasma lipoprotein transport molecules.

The situation is further complicated by the physical form of the vitamin E administered. Jansson *et al.*[37] found that a water dispersible form of *all-rac*-α-tocopheryl acetate is absorbed much more readily (even in infants with a gestational age of 32 weeks) than *all-rac*-α-tocopheryl acetate in a lipid carrier.

In contrast to the work of Melhorn and Gross,[35] Zipursky *et al.*[38] found that a 25 IU oral dose of *all-rac*-α-tocopherol was very effective in rapidly increasing (within 1 week) plasma tocopherol levels in infants with a mean gestational age of about 30 weeks and a mean body weight of 1210 g. This suggests VLBW infants have a better intestinal absorption of free tocopherol than tocopheryl acetate. Surprisingly, Zipursky *et al.*[38] found high levels of plasma vitamin E (i.e., 2.5 mg/dl) after only one week of supplementation with 25 IU/day. This unusual result may be an artifact resulting from the colorimetric assay used to measure vitamin E. In particular, the optical density was read at a wavelength where hemoglobin could produce a false reading.

Lipoproteins are the primary carriers of vitamin E (and cholesterol) in plasma and it is very likely that low levels of plasma lipoproteins can limit the ability of plasma to transport vitamin E. Desai *et al.*[39] have found that VLDL and LDL are very low in newborns. Moreover, the amount of tocopherol carried by the neonatal VLDL plus LDL fractions is only one-tenth that found in the VLDL plus LDL fraction of maternal or placental plasma. The low levels of VLDL and LDL in newborns may be due to either a decreased secretion of VLDL by the liver or a very rapid plasma clearance rate. Rapidly growing organisms have a very high expression of the apoB,E-receptors (which bind LDL and VLDL) in order to accommodate rapid synthesis of cellular membranes.

EVIDENCE FOR *IN VIVO* OXIDATIVE STRESS

Table 2 provides a summary of the experimental evidence for the existence of oxidative stress in premature infants. Each item in Table 2 will be discussed in detail.

Table 2

Evidence for Oxidative Stress in Premature Infants

- **Breath hydrocarbons from lipid peroxidation**
- **Malondialdehyde in urine and plasma**
- **Glutathione redox status low**
- **Oxidation of uric acid to allantoin**
- **Oxidation of proteins in lungs**

Breath Hydrocarbons

Perhaps the best evidence for *in vivo* oxidative stress in premature infants comes from measurement of breath hydrocarbons which are well-characterized chemical by-products of lipid peroxidation reactions. Ethane or pentane are formed during the *in vitro* peroxidation of ω-3 or ω-6 polyenoic fatty acids, respectively.[40] Rats fed diets deficient in vitamin E and/or selenium show increased *in vivo* evolution of ethane compared with rats fed diets supplemented with these antioxidant nutrients.[41] Lemoyne *et al.*[42] found a significant negative correlation of breath pentane in adults with plasma vitamin E levels. Moreover, breath pentane could be decreased with vitamin E supplementation.[42] Varsila *et al.*[43] measured levels of both breath pentane and ethane in 27 infants for the first 18 days of life and found that the levels of these hydrocarbons increased to a maximum after five days. The maximum levels were found to negatively correlate with both gestational age and birth weight. These researchers concluded that the degree of prematurity was the most important factor contributing to oxidative stress in premature infants and that therapeutic interventions to limit *in vivo* lipid peroxidation should begin at birth. Varsila *et al.*[43] did not, however, observe an association between the extent of oxygen therapy and the levels of expired ethane or pentane. Pitkanen[44] measured expired pentane and ethane in 19 VLBW infants and found that the maximal expired level of these hydrocarbons correlated with poor clinical outcome. In addition, on days 4 and 5 after birth, the levels of expired hydrocarbons correlated with fractional inspiratory oxygen. Drury *et al.*[45] have critically evaluated the use of pentane measurements in preterm infants and emphasized the importance of using a gas chromatography column capable of separating pentane from isoprene which is high in normal adult breath. These investigators found no correlation between exhaled pentane and fractional inspired oxygen concentration in premature infants but they did not specify the time at which (i.e., days after birth) the samples were collected.

Malondialdehyde Levels in Urine and Plasma

In addition to hydrocarbons, lipid peroxidation gives rise to aldehydes such as malondialdehyde (MDA) and 4-hydroxynonenal. Schlenzig *et al.*[46] have measured the levels of urinary MDA in 45 premature infants (25-35 weeks of gestation) by a sensitive and specific HPLC technique. A significant negative correlation was found between urinary MDA levels and both birth weight and gestational age. Urinary MDA levels in ELBW neonates were about twice those found in the VLBW or LBW neonates. Those neonates treated with supplementary oxygen had higher levels of urinary MDA than those infants not treated with oxygen. The premature infants in this study were receiving parenteral nutrition until enteral feeding could be established. It is possible, therefore, that MDA or a high amount of PUFA in the parenteral lipid emulsion could be a confounding variable. MDA levels in the lipid emulsions were, however, measured and found to be very low and unlikely to significantly contribute to the urinary levels. The antioxidant status of the neonates was not determined in this study.

Inder *et al.*[47] measured the levels of MDA in the plasma of 22 VLBW infants using an assay in which MDA forms an adduct with thiobarbituric acid (TBA). These investigators found that the number of days of oxygen treatment and the number of days of positive pressure support correlated with the plasma MDA levels. More recently, this group reported the results of a prospective study in which the plasma MDA levels of 61 VLBW infants were found to correlate (at seven days after birth) with adverse clinical outcomes.[48] The plasma MDA levels in VLBW infants were found to be significantly higher than those found in full-term infants.[48] It should be kept in mind, however, that the reaction between MDA and TBA is not specific and may be a measure of oxidative susceptibility rather than the actual levels of endogenous lipid oxidation products.

Glutathione Redox Status

Reduced glutathione (GSH) is a tripeptide (gamma-glutamyl cysteinylglycine) that is an important substrate for two key antioxidant enzymes, i.e., glutathione peroxidase and glutathione S-transferase. Oxidized glutathione (GSSG) is one of the products produced by both these enzymes. The ratio of oxidized to reduced GSH has been used, therefore, as a measure of oxidative stress in premature infants. Nemmeth and Boda[49] have measured this GSH redox ratio (GSSG/GSH) in whole blood from 25 neonates with RDS and 20 control neonates without RDS who were matched for gestational age and birth weight. Infants with RDS had lower blood levels of GSH and a higher GSH redox ratio than controls. A highly significant positive correlation was also found between GSH redox ratio and the fractional inspired air concentration necessary to maintain adequate arterial oxygen tension. In addition, oxidized GSH levels were highest in the most premature infants. Smith *et al.*[50] also observed increased GSSG levels in premature infants receiving oxygen therapy. These investigators found that the plasma GSSG levels in the premature infants were often an order of magnitude higher than those observed for normal adults. More recently, Jain *et al.*[27] also found that premature infants have a significant deficiency in plasma glutathione compared to term infants and that plasma levels reached a minimum at two days after birth. Moreover, plasma glutathione deficiency was more severe with increasing prematurity. Similarly, these investigators found that glutathione levels in the bronchoalveolar lavage fluid were markedly lower in premature infants compared with adult levels.[27]

Oxidation of Uric Acid to Allantoin

Uric acid is one of the major water soluble antioxidants in humans and allantoin is the major oxidation product of urate. The ratio of allantoin to urate is, therefore, a useful measure of oxidative stress in aqueous compartments. Ogihara *et al.*[51] found that the allantoin-to-urate ratio in plasma from premature infants who subsequently developed chronic lung disease was more than twice that of premature infants who did not develop this disease. All the infants in this study were treated with ventilation therapy and received surfactant. Those infants that developed chronic lung disease also received significantly more oxygen supplementation than those who did not. These data suggest that high levels of oxygen therapy are an important factor in oxidative stress in the plasma aqueous phase in premature infants.

Oxidation of Proteins in Neonatal Lungs

Oxidative modifications to proteins are associated with the introduction of carbonyl groups into the amino acid side chains. Gladstone et al.[52] measured the carbonyl content of lung lavage samples from 26 premature infants in their first 30 days of life. These infants were all receiving ventilation therapy, had a birth weight range of 450 to 3820 g and a gestational age range of 24 to 42 weeks. They found that the carbonyl content measured on the first day of life was relatively low and not related to birth weight, gestational age or oxygen therapy. However, the carbonyl content averaged over the first three days of life was significantly higher (by a factor of two) for infants receiving ventilation therapy for more than 72 hours compared with infants receiving ventilation therapy for less than 72 hours. It was interesting that those infants treated with the glucocorticoid, dexamethasone, showed a 50% reduction in lung lavage carbonyl content within 48 hours. In general glucocorticoids reduce oxidative stress and inflammatory responses.[53] Measurement of lung lavage carbonyl content appears to be a reliable indicator of oxidative damage to pulmonary proteins. In addition, it is possible that the oxidation and subsequent inactivation of key pulmonary proteins play a causal role in the development of chronic lung disease in premature infants. As suggested by Gladstone et al.,[52] identification of the specific lung lavage proteins damaged by oxidation should be a high research priority in the future.

ANTIOXIDANT THERAPY FOR PREMATURE INFANTS

Table 3 summarizes the potential antioxidant therapies that could be useful in treating the clinical problems arising from oxidative stress in premature infants. Tanswell and Freeman authored an excellent review on the theory and potential clinical applications of antioxidant therapy.[54] In general, the purposeful use of antioxidants to intervene in critical care medicine is not extensive. This situation is, however, rapidly changing and the clinical use of antioxidants to treat premature infants will likely accelerate in the near future.

Inhibitors of Xanthine Oxidase

In premature infants treated with hyperoxia there is a critical need to improve the antioxidant status of lung tissues and fluids and to decrease the generation of superoxide radicals from the hypoxanthine/xanthine oxidase system. Allopurinol and its active metabolite, oxypurinol, are inhibitors of xanthine oxidase. Although effective in a premature baboon model[55] enteral allopurinol did not provide prophylaxis in a recent randomized placebo control study with very preterm infants.[56] Similarly, allopurinol was not effective in reducing the abnormal morphogenesis of developing mouse lung explants exposed to hyperoxia.[57] The synthesis of new and more potent inhibitors of xanthine oxidase offers some hope that this strategy may yield positive results in future clinical trials.[58]

Table 3
Antioxidant Therapy for Premature Infants

- **Inhibitors of xanthine oxidase**
- **Surfactants to reduce the need for hyperoxia**
- **Antioxidant enzymes**
  - ⇒ **liposome encapsulation**
- **Vitamin E**
  - ⇒ **α-tocopherol**
  - ⇒ **non-α-tocopherols**
  - ⇒ **Natural RRR vs. synthetic *all-rac*-α-tocopherol**
- **interactions with polyunsaturated fatty acid**

Surfactants

Surfactants reduce oxidative stress in lung tissues because they rapidly improve oxygen delivery and thereby diminish the need for hyperoxia. In addition, preliminary data by Bharti *et al.*[59] suggest that ascorbate and urate levels in the bronchoalveolar lavage (BAL) of premature infants with respiratory distress syndrome (RDS) are significantly increased (by an unknown mechanism) after administration of surfactant (Exosurf® or Survanta®). In this study, a unique sodium dodecylsulfate-micellar electrokinetic chromatography method was developed to assay BAL levels of water soluble antioxidants. The method used theophylline as an internal standard for urate and isoascorbate as an internal standard for ascorbate. Pre- and post-surfactant urate levels (mean ± SEM) were 16.4 ± 10.6 μM and 64.4 ± 19.6 μM, whereas ascorbate levels were 2.5 ± 2.5 μM and 12.8 ± 8.3 μM.

Antioxidant Enzymes

The use of natural or recombinant antioxidant enzymes to minimize oxidative stress in the lungs of premature infants is a reasonable strategy but few clinical trials have been attempted. Native superoxide dismutase or catalase is not effective by either intravenous injection or by aerosolization because both their half-lives are very short and they have poor membrane permeability.[60] Nevertheless, Davis *et al.*[61] found that premature infants given multiple intratracheal doses of recombinant human CuZn superoxide dismutase (rhSOD) had increased activity of this enzyme in serum, BAL, and urine. Although BAL markers of acute lung injury were lower in the rhSOD group than the control group, there were no differences in clinical outcome. Perhaps rhSOD by itself is not sufficient to improve clinical outcome.

Antioxidant enzymes can also be encapsulated into liposomes or conjugated to polyethylene glycol.[62] Intratracheal administration of liposomes encapsulated with both Cu and Zn superoxide dismutase and catalase are effective in increasing the antioxidant activity of alveolar type II cells and protecting against oxidative stress in premature rabbits.[63] In addition, these antioxidant liposomes do not down regulate mRNA transcription of these enzymes.[64] Continued advances in the formulation of antioxidant liposomes may eventually result in a therapeutic treatment of oxygen toxicity in the lungs of premature infants. Briscoe *et al.*[65] have, for example, described a method for the delivery of superoxide to pulmonary epithelium using pH sensitive liposomes. Intraperitoneal administration of superoxide dismutase in polyethylene glycol modified liposomes with a long circulation time was also found to be beneficial in an animal model of retinopathy of prematurity.[66]

Vitamin E

The addition of antioxidants into the parenteral or enteral formulas used to feed high-risk premature infants is also a strategy with some promise. As mentioned above, cysteine which is required for the synthesis of glutathione is particularly important in the preterm infant.[67] Vitamin E is also a critical antioxidant nutrient (see discussion above) for premature infants. Excellent reviews are available on the role of vitamin E in infant nutrition.[68,69] In much of the early literature on vitamin E and infant nutrition, little attention was paid to the different chemical or stereochemical forms of vitamin E. Vitamin E is not a single molecule but is at least eight different molecules, i.e., four tocopherols (α, β, γ, and δ-tocopherol) and four tocotrienols (α β, γ, and δ-tocotrienols). In addition, natural α-tocopherol is a single stereoisomer (RRR-α-tocopherol) and synthetic α-tocopherol is a mixture of eight stereoisomers (*all-rac*-α-tocopherol) with only one-eighth being the natural RRR-α-tocopherol isomer. In adults, there has been considerable growth in our understanding of the bioavailability and mechanism of action of these different forms of vitamin E (reviewed by Stone and Papas[70] and in other chapters of this book). Moreover, it is now appreciated that tocopherols may have biological roles beyond that of being antioxidants.

In current clinical practice, premature infants usually receive vitamin E in a multivitamin preparation that is added to a parenteral formula at a level of 2–3 IU per kg of body weight.[71] The use of vitamin E to prevent problems associated with oxidative stress in premature infants has yielded conflicting information.[18,69] In a recent clinical study, the use of pharmacologic levels of α-tocopherol combined with cryotherapy was found to be superior to cryotherapy alone in decreasing the severity and sequelae of threshold retinopathy of prematurity in infants weighing less than 1250 gm.[72] Pharmacological use of vitamin E for either retinopathy of prematurity or bronchopulmonary dysplasia is not a generally accepted clinical practice.

In 1984 the use of a daily intravenous polysorbate emulsion of tocopheryl acetate (E-Ferol) in the U.S. was associated with the death of 38 infants. Recently, it was found that the rapid infusion of polysorbate-vitamin E into neonatal piglets resulted in the massive uptake of the polysorbate-emulsion into the phagocytic cells of the spleen and, to a lesser extent, in the liver and lungs.[73] It was speculated that this could result in increased susceptibility to sepsis and/or to damaging alterations in pulmonary functions.[73] In addition, tocopheryl acetate is not the optimal form for intravenous infusion; its active antioxidant 5'-hydroxyl group is blocked (see review by Bell[68] for an expanded discussion).

A Role of non-α-Tocopherols?

In many cases *all-rac*-α-tocopherol acetate is used as the supplement in parenteral vitamin preparation and, as discussed above, this may not be the optimal form of vitamin E. The intravenous lipid emulsions commonly used for the parenteral nutrition of premature infants are likely to have significant levels of non-α-tocopherols[74] but detailed information is lacking in this area. Concern has also been expressed with regard to the lipid emulsions used for total parenteral nutrition in premature infants. In particular, these emulsions could undergo peroxidation during storage and the resulting lipid hydroperoxides and aldehydes could be particularly toxic when administered intravenously to premature infants.[75-77]

Recent information suggests that γ-tocopherol has a unique ability to inhibit oxidative damage caused by reactive nitrogen species such as peroxynitrite.[78,79] This information is important in light of the potential damage caused by peroxynitrite in premature infants. The use of α-tocopherol alone may not be optimal in infant nutrition since this form of vitamin E does not form an adduct with peroxynitrite as does γ-tocopherol. Mixed tocopherols with both α-tocopherol and γ-tocopherol may be best but the optimal ratio of α-tocopherol to γ-tocopherol has not yet been determined. Stone and Papas have recently published a review article with a detailed summary of tocopherol biochemistry.[70]

Naturally Occurring (RRR) vs. Synthetic (all-rac) Forms of α-Tocopherol

Most vitamin E used in infant nutrition studies is the synthetic *all-rac*-α-tocopherol. When used for enteral feeding, the acetate ester, i.e., *all-rac*-α-tocopheryl acetate, is usually used because of its *in vitro* stability. Studies using deuterated forms of tocopherol have shown that adult humans have a greater biodiscrimination for RRR-α-tocopherol over *all-rac*-α-tocopherol than do rats.[80,81] There are, however, no similar studies in infants (term or preterm). This is an important issue and the adult data suggest that RRR-α-tocopherol may be superior to *all-rac*-α-tocopherol. Prenatal vitamin preparations usually contain *all-rac*-α-tocopheryl acetate. Recent studies by Acuff *et al.*[82,83] have shown that at low doses RRR-α-tocopheryl acetate has at least 3-fold better placental transfer into plasma than *all-rac*-α-tocopheryl acetate. Similar results were obtained by Schenker *et al.* (personal communication) who also found the RRR form to have a better placental transport than the *all-rac* form. Moreover, Schenker *et al.* found that the free form of vitamin E was transported better than the acetate form. The prenatal consumption of a multivitamin preparation with RRR-α-tocopheryl acetate or RRR-α-tocopherol may, therefore, be an ideal and cost-effective means of increasing the plasma alpha-tocopherol content of plasma in newborns.

In almost all cases, the vitamin E status of infants has been determined by measuring tocopherol levels in either red blood cells or plasma. In general, there is very little information on how dietary tocopherols influence either the levels or tocopherol content of tissues. Kaempf *et al.*[84] found that α-tocopherol levels in mononuclear leucocytes and buccal mucosal cells from premature infants were lower during the first week of life than corresponding levels found in control children (3-16 years old).

Vitamin E and Polyunsaturated Fatty Acids (PUFAs)

Increasing evidence supports the notion that dietary polyunsaturated fatty acids (PUFAs) such as arachidonate (20:4 ω-6) and docosahexaenoate (22:6 ω-3) are important for the growth and development of premature infants.[85] Attempts to increase the PUFA content of infant formula, especially with marine oils which have very low tocopherol levels, should be accompanied by careful consideration of both *in vitro* oxidation during the storage of the formula as well as the potential *in vivo* oxidative stress caused by the increased PUFA levels.

CONCLUSION

The literature provides a compelling argument for the role of oxidative stress in many of the diseases of prematurity. The lack of adequate chemical and enzymatic antioxidant defenses and the clinical requirements to use hyperoxia to treat respiratory distress syndrome are major contributors to this oxidative stress. The degree of this oxidative stress often correlates with poor clinical outcome. Rapid advances in the preparation of antioxidant formulations provide considerable hope for the treatment of oxidative stress-related diseases in premature infants. It is very likely that effective antioxidant formulations will have multiple components, e.g., chemical as well as enzymatic antioxidants. Antioxidant containing liposomes hold considerable promise in this respect since they can encapsulate water soluble chemical and enzymatic antioxidants in their aqueous domain and their hydrophobic domains can contain lipid soluble antioxidants. We are currently attempting to formulate and characterize such therapeutic antioxidant liposomes and testing is now underway in animal models.

REFERENCES

1. Sies H. Oxidative Stress: Introductory Remarks. In: Sies H, Ed. *Oxidative Stress*. London: Academic Stress, 1985:1.
2. Saugstad O. Oxygen toxicity in the neonatal period. *Acta Paediatr Scand* 1990;79:881-892.
3. Kelly F. Free radical disorders of preterm infants. *Br Med Bull* 1993;49:668-78.
4. Muller D. Free radical problems of the newborn. *Proceedings Nutr Soc* 1987;46:69-75.
5. Lewit E, Baker L, Corman H, Shiono P. The direct cost of low birth weight. In: Behrman RE, Ed. *The Future of Children: Low Birth Weight*. Los Altos, California: The David and Lucile Packard Foundation, 1995:35-56.
6. Popov IN, Lewin G. Photochemiluminescent detection of antiradical activity: II. Testing of nonenzymic water-soluble antioxidants. *Free Radic Biol Med* 1994;17:267-71.
7. Jain S, Wise R, Bocchini J, Jr. Vitamin E and vitamin E quinone levels in red blood cells and plasma of newborn infants and their mothers. *J Am Coll Nutr* 1996;15:44-48.
8. Chomitz V, Cheung L, Lieberman E. The role of lifestyles in preventing low birth weight. In: Behrman RE, Ed. *The Future of Children: Low Birth Weight*. Los Altos: The David and Lucile Packard Foundation, 1995:121-138.
9. Nordentoft M, Lou H, Hansen D, *et al.* Intrauterine growth retardation and premature delivery: the influence of maternal smoking and psychosocial factors. *Am J Public Health* 1996;86:347-54.
10. Reilly M, Delanty N, Lawson J, FitzGerald G. Modulation of oxidant stress *in vivo* in chronic cigarette smokers. *Circulation* 1996;94:19-25.
11. Rahman I, Morrison D, Donaldson K, MacNee W. Systemic oxidative stress in asthma, COPD, and smokers. *Am J Respir Crit Care Med* 1996;154:1055-60.
12. Church D, Pryor W. Free radical chemistry of cigarette smoke and its toxicological implications. *Environ Health Prospect* 1985;64:111.
13. Jendryczko A, Szpyrka G, Gruszczynski J, Kozowicz M. Cigarette smoke exposure of school children: effect of passive smoking and vitamin E supplementation on blood antioxidant status. *Neoplasma* 1993;40:199-203.
14. Freeman B, Topolosky M, Crapo J. Hyperoxia increases oxygen radical production in rat lung homogenates. *Arch Biochem Biophys* 1982;216:477-484.
15. Freeman B, Young S, Capro J. Liposome-mediated augmentation of superoxide dismutase in endothelial cells prevents oxygen injury. *J Biol Chem* 1983;258:12534-12542.
16. Kelly F, Lubec G. Hyperoxic injury of immature guinea pig lung is mediated via hydroxyl radicals. *Pediatr Res* 1995;38:286-91.
17. Saugstad O, Hallman M, Abraham J, B E, Cochrane C, Gluck L. Hypoxanthine and oxygen induced lung injury: a possible basic mechanism of tissue damage? *Ped Res* 1984;18:501-504.
18. Russell G. Antioxidants and neonatal lung disease. *Eur J Pediatr* 1994;153:S36-S41.
19. Supnet M, David-Cu R, Walther F. Plasma xanthine oxidase activity and lipid hydroperoxide levels in preterm infants. *Pediatr Res* 1994;36:283-7.
20. LeClair I, Stone W. A Sensitive Assay for Measuring Lipid Hydroperoxides in Low Density Lipoproteins. *FASEB J* 1991;5:A571.
21. Hayashi K, Noguchi N, Niki E. Action of nitric oxide as an antioxidant against oxidation of soybean phosphatidylcholine liposomal membranes. *FEBS Letters* 1995;370:37-40.
22. Radi R, Beckman J, Bush K, Freeman B. Peroxynitrite-induced membrane lipid peroxidation: The cytotoxic potential of superoxide and nitric oxide. *Arch Biochem Biophys* 1991;288:481-487.

23. Kikuchi K, Sudo M. Urinary nitrite/nitrate excretion in infancy: comparison between term and preterm infants. *Early Hum Dev* 1997;47:51-56.
24. Skimming J, Bender K, Hutchinson A, Drummond W. Nitric oxide inhalation in infants with respiratory distress syndrome. *J Pediatr* 1997;130:225-230.
25. Bazowska G, Jendryczko A. Antioxidant enzyme activities in fetal and neonatal lung: lowered activities of these enzymes in children with RDS. *Ginekol Pol* 1996;67:70-4.
26. Aliakbar S, Brown P, Bidwell D, Nicolaides K. Human erythrocyte superoxide dismutase in adults, neonates, and normal, hypoxemic, and chromosomally abnormal fetuses. *Clin Biochem* 1993;26:109-115.
27. Jain A, Mehta T, Auld P, *et al.* Glutathione metabolism in newborns: evidence for glutathione deficiency in plasma, bronchoalveolar lavage fluid, and lymphocytes in prematures. *Pediatr Pulmonol* 1995;20:160-6.
28. Zlotkin S, Bryan M, Anderson H. Cysteine supplementation to cysteine-free intravenous feeding regimens in newborn infants. *Am J Clin Nutr* 1981;34:914-923.
29. Naiman J, Oski E. *Hematological Problems in the Newborn*. 3rd ed. Philadelphia: WB Saunders, 1982.
30. Oski F, Barness L. Vitamin E deficiency: A previously unrecognized cause of hemolytic anemia in the premature infant. *J Pediat.* 1967;70:211-220.
31. Melhorn D, Gross S, Childers G. Vitamin E-dependent anemia in the premature infant. *J Pediat* 1971;79:569-580.
32. Williams M, Shott R, O'Neal P, Oski F. Role of dietary iron and fat on vitamin E deficiency anemia of infancy. *New Eng J Med* 1975;292:887-890.
33. Shahal Y, Bauminger E, Zmora E, *et al.* Oxidative stress in newborn erythrocytes. *Ped Res* 1990;29:119-122.
34. Gutcher G, Raynor W, Farrell P. An evaluation of the vitamin E status in premature infants. *Am J Clin Nutr* 1984;40:1078-1089.
35. Melhorn D, Gross S. Vitamin E-dependent anemia in the premature infant. II. Relationship between gestational age and absorption of vitamin E. *J Pediat* 1971;79:581-588.
36. Kelly F, Rodgers W, Handel J, Smith S, Hall M. Time course of vitamin E repletion in the premature infant. *Brit J Nutr* 1990;1990:631-638.
37. Jansson L, Lindroth M, Tyopponen J. Intestinal absorption of vitamin E in low birth weight infants. *Acta Paediatr Scand* 1984;73:329-332.
38. Zipursky A, Brown E, Watts J, *et al.* Oral vitamin E supplementation for the prevention of anemia in premature infants: a controlled trial. *Pediatrics* 1987;79:61-8.
39. Desai I, Martinez F, Dos Santos J, Dutra de Oliveria J. Transient lipoprotein deficiency at birth: a cause of low levels of vitamin E in the newborn. *Acta Vitaminol. Enzymol* 1984;6:71-76.
40. Dumelin E, Tappel A. Hydrocarbon gases produced during *in vitro* peroxidation of polyunsaturated fatty acids and decomposition of preformed hydroperoxides. *Lipids* 1977;12:894-900.
41. Hafeman D, Hoekstra W. Lipid peroxidation *in vivo* during vitamin E and selenium deficiency in the rat as monitored by ethane evolution. *J Nutr* 1977;107:666-672.
42. Lemoyne M, Van Gossum A, Kurian R, Ostro M, Axler J, Jeejeebhoy K. Breath pentane as an index of lipid peroxidation: a functional test of vitamin E status. *Am J Clin Nutr* 1987;46:267-272.
43. Varsila E, Pitkanen O, Hallman M, Andersson S. Immaturity-dependent free radical activity in premature infants. *Pediatr Res* 1994;36:55-9.
44. Pitkanen OM, Hallman M, Andersson SM. Correlation of free oxygen radical-induced lipid peroxidation with outcome in very low birth weight infants. *J Pediatr* 1990;116:760-4.

45. Drury J, Nycyk J, Cooke R. Pentane measurements in ventilated infants using a commercially available system. *Free Rad Biol Med* 1997;22:895-900.
46. Schlenzig JS, Bervoets K, von Loewenich V, Bohles H. Urinary malondialdehyde concentration in preterm neonates: is there a relationship to disease entities of neonatal intensive care? [published erratum appears in Acta Paediatr 1993 Jun-Jul;82(6-7):630]. *Acta Paediatr* 1993;82:202-5.
47. Inder T, Graham P, Sanderson K, Taylor B. Lipid peroxidation as a measure of oxygen free radical damage in the very low birthweight infant [see comments]. *Arch Dis Child Fetal Neonatal Ed* 1994;70:F107-11.
48. Inder T, Darlow B, Sluis K, *et al.* The correlation of elevated levels of an index of lipid peroxidation (MDA-TBA) with adverse outcome in the very low birthweight infant. *Acta Paediatr* 1996;85:1116-22.
49. Nemeth I, Boda D. Blood glutathione redox ratio as a parameter of oxidative stress in premature infants with IRDS. *Free Radic Biol Med* 1994;16:347-53.
50. Smith C, Hansen T, Martin N, McMicken H, Elliott S. Oxidant stress responses in premature infants during exposure to hyperoxia. *Pediatr Res* 1993;34:360-5.
51. Ogihara T, Okamoto R, Kim H, *et al.* New evidence for the involvement of oxygen radicals in triggering neonatal chronic lung disease. *Pediatr Res* 1996;39:117-9.
52. Gladstone I, Jr., Levine R. Oxidation of proteins in neonatal lungs. *Pediatrics* 1994;93:764-768.
53. Groneck P, Reuss D, Gotze-Speer B, Speer CP. Effects of dexamethasone on chemotactic activity and inflammatory mediators in tracheobronchial aspirates of preterm infants at risk for chronic lung disease. *J Pediatr* 1993;122:938-944.
54. Tanswell AK, Freeman BA. Antioxidant therapy in critical care medicine. *New Horiz* 1995;3:330-41.
55. Jenkinson S, Robets R, DeLemos R, *et al.* Allopurinol-induced effects in premature baboons with respiratory distress syndrome. *J Appl Physiol* 1991;70:1160-1167.
56. Russell G, Cooke R. Randomised controlled trial of allopurinol prophylaxis in very preterm infants. *Arch Dis Child Fetal Neonatal Ed* 1995;73:F27-31.
57. Wilborn A, Evers L, Canada A. Oxygen toxicity to the developing lung of the mouse: role of reactive oxygen species. *Pediatr Res* 1996;40:225-32.
58. Biagi G, Costantini A, Costantino L, *et al.* Synthesis and biological evaluation of new imidazole, pyrimidine, and purine derivatives and analogs as inhibitors of xanthine oxidase. *J Med Chem* 1996;39:2529-35.
59. Bharti D, Stone W, Tan Q, Huang T. The influence of surfactant on water soluble atioxidants in bronchoalveolar lavage from premature infants. *American Pediatric Society/ The Society for Pediatric Research* 1996:A12341.
60. Crapo J, DeLong D, Sjostrom K, Hasler G, Drew R. The failure of aerosolized superoxide dismutase to modify pulmonary oxygen toxicity. *Am Rev Respir Dis* 1977;115:1027-1033.
61. Davis J, Rosenfeld W, Richter S, *et al.* Safety and pharmacokinetics of multiple doses of recombinant human CuZn superoxide dismutase administered intratracheally to premature neonates with respiratory distress syndrome. *Pediatrics* 1997;100:24-30.
62. Walther FJ, Kuipers IM, Pavlova Z, Willebrand D, Abuchowski A, Viau AT. Mitigation of pulmonary oxygen toxicity in premature lambs with intravenous antioxidants. *Exp Lung Res* 1990;16:177-89.
63. Walther F, David-Cu R, Lopez S. Antioxidant-surfactant liposomes mitigate hyperoxic lung injury in premature rabbits. *Am J Physiol* 1995;269:L613-7.
64. Walther F, Mehta E, Padbury J. Lung CuZn-superoxide dismutase and catalase gene expression in premature rabbits treated intratracheally with antioxidant-surfactant liposomes. *Biochem Mol Med* 1996;59:169-73.

65. Briscoe P, Caniggia I, Graves A, *et al.* Delivery of superoxide dismutase to pulmonary epithelium via pH-sensitive liposomes. *Am J Physiol* 1995;268:L374-80.
66. Niesman M, Johnson K, Penn J. Therapeutic effect of liposomal superoxide dismutase in an animal model of retinopathy of prematurity. *Neurochem Res* 1997;22:597-605.
67. Neu J, Valentine C, Meetze W. Scientifically-based strategies for nutrition of the high-risk low birth weight infant. *Eur J Pediatr* 1990;150:2-13.
68. Bell E. History of vitamin E in infant nutrition. *Am J Clin Nutr* 1987;46:183-186.
69. Phelps D. Current perspectives on vitamin E in infant nutrition. *Am J Clin Nutr* 1987;46:187-191.
70. Stone W, Papas A. Tocopherols and the etiology of colon cancer. *J Nat Cancer Inst* 1997;89:1006-1014.
71. Committee on Nutrition AAoP. Nutritional needs of low-birthweight infants. *Pediatrics* 1985;75:976-986.
72. Johnson L, Quinn G, Abbasi S, Gerdes J, Bowen F, Bhutani V. Severe retinopathy of prematurity in infants with birth weights less than 1250 grams: incidence and outcome of treatment with pharmacologic serum levels of vitamin E in addition to cryotherapy from 1985 to 1991. *J Pediatr* 1995;127:632-9.
73. Hale T, Rais-Bahrami K, Montgomery D, Harkey C, Habersang R. Vitamin E toxicity in neonatal piglets. *J Toxicol Clin Toxicol* 1995;33:123-30.
74. Henton DH, Merritt RJ, Hack S. Vitamin E measurements in patients receiving intravenous lipid emulsions. *J Parenteral Enterol Nutr* 1992;16:133-135.
75. Pitkanen O, Hallman M, Andersson S. Generation of free radicals in lipid emulsion used in parenteral nutrition. *Pediatr Res* 1991;29:56-9.
76. Pitkanen OM. Peroxidation of lipid emulsions: a hazard for the premature infant receiving parenteral nutrition? *Free Radic Biol Med* 1992;13:239-45.
77. Helbock H, Motchnik P, Ames B. Toxic hydroperoxides in intravenous lipid emulsions used in preterm infants. *Pediatrics* 1993;91:83-7.
78. Cooney R, Franke A, Harwood P, Hatch-Pigott V, Custer L, Mordan L. Gamma-tocopherol detoxification of nitrogen dioxide: superiority to alpha-tocopherol. *Proc Natl Acad Sci U S A* 1993;90:1771-1775.
79. Christen S, Woodall A, Shigenaga M, Southwell-Keely P, Duncan M, Ames B. Gamma-tocopherol traps mutagenic electrophiles such as NOx and complements alpha-tocopherol: Physiological implications. *Proc Natl Acad Sci USA* 1997;94:3217-3222.
80. Acuff RV, Thedford SS, Hidiroglou NN, Papas AM, Odom Jr TA. Relative bioavailability of RRR- and *all-rac*-alpha-tocopheryl acetate in humans: studies using deuterated compounds. *Am J Clin Nutr* 1994;60:397-402.
81. Burton GW, Traber MG, Acuff RV, *et al.* Human plasma and tissue alpha-tocopherol concentrations in response to supplementation with deuterated natural and synthetic vitamin E. *Am J Clin Nutr* 1998;67:669-84..
82. Acuff R, Dunworth R, Webb L, Thedford S, Lane J, Kelley J. Transport of deuterium labeled tocopherols during pregnancy. *Am J Clin Nutr* 1998:67:459-64.
83. Acuff RV, Dunworth RG, Webb LW, Lane JR. Transport of deuterium-labeled tocopherols across the perfused placenta: Studies using deuterolabeled tocopherols. *J Am Dietetic Assoc* 1996:A11.
84. Kaempf D, Miki M, Ogihara T, Okamoto R, Konishi K, Mino M. Assessment of vitamin E nutritional status in neonates, infants and children -- on the basis of alpha-tocopherol levels in blood components and buccal mucosal cells. *Int J Vitam Nutr Res* 1994;64:185-91.
85. Carlson SE. Lipid requirements of very low birth weight infants for optimal growth and development. In: Dobbing J, Ed. Lipids, *Learning and the Brain: Fat in Infant Formulas.* Ohio: Ross Laboratories, 1992:188-214.

15

Alcoholism, Antioxidant Status, and Essential Fatty Acids

William E. M. Lands, Ph.D., Robert J. Pawlosky, Ph.D., and Norman Salem, Jr., Ph.D.,
NIAAA, National Institutes of Health, Rockville, Maryland, USA

INTRODUCTION

This chapter describes effects of alcohol abuse on cellular antioxidant status and on the essential fatty acids and nutrients that antioxidants help to preserve. Alcohol is a macronutrient for many people, ranging up to 30% of dietary calories, and it is usually metabolized to CO_2 within 6 to 12 hours of ingestion. Alcohol is a ready source of electrons to reduce oxidants, but paradoxically, chronic alcohol use is frequently reported to cause a loss of antioxidants linked to pathophysiology with oxidant stress. As a result, much research has examined metabolic interactions of alcohol with dietary nutrients to identify the disturbances among intra- and inter-cellular signals, which impair the ability of cells and tissues to regulate their antioxidant status and resist the effects of oxidants. Such disturbances can impair tissues either through necrotic, inflammatory processes with extensive extracellular oxidative stress or through apoptotic processes with only subtle intracellular oxidative signals.

In one sense, apoptosis provides a comparatively physiological, balanced, non-oxidative process of cell death as an alternative to the more pathological, highly oxidative process of inflammatory necrosis. Both types of cell death are executed by gene products that occur naturally in cells, although inflammatory signals recruit many new cells to the site. Cells avoid apoptotic death when activating NFκB, a factor that activates genes involved in oxidant stress, inflammation, and necrosis. Conversely, in shifting gene products rapidly toward apoptotic cell death, a single cell may diminish inflammatory conditions and prevent extensive oxidative damage to surrounding cells and tissues.[249] The effectiveness of nutritional and therapeutic antioxidant interventions for diminishing inflammatory signals, cell death processes, and overall harm to a tissue needs to be evaluated with an awareness of the ease with which one death process may merge into another.

A variety of positive feedback events enhance and amplify oxidant formation by tissues, and preventive actions to stop that amplification can preserve the antioxidant status of a cell or tissue in ways very different from a direct antioxidant removal of reactive oxygen species (ROS). For example, a major inhibitor of apoptosis, Bcl-2, has been regarded as an antioxidant by some researchers because it diminishes the production of ROS. However, Bcl-2 blocks loss of cytochrome c from mitochondria, preventing impairment of the electron transport system that would otherwise produce more ROS. Blocking cytochrome escape also prevents initiating a proteolytic caspase cascade that irretrievably commits the cell to apoptosis. The steady-state level of ROS, also called peroxide tone, can oxidize sulfhydryl groups essential for the active sites of caspases, protein tyrosine phosphatases, and the mitochondrial permeability pore, influencing whether the ROS act as indirect signals that trigger events or as direct mediators of oxidative damage. New information on these oxidative events may help design future interventions that shift cells away from necrosis to apoptosis. This chapter examines how the balance among oxidants, antioxidants, and nutrients modulate the intracellular signals that control cell survival and the character of cell death.

ALCOHOL EFFECTS ON ANTIOXIDANTS

Antioxidant status has been related to several alcohol-related illnesses including cancer,[22] liver pathology,[153,203] myopathy,[284] cerebellar atrophy,[24] testicular injury,[237] and immunosuppression.[287] Although many studies of moderate drinking show little impact of alcohol on nutrient intake,[148] chronic alcoholism may lead to a poor nutrient status through decreased dietary intake, decreased intestinal absorption, and altered vitamin metabolism.[170,177] When alcohol intake is increased, an accompanying decrease in the amount of energy derived from macro nutrients may decrease the nutritional quality of the diet.[103] Thus, alcoholics may exhibit decreased appetite, reduced storage of ingested vitamins, and a reduced ability to convert vitamins to their metabolically active form.[257]

In a population of middle-aged Scottish men, a mean alcohol intake of 66 g/day was associated with a significantly lower dietary intake of protein, fat, polyunsaturated fat, and linoleic acid.[269] For many of these nutrients, the intake was inversely related to alcohol consumption. Lower intakes of nonalcohol total calories was also found in a large study of U.S. adults with lower carbohydrate intake as the salient difference, particularly in women.[89,120] After alcoholics stop drinking, they may increase their intake of all of the major nutrients.[112] There have been several general reviews of the relationship of nutritional status with alcoholism.[85,176,185,201,291]

Vitamin A

The vitamin A content of the liver was decreased in rats fed ethanol as liquid diets.[90] This decrease was due to decreased hepatic storage of vitamin A and not to malabsorption of β-carotene or retinyl acetate or to altered enzyme activities. Also, a reduction in vitamin A was observed in rats consuming alcohol,[181] a finding subsequently confirmed and extended as an inverse correlation between zinc nutriture and vitamin A was found in these animals.[183] However, the combination of higher dietary levels of vitamin A with alcohol potentiated the hepatotoxicity of the vitamin alone, and this effect must be considered in designing supplemental regimens.[154] Nevertheless, of 26 patients with alcohol-associated cirrhosis, 14 had abnormalities in dark-adaptation which improved with vitamin A supplementation.[239]

Marked reductions occurred in liver vitamin A levels in both rats and baboons given 36 or 50 en% ethanol, respectively.[246] Kidney and testis vitamin A levels in the rats increased several-fold, suggesting a tissue redistribution of the vitamin due to ethanol. During β-carotene supplementation of alcohol-fed baboons, an increase in plasma and liver β-carotene resulted, but this did not correct the ethanol-induced loss of liver total carotenoids.[155] This rise in β-carotene levels was associated with increased ultrastructural lesions in the liver, leading the authors to suggest that alcohol interfered with the conversion of β-carotene to vitamin A. Employed Finnish men with a mean ethanol intake of 72 g/day had elevated serum retinol but reduced β-carotene.[233] No loss in plasma vitamin A was found in a study of 45 alcoholics receiving treatment in Prague,[270] but there was a negative correlation of plasma β-carotene and liver damage with an alcoholic cirrhotic group exhibiting an 80% loss.[284] In summarizing much of the existing evidence and controlling for dietary intake, Rimm and Colditz[231] suggested that both smoking and alcohol decreased plasma β-carotene. Alcohol consumption was a main determinant predicting increased plasma retinol and vitamin B_6 and decreased β-carotene in a multi-factorial study of an elderly population.[101] Smoking, a common habit of most alcoholics, was also related to a decreased level of plasma retinol, β-carotene, α-tocopherol, and ascorbic acid.

Vitamin E

Lower serum α-tocopherol (vitamin E) was observed in alcohol abusers in a series of papers by Bjorneboe, Drevon, and co-workers,[24,25,94] e.g., serum vitamin E of 15.2 μmoles per liter compared to 24.2 for controls.[25] The mean alcohol intake for the previous month (expressed in g/day) was about 218 versus 3.7 in alcoholics and controls, respectively. The pattern of drinking indicated about 26 weeks/yr of high alcohol intake (258 g/day) and 17 weeks/yr of moderate intake (49 g/day). Vitamin E intake was markedly reduced (1.1 mg/day) during the "hard drinking" periods relative to the periods of moderate drinking or abstinence (3.8 mg/day). In 34 alcoholics consuming a mean 167 g ethanol/day, serum vitamin E was 30% lower.[25] Another interesting observation was that half of the alcoholics with low serum vitamin E also had elevated neurological scores and cerebellar atrophy as tested by computer tomography.[24] The amount of alcohol intake may be a critical factor, as no difference in serum vitamin E was noted in a Finnish cohort of "employed problem drinkers" consuming an estimated mean of 72 g ethanol/day.[233] The daily intake of many vitamins and minerals were compared and few significant differences were found. However, there were differences in dietary patterns noted as the drinkers ate fewer meals, consumed more snacks and coffee as well as more meats such as sausage, but less fruits and vegetables and the same amounts of fish, grains, and dairy products. Only 19% of drinkers had a daily breakfast compared with 71% of control subjects.

The relationship of alcohol and circulating vitamin E has been studied in several other countries including France,[82] Czechoslovakia,[270] England,[284] and the United States.[231] Significantly lower levels of vitamin E were in both the plasma and erythrocytes of patients admitted for rehabilitation who had a mean intake of 253 g/day of alcohol for a mean of 11.8 years.[82] Vitamin E levels in both compartments remained about the same in these patients after 15 days of abstinence. Also, there was no significant decline of vitamin E in the plasma of patients undergoing inpatient therapy for alcohol abuse.[270] Plasma vitamin E in 20 alcoholics and 10 control subjects in London was significantly lower only in four cirrhotic patients, appreciably lower than in the five alcoholics with fibrosis.[284] Half of these alcoholics presented with Type II muscle fiber atrophy and the myopathic group lost about two-thirds of their plasma vitamin E relative to the non-myopathic alcoholics. In evaluating the contribution of malnutrition, the authors found the myopathic group had a lower body mass index score and a higher mean alcohol intake (294 versus 216 g/day). However, there were no differences in plasma β-carotene or hydroxy calciferol in these patients, and the authors suggested that the depletion of vitamin E in the myopathic patients was not merely due to malnutrition. A reduction in vitamin E was also found in a rat model of alcohol-induced chronic alcoholic myopathy.[215]

In relating plasma vitamin E levels in a population to factors which may modulate it, Rimm and Colditz[231] concluded that *among both men and women, no significant relation was observed between alcohol intake and either α-tocopherol or γ-tocopherol in the multi-variate analysis that controlled for age, plasma cholesterol and triglyceride levels, body mass index, energy intake, and vitamin E intake.* That analysis did not focus upon the subpopulation with a very high alcohol intake (as did most of the aforementioned studies), but a study focused on Norwegian "risk drinkers" consuming only 32 g ethanol/day versus control subjects matched for age, smoking, and cholesterol level, found a non-significant ($p<0.06$) difference for serum vitamin E.[232]

Cultured hepatocytes secreted less vitamin E when exposed to alcohol *in vitro.*[23] Also, cells isolated from animals given 35 en% alcohol for 5 weeks secreted 42% less vitamin E over a 20-hr incubation period relative to pair fed controls. Since the secretion of VLDL from the liver is also inhibited by alcohol, the authors suggested that this may account for the acute effects of alcohol, but, overall, they suggested that there is an increased turnover of vitamin E during chronic alcohol exposure. Examination of the liver vitamin E levels in various subcellular fractions indicated a decrease in the light mitochondrial fraction but an increase in the Golgi apparatus after chronic alcohol.[94]

Vitamin C

An early study of nutritional differences in patients with alcoholic liver disease, as well as a variety of other ailments, indicated a lower vitamin C as well as lower hematocrit, serum albumin, and hemoglobin levels.[27] No significant decline in vitamin C intake and no difference in mean plasma levels were found in a study of 29 drinkers consuming 72 g ethanol/day.[233] However, markedly lower (41%) plasma vitamin C and vitamin B_{12} (51%) was reported for other alcoholic patients.[270] Pawlosky *et al.* recently observed lower vitamin C in the plasma of rhesus monkeys after three years of alcohol consumption that was associated with liver fibrosis.[213] The intakes of vitamin C and other vitamins and minerals were controlled in this study at or above levels recommended by the National Research Council for this species. This study was important as it suggested that alcohol and low essential fatty acid intake could act synergistically to cause liver pathology as neither the alcohol (at 24 en%) nor the diet alone are expected to cause liver fibrosis.

Glutathione

Hepatic glutathione was lower in patients with alcoholic liver disease compared to patients with liver disease unrelated to alcohol, and this was accompanied by higher levels of diene conjugates, an index of lipid peroxidation.[253] No relationship was found between liver glutathione and the severity of liver disease nor indices of malnutrition as measured by recent weight losses and through a dietary questionnaire, serum albumin levels, and hematocrit; however, a greater number of patients may be required for testing these hypotheses. In a study of rats on a low-fat or high-fat diet where corn oil is used as the source of fat, hepatic glutathione was depressed either by ethanol consumption or by high dietary fat.[181] Animals with both high corn oil diets and ethanol had the lowest level of hepatic glutathione. It is noteworthy that although corn oil contains a high level of essential fatty acids, almost all are of the ω–6 type (60% is linoleic acid, 18:2 ω6) and little of the ω–3 type (1% is linolenic acid, 18:3 ω3). Thus the high-fat diet may not supply adequate support for liver long chain ω–3 polyunsaturates (discussed below).

Chronic alcohol exposure has long been known to deplete liver levels of reduced GSH in association with steatosis, inflammation, necrosis, fibrosis, and cirrhosis.[280] Associated with depressed GSH, high levels of diene conjugates indicate probable peroxidation of hepatic lipids.[253] Only 10-15% of cellular GSH is in mitochondria, where it is slightly more concentrated than in cytosol.[248] Chronic ethanol causes a modest (24%) decrease in cytosolic GSH and a marked (65%) decrease in mitochondrial GSH[70] due to impaired transport of GSH from cytosol into mitochondria.[68] Alcohol exposure led to a profound and selective loss of glutathione in liver mitochondria, but not in liver cytosol or renal mitochondria of rats.[69] The loss was attributed to decreased synthesis of glutathione in liver mitochondria (rather than the cytosol) after rats were fed alcohol and this result may also indicate impaired transport from cytosol to mitochondria (discussed below).

Selenium and Other Minerals

There have been many studies of selenium in relation to alcoholism. Early work by Valimaki *et al.*, suggested that serum selenium was lower (17%) in alcoholics and markedly lower in cirrhotic alcoholics (48%).[277] Lower whole blood, erythrocyte, and plasma selenium levels were found in alcoholics with mildly elevated aspartate aminotransferase along with lower tricep skin-fold thickness.[61] The mean selenium level in a group of nine alcoholics was lower and this may be accounted for, at least, in part, by a lower calculated selenium intake; however, a lower urinary excretion of selenium also occurred.[60] Korpela *et al.* reported that a group of 46 chronic alcoholics had significantly lower levels of selenium compared to 25 healthy controls.[129] Within the alcoholic group, selenium was inversely related to the severity of liver disease and those with decompensated liver disease had the lowest levels (45% decline). Lower selenium was also reported for erythrocytes, whole blood, and plasmas of alcoholics.[62] Alcoholics with severe liver disease had lower selenium in both whole blood and plasma compared with asymptomatic alcoholics, and selenium correlated directly with albumin levels and inversely with bilirubin. Lower selenium, zinc, and copper was also found in the serum of Norwegian alcoholics,[24,25] and lower plasma and whole blood selenium occurred in alcoholic patients without liver cirrhosis.[82] The selenium level in plasma continued to fall during 14 days of abstinence, but it recovered somewhat in whole blood. Corrigan *et al.*[46] studied alcoholics who were abstinent for from 2 weeks to 6 months or more and found that erythrocyte selenium was lower in the alcoholics and remained so for at least 6 months after the cessation of drinking. They also observed lower erythrocyte levels of lithium, cerium, boron, and zinc, but higher levels of cesium and manganese in the drinkers. Zinc deficiency in alcoholism has been reviewed by McClain and Su.[174] A loss of serum selenium was observed in moderate drinkers consuming a mean of 32 g ethanol/day.[232] In a study of 26 Finnish drinkers, serum selenium was lower in men consuming a mean of 72 g ethanol/day even though dietary surveys indicated that selenium intake was identical.[233] Analysis of 24-hr urinary excretion samples indicated lower output in the drinkers. The authors suggest that decreased intestinal absorption may be one important factor contributing to the loss of selenium in alcoholics. Control subjects in this study also had low selenium intakes, as dietary intake in Finland is among the lowest in the world.

When rats were given a 10% (v/v) ethanol/water solution as their sole drinking fluid for a period of 4 weeks, myocardial selenium decreased, but zinc increased.[230] Selenium losses were also observed in a rat model of chronic alcoholic myopathy.[215] In alcoholics with skeletal muscle myopathy, plasma selenium was decreased 41% relative to alcoholics without myopathy and 53% relative to a non-alcoholic group, but copper and zinc levels were not significantly different.[284] Other studies in larger populations have examined the influence of alcohol on selenium and other trace elements. In a random sample of 200 Danes, both selenium and zinc levels were negatively correlated with smoking; zinc was negatively correlated with alcohol use.[88] Blood mercury correlated with blood selenium but a relationship to fish intake could be established only for mercury. Selenium was the only mineral that was increased in subjects taking mineral supplements. In a Midwestern population of Americans,[255] half of the subjects were drinkers with a mean intake of about 10 drinks (estimated at 14 g ethanol/drink) per month (equivalent to about 5 g ethanol/day). A surprising result in this cross-sectional type of analysis was that the multiple regression analyses of 19 independent lifestyle variables showed a positive association of alcohol intake with both selenium and selenium-dependent glutathione peroxidase activity in whole blood and plasma. Caffeine intake and smoking were also positively related to blood selenium levels. In a related study, McAdam *et al.*[173] reported an inverse relationship between erythrocyte selenium and years of smoking and caffeine in white and black urban Georgians. Measurements of selenium in toenail clippings has been proposed as a method to get a time-integrated index of selenium intake over a period of several weeks with the nail forming up to a year prior to sampling.[111] Validity was established by these authors in that toenail selenium levels were correlated with selenium supplement use and was related to geographic variations of this element in forage crops. Their results indicated that toenail selenium declined with age and smoking, but it was not sensitive to alcohol consumption in a group of 677 women.

ALCOHOL EFFECTS ON ENZYMES

Loss of rat liver cells following ischemia-reperfusion[123] was recognized to have more controlled features than necrosis, and the term "apoptosis" was developed to describe the non-necrotic "programmed cell death" that became recognized in many tissues.[124] Both apoptotic and necrotic liver cell death occur following hypoxia or ischemia,[35] and such hypoxic injury is seriously exacerbated by prior chronic exposure to alcohol.[75] Oxygen free radical production is regarded as a major mechanism mediating this liver damage,[102,204,238,253] and chronic alcohol exposure increases oxidant stress during ischemic injury to brain, heart, liver, muscle, kidney, or immune cells. As a result, biomedical researchers are challenged to identify how alcohol-induced maladaptations increase inflammatory, necrotic conditions and to find appropriate ways to restore antioxidant status and minimize oxidant-mediated damage to tissues.

Many papers have extended the early report of DiLuzio[57] that antioxidants diminish ethanol-induced liver injury. The reports noted important interactions of ethanol with nutrients which produce much greater blood alcohol levels and tissue injury with a high-fat diet than a low-fat diet.[54,158,243,298] Also, increased carbohydrate intake at the time of ethanol consumption diminished ethanol cytotoxicity and ethanol-induced lipid peroxidation.[193] In general, indicators of nutritional imbalance have the strongest implications for survival during the acute hospitalization stage, and they are the best indicators of response to therapy during the recovery phase.[74] Such results are reminders of the years of research that produced many reports of alcohol-induced oxidant-related injury by diets with high ratios of fat/carbohydrate,[158,159,223] although mechanisms by which such nutrient imbalances enhance liver injury remain unsolved (reviewed recently).[214,218] A puzzling feature was that rats ingested more alcohol with little injury when macronutrient proportions favored carbohydrates, and a recent study assigned the deleterious effects of the Lieber-DiCarli diets to anorexic effects of ethanol rather than to ethanol toxicity *per se*.[184] The carbohydrate intermediate, pyruvate, exerts an anti-oxidant effect in decreasing free radical formation and anoxic injury by 50-60% for reperfused hepatocytes and in decreasing antimycin-induced formation of ROS.[29] A similar protective antioxidant action of pyruvate was reported for small intestine,[43] heart,[51] and brain.[55] The apparent antioxidant protection might be due to an unexpected ability of pyruvate to eliminate H_2O_2 directly by a non-enzymatic reaction,[55,81] but only careful, controlled studies will verify this suggestion. More research is needed to define how increased fat/carbohydrate ratios or decreased availability of pyruvate or Krebs cycle intermediates can exacerbate alcohol-induced oxidative damage to tissues.

Although ROS participate in initiating or activating programmed cell death, they are not required to carry out the multi-step death program.[116] As a result, rigorous proof of a causal role for ROS in signaling of cell death has been elusive. Low doses of H_2O_2[152] and ROOH[242] can initiate signaling, and it is important to distinguish between ROS in signaling apoptotic pathways and ROS causing direct cellular damage during necrotic, inflammatory conditions. Chronic alcohol increased 5-fold the number of apoptotic bodies in the first 2-3 cell layers around the hepatic central veins, and cessation of exposure reversed this effect.[84] The latest state-of-the-art study of alcohol-induced hepatocyte injury and death used a combination of several fluorescent probes with confocal imaging to display the pattern of ROS-related events.[141] The results help emphasize two features: (1) progressively severe effects occurred in a gradient from upstream periportal regions to the downstream pericentral regions, and (2) a loss of mitochondrial integrity associated with NADH accumulation and oxidant stress chronologically preceded cell death. Stability of periportal cells made it clear that 50 millimolar alcohol *per se* did not cause cell death. Future studies that combine these elegant methods with anterograde and retrograde perfusion of livers[171] seem likely to increase our understanding of the processes, mediators, and signals that promote alcohol-induced oxidative injury.

Apoptotic cell death is a major process for selectively and "silently" removing cells from tissues without disturbing the surrounding tissue during a time of tissue remodeling or repair. The overall programmed set of reactions ensures active destruction of mitochondria and phagocytic removal of the dying cell before its contents escape and trigger extracellular inflammatory processes.[133,134] For example, caspase-catalyzed destruction of poly(adenosine diphosphate ribose) polymerase (PARP) during apoptosis prevents the necrosis that would follow premature loss of ATP and NAD (in a futile cycle with the nicotinamide formed by PARP action on fragmented DNA).[286] This concept was confirmed by adding a PARP inhibitor which prevents H_2O_2-induced necrosis and shifts the response toward apoptotic cell death.[208] However, cleavage of PARP by caspase-3 is prevented when high peroxide tone oxidizes the active site sulfhydryl group, shifting the cell away from apoptotic events toward necrosis.[97] Some processes by which chronic alcohol exposure affects oxidant/antioxidant status of a tissue are noted below.

Increased Formation of Reactive Oxygen Species

Mitochondrial Electron Flux

Mitochondrial electron flux is the major route by which NADH transfers electrons from substrates through a series of intermediates, terminating in a four-electron transfer by cytochrome oxidase to form water (H_2O) from oxygen (O_2). However, this tightly controlled electron transport chain may still "leak" electrons in reactions to form H_2O_2 rather than H_2O, with nearly 4% of the oxygen consumed being incompletely reduced.[224] This shunting of electrons to form ROS becomes increasingly severe when steps between ubiquinone and cytochrome oxidase action are slowed (e.g., by ischemic hypoxia, by loss of cytochrome c, by inhibition with cyanide, antimycin, or adriamycin) or when uncoupling protein-2 interacts with GDP to raise mitochondrial membrane potential.[199] In that situation, reduced intermediates of the electron transport chain accumulate to facilitate one-electron transfers to oxygen. For this reason, much attention has been focused on the flow of electrons in the ubiquinone cycle and complex III as an important source of ROS. Ethanol metabolism creates a form of reductive stress that potentiates adriamycin toxicity by generating more NADH for redox cycling by the inhibited mitochondria.[162] In this manner, formation of ROS with oxidant stress paradoxically follows a form of reductive stress that gives accumulated reduced NADH and intermediates in the electron transport system of mitochondria.[49,202]

Interestingly, ethanol caused an accumulation of NADH with associated oxidant stress that was abundant in pericentral cells while not evident in periportal cells.[141] Thus, some factors (not fully characterized) make the downstream cells more vulnerable to an influx of ethanol that has little effect on the integrity of upstream cells. This difference occurred with pericentral ADH activity being only somewhat greater than periportal, and ALDH-1 activity similar in both regions.[167] The wide array of intercellular signaling cytokines[45] (e.g., TNFα or endothelin) and autacoids (e.g., PAF or thromboxane) that follow entry of alcohol and lipopolysaccharide through the portal vein[147] may reach progressively higher levels along the sinusoids and exert greater impact on downstream pericentral cells. Also, the potent action of PAF in elevating cytosolic Ca^{2+} could have important consequences in elevating respiratory rates and increasing hypoxic stress. Hepatic lipocytes (Ito cells) are sensitized to such alcohol-induced intercellular signals by high fat diets.[172] Alternatively, inactivation of Kupffer cells prevents much of the intercellular signaling, almost completely abrogates hepatic cell death,[31] and prevents the large oxygen gradient between periportal and pericentral regions.[12] Interestingly, inflammatory signaling induced by alcohol ingestion was more severe in female rats than males[113] suggesting that the rodent model may give useful insight into the apparently greater severity of alcohol-induced injury in women than men.

The decreasing oxygen gradient from periportal to pericentral regions may increase NADH and ubiquinone semiquinone levels in pericentral hepatocytes and thereby increase the peroxide tone (as evidenced by greater DCF fluorescence).[141] Ethanol at relatively high acute doses (5 g/kg versus 0.5 g/kg) caused apoptosis in 4 hours without increased necrotic release of transaminases or inflammatory events.[142] This apoptotic cell death was associated with increased dichlorofluorescein fluorescence (indicating higher ROS levels) but no change in monochlorobimane fluorescence (indicating unchanged GSH levels). These results suggest that acute ethanol created signaling levels of ROS without disturbing the overall glutathione level, even though prolonged chronic exposure to ethanol and ROS eventually does decrease mitochondrial GSH levels. Ethanol plus a sulfhydryl scavenger, diethyl maleate, but not ethanol alone, increased the number of hepatocytes with mitochondrial dysfunction and ROS production,[141,142] perhaps reflecting an ability of normal mitochondrial GSH-dependent scavenging to adequately restrain the moderate oxidant stress that occurs with ethanol alone.[297] A facilitative non-obligatory role of low peroxide tone in programmed cell death[133] may occur as chronic ethanol consumption decreased mitochondrial membrane potential and increased the proportion of low H_2O_2-producing thymocytes while increasing overall thymic apoptosis.[283]

Mitochondria have nearly 60% of the cellular NADH, and blocking mitochondrial respiration with 2 mM KCN and 0.5 mM iodoacetate caused a rapid increase in both cytosolic Ca^{2+} and ROS of hepatocytes.[28] Increased ROS in these circumstances eventually caused necrotic leakage of LDH that reflects a greater disruption of cell membranes than would have occurred during the more controlled processes of apoptosis and phagocytosis. The ability of elevated levels of Ca^{2+} to increase mitochondrial permeability is enhanced by either ROS, elevated phosphate, depleted adenine nucleotides, low membrane potential, or stabilization of the "c" conformation of the adenine nucleotide translocator.[95] These events interact to create a destabilizing positive feedback, and many disturbances of mitochondrial permeability involve Ca^{2+}, protein sulfhydryls, and oxidative stress.[47,225] Such disturbances may be cumulatively greater in downstream hepatocytes than in those upstream.

Peroxy radical damage to mitochondrial DNA transcription occurs in rat liver mitochondria prior to detectable evidence of lipid peroxidation.[132] Apparently, the natural abundance of antioxidants can protect membrane lipids against peroxidation, but they are inadequate to protect DNA transcription from damage. However, added antioxidants can reduce ROS-mediated inhibition of mt-DNA transcription and diminish the risk of forming more ROS from incompletely assembled mitochondria.[132] DNA strand cleavage is a very sensitive index of conditions that favor hydroxy ethyl radical formation,[135,136] and mitochondrial DNA damage is more extensive than nuclear DNA damage following oxidant stress.[294] Cells lacking mitochondrial DNA were unable to form functional respiratory systems that could produce ROS, and they did not develop apoptosis as cells with respiratory function did when treated with antimycin A.[290] This result indicates a pivotal role for functional mitochondria in producing apoptosis, and it suggests a need for further study of mitochondrial DNA integrity in alcohol-induced injury.

The conversion of NADH to ROS by ubiquinone/complex III could increase after loss of cytochrome c from mitochondria, an early step at which Bcl-2 may participate in the onset of apoptosis.[126,295] Also, cytochrome c in the cytosol activates the caspase cascade to create a commitment to cell death, while the absence of cytochrome c from the mitochondrial electron transport chain may act like antimycin A to enhance the production of ROS signals from reduced intermediates. An adapter protein, Apaf-1, functions as a facilitator during cytochrome c activation of caspase-3,[303] and its interactions with Bcl-2 and Apaf-3 remain important features in understanding the commitment to apoptotic cell death. In cell-free extracts from cells overexpressing Bcl-2, added cytochrome c and dATP activate caspase-mediated events characteristic of apoptosis independent of mitochondria being present.[64] During the early phase of thapsigargin-induced apoptosis in rat thymocytes, elevated cytosolic Ca^{2+} had no immediate effect on ROS production or mitochondrial membrane potential. Only after disruption of Bcl-2-protected mitochondrial membrane potential was a hyperproduction of ROS associated with rapid Ca^{2+} elevation.[166] Signaling levels of ROS have little influence on an initiated caspase cascade within an apoptotic cell, but when amplified enough they may promote membrane rupture with subsequent inflammatory sequelae, extending the signaling imbalance to other cells. Once Bcl-2 fails to control the integrity of Ca^{2+} and cytochrome c in the mitochondria, there is an apparent "race" between the caspase-mediated apoptotic process and the ROS-mediated inflammatory necrotic process in determining the nature of the inevitable cell death.

In contrast, Fas-mediated apoptosis occurs by specialized receptor-associated "death domains" activating caspase without mitochondrial release of cytochrome c[2] or mitochondrial production of ROS.[110] Fas-mediated apoptosis seems almost independent of ROS production. Nevertheless, treatment of JURKAT T lymphocytes with anti-Fas/APO-1 antibody stimulated specific glutathione efflux by a low-affinity/high-capacity GSH transporter like that on the hepatocyte canalicular plasma membrane.[58] Thus, a Fas-induced depletion of cellular GSH may not initially reflect an increased ROS production. However, it eventually would increase the probability that mitochondria would form ROS and lose ATP. The cytoprotective action of thiol antioxidants (N-acetyl-L-cysteine, dithiothreitol, mercaptopropionic acid, glutathione, thioredoxin)[247] in Fas-mediated death may occur by down-regulating the membrane-bound form of Fas (CD95) that mediates T cell apoptosis.[53] The Fas-induced activation of pro-CPP32 protease precursor is inhibited by Bcl-2,[9,110] but it is not diminished with antioxidants that do not contain a sulfhydryl group.[53] Rather, an elevated peroxide tone may actually delay apoptosis by oxidizing the active site sulfhydryl group of caspases, shifting cell death towards necrosis.[97]

Fatty acids stimulate production of H_2O_2 by liver tissue and homogenates, producing 2 to 3 times more H_2O_2 from the pericentral region of liver than the periportal region.[180] Also, chronic ethanol exposure gave 2-fold higher catalase activity and 30% lower glutathione peroxidase activity in both liver regions; enzyme levels unable to explain why increased H_2O_2 production occurred selectively with pericentral samples. Fatty acid oxidation was proposed to provide increased H_2O_2 in a manner inhibited by 4-methyl pyrazole, an inhibitor of fatty acyl-coenzyme A synthase as well as alcohol dehydrogenase.[30] Possibly a chronic lowering in pericentral cells of mitochondrial GSH or an elevation in Ca^{2+} created a vulnerability to oxidant imbalances. Also, three-hour incubations of hepatocytes with glycochenodeoxycholate induced 60% of cells to a type of apoptosis associated with appreciable oxidant stress,[212] as indicated by increased isoprostane formation (isoprostanes discussed below). A Trolox-like antioxidant, U83836, inhibited isoprostane formation and decreased the apoptosis by 70%. More research is needed to define how such fatty acids produce oxidant stress and induce apoptosis and how much of the cell death might be apportioned between apoptosis and necrosis. Here also, is an opportunity to employ retrograde perfusion with a series of fluorescent probes as noted above.

Ceramides induce hepatocellular death by necrosis rather than apoptosis,[11] and this action occurs by depolarizing mitochondria, depleting ATP, and inducing a mitochondrial membrane permeability transition. These disruptions may result from a direct inhibition of mitochondrial complex III by the ceramide.[91] Ceramide-induced production of low levels of H_2O_2 preceded a later loss of mitochondrial membrane potential, and it was exacerbated by antimycin A (blocking electron transport from ubiquinone) and diminished by ruthenium red (blocking mitochondrial Ca^{2+} flux). A mitochondrial uncoupler (p-(trifluoromethoxy)phenylhydrazone carbonyl cyanide; FCCP) caused a lower ATP level (30% of control) and higher cytosolic Ca^{2+} (250% of control) associated with greater tyrosine phosphorylation of ERK1 and ERK2 and with a shift from apoptosis to necrosis.[165] The importance of functioning mitochondria for ceramide-triggered cell death was evident in the lack of H_2O_2 formation by ρ^0 cells which lack mitochondrial DNA.[217] Similarly, the TNFα-induced production of ROS and activation of NFκB was less in cells lacking the mitochondrial respiratory chain.[252] Such results illustrate the importance of mitochondria in developing an intracellular peroxide tone that can either activate a kinase or inactivate a phosphatase, thereby controlling the amount of the phospho-isoform of IκB that suppresses NFκB activation[131] and the proportions of apoptotic and necrotic cells.

Microsomal Cytochrome P450 2E1 (CYP2E1)

CYP2E1 acts in a mixed function oxidase system that transfers electrons to oxygen from the reduced flavoprotein, cytochrome P450 reductase, and it can generate significant amounts of ROS. The increase in CYP2E1 activity during exposure to ethanol is apparently due to a stabilization of the protein, which decreases the formation of ubiquitin-CYP2E1 conjugates.[234] Stabilization of CYP2E1 by ethanol was recognized long ago,[258] and it has been repeatedly confirmed.[63,125] Also, turnover of CYP2E1 by proteolytic degradation in the proteasome pathway was confirmed to decrease in the presence of ethanol and other CYP2E1 substrates.[296] Blocking proteolytic degradation of CYP2E1 in the proteasome pathway increases CYP2E1 half-life and enhances the probability of oxidant stress with loss of antioxidant status.

The CYP2E1 is predominantly expressed by cells in the pericentral region around the hepatic central vein with little in cells in the periportal region around the portal vein.[109,114] However, glutamine synthase is also narrowly located in cells lining the central veins, but it has been assigned no role in alcohol-induced pericentral injury. New, useful insight into mechanisms of alcohol-induced pathology may come from the report that CYP2E1 induction and liver injury was similar accompanying either an alcohol-rich diet or a diet deficient in methionine and choline.[289] In both situations, an increase in CYP2E1 in the three to four cell-wide pericentral zone might play a role in the observed tissue injury. Combining these nutrient alterations with retrograde perfusions may help resolve the issue of differentiated cell topology from downstream signaling effects. Inhibiting the induction of CYP2E1 was associated with decreased formation of hydroxyethyl radical and lipid peroxidation products.[4] Human CYP2E1 appears to be especially "leaky" in allowing electrons to transfer from the reduced flavoprotein to molecular oxygen and thereby form reactive oxygen species.[48] A challenge remains to determine whether liver cell death is directly or indirectly linked to the oxidant species generated by the CYP2E1 and whether the presence of ethanol increases or decreases the generation of toxic radicals with CYP2E1.

An impact of the ROS "leaked" from CYP2E1 is evident in the report of arachidonate cytotoxicity in transfected HepG2 cells that no longer need ethanol to overexpress CYP2E1.[41] In these cells, arachidonic acid-induced apoptosis was diminished by adding an antioxidant, Trolox, whereas it was enhanced following depletion of cellular glutathione. Such results suggest that the presence of alcohol is not needed for arachidonate toxicity in hepatocytes already over expressing CYP2E1. In fact, adding ethanol did not increase the cell death mediated by ROS and lipid peroxides in this system.[41] Ironically, although arachidonate (and other fatty acids) exacerbate hepatic oxidant stress and form lipid radicals, the alcohol-induced decrease in arachidonate levels could not be attributed to CYP2E1 metabolism or to lipid peroxidation.[72]

The metabolism of ethanol (not merely its presence) seems important for a different model of ethanol toxicity in which inhibition of alcohol metabolism by added cimetidine prevented alcoholic hepatic injury.[97] Also, cytotoxicity of ethanol in transfected HepG2 cells that over-express CYP2E1[292] was prevented by adding antioxidant radical trapping agents, perhaps reflecting an ethanol-dependent formation of free radical products, such as the hydroxy ethyl radical[127] that is enhanced by dietary fats.[226] An effective removal of such carbon-centered radicals seems more likely if the abundance of cellular sulfhydryls is not compromised. Apparently, cytotoxicity from over-expression of CYP2E1 may not be due to the more common ROS *per se*, but to some radical products derived from an initial redox imbalance. Whatever action alcohol-induced CYP2E1 may have on hepatocytes, it depends upon high-fat, low-carbohydrate diets to create serious pathology,[159] because similar CYP2E1 induction with a high-carbohydrate diet gave little injury. Further experiments are needed to discern whether agents other than ethanol stabilize CYP2E1 levels and also cause injury similar to that seen for transfected HepG2 cells with constitutive CYP2E1.

Membrane NADH Oxidase (Generating $O_2^{\cdot}$ and H_2O_2)

A plasma membrane oxidoreductase system that includes NADH-ferricyanide reductase and NADH oxidase[33,263] was found in all eukaryotic cells studied. This system increases adaptively as cellular mitochondrial respiratory activity decreases.[149] Although the up-regulation of this system may aid the metabolism of cells that lose mitochondrial activity, it may also serve to produce ROS that trigger apoptotic and necrotic events.

Flavin-linked cytochrome b5 reductase activity that can oxidize the NADH derived from alcohol metabolism is found in most cellular membranes: nuclei, mitochondria, Golgi, microsomes, and plasma membrane. After chronic alcohol treatment, the ability of this activity to form lipid peroxides in the presence of ferric-ATP was increased two- to three-fold in nuclei, mitochondria, and microsomes.[135] Induction of such NADH reductases, along with the cytochromes P450 and b5 may increase ethanol-induced oxidant stress. Lipid peroxidation induced by NADH and ADP-iron is inhibited by other respiratory substrates (e.g., succinate) that might act by fully reducing ubiquinone and preventing semiquinone-mediated free radical attack on membrane lipids.[297] Alternatively, a GSH-dependent protection may occur via outer membrane-bound GSH S-transferase action preventing harmful accumulations of ROS and carbon-centered radicals in a way that is abolished by bromosulfo-phthalein that strongly inhibits the GSH S-transferase.

Amplification of Lipid Hydroperoxides

Fatty acid oxygenases, prostaglandin H synthases and lipoxygenases, require hydroperoxide activation as they catalyze the formation of prostaglandins and leukotrienes from essential polyunsaturated fatty acids.[137] Very small amounts of cellular hydroperoxides (ca. 10^{-8} for COX-1 and 10^{-9} for COX-2);[138] or micromolar levels of H_2O_2 can initially stimulate the enzymes to increase the intracellular peroxide tone and further activate other latent oxygenase molecules in an explosive, autocatalytic reaction. Such positive feedback permits a very rapid transition from an inactive basal state of low peroxide tone to an active cellular response to eicosanoid-producing stimuli. The resultant increase in intracellular peroxide tone can then promote oxidant-mediated signals associated with, but not directly involved in eicosanoid formation. Alternatively, the eicosanoids produced by rearrangement of the oxygenase products can activate specific receptors on nearby cells in an expanding set of inflammatory (and sometimes anti-inflammatory) signals. An interesting form of antioxidant action occurs when fatty acids that are ω–3 analogs compete with the common ω–6 fatty acid precursors, decreasing the intensity of formation and function of the ω–6 eicosanoids[139] and thereby diminishing the inflammatory conditions that would produce more oxidants. Recognition of the importance of peroxide tone in influencing inflammatory events helps interpret the mechanism of action of common therapeutic antioxidants, like acetamidophenol.[146]

Enhanced expression of COX-2 diminished an NO-induced apoptosis in a manner that was completely reversed by a selective COX-2 inhibitor.[281] Such abrogation of apoptosis parallels an action of COX-2 in promoting necrosis and inflammation of alcoholic liver disease,[196] and it illustrates complexities encountered in the different roles for peroxide tone in different forms of programmed cell death.

Lipoxygenase also catalyzes amplification of intracellular hydroperoxides which mediates activation of NFκB during the induction of IL-2 gene expression following stimulation of surface receptors on inflammatory cells via CD28.[164] Similarly, induction of c-Fos and c-Jun with activation of AP-1 follows release of arachidonic acid and its metabolism through the lipoxygenase pathway.[221] The hydroperoxides formed can also augment EGF receptor tyrosine kinase signaling by selectively inactivating a phosphatase that would otherwise inactivate the phosphorylated receptor.[83] H_2O_2 causes arachidonate release from smooth muscle cells by increasing MAP kinase and PKC activity in phosphorylating and activating $cPLA_2$.[219] During hypoxia, enhanced phospholipase activity may give intracellular fatty acids that enhance calpain protease action and contribute to hepatocyte necrosis and cell lysis.[10] Arachidonate and lipoxygenase have also been recognized to mediate the H_2O_2-initiated stimulation of mitogen-activated protein kinases, ERK and JNK.[271] Thus, fatty acid oxygenases act with the essential fatty acids to amplify peroxide tone and give signals that can influence both apoptosis and necrosis.

Signal Transduction for Expression of Oxidant-Producing Genes

Kinase and phosphatase signaling: The peroxide tone noted above modifies the network of signal transduction pathways[145] and alters the way that alcohol influences adaptive responses in gene expression. Many of these pathways are included in a diverse interactive web of kinases and phosphatases, and a major set of the signals involve accumulation of protein tyrosine phosphate derivatives that complex with Src homology (SH2) regions of other proteins within the cell. Accumulation of these signaling complexes is enhanced by activating specific protein tyrosine kinases, PTKs, and/or by inhibiting protein tyrosine phosphatases, PTPs. For example, long-term ethanol intake suppresses liver regeneration and interferes with EGF receptor tyrosine kinase autophosphorylation as well as with downstream PLC tyrosine phosphorylation and IP_3 formation.[245] Also, many reports of alcohol-induced enhancement of cellular protein kinase C (PKC) activity[179] may reflect an oxidant-enhanced accumulation of tyrosine phosphate residues on the various PKC isoforms.[128] Elevated peroxide tone inhibits PTP action by inactivating the essential cysteine sulfhydryl group in the active site[261] and oxidatively inactivating PTP activity permits kinases such as Syk and Erk2 to remain in an activated phosphorylated state.[130] Also, H_2O_2 strongly activates the kinase, Lck, by enhancing accumulation of the form phosphorylated at Tyr-394 in a manner that may relate to all Src family kinases.[98] However, sometimes the oxidative stress may be so strong that it also diminishes DNA binding by NFκB, creating a paradoxical requirement for some nuclear antioxidant to achieve maximal NF B response[130,194] (see below).

The ability of genistein to decrease H_2O_2-initiated tyrosine kinase-mediated signals might be due to either impaired kinase action (PTK) or enhanced phosphatase action (PTP) and antioxidant protection of the essential sulfhydryl at the PTP active site seems feasible. However, the greater efficacy of genistein over diadzein suggests that the protective effect might depend on some structurally selective interactions rather than only general antioxidant properties. In the case of d-α-tocopherol inhibition of H_2O_2-stimulated cell proliferation, an active phosphatase of the type 2A (sensitive to the inhibitor, okadaic acid) appears to suppress the cell response to oxidant.[44,266] Apparently, deactivation of PKC by this phosphatase is maintained by d-α-, but not d-β-tocopherol, making this structurally selective phenomenon also appear independent of general antioxidant properties. H_2O_2 causes activation of many PKC isoforms by phosphorylation of Tyr residues in their catalytic domains by tyrosine kinases (Lyk, Syk, Fyn, c-Src, growth factor receptor kinases).[128] Alternatively, inhibition of protein phosphatase-1 and -2A by okadaic acid increases both the degree of phosphorylation of IκB and the peroxide tone.[251] It will be useful to determine whether one of these events depends upon the other and whether okadaic acid exacerbates alcohol-induced hepatocyte injury.

Interleukin-1 and TNFα released in alcoholic liver disease stimulate the formation of ROS that activate cJun amino terminal kinases (JNKs) and enhance expression of c-jun, thereby enhancing the induction of genes by the jun-fos heterodimer, AP-1. The JNKs are a subgroup of mitogen-activated protein kinases (MAP kinases) characterized by activation with oxidant stress.[163] The activity of JNK1 leads to apoptosis, and it is increased by a wide variety of apoptotic stresses.[209] However, continued overstimulation of JNK action by H_2O_2 or NO may cause over-expression of c-jun and AP-1 activity followed by over-expression of matrix metalloproteinases and uncontrolled inflammatory, proliferative disorders such as arthritis, atherogenesis, metastatic proliferation, or alcoholic liver disease. Two distinct patterns of c-jun and c-fos expression occurred during liver response to ischemia-reperfusion: (1) coexpression of fos and jun at 1 to 3 hours post-perfusion in damaged regions undergoing early repair processes; (2) a decline in fos expression with sustained high levels of jun expression at 6 to 20 hours post-reperfusion in cells bordering regions of necrotic/apoptotic programmed cell death.[250]

The H_2O_2-triggered activation of another subgroup of MAP kinases (ERKs, p42 and p44), like that of Ras in vascular smooth muscle cells, led to an induced expression of c-fos and c-jun (and their heterodimer AP-1) which was blunted by adding the isoflavanoid, genistein.[222] Thus, this blunted expression may reflect a tonic action of PTP activity that is maintained by genistein but inactivated by ROS. The H_2O_2-induced activation of ERKs can be suppressed by genistein or by over-expression of a dominant-negative mutant of Ras or of a Raf-1 kinase, or of CSK (a negative regulator of Src PTKs).[3] These results illustrate the importance of maintaining PTP activity higher than PTK activity in the resting cell. In contrast to JNKs, ERKs seem to diminish apoptosis so that inhibiting the activity of ERKs increased the number of oxidatively induced apoptotic cells.[293] A rapid transient activation of ERK2 (10 to 20-fold) was blocked by NAC, suramin, or o-phenanthroline, indicating that a metal-catalyzed free radical mediated the signaling.[92] This oxidant-initiated signaling was abolished by expression of the dominant negative Ras-N-17 allele, making Ras and ERK appear pivotal in cell survival following oxidant stress.

Influx of extracellular Ca^{2+} was essential for oxidant-stimulated increases in c-jun and c-fos mRNA which also required PTK and PKC action.[19] The protein tyrosine kinase, Syk, is rapidly inactivated by H_2O_2 associated with increased influx of Ca^{2+} and release of Ca^{2+} from intracellular stores.[216] However, such a rise in Ca^{2+} during ROS-induced JNK activation did not occur in Syk(-) cells, and depletion of Ca^{2+} decreased the level of Syk activation produced by ROS. This result is one of many examples illustrating important interactions among peroxide tone, cytosolic Ca^{2+}, and kinase-mediated cellular responses. Alcohol-induced activation of PKC can occur by increased peroxide tone (noted above) or by increased cytosolic Ca^{2+}.[107]

The IκB of endothelial cells is phosphorylated and destroyed within 5 to 10 minutes of cell activation, leading to translocation of NFκB from the cytosol to the nucleus.[21] MEKK1 activates the IκB kinase (degrading I B and activating NFκB) and also the JNK pathway.[150] In turn, MEKK1 is activated by a caspase-catalyzed cleavage of an inhibitory N-terminal peptide, and activated MEKK1 activates more caspase (esp. caspase-7) providing a positive feedback loop that might drive the cell with increasing rapidity toward apoptosis.[37] However, that tendency is partially balanced by a shift toward necrosis exerted by NFκB and JNK.[14,18] In the TNFα-induced activation of NFκB, the degradation of IκB was mediated by MEK kinase (MEKK) action.[104] Signaling paths that include MEKK activity can produce apoptotic cell death.[119] The small GTP-binding protein, rac-1, mediates the increased peroxide tone leading to NFκB activation in response to inflammatory cytokines;[262] and this activation is inhibited by antioxidants such as N-acetyl cysteine (NAC) or pyrrolidine dithiocarbamate (PDTC).

Enhanced NFκB and AP-1 action: Increased ROS activation of NFκB initiates the transcription of inflammatory cytokines and other gene products that shift the cell away from apoptosis toward oxidant-rich necrotic death.[105,143,194] Prevention of NFκB action thus represents one way to maintain antioxidant status of the tissue while a cell continues to die by apoptosis. Anti-inflammatory steroids achieve this by inducing the transcription and formation of IκB, which suppresses NFκB action. In fact, NFκB itself activates transcription of IκB that eventually gives negative feedback to suppress transient NFκB action. However, prolonged sustained action of NFκB in promoting expression of the other genes leads to inflammatory, proliferative, and necrotic events and prevents the subtle, silent progress of apoptosis. A paradoxical response to 25 mM alcohol exposure gave preferential induction of NFκB as the inhibitory homodimer (p50/p50) rather than the active heterodimer (p50/p65) raising the possibility of alcohol disrupting inflammatory necrosis[168] and shifting the cells toward apoptosis.

The activity of factors activating gene transcription in a pre-monocytic cell line is both enhanced and inhibited by H_2O_2, with translocation from cytosol to nucleus favored by H_2O_2 and binding to nuclear DNA impaired by H_2O_2. There is a paradoxical aspect of active NFκB needing cytosolic ROS for release from IκB, while also needing a nuclear antioxidant such as thioredoxin[117] to prevent ROS from impairing NFκB action in the nucleus. Recent attention to oxidant stress during apoptosis noted that glutathione disulfide increased only after apoptotic changes had occurred, emphasizing the possibility of some thiols other than glutathione having even more critical roles during early signaling.[247]

Thioredoxin (TRX) is a protein that contains significant sulfhydryl groups that protect cells from Fas-mediated apoptosis and from the cytotoxic effects of TNFα, H_2O_2, activated neutrophils, and post-ischemic reperfusion injury. Also, TRX translocates into the nucleus where it regulates actions of redox factor-1 (Ref-1) on gene expression and other important interactions of proteins and nucleic acids. For example, TRX is required for optimal interaction between glucocorticoid receptor, AP-1, NFκB, and p53 with their corresponding DNA regulatory elements.[194] In a related manner, added thioredoxin diminished the induction of apoptotic death of lymphoid cells following a pro-oxidant state created by depleting GSH.[115] Intracellular oxidants can cause transcriptional activation of the thioredoxin gene that creates a negative feedback, because expression of the TRX gene product then prevents intracellular elevation of peroxide tone.[244] The eventual protective antioxidant actions of thioredoxin following a time-dependent induction of thioredoxin by H_2O_2 illustrate the complex timing encountered in balancing various signals during cellular responses to oxidant stress.[117] The timing of the thioredoxin response may be critical in determining whether a cell dies by apoptosis or necrosis. Recent research on regulating peroxide tone with thioredoxin noted that thioredoxin peroxidase activities in human tissues catalyze thioredoxin oxidation during peroxide removal in ways that permit dissociation of IκB from NFκB.[118] When thioredoxin peroxidase is overexpressed, it protects cells from apoptosis induced by serum deprivation, ceramide, or etoposide,[299] perhaps by preventing elevated peroxide tone.

Platelet activating factor (PAF) receptor signaling: Inflammatory processes are amplified by signal transduction from PAF receptors through G-protein-coupled signaling paths that increase cytosolic calcium, activate intracellular signaling by the α- and β-forms of PKC,[34,140] and increase the transcription of the inflammatory mediators like prostaglandin synthase-2, c-fos, c-jun.[15] The opposite effects may be attributed to Gi signals in the former transition and to Gq signals in the latter. Action of oxidized lipid mediators through PAF receptors was confirmed by the ability of a synthetic PAF-receptor antagonist to block the lipid-stimulated secretion of IL-8 and macrophage inflammatory protein-1 as well as leukocyte adhesion and aggregation in the microcirculation. The oxidized phospholipid formed from 1-palmitoyl-2-arachidonoyl-*sn*-glycero-3-phosphorylcholine, like those in mildly oxidized low-density lipoprotein[285] was reported to act as a PAF-mimic and increase cytosolic Ca^{2+}, which enhanced monocyte adhesion and transmigration at vascular walls[198] favoring local inflammatory oxidant stress and tissue injury.

Because inflammatory conditions produce increased amounts of oxidants, it is important to note that oxidized phospholipids derived from cellular[211,265] or plasma[100] phosphatidylcholines may act as PAF-mimics, activating inflammatory signals through PAF receptors, further enhancing Ca^{2+} flux, cell adhesion, and local inflammatory events.[143] Thus, an important consequence of local oxidant stress is a non-enzymatic formation of oxidized phospholipids that creates positive feedback in potent oxidant-related actions either as intact PAF mimics[301] or as the hydrolyzed isoprostane derivatives (noted above). Such PAF-like oxidized phospholipids (and their hydrolyzed isoprostanes) are produced *in vivo,* and they accumulate in plasma during putatively innocuous activities like cigarette smoking[151] or social drinking.[175] A productive area of research may combine PAF receptor blockers with retrograde and anterograde perfusions to assign a clearer role for this receptor-mediated increase in cytosolic Ca^{2+} in liver injury.

Decreased Removal of Reactive Oxygen Species

Decreased Mitochondrial GSH-Transporter Action

Normal movement of the GSH across mitochondrial membranes is via an ATP-stimulated transporter, RmGshT, whereas added Ca^{2+} and phosphate can permeabilize the inner mitochondrial membrane, equilibrating mitochondrial GSH and other small molecules with cytosolic levels. In contrast, GSH movement across plasma membranes occurs by two different transporters (RcGshT or RsGshT) at the canalicular or sinusoidal surfaces, respectively.[67,71] Ethanol impairment of the mitochondrial transporter gave significant selective depletion of mitochondrial GSH (discussed earlier) that appeared to precede mitochondrial dysfunction and alcoholic liver disease.[69] Alcohol-induced impairment of mitochondrial GSH transport was predominantly in the pericentral cells rather than the periportal cells,[67,78] and it paralleled the greater tendency for necrosis and fibrosis in the pericentral region. Thus, the result of alcohol-impairing mitochondrial transport was a decreased mitochondrial anti-oxidant status with an indirect effect of increased vulnerability to subsequent oxidant stress rather than a direct increase in oxidant stress. Such vulnerability is illustrated with antimycin-induced ROS, which is attributed mainly to an inhibition of complex III in the mitochondrial electron transport chain causing the ROS formed by the ubiquinone cycle.

Prior depletion of cytosolic and mitochondrial GSH to 10-20% of control values (by treatment with buthionine sulfoximine before mitochondria isolation or by adding diethyl maleate or ethacrynic acid to isolated mitochondria) led to increased formation of H_2O_2 and a 2 to 4-fold enhanced activation of NFκB, indicating an increased vulnerability for expressing inflammatory genes and causing still greater extracellular ROS signaling in the tissue.[77] Because inhibition of complex I and II of the mitochondrial electron transport chain prevented antimycin-induced oxidant stress, an excessive mitochondrial production of ROS by complex III seemed directly responsible for the activation of NFκB and subsequent inflammatory oxidative tissue damage. Prior depletion of mitochondrial GSH levels was directly proportional to the generation of oxidant stress indicated by dichlorofluorescein fluorescence, and it was an early, progressive event during the 16-week development of alcohol-induced liver injury.[67] Important features that need more detailed study are the mechanisms whereby ethanol impairment of mitochondrial GSH transport is greater in pericentral cells than periportal cells.

Feeding N-acetylcysteine raised cytosolic GSH, but did not prevent the mitochondrial GSH transport defect associated with alcohol feeding. In contrast, supplementing diets with S-adenosyl-L-methionine (SAM) raised mitochondrial GSH and preserved some mitochondrial integrity in periportal and pericentral regions of the liver.[79] Some of the protection by SAM may be due to an improved dietary supply of precursors of methylation that compensate for an alcohol-induced impairment of hepatic methyltetrahydrofolate:homocysteine methyltransferase that is associated in the micropig with deoxynucleoside triphosphate imbalance, increased apoptosis, and regenerative proliferation.[96] An imbalance in deoxynucleoside triphosphates is one enhancing feature in irreversibly committing model cell systems to apoptosis. Alcohol-induced loss of hepatic GSH and methyltransferase in the micropig gave increased apoptosis without the hepatic inflammation and zonal distribution of apoptotic cells seen in the alcohol-fed rat.

Decreased PAF Acetyl Hydrolase and Paraoxonase

Two enzymes, PAF acetyl hydrolase and paraoxonase, can improve antioxidant status by destroying certain phospholipids that provide potent inflammatory signals to disturb Ca^{2+} homeostasis and generate more ROS. The availability of PAF acetyl hydrolase from liver, tissue macrophages, platelets, and neutrophils[256,260] provides an important counterbalance to the pathophysiological roles for both enzymatically formed PAF and non-enzymatically formed PAF-mimics. Oxidant stress can both generate PAF mimics and also inactivate the human plasma acetyl hydrolase,[8] thereby potentiating and prolonging proinflammatory effects of PAF. Amplification of inflammatory stimuli occurs as entry of calcium to the cytosol increases formation of ROS and PAF-mimics. Calcium-stimulated phospholipase A_2 also provides substrate for enzymatic synthesis of PAF, which then facilitates still more entry of calcium and more formation of ROS with release of inflammatory cytokines.[147] Furthermore, the ROS formed can participate in non-enzymatic formation of oxidized phospholipids that bind at PAF receptors, act as PAF mimics, increase calcium entry into the cytosol, and cause still more ROS to appear. Blocking these positive feedback loops with enzymes such as PAF acetyl hydrolase and paraoxonase is an important physiologic process for maintaining the antioxidant status of a cell.[147]

High density lipoproteins (HDL) constitute a family of diverse particulate complexes, some of which contain PAF acetyl hydrolase in association with apoE (that may facilitate movement from HDL to LDL where it can inactivate oxidized phospholipids). Thus the HDL can diminish some inflammatory signals. Lecithin-cholesterol acyltransferase (LCAT) is another HDL-associated enzyme that can hydrolyze and inactivate oxidized PAF-mimics, although it apparently could not hydrolyze PAF.[87] Also, paraoxonase is another hydrolase associated with HDL particles, from which it may interact with oxidized LDL to prevent accumulation of oxidized PAF-mimics and diminish the pathological actions of oxidized LDL.[254]

Unfortunately, paraoxonase activity is also vulnerable to oxidant stress, and feeding rabbits an atherogenic diet lowered paraoxonase activity and decreased mRNA for paraoxonase 2.7-fold while it increased mRNA 2.4-fold for apoJ. Similarly, when oxidized LDL was injected into C57BL/6 mice, it lowered paraoxonase activity 59% and raised apoJ levels 3.6-fold.[198] This shift in apoJ/paraoxonase ratio did not occur with the C3H strain of mice, which differs dramatically from the C57Bl/6 strain in that it does not develop inflammatory responses to an atherogenic diet.[157] Clearly, the genetic background has a powerful influence on how nutrient interactions maintain antioxidant status in individuals.

Decreased SOD Activity

There are three forms of superoxide dismutase (SOD): the Mn-SOD found in mitochondria, a Cu,Zn-SOD found in cytosol, and a related Cu,Zn-SOD released into extracellular spaces.[76] Because mitochondria may be the major source of ROS during alcohol-induced oxidant stress, levels of Mn-SOD might be expected to be low, but serum levels in alcohol-dependent patients were almost twice as high as those for controls.[267] The increased Mn-

SOD released into serum may reflect either greater stress-induced synthesis or greater release from injured tissue. The latter event is indicated by finding that during abstinence of 1, 10, and 40 days, the serum Mn-SOD levels decreased from 150 to 120 to 95 μg/ml, approaching the 76 μg/ml value of the control group.[268] Alternatively, liver biopsies from 45 patients with alcoholic liver disease had Mn-SOD values similar to those for controls, but significantly lower Cu,Zn-SOD.[300] Apparently, alcohol-induced oxidant stress in liver is not likely due to inadequate mitochondrial Mn-SOD. Also, cultured rat hepatocytes exposed to alcohol had increased Cu,Zn-SOD (22%) and Mn-SOD (21%) indicating that ethanol-induced oxidant stress in these cells was not caused by impaired activities of these enzymes.[56] When mice were fed ethanol in liquid diets, levels of GSH, Mn-SOD, and Cu,Zn-SOD in liver were decreased, whereas glutathione peroxidase was unaffected and catalase and glutathione transferase were increased.[40] Interactions with nutrients remain poorly understood, and antioxidant defense was maintained at greater levels with the AIN-76A ethanol liquid diet than the Lieber-DeCarli ethanol liquid diet. Cell viability in aerobic conditions, ROS generation, and cell injury immediately after anoxia/reoxygenation were similar for steatotic and non-steatotic hepatocytes, but the anoxic injury was greater in the steatotic cells.[36]

Decreased Glutathione Peroxidase Activity

The seleno-glutathione peroxidase (GPX1) protects erythrocytes from oxidative hemolysis, and it is regarded as one of the major antioxidant enzymes (with SOD and catalase) that protect cells from ROS-mediated injury. However, results with engineered mouse strains with overexpression or no expression of GPX1 are rapidly changing researchers' perceptions of the importance of this gene product in maintaining antioxidant status of tissues. Deeper insight of a general physiological need for some ROS signaling was provided in showing that transgenic mice that overproduce GPX1 failed to carry out ROS-initiated induction of cytoprotective HSP70 and other cellular mechanisms regulating body temperature.[178] Again, researchers must recognize a balance between helpful ROS signaling and harmful ROS destruction of tissue integrity. Human T47D cell transfectants that overexpress GPX1 expressed normal contents of IκB and NFκB subunits (p65 and p50). However, the overexpressed peroxidase abolished the TNF-mediated transient accumulation of acidic, phosphorylated forms of IκB and NFκB failed to translocate into the nucleus.[131] The rapid burst of intracellular ROS induced by TNFα was abolished in the over-expressing cells, but restored when cells were grown in the absence of selenium. A balanced, transient (but not sustained) activation of NFκB is a necessary aspect of normal cellular adaptive responses. A related study of human endothelial cells over-expressing the phospholipid hydroperoxide glutathione peroxidase showed an inability of IL-1 to induce expression of NFκB, indicating the importance of peroxide tone in mediating the needed signaling.[32]

Further insight regarding GPX1 followed results from targeted gene disruption and development of GPX1(-) mice. Such "knockout" mice had no cellular GPX1 activity, but expressed normal levels of the plasma GPX, GPX3, and the GPX acting on phospholipid, GPX4.[42] Although selenium-deficient animals developed pulmonary injury following hyperoxic conditions, GPX1 knockout mice showed no increased sensitivity to hyperoxia.[106] Although some seleno-proteins appear to be important, it now seems likely that decreased levels of GPX1 activity may not have the pivotal role in tissue protection that they once were regarded to have. Again, combined use of anterograde and retrograde perfusion with fluorescent probes might provide useful results with livers from these mice.

ALCOHOL INCREASES LIPID PEROXIDATION

Aldehydes and Polyunsaturated Fatty Acids

Of the alcohol-mediated processes capable of generating reactive oxygen intermediates in the liver,[204] hydroxyl radicals produced from the metabolism of ethanol by the monooxygenase, P450 2E1, have a great potential to react rapidly with lipids, proteins, and nucleic acids.[5,73,186] These highly reactive compounds can cause the homolytic cleavage of the proton carbon bond of fatty acids to form carbon-centered radicals.[259] The methylene protons of polyunsaturated fatty acids are more susceptible to attacks by radicals than those of mono-unsaturated or saturated fatty acids owing to the resonance stabilization of the intermediate carbon radical. The resultant comparatively long-lived carbon radical species may undergo reactions with molecular oxygen to form hydroperoxy fatty acids which can decompose to form aldehydic products such as malonyldialdehyde (MDA), hydroxyalkenals (4-hydroxynonenal), 4-HNE and 4-hydroxyhexenal, 4-HHE and other aldehydes. Although both ω-3 and ω-6 fatty acids are substrates for the generation of the hydroxyalkenals, 4-HNE derived from ω-6 fatty acids appears to be more readily produced than is the ω-3 fatty acid derivative, 4-HHE.[16] Over a period of time, alcohol-induced lipid peroxidation may serve to reduce the concentrations of tissue polyunsaturated fatty acids.

Alcohol and Liver Aldehyde Accumulation

An accumulation of aldehydic compounds in liver mitochondria and microsomes has been observed in alcohol-exposed rodents[121,302] and confirmed in non-human primates.[161] Lipid peroxidation with aldehyde formation is also associated with decreased levels of liver antioxidants. An alcohol-induced production of MDA, for instance, was linearly correlated to decreased concentrations of liver α-tocopherol and glutathione.[238] The products of lipid peroxidation resulting from alcohol exposure has also been observed in fetal tissue, where 4-HNE accumulated in higher concentrations in the liver mitochondria of rat fetuses compared with the maternal levels.[39] A lower metabolism of 4-HNE in the fetuses suggested that the developing young animals have a prolonged exposure to the reactive compounds and therefore an increased susceptibility to the oxidative damage caused by alcohol metabolism.

Reactions of Aldehydes

The aldehydes resulting from lipid peroxidation are highly reactive compounds capable of forming covalent bonds with proteins[65,66,275] and nucleic acids.[38] Aldehydes, such as MDA and 4-HNE, bind to proteins in a synergistic manner, with a several-fold increase in acetaldehyde binding to bovine serum albumin in the presence of MDA compared with acetaldehyde alone.[274] This synergism suggested that MDA stimulated acetaldehyde binding to proteins, and it may form unexpected "hybrid" aldehyde-protein products. 4-HNE also competes for binding sites on acetaldehyde dehydrogenase, where it inhibits conversion of acetaldehyde to acetate.[99]

Aldehyde Determinations

In vivo assessments of aldehydic compounds have successfully demonstrated effects of alcohol consumption on lipid peroxidation.[73,93,272,276,278] The plasma concentrations of 4-hydroxynonenal were markedly increased in rhesus monkeys consuming alcohol[213] and MDA has been measured in the blood of humans following alcohol ingestion.[279] The metabolites of lipid peroxidation (MDA, acetaldehyde, formaldehyde, and acetone) have also been monitored in the urine of rodents during acute and chronic exposures to alcohol.[192]

The Effect of Aldehydes on Collagen Production

Both MDA and 4-HNE induce the expression of procollagen α-1 mRNA. Using an iron-ascorbate system to induce production of lipid peroxides, MDA, and 4-HNE in cultured human liver fat storing cells (stellate cells), an increase expression of procollagen α-1 mRNA was observed preceding a rise in the accumulation of extra-cellular protein.[210] Stellate cells, as a result of a chronic exposure to ethanol, are transformed into myofibroblasts that produce extra-cellular matrix collagen.[273] A similar aldehyde-mediated collagen production was observed in liver during metabolism of CCl_4 in rodents.[17] Aldehyde-bound protein products were found co-localized in regions of the liver that also had increased expression of the collagen gene. When cells were treated with allyl alcohol, which induces hepatic necrosis but not fibrosis, there was no increase in collagen mRNA synthesis.

Detoxification of 4-HNE in the Liver, P450 2E1 Inhibitors and Therapy

The liver diminishes 4-HNE toxicity by binding the alkenal to glutathione via glutathione-S-transferase,[6] by reductive metabolism via NADH-dependent alcohol dehydrogenase,[26] or by oxidation via aldehyde dehydrogenase.[182] Although P450 2E1 inhibitors, diallyl sulfide and phenethyl isothiocyante, effectively inhibit lipid peroxidation in alcohol-exposed rodents, only diallyl sulfide was also active in reducing liver pathology. Perhaps the lipid peroxidation products act in concert with other factors that affect fibrotic development.[187] An interesting report noted that a dietary supplement, polyenylphosphatidylcholine, dramatically decreased the level of 4-hydroxynonenal and the isoprostane, 8-epi-$F_{2\alpha}$ in liver of alcohol-exposed baboons below that of controls.[161] Currently a human trial is examining the effect of such dietary supplements in the treatment of alcoholic liver disease.

Isoprostanes

Isoprostane Formation and Biochemical Significance

Isoprostanes are generated *in vivo* in a non-enzymatic manner from reactions involving the bis-allylic carbon-centered radicals of a polyunsaturated fatty acid (e.g., arachidonic acid) and two molar equivalents of oxygen.[189] They can be synthesized from non-esterified arachidonic acid but they may also be formed on intact phospholipids prior to enzymatic excision and release.[190] Although structurally similar to prostaglandins, isoprostanes are optically inactive compounds, and many different stereoisomers may exist. For example, eight diastereomers of the four regioisomers of the F2 class of isoprostanes gives rise to 32 potentially distinct compounds that are derived from arachidonic acid.[191] The formation of E2 and D2 isoprostanes occurs less frequently than F2 compounds and, for reasons that are not completely clear, these compounds are not often detected in plasma.[235] Measurements of both urinary and plasma levels of the isoprostane, 8-epi F2-α, have been gaining acceptance as a useful index of free radical-mediated injury.[52] The biological activity conferred on isoprostanes is related to the prostanoid structure and several examples have been cited of potent biological activity. For example, 8-isoprostane-F2-α has been shown to be a potent renal[264] and pulmonary[122] vasoconstrictor and increases portal hypertension in the liver.[169] In an interesting series of studies, it has been suggested that vasoconstrictor properties associated with 8-iso-prostane-F2-α are mediated through a receptor-ligand binding site that is distinct from the thromboxane receptor.[235] Other prostanoids derived from DHA have been described from *in vitro* reactions of liposomes with transition metal complexes.[205]

Analysis of Isoprostanes

Both physical and immunological methods have been developed in order to analyze isoprostanes. An immunoassay method for 8-isoprostane F2-α was developed to determine isoprostanes in excretions.[282] This method, similar to other enzyme-linked assays, has a high degree of sensitivity but is hampered by cross-reactions with other prostanoids. Several gas chromatography mass spectrometric methods have been successfully developed to analyze for various isoprostanes.[188,191,288] Although analyses by these methods are expensive, the sensitivity and specificity are unrivaled. One such method has been successfully used to analyze for 8-isoprostane-F2-α in the plasma of rhesus monkeys[213] and in the livers of baboons[161] that were consuming alcohol. The development of a mass spectrometry method for the detection of urinary metabolites of 8-isoprostane-F2-α has led to the advancement of a non-invasive method for analyses of these products.[13,236]

Isoprostanes and Alcohol in the Liver

Alcohol consumption has been found to increase isoprostane formation in the liver, presumably through free radical-mediated mechanisms.[161,169] An increased concentration of isoprostane-reacting substances was detected in the plasma of rats exposed to alcohol[195] and the free 8-isoprostane-F2-α was measured in the plasma of rhesus monkeys consuming alcohol.[213] In the latter study, the plasma levels of 8-isoprostane-F2-α was correlated with the amount of alcohol that each individual animal consumed. In concert with this decline, it was also demonstrated that the plasma arachidonate concentration was negatively correlated with alcohol consumption.[213] Therefore, both the loss of hepatocyte membrane unsaturated phospholipids and the potent biological activity of isoprostanes and aldehydes may be potential factors underlying the development of liver fibrosis.[160,213]

ALCOHOL EFFECTS ON ESSENTIAL FATTY ACIDS

Increased lipid peroxidation and decreased levels of vitamins and minerals that maintain oxidative status may be expected to decrease the levels of highly unsaturated lipids. Alterations in essential fatty acid (EFA) status caused by alcohol have been recently reviewed[227-229,240,241] and this section will focus upon data from humans. Although the various animal studies had differences in many variables including the dose and duration of alcohol exposure, in the species, organ, and subcellular fraction studied as well as the lipid class or fraction determined, there was generally a loss of long-chain polyunsaturated fatty acids subsequent to alcohol exposure that was most pronounced in the liver but also observed in the blood stream, the brain, and other internal organs.

Several investigators have observed a loss in long-chain polyunsaturates in the bloodstream of alcoholics. Horrobin and Manku[108] reported less polyunsaturates, including arachidonate (AA) and docosahexaenoate (DHA), in the erythrocyte phospholipids of alcoholics compared to controls. Soon after, lower linoleic acid in erythrocyte phosphatidylcholine was reported.[144] In a Swedish population of alcoholics with a mean alcohol intake of 265 g for 19 years, Alling[7] found that the drinkers had less AA and DHA in erythrocyte phosphatidylcholine and phosphatidylethanolamine as well as less AA in plasma phosphatidylcholine. A group of alcoholics consuming at least 150 g/day of ethanol for more than a year and who had macrocytosis had profoundly lower AA and DHA.[20] Also, patients with a mean alcohol intake of 4.3 g/kg body weight who drank for about 35 days had less stearoyl, arachidonyl species of phosphatidylcholines and inositols in their platelets.[200] A group of Italian alcoholics consuming at least 200 g/day of ethanol for the five years previous to the study exhibited the same erythrocyte cholesterol and phospholipid distributions as controls but had low total lipid DHA.[80] Japanese patients consuming more than 100 g/day of ethanol for at least 10 years also have low erythrocyte AA and DHA.[1]

Patients with alcoholic liver disease had 40% less AA as well as less DHA in their erythrocytes,[59] and decompensated cirrhotic patients had less plasma polyunsaturates.[206] Addition of AA to a rat diet led to a decrease in the alcohol-induced rise in serum ALT.[207] These authors also noted that a similar supplement given to decompensated cirrhotics produced an increase in serum phospholipid AA after 24 hrs.[206] Cirrhotic patients with moderate or severe protein-energy malnutrition had lower DHA and about half of the plasma AA compared to controls.[86] A group of Chilean alcoholics with liver damage showed less total polyunsaturates and more oleic acid relative to alcoholics without liver damage.[50] In that study, mean AA and DHA seemed reduced in patients with liver damage, but statistical significance was not reached with six liver-damaged subjects. Preliminary evidence indicates that there is a selective loss of DHA relative to AA in alcoholic liver disease (Salem N, unpublished study). When liver samples from alcoholic liver disease patients at transplant were analyzed and compared to autopsy controls or patients with primary biliary cirrhosis, DHA was lower in the alcoholics. The brains of a small number of alcoholics who had "hepatocerebral degeneration" contained less than normal AA in the phosphatidylethanolamine fraction of cerebral gray matter, but not in the cerebral white matter, cerebellum or medulla.[156] Also, DHA was low in cerebral gray matter phosphatidylethanolamine from alcoholics, but it was high in the cerebral white matter, cerebellum and medulla.

SUMMARY

Ingested alcohol interacts with certain ratios of fat/carbohydrate nutrients to produce oxidative imbalances in pericentral hepatocytes which do not seem evident in the periportal cells that are upstream in the hepatic sinusoids. Differences in intra-cellular signals described in this chapter, as well as the extra-cellular microenvironment of the downstream cells in terms of cytokines and autacoids,[147] need careful evaluation in designing approaches to preventing the widely observed oxidative liver injury following alcohol intake. The injury involves both apoptotic and necrotic programmed cell death associated with loss of mitochondrial integrity and formation of reactive oxygen species. Important intra-cellular signaling altered during the oxidant-mediated death of hepatocytes includes essential sulfhydryls in protein tyrosine phosphatases, caspases, and mitochondrial permeability pores. Formation of oxidants is exacerbated by elevated cytosolic levels of Ca^{2+} which exerts positive feedback destabilization of mitochondria, favoring increasingly greater peroxide tone and more necrotic damage. The metabolic steps that initiate and propagate programmed cell death involve many redox events other than the steps commonly discussed in antioxidant actions of micronutrient vitamins and minerals in membrane lipid peroxidation. Selective interventions that diminish positive feedback in oxidant-mediated signaling loops need to evaluate how the balance of oxidants, antioxidants, and nutrients influence both cell survival and the character of cell death.

REFERENCES

1. Adachi J, Hojo K, Ueno Y, *et al.* Identification of cholesta-3,5-dien-7-one by gas chromatography-mass spectrometry in the erythrocyte membrane of alcoholic patients. *Alcoholism: Clin Exptl Res*, 20, 51A, 1996.
2. Adachi S, Cross AR, Babior BM and Gottlieb RA. Bcl-2 and the outer mitochondrial membrane in the inactivation of cytochrome c during Fas-mediated apoptosis. *J Biol Chem* 272, 21878, 1997.
3. Aikawa R, Komuro I, Yamazaki T, Zou Y, *et al.* Oxidative stress activates extracellular signal-regulated kinases through Src and Ras in cultured cardiac myocytes of neonatal rats. *J Clin Invest* 100, 1813, 1997.
4. Albano E, Clot P, Morimoto M, *et al.* Role of cytochrome P4502E1-dependent formation of hydroxyethyl free radical in the development of liver damage in rats intragastrically fed with ethanol. *Hepatology* 23, 155, 1996.
5. Albano E, Poli G, Tomasi A, *et al.* Study on the mechanisms responsible for ethanol-induced oxidative damages using isolated rat hepatocytes In: *Medical Biochemical and Chemical Aspects of Free Radicals.* Hayashi O, Niki E, Kondo M and Yoshikawa T, Eds, Elsevier Amsterdam The Netherlands 1988, pp 1389-1392.
6. Alin P, Danielson H and Mannervik B. 4-Hydroxyalk-2-enals are subtrates for glutathione transferase. *FEBS Lett* 179, 267, 1985.
7. Alling C, Gustavsson L, Kristensson-Aas A and Wallerstedt S. Changes in fatty acid composition of major glycerophospholipids in erythrocyte membranes from chronic alcoholics during withdrawal. *Scand J Clin Lab Invest* 44, 283, 1984.
8. Ambrosio G, Oriente A, Napoli C, *et al.* Oxygen radicals inhibit human plasma acetylhydrolase the enzyme that catabolizes platelet-activating factor. *J Clin Invest* 93, 2408, 1994.
9. Armstrong RC, Aja T, Xiang J, Gaur S, *et al.* Fas-induced activation of the cell death-related protease CPP32 is inhibited by Bcl-2 and by ICE family protease inhibitors. *J Biol Chem* 271, 16850, 1996.
10. Arora A, de Groen P, Emori Y and Gores GJ. A cascade of degradative hydrolase activity contributes to hepatocyte necrosis during anoxia. *Am J Physiol* 270, G238, 1996.
11. Arora A, Jones BT, Patel TC, *et al.* Ceramide induces hepatocyte cell death through disruption of mitochondrial function in the rat. *Hepatology* (April) 958,1997.
12. Arteel G, Raleigh J, Bradford B and Thurman R. Acute alcohol produces hypoxia directly in rat liver tissue *in vivo*: role of Kupffer cells. *Am J Physiol 271, Gastrointes Liver Physiol* 34, G494, 1996.
13. Bachi A, Zuccato E, Baraldi M, *et al.* Measurement of urinary 8-epi-prostaglandin F2-α, A novel index of lipid peroxidation *in vivo* by immunoaffinity extraction/gas chromatography-mass spectrometry. Basal levels in smokers and nonsmokers. *Free Rad Biol Med* 20, 619, 1996.
14. Barinaga M. Life-death balance within the cell. *Science* 274, 724, 1996.
15. Bazan NG, Fletcher BS, Herschman HR and Mukherjee PK. Platelet-activating factor and retinoic acid synergistically activate the inducible prostaglandin synthase gene. *Proc Natl Acad Sci USA*, 91, 5252, 1994.
16. Beckman JK, Howard MJ and Greene HJ. Identification of hydroxyalkenals formed from omega-3 fatty acids. *Biochem & Biophys Res Comm* 169, 75, 1990.
17. Bedossa P, Houglum K, Trautwein C, *et al.* Stimulation of collagen α-1 gene expression is associated with lipid peroxidation in hepatocellular injury: A link to tissue fibrosis? *Hepatology* 19, 1262, 1994.

18. Beg AA and Baltimore D. An essential role for NFκB in preventing TNF-α induced cell death. *Science* 274, 782, 1996.
19. Beiqing L, Hackshaw K and Whisler R. Calcium signals and protein tryosine kinases are required for the induction of c-*jun* in Jurkat cells stimulated by T cell-receptor complex and oxidative signals. *J Interferon Cytokine Res,* 16, 77, 1996.
20. Benedetti A, Birarelli AM, Brunelli E, *et al.* Modification of lipid composition of erythrocyte membranes in chronic alcoholism in *Pharmacol Res Comm* Vol 19, Paoletti R, Nicosia S, Eds, The Italian Pharmacological Society Italy 1987, pp 651.
21. Bennett BL, Lacson RG, Chen CC, *et al.* Identification of signal-induced IκB-α kinases in human endothelial cells. *J Biol Chem* 271, 19680, 1996.
22. Bjorneboe A and Bjorneboe G-EA. Antioxidant status and alcohol-related diseases. *Alcohol & Alcoholism* 28, 111, 1993.
23. Bjorneboe A, Bjorneboe G-EA, Hagen BF and Drevon CA. Acute and chronic effects of ethanol on secretion of α-tocopherol from primary cultures of rat hepatocytes. *Biochim Biophys Acta* 922, 357, 1987.
24. Bjorneboe G-EA, Johnsen J, Bjorneboe A, *et al.* Some aspects of antioxidant status in blood from alcoholics. *Alcoholism: Clin Exptl Res*, 12, 806, 1988.
25. Bjorneboe G-EA, Johnsen J, Bjorneboe A, *et al.* Diminished serum concentration of vitamin E in alcoholics. *Ann Nutr Metab* 32, 35, 1988.
26. Boleda MD, Saubi N, Farres J and Pares X. Physiological substrates for rat alcohol dehydrogenase classes: Aldehydes of lipid peroxidation ω–hydroxyfatty acids and retinoids. *Arch Biochem Biophys* 307, 85, 1993.
27. Bollet AJ and Owens S. Evaluation of nutritional status of selected hospitalized patients. *Am J Clin Nutr* 26, 931, 1973.
28. Borle AB and Barsic M. Chemical hypoxia increases cytosolic Ca^{2+} and oxygen free radical formation. *Cell Calcium* 17, 307, 1995.
29. Borle AB and Stanko RT. Pyruvate reduces anoxic injury and free radical formation in perfused rat hepatocytes. *Am J Physiol* 33, G535, 1996.
30. Bradford B, Forman D and Thurman R. 4-Methylpyrazole inhibits fatty acyl coenzyme synthetase and diminishes catalase-dependent alcohol metabolism: Has the contribution of alcohol dehydrogenase to alcohol metabolism been previously overestimated? *Mol Pharmacol 43, 115,* 1993.
31. Bremer C, Bradford B, Hunt K, *et al.* Role of Kupffer cells in the pathogenesis of hepatic reperfusion injury. *Am J Physiol* 267, (*Gastrointest Liver Physiol* 30 G630), 1994.
32. Brigelius-Flohe R, Friedrichs B, Maurier S, *et al.*. Interleukin-1-induced nuclear factor κB activation is inhibited by over-expression of phospholipid hydroperoxide glutathione peroxidase in a human endothelial cell line. *Biochem J* 328, 199, 1997.
33. Brightman AO, Wang J, Miu S-M, *et al.* A growth factor- and hormone-stimulated NADH oxidase from rat liver plasma membrane. *Biochim Biophys Acta* 1105, 109, 1992.
34. Bussolino F, Silvagno F, Garbarino G, *et al.* Human endothelial cells are targets for platelet-activating factor (PAF). *J Biol Chem* 269, 2877, 1994.
35. Caraceni P, Gasbarrini A, Nussler A, *et al.* Human hepatocytes are more resistant than rat hepatocytes to anoxia-reoxygenation injury. *Hepatology* 20, 1247, 1994.
36. Caraceni P, Ryu HS, Subbotin V, *et al.* Rat hepatocytes isolated from alcohol-induced fatty liver have an increased sensitivity to anoxic injury. *Hepatology* 25, 943, 1997.
37. Cardone MH, Salvesen GS, Widnamm C, *et al.* The regulation of anoikis: MEKK-1 activation requires cleavage by caspases. *Cell* 90, 315, 1997.
38. Chaudhary AK, Munetaka N, Reddy GR, *et al.* Detection of endogenous malondialdehyde-desoxyguanosine adducts in human liver. *Science* 265, 1580, 1994.

39. Chen JJ, Schenker S and Henderson GI. 4-hydroxynonenal levels are enhanced in fetal liver mitochondria by in utero ethanol exposure. *Hepatology* 25, 142, 1997.
40. Chen LH, Xi S and Cohen DA. Liver antioxidant defenses in mice fed ethanol and the AIN-76A diet. *Alcohol* 12, 453, 1995.
41. Chen Q, Galleano M and Cederbaum AI. Cytotoxicity and apoptosis produced by arachidonic acid in Hep G2 cells overexpressing human cytochrome P4502E1. *J Biol Chem* 272, 14532, 1997.
42. Cheng W, Ho Y, Ross DA, *et al.* Cellular glutathione peroxidase knockout mice express normal levels of selenium-dependent plasma and phospholipid hydroperoxide glutathione peroxidases in various tissues. *J Nutr* 127, 1445, 1997.
43. Cicalese L, Lee K, Schraut W, *et al.* Pyruvate prevents ischemia-reperfusion mucosal injury of rat small intestine. *Am J Surg* 171, 97, 1996.
44. Clement S, Tasinato A, Boscoboinik D and Azzi A. The effect of α-tocopherol on the synthesis phosphorylation and activity of protein kinase C in smooth muscle cells after phorbol 12-myristate 13-acetate down-regulation. *Eur J Biochem* 246, 745, 1997.
45. Colletti LM, Kunkel SL, Walz A, *et al.* The role of cytokine networks in the local liver injury following hepatic ischemia/reperfusion in the rat. *Hepatology* 506, 1996.
46. Corrigan FM, Besson JAO and Ward NI. Red cell caesium lithium and selenium in abstinent alcoholics. *Alcohol & Alcoholism* 26, 309, 1991.
47. Costantini P, Chernyak B, Petronilli V and Bernardi P. Modulation of the mitochondrial permeability transition pore by pyridine nucleotides and dithiol oxidation at two separate sites. *J Biol Chem* 271, 6746, 1996.
48. Dai Y, Rashba-Step J and Cederbaum AI. Stable expression of human cytochrome P4502E1 in HepG2 cells: Characterization of catalytic activities and production of reactive oxygen intermediates. *Biochemistry* 32, 6928, 1993.
49. Dawson TL, Gores GJ, Nieminen A, *et al.* Mitochondria as a source of reactive oxygen species during reductive stress in rat hepatocytes. *Am J Physiol* 264, C-961, 1993.
50. De la Maza MP, Hirsch S, Nieto S, *et al.* Fatty acid composition of liver total lipids in alcoholic patients with and without liver damage. *Alcoholism: Clin Exptl Res*, 20, 1418, 1996.
51. deGroot MJM, van Helden MAB, de Jong YF, *et al.*. The influence of lactate pyruvate and glucose as exogenous substrates on free radical defense mechanisms in isolated rat hearts during ischaemia and reperfusion. *Mol Cell Biochem* 146,147,1995.
52. Delanty N, Reilly D, Pratico D, *et al.* 8-epi PGF2-α: specific analysis of an isoeicosanoid as an index of oxidant stress *in vivo*. *Br J Clin Pharmacol* 42, 15, 1996.
53. Delneste Y, Jeannin P, Sebille E, *et al.* Thiols prevent Fas (CD95)-mediated T cell apoptosis by down-regulating membrane Fas expression. *Eur J Immunol* 26, 2981, 1996.
54. Derr RF, Porta EA, Larkin EC and Rao GA. Is ethanol per se hepatotoxic? *J Hepatol* 10, 381, 1990.
55. Desagher S, Glowinski J and Premont J. Pyruvate protects neurons against hydrogen peroxide-induced toxicity. *J Neurosci* 17, 9060, 1997.
56. Devi BG, Schenker S, Mazloum B and Henderson GI. Ethanol-induced oxidative stress and enzymatic defenses in cultured fetal rat hepatocytes. *Alcohol* 13, 327, 1996.
57. DiLuzio NR. Prevention of the acute ethanol-induced fatty liver by the simultaneous administration of antioxidants. *Life Sci,* 3, 113, 1964.
58. Dobbelsteen DJ van den, Nobel CSI, Schlegel J, *et al.* Rapid and specific efflux of reduced glutathione during apoptosis induced by anti-Fas/APO-1 antibody. *J Biol Chem* 271, 15420, 1996.
59. Driss F, Gueguen M, Delamaire D, *et al.* Abnormalities of erythrocyte deformability and membrane lipid composition in alcoholic liver diseases. *Clin Hemorheol* 5, 245, 1985.

60. Dutta SK, Miller PA, Greenberg LB and Levander OA. Selenium and acute alcoholism. *Am J Clin Nutr* 38, 713, 1983.
61. Dworkin BM, Rosenthal WS, Gordon GG and Jankowski RH. Diminished blood selenium levels in alcoholics. *Alcoholism: Clin Exptl Res,* 8, 535, 1984.
62. Dworkin B, Rosenthal WS, Jankowski RH, *et al.* Low blood selenium levels in alcoholics with and without advanced liver disease. Correlations with clinical and nutritional status. *Dig Dis Sci* 30, 838, 1985.
63. Eliasson E, Johanssen I and Ingelman-Sundberg M. Substrate-, hormone-, and cAMP-regulated cytochrome P450 degradation. *Proc Nat Acad Sci USA*, 87, 3225, 1990.
64. Ellerby HM, Martin SJ, Ellerby LM, *et al.* Establishment of a cell-free system of neuronal apoptosis: comparison of premitochondrial mitochondrial and postmitochondrial phases. *J Neurosc* 17, 6165, 1997.
65. Esterbauer H. Cytotoxicity and genotoxicity of lipid-oxidation products. *Am J Clin Nutr* 57(s) 779s, 1993.
66. Esterbauer H, Schaur RJ and Zollner H. Chemistry and biochemistry of 4-hydroxynonenal malonaldehyde and related aldehydes. *Free Rad Biol Med* 11, 81, 1990.
67. Fernandez-Checa JC, Kaplowitz N, Garcia-Ruiz C, *et al.* GSH transport in mitochondria: defense against TNF-induced oxidative stress and alcohol-induced defect. *Am J Physiol* 273, G7, 1997.
68. Fernandz-Checa JC, Garcia-Ruiz C, Ookhtens M and Kaplowitz N. Impaired uptake of glutathione by hepatic mitochondria from chronic ethanol-fed rats. *J Clin Invest* 397, 1991.
69. Fernandz-Checa JC, Hirano T, Tsukamoto H and Kaplowitz N. Mitochondial glutathione depletion in alcoholic liver disease. *Alcohol* 10, 469, 1993.
70. Fernandz-Checa JC, Ookhtens M and Kaplowitz N. Effect of chronic feeding on rat hepatocytic glutathion. *J Clin Invest* 80, 57, 1987.
71. Fernandz-Checa JC, Yi J, Ruiz CG, *et al.* Plasma membrane and mitochondrial transport of hepatic reduced glutathione. *Semin Liver Dis,* 2, 147, 1996.
72. French SW, Morimoto M, Reitz RC, Koop D, *et al.* Lipid peroxidation CYP2E1 and arachidonic acid metabolism in alcoholic liver disease in rats. *J Nutr* 127, 907S, 1997.
73. French SW, Wong K, Jui L, *et al.* Effect of ethanol on cytochrome P450 2E1 (CYP2E1). Lipid peroxidation and serum protein adduct formation in relation to liver pathology pathogenesis. *Exper Mol Path* 58, 61, 1993.
74. French S. Biochemistry of alcoholic liver disease. *Critical Reviews in Clinical Laboratory Sciences* 29, 83, 1992.
75. French S, Benson N, and Sun P. Centrilobular liver necrosis induced by hypoxia in chronic ethanol-fed rats. *Hepatology* 4, 912, 1984.
76. Fridovich I. Superoxide anion radical superoxide dismutases and related matters. *J Biol Chem* 272, 18515, 1997.
77. Garcia-Ruiz C, Colell A, Morales A, *et al.* Role of oxidative stress generated from the mitochondrial electron transport chain and mitochondrial glutathione status in loss of mitochondrial function and activation of transcription factor nuclear factor- κB: Studies with isolate mitochondria and rat hepatocytes. *Mol Pharmacol 48,*825, 1995.
78. Garcia-Ruiz C, Morales A, Ballesta A, *et al.* Effect of chronic ethanol feeding on glutathione and functional integrity of mitochondria in periportal and perivenous rat hepatocytes. *J Clin Invest* 94, 193, 1994.
79. Garcia-Ruiz C, Morales A, Colell A, *et al.* Feeding S-adneosyl-L-methionine attenuates both ethanol-induced depletion of mitochondrial glutathione and mitochondrial dysfunction in periportal and perivenous rat heaptocytes. *Hepatology* 21, 207, 1995.

80. Gatti P, Viani P, Cervato G, *et al.* Effects of alcohol abuse: Studies on human erythrocyte susceptibility to lipid peroxidation. *Biochemistry and Molecular Biology International* 30, 807, 1993.
81. Giandomenico AR, Cerniglia GE, Biaglow JE, *et al.* The importance of sodium pyruvate in assessing damage produced by hydrogen peroxide. *Free Rad Biol Med,* 3, 426, 1997.
82. Girre C, Hispard E, Therond P, *et al.* Effect of abstinence from alcohol on the depression of glutathione peroxidase activity and selenium and vitamin E levels in chronic alcoholic patients. *Alcoholism: Clin Exptl Res*, 14, 909, 1990.
83. Glasgow W, Hui R, Everhart A, *et al.* The linoleic acid metabolite (13*S*)-hydroperoxyoctadecadienoic acid augments the epidermal growth factor receptor signaling pathway by attenuation of receptor dephosphorylation. *J Biol Chem* 272, 19269, 1997.
84. Goldin R, Hunt N, Clark J, and Wickramasinghe S. Apoptotic bodies in a murine model of alcoholic liver disease: Reversibility of ethanol-induced changes. *J Pathol* 171, 73, 1993.
85. Goldsmith RH, Iber FL and Miller PA. Nutritional status of alcoholics of different socio-economic class. *J Am Coll Nutr* 2, 215, 1983.
86. Gonzalez J, Periago JL, Gil A, *et al.* Malnutrition-related polyunsaturated fatty acid changes in plasma lipid fractions of cirrhotic patients. *Metabolism* 41, 954, 1992.
87. Goyal J, Wang K, Liu M and Subbaiah PV. Novel function of lecithin-cholesterol acyltransferase hydrolysis of oxidized polar phospholipids generated during lipoprotein. *J Biol Chem* 272, 16231, 1997.
88. Grandjean P, Nielsen GD, Jorgensen PJ and Horder M. Reference intervals for trace elements in blood: significance of risk factors. *Scand J Clin Lab Invest* 1992, 52, 321, 1992.
89. Gruchow HW, Sobocinski KA, Barboriak JJ and Scheller JG. Alcohol consumption nutrient intake and relative body weight among U.S. adults. *Am J Clin Nutr* 42, 289, 1985.
90. Grummer MA and Erdman Jr. JW. Effect of chronic alcohol consumption and moderate fat diet on vitamin A status in rats fed either vitamin A or beta-carotene. *J Nutr* 113, 350, 1983.
91. Gudz T, Tserng KY and Hoppel C. Direct inhibition of mitochondrial respiratory chain complex III by cell-permeable ceramide. *J Biol Chem* 272, 24154, 1997.
92. Guyton KZ, Liu Y, Gorospe M, *et al.* Activation of mitogen-activated protein kinase by H_2O_2. *J Biol Chem* 271, 4138, 1996.
93. Hageman JJ, Bast A and Vermeulen NP. Monitoring of oxidative free radical damage *in vivo*: analytical aspects. *Chem-Biol Interactions* 82, 243, 1992.
94. Hagen BF, Bjorneboe A, Bjorneboe G-EA and Drevon CA. Effect of chronic ethanol consumption on the content of α-tocopherol in subcellular fractions of rat liver. *Alcoholism: Clin Exptl Res*, 13, 246, 1989.
95. Halestrap A, Woodfield KY and Connern C. Oxidative stress thiol reagents and membrane potential modulate the mitochondrial permeability transition by affecting nucleotide binding to the adenine nucleotide translocase. *J Biol Chem* 272, 3346, 1997.
96. Halsted CH, Villanueva J, Chandler CJ, *et al.* Ethanol feeding of micropigs alters methionine metabolism and increases hepatocellular apoptosis and proliferation. *Hepatology* (March) 497, 1996.
97. Hampton MB and Orrenius S. Dual regulation of caspase activity by hydrogen peroxide: implications for apoptosis. *FEBS Lett* 414, 552, 1997.
98. Hardwick JS and Sefton BM. The activated form of the Lck tyrosine protein kinase in cells exposed to hydrogen peroxide is phosphorylated at both Tyr-394 and Tyr-505. *J Biol Chem* 272, 25429, 1997.
99. Hartley DP and Petersen D. Co-metabolism of ethanol ethanol-derived acetaldehyde and 4-hydroxynonenal in isolated rat hepatocytes. *Alcoholism: Clin & Exp Res,* 21, 298, 1997.

100. Heery JM, Kozal M, Stafforini DM, *et al.* Oxidatively modified LDL contains phospholipids with platelet-activating factor-like activity and stimulates the growth of smooth muscle cells. *J Clin Invest* 96, 2322, 1995.
101. Herbeth B, Chavance M, Musse N, *et al.* Dietary intake and other determinants of blood vitamins in an elderly population. *Eur J Clin Nutr* 43, 175, 1989.
102. Higuchi H, Kurose I, Kato S, *et al.* Ethanol-induced apoptosis and oxidative stress in hepatocytes. *Alcoholism: Clin Exp Res* 20: 340A, 1996.
103. Hillers VN and Massey LK. Interrelationships of moderate and high alcohol consumption with diet and health status. *Am J Clin Nutr* 41, 356, 1985.
104. Hirano M, Osada S, Aoki T, *et al.* MEK Kinase is involved in tumor necrosis factor - induced NFκB activation and degradation of IκBα. *J Biol Chem* 271, 13234, 1996.
105. Hirota K, Matsui M, *et al.* AP-1 transcriptional activity is regulated by a direct association between thioredoxin and Ref-1. *Proc Natl Acad Sci USA*, 94, 3633, 1997.
106. Ho Y, Magnenat J, Bronson RT, *et al.* Mice deficient in cellular glutathione peroxidase develop normally and show no increased sensitivity to hyperoxia. *J Biol Chem* 272, 16644, 1997.
107. Hoek JB and Tarachi TF. Cellular adaptation to alcohol. *TIBS* 13, 269, 1988.
108. Horrobin DF, and Manku MS. Essential fatty acids in clinical medicine in *Nutrition and Health* Vol 2, A B Academic Pubs Great Britain 1983, pp 127.
109. Hu Y, Ingelman-Sundberg M and Lindros KO. Induction mechanisms of cytochrome P450 2E1 in liver: interplay between ethanol treatment and starvation. *Biochem Pharmacol* 50, 155, 1995.
110. Hug H, Enari M and Nagata S. No requirement of reactive oxygen intermediates in Fas-mediated apoptosis. *FEBS Lett* 351, 311, 1994.
111. Hunter DJ, Morris JS, Chute CG, *et al.* Predictors of selenium concentration in human toenails. *Am J Epidemiol* 132, 114, 1997.
112. Hurt RD, Higgins JA, Nelson RA, *et al.* Nutritional status of a group of alcoholics before and after admission to an alcoholism treatment unit. *Am J Clin Nutr* 34, 386, 1981.
113. Iimuro Y, Frankenberg M, Arteel G, *et al.* Female rats exhibit greater susceptibility to early alcohol-induced liver injury than males. *Am J Physiology 272, G1186,* 1997.
114. Ingelman-Sundberg M, Johansson I, Pentilla KE, *et al.* Centrilobular expression of ethanol-inducible cytochrome P-450(IIE1) in rat liver. *Biochem Biophys Res Commun* 157, 55, 1988.
115. Iwata S, Hori T, Sato N, *et al.*. Adult T cell leukemia (ATL)-derived factor/human thioredoxin prevents apoptosis of lymphoid cells induced by L-cystine and glutathione depletion: possible involvement of thiol-mediated redox regulation in apoptosis caused by pro-oxidant state. *J Immunol* 158, 3108, 1997.
116. Jacobson MD. Reactive oxygen species and programmed cell death. *TIBS* 21, 83, 1996.
117. Jacquier-Sarlin MR and Polla BS. Dual regulation of heat-shock transcription factor (HSF) activation and DNA-binding activity by H_2O_2: role of thioredoxin. *Biochem J* 318,187, 1996.
118. Jin DY, Chae H, Rhee S and Jeang KT. Regulatory role for a novel human thioredoxin peroxidase in NF-kappaB activation. *J Biol Chem* 272, 30952, 1997.
119. Johnson NL, Gardner AM, Diener KM, *et al.* Signal transduction pathways regulated by mitogen-activated/extracellular response kinase kinase kinase induce cell death. *J Biol Chem* 271, 3229, 1996.
120. Jones BR, Barrett-Connor E, Criqui MH and Holdbrook MJ. A community study of calorie and nutrient intake in drinkers and nondrinkers of alcohol. *Am J Clin Nutr* 35, 135, 1982.

121. Kamimura S, Gaal K, Britton RS, *et al.* Increased 4-hydroxynonenal levels in experimental alcoholic liver disease: Association of lipid peroxidation with liver fibrogensis. *Hepatology* 16, 448, 1992.
122. Kang KH, Morrow JD, Roberts LJ, *et al.* Airway and vascular effects of 8-epi-prostaglandin F2 α in isolated perfused rat lung. *J Appl Physiol* 74, 460, 1993.
123. Kerr JFR. A histochemical study of hypertrophy and ischemic injury of rat liver with special reference to changes in lysosomes. *J Pathol Bacteriol* 90, 419, 1965.
124. Kerr JFR, Wyllie AH and Currie AR. Apoptosis: a basic biological phenomenon with wide-ranging implications in tissue kinetics. *Br J Cancer* 26, 239, 1972.
125. Khani SC, Zaphiropoulos PG, Fujita VS, *et al.* cDNA and derived amino acid sequence of ethanol-inducible rabbit liver cytochrome P-450 isozyme 3a (P450ALC). *Proc Natl Acad Sci USA*, 84, 638, 1987.
126. Kluck RM, Bossy-Wetzel E, Green DR and Newmeyer DD. The release of cytochrome c from mitochondria: a primary site for Bcl-2 regulation of apoptosis. *Science* 275, 1132, 1997.
127. Knecht KT, Bradford BU, Mason RP and Thurman RG. *in vivo* formation of a free radical metabolite of ethanol. *Mol Pharmacol* 38, 26, 1990.
128. Konishi H, Tanaka M, Takemura Y, *et al.* Activation of protein kinase C by tyrosine phosphorylation in response to H_2O_2. *Biochemistry* 94, 11233, 1997.
129. Korpela H, Kumpulainen J, Luoma PV, *et al.* Decreased serum selenium in alcoholics as related to liver structure and function. *Am J Clin Nutr* 42, 147, 1985.
130. Krejsa CM, Nadler SG, Esselstyn JM, *et al.* Role of oxidative stress in the action of vanadium phosphotryosine phospatase inhibitors. *J Biol Chem* 27, 11541, 1997.
131. Kretz-Remy C, Mehlen P, Mirault ME and Arrigo AP. Inhibition of IκB-α phosphorylation and degradation and subsequent NF-kB activation by glutathione peroxidase over-expression. *J Cell Biology* 133, 1083, 1996.
132. Kristal BS, Park B and Yu BP. Antioxidants reduce peroxyl-mediated inhibition of mitochondrial transcription. *Free Rad Biol Med*, 16, 653, 1994.
133. Kroemer G, Petit P, Zamzani N, *et al.* The biochemistry of programmed cell death. *FASEB J*, 9, 1277, 1995.
134. Kroemer G. The proto-oncogene Bcl-2 and its role in regulating apoptosis. *Nat Med*, 3, 614, 1997.
135. Kukielka E and Cederbaum AI. DNA strand cleavage as a sensitive assay for the production of hydroxyl radicals by microsomes: role of cytochrome P4502E1 in the increased activity after ethanol treatment. *Biochem J*, 302, 773, 1994.
136. Kukielka E, Dicker E and Cederbaum AI. Inreased production of reactive oxygen species by rat liver mitochondria after chronic ethanol treatment. *Archives Biochem Biophys* 309, 377, 1994.
137. Kulmacz RJ and Lands WEM. Peroxide tone in eicosanoid signaling. In *Oxidative Stress and Signal Transduction* (Eds. HJ Forman & E Cadenas) Chapman & Hall New York pp134-156, 1997.
138. Kulmacz RJ, Chen W and Wang L-H. Differential control of cyclooxygenase catalysis in PGH synthase isoforms: Role of hydroperoxide initiator. In *Frontiers in Bioactive Lipids* (Ed. JY Vanderhoek) Plenum Press New York pp101-10, 1996.
139. Kulmacz RJ, Pendleton RB and Lands WEM. Interaction between peroxidase and cyclooxygenase activities in prostaglandin-endoperoxide synthase. *J Biol Chem* 269, 5527, 1994.
140. Kume K and Shimizu T. Platelet-activating factor (PAF) induces growth stimulation inhibition and suppression of oncogenic transformation in NRK cells overexpressing the PAF receptor. *J Biol Chem* 272, 22898, 1997.

141. Kurose I, Higuchi H, Kato S, *et al.* Oxidative stress on mitochondria and cell membrane of cultured rat hepatocytes and perfused liver exposed to ethanol. *Gastroenterology* 112, 1331, 1997.
142. Kurose I, Higuchi H, Miura S, *et al.* Oxidative stress-mediated apoptosis of hepatocytes exposed to acute ethanol intoxication. *Hepatology* 25, 368, 1997.
143. Kurose I, Saito H, Miura S, *et al.* CD18/ICAM-1-dependent oxidative NF-κB activation leading to nitric oxide production in rat kupffer cells cocultured with syngeneic hepatoma cells. *J Clin Invest* 99, 867, 1997.
144. La Droitte P, Lamboeuf Y, de Saint Blanquat G and Bezaury J-P. Sensitivity of individual erythrocyte membrane phospholipids to changes in fatty acid composition in chronic alcoholic patients. *Alcoholism: Clin and Exptl Res* 9, 135, 1985.
145. Lander H. An essential role for free radicals and derived species in signal transduction. *FASEB J*, 11, 118, 1997.
146. Lands W and Hanel A. Phenolic anticyclooxygenase agents in antiinflammatory and analgesic therapy. *Prostaglandins* 24, 271, 1982.
147. Lands WEM. Cellular signals in alcohol-induced liver injury: A review. *Alcohol Clin Exp Res*, 19, 928, 1995.
148. Lands WEM. Alcohol and energy intake. *Am J Clin Nutr* 62, 1101S, 1995.
149. Larm JA, Vaillant F, Linnane AW and Lawen A. Up-regulation of the plasma membrane oxidoreductase as a prerequisite for the viability of human Namalwa rho 0 cells. *J Biol Chem* 269, 30097, 1994.
150. Lee F S, Hagler J, Chen ZJ and Manatis T. Activation of the IkappaB alpha kinase complex by MEKK1, a kinase of the JNK pathway. *Cell* 88, 213, 1997.
151. Lehr A-H, Weyrich AS, Saetzler RK, *et al.* Vitamin C blocks inflammatory platelet-activating factor mimetics created by cigarette smoking. *J Clin Invest* 99, 2358, 1997.
152. Lennon SV, Martin SJ and Cotter TG. Dose-dependent induction of apoptosis in human tumor cell lines by widely diverging stimuli. *Cell Prolif* 24, 203, 1991.
153. Leo MA and Lieber CS. Hepatic fibrosis after long-term administration of ethanol and moderate vitamin A supplementation in the rat. *Hepatology* 3, 1, 1983.
154. Leo MA, Arai M, Sato M and Lieber CS. Hepatotoxicity of vitamin A and ethanol in the rat. *Gastroenterology* 82, 194, 1982.
155. Leo MA, Kim C-I, Lowe N and Lieber CS. Interation of ethanol with β-carotene: Delayed blood clearance and enhanced hepatotoxicity. *Hepatology* 15, 883, 1992.
156. Lesch P, Schmidt E and Schmidt FW. Effects of chronic alcohol abuse on the fatty acid composition of major lipids in the human brain. *Z Klin Chem Klin Biochem* 11, 159, 1973.
157. Liao F, Andalibi A, Qiao J, *et al.* Genetic evidence for a common pathway mediating oxidative stress inflammatory gene induction and aortic fatty streak formation in mice. *J Clin Invest* 94, 877, 1994.
158. Lieber CS and DiCarli LM. Quantitative relationship between amount of dietary fat and severity of alcoholic fatty liver. *Am J Clin Nutr* 23, 474, 1970.
159. Lieber CS, Lasker J, DiCarli LM, *et al.* Role of acetone dietary fat, and total energy intake in induction of hepatic microsomeal ethanol oxidizing system. *J Pharmacol Exp Ther* 247, 791, 1988.
160. Lieber CS, Leo MA, Mak KM, *et al.* Attenuation of alcohol-induced hepatic fibrosis by polyunsaturated lecithin. *Hepatology* 12, 1390, 1990.
161. Lieber C, Leo MA, Aleynik SI, *et al.* Polyenylphosphatidylcholine decreases alcohol-induced oxidative stress in the baboon. *Alcoholism: Clin & Exp Res*, 21, 375, 1997.
162. Liu Y and Thurman RG. Potentiation of adriamycin toxicity by ethanol in perfused rat liver. *J Pharm & Exper Ther* 263, 651, 1992.

163. Lo YY C, Wong JMS and Cruzz TF. Reactive oxygen species mediate cytokine activation of c-Jun NH_2-terminal kinases. *J Biol Chem* 271, 1703, 1996.
164. Los M, Schenk H, Hexel K, *et al.* IL-2 gene expression and NF-κB activation through CD2b requires reactive oxygen production by 5-lipoxygenase. *EMBO J*, 14, 3731, 1995.
165. Luo Y, Bond JD and Ingram VM. Compromised mitochondrial function leads to increased cytosolic calcium and to activation of MAP kinases. *Proc Natl Acad Sci*, 94, 9705, 1997.
166. Macho A, Hirsch T, Marzo I, *et al.* Glutathione depletion is an early and calcium elevation is a late event of thymocyte apoptosis. *J Immunology* 158, 4612, 1997.
167. Maly I and Sasse D. Intraacinar profiles of alcohol dehydrogenase and aldehyde dehydrogenase activities in human liver. *Gastroenterology* 101, 1716, 1991.
168. Mandrekar P, Catalano D and Szabo G. Alcohol-induced regulation of nuclear regulatory factor- in human monocytes. *Alcoholism: Clin Exptl Res,* 21, 988, 1997.
169. Marley R, Harry D, Anand R, *et al.* 8-Isoprostaglandin F2-α, a product of lipid peroxidation increases portal pressure in normal and cirrhotic rats. *Gastroenterology* 112, 208, 1997.
170. Marsano L. Alcohol and malnutrition. *Alcohol Health & Res World* 17, 284, 1993.
171. Matsumura T, Yoshihara H, Jeffs R, T *et al.* Hormones increase oxygen uptake in periportal and pericentral regions of the liver lobule. *Am J Physiol 262, Gastrointest Liver Physiol* 25 G645, 1992.
172. Matsuoka M, Zhang M and Tsukamoto H. Sensitization of hepatic lipocytes by high-fat diet to stimulatory effects of Kupffer cell-derived factors: Implication in alcoholic liver fibrogenesis. *Hepatology* 11, 173, 1990.
173. McAdam PA, Smith DK, Feldman EB and Hames. Effect of age, sex, and race on selenium status of healthy residents of Augusta, Georgia. *Biol Trace Elem Res*, 6, 3, 1984.
174. McClain CJ and Su L-C. Zinc deficiency in the alcoholic: A review. *Alcoholism: Clin Exptl Res*, 7, 5, 1983.
175. Meagher EA, Lucey MR and FitzGerald GA. Oxidant injury in social drinking and alcoholic cirrhosis. *Hepatology* 24, 444A, 1996.
176. Mezey E. Interaction between alcohol and nutrition in the pathogenesis of alcoholic liver disease. *Semin Liver Dis*, 11, 340, 1991.
177. Mezey E. Metabolic effects of alcohol. *Federation Proc* 44, 134, 1985.
178. Mirochnitchenko O, Palnitkar U, Philbert M and Inouye M. Thermosensitive phenotype of transgenic mice overproducing human glutathione peroxidases. *Proc Natl Acad Sci*, Cell Biology 92, 8120, 1995.
179. Mironov S and Hermann A. Ethanol actions on the mechanisms of Ca^{2+} mobilization in rat hippocampal cells are mediated by protein kinase C. *Brain Res,* 714, 27, 1996.
180. Misra UK, Bradford BU, Handler JA and Thurman RG. Chronic ethanol treatment induces H_2O_2 production selectively in pericentral regions of the liver lobule. *Alcohol Clin Exp Res,* 16 839, 1992.
181. Misslebeck NG, Campbell TC and Roe DA. Effect of ethanol consumed in combination with high or low fat diets on the postinitiation phase of hepatocarcinogenesis in the rat. *J Nutr* 114, 2311, 1984.
182. Mitchell DY and Petersen DR. The oxidation of α, β-unsaturated aldehydic products of lipid peroxidation by rat liver aldehyde dehydrogenase. *Toxicol Appl Pharmacol* 87, 403, 1991.
183. Mobarhan S, Layden TJ, Friedman H, *et al.* Depletion of liver and esophageal epithelium vitamin A after chronic moderate ethanol consumption in rats: Inverse relation to zinc nutriture. *Hepatology* 6, 615, 1986.

184. Monahan C, Padgett E, Biber K, *et al.* Dose response to ethanol-containing liquid diets for use in a murine model for studies of biological effects due to ethanol consumption. *Alcoholism: Clin Exptl Res,* 21, 1092, 1997.
185. Morgan MY. Alcohol and nutrition. *Br Med Bull* 38, 21, 1982.
186. Morimoto M, Hagbjork A-L, Nanji AA, *et al.* Role of cytochrome P4502E1 in alcoholic liver disease pathogenesis. *Alcohol* 10, 459, 1993.
187. Morimoto M, Hagbjork A-L, Wan Y-JY, *et al.* Modulation of experimental alcohol-induced liver disease by cytochrome P450 2E1 inhibitors. *Hepatology* 21, 1610, 1995.
188. Morrow JD and Roberts LJ. Mass spectrometry of prostanoids: F2-isoprostanes produced by non-cyclooxygenase free radical-catalyzed mechanism. *Methods Enzymol* 23, 163, 1994.
189. Morrow JD, Awad JA, Boss HJ, *et al.* Non-cycloxygenase-derived prostanoids (F2-isoprostanes) are formed *in situ* on phospholipids. *Proc Natl Acad Sci USA,* 89, 10721, 1992.
190. Morrow JD, Awad JA, Kato T, *et al.* Formation of novel non-cyclooxygenase-derived prostanoids (F2-isoprostanes) in carbon tetrachloride hepatotoxicity: an animal model of lipid peroxidation. *J Clin Invest* 90, 250, 1992.
191. Morrow JD, Harris TM and Roberts LJ. Noncyclooxygenase oxidative formation of a series of novel prostglandins: Analytical ramifications for measurements of eicosanoids. *Anal Biochem* 184, 1, 1990.
192. Moser J, Bagchi D, Akubue PI and Stohs JS. Excretion of malondialdehyde, formaldehyde, acetaldehyde and acetone in the urine of rats following acute and chronic administration of ethanol. *Alcohol & Alcoholism* 28, 287, 1993.
193. Nakajima T, Ikatsu H, Okino T, *et al.*. Enhancement of ethanol-induced lipid peroxidation in rat liver by lowered carbohydrate intake. *Biochem Pharm* 43, 245, 1992.
194. Nakamura H, Nakamura K and Yodoi J. Redox regulation of cellular activation. *Annu Rev Immunol* 15, 351, 1997.
195. Nanji AA, Khwaja S, Tahan SR and Hossein Sadrzadeh SM. Plasma levels of a novel non-cyclooxygenase-derived prostanoid (8-isoprostane) correlate with severity of liver injury in experimental alcoholic liver disease. *J Pharm Exp Ther* 269, 1280, 1993.
196. Nanji AA, Miao L, Thomas P, *et al.* Enhanced cyclooxygenase-2 gene expression in alcoholic liver disease in the rat. *Gastroenterology* 112, 943, 1997.
197. Nanji AA, Zhao S, Khwaja S, *et al.* Cimetidine prevents alcoholic hepatic injury in the intragastric feeding rat model. *J Pharm Exp Ther* 269 832, 1994.
198. Navab M, Hama-Levy S, Van Lenten BJ, *et al.* Mildly oxidized LDL induces an increased apolipoprotein J/paraoxonase ratio. *J Clin Invest* 99, 2005, 1997.
199. Negre-Salvayre A, Hirtz C, Carrera G, *et al.* A role for uncoupling protein-2 as a regulator of mitochondrial hydrogen peroxide generation. *FASEB J,* 11, 809, 1997.
200. Neiman J, Curstedt T and Cronholm T. Composition of platelet phosphatidylinositol and phosphatidylcholine after ethanol withdrawal. *Thrombosis Res,* 46, 295, 1987.
201. Neville JN, Eagles JA, Samson G and Olson RE. Nutritional status of alcoholics. *Am J Clin Nutr* 21, 1329, 1968.
202. Niknahad H, Khan S, and O'Brien PJ. Hepatocyte injury resulting from the inhibition of mitochondrial respiration at low oxygen concentrations involves reductive stress and oxygen activation. *Chem Biol Interact* 98, 27, 1995.
203. Nordmann R. Alcohol and antioxidant systems. *Alcohol & Alcoholism* 29, 513, 1994.
204. Nordmann R, Ribiere C and Rouach H. Implication of free radical mechanisms in ethanol-induced cellular injury. *Free Rad Biol Med* 12, 219, 1992.

205. Nrooz-Zadeh J, Liu ECL, Anggard EE and Halliwell B. F4-isoprostanes: A novel class of prostanoids formed during peroxidation of docosahexaenoic acid (DHA). *Biochem Biophys Res Commun* 242, 338, 1998.
206. Okita M, Miyamoto A, Wakabayashi H and Watanabe A. Improvement of polyunsaturated fatty acid deficiency in decompensated cirrhotic patients by arachidonic acid-rich oil capsules in *Advances in Polyunsaturated Fatty Acid Research* Yasugi T, Nakamura H and Soma M, Eds, Elsevier Science Pub, Tokyo 1993.
207. Okita M, Suzuki K, Sasagawa T, *et al.* Effect of arachidonate on lipid metabolism in ethanol-treated rats fed with lard. *J Nutr Sci Vitaminol* 43, 311, 1997.
208. Palomba L, Sestili P, Cattabeni F, *et al.* Prevention of necrosis and activation of apopotosis in oxidatively injured human myeloid leukemia U937 cells. *FEBS Lett* 390, 91, 1996.
209. Park J, Kim, I, Oh YJ, *et al.* Activation of c-Jun N-terminal kinase antagonizes an anti-apoptotic action of Bcl-2. *J Biol Chem* 272, 16725, 1997.
210. Parola M, Pinzani M, Casini A, *et al.* Stimulation of lipid peroxidation or 4-hydroxynonenal treatment increases procollagen-gene expression in human liver fat-storing cells. *Bioch Biophy Res Comm* 194, 1044, 1993.
211. Patel KD, Zimmerman GA, Prescott SM and McIntyre TM. Novel leukocyte agonists are released by endothelial cells exposed to peroxide. *J Biol Chem* 267, 15168, 1992.
212. Patel T and Gores GJ. Inhibition of bile-salt-induced hepatocyte apoptosis by the antioxidant lazaroid U83836E. *Tox & Appl Pharm* 142, 116, 1997.
213. Pawlosky RJ, Flynn BM and Salem NJr. The effects of a low essential fatty acid diet on alcohol-induced liver fibrosis in rhesus monkeys. *Hepatology* 26, 1387, 1997.
214. Porta EA. Symposium: Nutritional factors and oxidative stress in experimental alcoholic liver disease. *J Nutr* 127, 893S, 1997.
215. Preedy VR and Peters TJ. Alcohol and skeletal muscle disease. *Alcohol & Alcoholism* 25, 177, 1990.
216. Qin S, Minami Y, Kurosaki T and Yamamura H. Distinctive functions of syk and lyn in mediating osmotic stress- and ultraviolet c irradiation-induced apoptosis in chicken B cells. *J Biol Chem* 272, 17994, 1997.
217. Quillet-Mary A, Jaffrezou JP, Mansat V, *et al.* Implication of mitochondrial hydrogen peroxide generation in ceramide-induced apoptosis. *J Biol Chem* 272, 21388, 1997.
218. Rao GA and Larkin EC. Nutritional factors required for alcoholic liver disease in rats. *J Nutr* 127, 896S, 1997.
219. Rao GN, Runge MS and Alexander RW. Hydrogen peroxide activation of cytosolic phospholipase A_2 in vascular smooth muscle cells. *Biochim Biophys Acta* 1265, 67, 1995.
220. Rao G, Glasgow WC, Eling TE and Runge MS. Role of hydroperoxyeicosatetraenoic acids in oxidative stress-induced activation protein 1 (AP-1) activity. *J Biol Chem* 271, 27760, 1996.
221. Rao G. Hydrogen peroxide induces complex formation of SHC-Grb2-SOS with receptor tyrosine kinase and activates Ras and extracellular signal-regulated protein kinases group of mitogen-activated protein kinases. *Oncogene* 13, 713, 1996.
222. Rao G. Protein tyrosine kinase activity is required for oxidant-induced extracellular signal-regulated protein kinase activation and c-fos and c-jun expression. *Cell Signal* 9, 181, 1997.
223. Rao GA, Larkin EC, Derr RF. Biologic effects of chronic alcohol consumption related to a deficient intake of carbohydrate. *Alcohol* 21, 369, 1986.
224. Reed DJ and Savage MK. Influence of metabolic inhibitors on mitochondrial permeability transition and glutathione status. *Biochim Biophys Acta* 1271, 43, 1995.
225. Reed D. Status of calcium and thiols in hepatocellular injury by oxidative stress. *Semin Liver Dis* 10, 285, 1990.

226. Reinecke LA and McCay PB. Spin trapping studies of alcohol-initiated radicals in rat liver: Influence of dietary fat. *J Nutr* 127, 899S, 1997.
227. Reitz RC. The effects of ethanol ingestion on lipid metabolism. *Prog Lipid Res*, 18, 87, 1979.
228. Reitz RC, Wang L, Schilling RJ, *et al.* Effects of ethanol ingestion on the unsaturated fatty acids from various tissues. *Prog Lipid Res*, 20, 209, 1981.
229. Reitz RC. Dietary fatty acids and alcohol: effects on cellular membranes. *Alcohol* 28, 59, 1993.
230. Ribiere C, Hininger I, Rouach H and Nordmann R. Effects of chronic ethanol administration on free radical defence in rat myocardium. *Biochem Pharma* 44, 1495, 1992.
231. Rimm E and Colditz G. Smoking, alcohol, and plasma levels of carotenes and vitamin E. *Annals New York Acad Sci* 686, 323, 1993.
232. Ringstad J, Knutsen SF, Nilssen OR and Thomassen Y. A comparative study of serum selenium and vitamin E levels in a population of male risk drinkers and abstainers in *Biological Trace Element Research* Vol 36, The Humana Press Inc, Totowa, New Jersey, 1993.
233. Rissanen A, Sarlio-Lahteenkorva S, Alfthan G, *et al.* Employed problem drinkers: a nutritional risk group? *Am J Clin Nutr* 45, 456, 1987.
234. Roberts BJ, Song BJ, Soh Y, *et al.* Ethanol induces CYP2E1 by protein stabilization. *J Biol Chem* 270, 29632, 1996.
235. Roberts LJ and Morrow JD. The generation and actions of isoprostanes. *Biochim Biophys Acta* 1345, 121, 1997.
236. Roberts LJ, Moore KP, Zackert WE, O *et al.* Identification of the major urinary metabolite of the F2-isoprostane 8-isoprostaglandin F2-α in humans. *J Biol Chem* 271, 20617, 1996.
237. Rosenblum ER, Gavaler JS and Van Thiel DH. Lipid peroxidation: A mechanism for alcohol-induced testicular injury. *Free Rad Biol Med*, 7, 569, 1989.
238. Rouach H, Fataccioli V, Gentil M, *et al.* Effect of chronic ethanol feeding on lipid peroxidation and protein oxidation in relation to liver pathology. *Hepatology* 25, 351, 1997.
239. Russell RM, Morrison SA, Smith FR, *et al.* Vitamin-A reversal of abnormal dark adaptation in cirrhosis. *Annals of Internal Med,* 88, 622, 1978.
240. Salem NJr and Olsson NU. Abnormalities in essential fatty acid status in alcoholism in *Handbook of Essential Fatty Acid Biology: Biochemistry Physiology and Behavioral Neurobiology,* Yehuda S and Mostofsky DI, Eds, Humana Press Inc, Totowa New Jersey 1997, pp 67.
241. Salem N Jr and Ward G. The effects of ethanol on polyunsaturated fatty acid composition in *Alcohol Cell Membranes and Signal Transduction in Brain,* Alling C, *et al.* Eds, Plenum Press New York 1993, pp 33.
242. Sandstrom PA, Pardi D, Tebbey PW, *et al.* Lipid hydroperoxide-induced apoptosis: lack of inhibition by Bcl-2 over-expression. *FEBS Lett* 365, 66, 1995.
243. Sankaran H, Baba GC, Deveney CW, *et al.* Enteral macronutrients abolish high blood alcohol levels in chronic alcoholic rats. *Nutr Res,* 11, 217, 1991.
244. Sasada T, Iwata S, Sato N, *et al.* Redox control of resistance to *cis*-diamminedichloroplatinum (II) (CDDP). *J Clin Invest* 97, 2268, 1996.
245. Saso K, Moehren G, Higashi K and Hoek JB. Differential inhibition of epidermal growth factor signalling pathways in rat hepatocytes by long term ethanol treatment *Gastroenterology* 112, 2073, 1997.
246. Sato M and Lieber CS. Hepatic vitamin A depletion after chronic ethanol consumption in baboons and rats. *J Nutr* 111, 2015, 1981.
247. Sato N, Iwata S, Nakamura K, *et al.* Thiol-mediated redox regulation of apoptosis. *J Immunol* 154, 3194, 1995.

248. Savage MK and Rees DJ. Release of mitochondrial glutathione and calcium by a cyclosporin. A sensitive mechanism occurs without large amplitude swelling. *Arch Biochem Biophys* 315, 142, 1994.
249. Savill J. Apoptosis in resolution of inflammation. *J Leu Biol* 61, 375, 1997.
250. Schlossberg H, Zhang Y, Dudus L and Englehardt JF. Expression of c-fos and c-jun during hepatocellular remodeling following ischemia/reperfusion in mouse liver. *Hepatology* 23, 1546, 1996.
251. Schmidt K, Traenckner B, Meier B and Baeuerle P. Induction of oxidative stress by okadaic acid is required for activation of transcription factor NFκB. *J Biol Chem* 270, 27136, 1995.
252. Schulze-Osthoff K, Bakker AC, Vanhaesenbroeck B, *et al.* Cytotoxic activity of tumor necrosis factor is mediated by early damage of mitochondrial functions. Evidence for the involvement of mitochondrial radical generation. *J Biol Chem* 267, 5317, 1992.
253. Shaw S, Rubin KP and Lieber CS. Depressed hepatic glutathione and increased diene conjugates in alcoholic liver disease. *Dig Dis & Sci*, 28 585, 1983.
254. Shih DM, Gu L, Hama S, Xia Y-R, *et al.* Genetic-dietary regulation of serum paraoxonase expression and its role in atherogenesis in a mouse model. *J Clin Invest* 97, 1630, 1996.
255. Snook JT. Effect of ethanol use and other lifestyle variables on measures of selenium status. *Alcohol* 8, 13, 1991.
256. Snyder F. Platelet-activating factor and its analogs:metabolic pathways and related intracellular processes. *Biochim Biophys Acta* 1254, 231, 1995.
257. Somogyi JC and Kopp PM. Relation between chronic alcoholism drug addiction and nutrition with special reference to the thiamine status. *Bibl Nutr Dieta* 30, 131, 1981.
258. Song B-J, Gelboin HV, Park SS, *et al.* Complementary DNA and protein sequences of ethanol-inducible rat and human cytochrome P450s. *J Biol Chem* 261, 16689, 1986.
259. Spiteller G. Review: On the chemistry of oxidative stress. *I Lipid Mediat* 7, 199, 1993.
260. Stafforini DM, Satoh K, Atkinson DL, *et al.* Platelet-activating factor acetylhydrolase deficiency. *J Clin Invest* 97, 2784, 1996.
261. Stone RL and Dixon JE. Protein-tyrosine phosphatases. *J Biol Chem* 269, 31323, 1994.
262. Sulciner D, Irani K, Yu Z, *et al.* rac1 Regulates a cytokine-stimulated redox-dependent pathway necessary for NF-kappaB activation. *Mol Cell Biol* 16, 7115, 1996.
263. Sun IL, Sun EE, Crane FL, *et al.* Requirement for coenzyme Q in plasma membrane electron transport. *Proc Natl Acad Sci USA*, 89, 11126, 1992.
264. Takahashi K, Nammour TM, Fukunaga M, *et al.* Glomerular actions of a free radical-generated novel prostaglandin 8-epi-prostaglandin F2-α, in the rat. Evidence for interaction with thromboxane A2 receptors. *J Clin Invest* 90, 136, 1992.
265. Tanaka T, Minamino H, Unezaki S, *et al.* Formation of platlet activating factor-like phospholipids by Fe2+/ascorbate/EDTA-induced lipid peroxidation. *Biochim Biophys Acta* 1166, 264, 1993.
266. Tasinato A, Boscoboinik D, Bartoli G-M, *et al.* d-α-Tocopherol inhibition of vascular smooth muscle cell proliferation occurs at physiological concentrations correlates with protein kinase C inhibition and is independent of its antioxidant properties. *Proc Natl Acad Sci, USA*, 92, 12190, 1995.
267. Thome J, Foley P, Gsell W, *et al.* Increased concentrations of manganese superoxide dismutase in serum of alcohol-dependent patients. *Alcohol & Alcoholism,* 32, 65, 1997.
268. Thome J, Nara K, Foley P, *et al.* Time course of manganese superoxide dismutase concentrations in serum of alcohol-dependent patients during abstinence. *Drug Alcohol Depend* 44 151, 1997.
269. Thomson M, Fulton M, Elton RA, *et al.* Alcohol consumption and nutrient intake in middle-aged Scottish men. *Am J Clin Nutr* 47, 139, 1988.

270. Topinka J, Binkova B, Sram RJ and Fojtikova I. DNA-repair capacity and lipid peroxidation in chronic alcoholics. *Mutation Res*, 263, 133, 1991.
271. Tournier C, Thomas G, Pierre J, *et al.* Mediation by arachidonic acid metabolites of the H_2O_2-induced stimulation of mitogen-activated protein kinases (extracellular-signal-regulated kinase and c-Jun NH2-terminal kinase). *Eur J Biochem* 244, 587, 1997.
272. Tsuchida H, Miura T, Mitzutami K and Aibara K. Fluorescent substances in mouse and human serum as a parameter of *in vivo* lipid peroxidation. *Biochim Biophys Acta* 834, 196, 1985.
273. Tsukamoto H. Oxidative stress antioxidants and alcoholic liver fibrogenesis. *Alcohol* 10, 465, 1993.
274. Tuma DJ, Thiele GM, Xu D, *et al.* Acetaldehyde and malondialdehyde react together to generate distinct adducts in the liver during long-term ethanol administration. *Hepatology* 23, 872, 1996.
275. Uchida K and Stadtman ER. Modification of histidine residues in proteins by reaction with 4-hydroxynonenal. *Proc Natl Acad Sci USA*, 89, 4544, 1992.
276. Uchida K, Szweda LI, Chae H-Z and Stadtman E R. Immunochemical detection of 4-hydoxynonenal protein adducts in oxidized hepatocytes. *Proc Natl Acad Sci USA*, 90, 8742, 1993.
277. Valimaki MJ, Harju KJ and Ylikahri RH. Decreased serum selenium in alcoholics--a consequence of liver dysfunction. *Clin Chim Acta* 130, 291, 1983.
278. Van Kuijk FJ, Siakotos AN, Fong LG, *et al.* Quantitative measurement of 4-hydroxyalkenals in oxidized low density lipoprotein by gas chromatography-mass spectrometry. *Anal Biochem* 224, 420, 1995.
279. Vendemeiale G, Altomare E, Grattagliano I and Albano O. Increased plasma levels of glutathione and malondialdehyde after acute ethanol ingestion in humans. *J Hepatology* 9, 359, 1989.
280. Videla LA, and Valenzuela A. Alcohol ingestion liver glutathione and lipoperoxidation: metabolic interrelations and pathological implications. *Life Sciences* 31, 2395, 1982.
281. Von Knethen A and Brune B. Cyclooxygenase-2: an essential regulator of NO-mediated apoptosis. *FASEB J*, 11, 887, 1997.
282. Wang Z, Ciabattoni G, Creminon C, *et al.* Immunoassay of urinary 8-epi-PGF2-α. *J Pharmacol Exp Ther* 275, 94, 1995.
283. Wang JF and Spitzer JJ. Alcohol-induced thymocyte apoptosis is accompanied by impaired mitochondrial function. *Alcohol* 14, 99, 1997.
284. Ward RJ and Peters TJ. The antioxidant status of patients with either alcohol-induced liver damage or myopathy. *Alcohol & Alcoholism* 27, 359, 1992.
285. Watson AD, Leitinger N, Navab M, *et al.* Structural identification by mass spectrometry of oxidized phospholipids in minimally oxidized low density liprprotein that induce monocyte/endothelial interactions and evidence for their presence *in vivo*. *J Biol Chem* 272, 13587, 1997.
286. Watson AJM, Askew JN and Benson RSP. Poly(adenosine diphosphate ribose) polymerase inhibition prevents necrosis induced by H_2O_2 but not apoptosis. *Gastroenterology* 109, 472, 1995.
287. Watzl B and Watson RR. Role of alcohol abuse in nutritional immunosuppression. *J Nutr* 122, 733, 1992.
288. Waugh RJ and Murphy RC. Mass spectrometric analysis of four regioisomers of F2-isoprostanes formed by free radical oxidation of arachidonic acid. *J Am Soc Mass Spec* 7, 490, 1996.

289. Weltman MD, Farrell GC and Liddle C. Increased hepatocyte CYP2E1 expression in a rat nutritional model of hepatic steatosis with inflammation. *Gastroenterology* 111, 1645, 1996.
290. Wolvetang EJ, Johnson KL, Krauer K, *et al.* Mitochondrial respiratory chain inhibitors induce apoptosis. *FEBS Lett* 339, 40, 1994.
291. World MJ, Ryle PR and Thomson AD. Alcoholic malnutrition and the small intestine. *Alcohol & Alcoholism* 20, 89, 1985.
292. Wu D and Cederbaum AI. Ethanol cytotoxicity to a transfected hepG2 cell line expressing human cytochrome P4502E1. *J Biol Chem* 271, 23914, 1996.
293. Xia A, Dickens M, Raingeaud J, *et al.* Opposing effects of ERK and JNK-p38 MAP kinases on apoptosis. *Science* 270, 1326, 1995.
294. Yakes FM, and Van Houten B. Mitochondrial DNA damage is more extensive and persists longer than nuclear DNA damage in human cells following oxidative stress. *Proc Natl Acad Sci USA*, 94, 514, 1997.
295. Yang J, Liu X, Bhalla K, *et al.* Prevention of apoptosis by Bcl-2: release of cytochrome c from mitochondria blocked. *Science* 275, 1129, 1997.
296. Yang MX and Cederbaum AI. Characterization of cytochrome P4502E1 turnover in transfected hepG2 cells expressing human CYP2E1. *Arch Biochem Biophys* 341, 25, 1997.
297. Yonaha M and Tampo Y. Bromosulfophthalein abolishes glutathione-dependent protection against lipid peroxidation in rat liver mitochondria. *Biochem Pharmacol* 36, 2831, 1987.
298. Yonekura I, Nakano M and Sato A. Effects of carbohydrate intake on the blood ethanol level and alcoholic fatty liver damage in rats. *J Hepatol* 17, 97, 1993.
299. Zhang P, Liu B, Kang S, *et al.* Thioredoxin peroxidase is a novel inhibitor of apoptosis with a mechanism distinct from that of Bcl-2, *J Biol Chem* 272, 30615, 1997.
300. Zhao M, Matter K, Laissue JA and Zimmermann A. Copper/zinc and manganese superoxide dismutases in alcoholic liver disease: immunohistochemical quantitation. *Histol Histopathol* 11, 899, 1996.
301. Zimmerman GA, Prescott SM and McIntyre TM. Oxidatively fragmented phospholipids as inflammatory mediators: the dark side of polyunsaturated lipids. *J Nutr* 125(Suppl), 1661S, 1995.
302. Zloch Z. Temporal changes of the lipid peroxidation in rats after acute intoxication by ethanol. *Z Naturforsch* 49, 359, 1994.
303. Zou H, Henzel WJ, Liu X, *et al.* Apaf-1, a human protein homologous to C elegans CED-4, participates in cytochrome c-dependent activation of caspase-3. *Cell* 90, 405, 1997.

Part 5

Proposed Modes of Action of Antioxidants

- Low Density Lipoprotein Oxidation
- Immune Function
- Ultraviolet-Induced Nonmelanoma Skin Cancer
- Digesta and Colon Cancer
- Beyond Antioxidant Function: Other Biochemical Effects

16

Antioxidants and Low Density Lipoprotein Oxidation

Sampath Parthasarathy, Nalini Santanam, and Nathalie Augè
Department of Gynecology and Obstetrics
Emory University, Atlanta, Georgia USA

INTRODUCTION

α-Tocopherol and other antioxidants have long been suggested to be important preventative and/or therapeutic agents against a number of diseases including cancer and heart disease. Although the biochemical and pharmacological basis for such a role of α-tocopherol has not been questioned, its role in the physiological basis of the etiology of these diseases was, until recent years, not understood. Rapid advances in understanding the molecular mechanism(s) of atherosclerosis have now made it possible to suggest mechanism(s) by which antioxidants may retard progression of coronary artery disease.

0-8493-8009-X/98/$0.00+$.50

IS OXIDATION A RISK FACTOR?

Coronary heart disease (CHD) remains the number one killer in the Western society. Despite dramatic advances in treating CHD, its complete prevention remains elusive. Much of the progress made in our understanding of coronary artery disease or atherosclerosis can be traced to identification of several major risk factors.[1] These include elevated plasma cholesterol, diabetes, hypertension, and smoking. In addition, increased plasma Lipoprotein (a) Lp(a) levels, lack of physical activity, and elevated homocysteine levels may also affect progression of the disease. While these factors can be measured and quantified, "oxidative stress," which is neither measurable nor comparable among subjects, has emerged as a novel potential risk factor.[1] Researchers have tried to explain the impact of other risk factors on the basis of oxidation. While oxidation may be one of the mechanisms initiating atherosclerosis, oxidation as a risk factor remains to be established.

MOLECULAR BASIS OF ATHEROSCLEROSIS

Intracellular Accumulation of Lipids (Foam Cells)

One of the earliest events in atherogenesis is intracellular accumulation of lipids, particularly cholesterol esters, in the aortic intima. Lipids presumably come from uptake of plasma lipoproteins, particularly low density lipoproteins (LDL). The lipids are accumulated in foam cells, which are predominantly macrophages. *In vitro* incubation of macrophages with LDL does not lead to accumulation of cholesterol esters. Brown and his co-workers suggested that the charge on the particle may play a role in its uptake and demonstrated that acetylated LDL that bears an increased negative charge was taken up by macrophages.[2] Uptake was not mediated by the LDL receptor, but by a novel class of receptors, the scavenger receptor; the associated pathway was designated as the scavenger pathway. Acetylation to the degree required for scavenger receptor-mediated uptake, however, does not occur *in vivo*.

Role of Modified LDL

Fogelman and associates, realizing that formation of Schiff bases involving the amino groups of lysine and malondialdehyde (MDA), a product of lipid peroxidation, would also result in the acquisition of a net negative charge, generated MDA modified LDL and found it was readily taken up and degraded by macrophages.[3] They concluded that MDA could be generated *in vivo* during aggregation of platelets (from degradation of thromboxanes) or via lipid peroxidation.

Henriksen *et al.* reported that LDL incubated with endothelial cells was also internalized by macrophages.[4] Steinbrecher *et al.* demonstrated later that modification of LDL by endothelial cells occurred in Ham's F-10 medium (cell culture media which contains micromolar amounts of transition metals such as copper and iron) and was associated with production of large amounts of MDA.[5] They also showed that antioxidants inhibiting formation of MDA also inhibited modification of LDL. The rapid modification of LDL in Ham's F-10 medium was attributed to the presence of the prooxidant metals iron and copper, in the medium.

At the same time, the oxidation of LDL by endothelial cells was described. Heinecke *et al.* found that modification of LDL by smooth muscle cells was also related to lipid peroxidation.[6] Most of the earlier studies focused on generation of a modified LDL by an oxidative process that resulted in an increased uptake by macrophages. Since these initial studies, a number of cell types including fibroblasts, neutrophils, monocytes, macrophages, and others have been shown to oxidize LDL. However, serious doubts remain whether most of these cell types are indeed capable of initiating oxidation of LDL. Even though it was generally assumed that the actual uptake process was due to modification of apoprotein, it was not until several years later that studies by Parthasarathy *et al.*[7] using lipid-free, solubilized apoprotein established that the protein moiety was responsible for recognition by macrophages. For this reason, most of the earlier studies referred to oxidized LDL as oxidatively modified LDL. The term " modification" which originally referred to protein alterations, in later years included lipid alterations as well. Now modified LDL may simply refer to any LDL particle that has properties different from those of native, plasma LDL. A large number of review articles on oxidized LDL[8-12] have appeared in recent years. This chapter will focus on topics that have not been discussed in those reviews.

What is Oxidized LDL?

The term oxidized LDL (or oxidized lipoproteins, as similar modifications are feasible in other lipoproteins) has been used without any definition. There may not be a simple way to define an oxidized LDL. Oxidized LDL represents LDL exposed to an oxidant or LDL that may have lipid peroxides or products of lipid peroxidation associated with it. For example, the following may represent oxidized LDL (Figure 1):

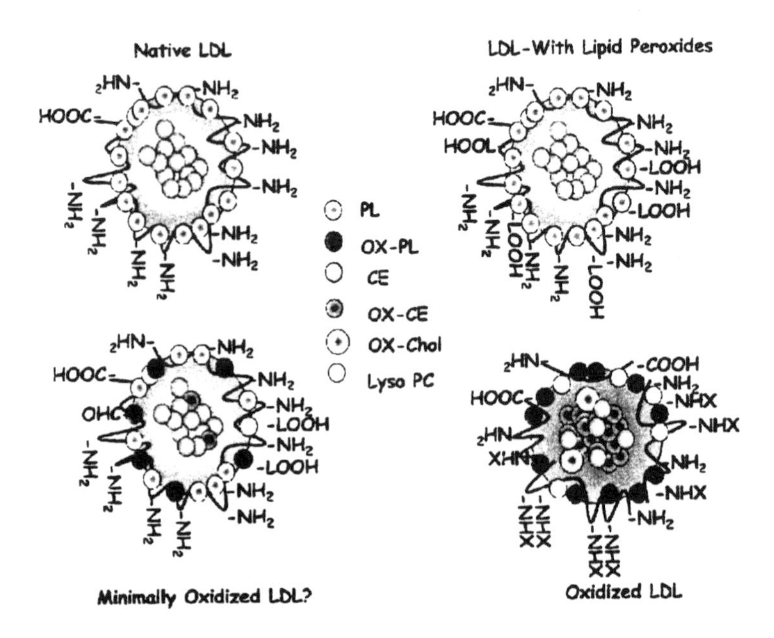

Figure 1. Native LDL, LDL with lipid peroxides, minimally oxidized LDL, and oxidized LDL. Each form is described in detail below.

1. LDL associated with lipid peroxides. Oxidized lipid does not always result from direct oxidation of LDL. Peroxidized lipids generated elsewhere in the system, besides the plasma compartment, may associate with LDL and generate particles that have altered physical and biological properties. This represents a "seeding" mechanism that may enhance susceptibility of LDL to further oxidation.
2. Oxidized LDL that contain limited amounts of lipid oxidation products. "Minimally modified LDL," as described by Berliner and associates meets these criteria.[13] A distinguishing characteristic may be the direct oxidation of LDL lipids.
3. Extensively oxidized LDL has changes in the apoprotein moiety that are recognized by macrophages.[14] This is also a poor definition. LDL can be oxidized by a variety of means and all of these methods may generate a particle that is avidly taken up by macrophages. However, the nature or extent of oxidation among these methods could be quite different. For example, oxidation of LDL by copper causes extensive fragmentation of oxidized lipids and production of very high thiobarbituric acid reactive

substance (TBARS).[15,16] On the other hand, oxidation of LDL by peroxidases, free radical generators, peroxynitrite or hypochlorous acid (HOCl) do not produce high (TBARS) levels, yet the oxidized LDL is rapidly degraded by macrophages. These methods can also directly affect the apoprotein. For example, treatment of LDL with Azobis amidino propane, hydrochloride (AAPH) at mM levels causes not just limited proteolysis, but extensive apoprotein degradation.[17] The majority of studies evaluating the oxidation of LDL by AAPH have overlooked the effects of such extensive damage to the apoprotein and it is very unlikely that such a particle could ever be generated *in vivo* regardless of how extensive the oxidation is.

Changes That Occur in the LDL Particle Caused by Oxidation

LDL undergoes rapid physicochemical changes during oxidation and some of these changes have been correlated with altered biological properties.

Electrophoretic Mobility

Alterations in electrophoretic mobility during oxidation have received considerable attention because of their potential role in the recognition by macrophages. Modifications of lysine residues of apoprotein B by-products of lipid peroxidation do not fully account for increased electrophoretic mobility. In addition to modification of lysine by aldehyde products generated from lipid peroxidation, direct oxidation of apoprotein B that results in formation of carboxylic acids and sulfonic acids should be considered. Presence of lipid peroxides does not necessarily mean that aldehydes are the only products involved in the modification of apoprotein B. For example, Fruebis *et al.* described a direct interaction between lysine residues of protein and peroxidized lipids that generated antigenic fluorescent adducts.[18] Kim *et al.*[19] and others[20,21] have developed antibodies to lipid peroxide-modified proteins and have shown the presence of such modified epitopes in oxidized LDL and in atherosclerotic lesions.

Change in Buoyant Density

Of all properties attributed to oxidized LDL, change in buoyant density attracted the least attention, yet this property might be the most important in determining the relevance of oxidation in the plasma. Oxidation gradually increases buoyant density distribution of the LDL particle and peak density increases from about 1.036 to as high as 1.06. This finding provides clues to the susceptibility of LDL of different density classes to oxidation.[4,22] There are, however, several compounding factors to be considered. Lipid distribution, particle size, fatty acid composition, and physical mapping of apoprotein at the surface might be important contributors without the need for particles that have undergone a milder degree of oxidation.

Chemical Changes

Chemical changes occurring during LDL oxidation include:

- loss of antioxidants
- loss of polyunsaturated fatty acids
- generation of lipid peroxidation products including lipid peroxides, hydroxides, aldehydes, ketones, and hydrocarbons
- generation of lysophospholipids and oxidatively tailored phospholipids
- oxidative scission of apoprotein
- oxidative loss of specific amino acids of the apoprotein
- oxidative conversion of one amino acid into another
- generation of protein carbonyls
- covalent modification of the protein involving products of lipid peroxidation including intact oxidized phospholipids and oxidized cholesterol esters
- modification of the apoprotein involving cross-links by products of lipid peroxidation
- modification of the apoprotein involving cross-links by the formation of dityrosine
- modification of the protein by products derived from the oxidation of amino acids
- products formed from the interaction of oxidized lipids and proteins with nitric oxide
- modified amino lipids.

Loss of Antioxidants and the Role of PUFA

One of the earliest changes that occur during oxidation of LDL is loss of antioxidants. Pioneering studies by Esterbauer and co-workers explained the temporal relationship between loss of antioxidants and rapid propagation of lipid peroxidation.[23-25] Antioxidants, such as vitamin E that reside in LDL, are lost within minutes after subjecting LDL particles to oxidation. Loss of PUFA during oxidation should be viewed with caution. A number of earlier studies have suggested the presence of decreased amounts of linoleic acid in adipose tissue and artery of atherosclerotic subjects.[26] This was viewed as deficiency. The oxidation hypothesis would suggest that this could be due to depletion. Deficiency and depletion would have different effects on supplemental fatty acids. If oxidation causes depletion, then adding more fatty acids would be equivalent to adding fuel to the fire and such may be the case with marine oil derived PUFA. There are excellent reviews on this topic and the majority of them concluded that fish oil has beneficial effects on atherosclerosis. Reported beneficial effects included lowering plasma lipids and and platelet aggregation. However, an analysis of the literature would clearly show the following differences: fish or crude fish oil had a clear protective effect as compared to refined, enriched, commercial preparations of fish oil that contain large amounts of eicosapentaenoic and docosahexaenoic acids. The effects of preparations of these specific fatty acids depended on the amount of cholesterol in the diet. When the diet contained very low amounts of cholesterol (0.5%), the preparations had, at least in some studies, a beneficial effect. With high (1-2%) cholesterol diets, these preparations increased the severity of atherosclerosis. In such cases increased levels of lipid peroxidation were also seen in plasma. Careful examination of the data leads to the following conclusions.

- Large amounts of highly unsaturated fatty acids may counteract the membrane rigidifying effect of cholesterol and prevent, among other things, generation of oxygen radicals. Under these conditions they affect platelet and monocyte functions.
- When there is severe hypercholesterolemia, the rate of oxidation is certainly enhanced, and fish oil-derived PUFA-enriched LDL may suffer an even greater degree of oxidation as compared to lipoprotein that is enriched in plant-derived PUFA.
- If the beneficial effects of these PUFA, or any PUFA are to be realized, regardless of the disease in question, they need to be protected from oxidation both *in vitro* and *in vivo*. There are clear indications from literature that a PUFA diet depletes antioxidants and a monounsaturated enriched diet conserves plasma antioxidants.

Very few studies have addressed the oxidizability of LDL enriched in fish oil-derived PUFA. Advocates of fish oil have not been receptive to the suggestion that these PUFA, regardless of origin, could enhance the oxidation of LDL and promote atherogenesis. In the past few years, a number of patients have been consuming large amounts of purified fish oil without adequate protection.

Protective Effect of Monounsaturated Fatty Acids

Fish oils also contain very large proportions of monounsaturated fatty acids and very little linoleic acid.[27] The protective effect of monounsaturated fatty acids on oxidation of LDL has been examined by Parthasarathy *et al.*[28]

in rabbits and by Reaven *et al.* [29,30] and by others in humans.[31,32] The availability of edible oils vastly enriched in oleic acid provided an opportunity to alter the fatty acid composition of LDL in normal and hypercholesterolemic subjects and results clearly established that the rate of oxidation of LDL enriched in oleic acid is much lower than that of LDL enriched in linoleic acid. This was not due to differences in the antioxidant content of lipoprotein although there is reason to suspect oleic acid itself could have acted as an "antioxidant." At present there are no published reports that consumption of large quantities of monounsaturated fatty acid may protect against atherosclerosis. Yet, epidemiological studies that point to the benefits of the Mediterranean diet, the cholesterol-lowering effect on monounsaturated fatty acid, and its effect on LDL oxidation should make monounsaturated fatty acids an attractive choice for replacing the saturated fat in the diet. Surprisingly, humans may have a protective mechanism that naturally increases the level of oleic acid in the lipoprotein. Studies by Grundy *et al.*[33] have shown that in humans a large proportion of stearic acid might be readily converted to oleic acid, which, in turn, might explain the difference between palmitic and stearic acid in their atherogenicity. There has been no study, however, demonstrating the beneficial effects of MUFA on experimental atherosclerosis. In contrast, PUFA have been shown by Rudel and co-workers to decrease the extent of atherosclerosis in monkeys.[34]

INHIBITORS OF LDL OXIDATION

The list of compounds that can inhibit LDL oxidation by virtue of their antioxidant properties is growing steadily (Table 1). In addition to probucol, vitamin E, ascorbic acid and other well-known antioxidants such as diphenylphenylenediamine (DPPD), estrogens, 21-amino steroids, RU-486, a spin trap, α-phenyl-n-tert-butylnitrone (PBN), calcium channel blockers, aminoguanidine, tamoxifen and catechin, isoflavones, and a number of natural as well as synthetic chemicals have been added to the list. Whether or not these compounds will have any value in preventing oxidation of LDL *in vivo* remains to be determined.

Amelioration of the severity of atherosclerosis by antioxidants in experimental animals has been established beyond doubt.[35-45] Some of the most commonly used antioxidants in animal studies are described in Table 2. These studies utilized several different antioxidants (Probucol, Vitamin E, BHT, and Diphenylphenylenediamine – DPDD) in three distinct species of animals (rabbits, mice, and monkeys) using naturally hypercholesterolemic

(WHHL rabbits), gene knockout, and cholesterol-fed animals. In addition, recent studies have shown the effectiveness of antioxidants in another model, ballooned and cholesterol-fed rabbits.[46] The remarkable efficacy of antioxidants in these models, yet unproved in human atherosclerosis, raises more questions than it answers. As mentioned before, some of the antioxidants are clearly toxic. The toxicity of BHT and DPPD and the multiple effects of probucol should be given serious consideration and taken as a reminder that the antioxidant controversy still lingers. It is also likely that many negative studies with antioxidants have not been reported. Moreover, in humans it still remains to be established that long-term intake of antioxidants has any long standing benefits against cardiovascular disease. The effects of antioxidants on human cardiovascular disease will be discussed elsewhere in this book.

Table 1
Inhibitors of LDL Oxidation *in vitro*

Simple phenols	Vitamin E, probucol and its analogs, BHT, estradiol, flavonoids, tocotrienol
Polyhydric phenols	Caffeic acid, nordihydroguairetic acid, polyphenols from plant extracts
Amino compounds	Diphenylphenylenediamine (DPPD), RU 486 and similar compounds, tamoxifen, aminoguanidine, nitric oxide
Metal chelators	EDTA and similar compounds, lazaroids (21-aminosteroids)
Antioxidant enzymes	Superoxide dismutase, catalase, paroxanase, PAF-acetyl hydrolase, GSH-peroxidase
Others	β-Carotene and other carotenoids, vitamin C, lipoic acid derivatives, lipoxygenase inhibitors, calcium channel blockers, nitric oxide donors, ebselen, carvedilol, captopril, dithiocarbamates
Interesting antioxidants	Oleic acid, bilirubin, boldine, uric acid, spin traps, quercetin, ubiquinol, dehydroepiandrosterone, fibrates, HMG-CoA reductase inhibitors, thiols including glutathione, garlic extract, curcumin, etya, cigarette smoke extract.

Table 2
Antioxidants and Experimental Atherosclerosis

Species	Experimental Design	Main Responses	Ref.
VITAMIN E			
WHHL rabbits	Vitamin E and probucol	↑ LDL resistance to oxidation, No ↓ in atherosclerosis	84,87,89
Rabbits	Restenosed lesions after angioplasty induced by cholesterol feeding +/- vitamin E 19 days before angioplasty	Vit E ↑ min luminal diameter of femoral arteries and restenosis after angioplasty. Vit E ↑ serum and lipoprotein vit E. LDL resistance to oxidation ↑. No effect on atherosclerotic lesions	42, 85, 86, 90, 91,93, 94, 96
Hypercholesterolemic hamsters	Diet deficient inantioxidants + corn oil and cholesterol during 10 weeks +/- vitamin E or probucol	Vitamin E and probucol decrease LDL oxidation *ex vivo* and foam cells formation	88
Cholesterol-fed Guinea pigs	Control, cholesterol and vitamin E group	Vitamin E ↓ intimal thickening; preserved the integrity of the vascular wall; inhibited progression of atherosclerosis	92
Male Primates	Basal or atherogenic diet +/- vitamin E before or after atherosclerosis	Vitamin E ↓ atherosclerotic lesions limits the lesion progression	43
Japanese quails	Diet with normal or oxidize cholesterol +/- BHT or vitamin E	Vitamin E ↓ lesion severity but no total prevention of atherosclerosis	95
DPPD			
Apo-E deficient mice	High fat diet and DPPD (0.5% w/w) was added to the diet of one subgroup for 6 months	DPPD ↑ LDL resistance to oxidation and lag time for conjugated dienes DPPD ↓ atherosclerosis by 36%	100
NZW rabbits	1. Diet containing 0.5% cholesterol and 10% corn oil (control group) 2. The same diet + 1% DPPD (DPPD-fed group) for 10 wks	DPPD ↓ TG (73%) and HDL (26%); ↑ LDL resistance to oxidation; ↓ thoracic aorta lesion 71%	35
BHT			
Rabbits	1% cholesterol, +/- 1% BHT, 1% BHT alone	Prevention of the early cholesterol-induced microcirculatory changes. Mean atherosclerotic involvement was reduced from 18.6% to 5.9%. No evidence of lipid peroxidation	42, 97, 98
Japanese quails	1. Cholesterol-free diet vs recrystallized (RCR) or oxidized (OXI) cholesterol 2. OXI, or plusBHT or d-α-tocopherol acetate/kg vs RCR 3. Same as 2 but no BH	1. OXI ↑ serum and liver cholesterol and atherosclerotic lesions 2. Vitamin E ↓ severity of OXI diet 3. Vitamin E did not completely prevent atherosclerosis	81

Table 2 (continued)

β-CAROTENE

Species	Experimental Design	Main Responses	Ref.
Rabbits	A. Fruit vegetables, and mustard oil B. Vitamin C and E plus β-carotene C. A high fat-day (5-10 g/d) D. A low fat diet (4-5 g/d)	1. Group B : HDL cholesterol ↑ and lipid peroxides ↓ 2. Aortic plaques were ↑ in groups C and D than in groups A and B	99
VITAMIN C/ASCORBIC ACID			
Healthy people aged < 25 years	1 g Vitamin C/day was added to normal diet	Cholesterol levels tended to fall Cholesterol ↑ with vitamin C supplements in atherosclerosis patients	101, 107
Guinea pigs	Fed both normal diet and atherogenic diet	High ascorbic ↓ cholesterol in liver and aorta compared to low dose Atherogenic diet ↓ cholesterol in the serum and liver but not in aorta	102
Rabbits	1. Injections of physiol. saline 2. Injections of L-ascorbic acid 3. Injections of L-ascorbate 2- sulfate	Plaque deposition, no effect. Ascorbic acid ↓ hype rcholesterolemia, peroxidation and atherosclerotic effect	103 -106
PROBUCOL			
Cholesterol-fed rabbits	0.5% probucol or 1% probucol to high cholesterol diet (2% wt/wt)	Probucol ↓ HDL, serum apo A-I, markedly ↓ atherosclerotic lesions in intimal aortic surface and total cholesterol in vascular tissue	40, 109, 114
WHHL rabbit	1. 1% probucol in the diet 2. 2. Plasma cholesterol matched controls	LDL degradation in macrophages, endothelial & smooth muscle cells only. Probucol ↓ total cholesterol, ↓ lesioned area analogue. Analogue had no effect	37, 38, 41, 44, 101, 110, 111, 113
LDL receptor rabbits	1% probucol or 0.05 % analogue	Probucol in LDL was 2x the analogue. Probucol ↓ lesion progression, lag time over control and analogue	82
Rhesus monkey	High fat, high cholesterol diet + cholestyramine and/or probucol	Probucol ↓ blood cholesterol and caused regression of plaques	108
Macaca nemestrina	High fat, high-cholesterol diet. plus probucol for 14 weeks	Probucol ↑ LDL resistance to oxidation, ↓ lipid accumulation in cells	112
Rats	1. Low-fat diet suppl. with cholesterol, cholic acid, 2-thiouracil 2. 5% Fish oil (MaxEPA) 3. Control with same FA as 2 4. Control oil and 1% probucol	Fish oil and probucol ↓ total cholesterol by 30%; Fish oil group ↓ cholesterol in VLDL fraction while probucol ↓ cholesterol in HDL	115

PEROXIDASE AND METAL-INDEPENDENT LDL OXIDATION

Most of the studies on oxidation suggested that a close association of the cell and the LDL is necessary and that perhaps a prooxidant molecule is transferred from the cell to the lipoprotein particle. Yet the requirement of metals such as copper in the medium has been of major concern. Metal-containing proteins such as hematin, hemin, ceruloplasmin, and hemoglobin can oxidize LDL under appropriate conditions, and such a mechanism may occur when damaged red blood cells are present in the lesion.[47-50] However, there is no evidence of necrosis in early atherosclerosis or under cell culture conditions.

Peroxidases

We observed that peroxidases such as horseradish peroxidase could readily modify LDL in the presence of H_2O_2 or lipid hydroperoxide (LOOH) in simple buffers and in the absence of added metals.[51] Furthermore, media conditioned in the presence of cells contained high levels of H_2O_2 and were capable of oxidizing LDL in the presence, but not in the absence of added peroxidase. As with simple heme-containing proteins, the requirement of an active enzyme did not appear to be necessary.

There is no horseradish peroxidase in the body. However, myeloperoxidase is found in abundance in neutrophils and monocytes and in somewhat less abundance in macrophages due probably to decrease in activity during differentiation of monocytes into macrophages. Myeloperoxidase has been localized in macrophage-rich atherosclerotic lesions[52] and studies by Hazan and Heinecke and co-workers have shown the presence of a number of metabolites in the atherosclerotic lesions that are formed as a result of myeloperoxidase action.[53-56] Several studies have shown that hypochlorous acid (a product of myeloperoxidase reaction) can oxidize lipoproteins, including LDL and HDL.[57-60] In addition to lipid peroxidation, these systems also induce oxidation of tyrosine residues and generate a different type of modified LDL. Lipoxygenases and prostaglandin H synthase activities also possess peroxidase activities and can generate intracellular and membrane bound peroxides.

One important caveat in the peroxidase-mediated oxidation of LDL is that the mechanism itself may include generation of a phenoxy radical, either from the apoprotein itself, from the antioxidant present in the LDL, or from extra cellular phenols, including phenol-red or tyrosine. If so, such a mechanism will rapidly deplete antioxidants from the lipoprotein and render the lipoprotein more readily oxidizable. In fact, under such conditions, a prooxidant function may be ascribed to the antioxidants when they are present at low concentrations, insufficient to inhibit the propagation.[61] However, contrary to expectations, the peroxidase-mediated oxidation of free fatty acids or lipids does not occur readily.

Smoking

Smoking increases death rates through its acceleration of atherosclerosis. Cigarette smoking is an independent causative factor, enhancing progression of coronary artery disease at any level of blood pressure or plasma cholesterol. Because cigarette smoke contains free radicals, several laboratories examined whether it accelerates atherogenesis through oxidative modification of LDL.[62,63] Direct exposure of LDL to cigarette smoke causes some oxidation (and perhaps a number of additional changes). *In vivo* cigarette smoke does not have direct access to plasma lipoproteins, so these *in vitro* effects of direct exposure may not fully reflect what actually happens *in vivo*.

Chronic cigarette smokers are known to differ in a number of respects from nonsmokers. Smokers have significantly lower blood levels of antioxidants such as vitamin C;[64] whether these differences are pertinent to increased risk of atherosclerosis remains inconclusive. LDL was isolated from plasma of smokers who refrained from smoking for a few days and then were asked to smoke 5 to 7 cigarettes in rapid succession, over a period of 90 minutes. Then a second sample was taken and LDL isolated and compared with the earlier, control sample. There was a dramatic, statistically significant increase in peroxidized products as indicated by the thiobarbituric acid reaction and an increased susceptibility of LDL to oxidation. These studies by Harats *et al.*[65] showed that high levels of vitamin C or vitamin E, taken prior to the smoking challenge, prevented the above changes.These studies provide the strongest direct evidence yet that smoking has a significant impact on oxidative modification of LDL and its susceptibility to further oxidation. However, these studies do not establish the mechanism(s) involved. Cigarette smoke also depletes cellular antioxidants and PUFA.

In contrast to the above findings, recent evidence indicates that cigarette smoke extracts may contain potent antioxidants. Pryor *et al.*[66] and Santanam *et al.*[67] observed that addition of cigarette smoke extracts to LDL in the presence of copper profoundly inhibited oxidation of LDL. This is not surprising, as cigarette smoke extract is also rich in polyphenols, which are known to have antioxidant properties. In the same study, Santanam *et al.* however, observed that addition of cigarette smoke extracts enhanced oxidation of LDL by peroxidases. Such apparent "prooxidant" effects of antioxidants in the peroxidase catalyzed oxidation of LDL have been noted before.[61,68,69] This finding raises the question whether copper-mediated oxidation of LDL that is used extensively to test the potency of antioxidants is appropriate. More important, since peroxidases (myeloperoxidase, heme, and others) may very well play a role in the oxidation of LDL *in vivo*, the prooxidant effects of antioxidants cannot simply be ignored. Whether such prooxidant effects actually contribute to the beneficial effects of the antioxidants on cardiovascular diseases remains to be explored.

MECHANISMS OF OXIDATION OF LDL

Since oxidized LDL was discovered, investigators focused their efforts on molecular mechanisms that may be involved in its generation. For reasons difficult to comprehend, most studies focused on cell-generated oxidants and cell- mediated oxidation. Early studies suggested that superoxide radicals might also play an important role in the oxidation of LDL.

Role of Superoxide Radicals

Studies by Heinecke and co-workers,[70] Steinbrecher,[71] and others,[72,73] suggested that superoxide radicals generated by cells might play an important role. This conclusion was supported by finding that addition of superoxide dismutase inhibited oxidation of LDL by cells. Furthermore, cells that are incapable of generating superoxide, e.g., monocytes from chronic granulamatous disease (CGD) subjects failed to oxidize LDL. This might suggest that the NADPH oxidase system may contribute to the generation of superoxide radicals. However, later studies by Heinecke and co-workers[74] and by Sparrow[75] showed that components of the extracellular media might also be involved in generating superoxide radicals. They showed that cells convert cystine into cysteine, which could react with redox metals in the media and generate superoxide radicals. While these mechanisms might suggest that superoxide and products derived from superoxide, for example, for hydrogen peroxide, may be involved in the oxidation of LDL, addition of either superoxide radicals or hydrogen peroxide to LDL failed to initiate oxidation of LDL in the absence of redox metals.

Role of Lipoxygenases

Studies by Parthasarathy and co-workers suggested that cellular enzymes such as lipoxygenase might contribute to oxidation of LDL.[76] This intracellular enzyme is suggested to provide and seed LDL with lipid peroxides. Initial studies suggested lipoxygenase could oxidize LDL when added to *in vitro* systems, and that lipoxygenase inhibitors could inhibit oxidation of LDL.[76] A number of studies also demonstrated that lipoxygenase, particularly 15-lipoxygenase, is quite active in atherosclerotic lesions, and both the enzyme as well as specific 15-lipoxygenase gene expression could be observed in macrophage rich atherosclerotic lesion.[77] Studies by Kuhn and others also established that specific products generated by lipoxygenase could be found in early stages of atherosclerosis.[78] Recently, animals with increased lipoxygenase expression or in which the lipoxygenase gene was knocked out were developed.[79] Studies by Chan *et al.*[79] showed that animals lacking in lipoxygenase actually developed increased atherosclerotic lesion thus contradicting the hypothesis. More recently, Harats[80] presented the exciting observation that animals overexpress 15-lipoxygenase enzyme activity and develop atherosclerosis at much earlier time periods as opposed to animals that process normal amounts of 15-lipoxygenase. It was also reported that animals that lack lipoxygenase expression were resistant to development of atherosclerosis. Studies by Sepo Yla Herttuala[81] also demonstrated that *in vivo* transfer of the lipoxygenase gene to the artery also resulted in enhanced generation of atherosclerosis. Whether lipoxygenase alone could be sufficient to initiate atherosclerosis still remains to be established. No specific inhibitors of 15-lipoxygenase reaction have been available until very recently. Doherty *et al.* described a specific 15-lipoxygenase inhibitor which decreased atherosclerosis when administered to susceptible animals given high-fat diets (personal communication).

Role of Peroxidases

In contrast to 15-lipoxygenase, metal catalyzed oxidation may not be relevant *in vivo*. For this reason, researchers looked at mechanisms that may oxidize LDL in the absence of redux metals. Peroxidases can oxidize LDL in the presence of hydrogen peroxide or lipid peroxide. Heinecke *et al.*[52] showed that myeloperoxidase can efficiently oxidize LDL and HDL. They also showed the presence of myeloperoxidase enzyme in the atherosclerotic artery and demonstrated products that could be generated by specific myeloperoxidase reaction. However, myeloperoxidase is lost during the differentiation of monocytes into macrophages. The presence of the myeloperoxidase gene in macrophages or in atherosclerotic lesion has not been demonstrated. One interesting aspect of the peroxidase catalysis of LDL oxidation is that these enzymes do not readily and directly cause oxidation of lipids. Formation of intermediate radicals have been suggested and these radicals include vitamin E or estradiol or other antioxidants that are usually associated with LDL. Such prooxidant nature of antioxidants, a paradox addressed by Santanam and Parthasarathy, should be viewed with caution as in humans there no direct correlation between the amount of antioxidants that are consumed and plasma concentration of antioxidants. Furthermore, studies by Steinberg and co-workers[82] have shown that oxidants or antioxidants in the plasma may not adequately define the oxidation condition that may prevail in the atherosclerotic artery.

Metal Catalyzed Oxidation

While the majority of the investigators shied away, Fox and co-workers[83] have described a unique mechanism by which ceruloplasmin could contribute to the oxidation of LDL. This copper binding protein has been found to process an additional easily displaceable copper atom that could contribute to oxidation of LDL. Fox and co-workers reported that macrophages could synthesize ceruloplasmin which could be an important mediator of further propagating oxidation in the atherosclerotic artery.

Thus a number of potential mechanisms of oxidation of LDL are still viable and could account for oxidized LDL formation *in vivo*. However, one has to remember that a number of components, for example, the formation of hydrogen peroxide, the seeding mechanisms that are involved in the seeding of LDL with lipid peroxides, the specific prooxidant enzymes such as peroxidases, the pro- or antioxidant components that are present in the atherosclerotic artery, etc., may all play a role in the oxidation of LDL. More important, the propagation could occur in the absence of any additional components, as the natural course of atherosclerotic lesion development takes several years and this process was duplicated *in vitro*.

Acknowledgment

This work was supported by NIH Grant HL 52628-01A3 "Molecular Mechanisms of Oxidation of LDL," and American Heart Association Grant "Benefits of Chronic Exercise May Involve Oxidative Clearance of Plasma LDL and Induction of Cellular Antioxidant Defenses," and generous start-up funds from the Department of Gynecology and Obstetrics at Emory University.

REFERENCES

1. Parthasarathy, S. 1994. *Modified Lipoproteins in the Pathogenesis of Atherosclerosis.* R. G. Landes Company, Austin, pp 1-125.
2. Brown, M. S., S. K. Basu, J. R. Falck, Y. K. Ho, and J. L. Goldstein. 1980. The scavenger cell pathway for lipoprotein degradation: specificity of the binding site that mediates the uptake of negatively-charged LDL by macrophages. *J. Supramol. Struct.* 13:67-81.
3. Haberland, M. E., C. L. Olch, and A. M. Fogelman. 1984. Role of lysines in mediating interaction of modified low density lipoproteins with the scavenger receptor of human monocyte macrophages. *J. Biol. Chem.* 259:11305-11311.
4. Henriksen, T., E. M. Mahoney, and D. Steinberg. 1983. Enhanced macrophage degradation of biologically modified low density lipoprotein. *Arteriosclerosis* 3:149-159.
5. Steinbrecher, U. P., S. Parthasarathy, D. S. Leake, J. L. Witztum, and D. Steinberg. 1984. Modification of low density lipoprotein by endothelial cells involves lipid peroxidation and degradation of low density lipoprotein phospholipids. *Proc. Natl. Acad. Sci. U.S.A.* 81:3883-3887.
6. Heinecke, J. W., H. Rosen, and A. Chait. 1984. Iron and copper promote modification of low density lipoprotein by human arterial smooth muscle cells in culture. *J. Clin. Invest.* 74:1890-1894.
7. Parthasarathy, S., L. G. Fong, D. Otero, and D. Steinberg. 1987. Recognition of solubilized apoproteins from delipidated, oxidized low density lipoprotein (LDL) by the acetyl-LDL receptor. *Proc. Natl. Acad. Sci. U.S.A.* 84:537-540.
8. Esterbauer, H., R. Schmidt, and M. Hayn. 1997. Relationships among oxidation of low-density lipoprotein, antioxidant protection, and atherosclerosis. *Adv. Pharmacol.* 38:425-456.
9. Westhuyzen, J. 1997. The oxidation hypothesis of atherosclerosis: an update. *Ann. Clin. Lab. Sci.* 27:1-10.
10. Devaraj, S. and I. Jialal. 1996. Oxidized low-density lipoprotein and atherosclerosis. *Int. J. Clin. Lab. Res.* 26:178-184.
11. Klatt, P. and H. Esterbauer. 1996. Oxidative hypothesis of atherogenesis. *J. Cardiovasc. Risk.* 3:346-351.
12. Grundy, S. M. 1995. Role of low-density lipoproteins in atherogenesis and development of coronary heart disease. *Clin. Chem.* 41:139-146.
13. Berliner, J. A., M. C. Territo, A. Sevanian, S. Ramin, J. A. Kim, B. Bamshad, M. Esterson, and A. M. Fogelman. 1990. Minimally modified low density lipoprotein stimulates monocyte endothelial interactions. *J. Clin. Invest.* 85:1260-1266.
14. Fogelman, A. M., B. J. Van Lenten, C. Warden, M. E. Haberland, and P. A. Edwards. 1988. Macrophage lipoprotein receptors. *J. Cell Sci. - Supplement* 9:135-149.
15. Patel, R. P., D. Svistunenko, M. T. Wilson, and V. M. Darley-Usmar. 1997. Reduction of Cu(II) by lipid hydroperoxides: implications for the copper-dependent oxidation of low-density lipoprotein. *Biochem. J.* 322:425-433.
16. Brown, A. J., R. T. Dean, and W. Jessup. 1996. Free and esterified oxysterol: formation during copper-oxidation of low density lipoprotein and uptake by macrophages. *J. Lipid Res.* 37:320-335.
17. Bjorkerud, B. and S. Bjorkerud. 1996. Contrary effects of lightly and strongly oxidized LDL with potent promotion of growth versus apoptosis on arterial smooth muscle cells, macrophages, and fibroblasts. *Arterioscl. Thromb. Vasc. Biol.* 16:416-424.

18. Fruebis, J., S. Parthasarathy, and D. Steinberg. 1992. Evidence for a concerted reaction between lipid hydroperoxides and polypeptides. *Proc. Natl. Acad. Sci. U.S.A.* 89:10588-1059.
19. Kim, J.G., F. Sabbagh, N. Santanam, J.N. Wilcox, R.M. Medford, and S. Parthasarathy. 1997. Generation of a Polyclonal Antibody against Lipid Peroxide-modified Proteins. *Free. Rad. Biol. Med.* 23(2):251-259.
20. Waeg, G., G. Dimsity, and H. Esterbauer. 1996. Monoclonal antibodies for detection of 4-hydroxynonenal modified proteins. *Free Radic. Res.* 25:149-159.
21. Itabe, H., H. Yamamoto, M. Suzuki, Y. Kawai, Y. Nakagawa, A. Suzuki, T. Imanaka, and T. Takano. 1996. Oxidized phosphatidylcholines that modify proteins. Analysis by monoclonal antibody against oxidized low density lipoprotein. *J. Biol. Chem.* 271:33208-33217.
22. Henriksen, T., E. M. Mahoney, and D. Steinberg. 1981. Enhanced macrophage degradation of low density lipoprotein previously incubated with cultured endothelial cells: recognition by receptors for acetylated low density lipoproteins. *Proc. Natl. Acad. Sci. U.S.A.* 78:6499-6503.
23. Jurgens, G., H. F. Hoff, G. M. Chisolm, and H. Esterbauer. 1987. Modification of human serum low density lipoprotein by oxidation — characterization and pathophysiological implications. *Chem. Phys. Lipids* 45:315-336.
24. Esterbauer, H., J. Gebicki, H. Puhl, and G. Jurgens. 1992. The role of lipid peroxidation and antioxidants in oxidative modification of LDL. *Free Radic. Biol. Med.* 13:341-390.
25. Esterbauer, H., G. Jurgens, O. Quehenberger, and E. Koller. 1987. Autoxidation of human low density lipoprotein: loss of polyunsaturated fatty acids and vitamin E and generation of aldehydes. *J. Lipid Res.* 28:495-509.
26. Hodgson J.M., M.L. Wahlqvist, and J.A. Boxall. 1993. Can linoleic acid contribute to coronary artery disease? *Am. J. Clin. Nutr.* 58:228-234.
27. Tichelaar H.Y. 1990. Eicosapentaenoic acid composition of different fish oil concentrates. *Lancet* 336:1450-1451.
28. Parthasarathy, S., J. C. Khoo, E. Miller, J. Barnett, J. L. Witztum, and D. Steinberg. 1990. Low density lipoprotein rich in oleic acid is protected against oxidative modification: implications for dietary prevention of atherosclerosis. *Proc. Natl. Acad. Sci. U.S.A.* 87:3894-3898.
29. Reaven, P. D., S. Parthasarathy, B. J. Grasse, E. Miller, D. Steinberg, and J. L. Witztum. 1993. Effects of oleate-rich and linoleate-rich diets on the susceptibility of low density lipoprotein to oxidative modification in mildly hypercholesterolemic subjects. *J. Clin. Invest.* 91:668-676.
30. Reaven, P. D., S. Parthasarathy, B. J. Grasse, E. Miller, F. Almazan, F. H. Mattson, J. C. Khoo, D. Steinberg, and J. L. Witztum. 1991. Feasibility of using an oleate-rich diet to reduce the susceptibility of low-density lipoprotein to oxidative modification in humans. *Am. J. Clin. Nutr.* 54:701-706.
31. Bonanome, A., A. Pagnan, S. Biffanti, A. Opportuno, F. Sorgato, M. Dorella, M. Maiorino, and F. Ursini. 1992. Effect of dietary monounsaturated and polyunsaturated fatty acids on the susceptibility of plasma low density lipoproteins to oxidative modification. *Arterioscler. Thromb.* 12:529-533.
32. Kleinveld, H. A., A. H. Naber, A. F. Stalenhoef, and P. N. Demacker. 1993. Oxidation resistance, oxidation rate, and extent of oxidation of human low-density lipoprotein depend on the ratio of oleic acid content to linoleic acid content: studies in vitamin E deficient subjects. *Free Radic. Biol. Med.* 15:273-280.
33. Denke M.A. and S.M. Grundy. 1991. Effects of fats high in stearic acid on lipid and lipoprotein concentrations in men. *Am. J. Clin. Nutr.* 54:1036-1040.

34. Thomas, M. J. and L. L. Rudel. 1996. Dietary fatty acids, low density lipoprotein composition and oxidation and primate atherosclerosis. *J. Nutr.* 126:1058S-62S.
35. Sparrow, C. P., T. W. Doebber, J. Olszewski, M. S. Wu, J. Ventre, K. A. Stevens, and Y. S. Chao. 1992. Low density lipoprotein is protected from oxidation and the progression of atherosclerosis is slowed in cholesterol-fed rabbits by the antioxidant N,N'-diphenyl-phenylenediamine. *J. Clin. Invest.* 89:1885-1891.
36. Mao, S. J., M. T. Yates, A. E. Rechtin, R. L. Jackson, and W. A. Van Sickle. 1991. Antioxidant activity of probucol and its analogues in hypercholesterolemic Watanabe rabbits. *J. Med. Chem.* 34:298-302.
37. Kita, T., Y. Nagano, M. Yokode, K. Ishii, N. Kume, S. Narumiya, and C. Kawai. 1988. Prevention of atherosclerotic progression in Watanabe rabbits by probucol. *Am. J. Cardiol.* 62:13B-19B.
38. Carew, T. E., D. C. Schwenke, and D. Steinberg. 1987. Antiatherogenic effect of probucol unrelated to its hypocholesterolemic effect: evidence that antioxidants *in vivo* can selectively inhibit low density lipoprotein degradation in macrophage-rich fatty streaks and slow the progression of atherosclerosis in the Watanabe heritable hyperlipidemic rabbit. *Proc. Natl. Acad. Sci. U.S.A.* 84:7725-7729.
39. Bjorkhem, I., A. Henriksson-Freyschuss, O. Breuer, U. Diczfalusy, Berglund, L, and P. Henriksson. 1991. The antioxidant butylated hydroxytoluene protects against atherosclerosis. *Arterioscler. Thromb.* 11:15-22.
40. Daugherty, A., B. S. Zweifel, and G. Schonfeld. 1989. Probucol attenuates the development of aortic atherosclerosis in cholesterol-fed rabbits. *Brit. J. Pharmacol.* 98:612-618.
41. Mao, S. J., M. T. Yates, R. A. Parker, E. M. Chi, and R. L. Jackson. 1991. Attenuation of atherosclerosis in a modified strain of hypercholesterolemic Watanabe rabbits with use of a probucol analogue (MDL 29,311) that does not lower serum cholesterol. *Arterioscler. Thromb.* 11:1266-1275.
42. Wilson, R. B., C. C. Middleton, and G. Y. Sun. 1978. Vitamin E, antioxidants and lipid peroxidation in experimental atherosclerosis of rabbits. *J. Nutr.* 108:1858-1867.
43. Verlangieri, A. J. and M. J. Bush. 1992. Effects of d-alpha-tocopherol supplementation on experimentally induced primate atherosclerosis. *J. Amer. Coll. Nutr.* 11:131-138.
44. Daugherty, A., B. S. Zweifel, and G. Schonfeld. 1991. The effects of probucol on the progression of atherosclerosis in mature Watanabe heritable hyperlipidaemic rabbits. *Brit. J. Pharmacol.* 103:1013-1018.
45. OBrien, K., Y. Nagano, A. Gown, T. Kita, and A. Chait. 1991. Probucol treatment affects the cellular composition but not anti-oxidized low density lipoprotein immunoreactivity of plaques from Watanabe heritable hyperlipidemic rabbits. *Arterioscler. Thromb.* 11:751-759.
46. Ferns, G. A., L. Forster, A. Stewart-Lee, M. Konneh, J. Nourooz-Zadeh, and E. E. Anggard. 1992. Probucol inhibits neointimal thickening and macrophage accumulation after balloon injury in the cholesterol-fed rabbit. *Proc. Natl. Acad. Sci. U.S.A.* 89:11312-11316.
47. Balla, G., H. S. Jacob, J. W. Eaton, J. D. Belcher, and G. M. Vercellotti. 1991. Hemin: a possible physiological mediator of low density lipoprotein oxidation and endothelial injury. *Arterioscler. Thromb.* 11:1700-1711.
48. Green, E. S., C. Cooper, J. Wrigglesworth, and C. A. Rice Evans. 1992. A novel hydrogen-donating drug suppresses heme damage from myoglobin mediated by oxidised low density lipoproteins. *Biochem. Soc. Trans.* 20:330S
49. Paganga, G., C. A. Rice Evans, R. Rule, and D. S. Leake. 1992. The interaction between ruptured erythrocytes and low-density lipoproteins. *FEBS Lett.* 303:154-158.

50. Dee, G., C. A. Rice Evans, S. Obeyesekera, S. Meraji, M. Jacobs, and K. R. Bruckdorfer. 1991. The modulation of ferryl myoglobin formation and its oxidative effects on low density lipoproteins by nitric oxide. *FEBS Lett.* 294:38-42.
51. Wieland, E., S. Parthasarathy, and D. Steinberg. 1993. Peroxidase-dependent metal-independent oxidation of low density lipoprotein *in vitro*: a model for *in vivo* oxidation? *Proc. Natl. Acad. Sci. U.S.A.* 90:5929-5933.
52. Daugherty, A., J. L. Dunn, D. L. Rateri, and J. W. Heinecke. 1994. Myeloperoxidase, a catalyst for lipoprotein oxidation, is expressed in human atherosclerotic lesions. *J. Clin. Invest.* 94:437-444.
53. Hazen, S. L., F. F. Hsu, K. Duffin, and J. W. Heinecke. 1996. Molecular chlorine generated by the myeloperoxidase-hydrogen peroxide-chloride system of phagocytes converts low density lipoprotein cholesterol into a family of chlorinated sterols. *J. Biol. Chem.* 271:23080-23088.
54. Hazen, S. L., F. F. Hsu, and J. W. Heinecke. 1996. p-Hydroxyphenylacetaldehyde is the major product of L-tyrosine oxidation by activated human phagocytes. A chloride-dependent mechanism for the conversion of free amino acids into reactive aldehydes by myeloperoxidase. *J. Biol. Chem.* 271:1861-1867.
55. Savenkova, M. L., D. M. Mueller, and J. W. Heinecke. 1994. Tyrosyl radical generated by myeloperoxidase is a physiological catalyst for the initiation of lipid peroxidation in low density lipoprotein. *J. Biol. Chem.* 269:20394-20400.
56. Jacob, J. S., D. P. Cistola, F. F. Hsu, S. Muzaffar, D. M. Mueller, S. L. Hazen, and J. W. Heinecke. 1996. Human phagocytes employ the myeloperoxidase-hydrogen peroxide system to synthesize dityrosine, trityrosine, pulcherosine, and isodityrosine by a tyrosyl radical-dependent pathway. *J. Biol. Chem.* 271:19950-19956.
57. Hazell, L. J. and R. Stocker. 1993. Oxidation of low-density lipoprotein with hypochlorite causes transformation of the lipoprotein into a high-uptake form for macrophages. *Biochem. J.* 290:165-172.
58. Carr, A. C., J. J. van den Berg, and C. C. Winterbourn. 1996. Chlorination of cholesterol in cell membranes by hypochlorous acid. *Arch. Biochem. Biophys.* 332:63-69.
59. Hu, M. L., S. Louie, C. E. Cross, P. Motchnik, and B. Halliwell. 1993. Antioxidant protection against hypochlorous acid in human plasma. *J. Lab. Clin. Med.* 121:257-262.
60. Van der Vliet, A., M. L. Hu, C. A. O'Neill, C. E. Cross, and B. Halliwell. 1994. Interactions of human blood plasma with hydrogen peroxide and hypochlorous acid. *J. Lab. Clin. Med.* 124:701-707.
61. Santanam, N. and S. Parthasarathy. 1995. Paradoxical actions of antioxidants in the oxidation of low density lipoprotein by peroxidases. *J. Clin. Invest.* 95:2594-2600.
62. Frei, B., T. M. Forte, B. N. Ames, and C. E. Cross. 1991. Gas phase oxidants of cigarette smoke induce lipid peroxidation and changes in lipoprotein properties in human blood plasma. Protective effects of ascorbic acid. *Biochem. J.* 277:133-138.
63. Kita, T., M. Yokode, H. Arai, M. Iiyama, Y. Ueda, K. Ueyama, and S. Narumiya. 1993. Cigarette smoke, LDL and cholesteryl ester accumulation in macrophages. Implications for atherosclerosis. *Ann. N.Y. Acad. Sci.* 686:91-6; discussion 97-8.
64. Harats, D., M. Ben-Naim, Y. Dabach, G. Hollander, E. Havivi, O. Stein, and Y. Stein. 1990. Effect of vitamin C and E supplementation on susceptibility of plasma lipoproteins to peroxidation induced by acute smoking. *Atherosclerosis* 85:47-54.
65. Harats, D., Y. Dabach, G. Hollander, M. Ben Naim, R. Schwartz, O. Stein, and Y. Stein. 1991. Fish oil ingestion in smokers and nonsmokers enhances peroxidation of plasma. *Atherosclerosis* 90:127-139.
66. Pryor, W.A. and K. Stone. 1993. Oxidants in Cigarette Smoke. Radicals, Hydrogen Peroxide, Peroxynitrate, and Peroxynitrite. *Ann. NY Acad. Sci.* 686:12-28.

67. Santanam, N., R. Sanzhez, S.Hendler, and S. Parthasarathy. 1997. Aqueous extracts of cigarette smoke promote the oxidation of low density lipoprotein by peroxidases. *FEBS Lett.* 414:549-551.
68. Santanam, N. and S. Parthasarathy. 1995. Cellular cysteine generation does not contribute to the initiation of LDL oxidation. *J. Lipid Res.* 36:2203-2211.
69. Kalyanaraman, B., V. Darley-Usmar, A. Struck, N. Hogg, and S. Parthasarathy. 1995. Role of apolipoprotein B-derived radical and alpha-tocopheroxyl radical in peroxidase-dependent oxidation of low density lipoprotein. *J. Lipid Res.* 36:1037-1045.
70. Hiramatsu, K., H. Rosen, J. W. Heinecke, G. Wolfbauer, and A. Chait. 1987. Superoxide initiates oxidation of low density lipoprotein by human monocytes. *Arteriosclerosis* 7:55-60.
71. Steinbrecher, U. P. 1988. Role of superoxide in endothelial-cell modification of low-density lipoproteins. *Biochim. Biophys. Acta* 959:20-30.
72. Jessup, W., J. A. Simpson, and R. T. Dean. 1993. Does superoxide radical have a role in macrophage-mediated oxidative modification of LDL? *Atherosclerosis* 99:107-120.
73. Wang, J. M., S. N. Chow, and J. K. Lin. 1994. Oxidation of LDL by nitric oxide and its modification by superoxides in macrophage and cell-free systems. *FEBS Lett.* 342:171-175.
74. Heinecke, J. W., M. Kawamura, L. Suzuki, and A. Chait. 1993. Oxidation of low density lipoprotein by thiols: superoxide-dependent and -independent mechanisms. *J. Lipid Res.* 34:2051-2061.
75. Sparrow, C. P. and J. Olszewski. 1993. Cellular oxidation of low density lipoprotein is caused by thiol production in media containing transition metal ions. *J. Lipid Res.* 34:1219-1228.
76. Rankin, S. M., S. Parthasarathy, and D. Steinberg. 1991. Evidence for a dominant role of lipoxygenase(s) in the oxidation of LDL by mouse peritoneal macrophages. *J. Lipid Res.* 32:449-456.
77. Folcik, V. A., R. A. Nivar-Aristy, L. P. Krajewski, and M. K. Cathcart. 1995. Lipoxygenase contributes to the oxidation of lipids in human atherosclerotic plaques. *J. Clin. Invest.* 96:504-510.
78. Kuhn, H., J. Belkner, S. Zaiss, T. Fahrenklemper, and S. Wohlfeil. 1994. Involvement of 15-lipoxygenase in early stages of atherogenesis. *J. Exp. Med.* 179:1903-1911.
79. Shen, J., H. Kuhn, A. Petho-Schramm, and. L., Chan. 1995. Transgenic rabbits with the integrated human 15-lipoxygenase gene driven by a lysozyme promoter: macrophage-specific expression and variable positional specificity of the transgenic enzyme. *FASEB J.* 9:1623-1631.
80. Harats, D. and A. Shaish. 1997. Lipoxygenase overexpression induces atheroclerosis in LDL-deficient mice. *Circulation.* 96: I-167
81. Yla Herttuala, S., M. E. Rosenfeld, S. Parthasarathy, C. K. Glass, E. Sigal, J. L. Witztum, and D. Steinberg. 1990. Colocalization of 15-lipoxygenase mRNA and protein with epitopes of oxidized low density lipoprotein in macrophage-rich areas of atherosclerotic lesions. *Proc. Natl. Acad. Sci. U. S. A.* 87:6959-6963.
82. Fruebis, J., D. Steinberg, H. A. Dresel, and T. E. Carew. 1994. A comparison of the antiatherogenic effects of probucol and of a structural analogue of probucol in low density lipoprotein receptor-deficient rabbits. *J. Clin. Invest.* 94:392-398.
83. Ehrenwald, E., G. M. Chisolm, and P. L. Fox. 1994. Intact human ceruloplasmin oxidatively modifies low density lipoprotein. *J. Clin. Invest.* 93:1493-1501.
84. O'Leary, V. J., L. Tilling, G. Fleetwood, D. Stone, and V. Darley-Usmar. 1996. The resistance of low density lipoprotein to oxidation promoted by copper and its use as an index of antioxidant therapy. *Atherosclerosis* 119:169-179.

85. Wiseman, S. A., J. N. Mathot, N. J. de Fouw, and L. B. Tijburg. 1996. Dietary non-tocopherol antioxidants present in extra virgin olive oil increase the resistance of low density lipoproteins to oxidation in rabbits. *Atherosclerosis* 120:15-23.
86. Shaish, A., A. Daugherty, F. O'Sullivan, G. Schonfeld, and J.W. Heinecke. 1995. Beta-carotene inhibits atherosclerosis in hypercholesterolemic rabbits. *J. Clin. Invest.* 96:2075-2082.
87. Fruebis, J., T.E.Carew, and W. Palinski. 1995. Effect of vitamin E on atherogenesis inLDL receptor-deficient rabbits. *Atherosclerosis* 117:217-224.
88. Parker, R. A., T. Sabrah, M. Cap, and B. T. Gill. 1995. Relation of vascular oxidative stress, alpha-tocopherol, and hypercholesterolemia to early atherosclerosis in hamsters. *Arterioscl. Thromb. Vasc. Biol.* 15:349-358.
89. Kleinveld, H. A., H. L. Hak-Lemmers, M. P. Hectors, N. J. de Fouw, P. N. Demacker, and A. F. Stalenhoef. 1995. Vitamin E and fatty acid intervention does not attenuate the progression of atherosclerosis in Watanabe heritable hyperlipidemic rabbits. *Arterioscl. Thromb. Vasc. Biol.* 15:290-297.
90. Lafont, A. M., Y. C. Chai, J. F. Cornhill, P. L. Whitlow, P. H. Howe, and G. M. Chisolm. 1995. Effect of alpha-tocopherol on restenosis after angioplasty in a model of experimental atherosclerosis. *J. Clin. Invest.* 95:1018-1025.
91. Morel, D. W., M. de la Llera-Moya, and K. E. Friday. 1994. Treatment of cholesterol-fed rabbits with dietary vitamins E and C inhibits lipoprotein oxidation but not development of atherosclerosis. *J. Nutr.* 124:2123-2130.
92. Qiao, Y., M. Yokoyama, K. Kameyama, and G. Asano. 1993. Effect of vitamin E on vascular integrity in cholesterol-fed guinea pigs. *Arterioscler. Thromb.* 13:1885-1892.
93. Prasad, K. and J. Kalra. 1993. Oxygen free radicals and hypercholesterolemic atherosclerosis: effect of vitamin E. *Amer. Heart J.*. 125:958-973.
94. Godfried, S. L., G. F. Combs, Jr., J. M. Saroka, and L. A. Dillingham. 1989. Potentiation of atherosclerotic lesions in rabbits by a high dietary level of vitamin E. *Brit. J. Nutr.* 61:607-617.
95. Donaldson, W. E. 1982. Atherosclerosis in cholesterol-fed Japanese quail: evidence for amelioration by dietary vitamin E. *Poult. Sci.* 61:2097-2102.
96. Brattsand, R. 1975. Actions of vitamins A and E and some nicotinic acid derivatives on plasma lipids and on lipid infiltration of aorta in cholesterol-fed rabbits. *Atherosclerosis.* 22:47-61.
97. Xiu, R. J., A. Freyschuss, X. Ying, L. Berglund, P. Henriksson, and I. Bjorkhem. 1994. The antioxidant butylated hydroxytoluene prevents early cholesterol-induced microcirculatory changes in rabbits. *J. Clin. Invest.* 93:2732-2737.
98. Bjorkhem, I., A. Henriksson Freyschuss, O. Breuer, U. Diczfalusy, L. Berglund, and P. Henriksson. 1991. The antioxidant butylated hydroxytoluene protects against atherosclerosis. *Arterioscler. Thromb.* 11:15-22.
99. Singh, R. B., M. A. Niaz, P. Agarwal, R. Begom, and S. S. Rastogi. 1995. Effect of antioxidant-rich foods on plasma ascorbic acid, cardiac enzyme, and lipid peroxide levels in patients hospitalized with acute myocardial infarction. *J. Am. Diet. Assoc.* 95:775-780.
100. Tangirala, R.K., F. Casanada, E. Miller, J.L. Witztum, D. Steinberg, and W. Palinski. 1995. Effect of the antioxidant N,N'-diphenyl 1,4-phenylenediamine (DPPD) on atherosclerosis in apoE-deficient mice. *Arterioscl. Thromb. Vasc. Biol.* 15:1625-1630.
101. Spittle, C.R. 1971. Atherosclerosis and vitamin C. *Lancet* 2:1280-1281.
102. Nambisan, B. and P.A. Kurup. 1975. Ascorbic acid and glycosaminoglycan and lipid metabolism in guinea pigs fed normal and atherogenic diets. *Atherosclerosis* 22:447-461.

103. Finamore, F.J., R.P. Feldman, and G.E. Cosgrove. 1976. L-ascorbic acid, L-ascorbate 2-sulfate, and atherogenesis. *Internat. J. Vit. Nutr. Res.* 46:275-285.
104. Verlangieri, A.J. and J.W. Stevens. 1979. L-ascorbic acid: effects on aortic glycosaminoglycan 35S incorproation in rabbit-induced atherogenesis. *Blood Vessels* 16:177-185.
105. Voskresenskii, O.N. and V.N. Bobyrev. 1979. Effect of ascorbic acid and rutin on the development of experimental peroxide atherosclerosis. [Russian]. *Farmakologiia i Toksikologiia* 42:378-382.
106. Altman, R.F., G.M. Schaeffer, C.A. Salles, A.S. Ramos de Souza, and P.M. Cotias. 1980. Phospholipids associated with vitamin C in experimental atherosclerosis. *Arzneimittelforschung.* 30:627-630.
107. Jialal, I. and S. M. Grundy. 1993. Effect of combined supplementation with alpha-tocopherol, ascorbate, and beta carotene on low-density lipoprotein oxidation. *Circulation* 88:2780-2786.
108. Wissler R.W. and D. Vesselinovitch. 1983. Combined effects of cholestyramine and probucol on regression of atherosclerosis in rhesus monkey aortas. *Appl. Pathol.* 1:89-96.
109. Tawara, K., M. Ishihara, H. Ogawa, and M. Tomikawa. 1986. Effect of probucol, pantethine and their combinations on serum lipoprotein metabolism and on the incidence of atheromatous lesions in the rabbit. *Jpn. J. Pharmacol.* 41:211-222.
110. Steinberg, D., S. Parthasarathy, and T. E. Carew. 1988. *In vivo* inhibition of foam cell development by probucol in Watanabe rabbits. *Am. J. Cardiol.* 62:6B-12B.
111. O'Brien, K., Y. Nagano, A. Gown, T. Kita, and A. Chait. 1991. Probucol treatment affects the cellular composition but not anti-oxidized low density lipoprotein immunoreactivity of plaques from Watanabe heritable hyperlipidemic rabbits. *Arterioscler. Thromb.* 11:751-759.
112. Sasahara, M., E. W. Raines, A. Chait, T. E. Carew, D. Steinberg, P. W. Wahl, and R. Ross. 1994. Inhibition of hypercholesterolemia-induced atherosclerosis in the nonhuman primate by probucol. I. Is the extent of atherosclerosis related to resistance of LDL to oxidation? *J. Clin. Invest.* 94:155-164.
113. Braesen, J. H., U. Beisiegel, and A. Niendorf. 1995. Probucol inhibits not only the progression of atherosclerotic disease, but causes a different composition of atherosclerotic lesions in WHHL-rabbits. *Virchows Arch. B. Cell Pathol. Incl. Mol. Pathol.* 426:179-188.
114. Keaney, J. F., Jr., A. Xu, D. Cunningham, T. Jackson, B. Frei, and J. A. Vita. 1995. Dietary probucol preserves endothelial function in cholesterol-fed rabbits by limiting vascular oxidative stress and superoxide generation. *J. Clin. Invest.* 95:2520-2529.
115. Barbeau, M.L., S.C. Whitman, and K.A. Rogers. 1995. Probucol, but not MaxEPA fish oil, inhibits mononuclear cell adhesion to the aortic intima in the rat model of atherosclerosis. *Biochem. Cell Biol.* 73:283-288.

17

Antioxidants and Immune Function

Dayong Wu, M.D. and Simin Nikbin Meydani, D.V.M., Ph.D.
USDA Human Nutrition Research Center on Aging at Tufts University, Boston, Massachusetts USA

INTRODUCTION

Immune cells contribute a substantial portion of the free radicals produced in the body as part of their normal host defense functions. On the other hand, immune cells are prone to oxidative insult because of the high content of polyunsaturated fatty acids in their plasma membranes. It has been well documented that the oxidant-antioxidant balance is an important determinant of immune cell function, not only for maintaining the integrity and functionality of membrane lipids, cellular proteins, and nucleic acids, but also for regulation of signal transduction and gene expression in immune cells. It is, therefore, conceivable that immune cells need more antioxidants to maintain optimal function. This is supported by the observation that immune cells in general have higher levels of antioxidant nutrients than do other cells.[1,2] Numerous animal experiments, clinical trials, and epidemiological investigations have provided evidence indicating a critical role for antioxidants in the regulation of immune cell function, as well as in the pathogenesis of immune-related diseases such as infection, inflammation, autoimmune, and neoplastic diseases. In general, deficiency of single or multi-antioxidant nutrients resulting in oxidant-antioxidant imbalance has been shown to correlate with impairment or abnormality of immune function. Supplementation with antioxidants can correct the deficiency and dysregulated balance, and consequently reverse the impaired or abnormal immune function. Of the antioxidants linked to the modulation of immune function, vitamin E, β-carotene, and GSH have been the subject of intensive investigation, and will be the focus of this review.

IMMUNE SYSTEM AND ASSESSMENT OF ITS FUNCTION

Immune system and immunity

The immune system is composed of cells and molecules responsible for host defense. The main function of the immune system is to eliminate foreign substances (including microbes and macromolecules), to clear damaged and aged tissues, and to monitor and destroy neoplasms in the body. Two types of immune function are present in healthy individuals: natural and acquired immunity.

Natural immunity includes physical barriers, phagocytic function of phagocytes (macrophages and neutrophils), and lysing activity of natural killer cells.

Acquired, or specific, immunity can be classified into two types, based on the components of the immune system that mediate the response, i.e., humoral immunity and cell-mediated immunity.

Humoral immunity is mediated by molecules called antibodies that are produced by B lymphocytes and are responsible for specific recognition and elimination of extracellular antigens. Cell-mediated immunity is mediated by cells of the immune system, particularly T lymphocytes. Cell-mediated immunity is responsible for delayed-type hypersensitivity (DTH) reactions, foreign graft rejection, resistance to many pathogenic microorganisms, and tumor immunosurveillance. Brief descriptions of some immunological tests referred to in this chapter are provided below.

Glossary

Antibody-dependent cellular (cell-mediated) cytotoxicity (ADCC)
A form of lymphocyte-mediated cytotoxicity that functions only if antibodies are bound to the target cells.

Cell-mediated (cellular) immunity
Adaptive immune responses which are initiated by T lymphocytes and mediated by T lymphocytes, macrophages, or both.

Cytotoxic T lymphocytes (CTL)
A group of T cells that kill other cells by recognizing their cell-surface antigens.

Delayed-type hypersensitivity (DTH)
A form of cell-mediated immune response elicited by antigens in the skin. It is so called because the reaction appears in hours to days instead of minutes as seen in immediate hypersensitivity.

Helper T cells
T cells that help B cells to make antibodies in response to antigenic challenge.

Hemagglutination
A process of red blood cell (RBC) clumping together. Hemagglutination takes place when RBC coated with antigen are exposed to the antibody specific for the antigen, and it can therefore be used to determine antibody level.

Humoral immunity
Specific immunity mediated by circulating antibodies produced by B lymphocytes in humoral immune response.

Interleukin (IL)
A generic name for cytokines, hormone-like small proteins secreted by many different cell types, which regulates intensity and duration of immune response.

Mitogen
A substance that stimulates mitosis and lymphocyte transformation, includes lectins such as Con A and PHA, and bacterial products such as lipopolysaccharide (LPS). Mitogenic proliferation of lymphocytes is the most commonly used *in vitro* index of immune response.

Natural killer (NK) cells
A group of non-T and non-B lymphocytes that kill virus-infected and tumor cells.

Suppressor T cells
T cells which, when mixed with naive or effector T cells, suppress their activity.

In vitro Indices of Immune Function

Immune cells are separated from the body and maintained *in vitro*. A variety of stimuli are applied to the cells to measure their proliferative activity and release of immunologically active molecules (cytokines, lipid mediators, etc.) or effector function on target cells (cytotoxic T lymphocyte activity, spontaneous or antibody-dependent cellular cytotoxicity, natural or activated killer activity). Phagocytes can be tested for their phagocytic ability.

1. Lymphocyte Proliferation Assay

Measurement of the proliferative response of lymphocytes is the most commonly used technique in evaluating cell-mediated immune response. Quantitating the proliferative response involves measuring the number of cells present in culture with or without addition of a stimulatory agent (such as mitogen). Measuring incorporation of [^{3}H]-thymidine into DNA is the most commonly used method to estimate changes in cell number. The proliferative assay is applied in clinical studies as an assessment of the overall immunologic competence of lymphocytes, as manifested by their ability to respond to proliferation signals. Decreased proliferation may indicate impaired cell-mediated immune function and has been observed in chronic diseases, cancer, HIV infection, and with aging.

2. Cytokine Production

Immune cells, particularly T cells, produce an array of protein mediators called cytokines. Cytokines are involved in the regulation of cell activation, growth and differentiation, inflammation, and immunity. Measurement of cytokine production has been used to estimate particular functions of immune system. Several techniques, including bioassay, radioimmunoassay, and ELISA has been employed to determine cytokine level. A brief description of interleukin (IL)-2 measurement is provided below as an example. For details of other cytokine measures, see *Protocols in Immunology.*[3]

IL-2 is a T cell growth factor produced by T helper type I (Th-1) cells. As autocrine and paracrine growth factor, IL-2 induces proliferation and differentiation of both T and B cells. IL-2 is responsible for progression of T lymphocytes from G_1 to S phase in the cell cycle, and also for stimulation of B cells for antibody synthesis. IL-2 stimulates the growth of NK cells and enhances their cytolytic function, producing so-called lymphokine-activated killer (LAK) cells. In addition, IL-2 can induce interferon (INF)-γ secretion by NK cells. IL-2 secreted in culture media or biological fluids can be measured by using a bioassay or an immunoassay. The most commonly used bioassay utilizes the IL-2 dependent cytotoxic T lymphocyte line (CTLL). The proliferation of CTLL cells largely reflects IL-2 activity. IL-2 activity in samples can be calculated according to a standard curve generated by adding different concentrations of recombinant IL-2. ELISA is also used often for IL-2 measurement. While ELISA is more specific in measuring IL-2 protein concentrations, it does not differentiate between biologically active and non-active proteins. Under most conditions the change in IL-2 production is associated with the change in lymphocyte proliferation, although in some cases these changes do not correlate with each other.

3. Cytotoxicity Assay

Activity of both cytotoxic T lymphocytes (CTL) and NK cells can be assessed by a cytotoxicity assay. CTL kill target cells on the basis of cell-surface antigen recognition. NK or LAK cells directly lyse tumor cells and virus-infected cells. In the CTL activity assay, target cells can be lymphoblasts, tissue culture cells, or tumor cells. In the NK or LAK activity assay, tumor cells serve as target cells. In both assays, the target cells are labeled with ^{51}Cr and then incubated with effector cells (stimulator cells-stimulated effector cells in CTL assay or IL-2-stimulated effector cells in LAK assay) at different ratios. The percentage of ^{51}Cr released is calculated to represent lysis of target cells which reflects the cytotoxic activity of effector cells. Both CTL and NK/LAK are important in the host response to tumor and virus infections.

4. Flow Cytometric Analysis

Immune cells bear specific markers (antigens) on their surface which can be used to identify different types of cells, i.e., lymphocytes, macrophages, etc., as well as sub-populations of cells, e.g., B and T lymphocytes. The same population of cells can be further classified into different sub-sets according to their surface markers. Different subsets of cells play varied roles in regulating immune response. For example, T cells can be classified as CD4+ or CD8+ subsets which, according to their function, are defined as helper T cells and suppressor T cells, respectively. Identifying the cells with different surface markers can provide a foundation for understanding the cellular basis of immune response. Flow cytometry, a fluorescence-activated cell sorter technology, has been widely used for characterizing and quantifying viable sub-populations of immune cells. Flow cytometric analysis involves three steps: 1) prepared cells are incubated with a specific antibody against a particular cell surface marker and labeled with fluorescent reagents, such as fluorescein isothiocyanate (FITC); 2) the stained cells are processed (identified and separated) by flow cytometry, and appropriate data are collected; and 3) the collected data are analyzed to obtain quantitative information on cell sub-populations. For additional details on flow cytometry methods, see Reference 3.

***In vivo* Indices of Immune Function**

Although measures of immune function rely predominantly on the *in vitro* methods, a limited number of *in vivo* methods are available which can provide information with more direct biological relevance taking into account other factors not present under *in vitro* conditions.

1. Delayed-Type Hypersensitivity Reaction

The DTH reaction is used as an *in vivo* assay to determine cell-mediated immune function. DTH has been widely used as a tool to assess immunocompetence *in vivo*. Several investigators have shown that a decrease in DTH is associated with greater mortality.[4-7] DTH is based on an antigen-specific, T cell-dependent, recall response manifested as an inflammatory reaction that reaches peak intensity approximately 24 to 48 h after antigenic challenge. In the DTH test, a small amount of soluble antigen is introduced into the epidermis and superficial dermal tissue by needle puncture. Circulating T cells sensitized to the antigen from prior contact react with the antigen in the skin and induce a specific immune response which includes mitosis (blastogenesis) and the release of soluble mediators. The reaction process involves antigen presentation by macrophages, release of IL-1 and tumor necrosis factor (TNF) from activated macrophages, release of IL-2 and INF-γ from activated T cells, as well as interaction between these mediators. In humans and guinea pigs, evaluation of DTH intensity is readily performed by measuring the redness and induration of an area of shaven skin exposed to the antigens.[8] However this method does not work well in mice. An alternative method has been developed in which antigens are injected subcutaneously into the footpad of a previously primed mouse. After 24 h, footpad swelling response is measured with a caliper.[9]

2. Antibody Response to Vaccine

Immunization with appropriate antigens (viral or bacterial) can elicit serum antibodies. Antibody production as a response to antigen challenge involves several cellular events that include antigen processing and presentation, recognition of presented antigen by helper T cells, T cell activation and production of cytokines that augment the response of memory B cells. Therefore, the qualitative and quantitative assays for antibodies provide information about B cell responsiveness and T cell cooperation. Antibody response to vaccine has been used as an index in evaluating the host resistance to infections.

EFFECT OF ANTIOXIDANTS ON IMMUNE RESPONSE

Antioxidant Deficiency and Immune Response

Several deficiency studies have been conducted with different species of experimental animals to determine the necessity of antioxidants in maintaining proper immune function. For obvious reasons, fewer human studies using a limited deficiency model have been performed. Primary severe deficiency of some antioxidants such as vitamin E rarely occurs in Western countries, while secondary deficiency is sometimes observed as a consequence of certain diseases. The available studies have demonstrated that deficiency in antioxidant nutrients impairs both humoral and cell-mediated immune functions.

Vitamin E

Tengerdy *et al.*[10] showed that mice fed a diet deficient in vitamin E had lower plaque forming cells and hemagglutination titer in response to sheep red blood cell injection than mice fed a diet sufficient in vitamin E. Decreases in antigen expression by macrophages,[11] phagocytic function of polymorphonuclear cells,[12] and lymphocyte proliferation[13] were observed in vitamin E-deficient rats. Depressed lymphocyte response to T cell mitogens were also reported in vitamin E-deficient dogs,[14] lambs.[15] and pigs.[16] Chickens fed a diet deficient in vitamin E and selenium showed a decreased proportion of peripheral T cells, especially $CD4^+$ cells, and impaired proliferative response to T cell mitogen concanavalin A (Con A) and phytohemagglutinin (PHA).[17] Neutrophils from pre-term infants[18] with vitamin E deficiency showed impaired phagocytic and bactericidal activity.[19] A study of 513 healthy Canadian children (3 years old) indicated that children with low serum vitamin E levels (<10th percentile) had lower levels of lymphocyte proliferation and serum IgM compared to those with high vitamin E levels (>90th percentile).[20] A case report[21] lent further support to this correlation by showing that severe vitamin E deficiency developed secondary to intestinal malabsorption in a 59-year-old woman and caused *in vivo* and *in vitro* impairment of T cell function. Supplementation with vitamin E improved plasma tocopherol levels as well as mitogenic response to T cell mitogen, IL-2 production, and DTH response.

β-Carotene

In contrast to antioxidant vitamins, there is no RDA established for β-carotene. It is therefore difficult to clearly define β-carotene deficiency. In a study reported by Daudu *et al.*,[22] nine healthy, pre-menopausal women were given a basal diet supplemented with 1.5 mg/d β-carotene for 4 days to attain baseline values. They were then fed a basal diet without β-carotene (depletion) for 68 days followed by a basal diet supplemented with 15 mg/d β-carotene (repletion) for 28 days. Results showed that neither β-carotene depletion nor repletion had a significant effect on altered peripheral blood mononuclear cells (PBMC) proliferative response to PHA or Con A, production of soluble IL-2 receptor, and number of lymphocytes and their subsets. In a recent study,[23] nine healthy pre-menopausal women were given a basal diet supplemented with 0.5 mg/d β-carotene for 120 days. During the final 20 days (days 101-120), subjects' diet was supplemented with three capsules of mixed carotenoids per day, which provided 10 mg/d β-carotene in addition to other carotenoids. Using whole blood, they examined lymphocyte proliferation and found that maximum mitogenic response to optimal dose PHA was reduced 60 and 100 days following consumption of a low carotenoid diet. But on day 120 (20 days after supplementation with 10 mg/day β-carotene), the decreased response was completely reversed, surpassing the levels observed on day 1.

Glutathione (GSH)

GSH is the most abundant non-protein thiol in the cells. Its deficiency associated with aging and disease will be reviewed later in this chapter. GSH, unlike vitamins, can be synthesized intracellularly through several enzymatic steps. As a metabolically important compound, tissue concentrations of GSH are highly regulated, and it is therefore difficult to see depletion or excess of GSH in the body. However, it is relatively easy to reduce GSH levels *in vitro* experimental models using GSH synthesis inhibitors or to replenish GSH using GSH- or thiol-containing compounds. Buthionine sulfoximine (BSO) is the most widely used GSH synthesis inhibitor, and 2-cyclohexene-1-one (2-CHX-1) is a compound that specifically interacts with GSH to conjugate the thiol group of GSH. Depletion of cellular GSH by these agents has been reported to suppress mitogenic response of lymphocytes,[24-30] prevent lymphocytes from entering the S phase in the cell cycle,[25,27,31] and inhibit blast transformation,[28,32] transferrin receptor expression, antibody-dependent cellular cytotoxicity and spontaneous cell-mediated cytotoxicity,[33,34] and IL-2-induced lymphokine-activated killer (LAK) activity.[35] Ifosfamide, an antineoplastic agent, has been shown to cause depletion of GSH in different cell types. Multhoff *et al.*[36] reported that incubation of human peripheral blood lymphocytes (PBL) with ifosfamide or BSO resulted in depletion of intracellular GSH which correlated with inhibition of PBL proliferation and lytic activity of $CD3^+$ cytotoxic T lymphocytes (CTL). Reconstruction of GSH levels with GSH ester restored CTL activity inhibited by ifosfamide and PBL proliferation inhibited by BSO. Ifosfamide-induced suppression of PBL proliferation was not restored by GSH repletion due to the irreversible inhibition of cell proliferation. There is little information available for *in vivo* GSH deficiency study. Robinson *et al.*[37] reported that rats depleted of GSH *in vivo* by diethyl maleate had decreased lymphocyte proliferation, decreased tumor necrosis factor (TNF), and IL-6 production, but unaltered IL-2 production.

Vitamin C

In a study determining non-scorbutic effects of moderate vitamin C deficiency reported by Jacob *et al.*,[38] healthy young men sequentially received ascorbic acid 250 mg/d (4 d), 5 mg/d (32 d), 10 or 20 mg/d (28 d), and 60 or 250 mg/d (28 d), in a total of 92 days. The results showed no changes in lymphocyte proliferation, but a significant depression in delayed type hypersensitivity (DTH) responses after 32 days of low vitamin C (5 mg/d) intake. The depressed DTH responses did not return to baseline after repletion with 250 mg/d vitamin C for 4 weeks.

Antioxidant Supplementation and Immune Response

Antioxidant repletion has been shown in most cases to successfully reverse this antioxidant level-associated depression in immune function. Either supplementing subjects *in vivo* or isolated immune cells *in vitro* with antioxidants can provide information on how immune function is affected by these antioxidants under "normal" instead of "deficient" status.

Vitamin E

As early as the 1950s, animal experiments showed that vitamin E supplementation improved antibody production after vaccination in rabbits.[39,40] Later, vitamin E-supplemented chickens were reported to have increased survival to Escherichia coli (E. coli) infection and faster clearance of E. coli from the blood.[41]

Dietary vitamin E supplementation has been shown to enhance T cell differentiation in rat thymus;[42] enhance lymphocyte proliferation in mice,[43,44] rats,[45,46] and pigs;[47] increase helper T cell activity;[48] increase IL-2 production but decrease IL-4 production in mice;[44] and increase NK activity and phagocytic ability of alveolar macrophages in rats.[45] Vitamin E supplementation *in vitro* was also shown to enhance mitogenic response of splenic lymphocytes in mice. In addition, these studies showed that vitamin E itself increases spontaneous proliferation of lymphocytes, indicating a mitogenic effect of vitamin E.[43,49,50] Meydani *et al.*[51] showed that dietary supplementation with 500 ppm vitamin E for 6 weeks increased DTH response and lymphocyte proliferation, and decreased PGE_2 (immuno-inhibitory factor) production in old mice. Recently, Beharka *et al.*[52] reported that *in vitro* addition of vitamin E increased Con A-stimulated cell proliferation when macrophages from old mice were co-cultured with purified T cells from either old or young mice, or when macrophages from young mice were co-cultured with purified T cells from old mice. In addition, vitamin E supplementation increased IL-2 production in co-cultures composed of macrophages from old mice and purified T cells from either old or young mice. Another recent study[53] confirmed the findings of Beharka *et al.* Sakai *et al.* reported that vitamin E supplementation (585 mg/kg diet) for 12 months reversed the age-associated suppression in cell-mediated immune response (mitogenic response and IL-2 production) observed in rats fed a control diet (containing 50 mg vitamin E/kg). Coculture experiments were conducted to determine the mechanism of the effect of vitamin E. The results indicated that vitamin E improved the age-associated decrease in cellular immune functions, and this improvement is due to enhanced responsiveness of both macrophages and lymphocytes. In another model, topical application of vitamin E was reported to reduce incidence of skin cancer in UV-irradiated mice and prevent UV irradiation-induced immunosuppression in these mice.[54]

Until recently, limited information on the effect of antioxidants on the immune response of humans was available. Baehner *et al.*[55] showed that administration of 1600 mg/d vitamin E for one week increased phagocytic rate but decreased bactericidal activity of PMN, which the authors believed to be a result of reduced H_2O_2 levels by vitamin E. In another study,[56] Prasad reported that young male subjects showed decreased bactericidal activity and mitogenic response to PHA, and unchanged DTH response after consuming 300 mg/d vitamin E for 3 weeks. A double-blind, placebo-controlled clinical trial reported by Meydani *et al.*[57] showed that healthy elderly subjects (60 y) supplemented with 800 mg/d vitamin E for 30 days had significantly higher DTH score, mitogenic response of PBMC to Con A, and IL-2 production. Decreased PGE_2 and unchanged IL-1 production by PBMC, and decreased plasma lipid peroxide levels were also observed. To further investigate the effect of long-term supplementation and optimal level of vitamin E on immune response of elderly persons, the same group conducted another trial in which eighty healthy elderly subjects (>65 y) received placebo, 60, 200, or 800 mg/d vitamin E. Immunologic and other laboratory indices were examined before and after 1 and 4.5 months of supplementation. Evaluation of the *in vivo* indices of immune response showed that after 4.5 months of supplementation, all three vitamin E-treated groups had increased DTH responses, with the largest increase being observed in 200 mg/d group. The subjects taking 200 mg/d vitamin E also had a significant increase in antibody titer to hepatitis B and tetanus vaccine. In addition, the vitamin E-supplemented subjects showed a trend for lower incidence of self-reported infections. Vitamin E supplementation did not have a significant effect on serum autoantibody levels or the ability of neutrophils to kill *Candida albicans.*[58] The data to date suggest that vitamin E supplementation is effective in enhancing immune response in the aged and is also safe at levels up to 800 mg consumed over a prolonged period of time (4.5 month).[58]

β-Carotene

β-Carotene supplementation has been substantially investigated for its putative impact on immune function. Bendich and Shapiro fed rats a diet containing β-carotene (0.2% by weight) and observed a significant enhancement in mitogenic response of splenocytes to both T and B cell mitogens after 20 weeks compared to control animals.[59] β-Carotene has also been reported to potentiate lymphocyte proliferation in other species of animals as reviewed by Chew.[60]

In human studies, T helper cells ($CD4^+$) were shown to be increased by 30% in healthy adults taking 180 mg/d β-carotene for 7 days[61] but unchanged in those taking 30 mg/d for 30 days.[62] In neither study, subjects showed changes in T suppressor cells ($CD8^+$) after β-carotene supplementation. Several other studies presented different results on the effect of β-carotene supplementation on total number of T cells and percentage of T cell subsets as reviewed by Meydani *et al.*[63]

Recently, in a β-carotene supplementation study of healthy male nonsmokers (18-60 y), Hughes *et al.*[64] showed that a 26-day dietary supplementation with 15 mg/day β-carotene increased the percentages of monocytes expressing the major histocompatibility complex class II molecule HLA-DR, intercellular adhesion molecule-1, and leukocyte function-associated antigen-3. These results suggest that β-carotene might enhance cell-mediated immune function by modulating the antigen-presenting and costimulatory functions of monocytes. Furthermore, this study observed an increased *ex vivo* secretion of tumor necrosis factor-α (TNF-α) from monocytes after β-carotene supplementation, indicating the possible anti-tumor potential of β-carotene.

In vitro addition of β-carotene to human PBMC caused an increase in percentage of NK cell and number of lymphocytes with surface markers for cell activation such as transferrin receptor, IL-2 receptor, and Ia antigen.[65] The same group obtained similar results in an *in vivo* study in which elderly human subjects received β-carotene supplementation at various doses for 2 months.[66] With regard to functional analysis of NK cells, increased NK activity has been observed after 3 months of oral β-carotene administration in male patients with precancerous lesions oral leukoplakia and Barrett esophagus.[67] In another study, however, healthy young male showed no change in NK activity and IL-2 production by blood lymphocytes, but an increase in lymphocyte proliferation, after taking 30 mg/d β-carotene for 30 days.[62] Recently, Santos *et al.*[68] examined the effect of 10 to 12 years of β-carotene supplementation (50 mg on alternate days) on NK activity in 59 (38 middle-aged men, 51-64 y; 21 elderly men, 65-86 y) Boston area participants in the Physicians' Health Study. Elderly subjects had lower NK activity than did middle-aged subjects, β-carotene supplementation reversed this age-related difference. There was no concomitant change in percentage of NK cells, IL-2 production and IL-2 receptor expression, or PGE_2 production. Similarly, Santos *et al.*[69] reported no effect of supplementation with 90 mg/d β-carotene for three weeks in healthy elderly women (60-80 y, mean 70 y). There was also no effect of short- or long-term supplementation with β-carotene on T cell-mediated function of elderly.[69] In a double-blind, placebo-controlled trial, β-carotene administration at 30 mg/d, however, prevented UV light-induced decrease of plasma β-carotene concentration and suppression of DTH test in healthy young volunteers.[70] Ringer *et al.*[71] examined the effect of various doses (15-300 mg/d) of β-carotene supplementation for 1 month on immune function in male and female subjects aged 18-54 y in a placebo-controlled but open-label trial. No significant change was found in any immune index measured including lymphocyte proliferation, IL-2 production, lymphocyte subsets, and immunoglobulin levels.

Taken together, the research for the putative effect of β-carotene in immunomodulation has thus far suggested that β-carotene supplementation may help reverse the impairment of certain, but not all, immune function seen in aging and diseases states, but it seems to have little effect in enhancing immune response of healthy young adults.

Numerous studies have accumulated a large body of evidence supporting the importance of intracellular GSH for immune cell function. In most studies, both experimentally induced and disease-caused decreases in intracellular GSH levels have been shown to be accompanied by suppressed immune response. On the other hand GSH supplementation has been shown to improve immune function.

Glutathione

In vitro GSH supplementation has been accomplished usually by adding GSH, or its mono-ester, or cysteine delivery agents to the culture system. The latter are a group of low molecular weight thiol compounds, including 2-oxothiazolidine-4-carboxylate (OTC), 2-mercaptoethanol (2-ME), and N-acetyl cysteine (NAC), etc. These compounds have been proven to successfully increase intracellular GSH and enhance primary antibody response and

LPS- (B cell mitogen) induced proliferation of murine spleen cells;[72] enhance antibody-dependent cellular cytotoxicity (ADCC) in human neutrophils and mononuclear cells;[73] enhance mitogenic response of splenocytes from mice,[24,25,74] young and old rats,[75,76] and human PBL;[26,31,77] potentiate the activity of lymphokine-activated killer cells;[78,79] increase transferrin receptor expression;[75] increase IL-2 production, decrease IL-4 production, and IL-4 mRNA transcription in human PBMC.[77] In addition, direct GSH supplementation of cell culture models has generated similar results. GSH supplementation enhanced lymphocyte proliferation in rats[75] and PBMC from young and old subjects,[29] increase IL-2 production and decrease calcium ionophore A23187-stimulated PGE_2 production by PBMC from young and old subjects,[29,77] enhance the binding of IL-2 to its high affinity receptor in IL-2-dependent T cell lines and increase the internalization and degradation of IL-2,[80] and decrease IL-4 production and IL-4-induced IgE and IgG4 production by human PBMC,[77] which may have the potential for attenuating T helper 2 (Th-2) cell-mediated diseases such as allergic diseases and AIDS.

Dietary GSH supplementation has been rarely reported. Furukawa *et al.* showed that dietary GSH supplementation increased intracellular GSH levels as well as improved *in vitro* and *in vivo* indices of immune response in old mice.[81] The importance of intracellular GSH status for immune cell activity was further highlighted by an interesting observation by Kavanagh *et al.*[82] When sorting human PBMC on the basis of GSH content by use of a flow cytometric assay, they found that a higher percentage of cells with high GSH concentrations were capable of entering the cell cycle than those with low GSH concentrations.

Mechanism for Immunostimulatory Effect of Antioxidants

The immuno-enhancing effect of antioxidants can be attributed to their antioxidant properties, i.e., protection of cells from oxidative damage. The immune system generates reactive oxygen metabolites as part of its regular defense functions. These reactive oxygen species are necessary for immune cells to kill pathogens and clear dead tissues, but chronic overproduction of them as seen in a variety of pathologic conditions can cause damage to the immune cells and compromise their functions.

Antioxidants, including water-soluble (such as vitamin C and GSH) and lipid-soluble (such as vitamin E and β-carotene), can reduce oxidative stress and thereby help immune cells maintain optimal functions, especially when they are challenged. However, a growing body of evidence suggests that immuno-regulatory effects of these antioxidants may not be mediated solely through their antioxidant function. Antioxidants have been shown to mediate a wide spectrum of cellular activities including cellular metabolism, signal transduction, gene activation, and transcription. Antioxidants possessing similar antioxidant capacity and mechanism may show different effects on these cellular processes. Studies have shown that some antioxidants are effective in modulating immune response but others are not, even though they all share common antioxidant properties, suggesting that some antioxidants have specific non-antioxidant-mediated effects in immunomodulation. Although the mechanism of these non-antioxidant functions have yet to be clearly elucidated, preliminary evidence is accumulating.

Protection of Cell Membranes

The cell membrane plays a critical role in immune cell activity. Immune cells require proper membrane activity to carry out the important functions including antigen recognition, receptor expression, secretion of antibodies and cytokines, lymphocyte transformation, and contact cell lysis. Lipid peroxidation can damage cell membranes as well as those membrane-associated functions. Lipid peroxidation is capable of reducing membrane fluidity, and loss of membrane fluidity has been implicated in decreased ability of lymphocytes to respond to challenges to the immune system.[83] The presence of lipid-soluble antioxidants such as vitamin E has the potential to affect the physical properties of membranes as well as membrane functions. It is therefore conceivable that antioxidants could maintain membrane fluidity by preventing membrane lipid peroxidation, which, in turn, maintains membrane-associated immunologic activity.

Effect on Production of Immunomodulators

Immune cells produce many active molecules that can regulate immune cell function. Antioxidants have been shown to affect production of some such molecules, and thus may contribute to their immunomodulatory effect. For example, IL-2 is a lymphocyte growth factor, and its importance in lymphocyte activation has been well documented. Suppressed IL-2 production has been related to oxidative stress and can be restored by antioxidant supplementation. Increased IL-2 production has been observed in mice[44,52] and in humans[57] supplemented with vitamin E. GSH supplementation was also reported to increase IL-2 production in human PBMC[29] and purified T cells.[77] Although β-carotene has not generally been shown to affect IL-2 production, some investigators observed an increase in percentage of cells expressing IL-2 receptor.[66,67] Increased production of plasma and PBMC TNF-α by β-carotene treatment may contribute to its enhancement of NK activity.[84,85]

Upon stimulation, immune cells, particularly macrophages, can produce a large amount of molecules that are suppressive to lymphocyte activation and proliferation. These molecules include oxygen-derived free radicals and active products of lipid metabolism. As mentioned above, one of the mechanisms for enhanced immune response by antioxidant treatment is their antioxidant function in attenuating oxidative stress and therefore restoring suppressed immune response. In addition, membrane lipid metabolites from arachidonic acid (AA) cascade have been shown in many studies to play an important role in immunomodulation. Membrane phospholipids release AA under action of phospholipase A_2, and released AA can then be catalyzed by cyclooxygenase or lipoxygenase into different eicosanoids (prostaglandins, leukotrienes, and hydroxyeicosatetraenoic acids). PGE_2 is a cyclooxygenase product of AA metabolism. At low concentrations, PGE_2 is believed to be necessary for certain aspects of cellular immunity as well as for a variety of normal cell functions. While at higher concentrations, PGE_2 is immunosuppressive for T cell-mediated immunity as demonstrated by decreased T cell proliferation and IL-2 production.[52,86-88] The age-associated decline in immune response has been linked to increased PGE_2 production, which is commonly observed in aged animals and humans.[51,52,57,86,89,90] In several studies, both *in vitro* and *in vivo* supplementation with vitamin E have resulted in the decreased PGE_2 production and concomitantly, enhanced lymphocyte proliferation, IL-2 production, and DTH responses.[51,52,57] This evidence has led to the hypothesis that the noted immuno-enhancing effect of vitamin E is partly mediated by its inhibition of PGE_2 production. In a recent study further investigating how vitamin E inhibits PGE_2 production, Wu *et al.*[91] showed that greater PGE_2 production in macrophages from old mice than those from young mice was reduced by dietary supplementation with 500 ppm vitamin E for 1 month. This reduction of PGE_2 synthesis resulted from decreased cyclooxygenase activity. Vitamin E may also decrease PGE_2 production through inhibiting phospholipase A_2 and therefore AA release from membrane phospholipids.[92]

In vitro supplementation with 5 mM GSH inhibited calcium ionophore A23187-stimulated PGE_2 production in PBMC from young and elderly human subjects.[29] The arachidonic acid lipoxygenase product leukotriene (LT) B_4 was also decreased under the same conditions in this study. LTB_4 was reported to inhibit lymphocyte proliferation in another study.[93] Mitogenic response of PBMC was suppressed in the presence of PGE_2, but this suppressed response was reversed by addition of 5 mM GSH.[29] This is in accordance with the previous observation reported by Yu *et al.*[94] that PGE_2 suppressed cell proliferation and release of soluble molecules of IL-2 receptor, CD4 and CD8 from human PBMC stimulated by PHA. Intracellular GSH was decreased when PBMC were stimulated in the presence of PGE_2. They suggested that the immunosuppressive effect of PGE_2 could be mediated by the decreased generation of intracellular GSH.

A trend toward lower PGE_2 production was also noted in subjects supplemented with β-carotene.[68] Thus, research to date supports the hypothesis that immune-enhancing effect of some antioxidants is mediated in part by their inhibiting production of immuno-suppressive factors.

Interactions and Sparing Effect of Antioxidants

Every individual antioxidant has its own independent antioxidant activity in protecting cells from oxidative damages. On the other hand, antioxidants can work interactively to compensate or improve each other's function. This is referred to as the "sparing effect," which refers to both overlap in antioxidant activity and regeneration of one antioxidant by the other. As reviewed by Winkler *et al.*,[95] GSH can regenerate ascorbic acid by reducing its oxidized form dehydroascorbic acid, and ascorbic acid itself, in turn, can reduce tocopherol radical to reduced tocopherol. This mechanism also makes it possible to transfer oxidative challenge between lipid and aqueous phases. Thus, for a given antioxidant, it is possible that the mechanisms of its immunomodulatory effect would be linked to its sparing effect on other antioxidants with immunomodulatory potential.

Effect on Apoptosis (Cell Death)?

Programmed cell death in both T and B lymphocytes has been suggested to regulate immune response. Reactive oxygen intermediates (ROI) have been shown to mediate activation-induced death in T cell blasts and hybridomas,[96,97] and mouse thymocytes.[98] Dysregulation of thiol redox status has been implicated in the loss of lymphocytes by apoptosis.[99-102] L-cysteine, NAC, GSH, and thioredoxin were shown to block apoptosis.[96-99] Therefore, potential involvement of antioxidants in the regulation of immune cell apoptosis might be another factor contributing to their immunomodulatory effect.

Effect on Signal Transduction

In the past few years, evidence has accumulated to show that reactive oxygen intermediates (ROI) may act as signal transduction messengers. At least two transcription factors, NF-κB and AP-1 have been identified to be regulated by redox status. Transcription factors play a central role by integrating the signals elicited by a variety of stimuli including growth factors, phorbol esters, cytokines, viruses, and bacterial LPS. Different stimuli use ROI as signaling messengers to activate transcription factors and induce those genes involved in inflammatory, immune, and acute phase responses. For example, many genes encoding cytokines, cytokine receptors, growth factors, and cell adhesion molecules, contain NF-κB binding sites in their promoter and enhancer regions.[103,104] Activation of NF-κB is shown to be inhibited by different antioxidants.[105-109] Vitamin E or its derivatives have been reported to inhibit NF-κB binding in mice[110] and human Jurkat T cells.[109,111] Droge *et al.*[112] indicated a thiol redox status-regulated NF-κB activation. At low glutathione disulfide (GSSG) levels, T cells cannot optimally activate NF-κB, whereas high GSSG levels inhibit its DNA binding activity. A moderate optimal level is required for effective NF-κB activation. Depletion of GSH and GSSG resulted in suppressed NF-κB activation.[112] Other thiol-containing antioxidants such as thioredoxin and NAC were reported to inhibit NF-κB activation.[105,113,114] A number of studies have demonstrated that AP-1 activation is enhanced by antioxidants[105,114-116] whereas some other studies showed that AP-1 activation was also enhanced by oxidants.[117,118] It has been observed that AP-1 is only moderately activated by the oxidant H_2O_2 but strongly activated by antioxidants.[116] Studies to date have suggested that NF-κB behaves primarily as an oxidative stress response factor while AP-1 acts as an antioxidant-responsive factor. Since redox-controlled transcription factors NF-κB and AP-1 are used extensively for signaling and gene induction in immune cells, the immunomodulatory effect of antioxidants can be partially attributed to their ability to regulate transcription factor activation. Further studies are needed to define the effect of different antioxidants on redox-regulated transcription process. Favorably regulated gene expression by selected antioxidants has the potential to modulate immune function, and therefore, immune-associated diseases.

POTENTIAL CLINICAL APPLICATIONS FOR THE IMMUNOMODULATORY EFFECTS OF ANTIOXIDANTS

Increased oxidative stress and its resultant damage to tissues has been shown to contribute to the pathology of several diseases including those associated with dysregulated immune function, e.g., infectious, inflammatory, autoimmune, and neoplastic diseases. Aging is associated with increased oxidative stress and dysregulated immune function. The incidence of most of the aforementioned diseases increases with age. Antioxidant supplementation has been shown to be beneficial in delaying or preventing the pathogenesis of some of these diseases.

Aging

There are several theories and numerous supportive studies linking aging with oxidative stress. Oxidative stress could be a consequence of excess reactive oxygen intermediates and/or deficit of antioxidants. Optimal levels of antioxidants are necessary for maintaining appropriate immunologic vigor across all age groups but particularly critical in the elderly. Age-associated dysregulation of the immune response, particularly T cell-mediated functions, has been intensively studied and well documented.[119,120] An impaired immune function predispose elderly population to infectious, neoplastic, autoimmune, and inflammatory diseases.[121]

Information about changes in antioxidant levels with aging is limited and sometimes controversial. Several reports on humans suggest that blood vitamin E concentrations do not change with age,[122,123] however, others suggested an age-associated decrease in platelets.[124] The immune cells were shown to have higher concentration of vitamin E than other cells,[1,2] but no difference in splenocyte vitamin E concentrations was observed between mice aged 4 and 24 months[86] while similar data from human immune cells are lacking. No age-associated difference in plasma and blood cell β-carotene concentrations was reported in several studies.[125-128] In contrast, GSH status has been suggested to relate inversely to aging and may serve as predictor of morbidity and mortality.[129] Lower GSH concentrations were observed in brain, liver, lens, lung, and spleen of old mice compared with young mice.[81,130-132] Lang *et al.*[129] showed that about one-half of healthy human subjects aged >60 y had lower blood GSH concentrations than young subjects. A positive correlation between tissue GSH concentrations and life span in mice[133] and mosquitoes[134] has been shown.

The effect of antioxidants on immune function in aged humans and animals has been already discussed as part of the evidence regarding the general immunomodulatory effect of antioxidants. The research results generated thus far indicate that aged subjects might benefit from certain antioxidant supplementation in terms of enhancement of the immune response. However, this is often not true or, at least, less pronounced for young subjects. This age-related difference in response to antioxidant supplementation reflects the increased requirement for antioxidants by aged subjects. This increased requirement for antioxidants may result from increased oxidative burden with aging or an increased sensitivity of aged tissues to the detrimental effect of oxidative stress, or both. Dietary intervention using antioxidants, especially vitamin E, has shown a promising potential in reversing suppressed immune response in the elderly.

Oxidant/Antioxidant Balance and Disease

Several diseases are associated with increased oxidative stress. Whether increased oxidant formation causes the disease or it is a consequence of the disease process is not clear. Regardless of the exact mechanism, reduction of oxidative stress by antioxidants might be beneficial.

Infection

As discussed above, antioxidants can, in general, enhance natural and specific immunity. This notion has also been supported by experimental, clinical, and epidemiological studies. Several animal studies indicated that the immunostimulatory effect of vitamin E is associated with increased resistance to infection such as Escherichia coli[41,135,136] and Pneumococcus pneumonia type I.[137] Meydani *et al.* recently observed a trend toward lower incidence of self-reported infections in elderly volunteers supplemented with vitamin E compared with those supplemented with a placebo.[58] Hayek *et al.*[138] recently showed that dietary supplementation with 500 ppm vitamin E significantly reduced lung viral titers in old mice infected with influenza virus. Epidemiological studies lend supports to the experimental data by showing that elderly subjects with high plasma vitamin E concentration had fewer infections.[139,140] In a mouse model of polymicrobial sepsis,[141] NAC was shown to improve mouse survival and reduce the liver toxicity. The effect was not related to the modulation of TNF, nitrites, or GSH generation, indicating a direct antioxidant effect. Transfection of the cell line (293 cells) by influenza virus hemagglutinin (HA) was reported to strongly activate NF-κB DNA binding and gene expression. Pre-incubation with antioxidant dithiothreitol inhibited HA-mediated NF-κB activation.[142]

HIV infection and AIDS

Human immunodeficiency virus (HIV) infection and acquired immune deficiency syndrome (AIDS) are a growing threat to human beings. HIV-induced immunosuppression results in high susceptibility of the host to a variety of infections. HIV infection causes defects in the immune system, especially cell-mediated immune function, as characterized by a decrease in CD4 lymphocytes. HIV infection is associated with increased production of ROI and deficiency in antioxidants, such as vitamin E,[143] GSH,[144,145] and β-carotene.[146] Supplementation with these antioxidants restored immune dysfunction and retarded the development of AIDS. For example, in a murine AIDS model, a 15-fold increase in dietary vitamin E levels restored mitogenic proliferation of splenic T and B cells, IL-2 and IFN-γ production of splenocytes, and NK cell activity, all of which were suppressed in murine AIDS.[147] Vitamin E supplementation also reduced the production of IL-6 and TNF-a, which are elevated in AIDS and contribute to inflammatory response and HIV replication.

It has been suggested that thiol depletion may be a general consequence of HIV infection. The anti-HIV drug azidothymidine (AZT), which has been shown to retard the progression of AIDS, was reported to cause a substantial recovery of the plasma thiol levels in AIDS patients.[144] NAC administration increased intracellular GSH level and inhibited HIV transcription and replication in *in vitro* model systems,[148,149] and the inhibited HIV activation was related to inhibited activation of transcription factor NF-κB by intracellular GSH.[150]

A double-blind, placebo-controlled study showed that β-carotene supplementation (180 mg/d for 1 m) in HIV-infected patients increased white blood cell count, percent CD4 and CD4/CD8 ratio compared with placebo group.[151] However, Coodley *et al.* later failed to replicate their result in a long-term study in which β-carotene supplementation at 180 mg/d for 3 m caused no significant change in any of the outcome variables other than an increased serum β-carotene concentration.[152] Even though the authors pointed out that the addition of multivitamin supplements to both arms of the study might have masked any difference between the two groups, they concluded that supplementation with high doses of β-carotene is not of benefit for HIV-infected patients.

Rheumatoid Arthritis (RA)

RA is discussed as an example to address the significance of the oxidant/antioxidant balance in inflammatory and autoimmune disorders. RA is a chronic illness characterized by inflammation of peripheral joints resulting in progressive destruction of articular tissues. About 1% of all populations are affected.[153] The cause is still unknown, but an autoimmune mechanism has been hypothesized. Major pathological change of RA is the thickened synovial membrane resulting from increased number and size of synovial lining cells and colonization by infiltrated lymphocytes and plasma cells. The lining cells produce collagenase, inflammatory cytokines, and prostaglandins. The colonizing lymphocytes produce IL-2, INF-γ, and immunoglobulins (such as rheumatoid factor). A wide spectrum of oxidation products have been shown to increase in the serum and synovial fluid of RA patients and experimental animals.[154,155] However, reports on antioxidant status in RA have been controversial. A consistent difference in plasma or serum vitamin E levels between RA patients and normal controls has not been demonstrated.[154] For example, Scherak and Kolarz reported that RA patients had normal plasma levels of vitamin E.[156] Honkanen *et al.* showed lower serum vitamin A and vitamin E levels in RA patients than in healthy controls.[157] Situnayake *et al.*[158] reported that the total radical-trapping antioxidant parameter (TRAP) values were lower in 20 RA patients than in healthy controls matched by age and sex. Serum ascorbic acid and vitamin E concentrations were also lower in RA patients compared with healthy controls. Heliovaara *et al.*[159] reported a case control study in a Finnish cohort of 1419 adult men and women. During a 20-year follow-up, 14 individuals developed RA. Authors matched each incident case with two controls for sex, age, and municipality. Serum vitamin E, β-carotene, and selenium concentrations were measured and antioxidant index was calculated as the product of the molar concentration of these three micronutrients. The results showed that elevated risks of RA were related to low levels of each of these micronutrients, but none of the associations was statistically significant. A significant association, however, was observed with a low antioxidant index. Some studies have provided evidence suggesting that impaired antioxidant status may be more likely to exist in synovial fluid than in serum. Fairburn *et al*[160] showed that synovial fluid concentrations of vitamin E were significantly lower in RA patients than those found in matched controls, but serum levels of vitamin E in these patients did not differ significantly from those in control subjects. The synovial fluid of RA patients was also shown to have lower antioxidant capacity[161] and ascorbate levels than those of controls.[162]

Vitamin E intervention in RA patients has been conducted in several studies, as summarized by Bendich and Cohen.[154] In most such studies, vitamin E appeared to ameliorate clinical symptoms, including pain scores and morning stiffness. Even when RA patients had normal baseline plasma vitamin E concentrations, vitamin E treatment at 1200 mg/day significantly increased plasma vitamin E concentrations and produced some clinical improvement.[156]

T cells in the inflamed joints of RA patients have been shown to be hyporesponsive.[163-165] Maurice *et al.*[166] reported that the T cells isolated from synovial fluid (SF) of RA patients had decreased proliferative responses to CD3 and CD28 stimulation compared with T cells from peripheral blood (PB). They found the decreased intracellular GSH levels in SF $CD4^+$ and $CD8^+$ compared with PB $CD4^+$ and $CD8^+$ T-cell subsets. Restoration of GSH levels in SF T cells with GSH precursor NAC enhanced T-cell proliferative responses and IL-2 production, whereas use of GSH synthesis inhibitor BSO markedly reduced the proliferation.

Although our knowledge of the relation between RA and other chronic inflammatory diseases, redox balance, and immune function is quite limited, the studies discussed so far indicate that antioxidants might be beneficial. Further studies are needed to substantiate the beneficial effect of antioxidants in prevention and/or treatment of these diseases.

Acknowledgments

The authors' work has been funded at least in part with Federal funds from the U.S. Department of Agriculture, Agricultural Research Service under contract number 53-K06-01; NIA grant #1R01 AG091 40-04; and USDA grant #94-37200-0489. The contents of this publication do not necessarily reflect the views or policies of the U.S. Department of Agriculture, nor does mention of trade names, commercial products, or organizations imply endorsement by the U.S. Government. The authors thank Timothy S. McElreavy, M.A., for preparation of this manuscript.

REFERENCES

1. Hatman, LJ, Kayden, HJ. A high-performance liquid chromatographic method for the determination of tocopherol in plasma and cellular elements of the blood. *J Lipid Res,* 20, 639, 1979.
2. Coquette, A, Vray, B, Vanderpas, J. Role of vitamin E in the protection of the resident macrophage membrane against oxidative damage. *Arch Int Physiol Biochem,* 94, 529, 1986.
3. Coligan, JE, Kruisbeek, AM, Margulies, DH, Shevach, EM, Strober W, Eds. *Current Protocols in Immunology*. New York: Greene Publishing Assoc 1994.
4. Roberts-Thomson, IC, Whittingham, S, Youngchaiyud, U, Mackay, IR. Ageing, immune response and mortality. *Lancet*, 2, 368, 1974.
5. Wayne, SJ, Rhyne, RL, Garry, PJ, Goodwin, JS. Cell-mediated immunity as a predictor of morbidity and mortality in the aged. *J Gerontol Ser A Biol Sci Med Sci*, 45, M45, 1990.
6. Cohn, JR, Hohl, CA, Buckley, CE. The relationship between cutaneous cellular immune responsiveness and mortality in a nursing home population. *J Am Geriatr Soc,* 31, 808, 1983.
7. Christou, NV, Tellado-Rodriguez, J, Chartrand, L, *et al.* Estimating mortality risk in preoperative patients using immunologic, nutritional, and acute-phase response. *Ann Surg*, 210, 69, 1989.
8. Kniker, WT, Anderson, CT, Roumiantzeff, M. The MULTITEST System: A standardized approach to evaluation of delayed hypersensitivity and cell mediated immunity. *Ann Allergy*, 43, 73, 1979.
9. Sunday, ME, Weinberger, JZ, Benacerraf, B, Dorf, ME. Hapten-specific T cell responses to 4-hydroxy-3-nitrophenyl acetyl. IV. Specificity of cutaneous sensitivity responses. *J Immunol*, 125, 1601, 1980.
10. Tengerdy, RP, Heinzerling, RH, Brown, GL, Mathias, MM. Enhancement of the humoral immune response by vitamin E. *Intern Arch Allergy*, 44, 221, 1973.
11. Gebremichael, A, Levy, EM, Corwin, LM. Adherent cell requirement for the effect of vitamin E on *in vitro* antibody synthesis. *J Nutr*, 114, 1297, 1984.
12. Harris, RE, Boxer, LA, Baehner, RL. Consequences of vitamin-E deficiency on the phagocytic and oxidative functions of the rat polymorphonuclear leukocytes. *Blood*, 55, 338, 1980.
13. Eskew, ML, Scholz, RW, Reddy, CC, Todhunter, DA, Zarkower, A. Effects of vitamin E and selenium deficiencies on rat immune function. *Immunol*, 54, 173, 1985.

14. Langweiler, M, Schultz, RD, Sheffy, BE. Effect of vitamin E deficiency on the proliferative response of canine lymphocytes. *Am J Vet Res, 42*, 1681, 1981.
15. Turner, R, Finch, J. Immunological malfunctions associated with low selenium-vitamin E diets in lambs. *J Comp Pathol*, 102, 99, 1990.
16. Jensen, M, Fossum, C, Ederoth, M, Hakkarainen, RV. The effect of vitamin E on the cell-mediated immune response in pigs. *J Vet Med*, 35, 549, 1988.
17. Chang, WP, Hom, JS, Dietert, RR, Combs, GFJ, Marsh, JA. Effect of dietary vitamin E and selenium deficiency on chicken splenocyte proliferation and cell surface marker expression. *Immunopharmacol Immunotoxicol*, 16, 203, 1994.
18. Oski, FA. Anemia in infancy: Iron deficiency and vitamin E deficiency. *Pediatr Rev*, 1, 247, 1980.
19. Miller, ME. Phagocytic function in the neonate: Selected aspects. *Pediatrics*, 64, 5709, 1979.
20. Vobecky, JS, Vobecky, J, Shapcott, D, Rola-Pleszczynski, M. Nutritional influences on humoral and cell-mediated immunity in healthy infants. *J Am Coll Nutr*, 3, 265, 1984.
21. Kowdley, KV, Mason, JB, Meydani, SN, Cornwall, S, Grand, RJ. Vitamin E deficiency and impaired cellular immunity related to intestinal fat malabsorption. *Gastroenterology*, 102, 2139, 1992.
22. Daudu, PA, Kelley, DS, Taylor, PC, Burri, BJ, Wu, MM. Effect of a low β-carotene diet on the immune functions of adult women. *Am J Clin Nutr*, 60, 969, 1994.
23. Kramer, TR, Burri, BJ. Modulated mitogenic proliferative responsiveness of lymphocytes in whole-blood cultures after a low-carotene diet and mixed-carotenoid supplementation in women. *Am J Clin Nutr*, 65, 871, 1997.
24. Fidelus, RK, Tsan, MF. Enhancement of intracellular glutathione promotes lymphocyte activation by mitogen. *Cellular Immunol, 97*, 155, 1986.
25. Fidelus, RK, Ginouves, P, Lawrence, D, Tsan, MF. Modulation of intracellular glutathione concentrations alters lymphocyte activation and proliferation. *Exp Cell Res, 170*, 269, 1987.
26. Smyth, MJ. Glutathione modulates activation-dependent proliferation of human peripheral blood lymphocyte populations without regulating their activated function. *J Immunol, 1*46, 1921, 1991.
27. Messina, JP, Lawrence, DA. Cell cycle progression of glutathione-depleted human peripheral blood mononuclear cells is inhibited at S phase. *J Immunol, 1*43, 1974, 1989.
28. Fischman, CM, Udey, MC, Kurtz, M, Wedner, HJ. Inhibition of lectin-induced lymphocyte activation by 2-cyclohexene-1-one: Decreased intracellular glutathione inhibits an early event in the activation sequence. *J Immunol, 1*27, 2257, 1981.
29. Wu, D, Meydani, SN, Sastre, J, Hayek, M, Meydani, M. *In vitro* glutathione supplementation enhances interleukin-2 production and mitogenic response of peripheral blood mononuclear cells from young and old subjects. *J Nutr,* 124, 655, 1994.
30. Walsh, AC, Michaud, SG, Malossi, JA, Lawrence, DA. Glutathione depletion in human T lymphocytes: analysis of activation-associated gene expression and stress response. *Toxicol Appl Pharmacol*, 133, 249, 1995.
31. Iwata, S, Hori, T, Sato, N. Thiol-mediated redox regulation of lymphocyte proliferation. *J Immunol*, 152, 5633, 1994.
32. Hamilos, DL, Wedner, H, J. The role of glutathione in lymphocyte activation. I. Comparison of inhibitory effects of buthionine sulfoximine and 2-cyclohexene-1-one by nuclear size transtormation. *J Immunol, 1*35, 2740, 1985.
33. MacDermott, RP, Bertovich, MJ, Bragdon, MJ, Nash, GS, Leusch, MS, Wedner, HJ. Inhibition of cell-mediated cytotoxicity by 2-cyclohexene-1-one: evidence for a role for glutathione and/or glutathione-protein interactions in cytolysis. *Immunology, 57*, 521, 1986.

34. Younes, M, Craig, G, Stacey, NH. Cell-mediated cytotoxicity by natural killer cells, lipid peroxidation and glutathione. *Experientia*, 42, 1257, 1986.
35. Yamauchi, A, Bloom, ET. Requirement of thiol compounds as reducing agents for IL-2 mediated induction of LAK activity and proliferation of human NK cells. *J Immunol*, 151, 5535, 1993.
36. Multhoff, G, Meier, T, Botzler, C, *et al*. Differential effects of ifosfamide on the capacity of cytotoxic T lymphocytes and natural killer cells to lyse their target cells correlate with intracellular glutathione levels. *Blood*, 85, 2124, 1995.
37. Robinson, MK, Rodrick, ML, Jacobs, DO, *et al*. Glutathione depletion in rats impairs T-cell and macrophage immune function. *Arch Surg*, 128, 29, 1993.
38. Jacob, RA, Kelley, DS, Pianalto, FS, *et al*. Immunocompetence and oxidant defense during ascorbate depletion of healthy men. *Am J Clin Nutr*, 54, 1302S, 1991.
39. Solana, G. Effects of vitamins on antibody production in rabbits to vibrio choleral. *Int Z Vitamin Forsch*, 27, 373, 1957.
40. Segagni, E. Vitamin E effect on vaccination. *Minerva Pediatr*, 7, 985, 1955.
41. Tengerdy, RP, Heinzerling, RH, Mathias, MM. Effect of vitamin E on disease resistance and immune response. In: *Tocopherol, Oxygen and Biomembranes,* de Dune C, Hayaishi O, Eds., Elsevier Science Inc, New York, 1978, 191.
42. Moriguchi, S, Miwa, H, Okamura, M, Maekawa, K, Kishino, Y, Maeda, K. Vitamin E is an important factor in T cell differentiation in thymus of F344 rats. *J Nutr Sci Vitaminol*, 39, 451, 1993.
43. Corwin, LM, Shloss, J. Influence of vitamin E on the mitogenic response of murine lymphoid cells. *J Nutr*, 110, 916, 1980a.
44. Wang, Y, Watson, RR. Vitamin E supplementation at various levels alters cytokine production by thymocytes during retrovirus infection causing murine AIDS. *Thymus*, 22, 153, 1994.
45. Moriguchi, S, Kobayashi, N, Kishino, Y. High dietary intakes of vitamin E and cellular immune functions in rats. *J Nutr*, 120, 1096, 1990.
46. Bendich, A, Gabriel, E, Machlin, LJ. Dietary vitamin E requirement for optimum immune response in the rat. *J Nutr*, 116, 675, 1986.
47. Larsen, HJ, Tollersrud, S. Effect of dietary vitamin E and selenium on the phytohaemagglutinin response of pig lymphocytes. *Res Vet Sci, 31*, 301, 1981.
48. Tanka, J, Fuyiwara, H, Torisu, M. Vitamin E and immune response: enhancement of helper T cell activity by dietary supplementation of vitamin E in mice. *Immunology*, 38, 727, 1979.
49. Roy, RM, Petrella, M, Ross, WM. Modification of mitogen-induced proliferation of murine splenic lymphocytes by *in vitro* tocopherol. *Immunopharmacol Immunotoxicol*, 13, 531, 1991.
50. Corwin, LM, Shloss, J. Role of antioxidants on the stimulation of the mitogenic response. *J Nutr*, 110, 2497, 1980b.
51. Meydani, SN, Meydani, M, Verdon, CP, Shapiro, AC, Blumberg, JB, Hayes, KC. Vitamin E supplementation suppresses prostaglandin E_2 synthesis and enhances the immune response of aged mice. *Mech Ageing Dev*, 34, 191, 1986.
52. Beharka, AA, Wu, D, Han, SN, Meydani, SN. Macrophage prostaglandin production contributes to the age-associated decrease in T cell function which is reversed by the dietary antioxidant vitamin E. *Mech Ageing Dev*, 93, 59, 1997.
53. Sakai, S, Moriguchi, S. Long-term feeding of high vitamin E diet improves the decreased mitogen response of rat splenic lymphocytes with aging. *J Nutr Sci Vitaminol*, 43, 113, 1997.
54. Gensler, HL, Magdaleno, M. Topical vitamin E inhibition of immunosuppression and tumorigenesis induced by ultraviolet irradiation. *Nutr Cancer*, 15, 97, 1991.

55. Baehner, RL, Boxer, LA, Allen, JM, Davis, J. Antooxidation as a basis for altered function of polymorphonuclear leukocytes. *Blood*, 50, 327, 1977.
56. Prasad, JS. Effect of vitamin E supplementation on leukocyte function. *Am J Clin Nutr*, 33, 606, 1980.
57. Meydani, SN, Barklund, MP, Liu, S, *et al.* Vitamin E supplementation enhances cell-mediated immunity in healthy elderly subjects. *Am J Clin Nutr, 52*, 557, 1990.
58. Meydani, SN, Meydani, M, Blumberg, JB, *et al.* Vitamin E supplementation and *in vivo* immune response in healthy elderly subjects. A randomized controlled trial. *JAMA*, 277, 1380, 1997.
59. Bendich, A, Shapiro, SS. Effect of β-carotene and canthaxanthin on the immune responses of the rat. *J Nutr*, 116, 2254, 1986.
60. Chew, BP. Role of carotenoids in the immune response. *J Dairy Sci, 76*, 2804, 1993.
61. Alexander, M, Newmark, H, Miller, RG. Oral beta-carotene can increase the number of OKT4+ cells in human blood. *Immunol Lett, 9*, 221, 1985.
62. Moriguchi, S, Okishima, N, Satoshi, S, Okamura, K, Doi, T, Kishino, Y. β–carotene supplementation enhances lymphocyte proliferation with mitogens in human peripheral blood lymphocytes. *Nutr Res*, 16, 211, 1996.
63. Meydani, SN, Wu, D, Santos, MS, Hayek, MG. Antioxidants and immune response in the aged: Overview of present evidence. *Am J Clin Nutr, 62* (Suppl), 1462S, 1995b.
64. Hughes, DA, Wright, AJA, Finglas, PM, *et al.* The effect of β-carotene supplementation on the immune function of blood monocytes from healthy male nonsmokers. *J Lab Clin Med*, 129, 309, 1997.
65. Prabhala, RH, Maxey, V, Hicks, MJ, Watson, RR. Enhancement of the expression of activation markers on human peripheral blood mononuclear cells by *in vitro* culture with retinoids and carotenoids. *J Leukoc Biol, 45*, 249, 1989.
66. Watson, RR, Prabhala, RH, Plezia, PM, Alberts, DS. Effect of beta-carotene on lymphocyte subpopulations in elderly humans: evidence for a dose-response relationship. *Am J Clin Nutr, 53*, 90, 1991.
67. Prabhala, RH, Garewal, HS, Hicks, MJ, Sampliner, RE, Watson, RR. The effects of 13-*cis* retinoic acid and beta-carotene on cellular immunity in humans. *Cancer*, 67, 1556, 1991.
68. Santos, MS, Meydani, SN, Leka, L, *et al.* Natural killer cell activity in elderly men is enhanced by β-carotene supplementation. *Am J Clin Nutr*, 64, 772, 1995.
69. Santos, MS, Leka, LS, Ribaya-Mercado, JD, *et al.* Short- and long-term β-carotene supplementation do not influence T cell-mediated immunity in healthy elderly. *Am J Clin Nutr*, 66, 917, 1997.
70. Fuller, CJ, Faulkner, H, Bendich, A, Parker, RS, Roe, DA. Effect of β-carotene supplementation on photosuppression of delayed-type hypersensitivity in normal young men. *Am J Clin Nutr, 56*, 684, 1992.
71. Ringer, TV, DeLoof, MJ, Winterrowd, GE, *et al.* Beta-carotene's effects on serum lipoproteins and immunologic indices in humans. *Am J Clin Nutr, 53*, 688, 1991.
72. Hoffeld, JT. Agents which block membrane lipid peroxidation enhance mouse spleen cell immune activities *in vitro*: relationship to the enhancing activity of 2-mercaptoethanol. *Eur J Immunol,* 11, 371, 1981.
73. Roberts, RL, Aroda, VR, Ank, BJ. N-acetylcysteine enhances antibody-dependent cellular cytotoxicity in neutrophils and mononuclear cells from healthy adults and human immunodeficiency virus-infected patients. *J Infect Dis*, 172, 1492, 1995.
74. Noelle, RJ, Lawrence, DA. Determination of glutathione in lymphcytes and possible association of redox state and proliferative capacity of lymphocytes. *Biochem J*, 198, 571, 1981.

75. Franklin, RA, Li, YM, Arkins, S, Kelley, KW. Glutathione augments *in vitro* proliferative responses of lymphocytes to Concanavalin A to a greater degree in old than in young rats. *J Nutr, 120*, 1710, 1990.
76. Lacombe, P, Kraus, L, Fay, M, Pocidalo, JJ. Lymphocyte glutathione status in relation to their Con A proliferative response. *FEBS, 91*, 227, 1985.
77. Jeannin, P, Delneste, Y, Lecoanet-Henchoz, S, *et al.* Thiols decrease human interleukin (IL) 4 production and IL-4-induced immunoglobulin synthesis. *J Exp Med*, 182, 1785, 1995.
78. Yim, C.-Y, Hibbs, JBL, McGregor, JR, Galinsky, RE, Samlowski, WE. Use of N-acetyl cysteine to increase intracellular glutathione during the induction of antitumor responses by IL-2. *J Immunol*, 152, 5796, 1994.
79. Liang, SM, Liang, CM, Hargrove, ME, Ting, CC. Regulation by glutathione of the effect of lymphocytes on differentiation of primary activated lymphocytes: influence of gluta thione on cytotoxic activity of CD3-AK˙. *J Immunol*, 146, 1909, 1991.
80. Liang, CM, Lee, N, Cattell, D, Liang, SM. Glutathione regulates interleukin-2 activity on cytotoxic T-cells. *J Bio Chem, 264*, 13519, 1989.
81. Furukawa, T, Meydani, SN, Blumberg, JB. Reversal of age-associated decline in immune responsivness by dietary glutathione supplementation in mice. *Mech of Aging and Dev*, 38, 107, 1987.
82. Kavanagh, TJ, Grossmann, A, Jaecks, EP, *et al.* Proliferative capacity of human peripheral blood lymphocytes sorted on the basis of glutathione content. *J Cell Physiol*, 145, 472, 1990.
83. Bendich, A, Phillips, M, Tengerdy, RP, Eds. *Antioxidant Nutrients and Immune Functions*. New York: Plenum, 1990.
84. Abdel-Fatth, G, Watzl, B, Huang, D, Watson, RR. Beta-carotene *in vitro* stimulates tumor necrosis alpha and interleukin 1 alpha secretion by human peripheral blood mononuclear cells. *Nutr Res*, 13, 863, 1993.
85. Probhala, RH, Braune, LM, Garewal, HS, Watson, RR. Influence of beta-carotene on immune functions. *Ann NY Acad Sci*, 691, 262, 1993.
86. Hayek, MG, Meydani, SN, Meydani, M, Blumberg, JB. Age differences in eicosanoid production of mouse splenocytes: Effects on mitogen-induced T-cell proliferation. *J Gerontol, 49*, B197, 1994.
87. Goodwin, JS, Ceuppens, J. Regulation of immune response by prostaglandins. *J Clin Immunol, 3*, 295, 1983.
88. Goodwin, JS, Ceuppens, J. Regulations of the immune reponse by prostaglandins. *J Exp Med, 155*, 943, 1982.
89. Bartocci, A, Maggi, FM, Welker, RD, Veronese, F. Age-related immunosuppression: Putative role of prostaglandins. In: *Prostaglandins and Cancer,* Backman RS, Honn XV, PR, Eds., Alan Riss, New York, 1982, 725.
90. Rosenstein, MM, Strauser, HR. Macrophage-induced T-cell mitogen suppression with age. *J Reticuloendoth Sc, 27*, 159, 1980.
91. Wu, D, Han, SN, Meydani, SN. Vitamin E (E) supplementation inhibits macrophage (Mf) cyclooxygenase (COX) activity of old mice. *FASEB J*, 10, A191, 1996.
92. Douglas, CE, Chan, AC, Choy, PC. Vitamin E inhibits platelet phospholipase A_2. *Biochim Biophys Acta*, 876, 639, 1986.
93. Shapiro, AC, Wu, D, Meydani, SN. Eicosanoids derived from arachidonic and eicosapentaenoic acids inhibit T cell proliferative response. *Prostaglandins*, 45, 229, 1993.
94. Yu, C.-L, Liu, C.-L, Tsai, C.-Y, *et al.* Prostaglandin E_2 suppresses phytogemagglutin-induced immune responses of normal human mononuclear cells by decreasing intracellular glutathione generation, but not due to increased DNA strand breaks or apoptosis. *Agents Actions*, 40, 191, 1993.

95. Winkler, BS, Orselli, SM, Rex, TS. The redox couple between glutathione and ascorbic acid: a chemical and physiological perspective. *Free Radic Biol Med*, 17, 333, 1994.
96. Williams, MS, Henkart, PA. Role of reactive oxygen intermediates in TCR-induced death of T cell blasts and hybridomas. *J Immunol*, 157, 2395, 1996.
97. Sandstrom, PA, Mannie, MD, Buttke, TM. Inhibition of activation-induced death in T cell hybridomas by thiol antioxidants: oxidative stress as a mediator of apoptosis. *J Leukoc Biol*, 55, 221, 1994.
98. Fernandez, A, Kiefer, J, Fosdick, L, McConkey, DJ. Oxygen radical production and thiol depletion are required for Ca^{2+}-mediated endogenous endonuclease activation in apoptotic thymocytes. *J Immunol*, 155, 5133, 1995.
99. Iwata, S, Hori, T, Sato, N, *et al.* Adult T cell leukemia (ATL)-derived factor/human thioredoxin prevents apoptosis of lymphoid cells induced by L-cystine and glutathione depletion. Possible involvement of thiol-mediated redox regulation in apoptosis caused by pro-oxidant state. *J Immunol*, 158, 3108, 1997.
100. Buttke, TM, Sandstrom, PA. Oxidative stress as a mediator of apoptosis. *Immunol Today*, 15, 7, 1994.
101. Sandstrom, PA, Roberts, B, Folks, TM, Buttke, TM. HIV gene expression enhances T cell susceptibility to hydrogen peroxide-induced apoptosis. *AIDS Res Hum Retroviruses*, 9, 1107, 1993.
102. Buttke, TM, Sandstrom, PA. Redox regulation of programmed cell death in lymphocytes. *Free Radic Res*, 22, 389, 1995.
103. Grilli, M, Chiu, J.-S, Lenardo, MJ. NF-κB and Rel: Participants in a multiform transcriptional regulatory system. *Int Rev Cytol*, 143, 1, 1993.
104. Baeuerle, PA, Henkel, T. Function and activation of NF-κB in the immune system. *Annu Rev Immunol*, 12, 141, 1994.
105. Schenk, H, Klein, M, Erdbrugger, W, Droge, W, Schulze-Osthoff, K. Distinct effects of thioredoxin and antioxidants on the activation of transcription factor NF-κB and AP-1. *Proc Natl Acad Sci USA*, 91, 1672, 1994.
106. Schreck, R, Rieber, P, Baeuerle, P. A. Reactive oxygen intermediates as apparently widely used messengers in the activation of the NF-kappa B. *EMBO J*, 10, 2247, 1991.
107. Schreck, R, Meier, B, Mannel, DN, Droge, W, Baeuerle, PA. Dithiocarbamates as potent inhibitors of nuclear factor kappa B activation in intact cells. *J Exp Med*, 175, 1781, 1992.
108. Schulze-Osthoff, K, Beyaert, R, Vandevoorde, V, Haegeman, G. Depletion of the mitochondrial electron transport abrogates the cytotoxic and gene-inductive effects of TNF. *EMBO J*, 12, 3095, 1993.
109. Suzuki, YJ, Packer, L. Inhibition of NF-kappa B DNA binding activity by alpha-tocopheryl succinate. *Biochem Mol Biol Int*, 31, 693, 1993.
110. Liu, SL, Degli Esposti, S, Yao, T, Diehl, AM, Zern, MA. Vitamin E therapy of acute CC14-induced hepatic injury in mice is associated with inhibition of nuclear factor kappa-B binding. *Hepatology*, 22, 1474, 1995.
111. Suzuki, YJ, Packer, L. Inhibition of NF-kappa B activation by vitamin E derivatives. *Biochem Biophys Res Commun*, 193, 277, 1993.
112. Droge, W, Schulze-Osthoff, K, Mihm, S, *et al.* Functions of glutathione and glutathione disulfide in immunology and immunopathology. *FASEB J*, 8, 1131, 1994.
113. Devary, Y, Rosette, C, DiDonato, JA, Karin, M. NF-κB activation by ultraviolet light not dependent on a nuclear signal. *Science*, 261, 1442, 1993.
114. Meyer, M, Schreck, R, Baeuerle, PA. H_2O_2 and antioxidants have opposite effects on activation of NF-κB and AP-1 in intact cells: AP-1 as secondary antioxidant-responsive factor. *EMBO J*, 12, 2005, 1993.

115. del Arco, PG, Martinez-Martinez, S, Calvo, V, Armesilla, AL, Redondo, JM. JNK (c-Jun NH_2terminal kinase) is a target for antioxidants in T lymphocytes. *J Biol Chem*, 271, 26335, 1996.
116. Meyer, M, Pahl, HL, Baeurele, PA. Regulation of the transcription factor NF-κB and AP-1 by redox changes. *Chem Biol Interact*, 91, 91, 1994.
117. Rao, GN, Glasgow, WC, Eling, TE, Runge, MS. Role of hydroperoxyeicosatetraenoic acids in oxidative stress-induced activating protein 1 (AP-1) activity. *J Biol Chem*, 271, 27760, 1996.
118. Pinkus, R, Weiner, LM, Daniel, V. Role of oxidants and antioxidants in the induction of AP-1, NF-κB, and glutathione S-transferase gene expression. *J Biol Chem*, 271, 13422, 1996.
119. Miller, RA. Aging and immune function. *Internat Rev Cytology*, 124, 187, 1991.
120. Miller, RA. Aging and immune function: Cellular and biochemical analyses. *Exp Gerontol*, 29, 21, 1994.
121. Makinodan, T, James, SJ, Inamizu, T, Chang, M.-P. Immunologic basis for susceptibility to infection in the aged. *Gerontology*, 30, 279, 1984.
122. Heseler, H, Schneider, R. Requirement and supply of vitamin C, E, and beta-carotene for elderly men and women. *Eur J Clin nutr*, *48*, 118, 1994.
123. Saccari, M, Garric, B, Ponteziere, C, Miocque, M, Cals, MJ. Influence of sex on vitamin A and E status. *Age and Ageing*, 20, 413, 1991.
124. Vatassery, GT, Johnson, GJ, Krezowski, AM. Changes in vitamin E concentrations in human plasma and platelets with age. *J Am Coll Nutr*, *4*, 369, 1983.
125. Murata, T, Tamai, H, Morinbu, T, *et al*. Determination of beta-carotene in plasma, blood cells, and buccal mucosa by electrochemical detection. *Lipids*, 27, 840, 1992.
126. Norkus, EP, Bhagavan, HN, Nair, PP. Relationship between individual carotenoids in plasma, platelets and red blood cells. *FASEB J*, *4*, A1174, 1990.
127. Meydani, M, Martin, A, Ribaya-Mercado, JD, Gong, J, Blumberg, JB, Russell, RM. β-Carotene supplementation increases antioxidant capacity of plasma in older women. *J Nutr*, 124, 2397, 1994.
128. Murata, T, Tamai, H, Morinobu, T, *et al*. Effect of long-term administration of β-carotene on lymphocyte subsets in humans. *Am J Clin Nutr*, *60*, 597, 1994.
129. Lang, CA, Naryshkin, S, Schneider, DL, Mills, EJ, Lindeman, RD. Low blood glutathione levels in healthy aging adults. *J Lab Clin Med*, *120*, 720, 1992.
130. Uejima, Y, Fukuchi, Y, Teramoto, S, Tabata, R, Orimo, H. Age changes in visceral content of glutathione in the senescence accelerated mouse (SAM). *Mech Ageing Dev*, *67*, 129, 1993.
131. Liu, J, Mori, A. Age-associated changes in superoxide dismutase activity, thiobarbituric acid reactivity, and reduced glutathione level in brain and liver senescence-accelerated mice (SAM): A comparison with ddY mice. *Mech Ageing Dev*, *71*, 23, 1993.
132. Chen, TS, Richie, JR, Lang, CA. Life span profiles of glutathione and acetaminophen detoxification. *Drug Metab Disposition*, 18, 882, 1990.
133. Abraham, EC, Taylor, JF, Lang, CA. Influence of mouse age and erythrocyte age on glutathione metabolism. *Biochem J*, *176*, 819, 1978.
134. Hazelton, GA, Lang, CA. Glutathione levels during the mosquito life span with emphasis on senescence. *Proc Soc Exp Biol Med*, *176*, 249, 1984.
135. Ellis, RP, Vorhies, MW. Effect of supplemental dietary vitamin E on the serologic response of swine to an Escherichia coli bacterin. *J Am Vet Med Assn*, *168*, 231, 1986.
136. Julseth, DR. Evaluation of vitamin E and disease stress on turkey performance. Fort Collins, CO. Colorado State University, 1984.

137. Heinzerling, RH, Tengerdy, RP, Wick, LL, Lueker, DC. Vitamin E protects mice against Diplococcus pneumonia type I infection. *Infect Immun, 10*, 1292, 1974.
138. Hayek, MG, Taylor, SF, Bender, BS, *et al.* Vitamin E supplementation decreases lung virus titers in mice infected with influenza. *J Infect Dis*, 176, 273, 1997.
139. Chavance, M, Brubacher, G, Herbert, B, *et al.* Immunological nutritional status among the elderly. In: *Nutritional Immunity and Illness in the Elderly,* Chandra RK, Ed., Pergamon Press, New York, 1985, 137.
140. Chavance, M, Herbeth, B, Fournier, C, Janot, C, Vernhes, G. Vitamin status, immunity and infections in an elderly population. *Euro J Clin Nutr, 43*, 827, 1989.
141. Villa, P, Ghezzi, P. Effect of N-acetyl-L-cysteine in sepsis in mice. *Eur J Pharmacol*, 292, 341, 1995.
142. Pahl, HL, Baeuerle, PA. Expression of influenza virus hemagglutinin activates transcription factor NF-κB. *J Virol*, 69, 1480, 1995.
143. Liang, B, S, C, Araghinidnam, M, Lane, LC, Watson, R. Vitamins and immunomodulation in AIDS. *Nutrition*, 12, 1, 1996.
144. Eck, HP, Gmünder, H, Hratmann, M, Petzoldt, D, Daniel, V, Drôge, W. Low concentrations of acid-soluble thiol (cysteine) in the blood plasma of HIV-1-infected patients. *Bio Chem Hoppe-Seyler, 3*70, 101, 1989.
145. Staal, FJ, Ela, SW, Roederer, M, Anderson, MT, Herzenberg, LA, Herzenberg, LA. Glutathione deficiency and human immunodeficiency virus infection. *Lancet*, 339, 909, 1992.
146. Sappey, C, Leclercq, P, Courdray, C, Faure, P, Micoud, M, Favier, A. Vitamin, trace element and peroxide status in HIV seropositive patients: asymptomatic patients present a severe beta carotene deficiency. *Clin Chim Acta*, 230, 35, 1994.
147. Wang, Y, Watson, RR. Is vitamin E supplementation a useful agent in AIDS therapy? *Prog Food Nutr Sci*, 17, 351, 1993.
148. Roederer, M, Staal, FJ, Raju, PA, Ela, SW, Herzenberg, LA, Herzenberg, LA. Cytokine-stimulated human immunodeficiency virus replication is inhibited by N-acetyl-L-cysteine. *Proc Natl Acad Sci USA*, 87, 4884, 1990.
149. Raju, PA, Herzenberg, LA, Herzenberg, LA, Roederer, M. Glutathione precursor and antioxidant activities of N-acetylcysteine and oxothiazoline carboxylate compared in *in vitro* studies of HIV replication. *AIDS Res Hum Retroviruses*, 10, 961, 1994.
150. Staal, FJ, Roederer, M, Herzenberg, LA, Herzenberg, LA. Intracellular thiols regulate activation of nuclear factor kappa B and transcription of human immunodeficiency virus. *Proc Natl Acad Sci USA*, 87, 9943, 1990.
151. Coodley, G, Nelson, H, Loveless, M, Folk, C. β-carotene in HIV infection. *J Acquir Immune Defic Syndr*, 6, 272, 1992.
152. Coodley, GO, Coodley, MK, Lusk, R, *et al.* β-Carotene in HIV infection: an extended evaluation. *AIDS*, 10, 967, 1996.
153. Merck & Co, I. *Rheumatoid Arthritis*. 16th Ed. Rahway. Merck & Co, Inc, 1992.
154. Bendich, A, Cohen, M. Vitamin E, rheumatoid arthritis, and other arthritic disorders. *J Nutr Immunol*, 4, 47, 1996a.
155. Bendich, A. Antioxidant vitamins and human immune response. *Vitam Horm*, 52, 35, 1996b.
156. Scherak, O, Kolaz, G. Vitamin E and rheumatoid arthritis. *Arthritis Rheum*, 34, 1205, 1991.
157. Honkanen, V, Konttinen, YT, Mussalo-Rauhamaa, MH. Vitamin A, E, zinc and retinol binding protein in rheumatoid arthritis. *Clin Exp Rheumatol*, 7, 465, 1989.
158. Situnayake, RD, Thurnham, DI, Kootathep, S, *et al.* Chain breaking antioxidant status in rheumatoid arthritis: Clinical and laboratory correlates. *Ann Rheum Dis*, 50, 81, 1991.

159. Heliovaara, M, Knekt, P, Aho, K, Aaran, RK, Alfthan, G, Aromaa, A. Serum antioxidants and risk of rheumatoid arthritis. *Ann Rheum Dis*, 53, 51, 1994.
160. Fairburn, K, Grootveld, M, Ward, R. J, *et al.* Alpha-tocopherol, lipids and lipoproteins in knee-joint synovial fluid and serum from patients with inflammatory joint disease. *Clin Sci*, 83, 657, 1992.
161. Gutteridge, JM, Hill, C, Blake, DR. Copper stimulated phospholipid membrane peroxidation: antioxidant activity of serum and synovial fluid from patients with rheumatoid arthritis. *Clin Chim Acta*, 139, 85, 1984.
162. Lunec, J, Blake, DR. The determination of dehydroascorbic acid and ascorbic acid in the serum and synovial fluid of patients with rheumatoid arthritis. *Free Rad Res Commun*, 1, 31, 1985.
163. Verwilghen, J, Vertessen, S, Stevens, EAM, Dequeker, J, Ceuppens, JL. Depressed T cell reactivity of recall antigens in rheumatoid arthritis. *J Clin Immunol*, 10, 90, 1990.
164. Kingsley, GH, Pitzalis, C, Panayi, GS. Abnormal lymphocyte reactivity to self-major histocompatibility antigens in rheumatoid arthritis. *J Rheumatol*, 14, 667, 1987.
165. Haraoui, B, Wilder, RL, Malone, DG, Allen, JB, Katona, IM, Wahl, SM. Immune function in severe, active rheumatoid arthritis: a relationship between peripheral blood mononuclear cell proliferation to soluble antigens and mononuclear cell subset profiles. *J Immunol*, 133, 697, 1984.
166. Maurice, MM, Nakamura, H, van der Voort, EAM, *et al.* Evidence for the role of an altered redox state in hyporesponsiveness of synovial T cells in rheumatoid arthritis. *J Immunol*, 158, 1458, 1997.

18

Oxidants and Antioxidants in Ultraviolet-Induced Nonmelanoma Skin Cancer

Maralee McVean, Ph.D., Kim Kramer-Stickland, Ph.D., and Daniel C. Liebler, Ph.D.
Department of Pharmacology, University of Arizona
Tuscon, Arizona, USA

OVERVIEW OF NONMELANOMA SKIN CANCER

Nonmelanoma skin cancers (NMSC), which include basal cell carcinomas (BCC) and squamous cell carcinomas (SCC), are the most common human cancers. Increasing incidence of NMSC has stimulated interest in both the mechanisms of ultraviolet light (UV)-induced skin carcinogenesis and its prevention. Here we review recent work on the mechanisms of skin carcinogenesis, with a particular emphasis on the roles of oxidants. We also discuss the roles of endogenous antioxidant defenses in preventing oxidative damage in the skin and the pharmacology of antioxidants in skin cancer prevention.

0-8493-8009-X/98/$0.00+$.50

The skin is a complex organ consisting of several layers and cell types. The epidermis contains keratinocytes in various stages of differentiation, hair follicles, melanocytes, sweat ducts, and cells involved in the immune response. The cellular origin of non-melanoma skin cancers remains unknown; however, evidence suggests a role for both follicular and interfollicular stem cells. Studies comparing chemically induced skin carcinogenesis in hairless and haired mice have shown that newborn hairless mice, which have follicles, developed papillomas and carcinomas when initiated with DMBA and promoted with croton oil.[1] Adult hairless mice, which no longer have hair follicles, developed significantly fewer papillomas and no carcinomas. Adult haired mice, like the newborn hairless mice, developed both papillomas and carcinomas, which implicated follicular stem cells as the original cancerous cells. Conversely, exposure of Oslo hr/hr hairless mice to 3-methylcholanthrene produced complete carcinogenesis, suggesting that intrafollicular stem cells were the site of initiation of the skin cancer. Histologic studies of tumors early in their formation have shown that chemically induced BCC in rats originate from follicular stem cells,[2] whereas SCC develop from interfollicular stem cells.[3] In humans, BCC have been shown to develop from either,[4] whereas actinic keratoses, a cancer precursor, were shown to form initially in interfollicular stem cells.[5] The origins of UV-induced skin cancers have not been established.

DEVELOPMENT OF UV-INDUCED SKIN CANCER

Overview

Although exposure to a variety of chemicals can induce carcinogenesis, exposure to solar radiation is the major cause of skin cancer. Sunlight contains many different wavelengths, but the ultraviolet portion has primarily been implicated in skin photocarcinogenesis. Much of the early work investigating UV-induced damage used UVC light (250-290 nm) sources. However, UVC is absorbed almost entirely by atmospheric ozone, calling into question the biological relevance of these wavelengths. UVA (320-400 nm)-induced oxidant formation has been postulated to contribute significantly to UV-induced lethality[6] and chronic exposure can result in carcinogenesis.[7] Although sunlight reaching the earth contains only 0.05%-0.3% UVB (290-320 nm), it is this portion of sunlight that is most effective in inducing tumors. Many UV induced events are wavelength dependent. Exposure to different UV sources can elicit widely variant responses, further underscoring the importance of carefully evaluating the light sources used in different studies.

UV induces a constellation of chemical, biochemical, and cellular effects, all of which contribute to photodamage and skin carcinogenesis. These effects include 1) induction of DNA photodamage, 2) induction of oxidative damage, 3) induction of an inflammatory response, and 4) perturbations of cellular signaling pathways with concomitant induction of stress response genes. Although these effects can be considered separate end-points, there is considerable evidence that they all are mechanistically interrelated. In the following sections, we consider the effects of UV on DNA photodamage, inflammation, and cellular signaling and stress responses. An expanded discussion of UV-induced oxidative damage then follows.

DNA Photodamage

There are many UV-induced cellular events that contribute to carcinogenesis. DNA absorbs well in the UVB and UVC range leading to the formation of DNA photoproducts, such as cyclobutane pyrimidine dimers and pyrimidine (6-4) pyrimidone dimers at dipyrimidine sites.[8] These lesions can disrupt a number of cellular functions including inhibition of DNA replication and protein synthesis,[9] transcription factor binding,[10] and RNA synthesis.[11] Both 6-4 photoproducts and pyrimidine dimers are also toxic to cells.[12,13] These DNA lesions are repaired by nucleotide excision repair mechanisms; however, if repair fails to remove these lesions, they can produce mutations.

Pyrimidine dimers have been implicated in characteristic C→T and CC→TT transition mutations[14] found in a variety of NMSCs. A number of factors may determine the sequences at which mutations occur. Hot spot codons containing runs of pyrimidines are frequently mutated[15,16] and the presence of the lesion on the transcribed strand of DNA as opposed to the nontranscribed also increases mutation frequency. The p53 tumor suppressor gene, which plays a role in cell cycle control, DNA repair, differentiation, and apoptosis,[17-19] is frequently mutated in NMSCs within runs of pyrimidines. These mutations are consistent with those caused by pyrimidine dimers.[20]

UV-Induced Signaling and Stress Responses

Early studies on UV-induced signal transduction pathways primarily used UVC lamps. These studies revealed that UVC exposure led to the activation of a number of genes involved in DNA repair and synthesis, transcription, and cell cycle regulation. These genes were generally termed UV-inducible or stress-response genes. Many of these genes contain a consensus binding sequence, TGACTA,[41,42] recognized by the transcription factor AP-1. AP-1 is composed of homo- and heterodimers of other gene products, c-*jun* and c-*fos*. Protein levels of c-*jun* and c-*fos* increase after UVC exposure.[43,44] Although levels of c-*jun* were higher than c-*fos*, further studies demonstrated the importance of c-*fos* in the UV-response. Murine fibroblasts lacking c-*fos* showed no increase in AP-1 binding activity and no induction of proteins normally induced by UV exposure such as collagenase I, stromelysin I, and stromelysin II.[45]

Coffer *et al.* reported that the initial UVC-induced signaling event was activation of the epidermal growth factor (EGF) receptor as evidenced by phosphorylation of key tyrosine residues in the receptor.[46] UV-induced activation of EGFR and Ha-*ras*[47] was shown to be an upstream event leading to activation of mitogen activated protein kinases (MAP kinases) such as extracellular-signal regulated kinases (ERK) and c-*jun* kinase (JNK).[48] In turn, JNK is responsible for the phosphorylation of c-*jun* and its subsequent activation in the AP-1 complex.[49-51]

While the EGF receptor has been implicated as the major membrane mediator in UVC-induced signal transduction, recent reports have noted differences in signaling induced by UVC and UVB. Exposure of both keratinocytes and skin to UVC caused robust activation of ERK and JNK. UVB, on the other hand, was an inefficient activator of MAP kinases,[48] suggesting that different molecular pathways could be activated by these different wavelengths. Other studies compared cells expressing wild type EGFR and cells devoid of EGFR. No differences in AP-1 activity after UVB exposure were noted, indicating that EGFR was not necessary for the UV-induced activation of AP-1.[52] On the other hand, Rosette *et al.* reported that exposure of HeLa keratinocytes to UVB-induced clustering of the IL-1, TNF, and EGF receptors and subsequent JNK activation. Inhibition of EGF clustering or receptor down-regulation reduced the UV response.[53] The authors believe that a concerted clustering of a number of cell surface receptors for growth factors and cytokines in the membrane is the initial signaling event leading to JNK activation.

UVA-induced AP-1 activation may be mediated through oxidative mechanisms.[54] N-acetylcysteine but not αTH inhibited AP-1 activation. Since αTH did prevent lipid peroxidation in this study, the authors suggest that UVA-dependent AP-1 activation is sensitive to redox states, but not to perturbations in the membrane caused by lipid peroxidation. Further studies will need to fully elucidate what molecular events ultimately mediate UV-induced AP-1 activation.

The role of protein kinase C (PKC) in UV signaling has also been investigated. In cells expressing a dominant negative mutant of an atypical PKC, PKCλ/i, UVB-induction of AP-1 activity was blocked.[52] AP-1 activity was not blocked, however, by down regulation of novel or conventional PKCs, suggesting a role for atypical PKCs in AP-1 activation. The atypical PKC isoforms also may play a role in suppressing UV-induced apoptosis.[55] Inhibition of atypical PKC activity preceded UV-induced apoptosis and decreased MAP kinase activity, suggesting that atypical PKCs may influence a variety of UV-induced signaling pathways.

Another UV-inducible transcription factor, NF-kB, modulates the expression of a number of immune and acute phase proteins. Direct activation of NF-kB has been demonstrated in enucleated cells after UVC exposure[56] and in nuclear extracts after UVB or UVA exposure.[57,58] NF-kB is activated by a number of oxidants[59] and is inhibited by water-soluble antioxidants.[57,59,60] Thus, the UV-dependent activation of NF-kB may result from oxidative stress generated by UV.

DNA damaging agents, including UV, activate the p53 tumor suppressor gene.[61] p53 mediates a G1 cell cycle arrest[62] via its downstream effector, p21,[63] allowing the cell time to repair DNA damage before entering S phase. It also appears to partially mediate apoptosis induction after UV.[17] UV exposure leads to increases in p53 expression[64] largely due to increases in the protein half-life.[65] Chronic sun exposure led to increased levels in human skin,[66] while UVA and UVC both induce elevations in p53 in discrete layers of the epidermis.[67] UVB was able to induce p53 expression throughout all layers of the epidermis.[67] This gene is frequently mutated in NMSC, primarily at dipyrimidine sites,[68,69] suggesting that changes in or loss of p53 function plays a major role in the progression of skin carcinogenesis.

MECHANISMS OF OXIDANT FORMATION IN SKIN

UV-Induced Oxidative Damage in the Skin

The skin is uniquely challenged by oxidants due to its role as a barrier. It is exposed to high oxygen tensions, which increase its vulnerability to oxidative damage. In addition to being exposed to ROS resulting from UV-radiation, skin is exposed to oxidants released from normal oxygen metabolism and to chemical irritants that can cause oxidative damage. The targets of UV-induced oxidative damage in the skin include lipid, proteins, and DNA. Oxidative damage to proteins can cause cross-linking, aggregation, or proteolysis, possibly leading to alteration of function of proteins involved in signaling pathways and antioxidant protection of the skin. Lipid peroxidation causes the formation of lipid radical species, resulting in membrane damage, release of inflammatory mediators,[70] activation of phospholipase A_2, prostaglandin formation, and inflammation.[71-73] UV-induced prostaglandin formation in the skin may also be mediated in part by oxidatively controlled phosphorylation of the EGF receptor.[74] The proinflammatory cytokines IL-1, IL-6, IL-8, and TNF-α are also induced by UV radiation in humans.[34,35,75-79] The resulting inflammatory infiltrate to the skin provides a further source of ROS and oxidative damage. Oxidative damage to DNA can lead to the formation of single and double strand breaks[80,81] and to mutagenic adducts, such as 8-oxo-deoxyguanosine. Oxidative damage to Langerhans cells, the resident macrophages of the epidermis, may be involved in the pathology of UVB induced immunosuppression, which allows for the escape of UV-induced tumors from immune surveillance.[82-85] ROS have also been implicated in the induction of transcription factors and growth factors via signaling pathways[86-89] that may be important in the unregulated cell growth seen in cancer.

Many studies have shown evidence of oxidative damage in the epidermis after UV irradiation. Products of lipid peroxidation, lipid radicals,[90,91] oxidatively damaged DNA bases,[92] and antioxidant depletion all have been found in UV-irradiated skin.[93,94] UV-induced oxidative damage has also been implicated in the formation of apoptotic keratinocytes (sunburn cells) and depletion of Langerhans cells in the epidermis.[83,85]

Endogenous Oxygen Metabolism and Oxidant Formation

During normal aerobic respiration, mitochondria reduce O_2 by sequential steps to produce H_2O. During this process, there is a leakage of electrons that leads to the partial reduction of O_2 to the superoxide anion (O_2^-), addition of another electron reduces O_2^- to H_2O_2, and addition of a third electron leads to the formation of the highly reactive hydroxyl radical ($^\bullet OH$).[95] $^\bullet OH$ reacts with surrounding molecules in a diffusion limited manner, whereas O_2^- may be able to escape from its site of production to elicit its effects elsewhere in the cell. H_2O_2 readily crosses biological membranes and is relatively stable in the absence of transition metal ions.[96] The toxicity of H_2O_2 resides primarily in its ability to be converted to more reactive species, such as $^\bullet OH$. NO synthases in the epidermis form NO, which may react with O_2^- to form the highly reactive oxidant peroxynitrite ($ONOO^-$). Photosensitization of the skin may involve production of singlet oxygen ($^1O_2$), a highly reactive nonradical oxidant. The half-lives, and thus the reactivities of these oxidant species are vastly different (Table 1).

Formation of ROS from the mitochondrial respiratory chain has been estimated to yield about 2 x 10^{10} O_2^- and H_2O_2 per cell per day.[98,99] In addition, in the presence of iron or copper, O_2^- and H_2O_2 can form $^\bullet OH$ via the Fenton reaction. H_2O_2 can also be produced by reduction of O_2^- by thioredoxin reductase, by superoxide dismutase, or by spontaneous dismutation of O_2^-. If the endogenous antioxidant defense of the skin is compromised, as may be the case in UVB-irradiated skin,[93,94] the skin becomes more susceptible to oxidative protein and DNA damage and lipid peroxidation by ROS resulting from endogenous oxygen metabolism.

Table 1
Estimate of the Half-Lives of Reactive Oxygen and Nitrogen Species (modified from Ref. 97)

Reactive Oxygen Species	Half Life (sec)
O_2^-	concentration dependent
$^{\bullet}OH$	10^{-9}
$RO^{\bullet}$	10^{-6}
$ROO^{\bullet}$	1-7
$^1O_2$	10^{-5}
NO	1-10
$ONOO^-$	0.05-1

UV-Induced Formation of Oxidants

Reactive oxygen species generated in the epidermis upon UVB irradiation include O_2^-, $^1O_2$, $^{\bullet}OH$, and lipid peroxyl ($LOO^{\bullet}$) and alkoxyl ($LO^{\bullet}$) radicals. Other oxidants generated in UVB irradiated epidermis include $ONOO^-$ and H_2O_2. The reaction of $^{\bullet}OH$ with biomolecules is diffusion-limited, whereas O_2^- and $ONOO^-$ may be able to escape from its site of production to elicit effects elsewhere in the cell. $^1O_2$ is much more reactive than O_2^- or H_2O_2 and reacts with polyunsaturated fatty acids in membranes to form lipid peroxides.[100] Production of $^1O_2$ has been shown to cause lipid peroxidation in human dermal fibroblasts,[101] collagen cross-linking,[102] and matrix metalloproteinase production in human dermal fibroblasts.[103] $^1O_2$ is formed from O_2 after absorption of energy from photoexcited photosensitizer molecules. Photosensitizers in the skin include protoporphyrins, NAD(P)H, flavins, melanins, and the tryptophan oxidation product N-formylkynurenine. O_2^-, $^1O_2$, $^{\bullet}OH$, and H_2O_2 all are generated directly or indirectly upon exposure of these molecules to UV-light.[101,103-107] Most UV-induced radicals are probably due to photosensitization reactions.

Lipid peroxidation can be initiated by UV irradiation directly, by causing photochemical cleavage of lipid hydroperoxides, forming reactive lipid alkoxyl $LO^{\bullet}$ or $LOO^{\bullet}$ radicals, which can initiate peroxyl radical chains. UV-induced $^{1}O_2$, O_2^{-}, $^{\bullet}OH$, and $ONOO^{-}$ all can initiate lipid peroxidation. It is thought that lipid peroxyl radicals probably cause most of the oxidative damage that occurs *in vivo*. This is due to the fact that many oxidants cause the formation of lipid peroxyl radicals, which then propagate the oxidative damage.

Inflammation secondary to UV-induced cytokine induction or lipid peroxidation brings with it a further oxidative insult to the skin. Infiltration of leukocytes and other phagocytic cells into the epidermis occurs, followed by a respiratory burst from the phagocytic cells due to an increase in activity of a plasma membrane NADPH oxidase, myeloperoxidase, and nitric oxide synthase. NADPH oxidase reduces O_2 to O_2^{-}.[108,109] H_2O_2 is formed from dismutation of O_2^{-} and hypochlorous acid (HOCl) is formed from the reaction of Cl^{-} and H_2O_2 via myeloperoxidase. The hypochlorous acid can then be reduced by O_2^{-} to form $^{\bullet}OH$.[108,110] The respiratory burst can also cause release of iron from storage molecules, providing a catalyst of the Fenton reaction (Eq. 1) and resulting in the generation of $^{\bullet}OH$.

$$H_2O_2 + Fe^{2+}\text{-ligand} \rightarrow {}^{\bullet}OH + OH^{-} + Fe^{3+}\text{-ligand} \qquad (1)$$

The free radical NO is also released from phagocytic cells[111,112] and can react with $O_2^{\bullet -}$ to form the powerful oxidant $ONOO^{-}$. NO, which is identical to endothelium-derived relaxing factor (EDRF), also causes vasorelaxation that may contribute to inflammation and edema. Membrane-bound NO synthase and xanthine oxidase in human keratinocytes are activated by UVB to release NO, O_2^{-}, and $ONOO^{-}$[113,114] $ONOO^{-}$ can exert cytotoxic effects in the epidermis by initiating lipid peroxidation, causing direct protein oxidation, or acting as a "hydroxyl radical-like" oxidant. $ONOO^{-}$ and NO may diffuse out to endothelial and smooth muscle cells, resulting in further vasodilation, erythema and inflammation.[113,115-117] Topical application of anti-inflammatory agents prior to UV-irradiation inhibits tumor formation[118] in mice. Oxidative DNA damage,[92,119,120] involves DNA base modification as well as strand breakage.[80,81]. $ONOO^{-}$ and $^{\bullet}OH$ are able to oxidize DNA bases *in vitro* and *in vivo*.[121] $^{\bullet}OH$ formed from the reaction of O_2^{-} with HOCl in the nucleus may be the source of $^{\bullet}OH$ involved in DNA adduct formation, since the highly reactive $^{\bullet}OH$ must be generated in the immediate vicinity of the DNA to elicit any effect. Metal ion dependent conversion of O_2^{-} and H_2O_2 to $^{\bullet}OH$ in the nucleus may also be a factor.[122,123] $ONOO^{-}$ has also been shown to have a hydroxyl radical-like activity when in the peroxynitrous acid form (ONOOH) and may be involved in modification of DNA bases. N_2O_3 formed from NO can nitrosate DNA base amino groups, leading to base deamination.[121] $^1O_2$, peroxyl ($ROO^\bullet$), and alkoxyl ($RO^\bullet$) radicals also are able to modify DNA bases, whereas O_2^- and H_2O_2 do not react directly with DNA bases.[122,123] Aldehyde products of lipid peroxidation are also able to form adducts with DNA bases.[124,125] $^\bullet OH$ forms primarily 8-oxo-G, but reacts with all four DNA bases, whereas $^1O_2$ reacts preferentially with guanine.[126,127] Levels of 8-oxo-G are increased[92, 128] in the nuclei of UVB-irradiated mouse epidermal cells.

Protein damage by UV-induced oxidants could lead to loss of function of important regulatory proteins in the cell.[116,129] Types of damage that could contribute to loss of function include protein cross-links, protein fragmentation, or site-specific lesions in proteins that may alter a critical protein function.[130,131] However, very little is known about protein oxidation *in vivo*, as appropriate evaluation of protein oxidation is difficult due to the complexity of protein secondary and tertiary structure. Enzyme inactivation, formation of protein carbonyls, oxidation of protein-SH, loss of tryptophan fluorescence, and enhanced protease degradation upon UV irradiation have been monitored as *in vitro* indicators of protein oxidation.[129] Knowledge of the basic chemistry of protein amino acids and amino acid sequence allows for prediction of possible oxidation "hot spots" in proteins. Amino acids that are susceptible to oxidation include tryptophan, methionine, and cysteine. Many enzymes contain critical cysteine thiols in the active site that are easily oxidized. Histidine, lysine, and tyrosine can also be oxidized.

ENDOGENOUS ANTIOXIDANT DEFENSES IN SKIN

Overview

The human skin contains a variety of enzymatic and non-enzymatic antioxidant defenses. Thiol containing molecules include glutathione (GSH) and thioredoxin. GSH is a ubiquitous cysteine-containing tripeptide capable of oxygen radical scavenging.[132] It plays an important role in reducing oxidized tissue components, such as lipid peroxides, and can regenerate other cellular antioxidants such as vitamin C.[133] Glutathione peroxidase (GPX) catalyzes the reduction of hydroperoxides to alcohols and of hydrogen peroxide to water (reviewed in Ref. 134), whereas glutathione reductase functions in the reduction of oxidized glutathione. Thioredoxin is a membrane-associated enzyme active in suppression of lipid peroxidation.[135] The thioredoxin system also acts as a disulfide reductase catalyzing the reduction of S-S bridges in a variety of proteins and may play a role in enzyme regulation (reviewed in Ref. 136). Catalase is a heme protein active in the conversion of hydrogen peroxide to water and oxygen (reviewed in Ref. 137). Superoxide dismutases (SOD) comprise a family of metalloproteins that catalyze the combination of superoxide and hydrogen ions to form hydrogen peroxide and oxygen. The active site may contain both copper and zinc or manganese. The different isoforms of SOD are localized to different cellular compartments,[138] suggesting different physiological roles for them.

The epidermis also contains many non-enzymatic antioxidants including vitamins A, E, and C. Vitamin A comprises a family of compounds, most of which probably have negligible importance as antioxidants. Vitamin A precursors, such as β-carotene, act as lipid soluble antioxidants, which can trap free radicals and quench singlet oxygen (reviewed in Ref. 139). Vitamin C, or ascorbic acid, is a water-soluble antioxidant active as a peroxyl and oxygen radical scavenger.[140] It may also regenerate the reduced form of vitamin E,[141] which emphasizes the interdependent relationships between antioxidant systems. Vitamin E, in the αTH form, is the primarily lipid soluble antioxidant in the body. It acts primarily as a peroxyl radical scavenger[142] but it is also important in maintaining membrane integrity.[143] αTH is the most biologically active of a family of tocopherol and tocotrienol compounds.[144] Its reaction with lipid peroxyl radicals yields relatively stable hydroperoxides and tocopheroxyl radicals, significantly protecting membranes against lipid peroxidation.

The epidermis is the first barrier of defense against UV oxidative processes and damage. Thus, it is not surprising that higher levels of all of these antioxidants were found in the human epidermis than in the dermis. SOD, GPX, and glutathione-reductase activities were significantly higher in the epidermis.[145] Catalase activity was notably higher by 720%. Hydrophilic antioxidants including ascorbic acid, reduced GSH, and total GSH were higher in the epidermis by 425%, 513%, and 471%, respectively. αTH was 90% higher in the epidermis also, lending support to the idea that the epidermis possesses greater defenses against oxidative stress than the dermis. Studies in mouse epidermis revealed that with the exclusion of SOD, all antioxidants measured were higher in the epidermis than the dermis.[94]

Effect of UV on Antioxidants in Epidermis

Irradiation of mice led to the depletion of many of these antioxidants in the epidermis, reflecting either their activity in free radical scavenging or their destruction by UV. Shindo[146] exposed hairless mice to solar simulated radiation (SSR) lamps emitting light in the wavelengths between 290-400 nm at doses ranging from 20-250 kJ/cm^2. A single exposure to between 20-50 kJ/m^2 solar simulated light resulted in the reduction of SOD and catalase to about 65% of their normal levels. GPX and glutathione reductase were less affected with depletion to 80-85% of normal, while ascorbate concentrations decreased to 66% of control in the epidermis. At higher doses of UV, GSH was decreased to less than 60% of control levels. αTH also required higher UV doses before depletion to 65% of control levels occurred. In other studies, UVA/vis light (>320 nm) exposure of hairless mice greatly reduced the activities of catalase and glutathione reductase but did not significantly affect GPX or SOD.[147]

Conversely, nonenzymatic antioxidants including GSH, αTH, ubiquinol, and ascorbate were slightly, but not significantly, decreased. Recent unpublished studies in our laboratory with FS20 UVB lamps (>285 nm) showed that αTH levels in C3H/HeNTac mouse epidermis were not affected by a single UVB exposure at a dose of 9000 J/m^2. Multiple exposures at a dose of 4500 J/m^2 actually increased αTH levels in mouse epidermis by 4-4.5-fold and also increased levels of the αTH oxidation products, tocopherol quinone and tocopherol hydroquinone. Other studies in cultured keratinocytes indicated that exposure to UVB led to an immediate increase in Cu-ZnSOD, whereas MnSOD levels declined only to recover 24 hours later.[148] Thus, these SOD isoforms may play a part in different phases of the antioxidant response to UV. Different wavelengths, different spectral distributions, and different intensities of light may all induce different amounts of oxidative stress and elicit different physiological responses. Collectively, these studies illustrate the importance of the interaction of antioxidants with UV-induced oxidants and how UV-induced oxidation and photochemistry modify antioxidant levels.

Although αTH is a potent antioxidant, it also absorbs in the UV, which suggests both antioxidant chemistry and photochemistry may be involved in its depletion. Exposure of αTH solutions in methanol to 25 kJ/m^2 SSR resulted in limited depletion of αTH levels to 70% of control.[146] Studies in our laboratory have shown, however, that αTH was rapidly depleted in soy phosphatidylcholine (SPC) liposomes irradiated with 10.8 kJ/m^2 UVB over a 30-min period.[149] Irradiation of a liposomal suspension containing 0.1 mol% αTH led to the depletion of approximately 90% of the αTH over the first 30-minutes and greater than 90% by 90 minutes. In liposomes containing 1.0 mol% αTH, approximately 70% of the αTH was depleted at 30 minutes and depletion was greater than 90% at 90 minutes. In contrast, UVB had no effect on levels of the αTH ester, αTAc. To assess the role of phospholipid peroxidation in αTH oxidation, αTH depletion was also monitored in dilinoleoyl phosphatidylcholine (DOPC) liposomes, which contain only singly unsaturated oleate chains and thus are largely resistant to lipid peroxidation. The time course of αTH depletion in DOPC liposomes was similar to that seen in SPC liposomes, indicating that peroxidation of liposomal lipid was not required for αTH depletion. Further evidence for the photochemical oxidation of αTH was seen in UVB irradiated solutions (acetonitrile:H_2O, 4:1 v/v), where depletion was greater than 90% after exposure to 32.4 kJ/m^2 UVB over 90 min.

PREVENTION OF UV-INDUCED PHOTODAMAGE

Inhibition of UV-Induced Damage

Antioxidants have been shown to inhibit many types of UV-induced damage. Preincubation of keratinocytes with vitamin C, sodium selenite (an essential cofactor for GPX function), or a water-soluble form of vitamin E, Trolox, prior to UVB irradiation resulted in a significant decrease in the formation of an oxidatively modified DNA product, 8-oxodeoxyguanosine.[150] Both GSH[151] and αTH[152] treatment inhibited UVB-induced cytotoxicity. Furthermore, GSH, catalase, and SOD have been shown to inhibit the formation of apoptotic sunburn cells, which are histological markers of UVB-induced epidermal cell injury.[153,154] Antioxidants including N-acetylcysteine, ascorbate, and αTH also inhibited UV-induced increases in p53 expression.[155] The generation of single strand breaks has been proposed as an important step leading to the increase in p53; these antioxidants may protect against oxidatively induced DNA strand breaks. Topically applied GSH has been shown to prevent UVB-induced immunosuppression in mice.[156] Thus, a role for antioxidants in protection against UV damage has been clearly established.

αTH acts directly as an antioxidant by inhibiting the propagation of oxygen radicals. Topically applied αTH-inhibited epidermal lipid peroxidation,[157] whereas αTH, αTAc, and α–tocopherol sorbate have been shown to decrease UV-induced radicals detected by spin-trapping and electron paramagnetic resonance spectroscopy (EPR).[158] Furthermore, αTH has been shown to suppress superoxide generation by activated neutrophils.[159] αTH treatment also resulted in the inhibition of oxidatively induced increases in ICAM-1 expression in human epidermal keratinocytes exposed to H_2O_2,[160] thus decreasing the ability of leukocytes and macrophages to destructively interact with epidermal cells. Thus, αTH may act to inhibit the influx of inflammatory cells, the release of free radicals from neutrophils and the deleterious effects of superoxide and other oxidants once formed.

Vitamin E Compounds and Sunscreens

αTH absorbs strongly in the UVB and can act as a sunscreen when topically applied. Both dietary supplementation and topical application of αTAc, an esterified derivative of αTH, prevented UV-induced increases in unscheduled DNA synthesis,[161] indicating protection against DNA damage. However, UVB-induced induction of cyclobutane thymine dimers is a more direct measure of DNA photodamage than increases in DNA synthesis. These lesions do not form through oxidative processes and directly reflect photodeposition of energy into DNA. Studies in our laboratory showed that application of a 1% dispersion of αTH inhibited thymine dimer formation in mouse epidermal DNA by approximately 50%.[162] Other tocopherol derivatives including αTAc, γTH, δTH, and α–tocopherol methyl ester and compounds found in commercial sunscreen products were also able to inhibit the formation of thymine dimers in mouse epidermal DNA when topically applied. αTH, however, was 5-10 times more potent than any of the other tocopherol derivatives or sunscreen compounds in its ability to protect against UVB induced DNA photodamage. These data strongly suggest that this is one mechanism by which αTH prevents UV-induced tumor formation.

Prevention of Other Effects of UV Photodamage by Vitamin E

Certain manifestations of UV-induced damage may result from both oxidative stress and photodestruction of cellular molecules. Edema, erythema, activation of inflammatory and immune responses, and photocarcinogenesis probably result from a combination of photodamage and oxidative damage. Topical αTH treatment has been shown to inhibit edema and erythema in UVB-irradiated mice.[163] αTH also completely prevented the suppression of the immune response that accompanied UVB exposure in mice[157,164] and partially protected against UVA-induced decreases in antigen-presenting function of Langerhans cells in human epidermal cell cultures.[165] αTH treatment also inhibited increases in PGE_2 levels and ornithine decarboxylase activity (ODC) occurring during urethane-induced lung tumorigenesis.[166] Since prostaglandins and ODC both play a role in skin tumor promotion,[167] this could constitute another anti-tumorigenic activity of αTH. Most important, topically applied αTH prevented the induction of skin tumors in mice exposed to UVB irradiation.[164] The photoprotective effects of αTH may be greater when αTH is topically applied than when orally supplemented. Although Gerrish *et al.*[168] showed that dietary αTAc protected against UVB-induced skin tumors in mice, studies in humans indicate that oral supplementation with αTAc did not significantly protect against UV-induced epidermal damage.[169]

Anti-carcinogenic effects of αTH may involve attenuation of a variety of UV-induced responses. Boscoboinik *et al.* showed that αTH specifically inhibited the growth of vascular smooth muscle cells.[170] The anti-proliferative effect of αTH was mediated through the inhibition of PKCα activity[171] and phosphorylation.[172] PKCs are a family of enzymes that play an important part in the signal transduction pathway leading to cell proliferation. Although the effect of αTH on the proliferation of epidermal cells has not been reported, similar mechanisms could be at work. Atypical PKCs, such as the UV-induced isoform PKCλ/*i*, appear to play a role in UV signaling[52] and it would be interesting to determine whether αTH inhibits this enzyme. The participation of αTH derivatives in the regulation of proliferative and signal transduction pathways has been demonstrated. The vitamin E derivatives αTAc and αTS, but not αTH, can inhibit activation of the transcription factor NF-kB.[173] αTH did, however, both inhibit and activate AP-1 binding to DNA in smooth muscle cells, depending on the experimental conditions.[174] Activation of other oxidatively regulated transcription factors such as p53 could also be modulated using αTH.

CHEMOPREVENTION OF SKIN CANCER BY VITAMIN E

Studies in Animal Models

In recent years, many researchers have been interested in the chemopreventive effects of antioxidants in skin cancer. Topical and dietary supplements of vitamin E,[164,168,175,176] tannic acid,[177] butylated hydroxytoluene (BHT),[178] ascorbate,[176] and antioxidant mixtures containing BHT, glutathione, ascorbate and αTH[178-181] have all been used to bolster the antioxidant defense in UV-irradiated epidermis. These antioxidants and others have been effective in animal models of oxidative skin damage,[158,161,182-184] inflammation,[185,186] and tumorigenesis (Table 2).

Much of the recent interest in the cancer chemoprevention by vitamin E has been generated from the results of a number of animal studies. These studies involve the monitoring of effects of topical and oral vitamin E on short and long-term endpoints of UV-damage in the skin. Short-term endpoints include skin erythema, edema, sunburn cell formation, immunosuppression, and lipid peroxidation. The effect of vitamin E supplementation on UV-induced DNA damage and medium- to long-term effects such as wrinkling (photoaging) and tumorigenesis have also been evaluated. The form of vitamin E used in most studies has been αTH, but the vitamin E esters αTAc and α–tocopherol succinate, as well as the water-soluble αTH analogue Trolox have also been utilized.

Table 2
Inhibition of UV-Tumorigenesis in Mice by Antioxidants

Strain	Agent	Endpoint	Ref.
BALB/c	Topical tannic acid	Inhibition of tumorigenesis, immunosuppression	177
C3H/HeN	Dietary αTAc	Inhibition of tumorigenesis	168
C3H/HeN	Topical αTH	Inhibition of tumorigenesis, immunosuppression	164
SKH:HR-1	Topical αTH or Ascorbate	Inhibition of tumorigenesis	176
SKH:HR-1	Topical or oral green tea polyphenols	Inhibition of tumorigenesis	187, 188
SKH:HR-1	Dietary BHT or glutathione	BHT: inhibition of tumorigenesis Glutathione: no inhibition	178
SKH:HR-1	Dietary BHT + glutathione +ascorbate + αTH	Increased tumor latency, inhibition of tumorigenesis	179-181 189

Oral Vitamin E Supplementation

The use of dietary supplements of antioxidant mixtures including αTH, ascorbate, BHT, and GSH has been shown to reduce UVB-induced skin cancers in mice.[178,180,181] However, the effectiveness of these supplements is dependent on antioxidant dose, dietary content of lipid, and UV dose.[179,189-191] Further studies utilizing oral supplements of αTH or αTAc in UVB-irradiated animals have provided both positive and negative results. UVB-induced tumorigenesis was inhibited in female C3H mice with high levels of dietary αTAc,[168] which is converted completely to αTH in the gut. However, supplementation with αTAc was also toxic to the mice that received UV.[168] A diet containing 1% αTH did not prevent UVB-induced skin wrinkling in female albino hairless SKH-HR1 mice,[176] and UVB/UVA-induced lipid peroxidation was not suppressed in mice fed low doses of αTAc for three weeks before irradiation.[161] This suggests large, potentially toxic dietary supplements of vitamin E may be needed to increase skin αTH to levels that are protective against photocarcinogenesis in mice. This effect may be specific to mice and other animals, as there is no evidence for toxicity in humans given large doses of αTAc.[192,193]

EFFECT OF TOPICAL VITAMIN E SUPPLEMENTATION

Studies with topical vitamin E provided a more direct supplementation of αTH to skin. The effects of topical supplements of αTH, αTAc, and other vitamin E derivatives on short-term endpoints of UV irradiation have been monitored in mouse and swine skin. Both αTH and αTAc absorb UV radiation directly and act as sunscreens. αTAc cannot act directly as an antioxidant in skin, and must first be hydrolyzed to αTH to elicit antioxidant effects. Topically applied αTH alone and in conjunction with ascorbic acid inhibited UVB-induced sunburn cell formation in swine skin.[194] In C3H/HeJ mice treated with αTH (5 mg dose before UV), there was a suppression in UVB/UVA induced lipid peroxidation. UV-induced immunosuppression was also inhibited, as was UV-induced decreases in Langerhans cell density.[157] Edema induced by a broad-band UV lamp in rabbit skin was inhibited by αTH, but not by αTAc.[195] Female SKH-1 hairless mice treated topically with αTAc before UVB/UVA irradiation showed a decrease in epidermal lipid peroxidation and a restoration of ^{3}H-thymidine incorporation into DNA to levels similar to unirradiated mice. UVB-induced skin wrinkling also was inhibited by topical αTH, αTAc, and Trolox (5% solutions) in female albino hairless SKH-HR1 mice.[176] Topically applied αTAc, α–tocopherol sorbate, and αTH protected against UVB-induced photoaging (wrinkling) in female albino hairless SKH-HR1 mice, and α–tocopherol sorbate significantly decreased UVB-induced radical formation in the mouse skin as measured by EPR.[158]

Topical αTH has been shown to inhibit tumorigenesis in UV-irradiated mice, whereas the αTH esters were unable to inhibit UV-induced tumors. UV-induced tumor formation, immunosuppression, and collagen damage was inhibited by topical αTH in female albino hairless SKH-HR1 and C3H/HeN mice.[164,176] UVB-induced photodamage in the C3H mice (in the form of thymine dimers) was also inhibited by topically applied αTH and αTAc, with αTH being the more potent sunscreening agent.[162] As noted above, these studies indicate a sunscreening effect against UV-induced photodamage to DNA for αTH and αTAc. However, topically applied αTAc and α–tocopherol succinate did not inhibit UVB-induced tumorigenesis or immunosuppression in female BALB/c mice, and actually enhanced the susceptibility to tumor challenge with a UV-induced squamous cell carcinoma cell line.[175] In this study, αTAc and α–tocopherol succinate were hydrolyzed to αTH in the skin, but perhaps not enough to confer protection against UVB-induced tumorigenesis. This suggests that the sunscreening ability of vitamin E alone may not confer protection against UVB tumorigenesis and that the antioxidant capabilities of αTH are necessary for inhibition of tumorigenesis.

These studies indicate that topical αTH is able to inhibit various indicators of UV-induced oxidative damage, photodamage, and UV-induced photocarcinogenesis in animal models. Also, topical application of vitamin E may be more effective and reliable than oral supplements in the prevention of photocarcinogenesis. Topical αTAc inhibits UV-induced lipid peroxidation most likely through its sunscreening actions and inhibits UV-induced photoaging most likely through a combination of its sunscreening actions and hydrolysis to αTH in the skin. The inability of αTAc to inhibit UVB-induced tumors in BALB/c mice is disturbing, as αTAc is the form of vitamin E in most commercially available sunscreens and lotions.

HUMAN CLINICAL STUDIES

Studies investigating the role of vitamin E supplementation in human skin have centered on the photoprotective effects of oral and topical vitamin E on short-term endpoints of UV-induced damage. Oral vitamin E (400 IU/day for 6 months) showed only a minor increase in plasma αTH and no increase in epidermal αTH.[196] There was no significant difference in the number of sunburn cells induced by UVB or in erythema induced by UVB in the vitamin E treated group. In contrast, topically applied αTH protected against erythema when applied before UVA-psoralen phototherapy.[185] However, the effects of topically applied vitamin E in UVB-irradiated human skin have not been measured.

Many commercially available skin products contain the ester αTAc, rather than αTH. Studies utilizing topical vitamin E in mouse skin have clearly shown that the antioxidant αTH is the most effective chemopreventive agent and that topical vitamin E esters may actually have deleterious effects in UV-irradiated skin. Few studies have been done in animals to monitor the extent of hydrolysis of αTAc to αTH in the skin, or the effect of UVB on hydrolysis. One recent study has reported epidermal and plasma levels of αTH in humans after topical vitamin E acetate supplementation. After four months of vitamin E acetate supplementation, there were no appreciable changes in plasma or skin αTH levels.[197]

These data collectively tend to indicate that topical vitamin E has a photoprotective effect in humans, that oral vitamin E has no photoprotective effect, and that topical αTAc is not hydrolyzed to the antioxidant αTH in significant quantities in human skin. However, this latter issue may require further investigation. Conversion of αTAc to αTH has been previously measured as increases in total plasma and epidermal αTH.[197] This does not measure hydrolysis of the topically applied αTAc, or effects of topical αTAc on distribution of dietary-derived tocopherols. The site of administration and dose of vitamin E and UVB are also important in interpreting results, as suggested by animal studies. The oral vitamin E study[197] employed histological data from UVB irradiated buttock skin, which is not normally sun exposed and may not represent the response in sun-exposed tissue that ultimately develops non-melanoma skin cancer. In addition, an oral dose of vitamin E was used in this study that did not increase plasma or skin vitamin E, so it was not surprising that no effect of vitamin E was found.

HUMAN EPIDEMIOLOGICAL STUDIES

Observational epidemiological studies have evaluated vitamin E and the risk of multiple cancers. Some clinical intervention trials have been started, but results are years away.[198] Very few of these studies, however, have monitored the effects of αTH on non-melanoma skin cancer. The majority of these studies are cross-sectional or longitudinal studies based on blood level of vitamin E. In nested case-control studies by Karagas *et al.*[199] and Breslow *et al.*[200] no statistically significant differences in plasma or prediagnostic serum αTH levels were seen between patients with SCC and control patients. However, cross-sectional studies have also related blood vitamin E levels to reduced skin cancer risk.[201,202] There seems to be no clear-cut relationship between cancer risk and plasma αTH in these studies. Again, there is a problem with interpreting many of these data, due to the use of improper control populations and small sample sizes. Other confounding factors include lifestyle factors of the participants (e.g., smoking and alcohol consumption), disease state of the patients, extent of UV exposure in each sample population, and modifying factors in the diet (e.g., other antioxidants, fats). Also, there was no estimation of dietary vitamin E intake or tissue vitamin E levels. In some studies, blood samples were stored for years before analysis, which raises doubts about the accuracy of αTH measurements reported.

CONCLUSION

A large body of evidence indicates that UV-induced skin cancer involves multiple consequences of UV photochemistry. In addition to promutagenic DNA photodamage, UV also induces oxidant formation, oxidative damage, an inflammatory response, and profound effects on cellular signaling pathways. All of these effects may be modulated by antioxidants, particularly αTH and other forms of vitamin E. Evidence for multiple anticancer mechanisms comes from both *in vitro* and *in vivo* studies and underscores the multiple roles of antioxidants. Studies with αTH and other vitamin E compounds suggest that these agents may be most effective as photoprotectants when applied topically. The contributions of specific photoprotective mechanisms remain to be established, as does the efficacy of topical vitamin E compounds in human skin cancer prevention. Nevertheless, widespread use, low toxicity, and compelling preliminary data make vitamin E compounds highly attractive agents for future studies of human skin cancer prevention.

REFERENCES

1. Giovanella, BC, Liegel, J, Heidelberger, C, The refractoriness of the skin of hairless mice to chemical carcinogenesis. *Cancer Res* 30, 2590-2597, 1970
2. Zackheim, HS, The origin of experimental basal cell epitheliomas in the rat. *J Invest Dermatol* 38, 57-64, 1961
3. Zackheim, HS, Evolution of squamous cell carcinoma in the rat. *J Invest Dermatol* 77, 434-444, 1964
4. Zackheim, HS, Origin of the human basal cell epithelioma. *J Invest Dermatol* 40, 283-297, 1962
5. Pinkus, H, Keratosis senilis. *Am J Clin Path* 29, 193-207, 1957

6. Danpure, HJ, Tyrrell, RM, Oxygen-dependence of near UV (365 nm) lethality and the interaction of near UV and x-rays in two mammalian cell lines. *Photochem Photobiol* 23, 171-177, 1976
7. De Laat, A, van der Leun, JC, de Gruijl, FR, Carcinogenesis induced by UVA (365-nm) radiation: the dose-time dependence of tumor formation in hairless mice. *Carcinogenesis*, 18, 1013-1020, 1997
8. Blackburn, GM, Davies, RJH, The structure of DNA-derived thymine dimer. *Biochem Biophys Res Comm* 22, 704-706, 1966
9. Brown, TC, Cerutti, P, Ultraviolet radiation inactivates SV40 by disrupting at least four genetic functions. *EMBO J* 5, 197-203, 1986
10. Tommasi, S, Swiderski, PM, Tu, Y, Kaplan, BE, Pfeifer, GP, Inhibition of transcription factor binding by ultraviolet-induced pyrimidine dimers. *Biochemistry*, 35, 15693-15703, 1996
11. Donahue, BA, Yin, S, Taylor, JS, Reines, D, Hanawalt, PC, Transcript cleavage by RNA polymerase II arrested by a cyclobutane pyrimidine dimer in the DNA template. *Proc Natl Acad Sci USA*. 91, 8502-8506, 1994
12. Mitchell, DL, The relative cytotoxicity of (6,4) photoproducts and cyclobutane dimers in mammalian cells. *Photochem Photobiol* 48, 51-57, 1988
13. Cleaver, JE, Cortes, F, Karentz, D, Lutze, LH, Morgan, WF, Player, AN, Vuksanovic, L, Mitchell, DL, The relative biological importance of cyclobutane and (6-4) pyrimidine-pyrimidone dimer photoproducts in human cells: Evidence from a Xeroderma Pigmentosum revertant. *Photochem Photobiol* 48, 41-49, 1988
14. Miller, JH, Mutagenic specificity of ultraviolet light. *J Mol Biol* 182, 45-68, 1985
15. Tornaletti, S, Rozek, D, Pfeifer, GP, The distribution of UV photoproducts along the human p53 gene and its relation to mutations in skin cancer. *Oncogene*, 8, 2051-2057, 1993
16. Dumaz, N, van Kranen, HJ, de Vries, A, Berg, RJW, Wester, PW, van Kreijl, CF, Sarasin, A, Daya-Grosjean, L, de Gruijl, FR, The role of UV-B light in skin carcinogenesis through the analysis of p53 mutations in squamous cell carcinomas of hairless mice. *Carcinogenesis* 18, 897-904, 1997
17. Ziegler, A, Jonason, AS, Leffell, DJ, Simon, JA, Sharma, HW, Kimmelman, J, Remington, L, Jacks, T, Brash, DE, Sunburn and p53 in the onset of skin cancer. *Nature*. 372, 773-776, 1994
18. Levine, AJ, Momand, J, Finlay, CA, The p53 tumour suppressor gene. *Nature*. 351, 453-456, 1991
19. Lane, DP, Benchimol, S, p53: oncogene or anti-oncogene. *Genes Dev* 4, 1-8, 1990
20. Drobetsky, EA, Grosovsky, AJ, Glickman, BW, The specificity of UV-induced mutations at an endogenous locus in mammalian cells. *Proc Natl Acad Sci USA* 84, 9103-9107, 1987
21. Valtonen, EJ, Janne, J, Siimes, M, The effect of the erythemal reaction caused by ultraviolet irradiation on mast cell degranulatin in the skin. *Acta Derm Venerol* 44, 269-272, 1964
22. Pentland, AP, Mahoney, M, Jacobs, SC, Holtzman, MJ, Enhanced prostaglandin synthesis after ultraviolet injury is mediated by endogenous histamine stimulation. *J Clin Invest* 86, 566-574, 1990
23. Black, AK, Fincham, N, Greaves, MW, Hensby, CN, Time course changes in levels of arachadonic acid and prostaglandins D_2, E_2, $F_{2\alpha}$ in human skin following ultraviolet B irradiation. *Br J Clin Pharmacol* 10, 453-457, 1980

24. Black, AK, Greaves, MW, Hensby, CN, Plummer, NA, Increased prostaglandins E_2 and $F_{2\alpha}$ in human skin at 6 and 24 h after ultraviolet B irradiation (290-320 nm). *Br J Clin Pharmacol* 5, 431-436, 1978
25. Gilchrest, BA, Soter, NA, Stoff, JS, Mihm, MC, The human sunburn reaction: Histologic and biochemical studies. *J Am Acad Dermatol* 5, 411-422, 1981
26. Hawk, JLM, Black, AK, Jaenicke, KF, Barr, RM, Soter, NA, Mallett, AI, Gilchrest, BA, Hensby, CN, Parrish, JA, Greaves, MW, Increased concentrations of arachidonic acid, prostaglandins E_2, D_2, and 6-oxo-F_{1a}, and histamine in human skin following UVA irradiation. *J Invest Dermatol* 80, 496-499, 1983
27. Miller, WS, Ruderman, FR, Smith, JG, Aspirin and ultraviolet light-induced erythema in man. *Arch Dermatol* 95, 357-358, 1967
28. Rheins, LA, Barnes, L, Amornsiripanitch, S, Collins, CE, Nordlund, JJ, Suppression of the cutaneous immune response following topical application of the prostaglandin PGE_2. *Cell Immunol* 106, 33-42, 1987
29. Needleman, P, Turk, J, Jakschik, BA, Morrison, AR, Lefkowith, JB, Arachidonic acid metabolism. *Ann Rev Biochem* 55, 69-102, 1986
30. Cornelius, LA, Sepp, N, Li, L-J, Degitz, K, Swerlick, RA, Lawley, TJ, Caughman, SW, Seclective upregulation of intercellular adhesion molecule (ICAM-1) by ultraviolet B in human dermal microvascular endothelial cells. *J Invest Dermatol* 103, 23-28, 1994
31. Rosario, R, Mark, GJ, Parrish, JA, and Mihm, MC, Histological changes produced in skin by equally erythemogenic doses of UV-A, UV-B, and UV-C and UV-A with psoralens. *Br J Dermatol* 101, 299-308.1979.
32. Kang, K, Hammerberg, C, Meunier, L, Cooper, KD, CD11b+ macrophages that infiltrate human epidermis after *in vivo* ultraviolet exposure potently produce IL-10 and represent the major secretory source of epidermal IL-10 protein. *J Immunol* 153, 5256-5264, 1994
33. Cooper, KD, Duraiswamy, N, Hammerberg, C, Allen, E, Dillon, WKAE, Thomas, D, Neutrophils, differentiated macrophages, and monocyte/macrophage antigen presenting cells infiltrate murine epidermis after UV injury. *J Invest Dermatol* 101, 155-163, 1993
34. Kupper, TS, Groves, RW, The interleukin-1 axis and cutaneous inflammation. *J Invest Dermatol* 105, 62S-66S, 1995
35. Kock, A, Schwarz, T, Kirnbauer, R, Urbanski, A, Perry, P, Ansel, JC, Luger, TA, Human keratinocytes are a source for tumor necrosis factor a: Evidence for synthesis and release upon stimulation. *J Exp Med* 172, 1609-1614, 1990
36. Cooper, KD, Oberhelman, L, Hamilton, TA, Baadsgaard, O, Terhune, M, LeVee, G, Anderson, T, Koren, H, UV exposure reduces immunization rates and promotes tolerance to epicutaneous antigens in humans: Relationship to dose, CD1-DR+ epidermal macrophage induction, and Langerhans cell depletion. *Proc Natl Acad Sci USA*. 89, 8497-8501, 1992
37. Tang, A, Udey, MC, Inhibition of epidermal Langerhans cell function by low dose ultraviolet B radiation. Ultraviolet B radiation selectively modulates ICAM-1 (CD45) expression by murine Langerhans cells. *J Immunol* 146, 3347-3355, 1991
38. Rivas, J, Ullrich, SE, Systemic suppression of delayed-type hypersensitivity by supernatants from UV-irradiated keratinocytes. *J Immunol* 149, 3865-3871, 1992
39. Streilein, JW, Taylor, JR, Vincek, V, Kurimoto, I, Shimizu, T, Tie, C, Golomb, C, Immune surveillance and sunlight-induced skin cancer. *Immunol Today* 15, 174-179, 1994
40. Fujisawa, H, Wang, H, Kondo, S, Shivji, GM, Sauder, DN, Costimulation with ultraviolet B and interleukin-1α dramatically increase tumor necrosis factor-α production in human dermal fibroblasts. *J Interferon Cytokine Res* 17, 307-313, 1997
41. Lee, W, Mitchell, P, Tjian, R, Purified transcription factor AP-1 interacts with TPA-inducible enhancer elements. *Cell.* 49, 741-752, 1987

42. Angel, P, Imagawa, M, Chiu, R, Stein, B, Imbra, RJ, Rahmsdorf, HJ, Jonat, C, Herrlich, P, and Karin, M, Phorbol ester-inducible genes contain a common cis element recognized by a TPA-modulated *trans*-acting factor. 729-739, 1987
43. Devary, Y, Gottlieb, RA, Lau, LF, Karin, M, Rapid and preferential activation of the c-*jun* gene during the mammalian UV response. *Mol Cell Biol* 11, 2804-2811, 1991
44. Hollander, MC, Fornace, AJ, Jr, Induction of *fos* RNA by DNA-damaging agents. *Cancer Res* 49, 1687-1692, 1989
45. Schreiber, M, Baumann, B, Cotten, M, Angel, P, Wagner, EF, *Fos* is an essential component of the mammalian UV response. *EMBO J* 14, 5338-5349, 1995
46. Coffer, PJ, Burgering, BM, Peppelenbosch, MP, Bos, JL, Kruijer, W, UV activation of receptor tyrosine kinase activity. *Oncogene* 1997
47. Davis, RJ, MAPKs: new JNK expands the group. *Trend Biochem Sci* 19, 470-474, 1994
48. Dhanwada, KR, Dickens, M, Neades, R, Davis, R, Pelling, JC, Differential effects of UV-B and UV-C components of solar radiation on MAP kinase signal transduction pathways in epidermal keratinocytes. *Oncogene*. 11, 1947-1953, 1995
49. Hibi, M, Lin, A, Smeal, T, Minden, A, Karin, M, Identification of an oncoprotein- and UV-responsive protein kinase that binds and potentiates the c-*Jun* activation domain. *Genes Dev* 7, 2135-2148, 1993
50. Derijard, B, Hibi, M, Wu, I, Barrett, T, Su, B, Deng, T, Karin, M, Davis, RJ, JNK1: A protein kinase stimulated by UV light and Ha-*ras* that binds and phosphorylates the c-*Jun* activation domain. *Cell* 76, 1025-1037, 1994
51. Kyriakis, JM, Banerjee, P, Nikolakaki, E, Dai, T, Rubie, EA, Ahmad, MF, Avruch, J, Woodgett, JR, The stress-activated protein kinase subfamily of *c-Jun* kinases. *Nature* 369, 156-160, 1994
52. Huang, C, Ma, W, Bowden, GT, Dong, Z, Ultraviolet B-induced activated protein-1 activation does not require epidermal growth factor receptor but is blocked by a dominant negative PKCl/*i*. *J Biol Chem* 271, 31262-31268, 1996
53. Rosette, C, Karin, M, Ultraviolet light and osmotic stress: Activation of the JNK cascade through multiple growth factor and cytokine receptors. *Science*. 274, 1194-1197, 1996
54. Djavaheri-Mergny, M, Mergny, J-L, Bertrand, F, Santus, R, Maziere, C, Dubertret, L, Maziere, J-C, Ultraviolet-A induces activation of AP-1 in cultured human keratinocytes. *FEBS Lett* 384, 92-96, 1996
55. Bera, E, Municio, MM, Sanz, L, Frutos, S, Diaz-Meco, MT, Moscat, J, Positioning atypical protein kinase C isoforms in the UV-induced apoptotic signaling cascade. *Mol Cell Biol* 17, 4346-4354, 1997
56. Devary, Y, Rosette, C, DiDonato, JA, and Karin, M. NF-kB activation by ultraviolet light not dependent on a nuclear signal. *Science* 261, 1442-1445, 1993
57. Mihm, S, Ennen, J, Pessara, U, Kurth, R, Droge, W, Inhibition of HIV-1 replication and NF-kappa B activity by cysteine and cysteine derivatives. *AIDS*. 5, 497-503, 1991
58. Vile, GF, Tanew-Iliitschew, A, Tyrrell, RM, Activation of NF-kB in human skin fibroblasts by the oxidative stress generated by UVA radiation. *Photochem Photobiol* 62, 463-468, 1995
59. Schreck, R, Rieber, P, Baeuerle, PA. Reactive oxygen intermediates as apparently widely used messengers in the activation of the NF-kB transcription factor and HIV-1. *EMBO J* 10, 2247-2258, 1991
60. Staal, FJT, Roederer, M, Herzenberg, LA. Intracellular thiols regulate activation of nuclear factor kB and transcription of human immunodeficiency virus. *Proc Natl Acad Sci USA*, 8 7, 9943-9947, 1990
61. Renzing, J, Hansen, S, Lane, DP. Oxidative stress is involved in the UV activation of p53. *J Cell Science*. 109, 1105-1112, 1996

62. Michalovitz, D, Halevy, O, Oren, M. Conditional inhibition of transformation and of cell proliferation by a temperature-sensitive mutant of p53. *Cell.* 62, 671-680, 1990
63. El-Deiry, WS, Tokino, T, Velculescu, VE, Levy, DB, Parsons, R, Trent, JM, Lin, D, Mercer, WE, Kinzler, KW, Vogelstein, B. *WAF*1, a poteintial mediator of p53 tumor suppression. *Cell.* 75, 817-825, 1993
64. Maltzman, W, Czyzyk, L. UV irradiation stimulates levels of p53 cellular tumor antigen nontransformed mouse cells. *Mol Cell Biol* 4, 1689-1694, 1984
65. Liu, M, Dhanwada, KR, Birt, DF, Hecht, S, Pelling, JC. Increase in p53 half-life in mouse keratinocytes following UV-B irradiation. *Carcinogenesis.* 15, 1089-1092, 1994
66. Barnadas, MA, Colomo, L, Curell, R, de Moragas, JM. Expression of the p53 protein in sun-damaged skin. *Acta Derm Venerol* 76, 203-204, 1996
67. Hall, PA, McKee, PH, Menage, HP, Dover, R, Lane, DP, High levels of p53 protein in UV-irradiated normal human skin. *Oncogene.* 8, 203-207, 1993
68. Ziegler, A, Leffell, DJ, Kunala, S, Sharma, HW, Gailani, M, Simon, JA, Halperin, AJ, Baden, HP, Shapiro, PE, Bale, AE, Brash, DE, Mutation hotspots due to sunlight in the p53 gene of nonmelanoma skin cancers. *Proc Natl Acad Sci USA*, 90, 4216-4220, 1993
69. Kanjilal, S, Pierceall, WE, Cummings, KK, Kripke, ML, Ananthaswamy, HN, High frequency of p53 mutations in ultraviolet radiation-induced murine skin tumors: Evidence for strand bias and tumor heterogeneity. *Cancer Res* 53, 2961-2964, 1993
70. Zimmerman, GA, Prescott, SM, McIntyre, TM, Oxidatively fragmented phospholipids as inflammatory mediators: the dark side of polyunsaturated lipids. *J Nutr* 125, 1661s-1665s, 1995
71. Hruza, LL, Pentland, A, Mechanisms of UV-induced inflammation. *J Invest Dermatol* 100, 35s-41s, 1993
72. Hanson, D, DeLeo, V, Long-wave ultraviolet light induces phospholipase activation in cultured human epidermal keratinocytes. *J Invest Dermatol* 95, 158-163, 1990
73. DeLeo, V, Hanson, D, Weinstein, IB, Harber, LC, Ultraviolet light stimulates the release of arachadonic acid from mammalian cells in culture. *Photochem Photobiol* 41, 51-56, 1984
74. Miller, CC, Hale, P, Pentland, A, Ultraviolet B injury increases prostaglandin synthesis through a tyrosine kinase-dependent pathway. *J Biol Chem* 269, 3529-3533, 1994
75. Strickland, I, Rhodes, L, Flanagan, BF, Friedmann, PS, TNF-α and IL-8 are upregulated in the epidermis of normal human skin after UVB exposure: correlation with neutrophil accumulation and E-selectin expression. *J Invest Dermatol* 108, 763-768, 1997
76. Walsh, LJ, Ultraviolet B irradiation of skin induces mast cell degranulation and release of tumor necrosis factor-α. *Immunol Cell Biol* 73, 226-233, 1995
77. Kramer, M, Sachsenmaier, C, Herrlich, P, Rahmsdorf, HJ, UV irradiation-induced interleukin-1 and basic fibroblast growth factor synthesis and release mediate part of the UV response. *J Biol Chem* 268, 6734-6741, 1993
78. Gahring, L, Baltz, M, Pepys, MB, Daynes, R, Effect of ultraviolet radiation on production of epidermal cell thymocyte-activating factor/interleukin 1 *in vivo* and *in vitro*. *Proc Natl Acad Sci USA*. 81, 1198-1202, 1984
79. Urbanski, A, Schwarz, T, Neuner, P, Krutmann, J, Kirnbauer, R, Kock, A, Luger, TA, Ultraviolet light induces increased circulating interleukin-6 in humans. *J Invest Dermatol* 94, 808-811, 1990
80. Birnboim, HC, Kanabus-Kaminska, M, The production of DNA strand breaks in human leukocytes by superoxide anion may involve a metabolic process. *Proc Natl Acad Sci USA*. 82, 6820-6824, 1985

81. Aruoma, OI, Halliwell, B, Dizdaroglu, M, Iron ion-dependent modification of bases in DNA by the superoxide radical-generating system hypoxanthine/xanthine oxidase. *J Biol Chem* 22, 13024-13028, 1989
82. Rattis, FR, Peguet-Navarro, J, Courtellemont, P, Redziniak, G, Schmitt, D, *In vitro* effects of ultraviolet B radiation on human Langerhan's cell antigen-presenting function. *Cell Immunol* 164, 65-72, 1995
83. El-Ghorr, AA, Norval, M, Lappin, MB, Crosby, J, The effect of chronic low-dose UVB radiation on Langerhans cells, sunburn cells, urocanic acid isomers, contact hypersensitivity and serum immunoglobulins in mice. *Photochem Photobiol* 62, 326-332, 1995
84. Murphy, GW, Norris, PG, Young, AR, Corbett, MF, Hawk, JLM, Low-dose ultraviolet-B irradiation depletes human epidermal langerhans cells. *Br J Dermatol* 129, 674-677, 1993
85. Axelrod, M, Serafin, D, Klitzman, B, Ultraviolet light and free radicals: an immunologic theory of epidermal carcinogenesis. *Plast Reconstr Surg* 86, 582-593, 1990
86. Meyer, M, Schreck, R, Baeuerle, PA, H2O2 and antioxidants have opposite effects on activation of NF-kB and AP-1 in intact cells: AP-1 as secondary antoxidant-responsive factor. *EMBO J* 12, 2005-2015, 1993
87. Goldstone, SD, Hunt, NH, Redox regulation of the mitogen-activated protein kinase pathway during lymphocyte activation. *Biochim Biophys Acta*, 1 355, 353-360, 1997
88. Sullivan, SG, Chiu, DT, Errasfa, M, Wang, JM, Qi, JS, Stern, A, Effects of H2O2on protein tyrosine phosphatase activity in HER14 cells. *Free Rad Biol Med* 16, 399-403, 1994
89. Xanthoudakis, S, Miao, G, Wang, F, Pan, YC, Curran, T, Redox activation of Fos-Jun DNA binding activity is mediated by a DNA repair enzyme. *EMBO J* 11, 3323-3335, 1992
90. Jurkiewicz, BA, Buettner, GR, Ultraviolet light-induced free radical formation in the skin: an electron paramagnetic resonance study. *Photochem Photobiol* 59, 1-4, 1994
91. Pelle, E, Maes, D, Padulo, GA, Kim, EK, Smith, WP, An *in vitro* model to test relative antioxidant potential: ultraviolet-induced lipid peroxidation in liposomes. *Arch Biochem Biophys* 283, 234-240, 1990
92. Hattori, Y, Nishigori, C, Tanaka, T, Uchida, K, Nikaido, O, Osawa, T, Hiai, H, Imamura, S, Toyokuni, S, 8-hydroxy-2'-deoxyguanosine is increased in epidermal cells of hairless mice after chronic ultraviolet B exposure. *J Invest Dermatol* 107, 733-737, 1997
93. Fuchs, J, Huflejt, ME, Rothfuss, LM, Wilson, DS, Carcamo, R, Packer, L, Impairment of enzymic and nonenzymic antioxidants in skin by UVB irradiation. *J Invest Dermatol* 93, 769-773, 1989
94. Shindo, Y, Witt, E, Packer, L, Antioxidant defense mechanisms in murine epidermis and dermis and their responses to ultraviolet light. *J Invest Dermatol* 100, 260-265, 1993
95. Frei, B, Reactive oxygen species and antioxidant vitamins: mechanisms of action. *Am J Med* 97, 5s-13s, 1994
96. Gutteridge, JMC, Lipid peroxidation and antioxidants as biomarkers of tissue damage. *Clin Chem* 41, 1819-1828, 1995
97. Sies, H, Strategies of antioxidant defense. *Eur J Biochem* 215, 213-219, 1993
98. Ames, BN, Shigenaga, MK, Hagen, TM, Oxidants, antioxidants, and the degenerative diseases of aging. *Proc Natl Acad Sci USA*. 90, 7915-7922, 1993
99. Chance, B, Sies, H, Boveris, A, Hydroperoxide metabolism in mammalian organs. *Physiol Rev* 59, 527-605, 1979
100. Stogner, SW, Payne, DK, Oxygen toxicity. *Ann Pharmacother* 26, 1554-1562, 1992

101. Vile, G, Tyrrell, RM, UVA radiation-induced oxidative damage to lipids and proteins *in vitro* and in human skin fibroblasts is dependent on iron and singlet oxygen. *Free Rad Biol Med* 18, 721-730, 1995
102. Kakehashi, A, Akiba, J, Ueno, N, Chakrabarti, B, Evidence for singlet oxygen-induced cross-links and aggregation of collagen. *Biochem Biophys Res Comm* 196, 1440-1446, 1993
103. Herrmann, G, Wlaschek, M, Bolsen, K, Prenzel, K, Goerz, G, Scharffetter-Kochanek, K, Photosensitization of uroporphyrin augments the ultraviolet A-induced synthesis of matrix metalloproteinases in human dermal fibroblasts. *J Invest Dermatol* 107, 398-403, 1996
104. Sato, K, Taguchi, H, Maeda, T, Minami, H, Asada, Y, Watanbe, Y, Yoshikawa, K, The primary cytotoxicity in ultraviolet-A-irradiated riboflavin solution is derived from hydrogen peroxide. *J Invest Dermatol* 105, 608-612, 1995
105. Torinuki, W, Miura, T, Seiji, M, Lysosome destruction and lipoperoxide formation due to active oxygen generated from haematoporphyrin and UV irradiation. *Br J Dermatol* 102, 17-27, 1980
106. Arakane, K, Ryu, A, Hayashi, C, Masunaga, T, Shinmoto, K, Mashiko, S, Nagano, T, Hirobe, M, Singlet oxygen (1δg) generation from coproporphyrin in propionibacterium acnes on irradiation. *Biochem Biophys Res Comm* 223, 578-582, 1996
107. Creed, D, The photophysics and photochemistry of the near-UV absorbing amino acids-I. tryptophan and its simple derivatives. *Photochem Photobiol* 39, 537-562, 1984
108. Darr, D, Fridovich, I, Free radicals in cutaneous biology. *J Invest Dermatol* 102, 671-675, 1994
109. Schallreuter, KU, Wood, JM, Free radical reduction in the human epidermis. *Free Rad Biol Med.* 6, 519-532,1989
110. Candeias, LP, Patel, KB, Stratford, MRL, Wardman, P, Free hydroxyl radicals are formed on reaction between the neutrophil-derived species superoxide anion and hypochlorous acid. *FEBS Lett* 333, 151-153, 1993
111. Stamler, JS, Singel, DJ, Loscalzo, J, Biochemistry of nitric oxide and its redox-activated forms. *Science.* 258, 1898-1902, 1992
112. Ischiropoulos, H, Zhu, L, Beckman, JS, Peroxynitrite formation from macrophage-derived nitric oxide. *Arch Biochem Biophys* 298, 446-451, 1992
113. Deliconstantinos, G, Villiotou, V, Stavrides, JC, Increase of particulate nitric oxide synthase activity and peroxynitrite synthesis in UVB-irradiated keratinocyte membranes. *Biochem J* 320, 997-1003, 1996
114. Deliconstantinos, G, Villiotou, V, Stavrides, JC, Alterations of nitric oxide synthase and xanthine oxidase activities of human keratinocytes by ultraviolet B radiation. *Biochem Pharmacol* 51, 1727-1738, 1996
115. Teixeira, MM, Williams, TJ, Helliwell, PG, Role of prostaglandins and nitric oxide in acute inflammatory reactions in guinea pig skin. *Br J Pharmacol* 110, 1515-1521, 1993
116. Radi, R, Beckman, JS, Bush, KM, Freeman, BA, Peroxynitrite oxidation of sulfhydryls. *J Biol Chem* 266, 4244-4250, 1991
117. Radi, R, Beckman, JS, Bush, KM, Freeman, BA, Peroxynitrite-induced membrane lipid peroxidation: the cytotoxic potential of superoxide and nitric oxide. *Arch Biochem Biophys* 258, 481-487, 1991
118. Bissett, DL, Chatterjee, R, Hannon, DP, Photoprotective effect of topical antiinflammatory agents against ultraviolet radiation-induced chronic skin damage in the hairless mouse. *Photodermatol Photoimmunol Photomed* 7, 153-158, 1990
119. Shacter, E, Beecham, EJ, Covey, JM, Kohn, KW, Activated neutrophils induce prolonged DNA damage in neighboring cells. *Carcinogenesis.* 9, 2297-2304, 1988

120. Yamashina, K, Miller, B, Heppner, GH, Macrophage-mediated induction of drug-resistant variants in a mouse mammary tumor cell line. *Cancer Res* 46, 239-2401, 1986
121. Spencer, JPE, Wong, J, Jenner, A, Aruoma, OI, Cross, CE, Halliwell, B, Base modification and strand breakage in isolated calf thymus DNA and in DNA from human skin epidermal keratinocytes exposed to peroxynitrite or 3-morpholinosydnonimine. *Chem Res Toxicol* 9, 1152-1158, 1996
122. Dizdaroglu, M, Chemical determination of free radical-induced damage to DNA. *Free Rad Biol Med* 10, 225-242, 1991
123. Wiseman, H, Kaur, H, Halliwell, B, DNA damage and cancer: measurement and mechanism. *Cancer Lett* 93, 113-120, 1995
124. Flagg, EW, Coates, RJ, and Greenberg, RS, Epidemiologic studies of antioxidants and cancer in humans. *J Am Coll Nutr.* 14(5), 419-427, 1995
125. Marnett, LJ, Burcham, PC, Endogenous DNA adducts: Potential and paradox. *Chem Res Toxicol* 6, 771-785, 1993
126. Dizdaroglu, M, Chemical determination of oxidative DNA damage by gas chromatography-mass spectrometry. *Methods in Enzymol* 234, 3-16, 1994
127. Cadet, J, Ravanat, JL, Buchko, GW, Yeo, HC, Ames, BN, Singlet oxygen DNA damage: chromatographic and mass spectrometric analysis of damage products. *Methods in Enzymol* 234, 79-88, 1994
128. Beehler, B, Przybyszewski, J, Box, HB, Kulesz-Martin, MF, Formation of 8-hydroxydeoxyguanosine within DNA of mouse keratinocytes exposed in culture to UVB and H_2O_2. *Carcinogenesis*, 1 3, 2003-2007, 1992
129. Hu, ML, Tappel, L, Potentiation of oxidative damage to proteins by ultraviolet-A and protection by antioxidants. *Photochem Photobiol* 56, 357-363, 1992
130. Floyd, RA, Role of free radicals in carcinogenesis and brain ischemia. *FASEB J* 4, 2587-2597, 1990
131. Wolff, S, Garner, A, Dean, RT, Free radicals, lipids, and protein degradation. *TIBS*, 1 1, 27-31, 1986
132. Connor, MJ, Wheeler, LA, Depletion of cutaneous glutathione by ultraviolet radiation. *Photochem Photobiol* 46, 239-245, 1987
133. Meister, A, Anderson, ME, Glutathione. *Annu Rev Biochem* 52, 711-760, 1983
134. Ursini, F, Bindoli, A, The role of selenium peroxidases in the protection against oxidative damage of membranes. *Chem Phys Lipids.* 44, 255-276, 1997
135. Schallreuter, KU, Wood, JM, The role of thioredoxin reductase in the reduction of free radicals at the surface of the epidermis. *Biochem Biophys Res Comm* 136, 630-637, 1986
136. Holmgren, A, Thioredoxin and glutaredoxin systems. *J Biol Chem* 264, 13963-13966, 1989
137. Calabrese, EJ, Canada, AT, Catalase: Its role in xenobiotic detoxification. *Pharmacol Ther* 44, 297-307, 1989
138. Kobayashi, I, Saito, N, Takemori, N, IIzuka, S, Suzuki, K, Taniguchi, N, IIzuka, H, Ultrastructural localization of superoxide dismutase in human skin. *Acta Derm Venerol* 73, 41-45, 1993
139. Bendich, A, Olson, JA, Biological actions of carotenoids. *FASEB J* 3, 1927-1932, 1989
140. Sies, H, Stahl, W, Vitamins E and C, β-carotene, and other carotenoids as antioxidants. *Am J Clin Nutr* 62(suppl), 1315S-1321S, 1995
141. Packer, JE, Slater, TF, Willson, RL, Direct observation of a free radical interaction between vitamin E and vitamin C. *Nature.* 278, 737-738, 1979
142. Wassall, SR, Wang, L, Yang McCabe, RC, Ehringer, WD, Stillwell, W, Electron spin resonance study of the interaction of alpha-tocopherol with phospholipid model membranes. *Chem Phys Lipids.* 60, 29-37, 1991

143. Kameda, K, Imai, M, Senjo, M, The effect of vitamin E deficiency on some erythrocyte membrane properties. *J Nutr Sci Vitaminol* 31, 481-490, 1985
144. Horwitt, MK, *Vitamin E Abstracts 1993*. LaGrange, IL, Veris, 1994.
145. Shindo, Y, Witt, E, Han, D, Epstein, W, Packer, L, Enzymic and non-enzymic antioxidants in epidermis and dermis of human skin. *J Invest Dermatol* 102, 122-124, 1994
146. Shindo, Y, Witt, E, Han, D, Packer, L, Dose-response effects of acute ultraviolet irradiation on antioxidants and molecular markers of oxidation in murine epidermis and dermis. *J Invest Dermatol* 102, 470-475, 1994
147. Fuchs, J, Huflejt, ME, Rothfuss, LM, Wilson, DS, Carcamo, G, Packer, L, Acute effects of near ultraviolet and visible light on the cutaneous antioxidant defense system. *Photochem Photobiol* 50, 739-744, 1989
148. Sasaki, H, Akamatsu, H, Horio, T, Effects of a single exposure to UVB radiation on the activities and protein levels of copper-zinc and manganese superoxide dismutase in cultured human keratinocytes. *Photochem Photobiol* 65, 707-713, 1997
149. Kramer, KA, Liebler, DC, UVB induced photoxidation of vitamin E. *Chem Res Toxicol* 10, 219-224, 1997
150. Stewart, MS, Cameron, GS, Pence, BC, Antioxidant nutrients protect against UVB-induced oxidative damage to DNA of mouse keratinocytes in culture. *J Invest Dermatol* 106, 1086-1089, 1996
151. Tyrrell, RM, Pidoux, M, Endogenous glutathione protects human skin fibroblasts against the cytotoxic action of UVB, UVA and near visible radiation. *Photochem Photobiol* 44, 561-564, 1986
152. Sakagami, H, Satoh, K, Makino, Y, Kojima, T, Takeda, M., Effect of α-tocopherol on cytotoxicity induced by UV irradiation and antioxidants. *Anticanc Res* 17, 1997
153. Miyachi, Y, Horio, T, Imamura, S, Sunburn cell formation is prevented by scavenging oxygen intermediates. *Clin Exp Dermatol* 8, 305-310, 1983
154. Hanada, K, Gange, RW, Connor, MJ, Effect of glutathione depletion on sunburn cell formation in the hairless mouse. *J Invest Dermatol* 96, 838-840, 1991
155. Vile, GF, Active oxygen species mediate the solar ultraviolet radiation-dependent increase in the tumour suppressor protein p53 in human skin fibroblasts. *FEBS Lett* 412, 70-74, 1997
156 Hemelaar, PJ, Beijersbergen van Henegouwen, GMJ, The protective effect of N-acetylcysteine on UVB-induced immunosuppression by inhibition of the action of *cis*-urocanic acid. *Photochem Photobiol* 63, 322-327, 1996
157. Yuen, KS, Halliday, GM, α-Tocopherol, and inhibitor of epidermal lipid peroxidation, prevents ultraviolet radiation from suppressing the skin immune system. *Photochem Photobiol* 65, 587-592, 1997
158. Jurkiewicz, BA, Bissett, DL, Buettner, GR, Effect of topically applied tocopherol on ultraviolet radiation-mediated free radical damage in skin. *J Invest Dermatol* 104, 484-488, 1995
159. Kanno, T, Utsumi, T, Kobuchi, H, Takehara, Y, Akiyama, J, Yoshioka, T, Horton, AA, Utsumi, K, Inhibition of stimulus-specific neutrophil superoxide generation by alpha-tocopherol. *Free Rad Res* 22, 431-440, 1995
160. Ikeda, M, Schroeder, KK, Mosher, LB, Woods, CW, Akeson, AL, Suppressive effect of antioxidants on intercellular adhesion molecule-1 (ICAM) expression in human epidermal keratinocytes. *J Invest Dermatol* 103, 791-796, 1994
161. Record, IR, Dreosti, IE, Konstantinopoulos, M, Buckley, RA, The influence of topical and systemic vitamin E on ultraviolet light-induced skin damage in hairless mice. *Nutr Cancer.* 16, 219-225, 1991

162. McVean, M, Liebler, DC, Inhibition of UVB induced DNA photodamage in mouse epidermis by topically applied a-tocopherol. *Carcinogenesis.* 18, 1617-1622, 1997
163. Trevithick, JR, Xiong, H, Lee, S, Shum, DT, Sanford, SE, Karlik, SJ, Norley, C, Dilworth, GR, Topical tocopherol acetate reduces post-UVB, sunburn-associated erythema, edema, and skin sensitivity in hairless mice. *Arch Biochem Biophys* 296, 575-582, 1992
164. Gensler, HL, Magdaleno, M, Topical vitamin E inhibition of immunosuppression and tumorigenesis induced by ultraviolet irradiation. *Nutr Cancer.* 15, 97-106, 1991
165. Clement-Lacroix, P, Michel, L, Moysan, A, Morliere, P, Dubertret, L, UVA-induced immune suppression in human skin: protective effect of vitamin E in human epidermal cells *in vitro. Br J Dermatol* 134, 77-84, 1996
166. Yano, T, Yano, Y, Uchida, M, Murakami, A, Hagiwara, K, Otani, S, Ichikawa, T, The modulation effect of vitamin E on prostaglandin E_2 level and ornithine decarboxylase activity at the promotion phase of lung tumorigenesis in mice. *Biochem Pharmacol* 53, 1757-1759, 1997
167. Verma, AK, Rice, HM, Boutwell, RK, Prostaglandins and skin tumor promotion: Inhibition of tumor promoter-induced ornithine decarboxylase activity in epidermis by inhibitors of prostanglandin synthesis. *Biochem Biophys Res Comm* 79, 1160-1166, 1977
168. Gerrish, KE, Gensler, HL, Prevention of photocarcinogenesis by dietary vitamin E. *Nutr Cancer.* 19, 125-133, 1993
169. Wernignhaus, K, Meydani, M, Bhawan, J, Margolis, R, Blumberg, JB, Gilchrest, BA, Evaluation of the photoprotective effect of oral vitamin E supplementation. *Arch Dermatol* 130, 1257-1261, 1994
170. Boscoboinik, D, Szewczyk, A, Hensey, C, Azzi, A, Inhibition of cell proliferation by α-tocopherol. *J Biol Chem* 266, 6188-6194, 1991
171. Chatelain, E, Boscoboinik, DO, Bartoli, G-M, Kagan, VE, Gey, FK, Packer, L, Azzi, A, Inhibition of smooth muscle cell proliferation and protein kinase C activity by tocopherols and tocotrienols. *Biochim Biophys Acta.* 1176, 83-89, 1993
172. Clement, S, Tasinato, A, Boscoboinik, D, Azzi, A, The effect of α-tocopherol on the synthesis, phosphorylation and activity of protein kinase C in smooth muscle cells after phorbol 12-myristate 13-acetate down-regulation. *Eur J Biochem* 246, 745-749, 1997
173. Suzuki, YJ, Packer, L, Inhibition of NF-kB activation by vitamin E derivatives. *Biochem Biophys Res Comm* 193, 277-283, 1993
174. Azzi, A, Boscoboinik, D, Chatelain, E, Ozer, NK, Stauble, B, *d*-α-Tocopherol control of cell proliferation. *Molec Aspects Med* 14, 265-271, 1993
175 Gensler, HL, Aickin, M, Peng, YM, Xu, M, Importance of the form of topical vitamin E for prevention of photocarcinogenesis. *Nutr Cancer.* 26, 183-191, 1996
176. Bisset, DL, Chatterjee, R, and Hannon, DP, Photoprotective effect of superoxide-scavenging antioxidants against ultraviolet radiation-induced chronic skin damage in the hairless mouse. *Photodermatol Photoimmunol Photomed*, 7, 56-62, 1990.
177. Gensler, HL, Gerrish, KE, Williams, T, Rao, G, Kittelson, J, Prevention of photocarcinogenesis and UV-induced immunosuppression in mice by topical tannic acid. *Nutr Cancer*, 22, 121-130, 1994
178. Black, H, Chan, JT, Brown, GE, Effects of dietary constituents on ultraviolet light-mediated carcinogenesis. *Cancer Res* 38, 1384-1387, 1978
179. Black, H, Lenger, W, McCann, V, Thornby, J, Relation of UV dose to antioxidant modification of photocarcinogenesis. *J Am Coll Toxicol* 2, 201-207, 1983
180. Black, H, Chan, JT, Suppression of ultraviolet light-induced tumor formation by dietary antioxidants. *J Invest Dermatol* 65, 412-414, 1975
181. Black, H, Effects of dietary antioxidants on actinic tumor induction. *Res Commun Chem Pathol Pharmacol* 7, 783-786, 1974

182. Fuchs, J, Packer, L, Photooxidative stress in the skin. In: *Oxidative Stress: Oxidants and Antioxidants*, Academic Press Ltd, 1991, p. 559
183 Reeve, VE, Bosnic, M, Rozinova, E, Boehm-Wilcox, C, A garlic extract protects from ultraviolet B (280-320 nm) radiation-induced suppression of contact hypersensitivity. *Photochem Photobiol* 58, 813-817, 1993
184. Kobayashi, S, Takehana, M, Tohyama, C, Glutathione isopropyl ester reduces UVB-induced skin damage in hairless mice. *Photochem Photobiol* 63, 106-110, 1996
185. Potapenko, A, Abijev, G, Pistsov, M, Roschchupkin, D, Vladimirov, Y, Pliquett, F, Ermolayev, A, Sarycheva, I, Evstigneeva, R, PUVA-induced erythema and mechanoelectrical properties of the skin. *Arch Dermatol Res* 276, 12-16, 1984
186. Kamimura, M, Antiinflammatory activity of vitamin E, *J Vitaminol* 18, 204-209, 1972
187. Mukhtar, H, Katiyar, SK, Agarwal, R, Green tea and skin-anticarcinogenic effects. *J Invest Dermatol,* 102, 3-7, 1994
188. Wang, ZY, Huang, MT, Lou, YR, Xie, JG, Reuhl, KR, Newmark, H, Ho, CT, Yang, CS, Conney, AH, Inhibitory effects of black tea, green tea, decaffeinated black tea, and decaffeinated green tea on ultraviolet B light-induced skin carcinogenesis in 7,12-dimethylbenz[a]anthracene-initiated SKH-1 mice. *Cancer Res* 54, 3428-3435, 1994
189. Black, H, Henderson, SV, Kleinhans, CM, Phelps, AW, Thornby, J, Effect of dietary cholesterol on ultraviolet light carcinogenesis. *Cancer Res* 39, 5022-5027, 1979
190. Black, H, Lenger, W, Phelps, AW, Thornby, JI, Influence of dietary lipid upon ultraviolet light-carcinogenesis. *J Environ Pathol Toxicol* 271-282, 1984
191. Forbes, PD, Photocarcinogenesis: an overview. *J Invest Dermatol* 77, 139-143, 1981
192. Meydani, SN, Meydani, M, Rall, LC, Morrow, F, Blumberg, JB, Assessment of the safety of high-dose, short-term supplementation with vitamin E in healthy older adults. *Am J Clin Nutr* 60, 704-709, 1994
193. Bendich, A, Machlin, LJ, Safety of oral intake of vitamin E. *Am J Clin Nutr* 48, 612-619, 1988
194. Darr, D, Dunston, S, Faust, H, Pinnell, SR, Effectiveness of antioxidants (vitamin C and E) with and without sunscreens as topical photoprotectants. *Acta Derm Venerol* 76, 264-268, 1996
195. Roschchupkin, D, Pistsov, M, Potapenko, A, Inhibition of ultraviolet light-induced erythema by antioxidants. *Arch Dermatol Res* 266, 91-94, 1979
196. Werninghaus, K, Meydani, M, Bhawan, J, Margolis, R, Blumberg, JB, Gilchrest, BA, Evaluation of the photoprotective effect of oral vitamin E supplementation. *Arch Dermatol* 130, 1257-1261, 1994
197. Alberts, DS, Goldman, R, Xu, MJ, Dorr, RT, Quinn, J, Welch, K, Guillen-Rodriguez, J, Aickin, M, Peng, YM, Loescher, L, Gensler, H, Disposition and metabolism of topically administered α-tocopherol acetate: a common ingredient of commercially available sunscreens and cosmetics. *Nutr Cancer.* 26, 193-201, 1996
198. Knekt, P. Epidemiological studies of vitamin E and cancer risk. In: Bendich, A, Butterworth, CE, Eds, *Micronutrients in Health and in Disease Prevention*, New York, Marcel Dekker, Inc, 1991, p. 141
199. Karagas, MR, Greenberg, ER, Nierenberg, D, Stukel, T, Morris, JS, Stevens, MM, Baron, JA, Risk of squamous cell carcinoma of the skin in relation to plasma selenium, α-tocopherol, β-carotene, and retinol: a nested case control study. *Cancer Epidemiology, Biomarkers & Prevention.* 6, 25-29, 1997
200. Breslow, RA, Alberg, AJ, Helzlsouer, KJ, Bush, TL, Norkus, EP, Comstock, GW, Serological precursors of cancer: malignant melanoma, basal and squamous cell skin cancer, and prediagnostic levels of retinol, β-carotene, lycopene, α-tocopherol, and selenium. *Cancer Epidemiology, Biomarkers & Prevention.* 4, 837-842, 1995

201. Knekt, P, Aromaa, A, Maatela, J, Aaran, RK, Nikkari, T, Hakama, M, Hakulinen, T, Peto, R, Teppo, L, Vitamin E and cancer prevention. *Am J Clin Nutr* 53, 283s-286s, 1991
202. Wald, NJ, Thompson, SG, Densem, JW, Boreham, J, Bailey, A, Serum vitamin E and subsequent risk of cancer. *Br J Cancer* 56, 69-72, 1987

19

Antioxidant Status of the Digesta and Colon Cancer: Is There a Direct Link?

Andreas M. Papas, Ph.D.
Health and Nutrition, Eastman Chemical Company
Kingsport, Tennessee, USA

INTRODUCTION

Currently, the antioxidant status of humans is considered almost exclusively in the context of blood and other body tissues. The digesta (a term defining the total contents of the digestive tract including food and drink, endogenous secretions, enzymes, bile, and the gut microflora) is largely ignored. Yet, the digesta is a very active biological system producing a large and diverse array of metabolic products and comes in direct contact with the very large surface area of our digestive system. A large number of metabolic

0-8493-8009-X/98/$0.00+$.50

products in the digesta may stimulate digestive diseases including colon cancer. These metabolic products include oxidation products formed during processing, storage and cooking of food, free radicals produced from metabolism of food components and interaction of bacteria with the contents of the colon, and reactive nitrogen species formed during intestinal inflammation. Antioxidants present in the digesta may protect the exposed surface or may enter the cells lining the digestive system and provide protection inside the cell.

The diet is probably the leading factor affecting the antioxidant status of the digesta and has a direct effect on diseases of the digestive system, especially cancer. For example, stomach cancer decreased dramatically in the last 60 years (Figure 1). This decrease is even more remarkable considering that the incidence of other cancers changed very little and, for lung cancer, it increased substantially. The primary reason for this decrease was probably the advent of refrigeration that made possible increased consumption of fresh fruits and vegetables and reduced consumption of preserved foods especially those producing nitrosamines. Another major development was the discovery and practical use of food antioxidants that reduced the lipid peroxides in our diets. We propose that the antioxidant status of the digesta plays a major role in colon cancer.[1]

This chapter will discuss the potential role of the antioxidant status of the digesta on health using tocopherols and colon cancer as examples of dietary antioxidants and digestive diseases, respectively.

COLON CANCER

Pathogenesis of Colon Cancer

Colon cancer starts in the epithelial cells (colonocytes), which line the bowel and come in direct contact with the contents of the lumen. It develops in a multi-step process, which involves somatic mutations and increased cell proliferation. Mutations in the p53 tumor suppressor gene, particularly deamination of 5-methylcytosine to thymidine, are common in colon cancer.[2] From the 130,000 cases of colorectal cancer diagnosed in the United States each year, about 15% have a hereditary component. Two well-defined syndromes, familial adenomatous polyposis and hereditary non-polyposis colorectal cancer, account for up to 5% of the total new cases. Truncating APC mutations are responsible for polyposis, and defective mismatch repair genes cause non-polyposis colon cancers. However, the genes responsible for most of the familial cases are unknown. A mutation (T to A at APC nucleotide

3920) found in 6% of Ashkenazi Jews and about 28% of Ashkenazim with a family history of colorectal cancer creates a small hypermutable region of the gene, indirectly causing predisposition to colon cancer.[3] While some people have a genetic predisposition, the mutations causing colon cancer are largely induced by dietary and environmental mutagens. It is widely believed that free radicals and other mutagens such as nitrosamines cause most mutations.

The free radical hypothesis as a major contributing factor for carcinogenesis is not limited to colon cancer.[4] Actually, free radicals have been implicated in the pathogenesis of practically all cancers. There are, however, some unique aspects for colon cancer arising from the direct contact of the colon epithelial cells with the digesta.

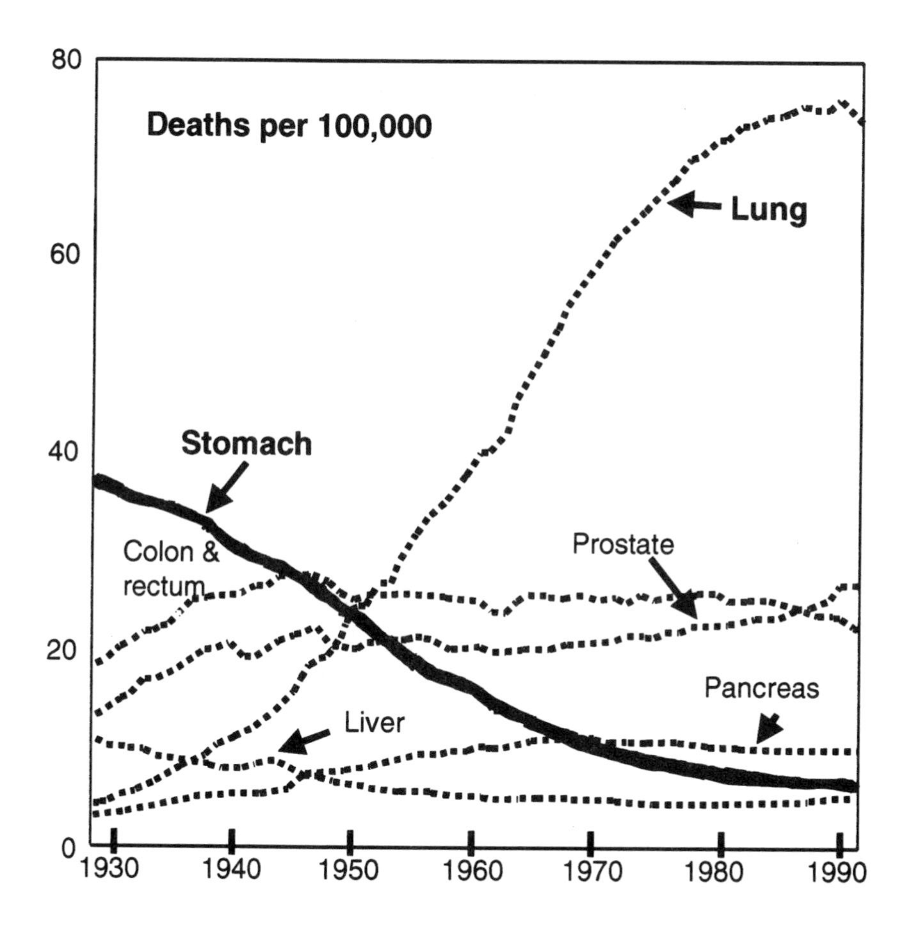

Figure 1. Deaths from cancer of men in the United States. Based on data from Reference 2.

Major Role of Diet in Colon Cancer — Epidemiological Evidence

Colon cancer varies approximately 20-fold internationally. It is the second most common cause of cancer deaths in the United States[5] and similar high rates are found in central northern Europe (Figure 2). In contrast, Mediterranean countries have lower rates and some Asian and African countries even lower.[6] Differences in diet account for the major part of this variability because it is estimated that 70-90% of colon cancer deaths are diet-related.[7] Low incidence is associated with diets rich in fiber, fruits, vegetables, and grains. In contrast, diets rich in saturated fat and low in fruits, vegetables, and fiber are associated with high rates.[8]

There is strong interest to identify and evaluate the specific components of the diet, in addition to fiber, which reduce colon cancer. Because fruits and vegetables are rich in antioxidants and fiber but low in fat, researchers have focused first on these components. While there is significant consensus on the benefit of high dietary fiber and low dietary saturated fat, the role of antioxidants remains rather controversial.

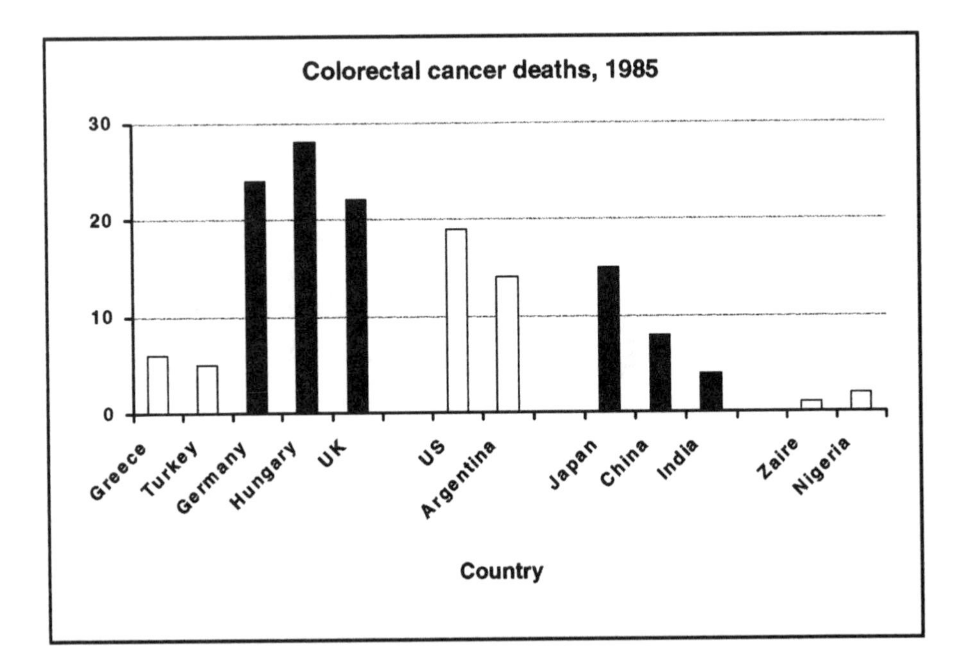

Figure 2. Deaths of men from colorectal cancer in selected countries showing major country- to-country variation. Data from the World Health Organization (WHO).

GUT MICROFLORA

The human colon contains an abundance of bacteria comprising about 40-55% of the dry weight of stool.[9] Actually the colon can be described as a complex microbial ecosystem of human tissue and secretions, food material, and several hundred bacterial species.[10] Some species are beneficial to the host and exhibit antimutagenic and anticarcinogenic properties.[11] Others contribute to the development of cancer.[12] Incidence of colon cancer is at least 30-fold higher than cancer of the small intestine.[13] While many factors account for this large difference, bacteria, whose numbers increase by six orders of magnitude between the ileum and the colon, probably play a partial role. Bacteria, in some cases convert environmental and dietary procarcinogens to carcinogens. For example, some intestinal bacteria deconjugate the bile acids secreted into the intestine and produce secondary bile acids that act as tumor promoters.[14,15]

Production of Free Radicals by Gut Microflora

Intestinal microflora produce free radicals, which generate fecal mutagens and genotoxins.[14] The respiratory activity of bacteria in feces produces superoxide radicals ($O_2^{\cdot-}$) which, in the presence of chelated iron, can generate hydroxyl radicals. Significantly, most dietary iron is not absorbed and is concentrated in feces at a level calculated to be 10-fold greater than in most tissues. Feces also have high levels of bile pigments (such as bilirubin, biliverdin) which can chelate iron in a form capable of supporting the superoxide driven Fenton reactions. Babbs calculated that the microflora in the fecal mass, adjacent to the mucosa, can generate hydroxyl free radicals ($^{\cdot}OH$) at a rate corresponding to that produced by over 10,000 rads of gamma irradiation per day.[4]

Effect of Diet on Total Number and Species in Gut Microflora

Diet has a major impact on the both the total number of bacteria and the dominating species in the digestive tract. The relationship of diet and gut microflora has been studied extensively in ruminant animals (such as cattle, sheep, goats, etc.) In these animals, the mostly anaerobic microbial population in the rumen (the largest component of their 4-compartment stomach) provides them with the unique ability to digest and utilize cellulose and non-protein nitrogen.[16] High-fiber diets promote the growth of cellulolytic bacteria, which produce short-chain fatty acids mostly acetic and butyric, and some propionic. In contrast, high-energy diets promote starch-digesting bacteria which produce the same fatty acids but significantly more propionic. Actually, high-energy diets with very low fiber content essentially eliminate some bacteria and protozoa species in the rumen. Some bacteria can hydrogenate fatty acids converting PUFA to partially or fully saturated fatty acids. In addition, bacteria can hydrolyze proteins and modify other nutrients and food components. The effect of diet on gut microflora is not limited to ruminants. It has also been shown in single-stomach animals such as rats[17] and swine.

While direct extrapolation from animals to humans is difficult, these findings are useful in evaluating the role of the colon microflora in humans. Studies on colon cancer using the rat model showed a major effect of diet on the gut microflora, and inhibition of induction of colon cancers by certain bacteria such as Bifidobacterium longum, a lactic acid-producing intestinal bacterium.[11,12,17-19] It is very intriguing that butyrate inhibits classical malignant behavior in cultured cells in clinically relevant concentrations. *In vivo*, however, colonocytes are able to grow in the environment of about 20 mM butyrate produced by bacterial fermentation on the luminal side of the colonic epithelium creating the so-called *in vivo* paradox of butyrate. While we do not understand fully the specific mechanisms involved, it appears that escape from butyrate-induced apoptosis is an essential prerequisite for the development of colorectal cancer. It also suggests that butyrate has a functional role in the growth, differentiation, and programmed cell death of colonic epithelial cells. Propionic acid may also play a role.[20-23]

DIETARY FAT

Lipid Oxidation in the Gut

As discussed in earlier chapters, fatty acids, particularly PUFA, are susceptible to free radical attack and form peroxyl radicals. Once formed, peroxyl radicals attack other fatty acids to form additional peroxyl radicals thus propagating a chain reaction. Ferrous iron and copper can reduce lipid hydroperoxides to yield lipid alkoxyl radicals. In blood and tissues these divalent metals are mostly bound to proteins and prevented from reacting with lipids and other compounds to produce free radicals. In the gut, however, these metals are available and can promote free radical production.

Lipid hydroperoxides and other oxidation products of unsaturated fatty acids induce proliferation of the colonic mucosa of rats. They also increase single and double strand DNA breaks while lipophilic antioxidants such as α-tocopherol, BHT, and BHA reduce DNA strand breaks.[24]

Peroxides in the diet and those formed in the digesta can be absorbed and transported by the chylomicrons to the liver and incorporated in the very low density lipoproteins.[25,26] Thus the oxidation products of lipids may have effects on the surface of the intestinal mucosa and systemic affects after they are absorbed and transported by chylomicrons and other lipoproteins.

Lipid hydroperoxides decompose to reactive aldehydes such as malondialdehyde and 4-hydroxynonenal. Malondialdehyde is a well-known mutagen that reacts with deoxyguanosine to form a major endogenous adduct found in the DNA of human liver.[27,28] Malondialdehyde levels and PUFA content of colon cancer tissues are significantly higher than in the surrounding normal mucosa.

PUFA Versus Saturated Fatty Acids

It is quite intriguing that consumption of vegetable oils, unlike animal fat, increases the risk of colon cancer only slightly or has no effect.[29,30] This is particularly significant because vegetable oils contain larger amounts of polyunsaturated fatty acids (PUFA), which are more prone to oxidation than saturated fatty acids common in animal fats. Actually diets rich in ω-3 PUFA appear to reduce the risk of colon cancer.[30-33] We examined the possibility that tocopherols, which are rather abundant in vegetable oils but not in animal fats, might explain the higher risk with saturated fat versus vegetable oils.[1] Tocopherols break the chain reaction of lipid oxidation. The protective effect of ω-3 PUFA is probably not related to their tocopherol content but rather to their antiinflammatory effects, as discussed below.

The fatty acids of the diet influence the fatty acid composition of the colonic mucosa. Colorectal tumors have higher levels of arachidonic acid (20:4, ω-6) and prostaglandins compared to the surrounding normal mucosa.[34-36] Peroxidation of ω-6 polyunsaturated fatty acids forms 4-hydroxyl-2-nonenal. This α,β-unsaturated aldehyde has the ability to increase oxidative stress in cultured fibroblasts by promoting cellular consumption of glutathione and by inactivating selenium-dependent glutathione peroxidase.[37] It is not known, however, if colonocytes exposed to 4-hydroxyl-2-nonenal *in vivo* experience a similar oxidative stress.

A Protective Effect of ω-3 Fatty Acids?

The protective effect of dietary ω-3 fatty acids may be related to decreased synthesis of prostaglandins from arachidonic acid. In a double-blind, crossover study, Bartram and his co-workers found that rectal mucosal cells of healthy individuals consuming fish oil rich in ω-3 fatty acids released less prostaglandin E_2 than a group consuming a corn oil supplement, which is low in ω-3 fatty acids.[38] Prostaglandin E_2 may promote colon cancer by increasing the proliferation rate of tumor cells[39] and by down-regulating the expression of HLA class II antigens thereby permitting malignant cells to escape immune surveillance.[40] A recent study in South Africa with fishermen indicated a lower incidence of colorectal cancer in fishermen than in urban cohorts despite lower intake of fiber, fruits, and vegetables and higher rate of smoking.[41] These researchers proposed that the higher consumption of ω-3 fatty acids reduced their risk.

BILE SALTS

Bile salts are produced in the liver and secreted in the digestive tract by the bile. Dietary fat stimulates production of bile salts. In studies with human volunteers, ingestion of 40% fat calories increased the concentration of bile acids in the colon more than lower levels of dietary fat.[42] The type of fat appears to influence the relative amounts of bile acids. Secondary bile acids, certain neutral sterols, and other metabolic products from bacterial enzyme activities appear to promote colon cancer.[14,18,42,43]

It has been proposed that bile acids activate phospholipases in colonocytes thereby liberating arachidonate and diacylglycerol. The released diacylglycerol activates a tumor promoter by activating protein kinase C which stimulates cell proliferation and also stimulates the respiratory burst of neutrophils to produce superoxide free radicals.[14,15]

VITAMIN E AND COLON CANCER

In vitro Studies

The role of vitamin E and other antioxidants in preventing cancer has been evaluated in cell culture systems. Most of these studies utilized fibroblast-like cell lines and are, therefore, of more relevance to sarcomas rather than carcinomas such as colon cancer. Incubation of C3H/10T1/2 fibroblasts with the α-tocopheryl succinate form of vitamin E, prior to exposure to X-rays or chemical carcinogens, reduced their transformation compared to control cells.[44] Surprisingly, and for reasons not well understood, α-tocopherol and α-tocopheryl acetate were not effective. It should be kept in mind, however, that α-tocopheryl succinate (like acetate) has its 6-hydroxyl group blocked and is ineffective as an antioxidant until its ester bond is hydrolyzed.

Animal Models

In general, animal studies strongly suggest that incidence of cancer was reduced when animals were supplemented with vitamin E doses ranging from 0.02 to 1.3%.[45,46] α-Tocopherol or α-tocopheryl acetate were the only forms of vitamin E tested and, for this reason, the efficacy of other tocopherols and tocotrienols is not known. Studies looking specifically at colon cancer induced by chemical carcinogens, also suggest a beneficial effect of vitamin E. For example, Wistar rats fed a diet with a low vitamin E content (less than 5 mg/kg diet) for 15 weeks developed a higher incidence of intestinal tumors induced by the chemical carcinogen 1,2 dimethylhydrazine (DMH) than rats fed an identical diet containing 100 mg of vitamin E/kg of diet. Nevertheless, by week 45 the incidence of tumors was the same in both groups.[47] In a similar study, it was found that mice fed a high vitamin E diet (600 mg/kg diet) for 28 weeks and treated with DMH showed a reduced production of colorectal tumors, fewer carcinomas, and fewer adenomas with marked atypia when compared with mice (DMH treated) fed a low vitamin E diet (10 mg/kg of diet).[48] In contrast to the above two studies, Toth and Patil reported that a diet with 40,000 mg of dl-α-tocopheryl acetate enhanced the intestinal tumorigenicity of DMH in mice.[49]

In a recent study, Coffey and his co-workers transplanted human colon cancer cells into mice and, after tumors developed, began treatment with the standard drug 5-fluorouracil (5FU) plus either vitamin E or a synthetic antioxidant (PDTC). Vitamin E attenuated the effect of 5FU over the six weeks of the study. The tumors disappeared when the animals were treated with 5FU plus PDTC. Based on *in vitro* tests, these researchers suggested that vitamin E and PDTC enhanced the action of the cancer drug 5FU by turning on the gene p21 in cancer cells thus inducing death of the cells by apoptosis.

Epidemiological and Clinical Studies

Clinical studies relating colon cancer to vitamin E produced inconsistent results. A metaanalysis of five prospective, nested case-control studies indicated that high plasma levels of α-tocopherol were associated with a modest decrease in the subsequent incidence of colorectal cancer.[50]

The Iowa Women's Health Study, a 4-year prospective study of 35,000 women between 55-66 years of age and without a prior history of cancer, indicated that a high vitamin E intake was associated with a reduced risk of colon cancer. The relative risk of colon cancer for the highest quintile of vitamin E intake was about one-third of the lowest quintile.[45] In a major multiyear intervention study, the Alpha-Tocopherol, Beta-Carotene Cancer Prevention Study of 29,000 male smokers from Finland (commonly known as the Finnish Study), a daily supplement of 50 mg of all-rac-α-tocopheryl acetate for 5-8 years, appeared to reduce colon cancer.[51]

Four other studies provided indirect support for a role of antioxidants, including vitamin E, in colon cancer. The first, a recent double-blind, placebo-controlled clinical study of 1312 patients with a history of basal or squamous cell carcinomas of the skin found that selenium supplementation, at 200 μg/day, reduced the incidence of lung, prostate and colorectal cancer.[52] Selenium is an essential component of antioxidant enzyme glutathione peroxidase and acts synergistically with vitamin E to inhibit *in vivo* lipid peroxidation.

The second study evaluated vitamin supplement use and colon cancer in a population-based case-control study among men and women aged 30-62 years in three counties in the Seattle metropolitan area.[53] The average daily intake of supplemental vitamins A, C, E, folic acid, calcium, and multivitamins during the reference period were each associated with reduced risk. The strongest associations were for use of vitamin E (odds ratio, 0.43; 95% confidence interval, 0.26-0.71 for intake of 200 IU/day or above versus none.

The third study, with 20 patients with colorectal adenomas, showed that an antioxidant supplement for 3 or 6 months decreased the index of cell proliferation in normal-appearing rectal mucosa.[54] The antioxidant supplement contained 30,000 IU vitamin A, 1000 mg ascorbate, and 70 mg all-rac-α-tocopheryl acetate. The fourth study evaluated the effect of various vitamin and mineral mixtures on esophageal/gastric cancer in Linxian, China, which has one of the world's highest incidence of such cancers. Although not focused on colorectal cancer, this study of 29,000 people indicated that supplementation with β-carotene, vitamin E (60 IU of all-rac-α-tocopheryl acetate), and selenium lowered cancer mortality, particularly stomach cancer.[55]

In contrast, the Polyp Prevention Study Group with 864 patients for 4 years indicated that antioxidants (vitamin E, β-carotene, and vitamin C) did not reduce the occurrence of new colonic adenomas in patients who had prior adenoma removed.[56] Another study also indicated that a supplement of 400 mg of vitamin C and 400 mg of α-tocopherol did not reduce the recurrence of colorectal polyps.[57]

ANTIOXIDANT STATUS OF THE DIGESTA AND COLON CANCER: A NEW PERSPECTIVE

Dietary antioxidants have a direct effect on the digesta by inhibiting lipid oxidation, quenching free radicals, and, possibly, influencing other metabolic processes including those of the gut microflora. In addition, they may protect the exposed surface of the mucosa or may enter the colonic cells and provide protection inside the cell. For this reason, antioxidants, which are not well absorbed or are secreted into the intestine, may help contribute to the antioxidant status of the digesta. For these reasons, we proposed that in evaluating the antioxidant status in humans we should include the antioxidant status of the digesta, particularly for colon cancer.[1]

The Role of Vitamin E in Colon Cancer — a New Look

The chemistry and biological function of vitamin E was discussed in Chapter 10. Briefly, vitamin E has become synonymous with α-tocopherol even though eight compounds, four tocopherols and four tocotrienols, have some vitamin E activity. α-Tocopherol is available commercially in the naturally occurring single stereoisomeric RRR or d form and the synthetic all-rac or dl form consisting of 8 stereoisomers.

The role of non-α-tocopherols and tocotrienols in nutrition and health has been largely ignored. Yet the typical American diet contains about 2 to 4 times more γ than α-tocopherol because commonly used vegetable oils (corn, soy, peanut, and palm) are rich in γ-tocopherol. Yet, plasma levels of γ are at least 2-3 times lower than α-tocopherol. It is now clear that α-tocopherol and γ-tocopherol are equally well absorbed. However, α-tocopherol is preferentially secreted by the liver into the blood lipoproteins. RRR and all-rac are equally well absorbed, yet the RRR causes higher levels of α-tocopherol in the blood and tissues. A tocopherol binding protein appears responsible for incorporating preferentially RRR-α-tocopherol over γ and other tocopherols into nascent VLDL resulting in higher levels in the blood and tissues.[58] It has been suggested that a large part of non-α-tocopherol and all-rac-α-tocopherol are secreted into the intestine via the bile[58] but this has not been confirmed.

A Significant Role of γ-Tocopherol?

It is intriguing to contemplate the role of γ-tocopherol in colon cancer. Recent research indicates that it may play a unique role in minimizing DNA damage caused by nitrogen radicals. In biological systems, nitrogen dioxide

(NO_2) forms from the reaction of nitrogen oxide (NO) with oxygen. The reactivity of γ and α-tocopherol with NO_2 are quite different. α-Tocopherol reacts with NO_2 to yield a nitrosating agent but this does not occur with γ-tocopherol. In contrast, γ-tocopherol reduces NO_2 to NO without generating a nitrosating species.[59,60] NO can act either as a pro-oxidant or an antioxidant depending on the relative rate of production of superoxide radicals. NO alone acts as a potent antioxidant by rapidly scavenging peroxyl radicals. NO acts as a pro-oxidant when the rate of $O_2^{\bullet -}$ production is greater than that of NO by reacting rapidly with the superoxide radical to yield peroxynitrite.

$$NO + O_2^{\bullet -} \longrightarrow ONOO^-$$

Christen and his co-workers,[61] reported that γ-tocopherol inhibited lipid hydroperoxide formation in liposomes (but not isolated low-density lipoprotein) exposed to peroxynitrite, more effectively than α-tocopherol. More important, α-tocopherol did not prevent nitration of the nucleophilic 5-position, which proceeded in both liposomes and human low-density lipoprotein at yields of approximately 50% and 75%. These researchers postulated that γ-tocopherol acts *in vivo* as a trap for membrane-soluble electrophilic nitrogen oxides and other electrophilic mutagens, forming stable carbon-centered adducts through the nucleophilic 5-position, which is blocked by α-tocopherol.

During inflammation, a known risk of cancer, neutrophils produce nitrogen oxides and nitrosamines from L-arginine.[62,63] Peroxynitrite is also a powerful mutagenic oxidant and nitrating species. The unique ability of γ-tocopherol to either reduce NO_2 or react with it to form a non-nitrosating agent may be particularly important in carcinogenesis since nitrosating agents can deaminate DNA bases causing mutations. It is significant, therefore, that γ-tocopherol may be more effective than other lipid soluble antioxidants in preventing DNA strand breaks mediated by NO_2. Endogenous production of nitric oxides is associated with the transformation of C3H/10T1/2 fibroblasts *in vitro* and γ-tocopherol was found to be superior to α in preventing transformation of this cell line.

The above data strongly suggest that the role of γ-tocopherol merits further attention. Of course α-tocopherol and other tocopherols and tocotrienols may play a significant role because their absorption is incomplete, especially for the portion embedded in plant material. In addition, metabolites secreted into the digesta via the bile may have an effect.

Tocotrienols appear to be absorbed in similar manner as tocopherols but blood levels are lower than tocopherols. It is not known whether they are secreted in the gut by the bile and if they have a role in colon cancer.

Non-Antioxidant Effects of Tocopherols

In addition to their antioxidant activity tocopherols may have distinct non-antioxidant functions. It is interesting, therefore, that RRR-α, but not RRR-β-tocopherol, can inhibit protein kinase C activity and thereby inhibit cell division in cultured smooth muscle cells. When added together, RRR-β blocks the effect of RRR-α-tocopherol. Since RRR-α and RRR-β-tocopherol are both antioxidants, their strikingly different effects are probably due to nonantioxidant mechanisms.[64,65] Cooney and his co-workers reported recently that γ-tocopherol was a more effective inhibitor than α in the transformation of C3H/10T1/2 murine fibroblasts incubated with the chemical carcinogen 3-methylanthrene.[59] The tocopherols were added after exposing the cells to the carcinogen, i.e., during the post-confluence promotional phase of the transformation assay. The reported effect of vitamin E, in combination with 5FU on human colon cancer cells transplanted in mice was attributed to an effect on gene p21, which induces apoptosis. It is not clear whether this is an antioxidant effect.

The non-antioxidant functions of tocopherols on colon cancer is not clearly understood. It is possible that a number of mechanisms may be involved.

Practical Implications

Antioxidants in fecal material may be particularly effective in preventing DNA damage to the epithelial cells lining the colon. Most colon cancer chemoprevention trials have, however, emphasized antioxidants, which are well absorbed into plasma rather than those that remain or are secreted into fecal material. While this review focused on the role of vitamin E and particularly γ-tocopherol, other agents, especially phytochemicals, probably contribute to the antioxidant status of the digesta. Many phytochemicals are only partially absorbed and a large part remains in the digesta. For example, absorption of some carotenoids in fresh vegetables is less than 50% and in some cases less than 10%. These compounds can have a major effect on the antioxidant status of the digesta.

Future studies should evaluate the role of antioxidants that remain or are secreted in the digesta. If non-absorbed antioxidants are effective in reducing the risk of colon cancer, we may need to reevaluate our current views of bioavailability as it relates to this effect.

We propose that both epidemiological and intervention studies on the role of vitamin E in colorectal cancer should consider all tocopherols and even tocotrienols.[1] In the past, the focus has been almost exclusively on α-tocopherol and, in some cases, without reference to its stereochemical form (all-rac or RRR). This may account, in part, for the conflicting results observed in clinical trials.

Supplementation with α-tocopherol depresses the levels of γ-tocopherol in blood and adipose tissue.[58] Currently, α-tocopherol is the most common form of vitamin E used to fortify foods and in nutritional supplements. If γ-tocopherol were found to reduce the formation of fecal mutagens and the risk of colorectal cancer, then mixed tocopherols would be a preferred vitamin E supplement.

CONCLUSION

The discussion above provided the basis for the following hypothesis:

1. The digesta constitutes a separate and important component of the overall antioxidant status of humans. The antioxidant status of the digesta plays a significant role in the development of colon cancer. The antioxidant status of the digesta is affected by factors different than tissues, including undigested material, bile secretions, intestinal microflora, and others. For this reason, strategies for reducing oxidative stress should be modified or expanded to include the digesta in addition to the tissues.
2. Antioxidant compounds, which are not absorbed or absorbed and secreted in the gut via the bile, reduce production of mutagens in the digesta and thus reduce colon cancer. Some of these antioxidants have been considered to be without apparent utility because they are poorly absorbed. γ-Tocopherol (and possibly other non-α-tocopherols and tocotrienols?) are examples of important antioxidants in the digesta.

REFERENCES

1. Stone WL, Papas AM. Tocopherols and the etiology of colon cancer. *J Natl Cancer Inst* 1997;89:1006-14.
2. Harris C. p53 tumor suppressor gene: from the basic research laboratory to the clinic--an abridged historical perspective. *Carcinogenesis* 1996;17:1187-1198.
3. Laken SJ, Petersen GM, Gruber SB, *et al.* Familial colorectal cancer in Ashkenazim due to a hypermutable tract in APC. *Nature Genetics* 1997;17:79-83.
4. Babbs CF. Free radicals and the etiology of colon cancer. *Free Radic Biol Med* 1990;8:191-200.

5. Parker SL, Tong T, Bolden S, Wingo PA. Cancer statistics, 1997. *CA Cancer J Clin* 1997;47:5-27.
6. Potter JD. Nutrition and colorectal cancer. *Cancer Causes Control* 1996;7:127-46.
7. Nelson NJ. Is chemoprevention overrated or underfunded? *J Nat Cancer Inst* 1996;88:947.
8. Giovannucci E, Willett WC. Dietary factors and risk of colon cancer. *Ann Med* 1994;26:443-52.
9. Stephen AM, Cummings JH. The microbial contribution to human faecal mass. *J Med Microbiol* 1980;13:45-56.
10. Gibson GR, Roberfroid MB. Dietary modulation of the human colonic microbiota: introducing the concept of prebiotics. *J Nutr* 1995;25:1401-1412.
11. Singh J, Rivenson A, Tomita M, Shimamura S, Ishibashi N, Reddy BS. Bifidobacterium longum, a lactic acid-producing intestinal bacterium inhibits colon cancer and modulates the intermediate biomarkers of colon carcinogenesis. *Carcinogenesis* 1997;18:833-41.
12. Onoue M, Kado S, Sakaitani Y, Uchida K, Morotomi M. Specific species of intestinal bacteria influence the induction of aberrant crypt foci by 1,2-dimethylhydrazine in rats. *Cancer Lett* 1997;113:179-86.
13. Chadwick RW, George SE, Claxton LD. Role of gastrointestinal mucosa and microflora in the bioactivation of dietary and environmental mutagens or carcinogens. *Drug Metabolism Rev* 1992;24:425-492.
14. Blakeborough MH, Owen RW, Bilton RF. Free radical generating mechanisms in the colon: their role in the induction and promotion of colorectal cancer? *Free Radic Res Commun* 1989;6:359-367.
15. DeLange RJ, Glazer AN. Bile acids: antioxidants or enhancers of peroxidation depending on lipid concentration. *Arch Biochem Biophys* 1990;276:19-25.
16. Swenson MJ. *Duke's Physiology of Domestic Animals.* 10th ed. Ithaca, N.Y.: Cornell University Press, 1984.
17. Maciorowski KG, Turner ND, Lupton JR, *et al.* Diet and carcinogen alter the fecal microbial populations of rats. *J Nutr* 1997;127:449-57.
18. Roberton AM. Roles of endogenous substances and bacteria in colorectal cancer. *Mutation Res* 1993;290:71-78.
19. Zarkovic M, Qin X, Nakatsuru Y, *et al.* Tumor promotion by fecapentaene-12 in a rat colon carcinogenesis model. *Carcinogenesis* 1993;14:1261-4.
20. Basson MD, Turowski GA, Rashid Z, Hong F, Madri JA. Regulation of human colonic cell line proliferation and phenotype by sodium butyrate. *Dig Dis Sci* 1996;41:1989-93.
21. Csordas A. Butyrate, aspirin and colorectal cancer. *Eur J Cancer Prev* 1996;5:221-31.
22. Gamet L, Daviaud D, Denis-Pouxviel C, Remesy C, Murat JC. Effects of short-chain fatty acids on growth and differentiation of the human colon-cancer cell line HT29. *Int J Cancer* 1992;52:286-9.
23. Velazquez OC, Lederer HM, Rombeau JL. Butyrate and the colonocyte. Implications for neoplasia. *Dig Dis Sci* 1996;41:727-39.
24. Yang MH, Schaich KM. Factors affecting DNA damage caused by lipid hydroperoxides and aldehydes. *Free Radical Biol Med* 1996;20:225-236.
25. Staprans I, Rapp JH, Pan XM, Feingold KR. Oxidized lipids in the diet are incorporated by the liver into very low density lipoprotein in rats. *J Lipid Res* 1996;37:420-30.
26. Staprans I, Pan XM, Miller M, Rapp JH. Effect of dietary lipid peroxides on metabolism of serum chylomicrons in rats. *Am J Physiol* 1993;264:G561-8.
27. Estabauer H, P. E, Ortner A. Possible mutagens derived from lipids and lipid precursors. *Mutation Res* 1990;238:223-233.

28. Chaudhary AK, Nokubo M, Reddy GR, *et al.* Detection of endogenous malondialdehyde-deoxyguanosine adducts in human liver. *Science* 1994;265:1580-1582.
29. Willett W, Stampfer M, Colditz G, Rosner B, Speizer F. Relation of meat, fat, and fiber intake to the risk of colon cancer in a prospective study among women. *N Engl J Med* 1990;323:1664-1672.
30. Hursting SD, Thornquist M, Henderson MM. Types of dietary fat and the incidence of cancer at five sites. *Prev Med* 1990;19:242-253.
31. Anti M, Marra G, Armelao F, *et al.* Effect of omega-3 fatty acids on rectal mucosal cell proliferation in subjects at risk for colon cancer. *Gastroenterology* 1992;103:883-91.
32. Eastwood G. Pharmacologic prevention of colonic neoplasms. Effects of calcium, vitamins, omega fatty acids, and nonsteroidal anti-inflammatory drugs. *Dig Dis* 1996;14:119-28.
33. Narisawa T, Fukaura Y, Yazawa K, Ishikawa C, Isoda Y, Nishizawa Y. Colon cancer prevention with a small amount of dietary perilla oil high in alpha-linolenic acid in an animal model. *Cancer* 1994;73:2069-2075.
34. Nicholson M, Neoptolemos J, Clayton H, Talbot I, Bell P. Increased cell membrane arachidonic acid in experimental colorectal tumors. *Gut* 1991;32:413-418.
35. Hendrickse C, Keighley M, Neoptolemos J. Dietary omega-3 fats reduce proliferation and tumor yields at colorectal anastomosis in rats. *Gastroenterology* 1995;109:431-9.
36. Hendrickse C, Kelly R, Radley S, Donovan I, Keighley M, Neoptolemos J. Lipid peroxidation and prostaglandins in colorectal cancer. *Br J Surg* 1994;81:1219-1223.
37. Kinter M, Roberts RJ. Glutathione consumption and glutathione peroxidase inactivation in fibroblast cell lines by 4-hydroxyl-2-nonenal. *Free Rad Biol Med* 1996;21:457-462.
38. Bartram HP, Gostner A, Kelber E, *et al.* Effects of fish oil on fecal bacterial enzymes and steroid excretion in healthy volunteers: implications for colon cancer prevention. *Nutr Cancer* 1996;25:71-8.
39. Qiao L, Kozoni V, Tsioulias G, *et al.* Selected eicosanoids increase the proliferation rate of human colon carcinoma cell lines and mouse colonocytes *in vivo*. *Biochim Biophys Acta* 1995;1258:215-223.
40. Arvind P, Papavassiliou E, Tsioulias G, *et al.* Prostaglandin E2 down-regulates the expression of HLA-DR antigen in human colon adenocarcinoma cell lines. *Biochemistry* 1995;34:5604-5609.
41. Schloss I, Kidd MS, Tichelaar HY, Young GO, O'Keefe SJ. Dietary factors associated with a low risk of colon cancer in coloured west coast fishermen. *S Afr Med J* 1997;87:152-8.
42. Weisburger JH. Dietary fat and risk of chronic disease: mechanistic insights from experimental studies. *J Am Diet Assoc* 1997;97:S16-23.
43. Reddy BS. Dietary fat and colon cancer: animal model studies. *Lipids* 1992;27:807-13.
44. Borek C, Ong A, Mason H, Donahue L, Biaglow JE. Selenium and vitamin E inhibit radiogenic and chemically induced transformation *in vitro* via different mechanisms. *Proc Natl Acad Sci U.S.A.* 1986;83:1490-1494.
45. Bostick RM, Potter JD, McKenzie DR, *et al.* Reduced risk of colon cancer with high intake of vitamin E: the Iowa Women's Health Study. *Cancer Res* 1993;53:4230-7.
46. Prasad KN, Edwards-Prasad J. Vitamin E and cancer prevention: recent advances and future potentials. *J. Am. Coll. Nutr.* 1992;11:487-500.
47. Sumiyoshi H. Effects of vitamin E deficiency on 1,2-dimethylhydrazine-induced intestinal carcinogenesis in rats. *Hiroshima J Med Sci* 1985;34:363-369.
48. Cook MG, McNamara P. Effect of dietary vitamin E on dimethylhydrazine-induced colonic tumors in mice. *Cancer Res* 1980;40:1329-1331.

49. Toth B, Patil K. Enhancing effect of vitamin E on murine intestinal tumorigensis by 1,2-dimethylhydrazine dihydrochloride. *J Natl Cancer Inst* 1983;70:1107-1111.
50. Longnecker M, Martin-Moreno J, Knekt P, *et al.* Serum alpha-tocopherol concentration in relation to subsequent colorectal cancer: pooled data from five cohorts. *J Natl Cancer Inst* 1992;84:430-5.
51. The Alpha-Tocopherol, Beta Carotene Cancer Prevention Study Group. The effect of vitamin E and beta carotene on the incidence of lung cancer and other cancers in male smokers. *N Engl J Med* 1994;330:1029-35.
52. Clark LC, Combs GF, Turnbull BW, *et al.* Effects of selenium supplementation for cancer prevention in patients with carcinoma of the skin. *JAMA* 1996;276:1957-1963.
53. White E, Shannon JS, Patterson RE. Relationship between vitamin and calcium supplement use and colon cancer. *Cancer Epidemiol Biomarkers Prev* 1997;6:769-74.
54. Paganelli GM, Biasco G, Brandi G, *et al.* Effect of vitamin A, C, and E supplementation on rectal cell proliferation in patients with colorectal adenomas. *J Natl Cancer Inst* 1992;84:47-51.
55. Blot W, Li J, Taylor P, *et al.* Nutrition intervention trials in Linxian, China: supplementation with specific vitamin/mineral combinations, cancer incidence, and disease-specific mortality in the general population. *J Natl Cancer Inst* 1993;85:1483-1492.
56. Group TPPS. A clinical trial of antioxidant vitamins to prevent colorectal adenoma. *N Eng J Med* 1994;331:141-147.
57. McKeown-Eyssen G, Holloway C, Jazmaji V, Bright-See E, Dion P, Bruce WR. A randomized trial of vitamins C and E in the prevention of recurrence of colorectal polyps. *Cancer Res* 1988;48:4701-4705.
58. Kayden HJ, Traber MG. Absorption, lipoprotein transport and regulation of plasma concentrations of vitamin E in humans. *J. Lipid Res.* 1993;34:343-358.
59. Cooney RV, Franke AA, Harwood PJ, Hatch-Pigott V, Custer LJ, Mordan LJ. Gamma-tocopherol detoxification of nitrogen dioxide: superiority to alpha-tocopherol. *Proc Natl Acad Sci U S A* 1993;90:1771-1775.
60. Cooney RV, Harwood PJ, Franke AA, *et al.* Products of gamma-tocopherol reaction with NO_2 and their formation in rat insulinoma (RINm5F) cells. *Free Radic Biol Med* 1995;19:259-269.
61. Christen S, Woodall AA, Shigenaga MK, Southwell-Keely PT, Duncan MW, Ames BN. Gamma-tocopherol traps mutagenic electrophiles such as NO(X) and complements alpha-tocopherol: physiological implications. *Proc Natl Acad Sci U S A* 1997;94:3217-22.
62. Cerutti PA, Trump BF. Inflammation and oxidative stress in carcinogenesis. *Cancer Cells* 1991;3:1-7.
63. Ohshima H, Bartsch H. Chronic infections and inflammatory processes as cancer risk factors: possible role of nitric oxide in carcinogenesis. *Mutat Res* 1994;305:253-264.
64. Azzi A, Boscoboinik D, Chatelain E, Özzer NK, Stäuble B. d-α-Tocopherol and cell proliferation. In: Pasquier C, Olivier RY, Auclair C, Packer L, Eds. *Oxidative Stress, Cell Activation and Viral Infection.* Basel: Birkhäuser Verlag, 1994:131-141.
65. Tasinato A, Boscoboinik D, Bartoli GM, Maroni P, Azzi A. d-alpha-tocopherol inhibition of vascular smooth muscle cell proliferation occurs at physiological concentrations, correlates with protein kinase C inhibition, and is independent of its antioxidant properties. *Proc Natl Acad Sci U S A* 1995;92:12190-4.

20

Beyond Antioxidant Function: Other Biochemical Effects of Antioxidants

Nesrin K. Özer, Ph.D.
Department of Biochemistry, Faculty of Medicine, Marmara University, Istanbul, TURKEY

Angelo Azzi, M.D.
Institute for Biochemistry and Molecular Biology, University of Bern, Bern, SWITZERLAND

ANTIOXIDANTS WITH ADDITIONAL FUNCTIONS

Molecules provided with an antioxidant function may have additional properties, the latter being sometimes of more importance than the former. Among the multiple examples that could be cited here only few will be discussed, which more clearly illustrate this notion.

0-8493-8009-X/98/$0.00+$.50

Estrogens

Estrogens such as estriol and 17-β-estradiol are naturally occurring antioxidants.[1] 2-Hydroxyestrone was found to posses an antioxidant activity 2.9-times higher than α-tocopherol as measured by the inhibition of lipid peroxidation. It was also found that the estrogens having an OH group at the aromatic ring have an ability to regenerate the tocopheroxyl to tocopherol with up to three orders of magnitude higher reactivity than ascorbic acid.[2] Exposure of LDL to physiological levels of 17-β-estradiol in a plasma milieu is associated with enhanced resistance to Cu^{2+}-mediated oxidation and incorporation of 17-β-estradiol derivatives into LDL. This antioxidant capacity could indeed be very important, being another means by which 17-β-estradiol limits coronary artery disease in women.[3] However, the most evident function of estrogens, responsible for the determination of secondary sexual characteristics, is unrelated to their antioxidant activity.

Retinol

all-Trans-retinol behaves as an effective antioxidant at low oxygen partial pressure and low retinol concentrations.[4-6]

Vitamin A in large doses increased the antioxidant potential of the tissues, and it was suggested that retinol also might be considered as a potential antioxidant similar to tocopherol in animal nutrition.[7] Low plasma concentrations of carotenoids or of other antioxidants increase the risk for age-related macular degeneration.[8] Also in this case, it appears obvious that the function of retinol in rhodopsin and vision is not related with its antioxidant properties.

Melatonin

Melatonin as a free radical scavenger that has been implicated in aging and age-related diseases.[9-10] This indole derivative may act as a potentially highly important antioxidant in the brain. *In vitro* melatonin is more effective than glutathione in scavenging the highly toxic hydroxyl radical and also more efficient than vitamin E in neutralizing the peroxyl radical.[10] In this sense, melatonin affords protection against gastric lesions induced by ischemia reperfusion possibly due to its antioxidant and mucosal microcirculatory effects.[11] All these events, however, are not associated with the sleep-propensity function of melatonin. Melatonin has been established to participate in the sleep-wake regulation in humans through a receptor-mediated signaling function.[12-16]

EFFECTS OF TOCOPHEROLS ON SMOOTH MUSCLE CELLS

α-Tocopherol at concentrations of 50 μM inhibits rat A7r5 smooth muscle cell proliferation, while β-tocopherol is ineffective. When α-tocopherol and β-tocopherol are added together, no inhibition of cell growth is seen. Both compounds are transported equally in cells and do not compete each other for the uptake.[17] The prevention by β-tocopherol of the proliferation inhibition by α-tocopherol suggests a site-directed event as the basis of α-tocopherol inhibition rather than a general radical scavenging reaction. The oxidized product of α-tocopherol, α-tocopherylquinone, is not inhibitory indicating that the effects of α-tocopherol are not related to its antioxidant properties.[17]

α-Tocopherol is not only responsible for the proliferation control of smooth muscle cells but it exhibits similar functions in a number of different cell lines (Table 1).

Table 1
Antiproliferative Effect of α-Tocopherol is Cell Specific

α-TOCOPHEROL SENSITIVE CELL LINES	
Origin of tissue	
Rat aorta smooth muscle	A10/A7r5
Human aorta smooth muscle	hAI
Human tendon fibroblasts	hTF
Human skin fibroblasts	CCD-SK
Mouse neuroblastoma	NB2A
Human pigmented retinal epithelial cells	hPRE
Human leukemia	U937
Human prostate tumor	DU-145
Mouse fibroblast	Balb/c-3T3
Glioma	C6
α-TOCOPHEROL NON-SENSITIVE CELL LINES	
Origin of tissue	
Cervix adenocarcinoma	HeLa
Chinese hamster lung	LR73
Chinese hamster ovary	CHO
Human osteosarcoma	Saos-2
Mouse macrophage	P388D1
Human hepatocarcinoma	HepG2
Human colon adenocarcinoma	CaCo2

Differences in the Effect of Tocopherols (α, β, γ, and δ), Tocotrienols and RRR- vs. all-rac-α-Tocopherols

δ-Tocopherol, α-tocopherol, and γ-tocopherol are, within experimental error, equally inhibitory.[18] On the other hand it appears that the inhibition by β-tocopherol is 10-fold less potent relative to the other compounds. Tocotrienols, although possessing a greater antioxidant activity than tocopherols,[19] inhibit cell proliferation to the same extent (Figure 1).[18]

Janero *et al.* have shown, in a series of 6-hydroxy-chroman-2-carbonitrile tocopherol derivatives, whose antioxidant properties strongly depend upon the nature and length of their side chains.[20] These compounds were tested in smooth muscle cells (A7r5) and their relative potency in inhibiting cell proliferation established. A Student t-test analysis between the two data sets (antioxidant and antiproliferative activity) has given a $p = 0.006$, indicating a lack of significant correlation between them.[18] Probucol, a potent hydrophobic antioxidant similar in its general properties to RRR-α-tocopherol, has been shown not to inhibit smooth muscle cell proliferation, but to prevent the inhibition by α-tocopherol, as was the case for β-tocopherol. The synthetic all-rac was half as effective as the naturally occurring RRR-α-tocopherol.

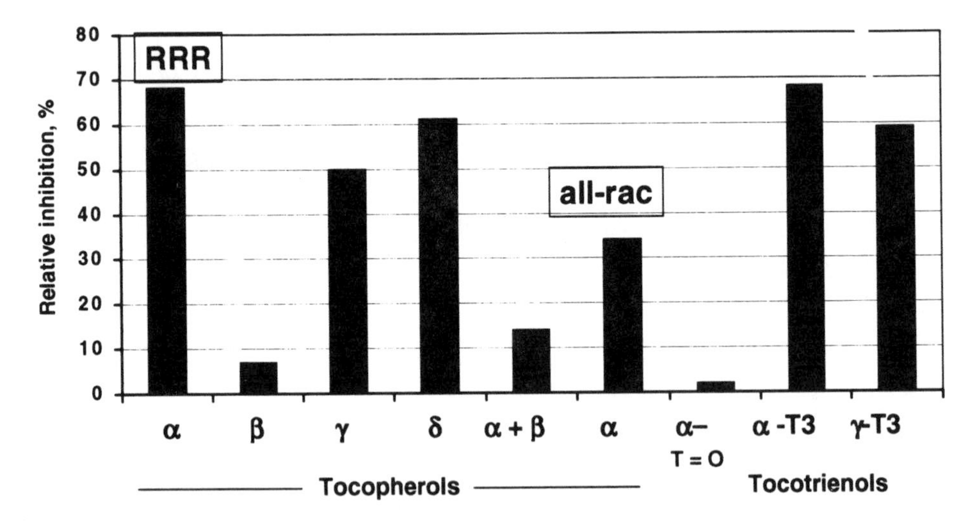

Figure 1. Relative inhibition of smooth muscle cells by antioxidants. The naturally occurring and synthetic α-tocopherols are designated as RRR and all-rac on their respective bars. A–T=O is α-tocopherylquinone. Conditions were as described in Reference 18.

EFFECTS OF α-TOCOPHEROL ON PROTEIN KINASE C

Protein kinase C has been originally suggested to be regulated, at a cellular level, by α-tocopherol.[18,21-23] A number of reports have subsequently confirmed this finding in different cell types, including monocytes, macrophages, neutrophils, fibroblasts, and mesangial cells.[24-35] Animal work has also confirmed the importance of protein kinase C inhibition by α-tocopherol *in vivo*.[36,37]

Effects on Protein Kinase C Not Related to Antioxidant Properties

The inhibitions by α-tocopherol of protein kinase C activity and of proliferation are parallel events in vascular smooth muscle cells. Inhibition is observed to occur at concentrations of α-tocopherol close to those measured in healthy adults.[18,21-23,38] While α-tocopherol inhibits protein kinase C activity, β-tocopherol is ineffective. When both are present, β-tocopherol prevents the inhibitory effect of α-tocopherol. The inhibition by α-tocopherol and the lack of inhibition by β-tocopherol of cell proliferation and protein kinase C activity shows that the mechanism involved is not related to the radical scavenging properties of these two molecules, which are essentially equal.[23,38]

Specificity of Action is Observed for Both Phytyl Chain Isomers and Chromanol Analogues

The measurements at both protein kinase C and proliferation level of the effect of the natural form of α-tocopherol relative to the racemic mixture of the phytyl chain isomers shows that the former is twice as potent as the latter.

POSSIBLE MECHANISMS

Inhibition by d-α-Tocopherol is Not Caused by a Direct Interaction With Protein Kinase C

Addition of α-tocopherol to protein kinase C in a test tube does not result in inhibition of protein kinase C. Inhibition of protein kinase C is obtained only at a cellular level. Protein kinase C activity increases during the cell cycle progression, reaching a maximum in the late G_1-phase. The time of addition of d-α-tocopherol during the cell cycle determines the extent of protein kinase C inhibition. If α-tocopherol is added in the G_o-phase of the cycle and incubated for 7 h, in the absence of fetal calf serum, no inhibition is observed. If, together with α-tocopherol, fetal calf serum is added and cells are stimulated to enter in the G_1-phase, after 7 hours of incubation inhibition of protein kinase C by α-tocopherol is observed. If α-tocopherol is added in the G_1-phase (and protein kinase C activity measured after 7 hours) d-α-tocopherol shows no inhibition.

α-Tocopherol Inhibits Protein Kinase C Activity in Smooth Muscle Cells but Not its Expression

When smooth muscle cells are supplemented in the G_0-phase with fetal calf serum a time-dependent α-tocopherol sensitive increase in protein kinase C activity is observed. A mRNA analysis carried out for the different isoforms (protein kinase C α, protein kinase C δ, protein kinase C ε, and protein kinase C ζ) did not show any significant changes. Similarly, the protein levels expressed during the transition were essentially the same. α-Tocopherol did not affect the mRNA of the protein kinase C isoforms. The protein level of protein kinase C after seven hours incubation with α-tocopherol was slightly increased (14%) rather than decreased.

α-Tocopherol Does Not Inhibit Protein Kinase C in the Presence of Gö 6976

Nanomolar concentrations of the indolocarbazole Gö 6976 are known to inhibit protein kinase Cα and β1, whereas even micromolar concentrations of Gö 6976 have no effect on the activity of protein kinase C δ, protein kinase C ε, and protein kinase C ζ.[39] After inhibition of protein kinase C α by Gö 6976, the residual protein kinase C activity was not sensitive to α-tocopherol. From this experiment it can be concluded that the isoforms of protein kinase C δ, ε, ζ, and μ are not involved in the α-tocopherol induced protein kinase C inhibition. The experiments suggest that protein kinase C α is the specific target of α-tocopherol.

α-Tocopherol Inhibits Protein Kinase C α Phosphorylation State and Activity

Protein kinase C was immunoprecipitated from cells incubated in the presence of ^{32}P and in the presence or absence of α-tocopherol, with antibodies specific for protein kinase C α. Treatment of smooth muscle cell with α-tocopherol resulted in inhibition of protein kinase C phosphorylation. β-Tocopherol was much less potent in inhibiting protein kinase C phosphorylation (Table 2). Pre-treatment of smooth muscle cells with α-tocopherol (but not with β-tocopherol) results in inhibition of the immunoprecipitated protein kinase Cα activity.

Table 2
Effect of α-Tocopherol and β-Tocopherol on Protein Kinase C α Phosphorylation State, Autophosphorylating Activity and Activity, Toward Histone III-S.

	^{32}P-protein kinase C, (%)	Autophosphorylating activity of protein kinase C α, (%)	Histone activity, (%)
PMA	100	100	100
α-tocopherol	18.5	36.4	56.0
β-tocopherol	74.1	84.9	79.0

Effects on PP_2A

The experiment presented above suggests that the protein kinase C activation occurring in the G_0 to G_1 transition was related with a change of phosphorylation of the enzyme. Moreover, the inhibitory effect of α-tocopherol has been correlated with a dephosphorylation of protein kinase Cα. PP_2A has been found *in vitro* to be activated by the treatment with α-tocopherol (Özer *et al.*, unpublished). This event may be crucial in the dephosphorylation of protein kinase C with its consequent diminution of activity.

Effect on Gene Expression

With the differential display technique we detected several candidate cDNAs of differentially expressed mRNAs. Sequence analysis of one of the cDNA fragments and comparison with DNA sequence databases has revealed 100% homology with the 3' region (exon 9b) of the α-tropomyosin isoform TMBr-2. The mRNA level increased transiently in the α-tocopherol treated, synchronously growing cells and reached a maximum after 2 h of restimulation. Maximum protein expression was observed after 4 h. At 7 h mRNA and protein levels returned to baseline levels. In the light of these observations, it might be possible that the induction of this tropomyosin isoform is an early event caused by α-tocopherol leading to cell proliferation inhibition.

OTHER NON-ANTIOXIDANT EFFECTS

α-Tocopheryl Hydroquinone and Blood Clotting

α-Tocopheryl hydroquinone is an oxidized product of α-tocopherol and an efficient antioxidant.[40] Vitamin E in the reduced, α-tocopherol form shows very modest anticoagulant activity. By contrast, vitamin E quinone is a potent anticoagulant as inhibitor of the vitamin K-dependent carboxylase that controls blood clotting. The newly discovered mechanism for the inhibition is unrelated to the antioxidant properties of the α-tocopheryl hydroquinone and requires attachment of the active site thiol groups of the carboxylase to one or more methyl groups on vitamin E quinone.[41]

γ-Tocopherol and Peroxynitrite

Peroxynitrite, a powerful oxidant and nitrating species, is formed by the near diffusion-limited reaction of NO and O^{2-}. Chronic inflammation induced by phagocytes is a possible source of peroxynitrite and a major contributor to cancer and other degenerative diseases. γ-Tocopherol at the nucleophilic 5-position is effectively scavenging peroxynitrite. These results suggest that γ-tocopherol effectively removes, by a non-antioxidant mechanism, the peroxynitrite-derived nitrating species.[42]

Carotenoids, Vitamin A, Retinoids, and Gene Expression

all-trans Retinoic acid is the major biologically active form of vitamin A, and nuclear retinoid receptors are the major mediators of its actions.[43,44] Retinoic acid metabolites of vitamin A are key regulators of gene expression involved in embryonic development and maintenance of epithelial tissues.[45] The absence of retinoic acid receptor gamma is associated with a loss of the retinoic acid-inducible expression of the Hoxa-1, Hoxa-3, laminin B1, collagen IV (alpha 1), GATA-4, and BMP-2 genes.[46] Furthermore, the loss of retinoic acid receptor gamma is associated with a reduction in the metabolism of *all-trans*-retinoic acid to more polar derivatives, while the loss of retinoic acid receptor alpha is associated with an increase in metabolism of retinoic acid.[47] Retinoic acid also induces osteopontin gene expression in concert with vitamin D[48] *all-trans*-retinoic acid 4-hydrolase[48] and suppresses that of collagenase.[49] Carotenoids both with and without provitamin A upregulate gap junctional communication and connexin[43] gene expression in human dermal fibroblasts and inhibit carcinogen-induced neoplastic transformation.[50-52] All the above effects are caused by antioxidant independent mechanisms.

Vitamin C

Calcineurin (protein phosphatase 2B) is an enzyme, which is inhibited by superoxide radicals that are capable of oxidizing the Fe^{2+} of the enzyme active center to Fe^{3+}. The enzyme can be activated by ascorbate but not by other strong reducing agents, such as dithiothreitol or mercaptoethanol indicating that ascorbate plays a more specific role than that of generic antioxidant.[53] Since inactivation of calcineurin (by cyclosporin A or FK506), results in the inhibition of interleukin-2 gene expression, its specific (not obtained by other reducing agents) activation by ascorbate may be at the basis of an immune response enhancement by vitamin C.[54]

PRACTICAL IMPLICATIONS

In the above discussion emphasis has been given to two notions. In general molecules can be provided with different properties, and the importance of one does not exclude the existence of a second and maybe of a third property. Research can certainly profit from the investigation of hidden properties of compounds provided with well-known functions. The second and more precise paradigm has been that of the identification of some antioxidants provided with different and more specific functions. One of the most important consequences of this concept is that through specific recognition interactions more precise and site-directed events could take place in a cell. This points to the uniqueness of some natural compounds, whose combination of antioxidant and non-antioxidant properties cannot be imitated or substituted for by simple synthetic antioxidants.

Acknowledgments

The present study has been supported by the Swiss National Science Foundation and by F. Hoffmann-La Roche, AG.

REFERENCES

1. Mooradian, AD, Antioxidant properties of steroids, *J Steroid Biochem Mol Biol*, 45, 509, 1993.
2. Mukai, K, Daifuku, K, Yokoyama, S, Nakano, M, Stopped-flow investigation of antioxidant activity of estrogens in solution, *Biochim Biophys Acta*, 1035, 348, 1990.

3. Shwaery, GT, Vita, JA, Keaney, JF, Jr, Antioxidant protection of LDL by physiological concentrations of 17 beta-estradiol. Requirement for estradiol modification, *Circulation*, 95, 1378, 1997.
4. Tesoriere, L, Ciaccio, M, Bongiorno, A, Riccio, A, Pintaudi, AM, Livrea, MA, Antioxidant activity of all-trans-retinol in homogeneous solution and in phosphatidylcholine liposomes, *Arch Biochem Biophys*, 307, 217, 1993.
5. Tesoriere, L, Bongiorno, A, Pintaudi, AM, D'Anna, R, D'Arpa, D, Livrea, MA, Synergistic interactions between vitamin A and vitamin E against lipid peroxidation in phosphatidylcholine liposomes, *Arch Biochem Biophys,* 326, 57, 1996.
6. Tesoriere, L, DArpa, D, Re, R, Livrea, MA, Antioxidant reactions of all-trans retinol in phospholipid bilayers: effect of oxygen partial pressure, radical fluxes, and retinol concentration, *Arch Biochem Biophys*, 343, 13, 1997.
7. Kartha, VN, Krishnamurthy, S, Antioxidant function of vitamin A, *Int J Vitam Nutr Res*, 47, 394, 1977.
8. Snodderly, DM, Evidence for protection against age-related macular degeneration by carotenoids and antioxidant vitamins, *Am J Clin Nutr*, 62, 1448S, 1995.
9. Reiter, RJ, Tan, DX, Poeggeler, B, Menendez-Pelaez, A, Chen, LD, Saarela, S, Melatonin as a free radical scavenger: implications for aging and age-related diseases, *Ann N Y Acad Sci*, 719, 1, 1994.
10. Reiter, RJ, Oxidative processes and antioxidative defense mechanisms in the aging brain, *FASEB J*, 9, 526, 1995.
11. Konturek, PC, Konturek, SJ, Majka, J, Zembala, M, Hahn, EG, Melatonin affords protection against gastric lesions induced by ischemia-reperfusion possibly due to its antioxidant and mucosal microcirculatory effects, *Eur J Pharmacol*, 322, 73, 1997.
12. Claustrat, B, Brun, J, Chazot, G, Melatonin in humans, neuroendocrinological and pharmacological aspects, *Int J Rad Appl Instrum [B]*, 17, 625, 1990.
13. Reppert, SM, Weaver, DR, Godson, C, Melatonin receptors step into the light: cloning and classification of subtypes, *Trends Pharmacol Sci*, 17, 100, 1996.
14. Lewy, AJ, Sack, RL, Blood, ML, Bauer, VK, Cutler, NL, Thomas, KH, Melatonin marks circadian phase position and resets the endogenous circadian pacemaker in humans, *Ciba Found Symp*, 183, 303, 1995.
15. Shochat, T, Luboshitzky, R, Lavie, P, Nocturnal melatonin onset is phase locked to the primary sleep gate, *Am J Physiol*, 273, R364, 1997.
16. Zhdanova, IV, Wurtman, RJ, Morabito, C, Piotrovska, VR, Lynch, HJ, Effects of low oral doses of melatonin, given 2-4 hours before habitual bedtime, on sleep in normal young humans, *Sleep*, 19, 423, 1996.
17. Azzi, A, Boscoboinik, D, Marilley, D, Özer, NK, Stäuble, B, Tasinato, A, Vitamin E: A sensor and an information transducer of the cell oxidation state, *Am J Clin Nutr,* 62 Suppl, 1337S, 1995.
18. Chatelain, E, Boscoboinik, DO, Bartoli, GM, Kagan, VE, Gey, FK, Packer, L, Azzi, A, Inhibition of smooth muscle cell proliferation and protein kinase C activity by tocopherols and tocotrienols, *Biochim Biophys Acta*, 1176, 83, 1993.
19. Serbinova, E, Kagan, V, Han, D, Packer, L, Free radical recycling and intramembrane mobility in the antioxidant properties of alpha-tocopherol and alpha-tocotrienol, *Free Radic Biol Med*, 10, 263, 1991.
20. Janero, DA, Cohen, N, Burghardt, B, Schaer, BH, Novel 6-hydroxychroman-2-carbonitrile inhibitors of membrane peroxidative injury, *Biochem Pharmacol,* 40, 551, 1990.
21. Azzi, A, Boscoboinik, D, Chatelain, E, Özer, NK, Stäuble, B, d-Alpha-tocopherol control of cell proliferation, *Mol Aspects Med,* 14, 265, 1993.

22. Tasinato, A, Boscoboinik, D, Bartoli, GM, Maroni, P, Azzi, A, *d*-α-Tocopherol inhibition of vascular smooth muscle cell proliferation occurs at physiological concentrations, correlates with protein kinase C inhibition, and is independent of its antioxidant properties, *Proc Natl Acad Sci USA*, 92, 12190, 1995.
23. Devaraj, S, Li, D, Jialal, I, The effects of alpha tocopherol supplementation on monocyte function decreased lipid oxidation, interleukin 1 beta secretion, and monocyte adhesion to endothelium, *J Clin Invest,* 98, 756, 1996.
24. Freedman, JE, Farhat, JH, Loscalzo, J, Keaney, JF, Jr, α-Tocopherol inhibits aggregation of human platelets by a protein kinase C-dependent mechanism, *Circulation*, 94, 2434, 1996.
25. Hehenberger, K, Hansson, A, High glucose-induced growth factor resistance in human fibroblasts can be reversed by antioxidants and protein kinase C-inhibitors, *Cell Biochem Funct*, 15, 197, 1997.
26. Kanno, T, Utsumi, T, Kobuchi, H, Takehara, Y, Akiyama, J, Yoshioka, T, Horton, AA, Utsumi, K, Inhibition of stimulus-specific neutrophil superoxide generation by alpha-tocopherol, *Free Radic Res,* 22, 431, 1995.
27. Kanno, T, Utsumi, T, Takehara, Y, Ide, A, Akiyama, J, Yoshioka, T, Horton, AA, Utsumi, K, Inhibition of neutrophil-superoxide generation by α-tocopherol and coenzyme Q, *Free Radic Res,* 24, 281, 1996.
28. Okada, S, Takehara, Y, Yabuki, M, Yoshioka, T, Yasuda, T, Inoue, M, Utsumi, K, Rapid reduction of nitric oxide by mitochondria, and reversible inhibition of mitochondrial respiration by nitric oxide, *Biochem J,* 315, 295, 1996.
29. Koya, D, Lee, IK, Ishii, H, Kanoh, H, King, GL, Prevention of glomerular dysfunction in diabetic rats by treatment with d-alpha-tocopherol, *J Am Soc Nephrol*, 8, 426, 1997.
30. Rattan, V, Sultana, C, Shen, YM, Kalra, VK, Oxidant stress-induced transendothelial migration of monocytes is linked to phosphorylation of PECAM-1, *Am J Physiol Endocrinol Metab,* 273, E453, 1997.
31. Skolnick, AA, Novel therapies to prevent diabetic retinopathy [news], *JAMA*, 278, 1480, 1997.
32. Studer, RK, Craven, PA, DeRubertis, FR, Antioxidant inhibition of protein kinase C-signaled increases in transforming growth factor-beta in mesangial cells, *Metabolism*, 46, 918, 1997.
33. Tada, H, Ishii, H, Isogai, S, Protective effect of D-alpha-tocopherol on the function of human mesangial cells exposed to high glucose concentrations, *Metabolism*, 46, 779, 1997.
34. Takehara, Y, Kanno, T, Yoshioka, T, Inoue, M, Utsumi, K, Oxygen-dependent regulation of mitochondrial energy metabolism by nitric oxide, *Arch Biochem Biophys,* 323, 27, 1995.
35. Özer, NK, Sirikci, Ö, Taha, S, San, T, Moser, U, Azzi, A, Effect of vitamin E and probucol on dietary cholesterol-induced atherosclerosis in rabbits, *Free Radic Biol Med,* 24:226-233, 1998.
36. Sirikci, Ö, Özer, NK, Azzi, A, Dietary cholesterol-induced changes of protein kinase C and the effect of vitamin E in rabbit aortic smooth muscle cells, *Atherosclerosis*, 126, 253, 1996.
37. Azzi, A, Boscoboinik, D, Hensey, C, The protein kinase C family, *Eur J Biochem,* 208, 547, 1992.
38. Pryor, AW, Cornicelli, JA, Devall, LJ, Tait, B, Trivedi, BK, Witiak, DT, Wu, M, A rapid screening test to determine the antioxidant potencies of natural and synthetic antioxidants, *J Org Chem,* 58, 3521, 1993.

39. Martiny Baron, G, Kazanietz, MG, Mischak, H, Blumberg, PM, Kochs, G, Hug, H, Marme, D, Schachtele, C, Selective inhibition of protein kinase C isozymes by the indolocarbazole Gö 6976, *J Biol Chem,* 268, 9194, 1993.
40. Neuzil, J, Witting, PK, Stocker, R, α-Tocopheryl hydroquinone is an efficient multifunctional inhibitor of radical-initiated oxidation of low density lipoprotein lipids, *Proc Natl Acad Sci USA*, 94, 7885, 1997.
41. Dowd, P, Zheng, ZB, On the mechanism of the anticlotting action of vitamin E quinone, *Proc Natl Acad Sci USA,* 92, 8171, 1995.
42. Christen, S, Woodall, AA, Shigenaga, MK, Southwell-Keely, PT, Duncan, MW, Ames, BN, gamma-Tocopherol traps mutagenic electrophiles such as NO_x and complements α-tocopherol: Physiological implications, *Proc Natl Acad Sci USA*, 94, 3217, 1997.
43. Ng, KW, Zhou, H, Manji, S, Martin, TJ, Regulation and regulatory role of the retinoids, *Crit Rev Eukaryot Gene Expr,* 5, 219, 1995.
44. Vieira, AV, Schneider, WJ, Vieira, PM, Retinoids: transport, metabolism, and mechanisms of action, *J Endocrinol,* 146, 201, 1995.
45. Fisher, GJ, Voorhees, JJ, Molecular mechanisms of retinoid actions in skin, *FASEB J,* 10, 1002, 1996.
46. Love, JM, Gudas, LJ, Vitamin A, differentiation and cancer, *Curr Opin Cell Biol,* 6, 825, 1994.
47. Harada, H, Miki, R, Masushige, S, Kato, S, Gene expression of retinoic acid receptors, retinoid-X receptors, and cellular retinol-binding protein I in bone and its regulation by vitamin A, *Endocrinology*, 136, 5329, 1995.
48. White, JA, Guo, YD, Baetz, K, Beckett Jones, B, Bonasoro, J, Hsu, KE, Dilworth, FJ, Jones, G, Petkovich, M, Identification of the retinoic acid-inducible all-trans-retinoic acid 4-hydroxylase, *J Biol Chem,* 271, 29922, 1996.
49. Pan, L, Eckhoff, C, Brinckerhoff, CE, Suppression of collagenase gene expression by all-trans and 9-cis retinoic acid is ligand dependent and requires both RARs and RXRs, *J Cell Biochem,* 57, 575, 1995.
50. Bertram, JS, Inhibition of chemically induced neoplastic transformation by carotenoids. Mechanistic studies, *Ann N Y Acad Sci,* 686, 161, 1993.
51. Zhang, LX, Cooney, RV, Bertram, JS, Carotenoids up-regulate connexin43 gene expression independent of their provitamin A or antioxidant properties, *Cancer Res,* 52, 5707, 1992.
52. Zhang, LX, Cooney, RV, Bertram, JS, Carotenoids enhance gap junctional communication and inhibit lipid peroxidation in C3H/10T1/2 cells: relationship to their cancer chemopreventive action, *Carcinogenesis*, 12, 2109, 1991.
53. Wang, XT, Culotta, VC, Klee, CB, Superoxide dismutase protects calcineurin from inactivation, *Nature*, 383, 434, 1996.
54. Klee, CB, Wang, X, Coupling between oxidative stress and calcium signaling, *FASEB J,* 11, A1120, 1997.

Part 6

Antioxidants and Disease

- Cardiovascular Disease
- Tocotrienols: Biological and Health Effects
- Cancer
- Diseases of the Eye
- Neurological Diseases
- Alpha-Lipoic Acid in Health and Disease

21

Antioxidant Vitamins and Cardiovascular Disease

Charles H. Hennekens, M.D.
Division of Preventive Medicine
Brigham and Women's Hospital, Boston, Massachusetts, USA

INTRODUCTION

Basic research has elucidated several plausible mechanisms for each of several different antioxidant vitamins on delaying or retarding atherosclerosis, and observational epidemiologic studies have suggested that individuals with high dietary intake or serum levels have 20 to 40% lower risk of coronary heart disease (CHD). Since CHD remains the leading cause of death in the United States as well as most developed countries, even small to moderate reductions in risk could yield substantial individual clinical as well as public health benefits. At present, however, the totality of evidence is insufficient to judge whether antioxidant vitamins reduce risk of CHD. Reliable evidence on this important and timely question will emerge over the next several years from ongoing randomized trials testing these agents in primary prevention among apparently healthy individuals as well as in secondary prevention among those with prior CHD.

0-8493-8009-X/98/$0.00+$.50

MECHANISMS OF ACTION

An accumulating body of research indicates that oxidative damage to low-density lipoprotein (LDL) cholesterol greatly enhances atherogenicity.[1] In basic research, oxidized LDL has been shown to accelerate several steps in atherosclerosis including endothelial damage, monocyte/macrophage recruitment, increased uptake of LDL by foam cells, alteration in vascular tone, induction of growth factors, as well as formation of autoantibodies.[2] Regarding postulated mechanisms of action, vitamin E inhibits oxidation of LDL cholesterol in plasma.[1] In contrast, β-carotene may protect endothelial damage by decreasing uptake into cells.[3] These data suggest that different antioxidant vitamins may have different primary mechanisms of action.

ANIMAL STUDIES

Three investigations have reported decreased formation of atheromatous lesions in animals assigned at random to vitamin E. One utilized restricted anovulatory hens, who are prone to hyperlipidemia and subsequent aortic intimal thickening. Those hens fed 1000 mg of vitamin E per kilogram of feed had reduced levels of plasma peroxides and less aortic intimal thickening compared to controls.[4] Second, in hypercholesterolemic mongrel rabbits, those fed 10 milligrams of vitamin E per kilogram body weight per day experienced a reduction in aortic atherosclerotic lesions compared to controls.[5] Third, in monkeys fed an atherogenic diet, a reduction in carotid ultrasound stenosis was reported among those assigned 108 IU of vitamin E per day compared to controls.[6] These findings were similar among monkeys who received vitamin E either prophylactically or therapeutically after atherosclerosis was established.

With respect to vitamin C, in guinea pigs dietary deficiency promotes atherosclerotic lesion formation.[7] Studies in deficient guinea pigs suggest that administration of vitamin C can lead to regression of early atherosclerotic lesions.[8]

As regards β-carotene, it inhibited atherosclerotic lesion formation[9] in hypercholesterolemic rabbits. β-Carotene was not detected in LDL of supplemented rabbits, providing support for the hypothesis that it may protect against atherosclerosis by means other than inhibition of LDL oxidation.

Probucol, an antioxidant with cholesterol-lowering properties, has been tested in several studies. In one, among Watanabe heritable hyperlipidemic rabbits, probucol's cholesterol-lowering effects were controlled for by having a lovastatin control.[10] The probucol group experienced a lower rate of aortic atherosclerosis than either the placebo or the lovastatin-treated group, suggesting that the observed benefit derives from antioxidant properties.

EPIDEMIOLOGIC STUDIES

Descriptive

Descriptive epidemiologic studies have contributed to the formulation of the hypothesis of an inverse relation of antioxidant vitamins and risk of cardiovascular disease (CVD) in humans. Two ecologic studies in Great Britain found significant inverse relationships of per capita consumption of fresh fruits and vegetables with CHD mortality.[11,12] Studies in Europe have reported inverse associations between plasma vitamin E levels standardized to plasma cholesterol levels and CVD mortality rates.[13,14] In a cross-sectional survey among Finnish men, no association was found between plasma levels of vitamin C or E and prevalent ischemic heart disease.[15] Finally, in another ecologic study in Europe, a trend for lower heart disease mortality with higher vitamin E levels was seen, but no consistent findings were observed for plasma vitamins A and C.[16] Thus, some, but not all, descriptive studies have suggested a correlation between dietary intake or plasma levels of antioxidant vitamins and CVD rates.

Analytic

1. Observational Investigations

Several large prospective cohort studies have examined the antioxidant vitamin/cardiovascular disease hypothesis. These include the Nurses' Health Study, the Health Professionals Follow-up Study, the Massachusetts Elderly Cohort Study, the First National Health and Nutrition Examination Survey (NHANES 1), the Iowa Women's Health Study, as well as three prospective blood-based investigations. Because these studies collect exposure and disease information from individuals prior to the onset of disease, they minimize the role of bias in the study findings. However, uncontrolled or uncontrollable confounding may nonetheless explain some or all of the observed associations. Results of the major prospective cohort studies are also summarized in Table 1.

Table 1
Summary of Results of Major Prospective Cohort Studies[a]

A. Nurses' Health Study
Antioxidant Vitamins and Risk of Coronary Heart Disease

Agent	Highest Daily Intake Quintile	Lowest Daily Intake Quintile	Relative Risk[b]	P-Trend
β-Carotene	≥11,404 IU	≤3850 IU	0.78	.02
Vitamin E	≥21.6 mg	≤3.5 mg	0.66	<.001
Vitamin C	≥359 mg	≤93 mg	0.80	.15

B. Health Professionals Follow-up Study
Antioxidant Vitamin Intake and Risk of Coronary Heart Disease

Agent	Relative Risk[b]	P-Trend
β-Carotene	0.71	.03
Vitamin E	0.60	.01
Vitamin C	1.25	.98

C. Massachusetts Elderly Cohort Study
β-Carotene Intake and Risk of Cardiovascular Disease (CVD)

Endpoint	Relative Risk[b]	95% CI[c]	P-Trend
CVD death	0.57	0.35-0.94	.02
Fatal MI	0.32	0.12-0.88	.02

D. NHANES 1
Vitamin C Intake and Risk of Cardiovascular Disease Death

Daily Vitamin C Intake	SMR[d]	95% CI[c]
0-49 mg	1.03	0.94-1.13
≥50 mg; no regular supplement use	0.90	0.82-0.99
≥50 mg and regular supplement use	0.66	0.53-0.82

E. Iowa Women's Health Study
Vitamin E and Coronary Heart Disease Mortality

Vitamin E Intake, IU/day	Relative Risk	95% CI[c]	P-Trend
Dietary, >9.6 vs. <4.9	0.38	0.18-0.80	0.004
Supplements, ≥250 vs. none	1.09	0.67-1.77	0.39

[a] The design and number of people in each study are provided in the text.
[b] Highest versus lowest quintile.
[c] CI: Confidence Interval.
[d] Standardized Mortality Ratio (SMR) compared with rates among U.S. whites.

Nurses' Health Study

The Nurses' Health Study (NHS) is the largest analytic observational study to evaluate antioxidant vitamins and CVD. The NHS is a prospective cohort of 121,700 U.S. female nurses, aged 30-55 at entry, established in 1976. In dietary intake studies, subjects are typically divided into quartiles or quintiles based on their intake of the variable being assessed, and the subsequent rate of disease occurrence in the highest intake category is then compared to that in the lowest. To estimate the intake of antioxidant vitamins, the Nurses' Health Study used dietary intake data provided on a semiquantitative food frequency questionnaire by 87,245 women free of prior CVD. The analyses were based on 552 incident cases of CHD (nonfatal myocardial infarction [MI] + fatal CHD) occurring over an 8-year period. For β-carotene, the relative risk for those in the highest intake quintile compared with lowest was 0.78, a 22% reduction, with a significant p-value for trend of 0.02. For vitamin E, the relative risk was 0.66, with a p-trend <0.001.[17] However, when vitamin E intake was examined separately from diet and supplements, the observed association was due almost entirely to use of supplements. For vitamin C, the relative risk was 0.80, but there was no clear trend across intake quintiles, with a p-trend of 0.15. All these estimates were adjusted for age, smoking, and a number of other CVD risk factors.

Health Professionals Follow-Up Study

Similar analyses have been performed among 39,910 participants in the Health Professionals Follow-Up Study, a prospective cohort study among 51,529 U.S. male health professionals, aged 40-75 at baseline in 1986. In this investigation, after adjusting for age, smoking, and other CVD risk factors, the relative risk of CHD (nonfatal MI + fatal CHD) for those in the highest β-carotene intake quintile was 0.71 (p-trend = 0.03).[18] For vitamin E, the relative risk was 0.60 (p-trend = 0.01). Although the relation was strongest for vitamin E supplement users, an association of borderline significance was still apparent for dietary vitamin E intake alone. Men with high intakes of vitamin C had no decreased risk of coronary heart disease.

Massachusetts Elderly Cohort Study

A prospective cohort study has evaluated the association between dietary β-carotene intake and subsequent CVD mortality among 1,299 elderly Massachusetts residents. After an average follow-up of 4.75 years, those in the highest β-carotene intake quartile had a relative risk of CVD death of 0.57 compared with those in the lowest intake category (p-trend = 0.016).[19] For fatal MI the corresponding relative risk was 0.32, with a p-value for trend of 0.02.

First National Health and Nutrition Examination Survey (NHANES 1)

The (NHANES 1) evaluated vitamin C intake among 11,348 U.S. adults, aged 25-74, whose mortality experience was followed for a median of 10 years and compared to that expected based on rates among US whites.[20] Among those with the highest vitamin C intake from diet and supplements, the standardized mortality ratio for cardiovascular death was 0.66 (95% confidence limits 0.53-0.83). The inverse relation of vitamin C from diet alone was of borderline statistical significance, so the overall association appeared to be explained by supplement use. This study, however, could not take into account use of other supplements, which, in both the Nurses' Health Study and Health Professionals Follow-Up Study, were highly correlated with use of vitamin C and reduced any association to nonsignificance.

Iowa Women's Health Study

Finally, the Iowa Women's Health Study evaluated the association between antioxidant vitamin intake and CHD mortality among 34,486 postmenopausal women with no history of CVD.[21] Based on approximately seven years of follow-up, there was an inverse relation of dietary vitamin E intake with CHD mortality among the subgroup of women who did not report any use of vitamin supplements, with those in the highest quintile of dietary vitamin E intake experiencing a relative risk of 0.38 in relation to those in the lowest intake quintile (p-trend = 0.004). Vitamin E supplement use, however, was not associated with a lower risk of CHD death, a finding in contrast to the Nurses' Health Study and Health Professionals Follow-up Study. Intake of vitamin A, carotenoids, and vitamin C in the Iowa study were not associated with risk of CHD death.

Prospective Blood-Based Investigations

Three blood-based studies of antioxidant vitamins and CVD have been conducted as nested case-control studies within larger prospective cohort investigations. In one, there was no significant association between serum vitamins A and E in frozen samples and subsequent coronary heart disease mortality.[22] Another study also reported no association between baseline levels of serum vitamins A and E and subsequent CVD mortality.[23] Both of these studies, however, stored samples at -20°C, a temperature at which antioxidant vitamin levels may not remain stable over time. A third study reported a significant inverse association between serum β-carotene in frozen samples and subsequent risk of myocardial infarction.[24]

For many, if not most, hypotheses, analytic observational studies, in conjunction with basic research findings, provide a sufficient totality of evidence upon which to base rational clinical decisions for individual patients and policy decisions for the health of the general public. However, for exposures postulated to confer small- to moderate-sized effects, as is the case with antioxidant vitamins, the amount of uncontrolled and uncontrollable confounding inherent in case-control and cohort studies is about as large as the most plausible benefits or risks.[25] It may be, for example, that greater dietary intake of antioxidant vitamins, measured by a diet assessment questionnaire or blood levels, is only a marker for other dietary practices that are truly protective. It is also possible that intake of antioxidant-rich foods is protective, but the benefits result not from their antioxidant properties, but other components these foods have in common. Finally, intake of antioxidant vitamins from food or supplements may simply be correlated with unmeasured or unknown non-dietary lifestyle behaviors that are protective against cardiovascular disease. In such circumstances, only randomized trials can provide reliable evidence. Such a conclusion was also reached in 1991 by a consensus conference convened by the National Heart, Lung, and Blood Institute, which supported the need for randomized clinical trials of β-carotene, vitamin E and/or vitamin C in primary and secondary prevention of cardiovascular disease.[26] However, only trials of sufficient sample size, dose, and duration to detect the postulated small to moderate effects can answer definitively whether or not there is any direct role for a given agent.

2. *Randomized Trials*

In primary prevention, four large-scale randomized trials of antioxidant vitamins have been completed, but their findings have not been consistent.

Chinese Cancer Prevention Study

The Chinese Cancer Prevention Study evaluated antioxidant and other micronutrient supplements among 29,584 residents of four communities in Linxian, a rural county in north-central China. This region suffers from one of the world's highest rates of esophageal and gastric cancer, and dietary intake of several micronutrients is very low. Four combinations of nine different agents were tested in the trial (retinol, zinc, riboflavin, niacin, vitamin C, molybdenum, β-carotene, vitamin E, and selenium). Subjects assigned to combined treatment with β-carotene (15 mg), vitamin E (30 mg), and selenium (50 μg) experienced a nonsignificant 10% decrease in cerebrovascular mortality compared with those not receiving this treatment (relative risk = 0.90; 95% confidence interval, 0.76-1.07).[27] Coronary heart disease is rare in this population and was not evaluated. In the primary analyses concerning cancer, among those assigned to the combination of β-carotene, vitamin E, and selenium there was a reduction in total cancer mortality of 13% of borderline statistical significance (relative risk = 0.87; 95% confidence interval, 0.75-1.00) due to a statistically significant 21% reduction in gastric cancer mortality (relative risk = 0.79; 95% confidence interval, 0.64-0.99). For total mortality, there was a significant 9% reduction among those allocated to this combination (relative risk = 0.91; 95% confidence interval, 0.84-0.99). Because the agents were evaluated in combined regimens, it is not possible to distinguish the separate effects of any one supplement. Moreover, these agents may well have effects in poorly nourished individuals that they would not have among those with adequate dietary intake of micronutrients.

Alpha-Tocopherol, β-Carotene Cancer Prevention Study (ATBC)

The ATBC study evaluated vitamin E (50 mg daily) and β-carotene (20 mg daily) among 29,133 male smokers in Finland, aged 50 to 69. After 6 years of randomized treatment, there were no overall benefits of either agent on cardiovascular disease. Those assigned β-carotene, in fact, experienced a statistically significant 11% increase in ischemic heart disease mortality, while those assigned vitamin E experienced a significant 50% increase in deaths due to cerebral hemorrhage.[28] Regarding lung cancer, the primary trial endpoint, unexpectedly, was a statistically significant 18% increase in the β-carotene group; there was no apparent effect of vitamin E. For vitamin E, a potential limitation of the ATBC trial was the 50 mg per day dose, which may have been inadequate to confer a benefit on cardiovascular disease risk, in light of the results seen in the observational studies that suggested benefits mainly or solely among those whose intakes exceeded 100 mg per day. Nevertheless, the ATBC findings were in contrast to the accumulating body of observational evidence, which indicated possible benefits for individuals with high intake of vitamin E or β-carotene. The results suggest that some of the apparent benefits seen in observational studies may have been overestimates, or even that these agents may have harmful effects not previously observed or even postulated.[29]

β-Carotene and Retinol Efficacy Trial (CARET)

The CARET randomized 18,314 men and women at high risk of lung cancer due to cigarette smoking history or occupational asbestos exposure to daily treatment with a combined supplement containing β-carotene (30 mg) and vitamin A (25,000 IU retinyl palmitate) or placebo. After an average duration of treatment of four years, CARET was terminated early, primarily because of an inability to detect a benefit, but also because of findings of a similar direction and magnitude to those in the ATBC trial. For cardiovascular disease mortality, there was a nonsignificant 26% increase among those assigned the supplement combination (relative risk = 1.26; 95% confidence interval, 0.99-1.61, p = 0.06).[30] There were statistically significant increases of 28% in lung cancer (relative risk = 1.28; 95% confidence interval, 1.04-1.57, p = 0.02) and 17% in total mortality (relative risk = 1.17; 95% confidence interval, 1.03-1.33, p = 0.02). However, it is important to note that the prespecified stopping boundary for early termination of the trial (p = 0.007) was not reached for any of these endpoints, and the finding for cardiovascular disease mortality did not even reach conventional statistical significance. In addition, as with the Chinese Cancer Prevention Study, independent effects of the study interventions cannot be established because the agents were given as a combined regimen.

Physicians' Health Study (PHS)

The PHS randomized 22,071 U.S. male physicians to alternate day β-carotene (50 mg), aspirin (325 mg), both active treatments, or both placebos. The aspirin component was terminated early, in 1988, due to the emergence of a statistically extreme 44% reduction in risk of a first myocardial infarction among participants assigned to aspirin.[31] Regarding β-carotene, after 12 years of treatment and follow-up — twice the duration of any other trial — there was no significant evidence of benefit or harm of β-carotene on risk of individual cardiovascular disease outcomes or on a combined endpoint consisting of nonfatal myocardial infarction, nonfatal stroke, and total cardiovascular death.[32] The relative risks in the β-carotene group were 0.96 for total myocardial infarction (95% confidence interval, 0.84-1.09), 0.96 for total stroke (95% confidence interval, 0.83-1.11), 1.09 for cardiovascular death (95% confidence interval, 0.93-1.27), and 1.0 for the combined endpoint (95% confidence interval, 0.91-1.08). There was also no significant effect of β-carotene on risk of total malignant neoplasms (relative risk = 0.98, 95% confidence interval, 0.91-1.06). Among the 11% of participants who were current smokers at baseline, there was no significant benefit or harm. Because the Physicians' Health Study has lasted far longer than any other trial of β-carotene, its findings of no significant benefit or harm in this general population are particularly reliable, and exclude the possibility of even small overall benefits or harm with a high degree of assurance.

Secondary Prevention and High-Risk Patients

Regarding randomized trial data in secondary prevention or among high-risk patients, a subgroup analysis in the Physicians' Health Study among the 333 participants with chronic stable angina or a prior coronary revascularization procedure at baseline indicated a possible 20-30% reduction in vascular disease events among those allocated to β-carotene.[33]

For vitamin E, three trials with very small samples have reported benefits among patients with claudication.[34-36] A fourth trial among patients with angina found no effect of vitamin E, but its six month treatment period may have been inadequate to observe an effect.[37] The largest completed trial of antioxidants in secondary prevention is the Cambridge Heart Antioxidant Study (CHAOS), which randomized 2,002 men and women with angiographically proven atherosclerosis to vitamin E (400 or 800 IU daily) or placebo for a median treatment duration of 1.4 years.[38] There was a significant benefit associated with vitamin E in the primary trial endpoint of nonfatal myocardial infarction plus cardiovascular death (relative risk = 0.53; 95% confidence interval, 0.34-0.83). This benefit was due entirely to a large and significant reduction in nonfatal myocardial infarction (relative risk = 0.23; 95% confidence interval, 0.11-0.47). There was also, however, a nonsignificant increased risk of cardiovascular death in the vitamin E group (relative risk = 1.18; 95% confidence interval, 0.62-2.27).

ONGOING LARGE-SCALE TRIALS

Several ongoing randomized trials should provide definitive data on the potential role of antioxidant vitamins in the primary and secondary prevention of cardiovascular disease (Table 2). In primary prevention, the Women's Health Study is assessing the benefits and risks of vitamin E (600 IU on alternate days) as well as low-dose aspirin (100 mg on alternate days) among 39,876 apparently healthy U.S. female health professionals, aged 45 and older.[39] The Physicians' Health Study will continue β-carotene treatment and utilize a factorial design to also evaluate the benefits and risks in cardiovascular disease, cancer, and eye diseases of vitamin E (400 IU on alternate days), vitamin C (500 mg daily), and multivitamins (daily). The SU.VI.M.AX study in France is evaluating a daily cocktail of β-carotene (6 mg), C (120 mg), vitamin E (30 mg), selenium (100 μg), and zinc (20 mg) among 15,000 apparently healthy men and women.

With respect to randomized trials in either secondary prevention or among high-risk patients, the Women's Antioxidant Cardiovascular Study will evaluate β-carotene (50 mg on alternate days), vitamin E (600 IU on alternate days), vitamin C (500 mg daily), and a combined daily regimen of folate (2.5 mg), vitamin B_6 (50 mg), and vitamin B_{12} (1 mg) among approximately 8,000 U.S. female health professionals, aged 45 and older, who are at high-risk due to a prior cardiovascular disease event or the presence of three or more coronary risk factors.[40] The Heart Outcomes Prevention Evaluation (HOPE) Study is testing vitamin E (400 IU daily) and an angiotensin con-

Table 2
Ongoing Large-Scale Trials of
Antioxidant Vitamins and Cardiovascular Disease

Trial Country	**Population**	**Agents, Dose, and Regimen**
1. **PRIMARY PREVENTION**		
Physicians' Health Study II U.S.A.	15,000 male physicians	β-Carotene 50 mg, vitamin E 400 IU every other day; vitamin C 500 mg, multivitamin - daily
SU.VI.M.AX Study France	15,000 men and women	Daily cocktail of β-carotene 6 mg, vitamin C 120 mg, vitamin E 30 mg, selenium 100 μg, zinc 20 mg
Women's Health Study U.S.A.	40,000 female health professionals	Vitamin E 600 IU, aspirin 100 mg - every other day
2. **SECONDARY PREVENTION**		
GISSI Prevention Trial Italy	11,000 men and women with recent myocardial infarction	Vitamin E 300 mg, ω-3 PUFA 1 g, pravastatin 20 mg - daily
Heart Outcomes Prevention Evaluation (HOPE) Study Canada, Europe, Mexico, South America and U.S.A.	9,000 high-risk men and women	Vitamin E 400 IU, ramipril titrated to 10 mg - daily
Heart Protection Study United Kingdom	20,000 high-risk men and women	Cocktail of β-carotene 20 mg, vit. C 250 mg, and vit. E 600 mg; simvastatin 40 mg - daily
Women's Antioxidant Cardiovascular Study U.S.A.	8,000 female health professionals with prior CVD events or 3 or more CVD risk factors	β-Carotene 50 mg, vitamin E 600 IU every other day; vitamin C 500 mg, and a combined regimen of folate 2.5 mg, vitamin B_6 50 mg, vitamin B_{12} 1 mg - daily

PUFA: Polyunsaturated fatty acids

CVD: Cardiovascular disease

verting enzyme (ACE) inhibiting drug among 9,000 high-risk patients in Canada and other countries,[41] while the Heart Protection Study is testing a daily cocktail of vitamin C (250 mg), vitamin E (600 mg), and β-carotene (20 mg), as well as the cholesterol-lowering drug simvastatin, among 20,000 high-risk patients in the United Kingdom.[42] Finally, in Italy, the GISSI Prevention Trial is evaluating vitamin E (300 mg daily) and fish oil supplements among 11,000 patients with a recent myocardial infarction.[42]

CONCLUSIONS

For β-carotene supplementation, the findings from completed large-scale randomized trials indicate no overall benefits in well-nourished populations. It remains possible, however, that β-carotene supplementation is beneficial among subgroups at high-risk due to prior coronary heart disease or those with low blood levels of antioxidants. Whether or not there is a true hazard of β-carotene supplementation among current cigarette smokers, as raised by the ATBC and CARET trials, will be evaluated by a collaborative overview of the post-publication results of continued follow-up in all completed trials of β-carotene. If the apparent excess risk observed in those trials is, in fact, real, it should persist with longer follow-up. Conversely, if, as is still possible, there is eventually some benefit from β-carotene supplementation, then this too may emerge with longer follow-up. A common protocol for a collaborative analysis of the post-publication results of all the β-carotene trials is therefore being devised, with the first analyses planned for sometime around the year 2000. This will provide the most reliable evidence on whether the long-term effects are favorable, unfavorable, or null.

For vitamin E, the totality of evidence from basic research and observational studies is consistent with a small to moderate benefit on coronary heart disease risk. However, the randomized trial data available to date are not conclusive, with the ATBC trial in primary prevention indicating no benefit on ischemic heart disease mortality using a relatively low dose of vitamin E, while the CHAOS trial among patients with prior CHD suggested benefits on subsequent nonfatal myocardial infarction (but not overall cardiovascular mortality).

The availability of data from ongoing major trials should allow rational clinical decision-making for individual patients and policy decisions for the health of the general public. In the meanwhile, antioxidant vitamins represent a promising, but unproven, means to lower risks of cardiovascular disease.

REFERENCES

1. Steinberg, D., Parthasarathy, S., Carew, T. E., *et al.* Beyond cholesterol: modifications of low-density lipoprotein that increase its atherogenicity. N Engl J Med 320:915, 1989.
2. Gaziano, J. M., Manson, J. E., Buring, J. E., Hennekens, C. H., Dietary antioxidants and cardiovascular disease, N Y Acad Sci, 669, 249, 1992.
3. Keaney, J. F., Jr., Gaziano, J. M., Xu, A., *et al.* Dietary antioxidants preserve endothelium-dependent vessel relaxation in cholesterol-fed rabbits, Proc Natl Acad Sci USA 90:11880, 1993.
4. Smith, T. L., Kummerow, F. A., Effect of dietary vitamin E on plasma lipids and atherogenesis in restricted anovulatory chickens. Atherosclerosis 75:105, 1989.
5. Wojcicki, J., Rozewicka, L., Barcew-Wiszniewska, B., *et al.*, Effect of selenium and vitamin E on the development of experimental atherosclerosis in rabbits, Atherosclerosis, 87, 9, 1991.
6. Verlangieri, A. J., Bush, M. Prevention and regression of atherosclerosis by alpha-tocopherol, J Am Coll Nutr, 11, 131, 1992.
7. Willis, G. C., An experimental study of the intimal ground substance in atherosclerosis, Can Med Assoc J, 69, 17, 1953.
8. Willis, G. C., The reversibility of atherosclerosis, Can Med Assoc J, 77, 106, 1957.
9. Shaish, A., Daugherty, A., O'Sullivan, F., *et al.*, Beta-carotene inhibits atherosclerosis in hypercholesterolemic rabbits, J Clin Invest, 96, 2075, 1995.
10. Carew, T., Schwenke, D., Steinberg, D., Antiatherogenic effect of probucol unrelated to its hypercholesterolemic effect: evidence that antioxidants *in vivo* can selectively inhibit low density lipoprotein degradation in macrophage-rich fatty streaks and slow the progression of atherosclerosis in the Watanabe heritable hypercholesterolemic rabbits, Proc Natl Acad Sci USA, 84, 7725, 1987.
11. Acheson, R. M., Williams, D. R. R., Does consumption of fruit and vegetables protect against stroke? Lancet 1, 1191, 1983.
12. Armstrong, B. K., Mann, J. L., Adelstein, A. M., Eskin, F., Commodity consumption and ischemic heart disease mortality, with special reference to dietary practices, J Chronic Dis, 36, 673, 1975.
13. Gey, K. F., Brubacher, G. B., Stahelin, H. B., Plasma levels of antioxidant vitamins in relation to ischemic heart disease and cancer, Am J Clin Nutr, 45, 1368, 1987.
14. Gey, K. F., Puska, P., Plasma vitamins E and A inversely correlated to mortality from ischemic heart disease in cross-cultural epidemiology, Ann N Y Acad Sci, 570, 268, 1989.
15. Salonen, J. T., Solonen, R., Seppanen, K., *et al.*, Relationship of serum selenium and antioxidants to plasma lipoproteins, platelet aggregability and prevalent ischemic heart disease in eastern Finnish men, Atherosclerosis, 70, 155, 1988.
16. Riemersma, R. A., Oliver, M., Elton, R. A., *et al.*, Plasma antioxidants and coronary heart disease: vitamins C and E, and selenium, Eur J Clin Nutr, 44, 143, 1990.
17. Stampfer, M. J., Hennekens, C. H., Manson, J. E., *et al.*, Vitamin E consumption and the risk of coronary disease in women, N Engl J Med, 328, 1444, 1993.
18. Rimm, E. B., Stampfer, M. J., Ascherio, A., *et al.*, Vitamin E consumption and the risk of coronary heart disease in men, N Engl J Med, 328, 1450, 1993.
19. Gaziano, J. M., Branch, L. G., Manson, J. E., *et al*, A prospective study of beta-carotene in fruits and vegetables and decreased cardiovascular mortality in the elderly, Ann Epidemiol, 5, 255, 1995.
20. Enstrom, J. E., Kanim, L. E., Klein, M. A., Vitamin C intake and mortality among a sample of the United States population, Epidemiol, 3, 194, 1992.

21. Kushi, L. H., Folsom, A. R., Prineas, R. J., *et al.*, Antioxidant vitamins and death from coronary heart disease in postmenopausal women, N Engl J Med, 334, 1156, 1996.
22. Salonen, J. T., Salonen, R., Penttila, I., *et al.*, Serum fatty acids, apolipoproteins, selenium and vitamin antioxidants and risk of death from coronary artery disease, Am J Cardiol, 56, 226, 1985.
23. Kok, F. J., de Bruijn, A. M., Vermeeren, R., *et al.*, Serum selenium, vitamin antioxidants and cardiovascular mortality: a 9 year follow-up study in the Netherlands, Am J Clin Nutr, 45, 462, 1987.
24. Street, D. A., Comstock, G. W., Salkeld, R. M., *et al.*, A population based case-control study of serum antioxidants and myocardial infarction, Am J Epidemiol, 134, 719, 1991.
25. Hennekens, C. H., Buring, J. E., *Epidemiology in Medicine*, Little, Brown and Company, Boston MA, 1987.
26. Steinberg, D., and workshop participants, Antioxidants in the prevention of human atherosclerosis: Summary proceedings of a National Heart, Lung, and Blood Institute Workshop: September 5-6, 1991; Bethesda, MD, Circulation, 85, 2337, 1992.
27. Blot, W. J., Li, J. Y., Taylor, P. R., Guo, W., Dawsey, S., Wang, G. Q., Yang, C. S., Zheng, S. F., Gail, M., Li, G. Y., Yu, Y., Liu, B. Q., Tangrea, J., Sun, Y. H., Liu, F., Fraumeni, J. F., Zhang, Y. H., Li, B., Nutrition intervention trials in Linxian, China: Supplementation with specific vitamin/mineral combinations, cancer incidence, and disease-specific mortality in the general population, J Natl Cancer Inst, 85, 1483, 1993.
28. Alpha-Tocopherol, Beta Carotene Cancer Prevention Study Group, The effect of vitamin E and beta carotene on the incidence of lung cancer and other cancers in male smokers, N Engl J Med, 330, 1029, 1994.
29. Hennekens, C. H., Buring, J. E., Peto, R., Antioxidant vitamins - benefits not yet proved, N Engl J Med, 330, 1080, 1994.
30. Omenn, G. S., Goodman, G. E., Thornquist, M. D., *et al.*, Effects of a combination of beta carotene and vitamin A on lung cancer and cardiovascular disease, N Engl J Med, 334, 1150, 1996.
31. Steering Committee of the Physicians' Health Study Research Group, Final report on the aspirin component of the ongoing Physicians' Health Study, N Engl J Med, 321, 129, 1989.
32. Hennekens, C. H., Buring, J. E., Manson, J. E., *et al.*, Lack of effect of long-term supplementation with beta carotene on the incidence of malignant neoplasms and cardiovascular disease, N Engl J Med, 334, 1145, 1996.
33. Gaziano, J. M., Manson, J. E., Ridker, P. M., Buring, J. E., Hennekens, C. H., Beta carotene therapy for chronic stable angina (abstract), Circulation 94,I-508, 1996.
34. Haeger, K., Long-time treatment of intermittent claudication with vitamin E, Am J Clin Nutr, 427, 1179, 1974.
35. Livingston, P. D., Jones, C., Treatment of intermittent claudication with vitamin E, Lancet, 2, 602, 1958.
36. Williams, H. T. G., Fenna, D., MacBeth, R. A., Alpha-tocopherol in the treatment of intermittent claudication, Surg Gynecol Obstet, 132, 662, 1971.
37. Gillilan, R. E., Mandell, B., Warbassee, J. R., Quantitative evaluation of vitamin E in the treatment of angina pectoris, Am Heart J, 93, 444, 1988.
38. Stephens, N. G., Parsons, A., Schofield, P. M., *et al.*, Randomised controlled trial of vitamin E in patients with coronary disease: Cambridge Heart Antioxidant Study (CHAOS), Lancet, 347, 781, 1996.
39. Buring, J. E., Hennekens, C. H., for the Women's Health Study Research Group, The Women's Health Study: Summary of the study design, J Myocardial Ischemia, 4, 27, 1992.

40. Manson, J. E., Gaziano, J. M., Spelsberg, A., *et al.*, A secondary prevention trial of antioxidant vitamins and cardiovascular disease in women: Rationale, design and methods, Ann Epidemiol, 5, 261, 1995.
41. The HOPE Study Investigators, The HOPE (Heart Outcomes Prevention Evaluation) Study. The design of a large, simple randomized trial of an angiotensin-converting enzyme inhibitor (ramipril) and vitamin E in patients at high risk of cardiovascular events, Can J Cardiol, 12, 127, 1996.
42. Jha, P., Flather, M., Lonn, E., Farkouh, M., Yusuf, S. The antioxidant vitamins and cardiovascular disease. A critical review of epidemiologic and clinical trial data, Ann Intern Med, 123, 860, 1995.

22

Tocotrienols: Biological and Health Effects

Tom R. Watkins, Ph.D. and Marvin L. Bierenbaum, M.D.
K. L. Jordan Heart Foundation, Montclair, New Jersey, USA

Angela Giampaolo, M.S.
Rangsit Biotech, Hadley, Massachusetts, USA

INTRODUCTION

The chemistry, absorption, transport of tocopherols and tocotrienols and their vitamin E activity was reviewed in Chapter 10. Several other chapters discussed the role of tocopherols and particularly α-tocopherol on basic biological processes, which have direct relationship to immunity, aging, exercise, heart disease, cancer, and diseases of the eye. This chapter focuses on

0-8493-8009-X/98/$0.00+$.50

tocotrienols and the emerging knowledge of their biological effects and potential health implications including clinical studies in humans. We will first discuss the physicochemical properties of tocopherols and tocotrienols as they affect their antioxidant properties.

ANTIOXIDANT PROPERTIES

Tocols (tocopherols and tocotrienols) vary in antioxidant potency. In a study by Olcott and van der Veen,[1] the ability of several tocopherols to prevent oxidative damage to menhaden oil was evaluated. The data showed that homologs lacking a methyl substituent at carbon 5, namely, the γ (7, 8-methyl) and δ (8-methyl) forms, were more effective antioxidants, in this system. In another experiment with squalene as the substrate, similar results were obtained, though the magnitude of the differences was even greater. Hence, the naturally more abundant γ form inhibited peroxidative damage on a molar basis better than any other form, including the α homolog, in this *in vitro* model.

The chroman system forms the basis for the antioxidant potency of the tocols. In general, unsubstituted phenols have little hydrogen-donating ability. The strength of the tocopherols and tocotrienols lies in their bearing ring substituents *ortho* and *para* to the OH group (at C6), and stereoelectronic effects based upon their orientation with respect to the plane of the aromatic ring, particularly with respect to C2-O. The electron-releasing substituents ortho and para to the OH increase its electron density, facilitating fission of the O-H bond and enhancing the stability of the phenoxy radical. Hence, the α form is expected to be more potent than β, γ, or δ, which lack one or more *ortho* methyls. Burton and Ingold[2] have proposed that the efficacy of tocopherols (which are on the order of 250 times as effective as butylated hydroxytoluene and other phenolic analogs) is attributable to the *para* oxygen in the chroman heterocycle. In this ring the lone p type electron pair of oxygen is kept nearly perpendicular to the plane of the ring. It overlaps with the semi-occupied molecular orbitals of the radical, thus stabilizing the phenoxyl radical by electron delocalization. The larger the orbital overlap (the dihedral angle θ), the greater the antioxidant activity. They found that when θ is a minimum, antioxidant activity is at a maximum, and when the angle approaches 90°, antioxidant acitivity is a minimum. The tocopherols have θs in the range of 17-21 degrees, whereas *para*-methoxy derivatives have $\theta s \approx 89°$, and low antioxidant activity. Studies in which a methyl at C2 replaced the side chain with antioxidant activity maintained have shown that activity is conferred by the chroman system.

The more complete methylation of the α form also enhances its lipophilicity, thus enhancing its effectiveness in lipid domains. Further, substitution *ortho* and *para* to the C6 OH decrease the tendency of reaction with atmospheric oxygen.[3]

In addition to inhibiting lipid autoxidation reactions, tocols inhibit oxidation by electronically excited singlet oxygen. Both physical and chemical quenching have been reported. Physical quenching (Kq) predominates, except in polar solvents in which more chemical quenching occurs.[4] In physical quenching, (singlet) oxygen in the excited state is deactivated to the ground (triplet) state, by a charge transfer mechanism. The tocol transfers an electron to the electron-lacking singlet oxygen, forming a charge transfer exiplex. This undergoes intersystem crossing, yielding the tocol and oxygen in the triplet state. The rates of the physical quenching by the tocopherols α, β, γ, and δ are 4.2, 2.3, 1.1, and 0.5 x $10^7/M^{-1}s^{-1}$, respectively. The quenching capability depends on a free phenolic H, since neither the ether nor the ester showed activity.[5] Over longer time courses, the γ and δ forms may prove more effective, as demonstrated for the tocopherols,[6] since they are more stable to photosensitized oxidation. Little evidence about physical quenching by tocotrienols has been published; similar behavior for the tocopherols would be expected, based upon the common chroman nucleus.

Chemical reaction of tocols with singlet oxygen leads to destruction via hydroperoxide intermediates going to the quinone and quinone-4α,5-epoxide.[7] Though not as effective as carotenoids (being about 50x slower), tocopherols have been reported able to deactivate about 40 - 120 singlet oxygens before being destroyed. Scant evidence exists regarding the chemical reactivity of the tocotrienols. The hydroperoxides of α-tocopherol resulting from reaction with singlet oxygen may generate free radicals leading to further PUFA autoxidation.[8] Medium polarity, temperature, viscosity, and other conditions of the milieu effect chemical quenching.[9,10]

BIOLOGICAL EFFECTS

Tocotrienol Distribution in Serum and Other Tissues

The fate of supplemental tocotrienols and the relationships between intestinal absorption, blood levels, and tissue distribution is still not fully understood. Even with relatively high doses of tocotrienols in animals or humans, sustained plasma levels of tocotrienols have not been observed.[11-15] Observations of rats fed atherogenic diets and high doses of α-tocotrienol for two weeks did not indicate significant differences in serum levels between treated and control groups.[16] The bioconversion of tocotrienols to tocopherols via methylation and reducing reactions has been suggested in plants, based on the notion that tocotrienols may be intermediates in the biosynthesis of α-tocopherol.[18,19] To date, the identification of the α-tocopherol binding protein may best explain the relatively lower plasma levels of tocotrienols seen during tocotrienol supplementation.

The appearance of the various tocol homologs in plasma appears to reflect their biological activity; however, the distribution of various forms in tissues remains to be explained. Absorptive uptake into the liver has been shown to be a direct response of the number of methyl groups attached to the chroman ring. In rats fed large doses of tocols by gavage, equal or greater amounts of tocotrienols were found in heart, muscle, and kidney, compared with the respective tocopherols.[20]

Tissue tocotrienol distribution appears to be based upon specific tissue need. In studies using hairless mice, tocotrienol levels were highest in skin, accounting for 15% of total body tocols, with kidney, liver, and heart containing 1% each.[20] Hayes[17] assessed the relative absorption and transport of tocopherols and tocotrienols in the hamster. He reported that the lymph contained four-fold more δ-tocotrienol than expected; similarly, proportionate levels of the α and γ homologs did not follow the dietary intake pattern or mucosal levels measured. Further, he noted that tocotrienols were not found in fasting plasma of the hamster and post-prandial patterns were related to lipoprotein transport patterns. At higher levels of tocotrienol supplementation (up to 223 ppm), only in adipose tissue did the tocotrienol exceed the tocopherol concentration. In control animals, the adipose tissue was the only site with detectable tocotrienol levels.

Non-Enzymatic Effects

Tocol effects of forms other than α-tocopherol, noted for its potency in the rat fetal resorption assay and other various anti-oxidation reactions, have been reported. *In vivo* studies by Goh[21] have shown that both γ- and δ-tocotrienol protected Raj lymphoblastoid cells in culture from EBV infection as assayed by synthesis of EBV Early Antigen, which appears soon after infection of the cell. In these human lymphoblastoid cells, induced by TPA, such protection was not conferred by α-, γ-tocopherol, or various dimers of them, and only marginally by δ-tocopherol or α-tocotrienol. The 5 position on the chroman ring was essential in this model study of the inhibition of tumor promotion. This is consistent with the importance of the C5 center of tocol as reported by Christen, *et al.*,[22] who aptly demonstrated that γ-tocopherol trapped mutagenic electrophiles such as NO_x, whereas the α form (with a methyl at C5) did not. This would also be expected to pertain in the case of γ-tocotrienol and thereby explain, in part, the protection conferred by isoprenoid substituted tocotrienols having an unsaturated side chain which gave markedly greater inhibition than did the phytol (saturated) substituted tocopherols. The fact that the bulkier dimers crosslinked at 5-5', though potent antioxidants, did not protect against tumor promotion re-emphasizes the importance of the γ form, and more particularly γ-tocotrienol. It further points toward the potential role of shape.

Along this same line, growth responses were evaluated in human breast cancer cell lines (MDA-MB-435 cells) in culture given tocotrienol supplements. Guthrie, *et al.*[23] showed that tocotrienols effectively inhibited growth of these cell lines; α-tocopherol had no effect. On further investigation, the authors measured protein kinase c activity (PKC) in order to infer a mechanism. The tocotrienols, α, γ, and δ, inhibited growth of the line by 50% at concentrations of 10, 4, and 8 μg/mL, respectively. In conclusion, the tocotrienols inhibited cell proliferation by inhibiting PKC activity. The tocopherols had no measurable inhibitory effect. All of the activity was observed only in the membrane fraction, when both cytosolic and membrane fractions were assayed. Here, then, we have seen modulation of membrane associated enzyme activity by the steric properties of tocotrienols incorporated into sensitive membrane domains. This one would have been predicted on the basis of earlier, exploratory work.

Enzymatic Effects

In addition to the well-known antioxidant effects of tocols, possible modulation of various enzyme activities has also been evaluated. Mahoney and Azzi[24] have reported studies of tocol influence on protein kinase C activity of bovine brain. Though the half-inhibitory concentration was 450 μM, about an order of magnitude greater than in plasma, the α-tocopherol tested is normally membrane associated. Protein kinase C has been implicated in tumor promotion, differentiation, the respiratory burst and platelet aggregation. Neither calcium ion nor vitamin K, another lipid soluble factor, influenced the kinase activity in these studies.

Some strong evidence of the distinct character of the tocotrienols over the tocopherols has appeared. Serbinova *et al.*[25] have evaluated tocols both in model membrane systems and organeller membranes. Not only did the presence of the tocotrienol decrease phase transition temperatures, but less clustering was observed, narrow line widths and faster rotational correlation times were seen for the tocotrienols, indicative of less ordering, when compared with the tocopherols. The authors also noted more rapid recycling of tocotrienols than tocopherols. Taken together, these emphasize the importance of the isoprenoid side chain, the molecule's shape, and its importance in altering membrane structure and membrane associated behavior.

Other enzyme activities implicated in cancer promotion respond to adequate levels of certain tocols in the tissue. To evaluate the potential value of γ-tocotrienol in a rat model of viral infection, Ngah[26] and colleagues fed a 'basal diet' doped with 2-acetylaminofluorene (AAF), a known hepatocarcinogen, with or without mixed palm tocotrienol supplement. [No composition data was given for the diet, including its tocopherol content. The reported composition of the palm-derived supplement was: α-tocopherol, 26%; α-tocotrienol, 26%; γ-tocotrienol, 36%; and δ-tocotrieniol, 12%.] Controls without tocols or AAF were also followed. Preneoplastic marker enzymes were assayed: γ-glutamyl transpeptidase (GGT) and uridyldiphosphate glucuronyl transferase (UDPGT). After treatment with AAF for 20 weeks, white patches appeared on the liver of unsupplemented animals. Though no significant effect was seen in liver microsomal GGT activity, the plasma GGT activity rose in the AAF treated group, but was normal in the group receiving both AAF and the palm extract. Similarly, the UDPGT activity was maintained at nearly normal levels in the AAF treated animals. The authors inferred that dietary mixed tocotrienols maintained hepatic membranes and protected DNA from AAF damage.

States of elevated tissue peroxides have been associated with viral activation. HIV proviral DNA has been examined. The long terminal repeat region of HIV-1 proviral DNA contains two binding sites for the transcription enhancer, nuclear factor-κB (NF-κB). Several compounds have been found to activate the NF-κB transcription enhancer, including protein kinase activators (e.g., TPA), protein synthesis inhibitors (e.g., cycloheximide, anisomycin), double stranded RNA; lectins (e.g., PHA, ConA), and cytokines (e.g., IL-1 and TNFα). Packer and Suzuki[27] have demonstrated that the pentamethyl-6-OH-chroman unit of the tocols (at 10 μM) effectively inhibited TNFα induced NF-κB activation, though α-tocopherol succinate inhibited only at much higher concentrations (1 mM). Whether this effect has been mediated directly or via inhibition of PLA_2 activity has not been clearly elucidated.

The shape of molecules has been well documented to be a modulator of membrane associated activity.[28] Consider cholesterol and its ordering effects. The influence of tocopherols and tocotrienols has been cited above in model membranes. Several reports have appeared documenting influence of tocols, tocotrienols primarily, on cholesterol clearance from the plasma. Some evidence, though limited, has also been reported by Wechter[29] in studies of renal membranes and natriuresis. Both natural and synthetic 2,7,8-trimethyl-2(carboxyethyl)-6-OH-chromane (LLU-α) have been shown to inhihibit the 70pS K^+ channel in the apical membrane of the thick ascending limb of the kidney. Further studies are awaited to provide more definitive evidence with respect to the role of tocols in renal sodium ion metabolism.

HEALTH EFFECTS

Animal Studies

Cardiovascular Disease

Extensive research *in vitro* and *in vivo* has been devoted to the potential of tocotrienols to suppress HMG-CoA reductase activity, the rate limiting enzyme of cholesterol biosynthesis, and subsequently, to decrease serum cholesterol levels. Some investigators have reported evidence that tocotrienols inhibit this activity in animal models.[14,29-35] Results of studies with HepG2 cells showed that both γ and δ homologs of tocotrienol were more effective in inhibiting HMG-CoA reductase activity.[36]

In animals, serum cholesterol levels of hypercholesterolemic chickens fed a diet containing approximately 20 ppm of palm oil tocotrienols decreased by 29% compared with controls,[35] as had been seen with d-α-tocotrienol given intra-peritoneally.[31] Larger decreases of 44 and 60% in total and LDL cholesterol, respectively, were reported in a swine model.[32] Hood[36] reported that inclusion of 50 ppm of palm oil 'tocotrienol rich fraction' in either young or old Japanese quail resulted in lower plasma and liver cholesterol levels. These data were clouded by possible attribution of these effects to guar gum (versus α-cellulose) in the ration, instead of the tocotrienol addendum.

In studies with the guinea pig, Khor[15] reported hypocholesterolemic effects with modest doses of tocotrienol. The lowest dose tested in these studies, 5 mg/kg/d, resulted in the lowest cholesterol levels. In studies with the male Wistar rat fed hypercholesterolemic (2% added cholesterol), AIN76A semisynthetic diets containing menhaden oil, an addendum of γ-tocotrienol (50 mg/kg) was accompanied by a significant decrease (-45%) in serum cholesterol.[37] Similar results were observed with α-tocopherol addenda at much higher levels (500 mg/kg), a 40% decrease in serum cholesterol level being recorded. Fed in combination, α-tocopherol and γ-tocotrienol resulted in no further hypocholesterolemic benefit in this animal model. In other models, some have reported that α-tocopherol stimulates HMG-CoA reductase activity.[31,33,38] Khor[15] has reported that dietary tocotrienol addenda in the guinea pig spared serum tocopherol.

In animals, other indices of cardiovascular disease have been reported to improve with tocotrienol addenda. The level of thromboxane A2, an indicator of platelet aggregation tendency, has been reported to decrease with tocotrienol supplementation.[31,33,39-41] Tocotrienol addendum has been reported to attenuate platelet aggregation tendency, indicative of thrombotic risk, in response to ADP, EPI, and collagen agonists. In one study, Holub[42] characterized δ-tocotrienol as significantly more potent than other homologs in inhibiting ADP-induced platelet aggregation. In Hayes' study,[17] he did not find an accumulation of δ-tocotrienol in the platelet.

Tocotrienol supplementation would be expected to limit accumulation of peroxidation products in plasma under conditions favoring peroxidation. In rats fed hypercholesterolemic diets with menhaden oil,[37] TBARS (thiobarbituric acid reactive substances, an *ex vivo* measure of lipid peroxidation) formation decreased 72% when γ-tocotrienol (50 mg/kg) was incorporated into the ration, whereas only 43% when α-tocopherol (500 mg/kg) was supplemented. A combination of both the tocotrienol and tocopherol resulted in no further improvement over γ-tocotrienol alone.

Cancer

Elson[43] has drawn interesting parallels between the IC_{50} values (half inhibitory concentration) of tocotrienols for HMG-CoA reductase and tumor growth suppression for several cell lines. The basis for this comparison lies in the essentiality of mevalonate both for HMG-CoA reductase and DNA synthesis and cell proliferation.[44-46] Further, mevalonate constitutes the key metabolite in the biosynthesis of cholesterol and other isoprenoid derivatives. Tocotrienols have been shown *in vitro* to inhibit the growth of several cell lines, including MDA-MB-435 and MCF-7 breast lines, and B16 melanoma.[21,47,48]

Animal models, particularly rodents, have been instrumental in broadening the understanding of these anti-cancer properties. In transplantable murine tumors, α- and γ-tocotrienol limited the life span of Sarcoma 180, Ehrlich carcinoma, and IMC carcinoma, though they had no effect against P388 leukemia cells.[49] In contrast, α-tocopherol had no measurable effect in these models. Mixed palm oil tocotrienols inhibited both chemically and virally induced skin cancers in HRS/J mice.[50] Tocotrienol addenda to the diet led to delayed onset of epithelial papilloma and subcutaneous lymphoma, and also resulted in longer survival times. In a rat model, Gould[51] showed that tocotrienol supplementation extended the latency of DMBA induced breast tumors, though it had no effect on multiplicity.

Tocotrienols may offer protection against early neoplasia. Marker enzymes, such as γ-glutamyl transpeptidase (GGT) and UDP-glucuronyl transferase (UDP-GT), have been used to assess pre-neoplastic changes. In rats given 2-acetylaminofluorene (AAF), incorporation of tocotrienols into the diet resulted in lower liver activities of both GGT and UDP-GT, and lower plasma GGT. From these data Ngah[25] inferred that tocotrienols decreased hepatocarcinogenesis. Results similar in nature for cytosolic glutathione dependent enzymes were observed in AAF-treated rats. Tocotrienols appeared to influence both glutathione-S-transferase (GST) and glutathione peroxidase (GPx). Both GST and GPx decreased with tocotrienol supplementation, suggesting less severe hepatocarcinogenesis.[52] In more recent work, Ngah[53] has suggested that α-tocopherol intervention must occur simultaneously with the carcinogen exposure to be effective in attenuating plasma enzyme activity.

Human Studies

Cancer

Extending animal studies to humans, it was noted[54] that the HMG-CoA activity in A549 tumor cells is higher than that of normal human fibroblasts. It was discovered that 40% of the reductase activity was devoted to non-sterol products, where, in contrast, normal fibroblasts exhibited only 15-20% reductase activity for such purposes. Also, Bennis showed that cholesterol as well as a non-sterol product are necessary for optimal cell growth of the A549 cell line. In conclusion, it was suggested that A549 cells produce more non-sterol substances, which may be indicative of increased requirement of mevalonate for unregulated cell growth, and that these cells need at least one of the non-sterol isoprenoids for growth. The isoprenylation of proteins for use in a signaling pathway of cell proliferation has also been offered as another regulatory mechanism.

Two human breast cancer cell lines were investigated[55] to determine their requirement for mevalonate. The Hs578T cell line is derived from an infiltrating primary breast tumor and MDA-231 from the pleural effusion of a metastasizing breast carcinoma. Mevinolin was used as an HMG-CoA reductase inhibitor. The effect of serum depletion on cellular proliferation differed considerably between the two cell lines. Thymidine labeling decreased by more than 75% in Hs578T cells whereas MDA-231 cells proliferated at the same rate as they did in serum. It was postulated that in the Hs578T cells, serum dependent mechanisms regulate the utilization of mevalonate in the formation of mevalonate derived growth regulating compounds. The authors inferred that the difference in mevalonate requirement was a reflection of the state of biological malignancy between the two cell lines. The fact that the MDA-231 cell line was metastatic may reflect the capacity of this particular cell to adapt and proliferate under changes in environment and physiological conditions.

Epidemiologically, γ-tocopherol and γ-tocotrienol have been shown to be of greater importance than the α forms. Serum γ-tocopherol levels are approximately two-fold higher in the population of Fiji compared to those from populations of the Cook Islands, while α-tocopherol levels are similar in the two populations.[56,57] However, lung cancer incidence rates in Fiji are 10-20 times lower than in the Cook Islands, despite similar patterns in smoking.

Extending observed effects of γ-tocotrienol as an HMG-CoA reductase inhibitor with anti-tumor activity to a possibly similar result utilizing lovastatin is a natural next stop forward. This was done[58] and similarities and differences found in the actions of lovastatin and tocotrienols, which enhanced the notion that tocotrienols may be an anti-cancer agent. The authors stated that drug concentrations which reached 3.9 μM were in the range associated with anti-proliferative activity *in vitro*. Ubiquinone administration was used as adjunctive therapy to combat lovastatin-induced muscle damage.

The published research substantiates the potential of tocotrienols as anti-cancer as well as anti-proliferative agents. Both *in vitro* and *in vivo* murine models have shown tocotrienols to be effective in the suppression of tumor growth. Collectively, the isoprenoid homologs have proven to be superior in this regard relative to the other homologs of vitamin E. More specifically, the cancer inhibiting potency of the various isomers is: δ-tocotrienol > γ-tocotrienol > α-tocotrienol > α-tocopherol. The extent of methylation on the ring as well as the isoprenoid tail have implications in anti-cancer properties.

The ability of the tocotrienols to inhibit the HMG-CoA reductase enzyme has been the attributed basis for their apparent success in arresting cell proliferation. Also, some cancer cell lines do exhibit markedly high HMG-CoA reductase activity as compared to normal cells. In a more specific analysis of the HMG-CoA reductase pathway, evidence suggests that the production of mevalonate, or a product thereof, regulates cell growth. Hence, the reduction in mevalonate deprives cells of a compound necessary for growth and proliferation. Additionally, there may be differences in the functional needs for mevalonate between young cancer cells and those that are metastatic. It has also been shown that tumor cells are not sensitive to sterol feedback mechanisms of this enzyme.

A phase 1 study of cancer patients has been conducted using the HMG-CoA reductase inhibitor lovastatin, initially introduced to lower serum cholesterol via the same enzymatic pathway. Lovastatin has been introduced as an anti-cancer agent because of its ability to inhibit mevalonate synthesis. In this primary research, high doses of lovastatin caused myopathy as a result of depletion of ubiquinone (CoQ_{10}). Also, *in vitro*, 50μM of lovastatin was shown to be cytotoxic to a human bladder carcinoma T24 cell line. It is evident that the use of lovastatin as an anti-cancer treatment may have drawbacks and the side effects must be weighed against the benefits in using it.

On the other hand, tocotrienol may succeed lovastatin as an anti-cancer treatment and/or adjunct to traditional treatment. The nature of the structure of tocotrienol is such that its isoprenoid tail may account for its inhibition of HMG-CoA reductase. Elson and his group[59] have focused their anti-proliferative/cytostatic research on such compounds. More important, tocotrienol has not been shown to be cytotoxic in either *in vitro* or *in vivo* models.

Further, the farnesylation (isoprenylation) of the p21ras protein may be the basis for suppression of cell growth. This may bring tocotrienols' isoprenyl unit in intimate contact with a cell signaling mechanism, a mechanism presently under investigation.

Tocotrienols may also have a significant role in the prevention or alleviation of breast/mammary cancer involvement with the lymphatic system. Tocotrienols have been shown to be effective in combating the onset of lymphatic tumorigenesis.

In a study of human breast cancer, no difference in antioxidant status was found with regard to proximity to the malignant tumor. Interestingly, there were only trace amounts of tocotrienols found in any of these tissue samples. This leaves one to speculate:

1. Was tocotrienol sacrificed in an attempt to combat tumor growth? Or
2. Was the absence of tocotrienol in adipose breast tissue a contributing factor in the onset of malignant breast cancer?

There may also be a site-specific action of tocotrienols with regard to cancer in the skin. This notion is substantiated by the fact that tocotrienols are preferentially deposited in the skin.[60] Thus it appears that avenues for research with tocotrienols are just beginning to open in the field of cancer.

Cardiovascular Disease

With evidence accumulating that antioxidants, particularly those containing tocotrienols, might be beneficial in ameliorating the arteriosclerotic process,[31,60] a randomized trial of 50 subjects with established cerebrovascular disease, including carotid stenosis ranging from 15-79%, was begun.[12] Risk factors were well balanced in the groups and the treatment group was started on a supplement of 64 mg α-tocopherol and 160 mg γ-tocotrienol daily (Figure 1).

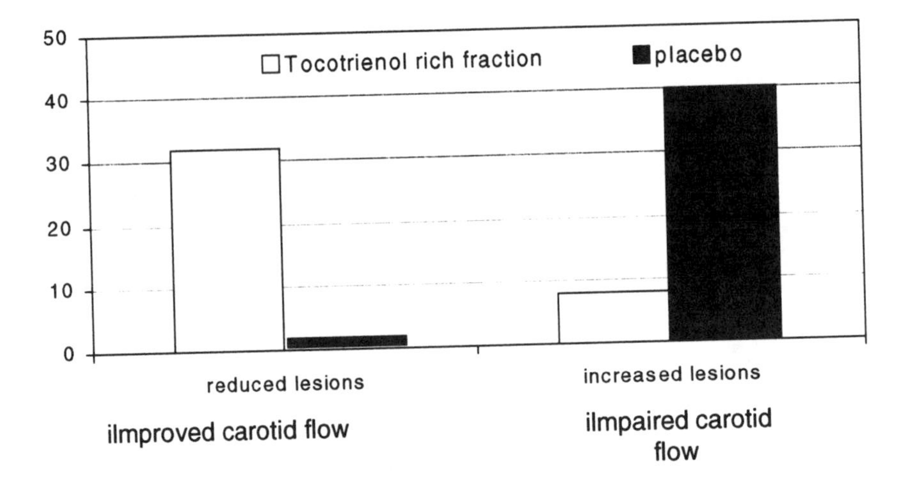

Figure 1. Interim results of an ongoing clinical, tocotrienol supplementation study with 50 stroke patients (<85 years of age). Subjects had suffered a hemispheric ischemic attack of 24 hours or less, a non-disabling hemispheric stroke within the past year, or monocular blindness of less than 24 hours. The data here (at three years) illustrate that none of the subjects taking placebo showed improvement in carotid blood flow, whereas in 40% carotid flow had decreased in this double blind trial. In subjects receiving a daily supplement of tocotrienol (240 mg) and tocopherol (96 mg), only 8% showed decreased blood flow, whereas in 32% carotid blood flow increased. No change in carotid blood flow was seen in 15 subjects of either the placebo or tocotrienol groups (data not shown). No serum lipid changes were observed in cholesterol, LDL- or HDL-cholesterol or triglycerides in either group. [See text and Ref. 12 for further details.]

It had been expected from earlier animal studies[36,37] and human studies[34] that the supplement would be hypolipidemic. This proved not to be so with this design, even when the dosage was increased to 96 mg α-tocopherol and 240 mg γ-tocotrienol daily. Similar results had been obtained by Wahlqvist[14] utilizing comparable dosage levels in hyperlipidemics. It was subsequently suggested[34] that a mixture of α-tocopherol and tocotrienol containing 30% or more of the former would negate this hypolipidemic effect. However, this did not appear to be applicable here, since the mixture derived from palm oil contained only 29% α-tocopherol. Despite the failure to reduce serum lipids in these subjects, the treatment group showed improvement over the placebo group ultrasonographically, both in regression and slowed progression of the disease. This appeared to be related specifically to significantly decreased levels of thiobarbituric acid reactive substances in the serum of the treated group, without a difference in platelet aggregability between the two groups. An anti-oxidation postulate for improvement appears tenable, since a number of other studies are supportive.[61,62] Additionally, the antioxidant supplement may inhibit protein kinase C stimulation and thus prevent the proliferation of smooth muscle cells,[63,64] further slowing the process.

With all of the pomp and ceremony associated with serum cholesterol as a risk factor in atherosclerosis, it was somewhat troublesome accepting the finding of improvement of carotid stenosis without cholesterol reduction. However, two recent meta analyses of randomized controlled trials[65,66] found that lowering the serum cholesterol did not reduce stroke morbidity or mortality in middle-aged men. Further substantiation of these results was made[67] in a Swedish report which showed no difference in carotid intimal media thickness or plaque status in a group with comprehensive risk factor reduction (including a 9% decrease in LDL cholesterol) after 3.5 years of observation. An earlier study[68] also showed that serum cholesterol was a poor predictor of carotid as opposed to coronary atherosclerosis. Attempting to reduce coronary risk with clofibrate and probucol over a 5-year period, they were unsuccessful, but no stroke cases were observed in the 1200-subject cohort. Subsequently, Mao[69] reported that attenuation of atherosclerotic lesions in Watanabi rabbits was demonstrated by a probucol analogue and was not contingent upon a concomitant reduction in serum cholesterol levels. Similarly, probucol[70] reduced the incidence of atherosclerotic lesions in a group of hypercholesterolemic Japanese quail without altering the plasma total or specific lipoprotein class cholesterol levels. Finally, as part of the EVA study,[71] it was found that lipid peroxidation and low antioxidant status were major players in the early phases of atherosclerosis, exclusive of serum lipid changes.

SUMMARY

Despite the emphasis upon α-tocopherol as an antioxidant and preventive in the rat fetal resorption assay over the past 70 years, newer evidence continues to show the excellence of the γ–homolog as an antioxidant and detoxifier of mutagenic electrophiles. The isoprenoid side chain confers distinct physicochemical properties, clearly manifested in the tocotrienols, which modulate membrane dynamics and protect the vascular system.

REFERENCES

1. Olcott, H. S. and Van der Veen, J. Comparison of antioxidant activities of tocol and its methyl derivatives. J. Am. Oil Chem. Soc. *35*: 161-164, 1958.
2. Burton, G. W. and Ingold, K. U. Vitamin E: application of the principles of organic chemistry to the exploration of its structure and function. Acc. Chem. Res. *19*: 194-201, 1986.
3. Kamal-Eldin, A. and Appelqvist, L.-A. The chemistry and antioxidant properties of tocopherols and tocotrienols. Lipids *31*: 671-701, 1996.
4. D'Ischia, M., Costantini, C. and Aprota, G. Dye-sensitized photoxidation of vitamin E revisited. New 7-oxaspiro-[4,5]-dec-1-ene-3,6-dione products or oxygenation and ring contraction of α-tocopherol. J. Am. Chem. Soc. *113*: 8353-8356, 1991.
5. Kaiser, S., DiMascio, P., Murphy, M. E. and Sies, H. Physical and chemical scavenging of singlet molecular oxygen by tocopherols. Arch. Biochem. Biophys. *277*: 101-108, 1990.
6. Yamauchi, R. and Matsushita, S. Products formed by photosensitized oxidation of tocopherols. Agric. Biol. Chem. *41*: 1425-1430, 1977.
7. Clough, R. L., Yee, B. G. and Foote, C. S. Chemistry of singlet oxygen. XXX. The unstable primary product of tocopherol photo-oxidation. J. Am. Chem. Soc. *101*: 683-686, 1979.
8. Terao, J. and Matsushita, S. The isomeric composition of monohydroperoxides produced by oxidation of unsaturated fatty acid esters with singlet oxygen. J. Food Proc. Preserv. *3*: 329-337, 1980.
9. Neely, W. C., Martin, J. M. and Barker, S. A. Products and relative reaction rates of the oxidation of tocopherols with singlet molecular oxygen. Photochem. Photobiol. 48:423-428, 1988.
10. Gorman, A. A., Gould, I. R., Hamblett, I. and Standen, M. C. Reversible exiplex formation between singlet oxygen ($^1O_2$) and vitamin E: solvent and temperature effects. J. Am. Chem. Soc. *106*: 6956-5959, 1984.
11. Stump, D. D. and Gilbert, H. S. The effect of dietary vitamin E supplementation on γ-tocopherol levels of human plasma and red blood cells. Ann. New York Acad. Sci. *435*: 497-498, 1984.
12. Bierenbaum, M. L., Watkins, T. R., Gapor, A., Geller, M. Tomeo, A. C. Antioxidant effects of tocotrienols in patients with hyperlipidemia and carotid stenosis. Lipids *30*: 1179-1183, 1995.
13. Kooyenga, D. K., Geller, M., Watkins, T. R., Gapor, A., Diakoumakis, E. and Bierenbaum, M. L. Palm oil antioxidants: Effects in patients with hyperlipemia and carotid stenosis: 2-year experience. Asia Pacific J. Clin. Nutr. *6*: 72-75, 1997.
14. Wahlqvist, M. L., Krivokuca-Bogetic, Z., Lo, C. S., Smith, R., Lukito, W. Differential serum responses of tocopherols and tocotrienols during vitamin supplementation in hypercholesterolaemic individuals without change in coronary risk factors. Nutr. Res. *12* (Suppl. 1): s181-s201, 1992.
15. Khor, H. T., Chieng, D. Y., Ong, K. K. Tocotrienols inhibit liver HMG-CoA reductase activity in the guinea pig. Nutr. Res. *15*: 537-544, 1995.
16. Hirahara, F. Effects of d-α-tocopherol, d-δ-tocopherol and d-α-tocotrienol on atherogenic diet fed rats after high-dose administration. Nutr. Rep. Int. *36*: 161-167, 1987.
17. Hayes, K. C., Pronczuk, A., Laing, J. S. Differences in the plasma transport and tissue concentrations of tocopherols and tocotrienols: observations in humans and hamsters. Proc. Soc. Exp. Biol. Med. *202*: 353-360, 1993.

18. Basynski, T. An attempt to explain the mechanism of the synthesis of α-tocopherol in the seedlings of *Pisum sativum L.* Acta Soc. Botan. Polon. *30*: 307-326, 1961.
19. Pennock, J. F., Hemming, F. W., Kerr, J. D. A reassessment of tocopherol chemistry. Biochem. Biophys. Res. Comm. *17*: 542-548, 1964.
20. Pearson, C. K. and Barnes, M. M. The absorption and distribution of the naturally occurring tocochromanols in the rat. Br. J. Nutr. *24*: 581-587, 1970.
21. Goh, S. H., Hew, N. F., Norhanom, A. W., and Yadav, M. Inhibition of tumour promotion by various palm-oil tocotrienols. Int. J. Cancer *57*: 529-531, 1994.
22. Christen, S., Woodall, A. A., Shigenaga, M. K., Southwell-Keely, P. T., Duncan, M. W. and Ames, B. N. γ-Tocopherol traps mutagenic electrophiles such as NO_x and complements α-tocopherol: physiological implications. Proc. Natl. Acad. Sci. U.S.A. *94*: 3217-3222, 1997.
23. Guthrie, N., Gapor, A., Chambers, A. F. and Carroll, K. K. Palm oil tocotrienols and plant flavonoids act with each other and with Tamoxifin in inhibiting proliferation and growth of estrogen receptor-negative MDA-MB-435 and -positive MCF-7 human breast cancer cells in culture. Asia Pacific J. Clin. Nutr. *6*: 41-45, 1997.
24. Mahoney, C. W. and Azzi, A. Vitamin E inhibits protein kinase c. Biochem. Biophys. Res. Comm. *154*: 694-697, 1988.
25. Serbinova, E., Kagan, V., Han, D. and Packer, L. Free radical recyling and intramembrane mobility in the antioxidant properties of alpha-tocopherol and alpha-tocotrienol. Free Rad. Biol. Med. *10*: 263-275, 1991.
26. Ngah, W. W., Jarien, Z., San, M. M., Marzuki, A., Top, G. M., Shamaan, N. A. and Kadir, K. A. Effect of tocotrienols on hepatocarcinogenesis induced by 2-acetylaminofluorene in rats. Am. J. Clin. Nutr. *53*: 1076S-1081S, 1991.
27. Packer, L. and Suzuki, Y. Vitamin E and α-lipoate: role in antioxidant recycling and activation of the NF-κB transcription factor. J. Molec. Aspects Med. *14*: 229-239, 1993.
28. Eletr, S., Williams, M. A., Watkins, T. and Keith, A. Perturbations of the dynamics of lipid alkyl chains in membrane systems: effect on the activity of membrane-bound enzymes. Biochim. Biophys. Acta *339*: 190-204, 1974.
29. Wechter, W. J., Kantoci, D., Murray, E. D., D'Amico, D. C., Jung, M. E. and Wang, W.H. A new endogenous natriuretic factor: LLU-α. Proc. Natl. Acad. Sci. USA *93*: 6002-6007, 1996
30. Packer, L., Podda, M., Weber, C., Traber, M. G. Simultaneous determination of tissue tocopherols, tocotrienols, ubiquinols, and ubiquinones. J. Lip. Res. *37*: 893-901, 1996.
31. Qureshi, A., Burger, W. C., Elson, C. E., Peterson, D. M. The structure of an inhibitor of cholesterol biosynthesis isolated from barley. J. Biol. Chem. *261*: 10544-10550, 1986.
32. Qureshi, A. A., Qureshi, N., Haslaer-Rapaez, J. O., Weber, F. E., Chaudhary, V., Crenshaw, T. D., Gapor, A., Ong, A., Chong, Y. H., Peterson, D., Rapaez, J. Dietary tocotrienols reduce concentrations of plasma cholesterol, apoB, thromboxane B_2, and platelet factor 4 in pigs with inherited hyperlipidemias. Am. J. Clin. Nutr. *53*: 1042s-1046s, 1991.
33. Qureshi, A. A., Peterson, D. M., Elson, C. E., Mangels, A. R., Din, Z. Z. Stimulation of avian cholesterol metabolism by α-tocopherol. Nut. Rep. Int. *40*: 993-1001, 1989.
34. Qureshi, A. A., Bradlow, B. A., Brace, L., Manganello, J., Peterson, D. M., Pearce, B. C., Wright, J. J. K., Gapor, A., Elson, C. E. Response of hypercholesterolemic subjects to administration of tocotrienols. Lipids *30*: 1171-1177, 1995.
35. Qureshi, A. A., Pearce, B. C., Nor, R. M., Gapor, A., Peterson, D. M., Elson, C. E. α-Tocopherol attenuates the impact of γ-tocotrienol on hepatic HMG-CoA reductase activity in chickens. J. Nutr. *126*: 389-394, 1996.
36. Hood, R. L. and Sidhu, G. S. Effect of guar gum and tocotrienols on cholesterol metabolism in the Japanese quail. Nut. Res. *12*: s117-s127, 1992.

37. Watkins, T. R., Lenz, P., Gapor, A., Struck, M., Tomeo, A. and Bierenbaum, M. L. γ-Tocotrienol as a hypocholesterolemic and antioxidant agent in rats fed atherogenic diets. Lipids *28*: 1113-1118, 1993.
38. Pearce, B. C., Parker, R. A., Deason, M. E., Qureshi, A. A., Wright, J. K. Hypocholesterolemic activity of synthetic and natural tocotrienols. J. Med. Chem. *35*: 3595-3606, 1992.
39. Parker, R. A., Pearce, B. C., Clark, R. W., Gordon, D. A., Wright, J. K. Tocotrienols regulate cholesterol production in mammalian cells by post-transcriptional suppression of 3-hydroxy-3-methylglutaryl coenzyme A reductase. J. Biol. Chem. *268*: 11230-11238, 1993.
40. Tan, D. T., Khor, H. T., Low, W. H., Ali, A., Gapor, A. Effect of palm oil vitamin E concentrate on the serum and lipoprotein lipids in humans. Am. J. Clin. Nutr. *53*: 1027s-1030s, 1991.
41. Qureshi, A. A., Bradlow, B. A., Salser, W. A. and Brace, L. D. Novel tocotrienols of rice bran modulate cardiovascular disease risk parameters of hypercholesterolemic humans. Nut. Biochem. *8*: 290-298, 1997.
42. Holub, B. J., Sicilia, F., Mahadevappa, V. G. Effect of tocotrienol derivatives on colagen and ADP induced human platelet aggregation. Intl. Palm Oil Conference, Abstract, Module 1, N9, 1989.
43. Elson, C. E. Suppression of mevalonate pathway activities by dietary isoprenoids: protective roles in cancer and cardiovascular disease. J. Nutr. *125*: 1666s-1672s, 1995.
44. Favre, G., Bennis, F., Gaillard, F. E., Soula, G. Importance of mevalonate-derived products in the control of HMG-CoA reductase activity and growth of human lung adenocarcinoma cell line A549. Int. J. Cancer *55*: 640-645, 1993.
45. Larsson, O., Blegen, H., Wejde, J. Requirement for mevalonate in the control of proliferation of human breast cancer cells. Anticancer Res. *12*: 317-324, 1992.
46. Siperstein, M. D., Wiley, M. H., Quesney-Huneus, V. Essential role for mevalonate synthesis in DNA replication. Proc. Natl. Acad. Sci. U.S.A. *76*: 5056-5060, 1979.
47. Mo, H., Peffley, D. M., Hentosh, P., Elson, C. E. Isoprenoid end products of plant mevalonate pathways induce tumor cell apoptosis. FASEB J. 11: A566, 1997.
48. Carroll, K. K., Chambers, A. F., Gapor, A., Guthrie, N. Inhibition of proliferation of estrogen-receptor-negative MDA-MB-435 and -positive MCF-7 human breast cancer cells by palm oil tocotrienols and Tamoxifen, alone and in combination. J. Nutr. *127*: 544s-548s, 1997.
49. Komiyama, K., Iuzuka, K, Yamaoka, M., Watanabe, H., Tsuchiya, N., Umezawa, I. Studies on the biological activity of tocotrienols. Chem. Pharm. Bull. *37*: 1369-1371, 1989.
50. Tan, B. Antitumor effects of palm carotenes and tocotrienols in HRS/J hairless female mice. Nut. Res. *12*: s163-s173, 1992.
51. Gould, M. N., Haag, J. D., Kennan, W. S., Tanner, M. A., Elson, C. E. A comparison of tocopherol and tocotrienol for the chemoprevention of chemically induced rat mammary tumors. Am. J. Clin. Nutr. *53*: 1068s-1070s, 1991.
52. Ngah, W. Z., Shamaan, N. A., Ibraham, R., Jarien, Z., Top, A. G., Kadir, K. A. Effect of tocotrienol on the activities of cytosolic glutathione-dependent enzymes in rats treated with 2-acetylaminofluorene. Biochem. Pharm. 45: 1517-1519, 1993.
53. Ngah, W. Z. Khalid, B. A. K., Top, A. G., Jarien, Z., Shamaan, N. A., and Makpol, S. Different starting times of α-tocopherol and γ-tocotrienol supplementation and tumor marker enzyme activities in the rat chemically induced with cancer. Gen. Pharm. *28*: 589-592, 1997.

54. Bennis, F., Favre, G., LeGaillard, F., and Soula, G. Importance of mevalonate-derived products in the control of HMG-CoA reductase activity and growth of human lung adenocarcinoma cell line A549. Int. J. Cancer *55*: 640-645, 1993.
55. Wejde, J., Blegen, H. and Larsson, D. Requirement for mevalonate in the control of proliferation of human breast cancer cells. Anticancer Res. *12*: 317-324, 1992.
56. Kolonel, L. N., Marchand, L., Hankin, J. H., Bach, F., Wilkins, L., Stacewicz, M., Bowen, P., Beecher, L. S., Lauden, F., Baques, P., Daniel, R., Serunatu, L. and Henderson, B. Relation of nutrient intakes and smoking in relation to cancer incidence in Cook Islanders. Proc. Am. Assoc. Can. Res. *32*: 472, 1991.
57. Henderson, B. E., Kolonel, L. N., Dworsky, R., Kerford, D., Mori, E., Singh, K. and Thevenot, H. Cancer incidence in the islands of the Pacific. Nat. Can. Inst. Monogr. *69*: 73-81, 1985.
58. Thibault, A., Samid, D., Tompkins, A. C., Figg, W. D., Cooper M. R., Hohl, R. I. Phase I study of lovastatin, an inhibitor of the mevalonate pathway, in patients with cancer. Clin. Can. Res. *2*: 483-491, 1996.
59. He, L., Mo, H., Hadisuslio, S., Qureshi, A. and Elson, C. E. Isoprenoids suppress the murine B16 melanomas *in vitro* and *in vivo*. J. Nutr. *127*: 668-674, 1997.
60. Traber, M. G., Podda, N., Weber, C., Thiele, J., Rallis, M. and Packer, L. Diet derived topically applied tocotrienols accumulate in skin and protect the tissue against uv light-induced oxidative stress. Asia Pacific J. Clin. Nutr. *6*: 63-67, 1997.
61. Kritchevsky, S. B., Shimakawa, T., Dennis, B., Eckfeldt, J. Carpenter, M., and Heiss, G. Dietary antioxidants and carotid artery wall thickness: ARIC study. Circulation *92*: 2142-2150, 1995.
62. Esterbauer, H., Dieber-Rotheneder, M., Striegel, G., Waeg, G. Role of vitamin E in preventing the oxidation of low-density lipoprotein. Am. J. Clin. Nutr. *53*: 314-321s, 1991.
63. Carew, T. E., Schwenke, D. C. and Steinberg, D. Antiatherogenic effect of probucol unrelated to its hypocholesterolemic effect: evidence that antioxidants *in vivo* can selectively inhibit low density lipoprotein degradation in macrophage-rich fatty streaks slowing the progression of atherosclerosis in the WHHL rabbit. Proc. Natl. Acad. Sci. U.S.A. *84*: 7725-7729, 1987.
64. Boscobornick, D., Szewczyk, A., Azzi, A. α-Tocopherol regulates vascular smooth muscle cell proliferation and protein kinase c activity. Arch. Biochem. Biophys. *286*: 264-269, 1991.
65. Atkins, D., Psaty, B. M., Koepsell, T. D., Longstreth, W. T., Larson, E. B. Cholesterol reduction and the risk of stroke in men. A meta-analysis of randomized, controlled trials. Ann. Intern. Med. *119*: 136-145, 1993.
66. Hebert, P. R., Gaziano, J. M. and Hennekens, C. H. An overview of trials of cholesterol lowering and risk of stroke. Arch. Int. Med. *155*: 50-55, 1995.
67. Suurbula, M., Agewall, S., Agerberg, B., Wendehag, I., Wikstrand, J. The Risk Intervention Study (RIS) Group. Multiple risk intervention in high-risk hypertensive patients. Arterioscl. Thromb. Vasc. Biol. *16*: 462-170, 1996.
68. Miettenen, T. A., Huttunen, J. K., Naukkaunien, V., Strandberg, T. and Watson, P. B. Long-term use of probucol in the multifactorial primary prevention of vascular disease. Am. J. Card. *57*: 49H-54H, 1986.
69. Mao, S. J. T., Yates, M. T., Parker, R. A., Chi, E. M. and Jackson, R. S. Attenuation of atherosclerosis in a modified strain of hypercholesterolemic Watanabe rabbit with use of a probucol analogue (MD29,311) that does not lower serum cholesterol. Art. and Thromb. *11*: 1266-1275, 1991.

70. Bocan, T. M. A., Mazur, M. J., Mueller, S. B., Charlton, G., Kieft, K. A. and Krause, B. R. Atherosclerotic lesion development in hypercholesterolemic Japanese quail following probucol treatment: a biochemical and morphological evaluation. Pharmacol. Res. *29*: 65-76, 1994.
71. Bonithan-Kopp, C., Coudray, C., Ben, C., Touboul, P., Feve, J., Favler, A., and Ducimetiere, P. Combined effects of lipid peroxidation and antioxidant status on carotid atherosclerosis in a population aged 49-71 y: The EVA study. Am. J. Clin. Nutr. *65*: 121-127, 1997.

23

Antioxidants and Cancer: Evidence from Human Observational Studies and Intervention Trials

Demetrius Albanes, M.D. and Terryl J. Hartman, Ph.D., M.P.H., R.D.
Division of Clinical Sciences, National Cancer Institute
Bethesda, Maryland, USA

INTRODUCTION

Cancer is one of the leading causes of morbidity and mortality throughout the world. In the West, its incidence is surpassed only by cardiovascular diseases. While important advances have been made in the area of cancer treatment and improved survival, it has been acknowledged that the greatest material gains against human cancer will continue to come from primary prevention strategies. Study of the relationship between human nutrition and risk of cancer has been undertaken as one of the major focus areas of prevention research, based in part on previous estimates of between one-third and two-thirds of all cancer deaths possibly being preventable through changes in dietary patterns alone.[1]

Toward this end, the past two decades have seen an explosion of research focused on the role played by antioxidant nutrients in human cancer. Most of the research has involved *observational epidemiology*, either prospective cohort investigations or case-control studies which explore and test associations between the dietary factor(s) of interest and risk of cancer. The former are generally considered scientifically stronger because information concerning personal characteristics that are risk factors or protective "exposures" (i.e., dietary and smoking habits, serologic parameters, family and medical histories, occupational settings, etc.) are ascertained well in advance of the onset or diagnosis of cancer, thereby reducing or eliminating altogether several biases inherent in case-control studies, including selection and recall bias.

Nutrient information in these investigations is available from dietary histories, food frequency, or other dietary questionnaires, whose food consumption data can be evaluated in terms of individual foods that are rich sources of antioxidants under study (e.g., citrus fruit and vitamin C or carrots and β-carotene) or total intake of specific antioxidant nutrients derived from the entire diet. In addition, nutrient biochemical status — usually plasma or serum micronutrient concentration — provides a more specific assessment, but is less commonly available in studies.

More recently, results have also become available from several large controlled trials of antioxidant nutrients that were initiated in the 1980s. These *randomized intervention trials* have provided highly relevant and specific evidence regarding the effects of micronutrients supplementation on the incidence of cancer. Specific nutrients or nutrient combinations, or in a some cases dietary interventions, are tested through randomized experimental designs devoid of most of the biases inherent in the observational epidemiological studies. Along with observational epidemiologic studies, they contribute to our knowledge regarding the potential effects of nutrition on cancer and continue to play a critical role in the development of nutrition-related public health recommendations.

ANTIOXIDANTS AND CARCINOGENESIS

Experimental data have established a wide range of biological effects of carotenoids, tocopherols/tocotrienols, ascorbic acid, and selenium, many of which are thought to influence processes involved in carcinogenesis.[2,3] These include effects on: tumor initiation, promotion, and progression; cell proliferation and differentiation; immune function; DNA repair; the *in vivo* formation of nitrosamines and other carcinogens; carcinogen detoxification/activation enzymes; cellular gap junction communication; and cell membrane stability. With respect to the biological function of carotenoids, it is important to bear in mind that in addition to their antioxidant, free-radical inactivation effects, β-carotene, α-carotene, and β-cryptoxanthin serve as precursors to vitamin A through their *in vivo* cleavage to retinoic acid both at the site of absorption in the small intestine and in other organs, particularly the liver.

β-CAROTENE AND OTHER CAROTENOIDS

Since the late 1970s, epidemiological studies in various populations throughout the world have demonstrated a relatively strong and consistent protective relationship between higher β-carotene intake or greater consumption of carotenoid-rich foods and lower risk of cancer.[4] This research is provided further specificity and support by the results of blood-based studies showing significant inverse associations between cancer risk and serum concentration of β-carotene, or in some instances, other carotenoids. The inverse relationship has been noted for nearly all cancer sites studied, with the most abundant evidence available for cancer of the lung, oropharynx, larynx, esophagus, stomach, and colon and rectum. These investigations can be divided into those assessing dietary intake of specific carotenoids, most commonly β-carotene intake (summarized in Table 1), and those evaluating levels of vegetable and fruit consumption, particularly those that are good sources of β-carotene and other carotenoids (Table 2).

It should be borne in mind when interpreting the latter studies of vegetable/fruit consumption that while the observed findings are consistent with a specific association for β-carotene or carotenoids, such attribution should be made cautiously, as other specific constituents of those foods (e.g., ascorbic acid, folic acid, etc.), the foods themselves, or an overall dietary pattern may underlie the relationship to cancer.

Carotenoids are yellow to dark orange/red colored pigments in plant cells associated with chlorophylls that serve a protective function in photoenergizing reactions involving, especially, singlet oxygen. Among the several hundred carotenoids identified, β-carotene and lutein are the most commonly available in the human diet from vegetable and fruit sources. As mentioned, β-carotene, α-carotene, and β-cryptoxanthin serve not only as antioxidants, but have vitamin A-related effects as a result of their metabolic conversion to retinoic acid.[5] This is particularly important in underdeveloped populations.

Table 1
Observational Epidemiologic Studies of β-Carotene, Carotenoid Intake or Biochemical Status and Cancer

Organ site	Number of studies	Studies suggesting protective association	References
Lung	36	32 (89%)	6-9 (reviews)
Upper aerodigestive	12	10 (83%)	14-16, 32-35, 44-48
Stomach	14	12 (86%)	69-82
Colorectum	9	6 (67%)	102-110
Pancreas	8	3 (38%)	80, 136-141, 143
Breast	32	21 (66%)	80, 112, 155-184
Ovary	4	3 (75%)	194-197
Endometrium	4	3 (75%)	200-203
Cervix	16	10 (63%)	206-221
Prostate	19	6 (32%)	80, 112, 177, 223-238
Bladder	11	3 (27%)	79, 80, 112, 244-251

Table 2
Observational Epidemiologic Studies of Vegetables/Fruit Consumption and Cancer

Organ site	Number of studies	Studies suggesting protective association	References
Lung	28	23 (82%)	6-9 (reviews)
Upper aerodigestive	45	38 (85%)	17-31,36-45,48-67
Stomach	26	20 (77%)	69,71,73-76,82-101
Colorectum	30	26 (87%)	90,102-4,107,111-35
Pancreas	14	10 (71%)	136,140,141,144-54
Breast	22	13 (57%)	112,155-8,161-2,164,167, 169,171,174-5,185-93
Ovary	6	6 (100%)	194-9
Endometrium	5	3 (60%)	201-5
Cervix	8	6 (75%)	206-10,212,213,218
Prostate	11	5 (45%)	112,223,235,236,239-43
Bladder	14	11 (79%)	112,245-250,253-9

Observational Epidemiologic Studies

Lung Cancer

Over 30 case-control and prospective cohort studies in various populations throughout the world have shown a strong protective association between greater consumption of carotenoid-rich foods (and, specifically, higher β-carotene intake) and lower risk of lung cancer. By most standards, their findings represent one of the most consistent associations in the cancer-nutritional epidemiologic literature. Several excellent reviews of these studies have been published.[6-9] While some early investigations demonstrated a protective role for diets having higher total vitamin A intake (i.e., both preformed retinol and pro-vitamin A carotene),[10] most subsequent studies link low self-reported consumption of vegetables or fruit (or both), derived from dietary histories, food frequency, or other dietary questionnaires, with increased risk of lung cancer. In many of the studies, the inverse relationship involves the consumption of carotenoid-rich foods specifically, such as dark green, yellow, or orange vegetables. In others, a protective association was demonstrated for higher β-carotene intake in particular, or for higher β-carotene biochemical status (usually serum concentration). Relative risk reductions of between 20% and 80% (i.e., RR = 0.8-0.2) have been reported typically for the highest β-carotene or vegetable/fruit categories compared to the lowest. They have been shown in studies of men and women, for several racial groups, and for current smokers, former smokers, and nonsmokers, and therefore appear quite generalized. In most investigations, statistical adjustment was made for the most important causal factor, cigarette smoking. A few studies demonstrate beneficial associations for dietary carotenoids in addition to β-carotene, such as α-carotene and lutein.[11-13] These investigations highlight the need for careful evaluation of the several highly correlated dietary carotenoids, in part made possible by improved food composition data.

It was in response to this growing evidence that several randomized intervention trials of β-carotene and cancer were initiated in the early 1980s, including those testing the efficacy of such supplementation in primary cancer prevention (see below).

Cancers of the Upper Aerodigestive Tract

Substantial data also exist supporting a protective role for β-carotene or carotenoid-rich diets in cancer of the oropharynx, larynx, and esophagus. Most investigations controlled for two of the more important etiologic factors for these sites, smoking and alcohol consumption. In a few studies of oropharyngeal cancer, increased carotenoid intake or serum concentrations were inversely related to risk.[14-16] Results from one cohort investigation[17] and 12 of 14 case-control studies[18-31] of oropharyngeal cancer have linked higher vegetable/fruit intake with substantial risk reductions, including among high-risk exposure populations (e.g., oral tobacco users).[21]

Similar strong associations have been reported for laryngeal cancer from the data available in 11 case-control studies, four involving carotenoid intake,[32-35] and seven related to vegetable consumption.[22,36-41] More limited information is available with respect to nasopharyngeal cancer, from studies conducted in China, showing an inverse relationship with vegetable intake.[42,43]

Cancer of the esophagus is another upper aerodigestive organ site where smoking and alcohol are believed to play a causative role and for which substantial evidence points to a risk-modifying effect for dietary carotenoids and other micronutrients. For example, five case-control studies have related higher β-carotene or carotenoid intake to lower esophageal cancer risk,[44-48] 20 investigations have made such a link for vegetable/fruit consumption,[45,49-67] and two studies found reduced risk for both increased β-carotene intake and vegetable consumption.[44,48] Approximately half of the latter studies were conducted in high-risk, non-Western regions of the world such as India, Iran, and China. In one of the latter areas affected by multiple nutrient deficiencies, a large, multifactorial nutritional supplementation trial[68] was undertaken in the 1980s along with several other trials. These studies are described later.

Stomach Cancer

Data from two cohort studies[69,70] and, with the exception of two,[71,72] all case-control studies revealed significant protective associations for dietary carotenoids.[73-78] In addition, four prospective analyses support an inverse relationship between serum β-carotene concentration and stomach cancer risk.[79-82] Vegetable consumption has also been heavily studied with respect to stomach cancer. Two[82,83] of five cohort studies,[69,82-85] and 18 of 21 case-control studies[71,73-76,86-101] reported significant inverse relationships for higher consumption of various vegetables. Green and yellow vegetables, raw vegetables, cooked vegetables, and all vegetables combined were most frequently ascertained and related to reduced risk.

Colorectal Cancer

β-Carotene and carotenoids have been less consistently related to large bowel cancer than has (low) vegetable consumption. Eight case-control and one cohort study assessed the relationship between β-carotene intake and colorectal cancer.[102-110] Protective associations were shown in six of these investigations,[103-106,109,110] although some showed a relationship for only colon or rectal cancer,[104,106] or suggested reduced risk for higher intake but did not achieve statistical significance (e.g., Ref. 110.) A large number of other investigations examined vegetable/fruit consumption and large bowel cancer, including four prospective studies[111-114] and over 20 case-control studies[90,102-104,107,115-135] of which the vast majority showed some degree of risk reduction for increased consumption. It should be kept in mind that, particularly for this cancer site, the evidence for a beneficial effect of diets rich in vegetables, including carotenoid-rich vegetables, is open to interpretation with regard to the responsible factor or substance(s). β-Carotene and other carotenoids are good candidates, especially with specific supportive β-carotene intake or serologic data, but dietary fiber and folic acid have had preventive effects ascribed to them for colorectal cancer.

Pancreatic Cancer

Evidence for the role of carotenoids in pancreatic cancer is not very strong. One prospective study[136] and two case-control studies[137,138] are consistent with a protective association for β-carotene intake, while three other case-control studies are not.[139-141] (A combined analysis of the latter four case-control studies yielded an estimated 30% lower risk for the highest quartile of β-carotene intake, however, with the suggestion of a dose-response trend that was not statistically significant.[142]) Two prospective serologic studies showed no significant inverse relations with pancreatic cancer for β-carotene status,[80,143] although one of these studies did find lower serum lycopene concentrations in pancreatic cancer cases compared to noncases.[143]

Investigations of pancreatic cancer and vegetable/fruit consumption have been more numerous and more consistent than those for β-carotene intake or biochemical status. Four cohort[136,144-146] and 10 case-control studies[140,141,147-154] in general demonstrate significant inverse relationships for various categories of vegetable and fruit use. In one of the prospective studies,[136] the β-carotene intake results were stronger than those for vegetable consumption.

Breast Cancer

The observational epidemiologic data regarding breast cancer and β-carotene and carotenoids are more consistent for food consumption (e.g., green vegetables) than for nutrient intake or serology. Relatively small (i.e., 10-20%) reductions in breast cancer risk have been observed within prospective dietary investigations of carotenoid intake.[112,155-157] In contrast, results from 18 case-control studies[158-175] are more supportive of a protective association for carotenoids, with most showing material risk reductions in both premenopausal and postmenopausal women. Serum β-carotene, other carotenoids, or total carotenoids have been studied in several prospective cohort analyses[80,176-181] and case-control studies.[159,163,170,182,183] In two of these,[163,176] a two-fold or greater breast cancer risk reduction was shown among women in the highest category of serum β-carotene, while in another, a significant protective relationship was found for serum lycopene, along with suggestive findings for β-cryptoxanthin and lutein-zeaxanthin.[181] Serum β-carotene was not similarly associated with breast cancer in this study, nor in the other studies of β-carotene biochemical status, with the exception of three showing higher blood levels to be associated with increased risk.[80,159,170] Consistent with these overall findings for carotenoid biochemical status is one other recent case-control investigation within the EURAMIC Study of adipose tissue antioxidant concentrations (i.e., β-carotene and α-tocopherol) in postmenopausal women that showed no association with risk of breast cancer.[184] Most of the studies cited controlled for at least some other important breast cancer risk factors such as reproductive or family breast cancer history, postmenopausal hormone use, and body weight and height.

There have been a large number of investigations of the relationship between breast cancer and vegetable/fruit consumption, with most supporting protective associations for various food groupings. Of the three cohort studies[112,156,157] and 19 case-control studies,[155,158,161,162,164,167,169,171,174,175,185-93] only nine failed to show statistically significant protective associations.[112,155,162,167,169,171,185,186,188] Results for vegetables and green, dark green, or green leafy vegetables specifically tended to be stronger overall.

Ovarian Cancer

Limited data exist regarding carotenoid intake and risk of ovarian cancer, including three case-control studies showing a protective relationship,[194-196] and one showing no association for β-carotene intake.[197] These studies did, however, find benefit for increased vegetable consumption, as did two other studies.[198,199]

Endometrial Cancer

Studies also suggest that higher carotenoid and vegetable intake are inversely related to endometrial cancer. Three[200-202] of four[200-203] case-control studies of β-carotene intake show an inverse relation, and three show protection for higher vegetable consumption,[201,202,204] while two did not.[203,205]

Cervical Cancer

A role for β-carotene in cervical cancer is supported by some of the available research. Of eight case-control investigations of carotenoid intake, four show protection for invasive disease,[206-209] three show no association with dysplasia,[210-212] and one shows a two-fold increased risk for higher intake.[213] Also, four β-carotene serologic studies have shown an inverse relationship to risk of invasive cervical cancer.[214-217] Regarding cervical intraepithelial neoplasia or carcinoma *in-situ*, there have been mixed results for carotenoid intake,[218,219] reduced risk for high lycopene intake,[220] and inverse relations demonstrated for several carotenoids.[221] Eight investigations evaluated vegetable/fruit consumption: six yielded protective associations,[206,207,210,212,213,218] and two showed no relationship.[208,209] Adjustment for sexual behavior history and smoking attenuated the risk relationships in some of these studies.

Prostate Cancer

Results from observational epidemiologic studies are more inconsistent for prostate cancer. Some case-control studies provide evidence of a protective or null association,[223-227] while others report a positive association between β-carotene intake and prostate cancer risk, particularly among older men.[228-232] Prospective cohort study findings are also mixed, with most showing no association;[112,233-237] however, in one of these, a protective relationship was seen for lycopene intake.[236] Serum β-carotene concentrations have been shown to be either inversely or unrelated to prostate cancer.[80,177,235,238]

Mixed results have also been observed with respect to vegetable/fruit consumption and prostate cancer. Of seven cohort studies, four had null or mixed findings,[112,236,239,240] two showed overall weak protection[235] or protection among younger men only,[233] and one found increased risk for higher consumption.[241] Case-control investigations have provided some evidence of a beneficial association for vegetables[223,230,242] or no association.[243]

Bladder Cancer

Most investigations of β-carotene intake and bladder cancer have shown little or no association,[244-247] while three other case-control studies suggest protection for higher intake,[248-250] and the one cohort study shows nonsignificantly increased risk for elderly men having the highest intake.[112] These reports are essentially corroborated by the four β-carotene biochemical investigations that gave null results as well.[79,80,249,251] In one of these, however, serum lycopene was found to be lower in cancer cases than in controls.[251]

Four cohort[112,253-255] and ten case-control studies[245-250,256-259] are generally supportive of a beneficial relationship with bladder cancer. These studies link higher vegetable/fruit consumption to decreased risk, with only three showing no association.[245,246,253]

Randomized Intervention Trials

Several large randomized, placebo-controlled primary prevention trials of β-carotene supplementation in human cancer have been conducted and their results published.[68,260-269] These completed studies are described in Table 3. They include the Alpha-Tocopherol, Beta-Carotene Cancer Prevention Study, the Beta-Carotene and Retinol Efficacy Trial, the Physicians' Health Study, and the Nutrition Intervention Trials I and II (NIT-I, NIT-II). Four smaller supplementation trials have also been reported, including the Skin Cancer Prevention Study, the Polyp Prevention Study, the Australian Polyp Prevention Project, and the Tyler Cancer Prevention Study. These β-carotene trials were initiated primarily in response to the overwhelming observational associations previously described, and in order to evaluate experimentally the public health significance of β-carotene.[4] Also shown in Table 3 is a recently reported selenium supplementation trial that will be discussed later.[270]

The Alpha-Tocopherol, Beta-Carotene (ATBC) Cancer Prevention Study

The ATBC Study was a large, double-blind, randomized placebo-controlled intervention trial testing the efficacy of daily supplementation with α-tocopherol (vitamin E) (50 mg) or β-carotene (20 mg), or both agents, for 5-8 years in the primary prevention of lung and other cancers.[260,261] It was conducted in southwestern Finland and included 29,133 50 to 69-year-old males who smoked ≥ 5 cigarettes daily at entry. Incident cancers were identified through the nation-wide cancer registry. Initial study findings were unexpected in that they provided no evidence for a cancer preventive effect from the β-carotene supplements, and instead suggested an adverse outcome for both lung cancer and overall mortality. Final lung cancer incidence was 16% greater for the β-carotene group, with a 95% confidence interval of between a 2% and 33% increase in incidence. Subgroup analyses suggested that the β-carotene effect might have been limited to the men with higher alcohol intake and in those who were heavier smokers (i.e., at least a pack of cigarettes daily).[261] Prostate and stomach cancer incidence were also 23% and 25% higher, respectively, in the β-carotene group.[260] These findings were not statistically significant, however.

Table 3
Large Randomized Cancer Prevention Trials of β-Carotene, Vitamin C, Vitamin E, and Selenium

Trial	Size	Cancer site	Dosage	Duration, yrs	Relative Risk (95% Confidence Interval)[1]
Nutrition Intervention Trial I (NIT-I)[68]	29,584	Esophagus, stomach, others	15mg β-carotene + vitamin E 30 mg + selenium 50 μg	5	RR 0.87 (0.75-1.00) (all sites) RR 0.96 (0.78-1.18) (esophagus) RR 0.79 (0.64-0.99) (stomach)
			vitamin C 120 mg+ molybdenum 30 μg		RR 1.16 (0.92-1.21) (all sites) RR 1.05 (0.85-1.29) (esophagus) RR 1.09 (0.88-1.36) (stomach)
Alpha-Tocopherol, Beta-Carotene Cancer Prevention Study (ATBC) [260,261,364]	29,133	Lung, prostate, colorectum, bladder, others	20 mg β-carotene ± vitamin E 50 mg	6	RR 1.18 (1.03-1.36) (β-carotene in lung) RR 1.03 (0.92-1.14) (β-carotene in others) RR 0.99 (0.87-1.13) (vitamin E in lung) RR 0.68 (0.53-0.88) (vitamin E in prostate) RR 0.78 (0.55-1.09) (vitamin E in colorectum)
Beta-Carotene and Retinol Efficacy Trial (CARET)[262,263]	18,314	Lung, breast, colorectum, prostate	25 mg β-carotene + vitamin A 25,000 IU	4	RR 1.18 (1.03-1.36) (lung) RR 0.78 (0.55-1.12) (breast) RR 1.01 (0.80-1.27) (prostate) RR 1.02 (0.70-1.51) (colorectum)

[1] Shown for active intervention group vs. placebo.

Table 3 (continued)
Large Randomized Cancer Prevention Trials of β-Carotene, Vitamin E, Vitamin C, and Selenium

Physicians' Health Study (PHS)[264]	22,071	Prostate, colorectum, lung, others	50 mg β-carotene every other day	12	RR 0.98 (0.91-1.06) (all sites) 520 vs. 527 cases (prostate) 167 vs. 174 cases (colorectum) 82 vs. 88 cases (lung)
Skin Cancer Prevention Study[266]	1,805	Nonmelanoma skin	50 mg β-carotene	5	RR 1.05 (0.91-1.22)
Nutrition Intervention Trial II (NIT II)[265]	3,318	Esophagus, stomach, others	15 mg β-carotene + multivitamin/ mineral supplement	6	RR 0.90 (0.70-1.16) (esophagus) RR 1.21 (0.90-1.64) (stomach) RR 0.99 (0.82-1.21) (all)
Polyp Prevention Study[267]	864	Colorectal adenoma	50 mg β-carotene ± vitamin C 1000 mg vitamin E 400 mg	4	RR 1.01 (0.85-1.20) (β-carotene) RR 1.08 (0.91-1.29) (vit C+vit E)
Australian Polyp Prevention Project[268]	306	Colorectal adenoma	20 mg β-carotene ± 25 g bran ± low-fat	4	RR 1.5 (0.9-2.5)
Tyler Cancer Prevention Study[269]	755	Sputum atypia (lung)	50 β-carotene + vitamin A 25,000 IU every other day	5	No effect on sputum atypia: 12% vs. 9% moderate or severe atypia in active vs. placebo group, resp.
Nutritional Prevention of Cancer Study[270]	1,312	Skin, lung, colorectal, prostate, breast	selenium 200 µg	4.5	RR 0.61 (0.46-0.82) (all sites) RR 0.56 (0.31-1.01) (lung) RR 0.35 (0.18-0.65) (prostate) RR 0.39 (0.17-0.90) (colorectal)

[1] Shown for active intervention group vs. placebo.

β-Carotene and Retinol Efficacy Trial (CARET)

ATBC Study results were published beginning in 1994, and were the first experimental data to conflict with the abundant observational epidemiologic data. Skepticism surrounding the generalizability of the findings was ameliorated, however, upon the announcement of similar results in the CARET.[262,263] CARET studied 18,314 men and women in the U.S. at elevated risk for lung cancer — smokers, former smokers, and workers exposed to asbestos. This study tested daily supplementation with β-carotene (30 mg) in combination with retinyl palmitate (25,000 IU), and halted intervention following an observed increase in lung cancer incidence (28%) and total mortality (17%) after 4 years. CARET data also indicated a somewhat greater excess in lung cancer incidence among heavier smokers and asbestos-exposed workers, and a modest relationship to higher alcohol consumption. The incidence of nearly all of the other major cancer sites did not differ significantly between active treatment and placebo arms in this study, with 1%, 2%, 8%, and 26% increased rates suggested for cancers of the prostate, large bowel, bladder, and oropharynx, and a 22% reduction in breast cancer (95% confidence interval, 45% reduction to a 12% increase).[263]

The Physicians' Health Study (PHS)

In contrast to the trial-based findings in the ATBC Study and CARET, the Physicians' Health Study (PHS), an intervention trial that enrolled 22,071 male, primarily nonsmoking, physicians in the U.S., showed no adverse or beneficial effects in its β-carotene (50 mg on alternate days) versus placebo group after 12 years of supplementation.[264] Specifically, no differences were observed for cancer of the prostate, large bowel, or lung, or for overall cancer incidence or mortality (386 vs. 380 deaths from cancer in the β-carotene and placebo groups, respectively).

Nutrition Intervention Trials I and II (NIT-I and II)

A general population trial conducted in Linxian, China, NIT-I, investigated the prevention of esophageal cancer and the lowering of overall cancer and total mortality in nearly 30,000 men and women (primarily nonsmokers).[68] It is the only large population trial to have demonstrated significant preventive effects — a 21% and 13% reduction in stomach and total cancer mortality, respectively — for β-carotene supplementation in the form of a combination of β-carotene (15 mg), α-tocopherol (30 mg), and selenium (50 ug) taken for over five years. Lower total mortality (by 9%) was also observed. In the NIT-II conducted among 3318 high-risk esophageal dysplasia patients, six years of supplementation with a high-dose multivitamin-multimineral supplement that included β-carotene 15 mg did not lead to a reduction in esophageal (or other) cancer incidence or mortality.[265]

Other Clinical Intervention Studies

Other trials that tested β-carotene separately included the Skin Cancer and Polyp Prevention Studies and the Australian Polyp Prevention Project. These studies showed no effect on nonmelanoma skin cancer[266] or colorectal adenoma[267,268], although in one of the latter studies,[268] slightly increased incidence was suggested for the β-carotene group. Results from one other placebo-controlled intermediate endpoint trial relevant to the lung cancer results mentioned above are from the Tyler Cancer Prevention Study which tested a combination of β-carotene (50 mg) and retinol (25,000 IU) on alternate days for 30 months in 755 men and women who were former asbestos workers (average age at entry was 52 years).[269] There was no reduction in incidence or prevalence of sputum atypia observed among those taking β-carotene and retinol.

In contrast to results from the ATBC, CARET, and PHS, several small, early clinical intervention studies of β-carotene and premalignant lesions in high-risk populations gave very promising results. In one study, a 66% reduction in frequency of buccal micronuclei was observed following nine weeks of supplementation (26 mg), although there was no such effect for canthaxanthin.[271] A similar 71% response was seen in patients with oral leukoplakia after six months of 30 mg β-carotene daily.[272] These findings were corroborated and extended in two subsequent investigations showing a reduction in micronuclei counts in response to β-carotene 30 mg daily,[273] and no progression of oral cancer in half the treated patients.[274] Mixed results were obtained in a three-month study of cervical dysplasia progression using 10 mg daily.[275] Rectal cell proliferation, as measured by ornithine decarboxylase (ODC) activity, was reduced 30-57% following six months of treatment with β-carotene 30 mg in one study,[276] while another failed to observe the same effect in the colonic mucosae.[277]

Several other trials are under way testing not only β-carotene, but vitamins E or C, selenium, or other antioxidants, either singly or in combinations, including the large Women's Health Study in the U.S. and the SU.VI.M.AX study in France. The future results from such controlled trials will continue to enhance our understanding of the role of various antioxidants in human carcinogenesis.

Conclusions

Observational epidemiologic data for some sites are fairly consistent and supportive of a beneficial association between β-carotene, or in a few instances, one or more other carotenoids or carotene-rich vegetables and human cancer. These include cancer of the lung, esophagus, stomach, colorectum, cervix, and oropharynx. For some other organ sites, notably, breast, larynx, pancreas, and bladder, the data are more convincing for a protective relationship with vegetable/fruit consumption than for β-carotene intake or biochemical status per se, while for others, such as prostate cancer, the evidence is very mixed and inconclusive for β-carotene, with a few studies even suggesting higher risk with increased intake. Most of this evidence is in the form of retrospective case-control studies rather than from prospective cohort investigations. As a result, the introduction of biases due to methods of participant selection, dietary recall, and the effects of cancer on various serologic markers is likely to have exaggerated some of the underlying beneficial relationships.

The prevention trial-based findings, on the other hand, do not substantiate a beneficial effect for β-carotene supplementation on cancer incidence or mortality. Although one trial in China showed a modest reduction in overall cancer rates from β-carotene combined with vitamin E and selenium, results from two other large randomized studies in Finland and the United States provide solid evidence for a relatively small adverse effect of β-carotene supplementation in lung cancer and overall mortality among cigarette smokers, and a fourth large trial in the United States observed no evidence for benefit or harm in primarily nonsmokers. These findings appear to contradict most of the case-control and cohort studies, and raise the issue of whether the results from the latter studies do in fact reflect a protective effect from β-carotene in the diet. They have also led to the exercise of some caution in recommendations concerning supplemental β-carotene.

Observational epidemiology is now reevaluating dietary carotenoids, plant foods, and related biochemical parameters in relation to human cancers. Newly available food composition data for the carotenoids has greatly facilitated this expanded hypothesis testing, and should help disentangle the component effects of the highly collinear dietary carotenoids and compare them to those of vegetables and fruits per se. Depending on the results from such studies, further experimental testing of supplemental carotenoids may be warranted in the future, as single agents, as combinations, or in factorial designs.

VITAMIN C

Vitamin C is a water-soluble vitamin. The Recommended Dietary Allowance (U.S.) for adults is 60 mg/day.[278] Mean intake of vitamin C by U.S. adult males and females is estimated at 119 and 92 mg/day, respectively.[279] This may be underestimated, as vitamin C added to processed foods as a preservative is not integrated in food composition tables, which generally include only L-ascorbic and not dehydroascorbic acid. The best sources of vitamin C are vegetables and fruits, such as broccoli, cabbage and other green leafy vegetables, peppers, tomatoes, citrus fruits, mangoes, papaya, and strawberries. Tubers, such as potatoes and yams, are also good sources. Vitamin C is relatively unstable; it is heat labile, prone to oxidation, and is lost as a result of cooking foods by immersing them in water. The well-known functions of vitamin C related to cancer prevention include trapping free radicals and reactive oxygen molecules and protecting against lipid peroxidation, reducing nitrates, and stimulating the immune system.

Epidemiologic studies of vitamin C and cancer have evaluated the association between both vitamin C and vitamin C-containing foods and cancer at various organ sites. In addition, some studies looked at the association between cancer and combinations of fruits and/or vegetables, including some known to be good sources of vitamin C. Studies are described below if they reported results for either vitamin C specifically or for foods known to be good sources of vitamin C, particularly some fruits. The reader should be cautious in interpreting these data, as in some cases the foods rich in vitamin C are also abundant in other dietary factors thought to protect against cancer. Studies that reported on the general categories of vegetables or green vegetables in particular are not included because of their high carotenoid content; most of these investigations were reviewed in the previous section.

A recent panel of experts[280] concluded that the evidence for a protective effect for vitamin C was strongest for stomach cancer, but that evidence also existed for protection in cancers of the upper aerodigestive tract, lung, pancreas, and cervix. The panel concluded that it was unlikely that vitamin C modified the risk of cancer of the prostate.

Lung Cancer

At least six prospective studies have examined the relationship between vitamin C and lung cancer. One study reported a strong protective association overall,[281] and two observed this within certain subgroups.[112,282] In one of these,[112] a weak protection was also suggested for users of vitamin C supplements. A prospective study of Swiss men found no differences in baseline plasma levels of vitamin C between non-cases and those who died of lung cancer during follow-up.[81] One study of 33 lung cancers reported that cases had lower intakes of vitamin C at baseline compared with controls, but the difference was not statistically significant.[283] Two other cohort studies found no association between vitamin C intake and lung cancer risk.[284,285] Of the 11 case-control studies that examined the relationship between lung cancer and vitamin C, five found statistically significant protective associations (odds ratio 0.2-0.7), two found protective associations which were not significant, and four studies reported no association.[280] Supplemental use of vitamin C was related to lower lung cancer risk among men and increased risk in women in one study,[286] and to nonsignificantly reduced risk in another.[287]

Seven prospective studies have examined fruit consumption in relation to lung cancer.[112,282,284-288] The relative risks ranged between 0.3 to 1.0, with two showing statistically significant protective associations.[281,285] The only study which looked at citrus fruits per se,[281] found that as compared to low consumers, high consumers had one-half the risk of lung cancer. At least 11 case-control studies examined the association between lung cancer and fruits[12,289-298] and although some have not found statistically significant effects, higher intakes have been consistently protective.

Cancers of the Upper Aerodigestive Tract

No prospective studies have reported on vitamin C or vitamin C-containing foods and cancers of the oropharynx, nasopharynx, larynx, or esophagus. Five case-control studies have examined the relationship between vitamin C intake and cancer of the oropharynx. Each of these has reported a statistically significant protective association, with intake in the uppermost category of vitamin C associated with approximately half the risk of cancer incidence (odds ratios between 0.3-0.6).[14,20,22,23,30] In one of these,[14] but not two others,[30,300] a protective relationship was also noted for supplemental vitamin C. To date, no case-control studies have reported on the relationship between vitamin C and nasopharyngeal cancer; however, one case-control study in China[43] reported a two-thirds risk reduction for weekly versus rarely consuming both tomatoes and citrus fruits in early life. Two case-control studies of laryngeal cancer found nonsignificant protective associations[34,301] and one found a statistically significant protective association[35] for the highest compared with the lowest quartile of intake of vitamin C. A recently completed European multi-center case-control study[302] reported that compared to those with intakes in the lowest quintile, those with the highest intakes were at a 40% lower risk for laryngeal cancer with a significant trend. Nine case-control studies found protective associations for fruit, vegetables and fruit, or specific vitamin C-containing vegetables or fruits and laryngeal cancer risk.[22,34-41,56] Protective associations for at least one vitamin C-rich source or vegetable and/or fruit category including a vitamin-C rich source, were seen in all of these investigations.

Several investigators have assessed the association between esophageal cancer and either vitamin C[44,45,48,51,52,54,59,305-307] or fruits.[22,37,44,45,48,49,51,52,55-59,61-63,65-67] and four of these studied citrus fruits specifically.[51,56,61,303] The evidence for a protective association has been consistent, with nearly all studies showing protective associations. The four latter studies showed statistically significant protective associations with between 40-90% lower risk suggested for the highest versus the lowest category of consumption of citrus fruits.

Stomach Cancer

There are several reasons why the association between vitamin C and stomach cancer is especially plausible. Vitamin C is known to block nitrosamine formation in the stomach, and supplementation with vitamin C has been shown in at least two studies to decrease the mutagenicity of gastric juice in humans.[308] Furthermore, studies have consistently found decreased stomach cancer risk with higher vitamin C intake or serum levels. The association for vitamin C intake has been evaluated in two cohort studies: one found no association,[69] the other, a 50% reduction in risk for those who consumed more vitamin C.[70] In a prospective study, baseline plasma levels of vitamin C were 20% lower among men subsequently diagnosed with stomach cancer compared to non-cases.[81] Of 13 case-control studies, 12 reported protective associations for vitamin C intake (odds ratios 0.3-0.6);[71-78,98,115,309,310] nine of these results were statistically significant. A total of 27 case-control studies examined the association between fruits and stomach cancer, with 14 specifically evaluating the association for citrus fruits.[280] The majority of these noted protective effects for greater consumption, and nine of the 14 studies found statistically significant protective associations (odds ratio = 0.1-0.8).[71-74,76-78,86,92,96,309-311]

No intervention trials have investigated the independent effect of vitamin C on the risk of stomach cancer; however, some intervention trials used vitamin C in a combination.[68,265,312,313] Investigators of a trial conducted in China (see Table 3) did not observe an effect for vitamin C (120 mg daily) combined with molybdenum (30 ug) on stomach cancer mortality or prevalence of gastric cardia dysplasia.[68,312] Another study found no effect on the vitamin C concentration of gastric juice from vitamin C supplementation.[313]

Colorectal Cancer

Of prospective studies, two reported decreased risk of colon cancer with higher vitamin C intake,[314] while in others, no association was found for dietary intake in an all-female cohort[110] or for supplemental vitamin C.[110,315] Case-control studies have also yielded inconsistent results. Seven of 11 case-control studies of colon or colorectal cancer[103,115,119,121,124,128,316] and four of eight rectal cancer studies[103,121,316,317] found no association with vitamin C intake. Protective effects were noted in three colon[122,123,317] (one of these for supplemental vitamin C also[123]) and three rectal studies,[105,123,314] and harmful effects were reported in one colon[318] and in one rectal cancer study.[119] Three case-control studies have examined the association between adenomatous polyps and vitamin C intake. One study found non-cases had higher intakes of vitamin C,[132] one found a non-significant protective effect of vitamin C consumption (odds ratio = 0.6),[123] and the last reported no association.[134]

The association between colorectal cancer and fruit alone or in combination with vegetables has been evaluated in two prospective cohort studies. The first reported relative risks of 1.1 and 0.5 for men and women, respectively, for high intake of fruits in relation to colon cancer,[112] and the other found no association for higher consumption of all vegetables and fruit.[114] A 50% reduction in risk for colorectal adenomatous polyps was reported among subjects with a high intake of vegetable and fruit fiber.[316] Case-control studies evaluating the association between colon or rectal cancer and fruit intake have generally not found protective effects of greater consumption, and in some cases, harmful associations have been reported for higher intake.[111,114]

Five clinical trials have tested the ability of vitamin C alone or in combination with other antioxidant vitamins to prevent colorectal adenoma, the precursors of invasive colorectal cancer. The largest and most recent study included 864 randomized subjects and found no preventive effect of supplementation with a combination of vitamin C and vitamin E (relative risk = 1.08; see Table 3).[263] From four much smaller studies (i.e., 19-143 subjects), a protective effect of vitamin C was seen for rectal polyps,[320] two studies reported no effects for a combination supplement of vitamins C and E,[321,322] and one study observed a statistically significant reduction in the incidence of adenomas for subjects receiving vitamins A, C, and E, as compared to those who received no treatment.[323]

Pancreatic Cancer

A recent review of pancreatic cancer and nutritional factors noted that one cohort and each of seven case-control studies has shown a weak to moderate protective association for vitamin C intake.[142] A U.S.-based cohort reported a non-significant relative risk of 0.8 and case-control investigations from several countries reported odds ratios ranging from 0.5 to 0.7 for higher as compared to lower intakes.

At least three prospective and ten case-control studies have examined fruit and vegetable consumption and risk of pancreatic cancer. One prospective study found a significant protective relationship for both fresh fruits and fresh citrus fruits.[144] The two other cohort analyses found no associations for fruits or vegetables and pancreatic cancer risk.[112,145] Overall, among nine of ten case-control studies, there is a consistent pattern of decreasing risk with increasing intake of fruits and vitamin C-rich fruits and vegetables.[142]

Breast Cancer

The association between vitamin C and breast cancer has been evaluated in four recent cohort studies, with relative risks ranging between 0.8-1.0 for either the highest compared to the lowest level of dietary intake or for supplemental intake.[155-157,324] In a pooled analysis of nine case-control studies, including some which had not reported on vitamin C separately, researchers reported 30% lower risk that was statistically significant for the highest compared to the lowest category of intake.[325] Results from individual case-control studies are, however, inconsistent. One study reported a statistically significant protective effect (odds ratio = 0.6),[169] another reported a non-significant protective association,[165] and four reported non-significant elevated risk of up to 50%.[158,188,326,327]

Fruit and vegetable consumption in relation to breast cancer risk has been evaluated in three prospective studies and 19 case-control studies. All three prospective studies failed to find an association for fruit intake.[112,156,157] One of these also examined the relationship between vegetables rich in vitamins A and C, and found a non-significant relative risk of 0.7 for the highest quintile of intake.[157] Of the 10 case-control studies which reported results for fruit or citrus fruits, two found significant protective effects,[193,328] five found non-significant protective effects,[161,174,192,329,330] and three found non-significant harmful effects.[167,188,331] One of these studies also reported no association for supplemental vitamin C use.[174]

Ovarian Cancer

Little evidence exists to support an important role for vitamin C for risk of ovarian cancer. Three case-control studies reported non-significant odds ratios ranging from 0.7-1.1 for the highest versus the lowest category of intake. [194,196,197] In addition, one case-control study reported no association between fruit intake and ovarian cancer.[198]

Endometrial Cancer

The evidence for an association between vitamin C and endometrial cancer is also limited and inconsistent. Only one[202] of four case-control studies reported a statistically significant protective association. The remaining three studies[201,203,205] reported odds ratios ranging from 0.7-1.4 for the highest versus the lowest category of intake or for supplemental vitamin C. Several case-control studies also examined the relationship between fruit and endometrial cancer.[201-205] Overall, although protective associations were seen for several vegetables in these studies, there was little evidence for a protective association for fruits rich in vitamin C.

Cervical Cancer

Four case-control studies[207,209,211,212] reported statistically significant protective associations between vitamin C intake and cervical cancer, including carcinoma *in-situ*; two others reported non-significant protective results for dietary or supplemental vitamin C.[208,218] One of the investigations also reported a significantly reduced risk for consumption of fruit juices, but found no association for fruits.[207] Two studies showed null associations between increasing consumption of fruit or fruit juices and cervical cancer risk.[208,209] Fruit and fruit juices and tomatoes are consistently associated with reduced risk for dysplastic lesions.

Prostate Cancer

In contrast to other sites, there appears to be little evidence for a protective effect of vitamin C or vitamin C-containing foods on prostate cancer. Two cohort studies[112,332] and five[225,227,229-231] of six case-control studies observed no association between vitamin C consumption and prostate cancer. Graham and colleagues[228] reported a statistically significant 3-fold risk increase for older men who had the highest intakes of vitamin C. In addition, no substantial protective effects were observed for fruit and vegetable intake and prostate cancer in seven cohort studies[112,236,239-241,333,334] and for vitamin C-rich fruits and vegetables in case-control studies.[280,335]

Bladder Cancer

The majority of observational epidemiologic studies have also reported no association between vitamin C intake and bladder cancer. Results from one prospective[112] and five case-control studies were essentially null,[244-246,248,249] while one case-control study reported a statistically significant protective association for higher vitamin C intake, either from the diet or as supplements.[247] The evidence for a protective association between fruit consumption and bladder cancer risk is more abundant. Two[112,255] of five prospective studies reported protective associations which were not significant; the three others reported no relationship.[245,254,255] Protective effects for fruit intake were observed in four[247,248,250,258] of seven case-control studies. One case-control study in Hawaii found a harmful association between papaya intake and bladder cancer,[249] and two other studies observed no association between fruit consumption and bladder cancer.[246,257] One cohort[112] and three case-control[245,247,249] investigations showed protective effects for vitamin C supplement use, and two of these were statistically significant.[112,247]

Conclusions

The evidence for a protective effect for vitamin C appears to be strongest for cancers of the stomach, upper aerodigestive tract, and pancreas. Fruit consumption has been associated with protective associations most consistently for lung, upper aerodigestive tract, stomach, and pancreatic cancers. For several sites, including cervical and bladder cancers, the results for both vitamin C and fruit consumption are inconsistent. There is little evidence to support a protective relationship between either vitamin C or vitamin C-rich fruits and cancer of the colon, breast, or prostate.

VITAMIN E

Vitamin E is a fat-soluble vitamin and functions as the major lipid-soluble antioxidant in cell membranes. Vitamin E is a free-radical scavenger, inhibits lipid peroxidation,[336,337] and has been reported to suppress chemically-initiated tumors in some,[338] but not all animal studies.[339,340] In addition, vitamin E acts to block the *in vivo* formation of N-nitroso compounds which have been associated with certain cancers.[341]

At least 8 different tocopherols and tocotrienols have vitamin E biological activity. The most active form of vitamin E, α-tocopherol, is also the most widely distributed in nature. For dietary purposes, vitamin E activity is expressed as α-tocopherol equivalents; i.e., biological effects equivalent to those from 1 mg of α-tocopherol. Vitamin E content of foods varies depending on the processing, storage, and preparation procedures during which losses may occur.[342] Vegetable oils and vegetable oil-containing products such as margarine and shortening are the richest sources in the U.S. diet.[343] Wheat germ or whole-wheat products and nuts are also good sources of vitamin E. The average vitamin E intake among men and women in the U.S. is estimated to be 9.8 mg/day and 7.1 mg/day, respectively.[344,345] The recommended dietary allowances are set at 10 mg for men and 8 mg for women daily.[278]

Lung Cancer

Most of the evidence regarding vitamin E and lung cancer suggests that vitamin E may have a role in decreasing risk of cancer at this site. Of the cohort studies that examined this relationship, four of six reported that prediagnostic serum vitamin E levels were lower for those who subsequently developed lung cancer compared to non-cases,[180] and one reported no differences in baseline dietary intake between cases and non-cases,[346] or a weakly protective association for supplemental vitamin E.[112] In the NHANES Followup Study, dietary vitamin E intake was protective only among current smokers in the lowest tertile of pack-years of smoking.[347] Repeated measurements of vitamin E intake was not associated with lung cancer incidence in the Zutphen Study.[348] Four of five case-control studies of lung cancer reported that blood levels of vitamin E were lower among cases than among controls, and one found no significant differences.[282] Lower or similar dietary vitamin E intakes among cases compared to controls were also observed in two investigations.[282]

In the ATBC Study previously described with respect to its findings for β-carotene, 5-8 years of vitamin E supplementation (50 mg daily) did not significantly affect the incidence of lung cancer overall in older male cigarette smokers (see Table 3).[260,261] Longer supplementation (i.e., for five or more years) did, however, suggest a modest beneficial reduction in incidence of between 10 and 15%.[261] Use of vitamin E supplements was also significantly associated with a reduced risk of lung cancer in a case-control study of nonsmokers.[298]

Cancers of the Upper Aerodigestive Tract

Relatively few studies have examined the association between vitamin E and upper aerodigestive tract cancers. As recently reviewed and reported,[280] in 12 investigations of the oral cancer, cases generally had lower serum vitamin E levels than controls. A significant protective association was reported for dietary vitamin E consumption and esophageal cancer in one case-control study,[280] and for supplemental vitamin E use in both esophageal[300] and oropharyngeal cancer (with relative risks of 0.5).[30,349]

Stomach Cancer

Two prospective cohort studies examined the relationship between stomach cancer and serum vitamin E, and six studies examined the association with vitamin E intake. No associations were found for vitamin E concentrations in the blood.[81,82] The dietary vitamin E studies found no association among Japanese men in Hawaii,[69] a non-significant 40% reduced risk for women in the highest tertile of vitamin E consumption compared to those with the lowest intakes,[70] statistically significant protective associations (also with odds ratio of 0.6),[76,78] and no significant associations.[73,77,98,310]

Two of the large randomized trials have reported findings relevant to vitamin E supplementation and stomach cancer (see Table 3);[68,260] however, in only one of these was the independent effect of vitamin E evaluable.[260] In the Nutrition Intervention Trial-I in China, the combination of vitamin E, β-carotene, and selenium resulted in 21% lower mortality from stomach cancer.[68] In contrast, slightly more incident cases were observed in the ATBC Study (70 versus 56) among men receiving vitamin E supplementation.[260]

Colorectal Cancer

Five prospective studies examined the association between serum α-tocopherol and colorectal cancer. In general, serum α-tocopherol levels were lower in those who subsequently developed colorectal cancer as compared to non-cases: a pooled estimate of 40% lower risk has been reported for the highest as compared to the lowest category of serum α-tocopherol concentration.[350] By contrast, three prospective studies reported no association between dietary vitamin E intake and incidence of colon or colorectal cancer,[110,317,351] although one of these among women in Iowa reported a protective association in colon cancer for vitamin E from supplements or diet and supplements,[110] and another showed no such association for supplemental vitamin E.[317] One case-control study conducted in Italy reported a significant inverse association for higher vitamin E intakes,[352] while the findings from several others reveal no substantive relationship with colorectal cancer.[105,127,129,108] In the large, randomized trial setting of the ATBC Study,[260] the group receiving α-tocopherol supplementation experienced a 16% reduction in the incidence of colorectal cancer.

Breast Cancer

Cohort and case-control investigations of vitamin E biochemical status and breast cancer are inconsistent, with reported risk estimates ranging from 0.5 to 4.2 for the highest compared to the lowest categories of vitamin E concentration.[353] The recent case-control analysis of adipose tissue antioxidants within the EURAMIC Study of postmenopausal women showed no association between α-tocopherol concentrations and breast cancer.[184] With regard to dietary intake, four prospective investigations reported non-significant associations ranging from 0.9 to 1.3 for higher compared to lower dietary intakes of vitamin E,[105,156,157,354] three of five case-control studies reported statistically non-significant protective effects (30-40% risk decreases),[165,166,170] and two others reported odds ratio of 1.0 and 1.3 for highest category of vitamin E intake.[167,188] Three of the cohort studies[156,157,324] and one case-control study[174] observed null associations for use of vitamin E supplements.

No vitamin E supplementation trial data are currently available with regard to breast cancer. The Women's Health Study, a trial involving 40,000 health professionals in the U.S., is currently underway testing the effects on cardiovascular disease and cancer of vitamin E (600 mg) and aspirin (100 mg) taken on alternate days. Two small intervention trials have reported no effect of vitamin E supplementation on benign breast disease.[355,356]

Cervical Cancer

Two prospective studies have evaluated the association between vitamin E biochemical status and risk of cervical cancer; one reported no association[221] and the other reported a protective association which was not statistically significant.[357] Two of three case-control studies have reported higher blood vitamin E levels to be protective[216,358] and one reported no association[217] for blood levels and cervical cancer risk. The relationship between dietary vitamin E and cervical cancer was examined in at least two case-control studies, one reporting a statistically significant 60% risk reduction,[207] and another a weaker protective association for women in the highest intake category.[211] Reduced risk has also been observed for supplemental vitamin E in both invasive disease,[208] and particularly carcinoma *in-situ*.[212]

Prostate Cancer

Observational studies are inconsistent with regard to a beneficial association between serum vitamin E and prostate cancer, and they offer little in the way of supportive data. Of the few prospective studies having a sufficient number of prostate cancers for analysis, two reported no association,[359,360] one reported a statistically significant protective association,[361] and one reported a protective effect in younger men and a harmful association in older men.[362] In a trial-based cohort analysis, the associations between prostate cancer and baseline α-tocopherol differed significantly according to the α-tocopherol intervention status, with the suggestion of a protective effect for total vitamin E intake among those who received the α-tocopherol intervention.[363] There were no significant associations between prostate cancer and baseline serum α-tocopherol in this study, however, and those for the intake of other tocopherols or tocotrienols were inconsistent. One case-control study reported no association between vitamin E intake and risk of prostate cancer.[227]

In contrast to the inconsistent results from the observational studies, controlled trial results from the ATBC Study demonstrated a significant 32% reduction in the incidence of prostate cancer following 5-8 years of supplementation with α-tocopherol 50 mg daily, with a somewhat greater reduction in prostate cancer mortality (e.g., 41%).[260,364] Clinical stages II-IV were most affected by vitamin E, and the results suggest inhibition of the progression from latent, subclinical tumors to more aggressive disease.

Bladder Cancer

Very few studies have evaluated the association between vitamin E and risk of bladder cancer. Two prospective analyses found no differences in serum vitamin E for cases as compared to controls.[249,252] Three case-control studies examining dietary vitamin E intake in relation to bladder cancer found no significant protective association,[246,247,250] although in one of these, the use of vitamin E supplements was related to 50% lower risk.[247] There was no material difference in the number of bladder cancer cases diagnosed between the α-tocopherol and no α-tocopherol arms in the ATBC Study.[260]

Conclusions

The evidence for a protective effect for vitamin E in human cancer is growing rapidly and varies in strength according to organ site. In general, the observational studies are most supportive of a protective role for vitamin E in lung, cervical, and colorectal cancer. For two of these sites (i.e., lung and colorectum), modest support is available from one of the large randomized trials that tested supplemental vitamin E (as α-tocopherol). In the same trial, a statistically significant 30-40% reduction in prostate cancer incidence and mortality was observed in the vitamin E group compared to placebo. For several other sites, there are still relatively few studies by which to judge the role played by vitamin E.

SELENIUM

A chemopreventive role for the essential trace element selenium was first proposed in the late 1960s as a result of the observed inverse relation between the geographic distribution of cancer mortality rates and soil selenium content in the United States.[365] Soon thereafter, cancer mortality rates were also found to be inversely associated with blood selenium concentrations.[366] Selenium is best-known for its presence at the active site of the enzyme glutathione peroxidase which catalyzes the oxidation of hydroperoxides.[367] Selenium may also inhibit the development of cancer through other mechanisms including inhibition of cell proliferation and stimulation of the immune system.[368] Selenium and vitamin E have been reported to compensate for deficiency of each other and to act synergistically to inhibit carcinogenesis.[369,370]

Seafoods, kidney, and liver, and other meats are consistently good sources of selenium. The selenium content of grains varies with the soil selenium content. The mean selenium intake for U.S. adults is estimated at 108 mcg/day.[371] The recommended dietary allowance for selenium is set at 70 and 55 ug/day for men and women, respectively.[278]

Epidemiologic studies of dietary selenium intake are problematic in that food composition values for selenium may be relevant only to the area from which the food was originally grown. Blood and toenail selenium concentrations are thought to be more valid measures of intake and status, reflecting relatively recent diets and those over a period of several months, respectively. They have been assessed in many etiologic studies.

All Cancers

There is evidence from prospective, case-control, and clinical trials that selenium may play a protective role against all cancers. A review in 1992 reported cancer cases as having lower prediagnostic serum selenium concentrations than controls in 17 out of 24 studies that included 10 cancer sites.[180] In the majority of these studies, however, the case-control differences in serum selenium were less than 10%. Two clinical trials have reported decreased overall incidence or mortality from cancer in response to selenium supplementation. In the Nutrition Intervention Trial-I in China conducted within a population known to have multiple micronutrient deficiencies, cancer mortality was reduced by 13% among those receiving a combination supplement of β-carotene, vitamin E, and selenium daily for 5 years compared to those given placebo.[68] Whether the effects resulted from selenium specifically, from one of the two other antioxidants, or from the unique combination is not known. Shedding some light on this is another recent randomized trial, the Nutritional Prevention of Cancer Study, that tested oral supplementation with 200 ug/day of selenium in 1312 men and women.[270] This study demonstrated a striking, statistically significant 39% reduction in overall cancer incidence resulting from effects on nearly all of the major cancer sites (Table 3).

Lung Cancer

Although far from conclusive, the majority of epidemiologic studies have reported protective associations between selenium and lung cancer risk. A total of 11 cohort and three case-control studies have evaluated the association between selenium and lung cancer. One recent study in a population-based serum bank found no association between selenium concentrations and risk of lung cancer.[372] In other large cohort studies examining serum selenium, relative risks have ranged between 0.3 to 1.4 for the highest selenium category.[178,373-375] Four of five smaller prospective studies reported that lung cancer cases had lower serum selenium at baseline than did non-cases.[376-379] There was no case-control difference in selenium concentrations in another study of only 18 lung cancer cases.[380] In a Dutch cohort, toenail selenium concentration was measured, with substantial risk reductions of 50% and 60% being observed for men and women, respectively.[381] Three case-control studies found protective associations between various biomarkers of selenium intake (i.e., blood, hair, urine, and toenails) and risk for lung cancer.[382-384] Further support for a protective role for selenium for lung cancer comes from the aforementioned prevention trial of supplemental selenium that reported approximately 50% lower incidence of lung cancer in the group receiving selenium.[270]

Stomach Cancer

The relationship between serum or toenail selenium concentration and stomach has been evaluated in three prospective studies. One study in Hawaii found no association,[373] while a Finnish study observed relative risks for higher as compared to lower serum selenium of 0.3 and 0.6 in men and women, respectively.[385] A third investigation showed a protective association among men only.[384] Prediagnositic serum selenium concentrations were also significantly lower in another study of gastrointestinal cancer cases as compared to matched controls.[380] The large multifactor trial in China reported 21% lower stomach cancer mortality for the β-carotene/vitamin E/selenium supplemented group, but this was of marginal statistical significance.[68] No protective effect was seen for selenium supplementation in stomach cancer risk in the Nutritional Prevention of Cancer Study.[270]

Colorectal Cancer

The association between selenium and colorectal cancer is unclear based on the evidence available from observational epidemiologic studies. At least five prospective studies have examined the relationship. In two reports from a cohort in Finland,[375,385] two U.S.-based cohorts,[386,387] and a report from The Netherlands,[388] serum selenium has not been materially associated with colorectal cancer risk. A marginally significant 44% reduction in colon cancer incidence was observed among Hawaiian Japanese men in the highest quintile of serum selenium,[373] and another study showed that patients with plasma selenium levels less than the population median were four times more likely to have one or more adenomatous polyps and had 250% more polyps per patient.[389] In the randomized trial of selenium supplementation,[270] 58% fewer colorectal cancers were observed among those receiving the active supplement.

Breast Cancer

A recent review concluded that the existing data do not support a protective effect of high selenium status in breast cancer.[353] Prospective studies have related both elevated risk[178,390] and reduced risk[382] with higher blood selenium levels. Three prospective studies of toenail selenium concentrations failed to find protective relationships with breast cancer,[391-393] and the results from two case-control studies were also inconsistent. A study with 38 cases reported a doubling of risk associated with high erythrocyte selenium concentrations,[394] while a larger study in The Netherlands reported 50% reduced risk for higher serum status.[395] Adipose tissue selenium-concentrations were unrelated to case-control status in the EURAMIC Study of breast cancer.[184] In the Nutritional Prevention of Cancer Study of selenium supplementation, six more breast cancers were diagnosed in the selenium-supplemented group than in the placebo group out of a total of only 12 cases, and these results were not statistically significant.[270]

Prostate Cancer

Prospective cohort studies offer little in the way of supportive data for an association between selenium and prostate cancer. No association was observed between serum selenium and prostate cancer in a Finnish cohort,[360] and prediagnostic serum selenium levels from among a small number of prostate cancer cases were somewhat lower than those for matched cases.[380] Regarding selenium intake, a recent analysis of older male smokers in Finland showed no association between dietary selenium and prostate cancer incidence,[363] and selenium intake was unrelated to risk in a large case-control study in Utah.[231] In contrast to available cohort and case-control results, the selenium supplementation trial reported a statistically significant 63% reduction in prostate cancer incidence for the selenium group.[270]

Conclusions

The association between selenium and cancer has been more difficult to study than for other antioxidant nutrients because of the variability in selenium content of foods even within single countries. As a result, most studies have relied upon either blood or toenail selenium concentrations as biomarkers of nutrient intake and status. Similar to the evidence surrounding vitamin E, results regarding selenium from human observational epidemiologic studies and experimental studies are not in complete agreement, with one randomized trial demonstrating large reductions in cancer incidence, particularly of the lung, colon, and prostate. The observational studies are most supportive of a protective role for selenium in cancer of the lung and stomach.

SUMMARY

Our knowledge concerning the role played by dietary patterns and nutritional status in human cancer has increased exponentially in the past two decades. This trend was stimulated by discoveries in experimental research and early leads from some observed protective associations (e.g., eating carrots and lung cancer) and some deleterious ones (e.g., high calorie-high fat diets and colon cancer). We know unequivocally that consuming diets replete with plant foods is related to lower cancer incidence, and that similar, more specific evidence exists for benefit from higher intake or biochemical status of several dietary antioxidants including carotenoids, vitamin C, vitamin E, and selenium. Large supplementation trials of the antioxidants are in agreement with some of these observed relationships, but have also provided solid evidence for lack of benefit or even harm, resulting in a conflicting picture of the appropriate role for such nutritional supplements on a population basis, particularly in certain higher-risk groups. Further, we still do not know whether, for example, certain antioxidant supplements are beneficial only in the setting of already adequate dietary intake or where there is sub-optimal nutriture, or if higher intake of these nutrients or their food sources need to be sustained over an entire lifetime to obtain a benefit. For the purposes of lowering cancer incidence, is optimum nutrient intake that which remains in the dietary range, but at the very high end? Are the beneficial diets and nutritional status indicative of higher intake of other beneficial phytochemicals or of reduced lifetime carcinogenic exposures? Current research is focused on these and other questions, including clarification of the cancer inhibitory mechanisms of action for the several antioxidants, and potential interactions between antioxidant intake and lifestyle factors such as smoking and alcohol consumption or specific genotypic markers of susceptibility or altered nutrient metabolism. The potential role of other dietary antioxidants (e.g., some flavonoids) is also under investigation. It is clear that while much is known about the role of antioxidants in cancer prevention, the final answers are not yet in.

REFERENCES

1. Doll R, Peto R. The causes of cancer: quantitative estimates of avoidable risks of cancer in the United States today. JNCI 66:1191-1308, 1981.
2. Weinberg RA. How cancer arises. Scientific American 189:62-70, 1996.
3. Couch DB. Carcinogenesis: basic principles. Drug Chem Toxicol 19:133-48, 1996.
4. Peto R, Doll R, Buckley JD, Sporn MB. Can dietary â-carotene materially reduce human cancer rates? Nature 290:201-8, 1981.
5. Bendich A, Olson JA. Biological actions of carotenoids. FASEB J 3:1927-32, 1989.
6. Willett WC. Vitamin A and lung cancer. Nutr Revs 48:201-11, 1990.
7. Steinmetz KA, Potter JD. Vegetables, fruit, and cancer. I. Epidemiology. Cancer Causes Control 2:325-57, 1991.
8. van Poppel G, Goldbohm RA. Epidemiologic evidence for â-carotene and cancer prevention. Am J Clin Nutr 62(suppl):1393S-1402S, 1995.
9. Ziegler RG, Mayne ST, Swanson CA. Nutrition and lung cancer. Cancer Causes Control 7:157-77, 1996.
10. Bjelke E. Dietary vitamin A and lung cancer. Int J Cancer 15:561-5, 1975.
11. Le Marchand L, Hankin JH, Kolonel LN, *et al.* Intake of specific carotenoids and lung cancer risk. Cancer Epidemiol Biomarkers Prev 2:183-7, 1993.
12. Ziegler RG, Colavito EA, Hartge P, *et al.* Importance of á-carotene, â-carotene, and other phytochemicals in the etiology of lung cancer risk. JNCI 88:612-5, 1996.
13. Candelora EC, Stockwell HG, Armstrong AW, *et al.* Dietary intake and risk of lung cancer in women who never smoked. Nutr Cancer 17:263-70, 1992.
14. Rossing MA, Vaughan TL, McNight B. Diet and pharyngeal cancer Int J Cancer 44:593-97, 1989.

15. Prasad MPR, Mukundan MA, Krishnaswamy K. Micronuclei and carcinogen DNA adducts as intermediate end points in nutrient intervention study on oral precancerous lesions. Oral Oncol Eur J Cancer 31B:155-9, 1995.
16. Ramaswamy G, Rao VR, Kumaraswamy SV, Anatha N. Serum vitamins' status in oral leucoplakias - a preliminary study. Oral Oncol Eur J Cancer 32B:120-2, 1996.
17. Hirayama T. A large scale cohort study on cancer risks by diet—with special reference to the risk reducing effects of green yellow vegetable consumption. Int Symp Princess Takamatsu Cancer Res Fund 16:41-53, 1985.
18. Graham S, Dayal H, Rohrer T, *et al.* Dentition, diet, tobacco and alcohol in the epidimiology of oral cancer. JNCI 59:1611-18, 1977.
19. Jafarey NA, Mahmood Z, Zavidi SH. Habits and dietary pattern of cases of carcinoma of the oral cavity and oropharynx. JPMA, 27:340-3, 1977.
20. Marshall J, Graham S, Mettlin C, *et al.* Diet in the epidemiology of oral cancer. Nutr Cancer 5:96-106, 1983.
21. Winn DM, Ziegler RG, Pickle LW, *et al.* Diet in the etiology of oral and pharyngeal cancer among women from Southern United States. Cancer Res 44:1216-22, 1984.
22. Notani PN, Jayant K, Role of diet in upper aerodigestive tract cancers, Nutr Cancer 10:103-13, 1987.
23. McLaughlin JK, Gridley G, Block G *et al.* Dietary factors in oral and pharyngeal cancer, J Natl Cancer Int, 80:1237-43, 1988.
24. Franco EL, Kowalski LP, Oliveira BV, *et al.* Risk factors for oral cancer in Brazil: A case control study. Int J Cancer 43:992-1000, 1989.
25. Zheng TZ, Boyle P, Hu HF, *et al.* Tobacco smoking alcoholic consumption and risk of oral cancer: A case study in Beijing, People's Republic of China. Cancer Causes Control 1:173-9, 1990.
26. Franceschi S, Bidoli E, Baron AE, *et al.* Nutrition and cancer of the oral cavity and pharynx in north-east Italy. Int J Cancer 47:20-5, 1991.
27. Franceschi S, Barro S, La Vecchia C, *et al.* Risk factors for cancer of the tongue and the mouth. A case control study from Northern Italy. Cancer 70:2227-33, 1992.
28. La Vecchia C, Negri E, D'Avanzo B, *et al.* Dietary indicators of oral and pharyngeal cancer. Int J Epidemiol 20:39-44, 1991.
29. Oreggia F, De Stefani E, Correa P, Fierro L. Risk factors for cancer of the tongue in Uruguay. Cancer 67:180-3, 1991
30. Gridley G, McLaughlin JK, Block G, *et al.* Vitamin supplement use and reduced risk of oral and pharyngeal cancer. Am J Epidemiol 135:1083-92, 1992.
31. Prasad MPR, Krishna TP, Pasricha S, *et al.* Diet and oral cancer - A case control study. Nutr Cancer 18:85-93, 1992.
32. Mackerras D, Buffer PA, Randall DE, *et al.* Carotene intake and the risk of laryngeal cancer in coastal Texas. Am J Epidemiol 128:980-8, 1988.
33. Freudenheim JL, Graham S, Byers TE, *et al.* Diet, smoking and alcohol in cancer of the larynx: a case control study. Nutr Cancer 17:33-45, 1992.
34. Zheng W, Blot WJ, Shu X, *et al.* Diet and other risk factors for laryngeal cancer in Shanghai, China. Am J Epidemiol 136:178-91, 1992.
35. Esteve J, Riboli E, Pequignot G, *et al.* Diet and cancers of the larynx and hypopharynx: the IARC multi-center study in southwestern Europe. Cancer Causes Control 7:240-52, 1996.
36. Graham S, Mettlin C, Marshall J, *et al.* Diet in the epidemiology of cancer of the larynx. Am J Epidemiol 113:675-80, 1981.
37. DeStefani E, Correa P, Oreggia F, *et al.* Risk factors in laryngeal cancer. Cancer 60:3087-91, 1987.

38. Zemla B, Day N, Swiatnicka J, Banasik R. Larynx cancer risk factors. Neoplasm 34:223-33, 1987.
39. La Vecchia C, Negri E, D'Avanzo B, *et al.* Dietary indicators of laryngeal cancer risk. Cancer Res 50:4497-500, 1990.
40. Zatonski W, Becher H, Lissowska J, *et al.* Tobacco, alcohol, diet and occupational exposure in etiology of laryngeal cancer - a population based case-control study. Cancer Causes Control 2:3-10, 1991.
41. Maier W, Beck C. Larynxkarzinom nach schussverletzung und paraffinenjektion. Laryngorhinootologie 71:83-5, 1992.
42. Ning JP, Yu MC, Wang QS, Henderson BE. Consumption of salted fish and other risk factors for nasopharyngeal carcinoma (NPC) in Tianjin, a low risk region for NPC in the People's Republic of China. JNCI 82:291-6, 1990.
43. Yu MC, Huang TB, Henderson BE. Diet and nasopharyngeal carcinoma: a case control study in Guangzhou, China. Int J Cancer 43:1077-82, 1989.
44. Ziegler R, Morris L, Blot W, *et al.* Esophageal cancer among black men in Washington D.C. II. Role of nutrition. JNCI 67:1199-206, 1981.
45. DeCarli A, Liati P, Negri E, *et al.* Vitamin A and other dietary factors in the etiology of esophageal cancer. Nutr Cancer 10:29-37, 1987.
46. Graham S, Marshall J, Haughey B, *et al.* Nutritional epidemiology of cancer of the esophagus. Am J Epidemiol 131:454-67, 1990.
47. Valsecchi MG. Modelling the relative risk of esophageal cancer in a case control study. J Clin Epidemiol 45:347-55, 1992.
48. Hu J, Nyren O, Wolk A, *et al.* Risk factors for oesophageal cancer in northeast China. Int J Cancer 57:38-46, 1994.
49. Wynder EL, Bross IJ. A study of etiological factors in cancer of the esophagus. Cancer 14:389-413, 1961.
50. DeJong UW, Breslow N, Hong J, *et al.* Aetological factors in oesophageal cancer in Singapore Chinese. Int J Cancer 13:291-303, 1974.
51. Cook-Mozaffari PJ, Azordegan F, Day NE, *et al.* Oesophageal cancer studies in the Caspian Littoral of Iran: results of a case control study. Br J Cancer 39:293-309, 1979.
52. Mettlin C, Graham S, Priore R, *et al.* Diet and cancer of the esophagus, Nutr Cancer 2:143-7, 1980.
53. Hirayama T. Nutrition and cancer— a large scale cohort study. Prog Clin Biol Res 206:299-311, 1986.
54. Tuyns AJ, Riboli E, Doornbos G, *et al.* Diet and oesophageal cancer in Cavador (France). Nutr Cancer 9:81-92, 1987.
55. Victora CG, Munoz N, Day NE, *et al.* Hot beverages and oesophageal cancer in southern Brazil: A case control study. Int J Cancer 39:710-16, 1987.
56. Brown LM, Blot WJ, Schuman SH, *et al.* Environmental factors and high risk of esophagaeal cancers among men in coastal South Carolina. JNCI 80:1620-5, 1988.
57. Wahrendorf J, Chang-Cluaude J, Liang QS, *et al.* Precursor lesions of oesophageal cancer in young people in a high risk population in China, Lancet 2:1239-41, 1988.
58. Yu MC, Garabrant DH, Peters JM, Mack TM. Tobacco, alcohol, diet, occupation, and carcinoma of the esophagus. Cancer Res 48:3843-48, 1988.
59. Li JY, Ershow AG, Chen ZJ, *et al.* A case control study of cancer of the esophagus and gastric cardia in Linxian. Int J Cancer 43:755-61, 1989.
60. DeStefani E, Munoz N, Esteve J, *et al.* Mate drinking, alcohol, tobacco, diet and esophageal cancer in Uruguay. Cancer Res 50:426-31, 1990.
61. Cheng KK, Day NE, Duffy SW, *et al.* Pickled vegetable in the aetiology of oesophageal cancer in Hongkong Chinese, Lancet, 339:1314-8, 1992.

62. Guo WD, Li JY, Blot WJ, *et al.* Correlations of dietary intake and blood nutrient levels with oesophageal cancer mortality in China, Nutr Cancer 13:121-7, 1990.
63. Prasad MPR, Krishna TP, Pasricha S, *et al.* Esophageal cancer: a case-control study. Nutr Cancer 18:85-93, 1992.
64. Wang LD. Preliminary study on nutrition and precancerous lesions of the esophagus in adolescents. Chung Hua Chung Liu Tsa Chih 14:94-7, 1992.
65. Gao YT, McLaughlin JK, Gridley G, *et al.* Risk factors for esophageal cancer in Shanghai, Role of diet and nutrients. Int J Cancer 58:197-202, 1994.
66. Tavini A, Negri E, Franceschi S, La Vecchia C. Risk factors for esophageal cancer in life-long nonsmokers. Cancer Epidemiol Biomarkers Prev, 3:87-92, 1994.
67. Tomuyuki H, Tsugane S, Ando N, *et al.* Alcohol consumption and risk of cancer in Japan: A case-control study in seven hospitals. Jpn J Clin Oncol 24:241-6, 1994.
68. Blot WJ, Li JY, Taylor PR, *et al.* Nutrition intervention trials in Linxian, China: supplementation with specific vitamin/mineral combinations, cancer incidence, and disease-specific mortality in the general population. JNCI 85:1483-92, 1993.
69. Chyou PH, Nomura A, Hankin JH, Stemmermann GN. A case-control study of diet and stomach cancer. Cancer Res 50:7501-4, 1990.
70. Zheng W, Sellers TA, Doyle TJ, *et al.* Retinol, antioxidant vitamins, and cancers of the upper digestive tract in a prospective cohort study of postmenopausal women. Am J Epidemiol 142:955-60, 1995.
71. Correa P, Fontham E, Pickle LW, *et al.* Dietary determinants of gastric cancer in south Louisiana inhabitants. JNCI 75:645-54, 1985.
72. Boeing H, Frentzel-Beyme R, Berger M, *et al.* Case-control study on stomach cancer in Germany. Int J Cancer 47:858-64, 1991.
73. Risch HA, Jain M, Choi NW, *et al.* Dietary factors and the incidence of cancer of the stomach. Am J Epidemiol 122:947-59, 1985.
74. La Vecchia C, Negri, E, DeCarli A, *et al.* A case-control study of diet and gastric cancer in northern Italy. Int J Cancer 40:484-9, 1987.
75. You WC, Blot WJ, Chang YS, *et al.* Diet and high risk of stomach cancer in Shandong, China. Cancer Res 48:3518-23, 1988.
76. Buiatti E, Palli D, DeCarli A, *et al.* Case-control study of gastric cancer and diet in Italy. Int J Cancer 44:611-6, 1989.
77. Ramon JM, Serra L, Cerdo C, Oromi J. Nutrient intake and gastric cancer risk: a case-control study in Spain. Int J Epidemiol 22:983-8, 1993.
78. Hansson LE, Baron J, Nyren O, *et al.* Nutrients and risk of gastric cancer: a population-based case-control study in Sweden. Int J Cancer 57:638-44, 1994.
79. Wald NJ, Thompson SG, Densem JW, *et al.* Serum beta-carotene and subsequent risk of cancer: results from the BUPA study. Br J Cancer 57:428-33, 1988.
80. Knekt P, Aromaa A, Maatela J, *et al.* Serum vitamin A and subsequent risk of cancer: cancer incidence follow-up of the Finnish mobile clinic health examination survey. Am J Epidemiol 132:857-70, 1990.
81. Stahelin HB, Gey KF, Eicholzer M, *et al.* Plasma antioxidant vitamins and subsequent cancer mortality in the 12-year follow-up of the prospective Basel Study. Am J Epidemiol 133:766-75, 1991.
82. Nomura AM, Stemmermann GN, Chyou PH, Gastric cancer among the Japanese in Hawaii. Jpn J Cancer Res 86:916-23, 1995.
83. Hirayama T. A large-scale study on cancer risks by diet—with special reference to the risk reducing effects of green-yellow vegetable consumption. In Hayashi Y, Magao M, Sugimura T, *et al.* ed. Diet, Nutrition and Cancer Tokyo, Japan:Scientific Societies Press, 41-53, 1986.

84. Kneller RW, McLaughlin JK, Bjelke E, *et al.* A cohort study of stomach cancer in a high-risk American population. Cancer 68:672-8, 1991.
85. Kato I, Tominaga S, Matsumoto K. A prospective study of stomach cancer among a rural Japanese populalation: a 6-year survey. Jpn J Cancer Res 83:568-75, 1992.
86. Acheson ED, Dolt R. Dietary factors to carcinoma of the stomach: a study of 100 cases and 200 controls. Gut 5:126-31, 1964.
87. Higginson J. Etiological factors in gastrointestinal cancer in man. JNCI 37:527-45, 1966.
88. Graham S, Scbotz W, Martino P. Alimentary factors in the epidemiology of gastric cancer. Cancer. 30:927-38, 1972.
89. Haenszel W, Kurihara M, Segi M, Lee RK. Stomach cancer among Japanese in Hawaii. JNCI 49:969-88, 1972.
90. Bjelke E. Case-control study in Norway. Scand J Gastroenterol 9(suppl 31):42-8, 1974.
91. Bjelke E. Case-control study in Minnesota. Scand J Gastroenterol 9(suppl 31):49-53, 1974.
92. Trichopoulos D, Ouranos C, Day NE, *et al.* Diet and cancer of the stomach: a case-control study in Greece. Int J Cancer 36:291-7, 1986.
93. Tajima K, Tominaga S. Dietary habits and gastro-intestinal cancers: a comparative case-control study of stomach and large intestinal cancers in Nagoya, Japan. Jpn J Cancer Res 76:705-16, 1985.
94. Jedrychowski W, Wahrendorf J, Popiel T, *et al.* A case-control study of dietary factors and stomach cancer risk in Poland. Int J Cancer 37:837-42, 1986.
95. Hu J, Zhang S, Sin S, *et al.* Diet and cancer of the stomach: a case-control study in China. Int J Cancer 41:331-5, 1988.
96. Kono S, Ikeda M, Tokudome S, Kuratsune M. A case-control study of gastric cancer and diet in northern Kyushu, Japan. Jpn J Cancer Res 79:1067-74, 1988.
97. Demirer T, Icli F, Uzunalimoglu C, Kucuk O. Diet and stomach cancer incidence. A case-control study in Turkey. Cancer 65:2344-8, 1990.
98. Graham S, Haughey B, Marshall J, *et al.* Diet in the epiedemiology of gastric cancer. Nutr Cancer 13:19-34, 1990.
99. Kato I, Tominaga S, Ito Y, *et al.* A comparative case-control analysis of stomach cancer and atrophic gastritis. Cancer Res 50:6559-64, 1990.
100. Boeing H, Jedrychowski W, Wahrendorf J, *et al.* Dietary risk factors in intestinal and diffuse types of stomach cancer: a multicenter case-control study in Poland. Cancer Causes Control 2:227-33, 1991.
101. Lee, JK, Park BJ, Yoo KY, Yo A. Dietary factors and stomach cancer: a case-control study of diet and gastric cancer in Korea. Int J Epidemiol 24:33-41, 1995.
102. Tuyns AJ, Kaaks P, Haelterman M. Colorectal cancer and the consumption of foods: a case-control study in Belgium. Nutr Cancer 11:189-204, 1988.
103. La Vecchia C, Negri E, DeCarli A, *et al.* A case-control study of diet and colorectal cancer in northern Italy. Int J Cancer 41:492-8, 1988.
104. Lee HP, Gourley L, Duffy SW, *et al.* Colorectal cancer and diet in an Asian population study among Singapore Chinese. Int J Cancer 43:1007-16, 1989.
105. Freudenheim JL, Graham S, Horvath PJ, *et al.* Risks associated with source of fiber components in cancer of the colon and rectum. Cancer Res 50:3295-300, 1990.
106. Whittemore AS, Wu-Williams AH, Lee M, *et al.* Diet, physical activity, and colorectal cancer among Chinese in North America and China. JNCI 82:915-26, 1990.
107. Peters PR, Pike MC, Garabrant P, Mack TM. Diet and colon cancer in Los Angeles County, California. Cancer Causes Control 3:457-74, 1992.
108. Meyer F, White E. Alcohol and nutrients in relation to colon cancer in middle-aged adults. Am J Epidemiol 136:225-36, 1993.

109. Zaridze, D, Filipchenko V, Kustov V, *et al.* Diet and colorectal cancer: results of two case-control studies in Russia. Eur J Cancer 29A:112-5, 1993.
110. Bostick RM, Potter JD, McKenzie DR, *et al.* Reduced risk of colon cancer with high intake of vitamin E: the Iowa Women's Health Study. Cancer Res 53:4230-7, 1993.
111. Phillips RL, Snowdon DA. Dietary relationships with fatal colorectal cancer among Seventh-Day Adventists. JNCI 74:307-17, 1985.
112. Shibata A, Paganini-Hill A, Ross RK, Henderson BE. Intake of vegetables, fruits, beta-carotene, vitamin C and vitamin supplements and cancer incidence among the elderly: a prospective study. Br J Cancer 66:673-9, 1992.
113. Thun MJ, Calle EE, Nambodiri MM, *et al.* Risk factors for fatal colon cancer in a large prospective study. JNCI 84:1491-1500, 1992.
114. Steinmetz KA, Kushi LH, Bostick M, *et al.* Vegetables, fruit and colon cancer in the Iowa Women's Health Study. Am J Epidemiol 139:1-15, 1994.
115. Bjelke E. Epidemiologic studies of cancer of the stomach, colon, and rectum; with special emphasis on the role of diet. Scand. J Gastroenterol, 9:124-9, 1974.
116. Modan B, Cuckle H, Lubin F. A note on the role of dietary retinol and carotene in human gastro-intestinal cancer. Int J Cancer 28:421-4, 1981.
117. Phillips RL. Role of life-style arid dietary habits in risk of cancer among Seventh-Day Adventists. Cancer Res 35:3513-22, 1975.
118. Graham S, Dayal H, Swanson M, *et al.* Diet in the epidemiology of cancer of the colon and rectum. JNCI 61:709-14, 1978.
119. Jain M, Miller AB, To T. A case-control study of diet and colorectal cancer. Int J Cancer 26:757-68, 1980.
120. Miller AB, Howe GR, Jain M, Craib KJ, Harrison L. Food items and food groups as risk factors in a case-control study of diet and colorectal cancer. Int J Cancer 32:155-61, 1983.
121. Pickle LN, Green MH, Ziegler RG, *et al.* Colorectal cancer in rural Nebraska. Cancer Res 44:363-9, 1984.
122. Macquart-Moulin G, Riboli E, Corneci, Charnay B, Berthezene P. Case-control study an colorectal cancer and diet in Marseilles. Int J Cancer 38:183-91, 1986.
123. Kune S, Kune GA, Watson LE. Case-control study of dietary etiological factors: the Melbourne Colorectal Cancer Study. Nutr Cancer 9:21-42, 1987.
124. Graham S, Marshall J, Haughey B, *et al.* Dietary epidemiology of cancer of the colon in western New York. Am J Epidemiol 128:490-503, 1988.
125. Slattery ML, Sorenson AW, Mahoney AW, *et al.* Diet and colon cancer: assessment of risk by fiber type and food source. JNCI 80:1474-80, 1988.
126. Young TB, Wolf DA. Case-control study of proximal and distal colon cancer and diet in Wisconsin. Int J Cancer 42:167-75, 1988.
127. Lee HP, Gourley L, Duffy SW, *et al.* Colorectal cancer and diet in an Asian population study among Singapore Chinese. Int J Cancer 43:1007-16, 1989.
128. West DW, Slattery ML, Robison LM, *et al.* Dietary intake and colon cancer: sex and anatomic site-specific associations. Am J Epidemiol 130:883-94, 1989.
129. Benito E, Obradar A, Stiggelbout A, *et al.* A population-based case-control study of colorectal cancer in Majorca, I: dietary factors. Int J Cancer 45:69-76, 1990.
130. Hu J, Liu Y, Zhao T, *et al.* Diet and cancer of the colon and rectum a case-control study in China. Int J Epidemiol 20:362-67, 1991.
131. Bidoli S, Franceschi S, Talamini R, Barra S, La Vecchia C. Food consumption and cancer of the colon and rectum in northeastern Italy. Int J Cancer 50:223-9, 1992.
132. Iscovich JM, L'Abby KA, Castello P, *et al.* Colon cancer in Ageunna, I: risk from intake of dietary items. Int J Cancer 51:851-7, 1992.

133. Steinmetz KA, Potter JD. Food-group consumption and colon cancer in the Adelaide Case-Control Study, I: vegetables and fruit. Int J Cancer 53:711-9, 1993.
134. Olsen J, Kronborg O, Lynggard J, Ewertz, M. Dietary risk factors for cancer and adenomas of the large intestine: a case-control study within a screening trial in Denmark. Eur J Cancer 30:53-60, 1994.
135. Kampman E, Verhoeven D, Sloots L, van't Veer P. Vegetable and animal products as determinants of colon cancer risk in Dutch men and women. Cancer Causes Control 6:225-34, 1996.
136. Mack TM, Yo MC, Hanisch R, *et al.* Pancreas cancer and smoking, beverage consumption, and past medical history. JNCI 76:49-60, 1986.
137. Falk RT, Pickle LW, Pontham ET, *et al.* Life-style risk factors for pancreatic cancer in Louisiana: a case-control study. Am J Epidemiol 128:324-36, 1988.
138. Ghadirian P, Simard A, Baillargeon J, *et al.* Nutritional factors and pancreatic cancer in the francophone community in Montreal, Canada. Int J Cancer 47:1-6, 1991.
139. Howe GR, Jain M, Miller AB. Dietary factors and risk of pancreatic cancer: results of a Canadian population-based case-control study. Int J Cancer 45:604-8, 1990.
140. Baghurst PA, McMichael AJ, Slavotinek AH, *et al.* A case-control study of diet and cancer of the pancreas. Am J Epidemiol 134:167-79, 1991.
141. Bueno de Mesquita HB, Maisonneuve P, Runia S, *et al.* Intake of foods and nutrients and cancer of the exocrine pancreas: a population-based case-control study in The Netherlands. Int J Cancer 48: 540-9, 1991.
142. Howe GR and Burch JD. Nutrition and pancreatic cancer. Cancer Causes Control 7:69-82, 1996.
143. Burney PG, Comstock GW, and Morris JS. Serologic precursors of cancer: serum micronutrients and subsequent risk of pancreatic cancer. Am J Clin Nutr 49:895-900, 1989.
144. Mills PK, Beeson L, Abbet DE, *et al.* Dietary habits and past medical history as related to fatal pancreas cancer risk among Adventists. Cancer 61:2578-85, 1988.
145. Zheng W, McLaughlin JK, Gridley G, *et al.* A cohort study of smoking, alcohol and dietary factors for pancreatic cancer (United States). Cancer Causes Control 4:477-82, 1993.
146. Shibata A, Mack TM, Paganini-Hill A, *et al.* A prospective study of pancreatic cancer in the elderly. Int J Cancer 58:46-9, 1994.
147. Gold EB. Epidemiology of and risk factors for pancreatic cancer. Surg Clinics North Am 75:819-45, 1985.
148. Norell SE, Ahlbom A, Erwald R, *et al.* Diet and pancreatic cancer: a case-control study. Am J Epidemiol 124:894-902, 1986.
149. Olsen GW, Mandel JS, Gibson RW, *et al.* A case-control study of pancreatic cancer and cigarettes, alcohol, coffee and diet. Am J Public Health 79:101-9, 1989.
150. Goto IL, Masuola H, Yoshida K, *et al.* A case-control study of cancer of the pancreas. Japanese J Cancer Clinics 36:344-50, 1990.
151. La Vecchia C, Negri E, D'Avanzo B, *et al.* Medical history, diet and pancreatic cancer. Oncology 47:463-6, 1990.
152. Raymond L, Bouchardy C. Les facteurs de risque du cancer du pancreas d'apres les etudes epidemiologiques analytiques. Bull Cancer 77:47-68, 1990.
153. Negri E, La Vecchia C, Pranceschi S, *et al.* Vegetable and fruit consumption and cancer risk. Int J Cancer 48:350-4, 1991.
154. Lyon JL, Slattery ML, Mahoney AW, Robison TM. Dietary intake as a risk factor for cancer of the exocrine pancreas. Cancer Epidemiol Biomark Prev 2:513-8, 1993.
155. Graham S, Zielerny M, Marshall J, *et al.* Diet in the epidemiology of postmenopausal breast cancer in New York State. Am J Epidemiol 136:1317-37, 1992.

156. Hunter DJ, Manson JE, Colditz GA, *et al.* A prospective study of the intake of vitamins C, E, and A and the risk of breast cancer. N Engl J Med 329: 234-40, 1993.
157. Rohan TE, Howe GR, Friedenreich CM, *et al.* Dietary fiber, vitamins A, C, and E, and risk of breast cancer: a cohort study. Cancer Causes Control 4:29-37, 1993.
158. Katsouyanni K, Willett W, Trichopoulos D, *et al.* Risk of breast cancer among Greek women in relation to nutrient intake. Cancer 61:181-5, 1988.
159. Marubini E, DeCarli A, Costa A, *et al.* The relationship of dietary intake and serum levels of retinol and beta-carotene with breast cancer. Results of a case-control study. Cancer 61:173-80, 1988.
160. Rohan TE, McMichael AJ, Baghurst, PA. A population-based case-control study of diet and breast cancer in Australia. Am J Epidemiol 123: 478-89, 1988.
161. Iscovich JM, Iscovich RB, Howe G, *et al.* A case-control study of diet and breast cancer in Argentina. Int J Cancer 44:770-6, 1989.
162. Ewertz M, Gill C. Dietary factors and breast-cancer risk in Denmark. Int J Cancer 46:779-84, 1990.
163. Potischman N, McCulloch CE, Byers T, *et al.* Breast cancer and dietary and plasma concentrations of carotenoids and vitamin A. Am J Clin Nutr 52:909-15, 1990.
164. van 't Veer P, Kolb CM, Verhoef P, *et al.* Dietary fiber, beta-carotene and breast cancer: results from a case-control study. Int J Cancer 45:825-8, 1990.
165. Graham S, Hellman R, Marshall J, *et al.* Nutritional epidemiology of postmenopausal breast cancer in western New York. Am J Epidemiol 134:532-46, 1991.
166. Lee HP, Gourley L, Duffy SW, *et al.* Dietary effects on breast-cancer risk in Singapore. Lancet 337:1197-200, 1991.
167. Richardson S, Gerber M, Cenee S. The role of fat, animal protein and some vitamin consumption in breast cancer: a case-control study in southern France. Int J Cancer 48:1-9, 1991.
168. van't Veer P, van Leer EM, Rietdijk A, *et al.* Combination of dietary factors in relation to breast cancer occurrence. Int J Cancer 47:649-53, 1991.
169. Zaridze D, Lifanova Y, Maximovitch D, *et al.* Diet, alcohol consumption and reproductive factors in a case-control study of breast cancer in Moscow. Int J Cancer 48:493-501, 1991.
170. London SJ, Stein BA, Henderson IC, *et al.* Carotenoids, retinol, and vitamin E and risk of proliferative benign breast disease and breast cancer. Cancer Causes Control 3:503-12, 1992.
171. Holmberg L, Ohlander EM, Byers T, *et al.* Diet and breast cancer risk. Results from a population-based, case-control study in Sweden. Arch Intern Med 154:1805-11, 1994.
172. Ambrosone CB, Marshall JR, Vena JE, *et al.* Interaction of family history of breast cancer and dietary antioxidants with breast cancer risk (New York, United States). Cancer Causes Control 6:407-15, 1995.
173. Yuan JM, Wang QS, Ross RK, Henderson BE, Yu MC. Diet and breast cancer in Shanghai and Tianjin, China. Br J Cancer 71; 1353-8, 1995.
174. Freudenheim, JL, Marshall JR, Vena JE, *et al.* Pre-menopausal breast cancer risk and intake of vegetables, fruit, and related nutrients. JNCI 88:340-8, 1996.
175. Negri E, La Vecchia C, Franceschi S, *et al.* Intake of selected micronutrients and the risk of breast cancer. Int J Cancer 65:140-4, 1996.
176. Wald NJ, Boreham J, Hayward JL, Bulbrook RD. Plasma retinol, beta-carotene and vitamin E levels in relation to the future risk of breast cancer. Br J Cancer 49:321-4, 1984.
177. Willett WC, Polk BF, Underwood BA, *et al.* Relation of serum vitamins A and E and carotenoids to the risk of cancer. New Eng J Med 310:430-4, 1984.

178. Coates RJ, Weiss NS, Daling JR, *et al.* Serum levels of selenium and retinol and the subsequent risk of cancer. Am J Epidemiol 128:515-23, 1988.
179. Russell MJ, Thomas BS, Bulbrook RD. A prospective study of the relationship between serum vitamins A and E and risk of breast cancer. Br J Cancer 57:213-5, 1988.
180. Comstock GW, Bush TL, Helzlsouer K. Serum retinol, beta-carotene, vitamin E, and selenium as related to subsequent cancer of specific sites. Am J Epidemiol 135:115-21, 1992.
181. Dorgan JF, Sowell A, Swanson CA, *et al.* Relationships of serum carotenoids, retinol, á-tocopherol, and selenium with breast cancer risk: results from a prospective study in Columbia, Missouri (United States). Cancer Causes Control 9 (in press) 1998.
182. Gerber M, Cavallo F, MarubiniE, *et al.* Lipid-soluble vitamins and lipid parameters in breast cancer. A joint study in Northern Italy and Southern France. In J Cancer 42:489-94, 1988.
183. Smith AH, Waller KD. Serum beta-carotene in persons with cancer and their immediate families. Am J Epidemiol 133:661-71, 1991.
184. van't Veer P, Strain JJ, Fernandez-Crehuet J, *et al.* Tissue antioxidants and postmenopausal breast cancer: The European Community Multicenter Study of Antioxidants, Myocardial Infarction, and Cancer of the Breast (EURAMIC). Cancer Epidemiol Biomarkers Prev 5:441-7, 1996.
185. Zemla B. The role of selected dietary elements in breast cancer risk among native and migrant populations in Poland. Nutr Cancer 6:187-95, 1984.
186. Hislop TG, Coldman AJ, Elwood JM, *et al.* Childhood and recent eating patterns and risk of breast cancer. Cancer Detection Prev 9:47-58, 1986.
187. Simard A, Vobecky J, Vobecky JS. Nutrition and life-style factors in fibrocystic disease and cancer of the breast. Cancer Detection Prev 14:567-72, 1990.
188. Toniolo P, Riboli E, Protta F, *et al.* Calorie-providing nutrients and risk of breast cancer. JNCI 81:126-31, 1989.
189. Young TB. A case-control study of breast cancer and alcohol consumption habits. Cancer 64:551-8, 1989.
190. Kato I, Miura S, Kasumi F, *et al.* A case-control study of breast cancer among Japanese women: with special reference to family history and reproductive and dietary factors. Breast Cancer Res Treat 24:51-9, 1992.
191. Pawlega J. Breast cancer and smoking, vodka drinking and dietary habits. Acta Oncologica 31:387-92, 1992.
192. Levi F, La Vecchia C, Gulie C, Negri E. Dietary factors and breast cancer risk in Vaud, Switzerland. Nutr Cancer 19:327-35, 1993.
193. Trichopoulou A, Katsouyanni K, Stuver S, *et al.* Consumption of olive oil and specific good groups in relation to breast cancer risk in Greece. JNCI 87:110-6, 1995.
194. Byers T, Marshall J, Graham S, *et al.* A case-control study of dietary and nondietary factors in ovarian cancer. JNCI 71:681-6, 1983.
195. Engle A, Muscat JE, Harris RE. Nutritional risk factors and ovarian cancer. Nutrition Cancer 15:239-47, 1991.
196. Slattery ML, Schuman KL, West DW, *et al.* Nutrient intake and ovarian cancer. Am J Epidemiol 130:497-502, 1989.
197. Shu XO, Gao YT, Yuan JM, *et al.* Dietary factors and epithelial ovarian cancer. Br J Cancer 59:92-6, 1989.
198. La Vecchia C, DeCarli A, Negri E, *et al.* Dietary factors and the risk of epithelial ovarian cancer. JNCI 79:663-9, 1987.
199. Risch HA, Jain M, Marrett LD, *et al.* Dietary fat intake and the risk of epithelial ovarian cancer. JNCI 86:1409-15, 1994.

200. La Vecchia C, DeCarli A, Fasoli M, *et al.* Nutrition, diet in the etiology of endometrial cancer. Cancer 57:1248-53, 1986.
201. Barbone F, Austin H, Partridge EE. Diet and endometrial cancer: A case-control study. Am J Epidemiol 137:393-403, 1993.
202. Levi F, Franceschi S, Negri E, *et al.* Dietary factors and the risk of endometrial cancer. Cancer 71:3575-81, 1993.
203. Shu XO, Zheng W, Potischman N, *et al.* A population-based case-control study of dietary factors in endometrial cancer in Shangai, Peoples Republic of China. Am J Epidemiol 137:155-65, 1993.
204. Zemla B, Guminski S, Banasik R. Study of risk factors in invasive cancer of the corpus uteri. Neoplasma 33:621-9, 1986.
205. Potischman N, Swanson CA, Brinton LA, *et al.* Dietary associations in a case-control study of endometrial cancer. Cancer Causes Control 4:239-50, 1993.
206. Marshall J, Graham S, Byers T. Diet and smoking in the epidemiology of cancer of the cervix. JNCI 70:847-51, 1983.
207. Verreault R, Chu J, Mandelson M, Shy K. A case-control study of diet and invasive cervical cancer. Int J Cancer 43:1050-4, 1989.
208. Ziegler R, Brinton LA, Hamman R, *et al.* Diet and risk of invasive cervical cancer among white women in the United States. Am J Epidemiol 132:432-45, 1990.
209. Herrero R, Potischman N, Brinton LA, *et al.* A case-control study of nutrient status and invasive cervical cancer: dietary indicators. Am J Epidemiol 134, 1335-46, 1991.
210. La Vecchia C, DeCarli A, Fasoli M, *et al.* Dietary vitamin A and the risk of intraepithelial and invasive cervical neoplasia. Gynecol Oncol 30:187-95, 1988.
211. Slattery M, Abbott T, Overall J, *et al.* Dietary vitamin A, C, and E and selenium and as risk factors for cervical cancer. Epidemiol 1:8-15, 1990.
212. Ziegler RG, Jones CI, Brinton LA, *et al.* Diet and risk of *in situ* cervical cancer among white women in the United States. Cancer Causes Control 2:17-29, 1991.
213. deVet H, Knipschild P, Grol M, *et al.* The role of beta-carotene and other dietary factors in the aetiology of cervical dysplasia: results of case-control study. Int J Epidemiol 20:603-10, 1991.
214. Harris R, Forman D, Doll R *et al.* Cancer of the cervix uteri and vitamin A. Br J Cancer 53:653-9, 1986.
215. Palan P, Romney S, Mikhail M, *et al.* Decreased plasma BC levels in women with uterine cervical dysplasias and cancer. JNCI 80:454-5, 1988.
216. Palan P, Mikhail M, Basu J, *et al.* Plasma levels of antioxidants BC and AT in uterine cervix dysplasias and cancer. Nutr Cancer 15:13-20, 1991.
217. Potischman N, Herrero R, Brinton LA, *et al.* A case-control study of nutrient status and invasive cervical cancer. Am J Epidemiol 134:1347-55, 1991.
218. Brock K, Berry G, Mock P, *et al.* Nutrients in diet and plasma and risk of in situ cervical cancer. JNCI 80:580-5, 1988.
219. Butterworth C, Hatch K, Macaluso M, *et al.* Folate deficiency and cervical dysplasia. JAMA 267:528-33, 1992.
220. VanEenwyk J, Davis F, Bowen P. Dietary and serum carotenoids and cervical intraepithelial neoplasia. Int J Cancer 48:34-8, 1991.
221. Batieha A, Armenian H, Norkus E, *et al.* Serum micronutrients and the subsequent risk of cervical cancer in a population-based nested case-control study. Cancer Epidemiol Biomarkers Prevention 2:335-9, 1993.
222. La Vecchia C, DeCarli A, Fasoli M, *et al.* Dietary vitamin A and the risk of intraepithelial and invasive cervical neoplasia. Gynecol Oncol 30:187-95, 1988.

223. Schuman LM, Mandel JS, Radke A, *et al.* Some selected features of the epidemiology of prostate cancer: Minneapolis-St. Paul, Minnesota case-control study, 1976-1979. In: Magnus K, Ed. *Trends in Cancer Incidence: Causes and Practical Implications.* Washington D.C.: Hemisphere, 1982; 345-54.
224. Ross RK, Shimizu H, Paganini-Hill A, Honda G, Henderson BE. Case-control studies of prostate cancer in blacks and whites in southern California. JNCI 78:869-74, 1987.
225. Ohno Y, Yoshida O, Oishi K, Okada K, Yamabe H, Schroeder FH. Dietary â-carotene and cancer of the prostate: a case-control study in Kyoto, Japan Cancer Res 48:1331-6, 1988.
226. Mettlin C, Selenskas S, Natarajan N, Huben R. Beta-carotene and animal fats and their relationship to prostate cancer risk. Cancer 64:605-12, 1989.
227. Rohan TE, Howe GR, Burch ID, *et al.* Dietary factors and risk of prostate cancer: a case-control study in Ontario, Canada. Cancer Causes Control 6:145-54, 1995.
228. Graham S, Haughey B, Marshall J, *et al.* Diet in the epidemiology of carcinoma of the prostate gland. JNCI 70:687-92, 1983.
229. Kolonel LN, Yoshizawa CN, Hankin B. Diet and prostate cancer: a case-control study in Hawaii. Am J Epidemiol 127:999-1012, 1988.
230. Heshmat MY, Kaul L, Kovi J, *et al.* Nutrition and prostate cancer: a case-control study. Prostate 6:7-17, 1985.
231. West DW, Slattery ML, Robison LM, *et al.* Adult dietary intake and prostate cancer risk in Utah: a case-control study with special emphasis on aggressive tumors. Cancer Causes Control 2:85-94, 1991.
232. Talamini R, Franceschi S, La Vecchia C, Serraino D, Barra S, Negri F. Diet and prostate cancer: a case-control study in northern Italy. Nutr Cancer 18:277-86, 1992.
233. Hirayama T. Epidemiology of prostate cancer with special reference to the role of diet. Natl Cancer Inst Monogr 53:149-55, 1979.
234. Paganini-Hill A, Chao A, Ross RK, Henderson BE. Vitamin A, â-carotene, and the risk of cancer: a prospective study. JNCI 79:443-8, 1987.
235. Hsing AW, McLaughlin JK, Schuman LM, *et al.* Diet, tobacco use, and fatal prostate cancer: results from the Lutheran brotherhood cohort study. Cancer Res 50:6836-40, 1990.
236. Giovannucci E, Ascherio A, Rimm EB, *et al.* Intake of carotenoids and retinol in relation to risk of prostate cancer. JNCI 85:1571-9, 1995.
237. Daviglus ML, Dyer AR, Persky V, *et al.* Dietary beta-carotene, vitamin C, and risk of prostate cancer: results from the Western Electric Study. Epidemiology 7:472-7, 1996.
238. Hayes RB, Bogdanovicz JF, Schroeder FH, *et al.* Serum retinol and prostate cancer. Cancer 62:2021-6, 1988.
239. Snowdon DA, Phillips RL, Choi W. Diet, obesity, and risk of fatal prostate cancer. Am J Epidemiol 120:244-50, 1984.
240. Mills PK, Beeson WL, Phillips RL, *et al.* Cohort study of diet lifestyle, and prostate cancer in Adventist men. Cancer 64:598-604, 1989.
241. Severson RK, Nomura A, Grove JS, *et al.* A prospective study of demographics, diet and prostate cancer among men of Japanese ancestry in Hawaii. Cancer Res 49:1857-60, 1989.
242. Walker AR, Walker BF, Tsotetsi NG, *et al.* Case-control study of prostate cancer in black patients in Soweto South Africa. Br J Cancer 65:438-41, 1992.
243. Talamini R, La Vecchia C, DeCarli A, *et al.* Nutrition, social factors and prostatic cancer in a Northern Italian population. Br J Cancer 53:817-21, 1986.
244. Risch HA, Burch JD, Miller AB, *et al.* Dietary factors and the incidence of cancer of the urinary bladder. Am J Epidemiol 127:1179-91, 1988.

245. Steineck G, Hagman U, Gerhardsson M, *et al.* Vitamin A supplements, fried foods, fat and urothelial cancer: A case-referent study in Stockholm in 1985-87. Int J Cancer 45:1006-11, 1990.
246. Riboli E, Gonzalex CA, Lopez-Abente G, *et al.* Diet and bladder cancer in Spain: a multi-center case-control study. Int J Cancer 49:214-9, 1991.
247. Bruemmer B, White E, Vaughan TL, *et al.* Nutrient intake in relation to bladder cancer among middle-aged men and women. Am J Epidemiol 144:485-95, 1996.
248. La Vecchia C, Negri E, DeCarli A, *et al.* Dietary factors in the risk of bladder cancer. Nutr Cancer 12:93-101, 1989.
249. Nomura AM, Kolonel LN, Hankin JH *et al.* Dietary factors in cancer of the lower urinary tract. Int J Cancer 48:199-205, 1991.
250. Vena JE, Graham S, Freudenheim J, *et al.* Diet in the epidemiology of bladder cancer in western New York. Nutr Cancer 18:255-64, 1992.
251. Helzlsouer KJ, Comstock GW, Morris JS. Selenium, lycopene, á-tocopherol, BC, retinol, and subsequent bladder cancer. Cancer Res 49:6144-48, 1989.
252. Steineck G, Norell SE, Feychting M. Diet, tobacco and urothelial cancer. Acta Oncol 27:323-7, 1988.
253. Hirayama T. *Life-style and Mortality*. Karger, Basel, 1990.
254. Mills PK, Beeson WL, Phillips RL, *et al.* Bladder cancer in a low-risk population: results from the Adventist health study. Am J Epidemiol 133:230-9, 1991.
255. Chyou PH, Nomura AM, Stemmermann GN. A prospective study of diet, smoking, and lower urinary tract cancer. Ann Epidemiol 3:211-6, 1993.
256. Mettlin C, Graham S. Dietary risk factors in human bladder cancer. Am J Epidemiol 110:255-63, 1979.
257. Claude J, Kunze E, Frentzel-Beyme R, *et al.* Life-style and occupational risk factors in cancer of the lower urinary tract. Am J Epidemiol 124:578-89, 1986.
258. DeStefani E, Correa P, Fierro L, *et al.* Black tobacco, mate and bladder cancer: a case-control study from Uraguay. Cancer 67:536-40, 1991.
259. Momas I, Daures JP, Festy B, *et al.* Relative importance of risk factors in bladder carcinogenesis: some new results about Mediterranean habits. Cancer Causes Control 5:326-32, 1994.
260. The ATBC Cancer Prevention Study Group. The effect of vitamin E and beta carotene on the incidence of lung cancer and other cancers in male smokers. N Engl J Med 330:1029-35, 1994.
261. Albanes D, Heinonen OP, Taylor PR, *et al.* á-Tocopherol and â-carotene supplements and lung cancer incidence in the Alpha-Tocopherol, Beta-Carotene Cancer Prevention Study: effects of baseline characteristics and study compliance. JNCI 88:1560-70, 1996.
262. Omenn GS, Goodman GE, Thornquist MD, *et al.* Effects of the combination of beta-carotene and vitamin A on lung cancer incidence, total mortality, and cardiovascular mortality in smokers and asbestos-exposed workers. N Engl J Med 334:1150-5, 1996.
263. Omenn GS, Goodman GE, Thornquist MD, *et al.* Risk factors for lung cancer incidence and intervention effects in CARET, the Beta-Carotene and Retinol Efficacy Trial. JNCI 88:1550-9, 1996.
264. Hennekens CH, Buring JE, Manson JE, Stampfer M, Rosner B, Cook NR, *et al.* Lack of effect of long-term supplementation with beta carotene on the incidence of malignant neoplasms and cardiovascular disease. N Engl J Med 334:1145-9, 1996.
265. Li JY, Taylor PR, Li B, *et al.* Nutrition intervention trials in Linxian, China: multiple vitamin/mineral supplementation, cancer incidence, and disease-specific mortality among adults with esophageal dysplasia. JNCI 85:1492-8, 1993.

266. Greenberg ER, Baron JA, Stukel TA, *et al.* A clinical trial of beta carotene to prevent basal-cell and squamous-cell cancers of the skin. N Engl J Med 323:789-95, 1990.
267. Greenberg ER, Baron JA, Tosteson TD, *et al.* A clinical trial of antioxidant vitamins to prevent colorectal adenoma. N Engl J Med 331:141-7, 1994.
268. MacLennan R, Macrae FA, Bain CV, *et al.* Randomized trial of intake of fat, fiber, and beta carotene to prevent colorectal adenomas. JNCI 87:1760-6, 1995.
269. McLarty JW, Holiday DB, Girard WM, *et al.* β-Carotene, vitamin A, and lung cancer chemoprevention: results of an intermediate endpoint study. Am J Clin Nutr 1995;62(suppl. 6):1431S-8S.11.
270. Clark LC, Combs GF, Turnbull BW, *et al.* Effects of selenium supplementation for cancer prevention in patients with carcinoma of the skin. A randomized controlled trial. JAMA 276:1957-63, 1996.
271. Stich HF, Rosin MP, Vallejera MO. Reduction with vitamin A and beta-carotene administration of proportion of micronucleated buccal mucosal cells in Asian betel nut and tobacco chewers. Lancet i:1206-6, 1984.
272. Garewal HS, Meyskens FL, Killen D. Response of oral leukoplakia to beta-carotene. J Clin Oncol 8:1715-20, 1990.
273. Benner SE, Lippman SM, Wargovich MJ, *et al.* Micronucleii, a biomarker for chemoprevention trials: results of a randomized study in oral-premalignancy. Int J Cancer 59:457-9, 1994
274. Lippman SM, Batsakis JG, Toth BB, *et al.* Comparison of low-dose isotretinoin with beta carotene to prevent oral carcinogenesis. N Engl J Med 328:15-20, 1993.
275. deVet HCW, Knipschild PG, Willebrand D, *et al.* The effect of beta-carotene on the regression and progression of cervical dysplasia: a clinical experiment. J Clin Epidemiol 44:273-83, 1991.
276. Phillips RW, Kikendall JW, Luk GD, *et al.* BC inhibits rectal mucosal ornithine decarboxylase activity in colon cancer patients. Cancer Res 53:3723-5, 1993.
277. Frommel TO, Mobarhan S, Doria M, *et al.* Effect of BC supplementation on indices of colonic cell proliferation. JNCI 87:1781-7, 1995.
278. National Research Council (NRC), Recommended Dietary Allowances, 10th edition. National Academy Press, Washington, D.C., 1989.
279. Federation of American Societies for Experimental Biology (FASEB), Life Sciences Research Office. Third Report on Nutrition Monitoring in the United States: Volume 2. U.S. Government Printing Office, Washington D.C., 1995.
280. World Cancer Research Fund/American Institute for Cancer Research (WCRF). Food, Nutrition and the Prevention of Cancer a Global Perspective. American Institute for Cancer Research, Washington, D.C., 1997.
281. Kromhout D. Essential micronutrients in relation to carcinogenesis. Am J Clin Nutr 45:1361-7, 1987.
282. Knekt P, Jarvinen R, Seppanen R, *et al.* Dietary antioxidants, and the risk of lung cancer. Am J Epidemiol 134:471-9, 1991.
283. Shekelle RB, Lepper M, Liu S, *et al.* Dietary vitamin A and risk of cancer in the Western Electric Study. Lancet 2:1186-90, 1981.
284. Kvale G, Bjelke E, Gart JJ. Dietary habits and lung cancer risk. Int J Cancer 31:397-405, 1983.
285. Steinmetz KA, Potter JD, Folsom AR. Vegetables, fruit, and lung cancer in the Iowa Women's Health Study. Cancer Res 53:536-43, 1993.
286. Le Marchand L, Yoshizawa CN, Kolonel LN, *et al.* Vegetable consumption and lung cancer risk: a population-based case-control study in Hawaii. JNCI 81:1158-64, 1989.

287. Long-de W, Hammond EC. Lung cancer, fruit, green salad, and vitamin pills. Chin Med J 98:206-10, 1985.
288. Hirayama T. Does daily intake of green-yellow vegetables reduce the risk of cancer in man? An example of the application of epidemiologic methods to the identification of individuals at low risk. IARC Sci. Publ, 39:531-40, 1986.
289. Fraser GE, Beeson WL, Phillips RL. Diet and lung cancer in California Seventh Day Adventists. Am J Epidemiol 133:683-93, 1991.
290. Ziegler RG, Mason TJ, Stemhagen A, *et al.* Carotenoid intake, vegetables, and the risk of lung cancer among white men in New Jersey. Am J Epidemiol 123:1080-1093, 1986.
291. Koo LC. Dietary habits and lung cancer risk among Chinese females in Hong Kong who never smoked. Nutr Cancer 11:155-172, 1988.
292. Fontham ET, Pickle LW, Haenszel W, *et al.* Dietary vitamin A and C and lung cancer risk in Louisiana. Cancer 62:2267-73, 1988.
293. Jain M, Burch JD, Howe GR, *et al.* Dietary factors and risk of lung cancer: results from a case-control study, Toronto, 1981-1985. Int J Cancer 45:287-93, 1990.
294. Kalandidi A, Katsouyanni K, Voropoulou N, *et al.* Passive smoking and diet in the etiology of lung cancer among non-smokers. Cancer Causes Control 1:15-21, 1990.
295. Harris RW, Key TJ, Silcocks PB, *et al.* A case-control study of dietary carotene in men with lung cancer and in men with other epithelial cancers. Nutr Cancer 15:63-8, 1991.
296. Swanson CA, Mao BL, Li JY, *et al.* Dietary determinants of lung-cancer risk: results from a case-control study in Yunnan Province, China. Int J Cancer 50:876-80, 1991.
297. Gao C, Tajima K, Kuroishi T, *et al.* Protective effects of raw vegetables and fruit against lung cancer among smokers and ex-smokers: a case-control study in the Tokai area of Japan. Jpn J Cancer Res 84:594-600, 1993.
298. Dorgan JF, Ziegler RG, Schoenberg JB, *et al.* Race and sex differences in associations of vegetables, fruits, and carotenoids with lung cancer risk in New Jersey (U.S.A). Cancer Causes Control 4:273-81, 1993.
299. Mayne ST, Janerick DT, Greenwald P, *et al.* Dietary beta-carotene and lung cancer risk in U.S. nonsmokers. JNCI 86:33-8, 1994.
300. Barone J, Taioli E, Hebert JR, Wynder EL. Vitamin supplement use and risk for oral and esophageal cancer. Nutr Cancer 18:31-41, 1992.
301. Freudenheim JL, Graham S, Byers TE, *et al.* Diet, smoking, and alcohol in cancer of the larynx. Am J Epidemiol 113:675-80, 1992.
302. Esteve J, Riboli E, Pequignot G, *et al.* Diet and cancers of the larynx and hypopharynx: the IARC multi-center study in southwestern Europe. Cancer Causes Control 7:240-52, 1996.
303. Tuyns AJ. Oesophageal cancer in non-smoking drinkers and in non-drinking smokers. Int J Cancer 32:443-4, 1983.
304. Hirayama T. Diet and cancer. Nutr Cancer 1:67-81, 1979.
305. Bjelke E. Case-control study of cancer of the stomach, colon, and rectum. In: Clark R, Cumley RW, McCay JE, Copeland MM, Eds. *Oncology 1970: Proceedings of the Tenth International Cancer Congress,* Volume V, Chicago, IL, Yearbook Medical Publishers, Inc, 320-4, 1971.
306. Martinez I. Factors associated with cancer of the oesophagus, mouth and pharynx in Puerto Rico. JNCI 42:1069-94, 1969.
307. Chen J, Geissler C, Parapia B, *et al.* Antioxidant status and cancer mortality in China. Int J Epidemiol 22:625-35, 1992.
308. Singh VN, Gaby SK. Premalignant lesions: role of antioxidant vitamins and beta-carotene in risk reduction and prevention of malignant transformation. Am J Clin Nutr 53(1 Suppl):386S-90S, 1991.

309. Palli D, Bianchi S, DeCarli A, *et al.* A case-control study of cancers of the gastric cardia in Italy. Int J Cancer 65:263-6, 1992.
310. Gonzalez CA, Sanz JM, Marcos G, *et al.* Dietary factors and stomach cancer in Spain: a multi-centre case-control study. Int J Cancer 49:513-9, 1991.
311. Tuyns AJ, Kaaks R, Haelterman M, Riboli E. Diet and gastric cancer: a case-control study in Belgium. Int J Cancer 51:1-16, 1992.
312. Taylor PR, Li JY, Li B, Blot WJ. Nutritional intervention trial in Linxian, China: supplementation with specific vitamin/mineral combinations, cancer incidence, and disease-specific mortality in the general population. JNCI 86:1647-48, 1994.
313. De Sanjose, S, Munoz, N, Sobala, G, *et al.* Antioxidants, helicobacter pylori, and stomach cancer in Venezuela. Eur J Cancer Prev 5:57-62, 1996.
314. Stemmermann GN, Nomura A, Heinbrun LK. Dietary fat and risk of colorectal cancer. Cancer Res 44:4633-7, 1984.
315. Tuyns AJ, Haelterman M, Kaaks R. Colorectal cancer and the intake of nutrients: a case-control study in Belgium. Nutr Cancer 10:181-96, 1987.
316. Heilbrun LK, Nomura A, Hankin JH, Stemmermann GN. Diet and colorectal cancer with special reference to fiber intake. Int J Cancer 44:1-6, 1989.
317. Wu AH, Paganini-Hill A, Ross RK, Henderson BE. Alcohol, physical activity and other factors for colorectal cancer: a prospective study. Br J Cancer 55:687-94, 1987.
318. Potter JD, McMichael AJ. Diet and cancer of the colon and rectum: a case-control study. JNCI 76:557-69, 1986.
319. Giovannucci E, Stampfer MJ, Colditz GA, *et al.* Relationship of diet to risk of colorectal adenoma in men. JNCI 84:91-8, 1992.
320. Bussey HJ, De Cosse JJ, Deschner EE, *et al.* A randomized trial of ascorbic acid in polyposis coli. Cancer 50:1434-9, 1980.
321. De Cosse JJ, Miller HH, Lesser ML. Effect of wheat fiber and vitamins C and E on rectal polyps in patients with familial adenomatous polyposis. JNCI 81:1290-7, 1989.
322. McKeown-Eyssen G, Holloway C, Jazmaji V, *et al.* A randomized trial of vitamins C and E in the prevention of recurrence of colorectal polyps. Cancer Res 48:4701-5, 1988.
323. Ronucci L, Di Donato P, Carati L, *et al.* Antioxidant vitamins or lactulose for the prevention of the recurrence of colorectal adenomas. Dis Colon Rectum 36:227-34.
324. Kushi LH, Fee RM, Sellers TA, *et al.* Intake of vitamins A, C, E and postmenopausal breast cancer. Am J Epidemiol 144:165-74, 1996.
325. Howe GR, Hirohata T, Hislop TG, *et al.* Dietary factors and risk of breast cancer; combined analysis of 12 case-control studies. JNCI 82:561-9, 1990.
326. Graham S, Marshall J, Mettlin C, *et al.* Diet in the epidemiology of breast cancer. Am J Epidemiol 116:68-75, 1982.
327. Ingram DM, Nottage E, Roberts T. The role of diet in the development of breast cancer; a case-control study of patients with breast cancer, benign epithelial hyperplasia and fibrocystic disease of the breast. Br J Cancer 64:187-91, 1991.
328. Katsouyanni K, Trichopoulos D, Boyle P, *et al.* Diet and breast cancer: a case-control study in Greece. Int J Cancer 38:815-20, 1986.
329. van't Veer P, Kalb CM, Verhoef P, *et al.* Dietary fiber, beta-carotene and breast cancer: results from a case-control study. Int J Cancer 45:825-8, 1990.
330. Holmberg L, Ohlander EM, Byers T, *et al.* Diet and breast cancer risk: results from a population-based, case-control study in Sweden. Arch Internal Med 154:1805-11, 1994.
331. La Vecchia C, DeCarli A, Parazzini F, *et al.* General epidemiology of breast cancer in Northern Italy. Int J Epidemiol 16:347-55, 1987.
332. Fincham SM, Hill GB, Hanson J, *et al.* Epidemiology of prostatic cancer: a case-control study. Prostate 17:189-206, 1990.

333. Severson RK, Nomura A, Grove JS, *et al.* A prospective analysis of physical activity and prostate cancer among men of Japanese ancestry in Hawaii. Am J Epidemiol 130:522-9, 1989.
334. Mills PK, Beeson WL, Phillips RL, *et al.* Cohort study of diet lifestyle, and prostate cancer in Adventist men. Cancer 64:598-604, 1989.
335. Block G. Vitamin C and cancer prevention: the epidemiologic evidence. Am J Clin Nutr 53:270S-82S, 1991.
336. Burton GW, Ingold KU. Autoxidation of biological molecules. 1. The antioxidant activity of vitamin E and related chain-breaking phenolic antioxidants *in vitro*. J Am Chem Soc 103:6472, 1981.
337. Burton GW, Cheeseman KH, Doba T, Ingold U. Vitamin E as an antioxidant *in vitro* and *in vivo*. In: R. Porter, J. Whelan (Eds.), *Biology of Vitamin E*. London: Pitman, 1983.
338. Cook MG, McNamara P. Effect of dietary vitamin E on dimethylhydrazine-induced colonic tumors in mice. Cancer Res 40:1329-31, 1980.
339. Reddy BS, Tanaka T. Interactions of selenium deficiency, vitamin E, polyunsaturated fat, on azoxymethane-induced colon carcinogenesis in male F344 rats. JNCI 76:1157-62, 1986.
340. Toth B, Patil K. Enhancing effect of vitamin E on murine intestinal tumorigenesis by 1,2-dimethylhydrazine dihydrochloride. JNCI 70:1107-11, 1983.
341. Mirvish SS. Effects of vitamins C and E on N-nitroso compound formation, carcinogenesis, and cancer. Cancer 58:1842-50, 1986.
342. Bauernfeind J. Tocopherols in foods, In L. J Machlin, Ed. *Vitamin E: A comprehensive treatise*, Marcel Decker, New York, 1980.
343. USDA (U.S. Department of Agriculture). Oil crops: outlook and situation report, OCS-4. Economic Research Service, U. S. Department of Agriculture, Washington, D.C, 1984.
344. USDA (U.S. Department of Agriculture). Nationwide food consumption survey continuing survey of food intake by individuals: women 19-50 years and their children 1-5 years, 4 days, 1985, Report No. 85-4, Nutrition and Monitoring Division, Human Nutrition Information Economic Research Service, U. S. Department of Agriculture, Hyattsville, MD, 1987.
345. USDA (U.S. Department of Agriculture). Nationwide food consumption survey continuing survey of food intake by individuals: men 19-50 years 1 day, 1985, Report No. 85-3, Nutrition and Monitoring Division, Human Nutrition Information Economic research Service, U. S. Department of Agriculture, Hyattsville, MD, 1987.
346. Connett JE, Kuller LH, Kjelsberg MO, *et al.* Relationship between carotenoids and cancer; the Multiple Risk Factor Intervention Trial (MRFIT) Study. Cancer 64:126-34, 1989.
347. Yong LC, Brown CC, Schatzkin A, *et al.* Intake of vitamins E, C, and A and risk of lung cancer: The NHANES I Epidemiologic Follow-up study. Am J Epidemiol 146:231-43, 1997.
348. Ocke MC, Bueno-de-Mesquita HB, Feskens EJ, *et al.* Repeated measurements of vegetables, fruits, â-carotene, and vitamins C and E in relation to lung cancer: The Zutphen study. Am J Epidemiol 145:358-65, 1997.
349. Day GL, Blot WJ, Austin DF, *et al.* Racial differences in risk of oral and pharyngeal cancer: alcohol, tobacco, and other determinants. JNCI 85:465-73, 1993.
350. Longnecker MP, Martin-Moreno JM, Knekt P, *et al.* Serum alpha-tocopherol concentration in relation to subsequent colorectal cancer: Pooled data from five cohorts. JNCI 84:430-5, 1992.
351. Willett WC, Stampfer MJ, Colditz GA, *et al.* Relation of meat fat and fiber intake to the risk of colon cancer in a prospective study among women. N Engl J Med 323:1664-72, 1990.

352. Ferraroni M, La Vecchia C, D'Avanzo B, *et al.* Selected micronutrient intake and the risk of colorectal cancer. Br J Cancer 70:1150-5, 1994.
353. Garland M, Willett WC, Manson JE, Hunter DJ. Antioxidant micronutrients and breast cancer. J Am Coll Nutr 12:400-11, 1993.
354. Verhoeven DT, Assen N, Goldbohm RA, *et al.* Vitamins C and E, retinol, beta-carotene and dietary fibre in relation to breast cancer risk: a prospective cohort study. Br J Cancer 75:149-55, 1997.
355. Ernster VL, Goodson WH, Hunt TK, *et al.* Vitamin E and benign breast "disease"; A double-blind, randomized clinical trial. Surgery 97:490-94, 1985.
356. London RS, Sundaram GS, Murphy L, *et al.* The effect of vitamin E on mammary dysplasia: a double-blind study. Obstet Gynecol 65:104-6, 1985.
357. Knekt P. Serum vitamin E level and risk of female cancers. Int J Epidemiol 17:281-6, 1988.
358. Cuzick J, De Stavola B, Russell J, Thomas B. Vitamin A, vitamin E and the risk of cervical intraepithelial neoplasia. Br J Cancer 62:651-2, 1990.
359. Comstock GW, Helzlsouer KJ, Bush TL. Prediagnostic serum levels of carotenoids and vitamin E as related to subsequent cancer in Washington county, Maryland. Am J Clin Nutr 53:260S-64S, 1991.
360. Knekt P, Aromaa A, Maatala J, *et al.* Serum vitamin E and risk of cancer among Finnish men during a 10-year follow-up. Am J Epidemiol 127:28-41, 1988.
361. Eichholzer M, Stahelin HB, Gey FK, *et al.* Prediction of male cancer mortality by plasma levels of interacting vitamins: 17-year follow-up of the prospective Basel study. Int J Cancer 55:145-50, 1996.
362. Hsing AW, Comstock GW, Abbey H, Polk BF. Serologic precursors of cancer; retinol, carotenoids, and tocopherol and risk of prostate cancer. JNCI 82:941-6, 1990.
363. Hartman TJ, Albanes D, Pietinen P, *et al.* The association between baseline vitamin E, selenium, and prostate cancer in the Alpha-Tocopherol, Beta-Carotene Cancer Prevention Study. Cancer Epidemiol Biomarkers Prev 7:335-40, 1998.
364. Heinonen OP, Albanes D, Virtamo J, *et al.* Prostate cancer and supplementation with á-tocopherol and â-carotene: incidence and mortality in a controlled trial. JNCI 90:440-6, 1998.
365. Shamberger RJ, Frost DV. Possible protective effect of selenium against human cancer. Can Med Assn J 100:682, 1969.
366. Shamberger RJ, Willis CE. Selenium distribution of human cancer mortality. CRC Crit Rev Clin Lab Sci 2:211-21, 1971.
367. Hoekstra WG. Biochemical function of selenium and its relation to vitamin E. Fed Proc 34:2083-9, 1975.
368. Medina D. Mechanisms of selenium inhibition of tumorigness. Adv Exp Med Biol 206:465-72, 1986.
369. Flohe L, Beckmann R, Girtz H, Loschen G. Oxygen-centered free radicals as mediators of inflammation. *In Oxidative Stress*, Sies, H, Ed. New York, Academic, 1985.
370. Parker RS. Dietary and biochemical aspects of vitamin E. Adv. Food Nutr Res 33:157-232, 1989.
371. Pennington JA, Wilson DB, Newell RF. Selected minerals in food surveys, 1974 to 1981/82. J Am Diet Assoc 84:771-80, 1984.
372. Comstock GW, Alberg AJ, Huang HY, *et al.* The risk of developing lung cancer associated with antioxidants in the blood: ascorbic acid, carotenoids, α-tocopherol, selenium, and total peroxyl radical absorbing capacity. Cancer Epidemiol Biomarkers Prev 6:907-16, 1997.

373. Nomura A, Heilbrun LK, Morris JS, Stemmermann GN. Serum selenium and the risk of cancer, by specific sites; case-control analysis of prospective data. JNCI 79:103-8, 1997.
374. Menkes MS, Comstock GW, Vuilleumier JP, *et al.* Serum beta-carotene, vitamins A and E, selenium, and the risk of lung cancer. N Engl J Med 315:1250-4, 1986.
375. Knekt P, Aromaa A, Maatela J, *et al.* Serum selenium and subsequent risk of cancer among Finnish men and women. JNCI 32:864-8, 1990.
376. Salonen JT, Alfthan G, Huttunen JK, Puska P. Association between serum selenium and the risk of cancer. Am J Epidemiol 120:342-9, 1984.
377. Peleg I, Morris S, Hames CG. Is serum selenium a risk factor for cancer? Med Oncol Tumor Pharmacol 2:157-63, 1985.
378. Virtamo, J, Valkeila, E, Alfthan G. Serum selenium and risk of cancer. Cancer 60:145-8, 1987.
379. Ringstad J, Jacobsen BK, Tretlik S, *et al.* Serum selenium concentration associated with risk of cancer. J Clin Pathol 41:454-7, 1988.
380. Willett WC, Polk BF, Morris JS, *et al.* Prediagnostic serum selenium and risk of cancer, Lancet 2:130-4, 1983.
381. van den Brandt PA, Goldbohm RA, van't Veer P, *et al.* A prospective cohort study on selenium status and the risk of lung cancer. Cancer Res 53:4860-5, 1993.
382. Poole C. Cancer and high selenium intake. Doctoral thesis, Harvard School of Public Health, 1989.
383. Bratakos MS, Vouterakos TP, Iouannou PV. Selenium status of cancer patients in Greece. Sci Total Environ 92:207-22, 1990.
384. Tominga K, Saito Y, Mori K, *et al.* An evaluation of serum microelement concentrations in lung cancer and matched non-cancer patients to determine the risk of developing lung cancer; a preliminary study. Jpn J Clin Oncol 22:96-101, 1992.
385. Knekt P, Aromaa A, Maatela J, *et al.* Serum vitamin E, serum selenium and the risk of gastrointestinal cancer. Int J Cancer 42:846-50, 1988.
386. Schober SE, Comstock GW, Helzlsouer KJ, *et al.* Serologic precursors of cancer. Am J Epidemiol 126:1033-41, 1987.
387. Garland M, Morris JS, Stampfer M, *et al.* Prospective study of toenail selenium levels and cancer among women. JNCI 87:497-505, 1995.
388. van den Brandt PA, Goldbohm RA, van't Veer P, *et al.* A prospective cohort study on toenail selenium levels and risk of gastrointestinal cancer. JNCI 85:224-9, 1993.
389. Clark L, Hixon L, Combs GF, Jr, *et al.* Plasma selenium concentration predicts the prevalence of colorectal adenomatous polyps. Cancer Epidemiol Biomarkers Prev 2:41-6, 1993.
390. Overvad K, Wang DY, Olsen J, *et al.* Selenium in human mammary carcinogenesis: a case-cohort study. Eur J Cancer 27:900-2, 1991.
391. Hunter DJ, Morris JS, Stampfer MJ, *et al.* A prospective study of selenium status and breast cancer risk. JAMA 264:1128-31, 1990.
392. van Noord PA, Collette HJ, Maas MJ, de Waard F. Selenium levels in nails of premenopausal breast cancer patients assessed prediagnostically in a cohort-nested case-referent study among women screened in the DOM project. Int J Epidemiol 16:318-22, 1987.
393. van den Brandt PA, Goldbohm RA, van't Veer P. Toenail selenium levels and the risk of breast cancer. Am J Epidemiol 140:20-6, 1993.
394. Meyer F, Verreault R. Erythrocyte selenium and breast cancer risk. Am J Epidemiol 125:917-9, 1987.
395. van't Veer P, van der Wielen RP, Kok FJ, *et al.* Selenium in diet, blood, and toenails in relation to breast cancer: a case-control study. Am J Epidemiol 131:987-94, 1990.

24

Antioxidants and Diseases of the Eye

John R. Trevithick, Ph.D.
University of Western Ontario, London, Ontario, CANADA

Kenneth P. Mitton, Ph.D.
University of Michigan Medical Center, Ann Arbor, Michigan, USA

VISION AND EYE DISEASE: AGE AND OXIDATION

The Basics of Vision

Light enters at the corneal surface of the eye where the major refraction or bending occurs. After passing through the liquid aqueous humor which bathes the lens front surface, it is refracted again by the lens, passes through the vitreous humor and is focused as an image on the retina (Figure 1). The light first passes through the neural retinal layers, which conduct the nerve Impulses to the brain, then reaches the rod and cone photoreceptor cells which permit fine details and color to be perceived (Figure 2). To maintain the rods and cones, their outer segments including polyunsaturated fatty acids and retinol (vitamin A) are engulfed by the cells of the retinal pigment epi-

0-8493-8009-X/98/$0.00+$.50

thelium, digested, and recycled in a process initiated each morning. In contrast to the photoreceptor outer segments, which turn over, the lens continues to build up new fiber cell layers like tree rings, approximately one cell layer per day, resulting in the loss of flexibility and the onset of middle-aged farsightedness (Figure 3). These new cells come into being by a remarkable example of cell differentiation. Lens epithelial cells move to the lens equator, and as they change to internal lens fiber cells, turn right around 180°, so that the new fiber cell apex is oriented apex to apex with the overlying epithelial cells from which they differentiate; then they elongate up to 1000 times. This elongation gives a characteristic appearance to histological sections of the lens, in which the displaced nuclei form a regular curve called the lens bow. Along with this elongation, new classes of proteins, the γ- and β-crystallins, are synthesized in large quantities in the fiber cells. The signals for this differentiation are proteins called basic fibroblast growth factor (β-FGF), which apparently comes to the lens across the vitreous from the retina, and insulin-related growth factor[1] (IGF).

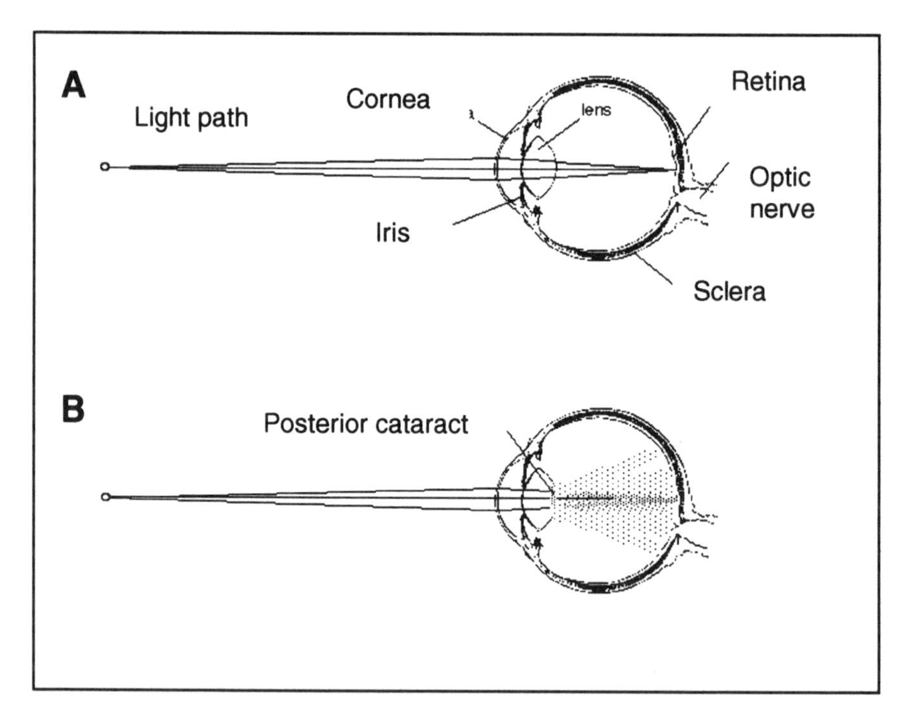

Figure 1. A. Normal light paths in the human eye. The cornea, aqueous humor, and lens form an adjustable compound lens for focusing light rays from near or far objects onto the retina.
B. Cataracts, lens opacities, can completely block light or scatter light leading to vision as if through a dense fog. Cataracts on the central optical axis of the lens will interfere with the most important field of vision, the central visual field, used for reading and other visual tasks.

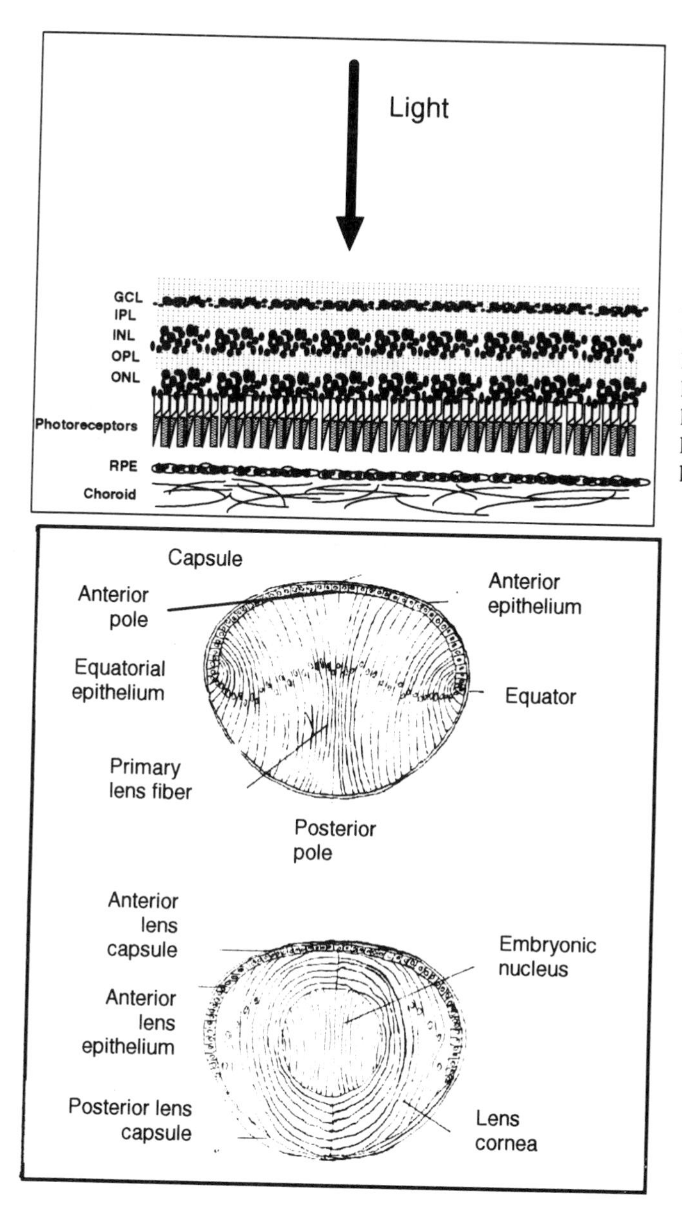

Figure 2. Diagram of the layers of the human retina and the retinal pigment epithelium (RPE). Ganglion cell layer (GCL), inner plexiform layer (IPL), inner nuclear layer (INL), outer plexiform layer (OPL), outer nuclear layer (ONL).

Figure 3. Cross-section of eye lens to show its structural organization in embryo (upper) and adult (lower).

Factors Causing Oxidative Stress

The eye, by its very sensory nature, is in an oxidation-prone environment. The cornea, lens, and retinal tissues are exposed to extensive ambient ultraviolet radiation (UV, mostly absorbed by the cornea). Even though the lens and retina see little of the external UV radiation impinging on the cornea, they transmit and absorb visible light, which can interact with photosensitizing biomolecules of the tissue. The retina is potentially sensitive to lipid peroxidation because of the high content of unsaturated fatty acids in the photoreceptor cells. The lens is mostly composed, by weight, of specialized crystallin proteins that are long-lived (little if any turn-over) yet essential for clarity. Such long-lived macromolecules are targets that accumulate the normal ravages of chemical aging in the form of sulfhydryl loss, glycation, and protein crosslinking. All of these processes involve reactive oxygen species.

While oxidation can be used to induce degenerative eye diseases in animal models, we do not know how much oxidative stress contributes to cataract, retinal disease, or even elevated intraocular pressure (IOP). However, evidence from human studies indicated that oxidation and antioxidant compromise are part of these progressive ocular diseases.

This chapter will provide an overview, highlighting the mechanism and the role of oxidation and antioxidants in the three major causes of blindness namely, cataract, age related macular degeneration (AMD), and glaucoma.

CATARACT

Cataract refers to opacities of the lens, which interfere with vision. Cataract occurs in the outer layer or cortex of the lens (cortical), the central region or nucleus of the lens (nuclear), or may be mixed (cortical and nuclear). In general, problems with vision arise when the cataract is located on the visual axis, since the scattering of light results in a foggy image. Cataract is a major chronic disease and its prevalence increases from 5% at age 55-65 years, to 15% at age 65-75, to 43% at age 75-85.[2] Cataract operations in the United States currently exceed by 450,438 the sum of the next 9 major operations combined.[3]

By our mid-40s we become progressively more far-sighted as our eye lens grows and becomes less flexible. This is called presbyopia. As a consequence, many of us require glasses to read print, although we may see well at longer distances. Loss of flexibility of the lens is followed by progressive opacities or clouding in the central nucleus and outer layer or cortex. Aging of the lens appears to be a good indicator of general aging, since persons having early cataract operations are also at increased risk for early death.[4]

Because cells in the equator area are changing rapidly, they are most easily affected by stress. Such effects may be expressed years later when the cells have entered into the body of the lens. One report[5] describes a cataract, which arose 20 years after exposure of an X-ray technician to radium irradiation (α-particles) while carrying radium needles in his shirt pocket. This illustrates the fact that the lens carries its entire life history with it.

Pathogenesis

Cortical opacities usually occur at the lens periphery or equatorial edge. They spread like the points of a star, growing towards the center of the lens. Facing oncoming headlights at night becomes difficult since these opacities scatter light. When an opaque area grows across the visual axis of the lens, it interferes with vision by obscuring images in the area of fine focusing — the macula. Figure 1 illustrates scattering of light by a posterior cortical lens cataract. Nuclear cataracts have been attributed to protein aggregation into large, light-scattering entities.[6] Any cataracts that form in the central area or along the optical axis of the lens can potentially scatter a large amount of light and interfere with vision.

Role of Oxidation in Globular Degeneration and Protein Aggregation

Opaque lens contain in the nucleus or central area aggregates of proteins which are believed to cause scattering of the light.[6] This phenomenon is similar to small protein particles of casein making milk white. Phase change of protein solutions in the cells of the lens can also result in light scattering entities.[7]

Opacities in the cells of the cortex or the outer area of the lens, examined by electron microscopy and scanning electron microscopy (SEM), are found to have a characteristic globular degeneration, disrupting the normal regular fiber cell structure.[8] The light is scattered by the globules and by fibrous proteins and membranes left when the cell cytoplasm leaks out as the cells die. How do these globules form? Lens cells normally have an internal cytoskeleton which maintains their characteristic hexagonal cross-sectional shape. When the cells are stressed or in the process of dying this cytoskeleton disaggregates, allowing the cell membrane to herniate outward into globules containing cytoplasm. This disrupted area of the lens scatters light, and also prevents the lens from focusing light on to the retina as shown by the shadowgram images shown in Figure 4. In an organ culture diabetic model such globular degeneration increases with increased sugar concentration. Similar increases are found, with time, in diabetic rats.[9] Recently Srivastava's group modeled the process of globule formation at the cellular level using isolated lens fiber cells.[10]

Klintworth and Garner[11] proposed the following as contributing factors to cataract formation: ultraviolet light,[12-14] oxidation, heat, radiation including microwave x- and γ-irradiation, neutron and α-irradiation, aminoglycoside antibiotics, agricultural chemicals (paraquat), diarrhea (osmotic stress),[12] diabetes, and pharmaceuticals (steroid drugs). To these we add another: vitamin deficiency.[9,15]

Recently, Ortwerth's group[16] demonstrated increased superoxide and peroxide formation following UV radiation A 369 nm peak irradiation of a lens protein fraction. Although UV light has been implicated as a possible contributing factor some controversy remains as to its actual role.[12] Other researchers, using a variety of tests, indicate that oxidative stress increases with age. We used a luminescent assay to measure reactive oxygen species[17] in rats and found that the concentration of luminescent species per unit protein increased with age for retina, lens, and vitreous and aqueous humors.[18]

Role of Dietary Antioxidants

In Vitro, Animal and Basic Clinical Human Studies

Vitamin E prevents or reduces globular degeneration[19] and even after 6 weeks can still reverse many changes in the rat lens (Figure 4). We confirmed this hypothesis in diabetic cataract using ^{60}Co-γ-irradiation to produce free radicals. Figure 4 illustrates the globular degeneration observed after irradiation and its reduction associated with treatment with vitamin E.

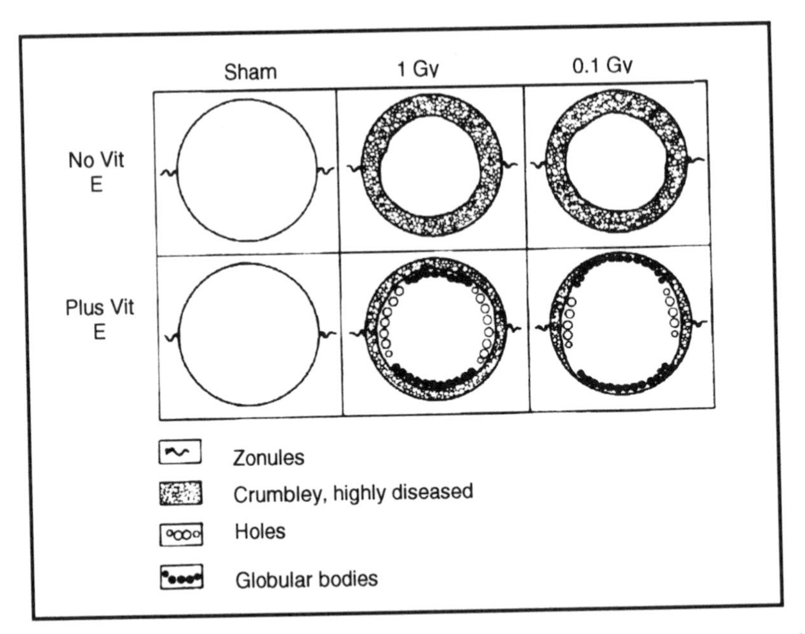

Figure 4. Cataractous damage (schematic) and the protective influence of vitamin E (2.4 micromolar) observed by SEM after 24-hr incubation at 35.5 °C following 0.1 Gy, 1.0 Gy, or sham irradiation. With permission of Academic Press.[20]

Low plasma vitamin E may increase risk of cortical cataracts.[21] Liquidators of the Chernobyl nuclear accident have increased risk[22] for both cataract and retinal angiopathy (blood vessel growth similar to that found in macular degeneration). Recently we showed that antioxidants such as vitamin E and R-α-lipoate reduce lens damage from low level radiation in a model of astronaut, jet crew, and radiation clean-up workers.[23]

Natural defenses of the lens include endogenous antioxidants such as cysteine, glutathione, taurine, and ascorbate[24-26] and antioxidant enzyme systems such as superoxide dismutase, catalase, and glutathione peroxidase. Several exogenous antioxidants have been suggested to reduce cataract risk: taurine,[25,26] butylated hydroxytoluene (BHT),[27] vitamin C,[28,29] vitamin E,[19,30-32] vitamin A,[33] R-α-lipoic acid,[34] carotenoids, rutin and venoruton,[35-38] and melatonin.[39] *In vivo* studies support the role of antioxidants.[31-33,35-38]

It is useful to consider the paradigm of animal and test-tube experiments with a high stress level produced by glucose or short-term radiation, with treatment by very high levels of antioxidants. We hypothesized that at the lower stress levels which occur in the aging human, treatment with lower levels of antioxidants obtained by supplementation with vitamin E or C might result in lower risk of cataracts.[30,31] We found that persons taking supplemental vitamins E (~400 IU/day) and/or vitamin C (~500 mg/day) had reduced risk of cataracts: 56% for E, and 70% for C alone or in combination with E. Vitamins C is believed to regenerate oxidized vitamin E.[40]

Epidemiological and Clinical Studies

Taylor and Nowell[41] reviewed the evidence for vitamins E and C and carotenoids in reducing the risk of human cataract. They expressed the opinion that the best evidence exists for vitamins C and E, while for carotenoids the evidence is less persuasive. Several clinical studies including our own[30,31,42-45] suggested benefits of vitamins E and C, and even of other vitamin supplements.[45]

Several studies evaluating low levels of vitamin E showed no benefit. The Linxian study in China[45] did not report any beneficial effect of vitamin E, although an effect for riboflavin was noted and was also reported for the population of India by Bhat.[15] Several vitamin E intervention studies are now in progress. A common problem with these studies, in our opinion, is the short period of intervention. Cataract develops over a long period of time, so a minimum of 5 years treatment should be anticipated before any difference between control and treated groups becomes measurable even for a cohort aged 50-55 years of age at the beginning of the study.

Other Observations

Glutathione (GSH), which falls in many cataracts, may partially be taken up intact from the diet.[46] Taurine[47] (also high in the retina) and N-acetyl carnosine[48] appear to function, as precursors of the antioxidant carnosine. Cysteine is an important precursor of GSH. Vitamin C is actively taken up by the lens and is present at millimolar levels. Vitamin A and its precursor β-carotene are both antioxidants. Vitamin A is necessary for the lens epithelium, helps reduce risk in model diabetic cataracts,[33] and recently has been associated with reduced risk of human cortical cataracts.[49,50] The carotenoids zeaxanthin and lutein may also play an antioxidant role. Bioflavonoids such as rutin, quercetin and quercitrin and their derivatives such as venoruton appear to reduce the risk of cataracts in model systems.[35,37,38] Curcumin, the spice of curry, has anticataract activity.[51] BHT[27] appears effective in reducing oxidative damage to the lens. R-α-lipoic acid, but not the unnatural isomer S-α-lipoate, is active in reducing cataract damage in model systems whether stress is induced by diabetes[34] or radiation (astronaut cataract model),[23] and seems to be important in reducing mitochondrial damage.[23] In a cataract model in which cell membrane damage follows cytoskeletal disruption, vitamin C reduces lactate dehydrogenase leakage.[52] Recently tests of lazaroids[53] and viscoelastic molecules such as sodium hyaluronate[54] show promise as antioxidants. Alcohol, a hydroxyl radical scavenger[55] at a consumption level of one drink/day, was correlated with significant reduction (>50%) in cataract risk.[14] Another study showed that cataract risk increased from this minimum in a U-shaped curve, to 100% or more at either zero alcohol intake or two or more drinks each day.[56]

Recommendation

We propose providing aging persons with supplemental antioxidants to reduce cataract risk. Although surgery is very safe, with less than a 1% rate of complications leading to blindness, the number of operations is very large and the cost extremely high. Even a 10% reduction in the incidence of cataracts will reduce by 130,000 the number of operations in the United States and 13,000 in Canada.

AGE-RELATED MACULAR DEGENERATION

Occurrence

AMD is a disease that affects the central vision. It is a common cause of vision loss among people over age of 60. AMD destroys the important central area of vision. However, AMD can sometimes make it difficult to read, drive, or perform other daily activities that require fine, central vision. AMD is associated with cataract[61] and is now recognized as the major cause of blindness in England, Wales, Western Scotland, Canada, and the United States.[65] As with cataract, prevalence is age-dependent (Table 1).

Table 1
Prevalence of Macular Degeneration in Eyes (Framingham Study)

Age	All	Males	Females
	% eyes affected		
<65	0.6	0.4	0.8
65 - 74	4.1	2.5	5.2
75$^+$	15.4	12.5	17.4
Total	4	2.8	4.8

Pathogenesis

The retina, like the lens, is unique as the only part of the human brain that exists outside the cranium. Ganglion cells of the neural retina make their connections through the optic nerve all the way to the brain. Like other neural tissues in humans, loss of these cells or their normal connectivity means a permanent loss of signal transduction to the brain and thus permanent vision loss.

The macula is located centrally in the retina and has a high concentration of photoreceptors located in its central foveal region. This area is required for the detailed central visual field upon which we rely for our everyday tasks. This is the region damaged by AMD. AMD is divided into two types. Dry AMD is about 90% of this disease and is a slowly progressing loss of viable photoreceptors in the macula. Wet AMD is found in the remaining 10% of persons with AMD, but it is responsible for 90% of the blindness caused by AMD. New blood vessels begin to grow behind the retina and move into the macula where they are usually not seen. These vessels are not as robust as vessels laid down in early normal retinal development, and they tend to leak blood and fluid under the macular region. This process quickly damages the normal macular function and can cause loss of vision. The progress of wet AMD can even physically lift the macula forward in uneven ridges causing the patient to have a distorted and stretched visual field. Distortion of parallel lines while viewing a tiled test pattern may indicate changes to the retina of the type found in macular degeneration.

Diabetic retinopathy also results in similar but not exactly identical changes, particularly angiogenesis.[66,67] The vessel proliferation is often treated by laser photocoagulation to destroy the retinal tissue and reduce angiogenesis.

Diagnosis

Standard fundus photography through the cornea and pupil shows several characteristic features: (1) Drusen (a German word meaning sediment) — lipid deposits or drops at the retinal pigment epithelium — Bruch's membrane border composed heavily of lipofuscin, a non-metabolizable side product of lipid peroxidation; (2) irregular macular pigmentation; (3) in advanced cases, neovascularization or growth of new blood vessels; (4) in most severe, irreversible blindness, disciform lesions. Fundus photographs and fluorescein angiogram photos may show blood vessels and blood pooling in leaky areas. In the normal fundus photo, the central area or fovea has no vessels — the vessels terminate just outside the central circular area, the macula. In macular degeneration yellow drusen are seen in treatable neovascularization, while areas of stronger fluorescence can be seen in the vicinity of the drusen. Progression occurs from drusen without neovascularization, with pooling of the fluorescent dye in small areas of retinal lesions, to the final stage of neovascularization which cannot be treated by laser.

Mechanism and Role of Oxidation: Loss of Fovea and Macular Pigment

At this time we can only hypothesize about mechanisms. Based on careful electron microscopy, Dr. Richard Young[4,65] suggested a sequence of events in which drusen prevent the exchange of nutrients through the Bruch's membrane between the retinal pigment epithelial cells and the choriocapillaris — the capillaries that supply nutrients to the retina. As lipid droplets form under the retinal pigment epithelium cells, the cells over the drusen die, while those around the drusen may grow and proliferate resulting in low concentrations of pigment over the drusen, and high concentration at the edges. The net result at this early stage is very irregular patterns of pigment concentration. As the damage becomes greater, chemoattractants are released possibly by the retinal pigment epithelium and retina. These can lead to neovascularization — growth of new but abnormal blood vessels into the area. As the pigment epithelium does this, its cells may die in areas directly over the drusen, attracting macrophages, which produce many oxidizing species during their phagocytosis of dead cells. This in turn can induce more neovascularization of the area. These abnormal blood vessels are leaky and bleeding from small hemorrhages may occur. This blood releases iron which can also potentiate oxidizing Haber-Weiss reactions, resulting in an increase of damaging hydroxyl radicals in the area of the bleed. If the bleed is large, as can occur prior to disciform lesion formation, it can form in a fan shape with a rounded leading edge (as found in a blister or blood blister in the skin). This can also mechanically lift the retinal pigment epithelium cells and the rod and cone cells, which depend on them. This destroys the rods and cones as they lose physical contact and metabolic exchange with the Bruch's membrane and its underlying capillaries.

The central macular region, fovea, has a distinct yellow color which is due to the high content of the macular pigmentation comprised of compounds called xanthophylls. Two of these compounds are zeaxanthin and lutein.[68] There is good evidence that these compounds are generally deficient in the retinas of persons with macular degeneration compared to normal retinas of the same age[69] and that antioxidants are useful in protecting against their loss and the resulting macular degeneration. Because the layers of macular pigments are above the photoreceptor cells, all light entering the eye must pass through this pigmented layer. In plants these pigments adsorb and aid the funneling of light energy to chlorophyll and protect the plant from photo-oxidative stress, like a filter. It is believed that the macular pigment has the same protective filtering role for the fovea.[69] It is not known whether lower macular pigment levels of AMD retinas cause photo-oxidative damage to the retina or whether the pigment content is lower just because of damage to the normal retina.

AMD may be multifactorial, influenced by dietary intake of pigments, light exposure, and unknown genetic predispositions to this pathology. Recently, a mutation of the Stargardt disease gene (ABCR) was linked to some families with AMD.[70] The possible functional consequences of this mutation are not known at this time, but will be very informative as future studies determine if this mutation alters macular pigment distribution directly or causes retinal degeneration independent of pigment metabolism. In the later scenario, it is still possible that the ensuing loss of the macular pigment content would lead to increased photo-oxidative damage that would act in a vicious cycle to accelerate damage to the retina. It is this damage which antioxidants appear to prevent or reduce.[6]

Role of Dietary Antioxidants in Prevention

Vitamin A is necessary as part of the visual pigment rhodopsin. Deficiency of vitamin A or its precursor, beta-carotene or other carotenoids which can be cleaved to vitamin A (such as γ-carotene, etc.) can cause night blindness as well as corneal weakness. Retinal ischemia induces free radicals in the postischemic recovery period.[71] Free radical scavengers may reduce the formation of post-ischemic lesions. Preliminary experiments by Muller *et al.*[53] indicate that lazaroids may reduce damage at reperfusion. Inflammation of the vitreous and uveitis are uncommon, but if they occur they contribute to oxidative stress.[71]

Vitamin E has been shown to be effective in treating retinopathy of prematurity in a meta-analysis of all available studies.[72] West *et al.*[73] showed that vitamin E reduced the risk of AMD and it seems likely that it would also reduce the risk of onset of diabetic retinopathy, in which retinal ischemia also seems to induce retinal neovascularization — the growth of sprouting retinal blood vessels which interfere with vision. In the Beaver Dam Eye Study, data weakly supported a protective role for zinc in reducing early stages of age-related maculopathy.[74] Currently there is no treatment for Dry AMD, but this form progresses slowly. Many patients do not lose their vision completely, and only one eye may be affected. Early treatment of Wet AMD is possible using laser surgery, preferably to stop newly forming vessels before they extend into the central fovea.

The possible involvement of free radicals has prompted intervention studies with antioxidants. West and the Hopkins (Wilmer Eye Institute) group[73] found that persons with elevated antioxidants and β-carotene levels have significantly lower risk for senile macular degeneration. Their data suggest a rationale for prevention of oxidized lipids which get into the drusen, as well as reduction of damage from inflammation. This preventive strategy may supplement the conventional laser treatment, to prevent new blood vessel growth and, occasionally, surgical intervention.

Another antioxidant, the hormone melatonin, may be involved in protection of retinal neurons.[75] Osborne's group[76] showed that it reduces forskolin-stimulated ATP hydrolysis in human and rat retinal pigment epithelium (RPE), which was attenuated by pertussis toxin. This indicated that the RPE cells contain melatonin receptors negatively coupled to adenylate cyclase and sensitive to pertussis toxin.

Vitamin E reduced the severity of diabetic retinopathy[77] (due probably to chronic ischemia of the retina).

Relationship Between Cataract and Macular Degeneration

The almost parallel rise with age in prevalence of cataract and macular degeneration, taken together with the increased risk of both conditions in women, suggests that there may be a common factor linking the two conditions.[78-82] Similar elevation in cataract and retinal angiopathy in the Chernobyl liquidators[22] further support this concept.

Using the animal model of retinal degeneration in the Royal College of Surgeons (RCS) rat we showed an inverse relation between the integrity of the retina and the occurrence of cataracts.[81] Zigler and Hess[82] suggested that lipoperoxides arising from the congenital retinal degeneration reach the lens by diffusion from the degenerating retina across the vitreous to the posterior part of the lens. Antioxidants may prevent damage to the retina and also reduce the incidence of cataracts by reducing the amount of damaging lipoperoxides and other oxidative species produced in the retina from reaching the lens. The fact that macrophages, which also emit reactive oxygen species, are found in the degenerating retina further suggest that macular degeneration could be contributing to the damage to the lens. Consistent with this hypothesis, Hess and co-workers[83] have observed several hundred-fold elevations of vitreal macrophages in the RCS rat during the peak of the retinal degeneration. Thus a possible scenario linking the two processes would be damage to the retina resulting in the degeneration, releasing lipoperoxides which act as chemoattractants for macrophages which emit ROS in the vitreous. Protection of both tissues by antioxidants is consistent with this hypothesis.

GLAUCOMA

Prevalence and Pathogenesis

Glaucoma is a group of diseases that can cause permanent blindness by damaging the optic nerve of the eye which contains over 1 million nerve fibers. The most prevalent form of this disease is open-angle glaucoma. The major risk factor for open-angle glaucoma is increased intraocular pressure (IOP) killing the retinal cells beginning in the peripheral visual field. The exact mechanism of this cell death is not completely understood. This disease is described as "silent" because it occurs insidiously without the victim's awareness until it is too late, and currently affects at least 3 million Americans.

IOP is most affected by two factors: the rate of production of aqueous humor in the front segment of the eye by the ciliary body and the rate of outflow though the trabecular meshwork (TM) into Schlemm's canal (80%) and uveal-scleral outflow though the ciliary muscle (20%). Elevated IOP arises from decreased drainage though the TM facility as a result of increased resistance to the aqueous outflow (Figure 5). Most treatments of glaucoma start with use of therapeutic agents that reduce the production of aqueous humor. Therapeutic agents include beta-blockers and carbonic anhydrase inhibitors that often have side effects that are not tolerated by all patients. Research studies under way will clarify the use of early laser surgery to manage IOP safely. It appears that this option will become more popular. Laser trabeculoplasty may help control IOP in some patients, but some antiglaucoma drug therapy is still used after surgery. Unfortunately, most laser surgery lasts for only a couple of years and may be repeated, but often further treatment will not be as effective as the first.

Glaucoma and Antioxidants

Several papers by Russian workers[84-89] have suggested beneficial effects of antioxidants. Others including Shumer and Podos[90] in the United States, Bonne[91] in France, and Osborne *et al.*[92] in Great Britain suggested the need for further research on the role of antioxidants in reducing the risk of glaucoma.

There is some indication in the literature that high levels of antioxidants such as vitamin E may be necessary for the permeability of the trabecular meshwork, through which the aqueous humor exits the eye. Filina *et al.*[88] showed that, of patients administered a daily dose of 0.15 g lipoic acid, improvement was noted in approximately 45-47%.

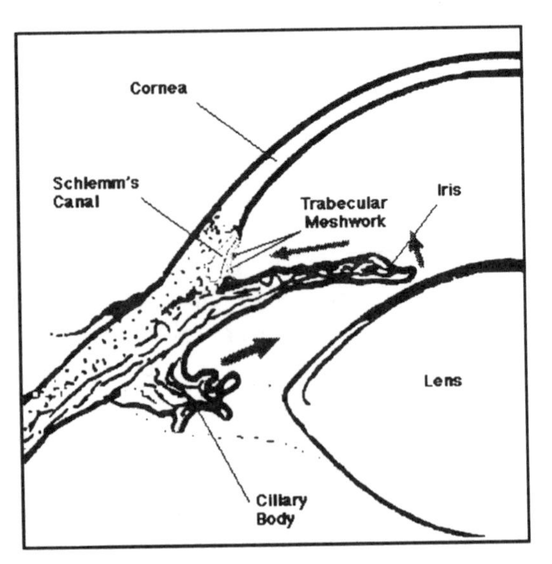

Figure 5. Intraocular pressure (IOP) is a function of aqueous humor production from the ciliary body and aqueous outflow, most of which is through the trabecular meshwork into Schlemm's canal (path shown by arrows). Aqueous humor is optically clear and carries important nutrient supplies to the lens and cornea, which do not have a direct blood supply.

TRABECULAR MESHWORK AND OXIDATION

The TM of the eye is physically composed of trabecular beams; an extracellular matrix (ECM) composed of collagens, elastin, laminin, and other extracellular glycoprotein classes. This extracellular matrix is formed and maintained by the TM cells that are anchored in a monolayer that ensheaths the trabecular beams. These special cells are epithelial-like, yet also have the ability to phagocytose material and migrate to new positions in the meshwork. TM cells display evidence of both inside-out and outside-in signal transduction via integrin receptors and their production of extracellular matrix is influenced by the ECM composition itself.[93]

It is known that ECM deposition is altered and elevated above normal in glaucomatous donor eyes compared to age-matched normal donor eyes. Diurnal variation as well as longer term variation in IOP alters the diameter and compactness of the meshwork and therefore must stretch TM cell basal membranes as each eye contains a finite number of these cells that are lost throughout life.

Recently it has been demonstrated that human TM cells can respond to mechanical stretch through their basal attachments, causing modulation of α-B-crystallin and signal transduction events.[94] Both the aging stresses on the finite TM cell population as well as the composition and maintenance of the ECM are factors which may be influenced directly by antioxidant and nutritional status. Human TM tissue does contain large quantities of glutathione reductase as well as other antioxidant enzymes.[95]

Ascorbate is essential for the synthesis of collagen, a major component of the ECM of the TM. It has been demonstrated that external ascorbate concentration effects collagen synthesis in human trabecular meshwork.[93] Agents that affect the cytoskeleton of TM cells are known to alter the resistance to aqueous outflow in the eye.[96] Therefore, the general tensegrity of the TM may affect the outflow resistance and, therefore, in turn, be influenced by any factors that alter the cytoskeleton/ECM network. The importance of antioxidant status to normal ECM production and remodeling is an area that requires attention in future research on the trabecular meshwork, Schlemm's canal, and aqueous outflow.

CORNEA

The cornea is the transparent tissue that covers the front of the eye. Because the cornea is as smooth and clear as glass but as strong and durable as plastic, it provides a protective physical barrier. It acts as the eye's outermost lens.

Vitamin A or its precursor carotenoids are necessary for corneal health in childhood. In some developing countries vitamin A deficiency causes corneal conditions, xerophthalmia and kerotomalacia in children. These conditions result in loss of corneal clarity and thus loss of vision and may also potentiate earlier cataract onset. In Nigeria, for instance, the northern population which uses white, vitamin A-poor palm oil exhibits earlier cataract onset than the southern population which cooks with vitamin A-rich red palm oil.[97] The new refraction correction procedure, photorefractive keratotomy (PRK), uses an excimer laser ablation procedure. This has recently been shown to produce free radicals.[98] Furthermore this procedure, using rabbit eyes, has been recently shown to cause a transient, yet long-term decrease in concentrations of glutathione and ascorbate in various anterior chamber tissues separate from the cornea itself such as lens and iris. This shows that oxidation type stress is a potential problem with possible long-term effects that are not known at this time. The corneal endothelial cell monolayer is similar to the TM cell layer in that there is a finite population of these important cells that decreases throughout our lifetime. The endothelial cells are the site of energy-intensive ion and water pumping that must be maintained constantly to prevent corneal swelling due to influx of water.

At risk because of its direct contact with the oxygen of air, the cornea has well-developed defense systems. Use of oxidizing disinfectants for contact lenses requires rigorous post-disinfection washing to prevent the potentially damaging oxidants reaching the cornea. Corneal inflammation and infections are also a potential source of oxidant stress as leucocytes fight the infection. This cellular response produces hydrogen peroxide and hypochlorite. Previously reviewed data[72] indicate that vitamin E may be useful for treating the corneal weakening in keratoconus.

HUMAN CLINICAL STUDIES IN PROGRESS

The VECAT Study in Melbourne, Australia, the U.S. Age-Related Eye Diseases Study (AREDS),[99] and the U.S. Beaver Dam study are longitudinal studies in progress. The VECAT Study is studying the cataract reduction associated with supplemental use of 400 IU of vitamin E per day, and is expected to be finished by the year 2000. The Beaver Dam study is a descriptive noninterventional study, while the antioxidant doses in the AREDS study are at the level commonly used for antioxidant supplements (for ascorbate ca. 8 times the RDA, for tocopherol 40 times the RDA, and for β-carotene, approximately 6 times the RDA). Compliance, a problem in most intervention studies, is being monitored by spot checks in the AREDS study.

REFERENCES

1. Chamberlain CG, McAvoy JW. Evidence that fibroblast growth factor promotes lens fibre differentiation. Curr Eye Res 6:1165-9, 1987.
2. Leibowitz HM, Krueger DE, Maunder LR, Milton RC, Kini MM, Kahn HA *et al.* Framingham eye study monograph. Surv Ophthalmol. 24 (suppl):335-610, 1980.
3. Young RW. The family of sunlight-related eye diseases. Optometry and Vision Sci 71:125-144, 1994.
4. Thompson JR, Sparrow JM, Gibson JM, Rosenthal AR. Further follow up in the Leicester cataract and survival study. Invest Ophthalmol Visual Science 35:1990, 1994.
5. Hayes RP, Fisher RF. Influence of a prolonged period of low dosage x-rays on the optic and ultrastructural appearance of cataract of the human lens. Brit J Ophthalmol 63:457-464, 1979.
6. Benedek GB. Theory of transparency of the eye. Appl Optics 10:459-473, 1971.
7. Clark JI, Livesey JC, Steele JE. Phase separation inhibitors and lens transparency. Optom Vis Sci 70:873-9, 1993.

8. Creighton MO, Trevithick JR, Mousa GY, Percy DH, McKinna AJ, Dyson C, Maisel H, Globular bodies: A primary cause of the opacity in senile and diabetic posterior cortical subcapsular cataracts? Can J Ophthalmol 13:166-181, 1978.
9. Trevithick JR, Creighton MO, Ross WM, Stewart DeHaan PJ, Sanwal M. Modelling cortical cataractogenesis 2. *In vitro* effects on the lens of agents preventing glucose- and sorbitol-induced cataracts. Can J Ophthalmol. 16:32-38, 1981.
10. Bhatnagar A, Ansari NH, Wang L, Khanna P, Wang C, Srivastava SK. Calcium-mediated disintegrative globulization of isolated lens fibers mimics cataractogenesis. Exp Eye Res. 61:303-310, 1995.
11. Klintworth GK, Garner A. The Causes, Types and Morphology of Cataracts pp 1223-1272 in *Pathobiology of Ocular Disease*, Garner A, Klintworth GK, Eds, Marcel Dekker, New York, 1982.
12. Harding JJ. Cataract:sanitation or sunglasses? Lancet 1(8262):39, 1982.
13. Sasaki H, Kojima M, Shui YB, Chen HM, Nagai K, Kasuga T, Katoh N, Jin CS, Sasaki K. The Singapore-Japan Cooperative Eye Study. Abstracts U.S.-Japan Cooperative Cataract Research Group Meeting, Kona HI, November 16-19, 1997 pp. 66.
14. Katoh N, Kojima M, Sasaki H, Jonasson F, Ono M, Nagata M, Sasaki K. UV-Light exposure and pure cortical cataract: a population bases case-control study in Iceland. Abstracts U.S.-Japan Cooperative Cataract Research Group Meeting, Kona HI, November 16-19, 1997 pp. 65.
15. Bhat KS. Nutritional status of thiamine riboflavin and pyridoxine in cataract patients. Nutr. Reports International 36:685-692, 1987.
16. Linetsky M, James HL, Ortwerth BJ. The generation of superoxide anion by the UVA irradiation of human lens proteins. Exper Eye Res 63:67-74, 1996.
17. Trevithick JR, Dzialoszynski T. A new technique for enhancing luminol luminescent detection of free radicals and reactive oxygen species. Biochem Mol Biol Internat 33:1179-1190, 1994.
18. Trevithick JR, Dzialoszynski T. Endogenous superoxide-like species and antioxidant activity in ocular tissues detected by luminol luminescence. Biochem Mol Biol Internat 41:695-705, 1997.
19. Ross WM, Creighton MO, Stewart-DeHaan PJ, Sanwal M, Hirst M, Trevithick JR. Modelling cortical cataractogenesis 3. *In vivo* effects of vitamin E on cataractogenesis in diabetic rats. Can J Ophthalmol 17, 61-66, 1982.
20. Ross WM, Creighton MO, Inch WR, Trevithick JR. Radiation cataract *in vitro* reduced by vitamin E. Exper Eye Research 36,645-653, 1983.
21. Rouhiainen P, Rouhiainen H, Salonen JT. Association between low plasma vitamin E concentration and progression of early cortical lens opacities. Amer J Epidemiol 144:496-500, 1996.
22. Eglite A, Ozola G, Curbakova E. The incidence of eye disorders among Chernobyl clean-up workers. Abstracts NATO Advanced Research Workshop: Ocular radiation risk assessment in populations exposed to environmental radiation contamination. p. 34, 1997.
23. Bantseev V, Bhardwaj R, Rathbun W, Nagasawa H, Trevithick JR. Antioxidants and cataract: (cataract induction in space environment and application to terrestrial aging cataract) Biochem Molec Bio. Internat. 42:1189-1197, 1997.
24. Mitton KP, Dzialoszynski T, Sanford SE, Trevithick JR. Cysteine and ascorbate loss in the diabetic lens prior to hydration changes. Curr Eye Res 16:564-571, 1997.
25. Linklater H. *Nutritional Studies in Diabetic Cataract Prevention.* Ph.D. thesis, University of Western Ontario, 1985.
26. Kilic F. *Using Model Systems to Study Rat Lens Membrane Damage During Cortical Cataract Formation.* Ph.D. thesis, University of Western Ontario, 1995.
27. Linklater HA, Dzialoszynski T, McLeod HL, Sanford SE, Trevithick JR. Modelling cortical cataractogenesis VII. Effects of butylated hydroxy toluene (BHT) on protein leakage from lenses in diabetic rats. Exper Eye Res 43, 305-313, 1986.

28. Linklater HA, Dzialoszynski T, McLeod HL, Sanford SE, Trevithick JR. Modelling cortical cataractogenesis XI. Vitamin C treatment reduces γ-crystallin leakage from lenses in diabetic rats. Exper Eye Res 51:247-247, 1990.
29. Kilic F, Trevithick JR. Modelling Cortical Cataractogenesis 16. Leakage of Lactate Dehydrogenase: A New Method For Following Cataract Development in Cultured Lenses. Biochemistry and Molecular Biology International 35:1143-1152, 1995.
30. Robertson J McD, Donner AP, Trevithick JR. Vitamin E intake and risk of cataracts in humans. Ann NY Acad Sci 570:372-382, 1989.
31. Robertson J McD, Donner AP, Trevithick JR. A possible role for vitamins C and E in cataract prevention. Amer J Clin Nutr 53:3465-515, 1991.
32. Chylack L. Nutritional risk factors for progression of age-related nuclear cataract. Abstracts U.S.-Japan Cooperative Cataract Research Group Meeting, Kona HI, November 16-19, 1997 pp. 67.
33. Linklater HA, Dzialoszynski T, McLeod HL, Sanford SE, Trevithick JR. Modelling Cortical Cataractogenesis XII Supplemented Vitamin A Treatment Reduces γ-Crystallin Leakage from Lenses in Diabetic Rats. Lens & Eye Toxicity Res 9:115-126, 1992.
34. Kilic F, Handelman G, Serbinova E, Packer L, Trevithick JR. Modelling cortical cataractogenesis 17: *in vitro* effect of alpha-lipoic acid on glucose-induced lens membrane damage, a model of diabetic cataractogenesis. Biochemistry and Molecular Biology International. 37:361-370, 1995.
35. Trevithick JR, Linklater HA, Dzialoszynski T, McLeod HL, Sanford SE, Robertson J McD. Modelling Cortical Cataractogenesis 15: Use of combined dietary antioxidants to reduce cataract risk. Develop Ophthal 26:72-82, 1994.
36. Knekt P, Heliovaara M, Rissanen A, Aromaa A, Aaran R. Serum antioxidant vitamins and risk of cataract. Brit Med J 305:1392-1394, 1992.
37. Kilic F, Mitton K, Dzialoszynski T, Sanford SE, Trevithick JR. Modelling Cortical Cataractogenesis 14: Reduction in Lens Damage in Diabetic Rats by a Dietary Regimen Combining Vitamins C and E and Beta-Carotene. Develop Ophthalm 26:63-71, 1994.
38. Kilic F, Bhardwaj R, Trevithick JR. Modelling cortical cataractogenesis 18: *In vitro* diabetic cataract reduction by venoruton. Acta Ophthalmol Scand 74:372-376, 1996.
39. Li ZR. Reiter RJ, Fujimori O, Oh CS. Duan YP. Cataractogenesis and lipid peroxidation in newborn rats treated with buthionine sulfoximine: preventive actions of melatonin. J Pineal Res 22:117-23, 1997.
40. Niki E, Tsuchiya J, Tanimura R, Kamiya Y. Regeneration of vitamin E from α-chromanoxyl radical by glutathione and vitamin C. Chemistry Letters pp 789-792, 1982.
41. Taylor A, Nowell T. Oxidative stress, antioxidant function in relation to risk for cataract. Advances in Phanmacol 38:515-535, 1997.
42. Jacques PF, Chylack LT, McGandy RB, Harts SC. Antioxidant status in persons with and without senile cataract. Arch Ophthalmol. 108, 337-340, 1988.
43. Leske MC, Chylack LT Jr, Wu SY. the LOCS Research Group. The lens opacities case-control study. Arch Ophthalmol 109:244-251, 1990.
44. Schoenfeld ER, Leske MC. Wu SY. Recent epidemiologic studies on nutrition and cataract in India, Italy and the United States. J Am Coll Nutr. 12:521-6, 1993.
45. Sperduto RD, Hu TS, Milton RC, Zhao JL, Everett DF, Cheng QF, Blot WJ, Bing L, Taylor PR, Li JY, *et al.* The Linxian cataract studies. Two nutrition intervention trials. Arch Ophthalmol 111:1246-1253, 1993.
46. Hagen TM, Wierzbicka GT, Sillau AH, Bowman BB, Jones DP. Fate of dietary glutathione:disposition in the gastrointestinal tract. Am J Physiol 259:G524-529, 1990.
47. Caulfeild J, personal communication, 1997.

48. Babizhayev MA, Yermakova VN, Sakina NL, Evstigneeva RP, Rozhkova EA, Zheltukhina GA. N alpha-acetylcarnosine is a prodrug of L-carnosine in ophthalmic application as antioxidant. Clin Chem Acta 254:1-21, 1996.
49. McCarty C, Lloyd-Smith W, Livingston P, Jin C, Stanislavsky Y, Taylor H. Risk factors for cataract in the Melbourne Visual Impairment Project. Abstract S5-3, pp. 27 in program book for "Cataract and Posterior Opacification," a conference held at Het Trippinhuis, Amsterdam, Netherlands, Sept 29-Oct 2, 1997.
50. Delcourt C, Cristol JP, Gourgou S, Leger C, Papoz L. Association between cataract and antioxidant enzymes in the POLA study. Vision Research 36(suppl):S120, 1996.
51. Awasthi S, Srivatava SK, Piper JT, Singhal SS, Chaubey M, Awasthi YC. Curcumin protects against 4-hydroxy-2-trans-nonenal induced cataract formation in rat lenses. Am J Clin Nutr 64:761-6, 1996.
52. Kilic F, Trevithick JR. Vitamin C reduces cytochalasin D cataractogenesis. Current Eye Res 14:943-949, 1995.
53. Muller A, Villain M, Favreau B, Sandillon F, Privat A, Bonne C. Differential effect of ischemia/reperfusion on pigmented and albino rabbit retina. Ocular Pharmacol Therapeut 12 :337-342, 1996.
54. Artola A, Alio JL, Bellot JL, Ruiz JM. Lipid peroxidation in the iris and its protection by means of viscoelastic substances (sodium hyaluronate and hydroxypropylmethylcellulose). Ophthalmic Res 25:172-6, 1993.
55. Worm KH, Klimczak U, Schulte-Frohlinde D. Radiosensitization and radioprotection of E. coli by alcohols. Int J Radiat Biol 64:485-95, 1993.
56. Clayton RM, Cuthbert J, Duffy J, Seth J, Phillips CI, Bartholomew RS, Reid JMcK. Some risk factors associated with cataract in SE. Scotland: a pilot study. Trans Opthalmol Soc UK. 102, 331-336, 1982.
57. Stark WJ, Worthern DN, Holladay JT, Bath PE, Jacobs ME, Murray GC, *et al.* The FDA report on intraocular lenses. Ophthalmol 90:311-7, 1983.
58. Steinberg EP *et al.* National study of cataract surgery outcomes: Variation in 4-month postoperative outcomes as reflected in multiple outcome measures. Ophthalmol 101:1131-1141, 1994.
59. Javitt JC, Tielsch JM, Canner JK, Kolb MM, Sommer A, Steinberg EP. National outcomes of cataract extraction, Increased risk of retinal complications associated with Nd: YAG laser capsulotomy. Ophthalmol 99:1487-1498, 1992.
60. van der Schaft TL, Mooy CM, de Bruijn WC, Mulder PGH, Pameyer JH, de Jong PTVM. Increased prevalence of disciform macular degeneration after cataract extraction with implantation of an intraocular lens. Brit J Ophthalmol 78:441-445, 1994.
61. Bourne WM, Nelson LR, Hodge DO. Continued endothelial cell loss ten years after lens implantation. Ophthalmol 101:1014-1023, 1994.
62. Tunstall-Pedoe H, Kuulasmaa K, Amouyel P, Arveiler D, Rajakangas AM, Pajak A. Myocardial infarction and coronary deaths in the World Health Organization MONICA Project. Registration procedures, event rates, and case-fatality rates in 38 populations from 21 countries in four continents. Circulation 90:583-612, 1994.
63. Street DA, Javitt JC, Wang O, Tieloch JM, Steinberg EP, 1993 Morbidity and mortality in patients undergoing cataract extraction: A nationwide case-control study. Invest. Ophthalmol Visual Sci 34:1065, 1993.
64. Liu IY, White L, LaCroix AZ. The association of age-related macular degeneration and lens opacities in the aged. Am J Public Health 79:765-9, 1989.
65. Young RW. Pathophysiology of age-related macular degeneration. Surv Ophthalmol 31:291-305, 1987.

66. Garner A. Pathology of macular degeneration in the elderly. Trans Ophthalmol Soc U.K. 95:54-61, 1975.
67. Garner A. Diabetic retinopathy in Pathobiology of Ocular Disease, Garner A, Klintworth GK, Eds, Marcel Dekker, New York, pp. 1539-1556, 1982.
68. Snodderly DM. Evidence for protection against age-related macular degeneration by carotenoids and antioxidant vitamins. Am J Clin Nutr 62(Suppl):1448S-1461S, 1995.
69. Landrum JT, Bone RA, Kilburn MD. The macular pigment: a possible role in protection from age-related macular degeneration. Adv Pharmacol 38:537-56, 1997.
70. Allikmets R, Singh N, Sun H, Shroyer NF, Hutchinson A, Chidambaram A, Gerrard B, Baird L, Stauffer D, Peiffer A, Rattner A, Smallwood P, Li Y, Anderson KL, Lewis RA, Nathans J, Leppert M, Dean M, Lupski JR. A photoreceptor cell-specific ATP-binding transporter gene (ABCR) is mutated in recessive Stargardt macular dystrophy. Nat Genet 15:236-46, 1997.
71. Menerath JM, Cluzel J, Droy-Lefaix MT, Doly M. Experimental electroretinographic exploration of retinal ischemia: preventive use of free radical scavengers and anti-PAF agents. J Ocul Pharmacol Ther 13:81-8, 1997.
72. Trevithick JR, Robertson JM, Mitton KP. Vitamin E and the eye, in *Vitamin E in Health and Disease*, Packer L, Fuchs J, Eds pp. 873-926, Marcel Dekker, New York, 1993.
73. West S, Vitale S, Hallfrisch J, Munoz B, Muller D, Bressler S, Bressler NM. Are antioxidants or supplements protective for age-related macular degeneration? Arch Ophthalmol 112:222-227, 1994.
74. Maresperlman JA, Klein R, Klein BEK, Greger JL, Brady WE, Palta M, Ritter LL. Association of zinc and antioxidant nutrients with age-related maculopathy. Arch Ophthalmol 114:991-997, 1996.
75. Cazevieille C, Osborne NN. Retinal neurones containing kainate receptors are influenced by exogenous kainate and ischaemia while neurones lacking these receptors are not — melatonin counteracts the effects of ischaemia and kainate. Brain Res 755:91-100, 1997.
76. Nash MS, Osborne NN. Agonist-induced effects on cyclic AMP metabolism are affected in pigment epithelial cells of the Royal College of Surgeons rat. Neurochem Int 27:253-62, 1995.
77. Bursell S-E, Clermont A, Aiello LM, Aiello LP, King GL. Vitamin E treatment and diabetic microvascular disease in diabetic patients. U.S. -Japan Nutrition and Metabolism Panel-1997. Abstract presented at meeting, Sept. 1997.
78. Gjessing HGA. Gibt es einen antagonismus zwischen cataracta senilis und haabscher seniler makula verlndergungen? Acta Ophthalmol 31:401-21, 1953.
79. Klein BE, Klein R. Cataracts and macular degeneration in older Americans. Arch Ophthalmol 100:571-3, 1982.
80. Van de Hoeve J. Senile makuladegeneration und senile linsentrbung. Grafes Arch Ophthalmol 98:1-6, 1918.
81. Clarke IS, Dzialoszynski T, Sanford SE, Chevendra V, Trevithick JR. Dietary prevention of damage to retinal proteins in RCS rats. *Ocular Toxicity*. Lerman S, Tripathi R. Eds. Marcel Dekker, New York pp. 253-272, 1989.
82. Zigler JS, Hess HH. Cataracts in the Royal College of Surgeons Rat: evidence for initiation by peroxidation products. Exper Eye Res 1985; 41:67-76, 1985.
83. O'Keefe TL, Hess HH, Zigler JS Jr, Kuwabara T, Knapka JJ. Prevention of cataracts in pink-eyed RCS rats by dark rearing. Exper. Eye Res. 51:509-517, 1990.
84. Alekseev VN, Ketlinskii SA, Sharonov BP, Martynova EB, Lauta VF. Lipid peroxidation in experimental glaucoma and the possibilities for its correction. [Russian] Vestn Oftalmol. 109:10.
85. Kurysheva NI, Vinetskaia MI, Erichev VP, Demchuk ML, Kuryshev SI. Contribution of free-radical reactions of chamber humor to the development of primary open-angle glaucoma. [Russian] Vestn Oftalmol. 112:3-5, 1996.

86. Lebedev OI, Dumenova NV, Kovalevskii VV. Laser irradiation: study of total effect of irradiation of the eyeball. A clinical study. [Russian] Vestn Oftalmol 111:17-9, 1995.
87. Popova ZS, Kuz'minov OD. Treatment of primary open-angle glaucoma by the method of combined use of hyperbaric oxygenation and antioxidants. [Russian] Vestn Oftalmol 112:4-6, 1996.
88. Filina AA, Davydova NG, Endrikhovskii SN, Shamshinova AM. Lipoic acid as a means of metabolic therapy of open-angle glaucoma. Vestn Oftalmol 111:6-8, 1995.
89. Bunin AI, Ermakov VN, Filina AA. New directions in the hypotensive therapy of open-angle glaucoma. [Russian] Vestn Oftalmol. 109:3-6, 1993.
90. Schumer RA, Podos SM. The nerve of glaucoma. Arch Ophthalmol. 112:37-44, 1994.
91. Bonne C. New perspectives in the pharmacological treatment of glaucoma. Therapie 48:559-65, 1993.
92. Osborne NN. Serotonin and melatonin in the iris/ciliary processes and their involvement in intraocular pressure. Acta Neurobiol Exp (Warsz). 54 (Suppl):57-64, 1994.
93. Yue BY. The extracellular matrix and its modulation in the trabecular meshwork. Surv Ophthalmol 40:379-390, 1996.
94. Mitton KP, Tumminia SJ, Arora J, Zelenka P, Epstein DL, Russell P. Transient loss of αB-crystallin and early cellular response to mechanical stretch. Biochem Biophys Res Commun 235:69-73, 1997.
95. Russell P, Johnson DH. Enzymes protective of oxidative damage present in all decades of life in the trabecular meshwork as detected by two-dimensional gel electrophoresis protein maps. J Glaucoma 5:317-24, 1996.
96. O'Brien ET, Perkins SL, Roberts BC, Epstein DL. Dexamethasone inhibits trabecular cell retraction. Exp Eye Res 62:675-88, 1996.
97. Imafidon C. Personal communication, 1995.
98. Hayashi S, Ishimoto S, Wu GS, Wee WR, Rao NA, Mcdonnell PJ. Oxygen free radical damage in the cornea after excimer laser therapy. Brit J Ophthalmol 81:141-144, 1997.
99. Sperduto RD, Ferris FL, Kurinij N. Do we have a nutritional treatment for age-related cataract of macular degeneration? Arch Ophthalmol 108:1403-5, 1997.

25

Antioxidants and Neurological Diseases

Ronald J. Sokol, M.D.
Department of Pediatrics
University of Colorado School of Medicine, Denver, Colorado, USA

Andreas M. Papas, Ph. D.
Health and Nutrition
Eastman Chemical Company, Kingsport, Tennessee, USA

INTRODUCTION

Interest in the role of antioxidants in neurological disease has recently expanded, however, vitamin E was linked directly to the function of the nervous system many decades ago. In 1928, paralysis was observed in suckling offspring of vitamin E-deficient female rats.[1] Subsequently, nutritional encephalomalacia was reported in the chick and nutritional muscular dystrophy in guinea pigs and rats fed vitamin E-deficient diets.[2,3] In 1965, Kayden *et al.* proposed that neurologic abnormalities in abetalipoproteinemia, a very rare human disease characterized by chronic fat malabsorption and the absence of circulating beta-lipoproteins, were caused by malabsorption and deficiency of vitamin E.[4] Subsequently, it has been well demonstrated that chil-

0-8493-8009-X/98/$0.00+$.50

dren and adults with a variety of diseases causing chronic lipid and vitamin E malabsorption develop a characteristic neurologic disorder similar in nature to that observed in abetalipoproteinemia.[5] The isolated vitamin E deficiency syndrome, in the absence of lipid malabsorption and its strong association with neurologic dysfunction, further confirmed the neurologic role of vitamin E in man.[6]

While earlier studies focused on vitamin E, lipid malabsorption disorders may also impair the absorption of other fat-soluble nutrients and food components, including other antioxidants. For example, cholestatic children have low blood levels of vitamins A, D, E, K and β-carotene,[7,8] and cystic fibrosis patients have low blood levels of β-carotene.[9-11] In addition to the antioxidant nutrients, a large number of phytochemicals have antioxidant activity and, as discussed in other chapters, may play an important role in nutrition and health.[12] Several studies documented serious oxidative stress associated with vitamin E deficiency, which is probably accentuated further by poor absorption of other fat-soluble antioxidants.[10,13-17] All major indicators of oxidative stress were observed, including reduced resistance of low density lipoprotein (LDL) and fatty acids to oxidation, increased production of malondialdehyde and thiobarbituric reactive substances (TBARS), and hemolysis.

For other major neurologic diseases such as Alzheimer's disease, Parkinson's disease, Huntington's disease, and amyotrophic lateral sclerosis (ALS), genetic defects, not related to vitamin E deficiency, are believed to be the cause. Oxidative stress may play a role either in triggering the defect when it is not inherited, or accelerating the onset of the disease after the defect occurs. Extensive postmortem and other studies support the involvement of oxidative stress in the development of these diseases probably due, at least in part, to impaired mitochondrial function. Evidence supporting oxidative stress includes increased brain iron content, decline of superoxide dismutase (SOD) and glutathione (GSH), and oxidative damage to lipids, proteins, and DNA.[18-25] In familial forms of ALS, genetic defects in cytosolic SOD have been demonstrated. In addition, neuroleptic drugs such L-beta-3,4-dihydroxyphenylalanine hydrochloride (L-DOPA), used in the treatment of Parkinson's disease, may increase the production of free radicals.[26,27] In the last decade, several epidemiological and clinical studies evaluated the role of antioxidants, primarily vitamin E, in delaying the onset or for treatment of these diseases with mixed results.[28-30]

In this review, we will describe the major features of the vitamin E deficiency neurologic syndrome. We will also discuss the role of oxidative stress in the pathogenesis of other major neurologic degenerative disorders. Finally, we will critically discuss the possible use of vitamin E and antioxidants as nutritional and pharmacological agents in delaying the onset and management of these diseases.

NEURODEGENERATIVE DISEASES ASSOCIATED WITH VITAMIN E DEFICIENCY

Deficiency Due to Malabsorption

Malabsorption is the most common cause of serious vitamin E deficiency because tocopherols are ubiquitous in grains, vegetable oils, and animal fat. As discussed in the earlier chapter on vitamin E (Papas), ingested tocopherols are incorporated into micelles in the intestinal lumen with the aid of pancreatic secretions and bile acids produced in the liver. They are absorbed from the small intestine and secreted into lymph in chylomicrons synthesized in the intestinal epithelium. Lipoprotein lipases catabolize circulating chylomicrons rapidly and a small amount of tocopherol may be transferred from chylomicron remnants to other lipoproteins or tissues during this process, and apolipoprotein E is transferred to chylomicron remnants. Because the liver has specific apolipoprotein E receptors, it retains and clears the majority of the chylomicron remnants. Tocopherols are then released within the hepatocyte where they are bound to hepatic tocopherol transfer protein, which is involved in the preferential secretion of alpha tocopherol by the hepatocyte into very low-density lipoproteins (VLDL) that then circulate in the plasma. VLDL is hydrolyzed by lipoprotein lipase to low-density lipoproteins (LDL) which carry the largest part of plasma tocopherols and appears to exchange them readily with high-density lipoproteins (HDL) and with tissues.[31]

Gastrointestinal, pancreatic, and hepatic disorders that interfere with the digestion or absorption of lipid impair vitamin E absorption (Figure 1). Indeed, low serum concentrations have been observed in patients with a variety of steatorrheic disorders;[32] an inverse relationship was evident between the serum vitamin E concentration and the severity of impairment of fat absorption. Chronic conditions causing symptomatic vitamin E deficiency include abetalipoproteinemia and other disorders of lipoprotein secretion, chronic cholestatic hepatobiliary diseases, cystic fibrosis and other causes of pancreatic insufficiency, short bowel syndrome, radiation enteritis, congenital hymphangiectasia, intestinal pseudo-obstruction, and others.[5] The isolated vitamin E deficiency syndrome, a genetic defect in the structure of the tocopherol transfer protein, is a major exception because it causes symptomatic vitamin E deficiency despite normal intestinal absorption of vitamin E.[33,34]

Symptoms of Vitamin E Deficiency

Early recognition of vitamin E deficiency in patients with neurological disease is important because it may be possible to reverse, stabilize, or prevent neurological deterioration by correcting the deficiency.[35,36] For this reason, a high index of suspicion for vitamin E deficiency is obligatory when evaluating patients with movement disorders, ataxia, neuropathy, or retinopathy. The characteristic clinical findings of this neurologic syndrome include loss of deep tendon reflexes, truncal and limb ataxia, impaired position and vibratory sensations, ophthalmoplegia, muscle weakness, and, if severe, dystonic facial appearance, pes cavus, and scoliosis (Figure 2). In advanced cases, the child or adult may be confined to a wheel chair and be unable to care for him(her)self. These findings are corroborated by electrophysiologic tests that show decreased action potential of sensory nerves, mild denervation of muscles, delayed conduction through the posterior columns of the spinal cord, abnormal visual evoked response, and abnormal electroretinograms.

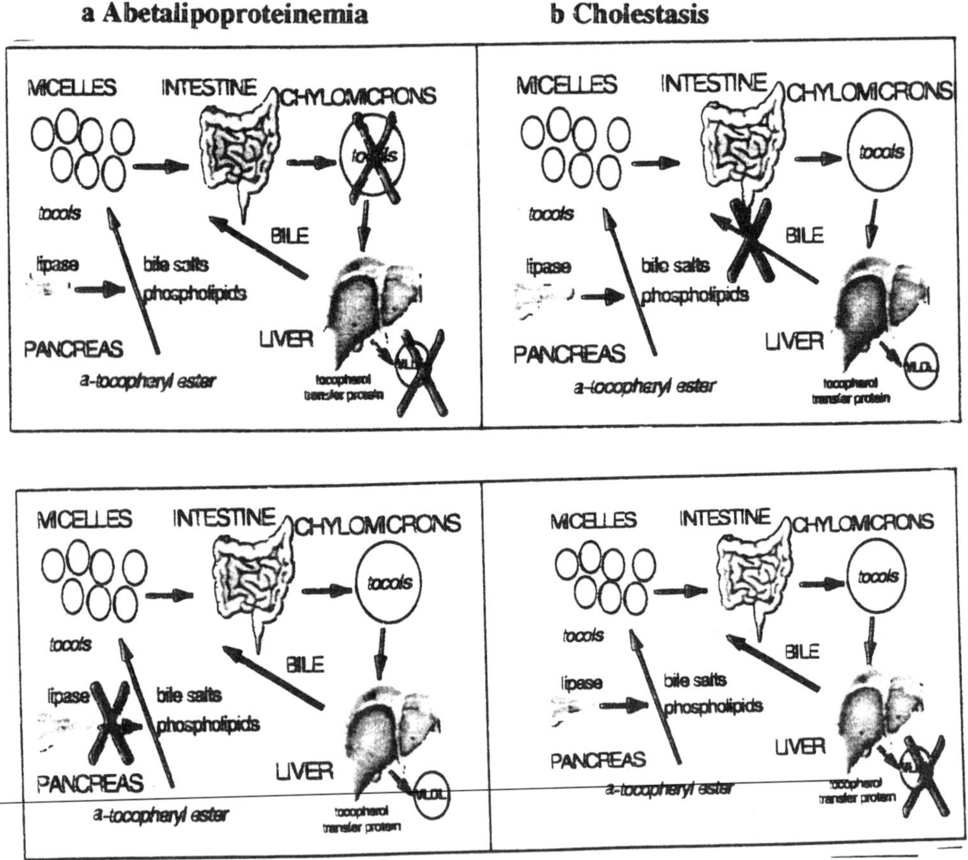

Figure 1. Absorption and transport of vitamin E and defects (shown by large X) causing abetalipoproteinemia (panel a), cholestasis (b), cystic fibrosis (c), and familial isolated vitamin E (FIVE) deficiency (d).

Abetalipoproteinemia and Other Defects of Beta-Lipoprotein Secretion

Abetalipoproteinemia is a rare autosomal recessively inherited disease characterized by failure to assemble and secrete normal apolipoprotein B-containing lipoproteins. The defect is caused by a deficiency of the microsomal triglyceride transfer protein that is involved in translocation of apolipoprotein B-containing lipoproteins across the endoplasmic reticulum. This defect prevents the intestinal and hepatic secretion of chylomicrons and VLDL, which are essential for transport of vitamin E (Figure 1a).[31] The inability of the intestinal mucosal cell to transport absorbed dietary fat into the mesenteric lymphatic circulation causes steatorrhea from birth. These two perturbations of normal tocopherol metabolism result in serum vitamin E levels that are almost undetectable and adipose tissue stores that are extremely low.[37] The resulting vitamin E deficiency leads to progressive ataxia and pigmented retinopathy (Figure 2); acanthocytosis of red blood cells occurs because of the abnormal lipid composition of the red cell membrane. Long-term treatment trials with massive supplements of vitamin E have conclusively demonstrated that neurological function can be preserved if vitamin E deficiency is corrected at an early age.[35,36,38,39]

Identical neurological findings have been described in homozygous hypobetalipoproteinemia patients who fail to synthesize adequate amounts of apolipoprotein B and consequently malabsorb lipid and vitamin E.[40] Other disorders in which apolipoprotein B synthesis is intact but some other chylomicron-processing defect is present, such as chylomicron retention disease (Anderson's disease), are associated with vitamin E malabsorption and deficiency and neurological degeneration.[41]

Treatment

Serum vitamin E measurements do not accurately reflect vitamin E status in abetalipoproteinemia because the underlying problem is the absence of beta-lipoproteins, the major carrier of tocopherol. Rather, adipose tissue vitamin E content is a better indicator.[37] Patients with abetalipoproteinemia should be assumed to be vitamin E deficient, unless they receive adequate α-tocopherol in parenteral nutrition infusates or with chronic intramuscular injection. Otherwise, they should all receive 100-200 mg/kg/day of α-tocopherol or α-tocopheryl acetate in two or three divided oral doses with meals and their status monitored by neurologic examination, serial needle aspirate biopsies of adipose tissue for analysis of repletion of vitamin E stores, or serial electrophysiological studies (SEP or visual evoked response). In addition, most authorities recommend concomitant treatment with vitamin A monitored by its serum concentration.[38,39] This therapeutic regimen stabilized neurological abnormalities, as well as retinal dysfunction, in older patients and completely prevented their development if therapy was started early in life. Patients have now been treated in this way for 19-26 years without development of significant visual impairment or appreciable neuropathy.

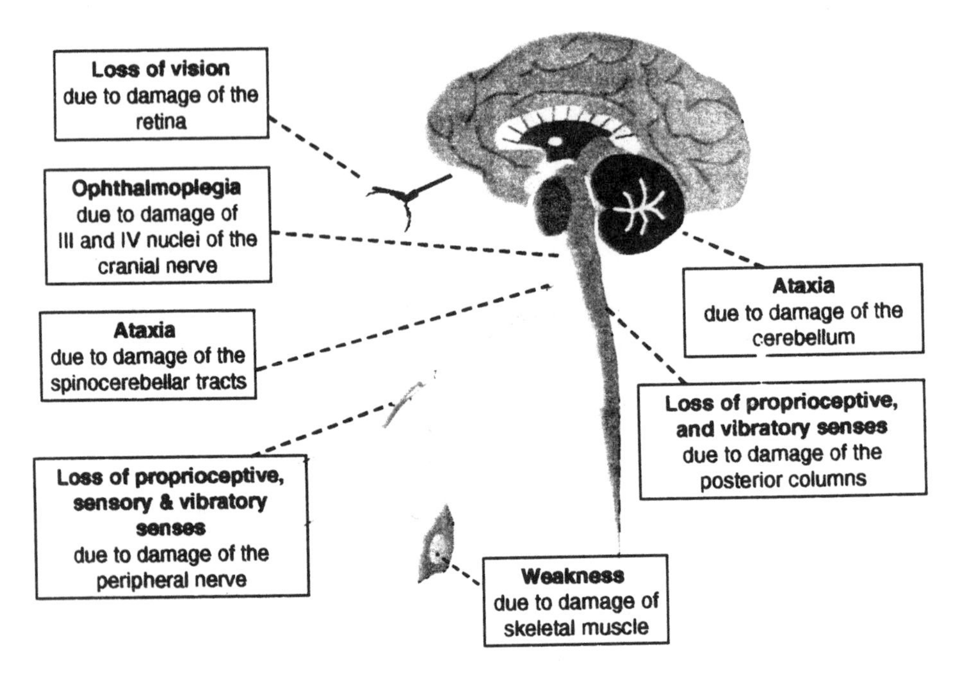

Figure 2. Symptoms of neurological diseases associated with vitamin E deficiency.

Chronic Cholestatic Hepatobiliary Disorders

Chronic cholestatic hepatobiliary disorders include diseases of the liver (idiopathic neonatal hepatitis, chronic hepatitis, metabolic liver diseases, and familial cholestatic syndromes), of the intrahepatic bile ducts (Alagille syndrome, paucity of interlobular bile ducts, primary biliary cirrhosis, graft vs. host disease), and of the extrahepatic bile duct (extrahepatic biliary atresia, primary and secondary sclerosing cholangitis).[2,3,5,6] Children, and rarely adults, suffering from chronic forms of these diseases develop degenerative neurological disorders. In 1981, these disorders were linked to vitamin E deficiency. The reduction in bile flow from the liver to the intestine in cholestasis leads to diminished concentrations of bile acids in the intestinal lumen, causing failure of micellar solubilization and impairment of absorption of dietary lipids, including fat-soluble nutrients and antioxidants (Figure 1b).

dietary lipids, including fat-soluble nutrients and antioxidants (Figure 1b). Severe cholestasis results in biochemical (low serum vitamin E concentrations and low serum vitamin E: total lipid ratios) and functional (elevated hydrogen peroxide hemolysis) evidence of vitamin E deficiency, as well as depleted adipose tissue, muscle, and nerve concentrations. Supplementation with common oral forms of vitamin E does not correct the biochemical deficiency in 50-75% of children with these disorders.[44] Neurological abnormalities, which develop as early as the second year of life, may lead to irreversible, devastating consequences if the vitamin E deficiency is not corrected by the second decade of life.[45] Neurological symptoms occur much more commonly in vitamin E-deficient children with chronic cholestasis compared to those with cystic fibrosis. Biochemical evidence of vitamin E deficiency has also been described in approximately 20-50% of adults with chronic cholestasis due to primary biliary cirrhosis,[46] although a direct relationship to neurological symptoms was observed in only one patient. However, the majority of patients with primary biliary cirrhosis have severe malabsorption of vitamin E even when serum indices indicate vitamin E sufficiency.[47]

Treatment

In childhood and adult cholestasis, biliary lipids are regurgitated into the systemic circulation and, in combination with poor clearance of lipoproteins, may elevate serum vitamin E concentrations thus masking the underlying vitamin E deficiency.[6] Therefore, serum vitamin E concentrations alone do not accurately reflect vitamin E status during cholestasis and the ratio of serum vitamin E to total serum lipid concentration has been advocated to compensate for the hyperlipidemia of cholestasis. Ratios below 0.8 mg tocopherol/g total lipids indicate biochemical deficiency, and ratios below 0.4 mg/g denote severe deficiency. Other assays, such as hydrogen peroxide hemolysis or malondialdehyde release from red blood cells, can be used to confirm the deficiency state if there is a question; however, these assays have not been validated during hyperlipidemia. Although adipose tissue levels of vitamin E are usually low in these patients, there is no clinical need to obtain tissue levels.

Reversing the vitamin E deficiency state during cholestasis is beneficial. After initial reports of improvement from small observational trials,[48,49] five larger treatment trials of over 50 children have been reported.[50] Vitamin E therapy for 1-4 years prevented neurological abnormalities in 25% of the patients, stabilized function in another 25%, and resulted in improvement in 50% of the patients. The magnitude of the response to vitamin E repletion was age-dependent. Children under age 3 years showed complete reversal or prevention of development of neurologic symptoms, whereas older patients with more advanced disease had stabilization or more limited and gradual improvement; the most severely affected patients continued to have significant neurological handicaps despite vitamin E therapy. The better outcome in young children underscores the need to determine very early in life if vitamin E deficiency exists and initiate therapy, or to prevent its development by early vitamin E supplementation in cholestatic infants predisposed to vitamin E malabsorption.

Treatment of vitamin E deficiency should be started with large oral doses of standard vitamin E preparations, starting with 25-50 IU/kg/day and advancing by 50 IU/kg/day increments up to 150-200 IU/kg/day if the ratio of serum E to total lipids does not normalize (>0.8 mg/g) within 2-3 weeks. Vitamin E capsules can be opened and the contents put in formula or on food that is ingested followed by formula or milk. It is advisable to keep serum vitamin E below 25-30 μg/ml, unless serum lipids are extremely high in which case the serum vitamin E:total lipid ratio should be the index that must be corrected. We prefer using α-tocopherol instead of esterified preparations because of the theoretical requirement of intraluminal bile acids to stimulate the mucosal tocopheryl ester hydrolytic enzyme before intestinal absorption of tocopheryl esters can occur. In addition, the RRR-isomer (d-α-tocopherol) is more bioactive than the *all-rac* form (d,1-α-tocopherol) and exhibits efficient transport and uptake by the nervous system.[31,51,52] Alternatively, the liquid form of water-soluble vitamin E (see below) can be administered from the onset. The vitamin E is given at the time of maximal bile flow, as a single morning dose with breakfast several hours before administration of any medication that may interfere with vitamin E absorption, such as cholestyramine, vitamin A, or ferrous sulfate.

Dosage adjustments are dictated by the ratio of serum vitamin E to total lipids. In patients with severe cholestasis, intraluminal bile acid concentrations are well below the critical micellar concentration resulting in failure of absorption of standard oral vitamin E preparations regardless of the size of the dose.[42] These patients usually have serum direct bilirubin above 3-4 mg/dl and serum bile acid levels at least 10-fold elevated. However, patients may be anicteric (yet have very high serum bile acid concentrations) and be incapable of absorbing vitamin E. For this reason it is absolutely essential to monitor vitamin E status before and during therapy, not to assume that the recommended dose will be absorbed and correct the deficiency. If vitamin E status does not normalize after several months of the maximal oral dose, therapy should be started with the water-soluble oral form of vitamin E (see later). Rarely is parenteral vitamin E therapy necessary with the availability of the water-soluble vitamin E. In the United States, there is no available form of parenteral vitamin E. Elsewhere, parenteral d,1-α–tocopheryl acetate (100 mg/ml) is available from Hoffman-LaRoche (Basel, Switzerland; Ephynal), without limitations on its use. One ampule is administered intramuscularly per dose and the interval between doses is calculated to provide the approximately 1.0 mg/kg/day. In small children, the ampule is divided into two 0.5 ml injections to prevent subcutaneous leakage that can cause erythema and induration.[44] A French group has successfully used a slightly lower dose of Ephynal.[53] Use of any other parenteral vitamin E preparation intramuscularly is discouraged unless vigorous safety testing in children and adults has been adequately performed and reviewed by the appropriate regulatory agencies.

Recent studies now indicate that a water-soluble ester of vitamin E, d-α-tocopheryl polyethylene glycol-1000 succinate (TPGS: Eastman Chemical Company, Kingsport, TN; Figure 3), is absorbed after oral administration in children with severe cholestasis, corrects the biochemical vitamin E deficiency state at a dose of 15-30 IU/kg/day, appears to be nontoxic, and reverses and prevents neurological dysfunction.[54] Inasmuch as a small portion of the polyethylene glycol present in TPGS is absorbed and excreted in the urine, the potential is present for inducing a hyperosmolar state if the patient suffers from renal failure or dehydration. More than 50 children with severe cholestasis, who were unresponsive to other forms of vitamin E, received TPGS in a multicenter trial, all children showing correction of vitamin E deficiency without adverse effects.[50] A commercial product in the United States [Liqui-E; Twin Laboratories, Ronkonkoma, NY contains 26.6 IU TPGS per ml (as well as lecithin, glycerol, and sorbitol)] is available for over-the-counter use and is well tolerated by cholestatic children.

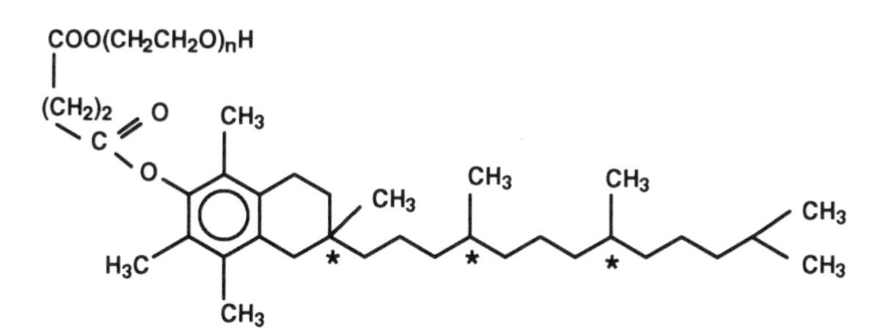

Figure 3. d-α-Tocopheryl polyethylene glycol-1000 succinate (TPGS) is a water-soluble form of vitamin E which forms its own micelles and is absorbed by cholestatic patients.

Although biochemical vitamin E deficiency may be present in over 50% of adults with primary biliary cirrhosis, neurological dysfunction is rarer.[46,47]

Therefore, the aggressiveness with which vitamin E deficiency should be corrected in adults with cholestasis is controversial. In the absence of neurological indications, it has been recommended that vitamin E therapy be started to prevent possible additional hepatic injury caused by copper accumulation and ongoing oxidant stress associated with cholestasis and to correct possible impaired neutrophil function. Criteria for defining vitamin E deficiency and treatment modalities should be similar to those used in cholestatic children. The availability of TPGS increases the ease by which vitamin E deficiency can be corrected in these patients.

Other antioxidants may further improve the antioxidant status. A recent study with cholestatic children reported that the resistance of LDL to oxidation remained unchanged even though TPGS supplementation improved their vitamin E and neurologic status.[55] As discussed below, β-carotene improves the resistance to oxidation of LDL in cystic fibrosis patients. Thus a combination of TPGS and other antioxidants might reduce further oxidative stress. TPGS may play a useful role in such studies because it enhances the absorption of other fat-soluble materials by providing micelle-like vehicles. For example, TPGS enhanced the absorption of vitamin D in cholestatic children and cyclosporin in children who received liver transplants.[7,56]

Cystic Fibrosis and Pancreatic Insufficiency

Cystic fibrosis is the most common lethal autosomal recessive disease among Caucasians. In cystic fibrosis, increased viscosity of pancreatic secretions causes obstruction of pancreatic ducts, leading ultimately to destruction and fibrosis of the exocrine pancreas in 85% of patients. The resulting failure of secretion of pancreatic digestive enzymes (Figure 1c) causes steatorrhea and malabsorption of vitamin E and possibly other fat-soluble antioxidants, even when pancreatic enzyme supplements are administered orally.[9,10,57,58] In addition, a diminished bile acid pool size caused by increased fecal excretion of bile acids may contribute to the impairment of absorption of fat-soluble antioxidants. Low serum vitamin E and β-carotene concentrations are common in unsupplemented cystic fibrosis patients.[9,10,57-59] In contrast, vitamin C levels are similar[60] or sometime higher than in normal controls.[9] Several studies documented oxidative stress in cystic fibrosis patients and particularly increased lipid and lipoprotein oxidation.[13,15,58] Supplementation with vitamin E or β-carotene reduced indices of oxidative stress such as blood malondialdehyde and lipid peroxides.[9,58,59]

Treatment

Patients receiving oral replacement of pancreatic enzymes respond well to 5-10 IU/kg/day of oral vitamin E if there is no serious liver involvement.

Cystic fibrosis patients with pancreatic insufficiency who receive pancreatic enzymes supplements should be routinely treated with this dose of vitamin E even if not deficient. Cystic fibrosis or alcoholic patients with cholestatic liver disease or cirrhosis should be evaluated and treated in the same manner as the other patients with chronic cholestasis. In the absence of hyperlipidemia, once treatment has been initiated, serum vitamin E concentrations above 5 μg/ml reflect successful vitamin E repletion and normal vitamin E status in patients with cystic fibrosis. Supplementation should continue for life. Serum vitamin E concentrations and neurological function should be monitored at least yearly to assure adequate absorption and compliance. Occasional patients do not respond to this dose of vitamin E and larger doses may be needed.

Recently, several studies evaluated the role of β-carotene in cystic fibrosis patients for periods up to 16 months.[9,10,58] Doses in the range of approximately 0.5-1.0 mg/kg, normalized β-carotene status within 2-3 weeks and improved several circulating markers of oxidative stress such as LDL oxidation and malondialdehyde production. In addition, one study reported that β-carotene improved vitamin A status.[10] It is likely that many factors contribute to oxidative stress in cystic fibrosis since multiple organs are involved. Investigation of the role of antioxidant therapy in improving lung and hepatic function is now in progress.

Other Fat Malabsorption Disorders

In adults, vitamin E deficiency can result from chronic dysfunction or resection of the small bowel.[33,61-64] Lengthy intestinal resections (creating a short bowel syndrome) for treatment of Crohn's Disease, mesenteric vascular thrombosis, or intestinal pseudoobstruction have been associated with vitamin E deficiency and neurological degeneration. These conditions require vitamin E supplementation, which may be provided intravenously in the multiple vitamin supplement in the patient's parenteral nutrition infusates or as an oral supplement. Other medical conditions in adults that may cause vitamin E malabsorption and deficiency include the blind loop syndrome, intestinal lymphangiectasia,[65] celiac disease,[66] and chronic pancreatitis leading to pancreatic insufficiency.[62,67] Frequently these conditions are associated with the deposition of lipofuscin pigment in smooth muscle cells of the digestive tract ('brown bowel syndrome' and intestinal ceroidosis) presumably due to accumulation of peroxidized membrane lipid. Serum vitamin E levels may fall within 1-2 years of acquired lipid malabsorption in adolescents and adults; neurological and ophthalmologic symptoms, however, develop 5-20 years later in adults as opposed to after 1-2 years of vitamin E deficiency in young children. This difference in rapidity of development of neurological injury is most likely related to the increased susceptibility of the young developing nervous system, the time required to deplete nervous tissue stores of vitamin E in the adult, and age-related differences in other antioxidant protective mechanisms.

Treatment

Most patients with short bowel syndrome or other chronic fat malabsorption disease, who are found to be vitamin E deficient, respond to large supplemental oral doses of vitamin E (200-3600 mg/day).[33,61-63] The water soluble TPGS may be used in patients not responding to the standard forms of vitamin E.[68] Intramuscular injections of vitamin E are only rarely necessary. Because 5-20 years of deficiency appear to be necessary before overt neurological symptoms develop in adolescents and adults with long-standing Crohn's disease, gluten-sensitive enteropathy, radiation enteritis, and short bowel syndrome, asymptomatic vitamin E deficiency is more common than previously appreciated. Therefore, periodic serum vitamin E concentrations and neurological examinations should be incorporated into the standard clinical monitoring of patients with ongoing steatorrhea. The neurological response to vitamin E repletion has been dramatic in many of these patients.

Isolated Vitamin E Deficiency Syndrome

This syndrome is also known as familial isolated vitamin E (FIVE) deficiency because it has been observed in families and siblings.[9,31] It is also referred to as ataxia with vitamin E deficiency (AVED). It has been described in several dozen patients worldwide. This syndrome is unique because it causes deficiency of vitamin E despite normal lipid and vitamin E absorption.[33,34,61,63,64,70,71] It is associated with neurological deterioration, (generally ataxia, head titubation, and clumsiness) similar to that observed in cases of vitamin E deficiency resulting from malabsorption; however, impairment of eye movements and retinal degeneration are very unusual. Instead, decreased vibratory sensation, ataxia, head titubation, and muscle weakness are the predominant symptoms. These differences may result from adequate absorption of dietary lipid in contrast to the lipid malabsorption diseases. As a result, tissues contain higher levels of polyunsaturated fatty acids, which, in the absence of vitamin E, are more likely to be oxidized to harmful products.

This syndrome is an inborn error in vitamin E metabolism with autosomal recessive inheritance in most cases. It was first postulated that selective impairment of intestinal absorption of vitamin E was causing this disorder. In contrast, our investigations using deuterated α-tocopherol (a stable isotope) in physiological doses have demonstrated normal intestinal absorption and chylomicron transport of ingested vitamin E, but defective hepatic resecretion of absorbed tocopherol into lipoproteins in the liver.[31,72] The most logical explanation for these findings was a structurally or functionally abnormal hepatic tocopherol transfer protein (Figure 1d). As discussed in earlier chapters, this protein has been identified and characterized.[73-75] Further studies by Traber *et al.* using stable vitamin E isotopes showed that some FIVE patients did not biodiscriminate at all between the naturally occurring RRR and synthetic all-rac-α-tocopherol, while others were intermediate between non-discriminators and controls. These researchers suggested that the non-discriminators are lacking this protein, or have a marked defect in the binding region of the protein; and that patients who discriminate, but have difficulty maintaining plasma RRR-α-tocopherol concentrations, have a less severe defect, or perhaps a defect in the transfer function of the protein.[72] All patients with the isolated vitamin E deficiency syndrome have mutations in the gene for this protein, thus confirming that this defect causes this inherited form of vitamin E deficiency.[31,74-78]

The incidence of this disorder may be higher than initially estimated, stressing the need to investigate the vitamin E status in patients of any age with movement disorders, ataxia, or peripheral neuropathy, even in the absence of lipid malabsorption and apparently normal blood levels. Two surveys of patients with cerebellar ataxia failed to demonstrate vitamin E deficiency in 95 patients, however, in Tunisia a high proportion of patients previously diagnosed with Friedreich's ataxia were found to have the isolated Vitamin E deficiency syndrome.[64,76,79,80] Larger prospective evaluation of these types of disorders is needed to determine the true frequency of isolated vitamin E deficiency in different populations around the world.

Treatment

Vitamin E deficiency in this disorder is determined by low serum vitamin E and ratios of serum vitamin E and total lipids. Patients respond to 800-1200 mg/day of oral *all-rac*-α-tocopherol, RRR-α-tocopherol, or α-tocopheryl acetate, most patients requiring the lower dose.[33,61,64,71,79,80] Patients need to be continuously treated for life, since serum vitamin E levels will fall rapidly if therapy is discontinued. Patients with more advanced neurological deterioration show a more limited neurological response. If vitamin E deficiency is identified, thorough evaluation for fat malabsorption, liver disease, and lipoprotein abnormalities should be performed and all first-degree relatives screened for vitamin E deficiency. Asymptomatic relatives who have evidence of biochemical vitamin E deficiency should also be treated after a thorough neurological evaluation. Serum vitamin E levels should be monitored and doses adjusted accordingly. Neurological status should be serially evaluated during therapy as in all patients undergoing vitamin E repletion.

OTHER MAJOR NEURODEGENERATIVE DISEASES

Alzheimer's Disease

Alzheimer's disease is the most common neurodegenerative disorder. It is characterized by loss of neurons, accumulation of neurofibrillary tangles, deposition of amyloid (amorphous aggregates of protein), senilic plaques (consisting of amyloid and cellular debris), and impaired synaptic function. Major symptoms of the disease include loss of memory and other cognitive abilities. As with other neurodegenerative diseases, the process of the disease probably starts decades before it is diagnosed. Mutations of gene PS1 on chromosome 14, PS2 on chromosome 1, and APP in chromosome 21 have been associated with familial cases of Alzheimer's disease.[81] Most notable is mutation E280A of this gene identified recently in the Antioquia families in Colombia.[82] Inheritance of the apolipoprotein E epsilon 4 gene is associated with a higher risk for development of Alzheimer's disease and for occurrence of this illness at a younger age. Inherited forms of Alzheimer's disease, however, make up only about 5 percent of cases. Two reports suggesting that point mutations in the mitochondrial CO1 and CO2 genes encoding for cytochrome c oxidase, contribute to the pathogenesis of non-familial Alzheimer's disease were attributed to artifact arising from the amplification of nuclear encoded mitochondrial DNA.[83]

Role of Oxidative Stress and Antioxidants

Defects in cytochrome c oxidase disrupt the normal mitochondrial electron transport and oxidative phosphorylation and causes electrons to be diverted from the electron transport chain to produce reactive oxygen species and significant oxidative stress. Evidence of oxidative stress includes increased lipid oxidation in the frontal cortex, oxidative damage of glutamine oxidase, and increased concentration of aluminum.[20,22,24,25,84,85] Alzheimer's patients have lower blood levels of antioxidants but tocopherol levels in the brain cortex are as in controls. The level of α-tocopheryl quinone, however, is severalfold higher indicating increased oxidation or decreased breakdown of this compound.[84,86,87]

The first major clinical trial evaluating an antioxidant in this disease indicated that high vitamin E delayed the progression of the Alzheimer's disease. A double-blind, placebo-controlled, randomized, multicenter trial with 341 patients of moderate severity evaluated the selective monoamine oxidase inhibitor selegiline (10 mg/day), vitamin E (all-rac-α-tocopherol, 2000 IU/day), both selegiline and vitamin E, or placebo for two years.[29] The primary outcome was the time to the occurrence of any of death, institutionalization, loss of the ability to perform basic activities of daily living, or severe dementia. Both selegiline and α-tocopherol slowed the progression of disease by approximately seven months. Whether earlier introduction of vitamin E, larger doses, or combination with other antioxidants will result in a better clinical outcome must await further clinical trials.

Parkinson's Disease

After Alzheimer's, Parkinson's disease is the second most common neurodegenerative disorder affecting about 10% of people over 65 years old. Although clinical symptoms of Parkinson's disease appear at the mean age of 60, the disease process probably begins decades earlier. It is estimated that 75-80% of the function of substantia nigra, the principal dopaminergic nucleus of the brain, is lost before Parkinson's disease is diagnosed. Symptoms progress from resting tremor and stiffness or slowness in the use of one hand to loss of postular stability, lessening of manual dexterity, softening of the voice and, in a significant minority, some dementia. Patients become chair-bound 5-7 years later and die 10-15 years after the onset of the disease.

Role of Oxidative Stress and Antioxidants

The pathogenesis of the disease is not understood. Genetic factors may be involved especially in familial cases. A mutation in the α-synuclein gene on chromosome 4, which codes for a presynaptic protein thought to be involved in neuronal plasticity with autosomal dominant inheritance for the phenotype, was identified in familial occurrence of the disease in Italian and Greek families.[88] This mutated gene was not present in patients with no family history of the disease.

There are strong indications that oxidative stress is involved, although it is not clear whether it is part of the cause or a consequence of the disease.[19,21,23-25,89] Metabolic products of dopamine, which include hydrogen peroxide, aldehydes, and quinones, may contribute to oxidative stress.[26,27,90] Monoamine oxidase type B (MAO-B), one of the enzymes hydrolyzing dopamine, activates 1-methyl-4-phenyl-1,2,3,6-tetrahydropyridine to 1-methyl-4-phenyl-pyridinium ion, for a component of the enzymatic conversion of dopamine to hydrogen peroxide, and for the activation of other potential toxins such as isoquinolines and beta-carbolines.[21] The normal brain scavenges hydrogen peroxide with GSH and catalase. In patients with Parkinson's disease production of dopamine is probably increased to compensate for the reduced number of nigral neurons thus increasing the amount of oxidation products. Specific indications of oxidative stress include increased brain iron content, impaired mitochondrial function, decline of superoxide dismutase (SOD) and glutathione (GSH), and oxidative damage of lipids, proteins, and DNA. The α-tocopherol and GSH in the cerebrospinal fluid remains within normal levels but the levels of both oxidized glutathione and α-tocopheryl quinone (oxidized α-tocopherol) increase.[91]

The role of antioxidants in reducing the risk or delaying the onset of Parkinson's disease is not clear. Some studies showed significant benefit but others did not. The community-based Rotterdam Study,[30] of 5342 individuals without dementia between 55 and 95 years of age, suggested that a high intake of dietary vitamin E might have a protective effect. A positive but statistically not significant trend was observed for β-carotene but not for vitamin C and flavonoid intake. A pilot intervention study[92] suggested that vitamin E, or vitamin E plus vitamin C, may have beneficial effects. The time when levodopa became necessary was extended by 2.5 years in the group receiving α-tocopherol and ascorbate. In contrast to these findings, two other studies showed no association of higher dietary vitamin E or other antioxidants and lower incidence of the disease.[93,94] A beneficial association was observed with higher consumption of legumes.[93]

Vitamin E does not delay the progress of the disease after it is diagnosed. In a multicenter controlled clinical trial (DATATOP)[28] of deprenyl (a monoamine oxidase inhibitor, 10 mg/day) and vitamin E (all-rac-α-tocopherol, 2000 IU/day) 800 patients in early Parkinson's disease were assigned to one of four treatments: placebo, active tocopherol and deprenyl placebo, active deprenyl and tocopherol placebo, or both active drugs. The primary end point was the onset of disability prompting the clinical decision to begin administering levodopa. Deprenyl delayed the end point but vitamin E did not.

Tardive Dyskinesia

L-DOPA, the most useful drug in the symptomatic treatment of Parkinson's disease, has been associated with involuntary movement, a neurologic condition defined as tardive dyskinesia. Orofacial movements are most frequent, although other body areas, limbs, neck, and trunk, may be involved. Other neuroleptic drugs may cause this condition, which in some cases causes more severe symptoms than those of the disease affecting about 20% of the patients on long-term therapy.

Role of Oxidative Stress and Antioxidants

Although the pathophysiology of tardive dyskinesia remains poorly understood, oxidative stress has been proposed as a contributing factor.[95] Early studies showed that vitamin E attenuated the effect of 6-hydroxydopamine injected intrastriatally in rats.[95] This compound damages selectively the catecholaminergic nerve cells and may simulate damage from dopamine oxidation products. A number of studies with humans indicate that large doses of vitamin E, usually above 800 IU/day, reduce the symptoms of tardive dyskinesia.[96-101] The National Veterans Affairs Cooperative Study (CS #394), involving nine sites, now in progress, may help obtain a conclusive answer regarding the benefits of vitamin E.[102]

Amyotrophic Lateral Sclerosis (ALS) and Huntington's Disease

ALS, also known as Lou Gehrig's disease and motor neuron disease, is characterized by degeneration of the motor neurons of the spinal cord, brain stem, and cerebral cortex. In familial ALS, which represents about 10% of cases, the genetic defect has been linked to the SOD1 gene encoding Cu, Zn superoxide dismutase.[103] Huntington's disease is a hereditary type of brain atrophy. Changes occur in a group of nerve cells in the middle of the part of the brain called the basal ganglia/caudate nucleus. In 1993, the Huntington gene was localized on chromosome 4; the mutation results in excessive activation of glutamate-gated ion channels, which damages neurons by oxidative stress.[18,104] Very recently, British researchers reported a major breakthrough in understanding the pathogenesis of this disease. They discovered that molecules of the huntingtin protein that normally reside in the cytoplasm, outside the nucleus, migrated into the nucleus and accumulated into clumps.[105] This phenomenon is similar to the accumulation of amyloid found in the brains of Alzheimer's patients and also in scrapie, an infectious neurodegenerative disease of sheep.

Role of Oxidative Stress and Antioxidants

The oxidative stress mechanisms proposed for Parkinson's and Alzheimer's diseases are believed to play a contributory role in these diseases.[18,20] Particularly interesting is the hypothesis of an adverse effect on the electron transport system in the mitochondria leading to leakage of free radicals.[106]

Studies on the role of antioxidants in these diseases have been limited. A prospective, double-blind, placebo-controlled study of high-dose of vitamin E (RRR-α-tocopherol) treatment was conducted in a cohort of 73 patients with Huntington's. Although vitamin E had no effect on neurologic and neuropsychiatric symptoms in the treatment group overall, post hoc analysis revealed a significant selective therapeutic effect on neurologic symptoms for patients early in the course of the disorder.[104] In another study, treatment with coenzyme Q10 (an essential cofactor of the electron transport chain and an antioxidant) decreased cortical lactate concentrations in 18 patients, which reversed when the treatment stopped.[106]

Diabetic Neuropathy

This disease is common long-term complication of diabetes and is characterized by degeneration of the peripheral nerves. Alpha-lipoic acid and other antioxidants is currently used in Germany for treatment of this disease. The role of alpha-lipoic acid in diabetes and other diseases is discussed in Chapter 26.

CONCLUSIONS AND FUTURE RESEARCH

The neurodegenerative diseases associated with lipid malabsorption and the Isolated Vitamin E Deficiency syndrome have striking clinical and histopathological similarities to animal models of vitamin E deficiency. Correction of the vitamin E deficiency resulting from lipid malabsorption in patients with chronic cholestasis, disorders of β-lipoprotein secretion, short bowel syndrome, and other steatorrheic conditions, prevents, reverses, or at least stabilizes the condition, generally improving the quality of life. There is continuing progress in identifying the best route and form of vitamin E therapy for each disease.

For other neurodegenerative diseases such as Parkinson's, Alzheimer's, ALS, and Huntington's, research on the role of vitamin E and other antioxidants is at its early stages. There are promising results with vitamin E for Alzheimer's, tardive dyskinesia, and Huntington's diseases (albeit limited and preliminary) and disappointing results for Parkinson's from the DATATOP study. In these studies the focus has been on treatment of symptomatic patients. Because the disease process starts decades before it is diagnosed, the effect of antioxidants in preventing or delaying the onset of the disease remains to be evaluated. A common characteristic of these diseases is impaired energy metabolism in the mitochondria of brain cells, which disrupts the normal oxidation of respiratory substrates and causes electrons to be diverted and produce free radicals. The excessive production of free radicals suggests a potential for antioxidants for reducing the risk or delaying the onset of these diseases.

The early focus has been on vitamin E due to its unique role as a biological antioxidant and its direct link to several neurodegenerative diseases. Other antioxidants may play a very important role due to the close interdependence of the human antioxidant system, the additive or synergistic effect of dietary antioxidants, and especially the ability of some antioxidants to spare others. Some of the lipid malabsorption conditions impair absorption of other fat-soluble nutrients and food components including antioxidants. Thus, the oxidative stress due to vitamin E deficiency is probably accentuated further. For example, in cystic fibrosis patients, β-carotene appears to improve antioxidant status. There is a need to determine whether other antioxidants are beneficial. Other tocopherols such as γ-tocopherol may be of particular interest based on new findings on their role in neutralizing nitrogen radicals, which have been implicated in the pathogenesis of some diseases. Antioxidants, which play a key role in mitochondrial respiration, such as coenzyme Q_{10}, may also have a role.

Finally, we would like to emphasize a very important consideration in evaluating the role of antioxidants. While it is universally accepted that the damage leading to neurodegenerative diseases develops over years and even decades, there is little consideration for the slow process of enrichment of nerve tissue. As discussed in earlier chapters, uptake (and probably depletion) of vitamin E by nerve tissue is slower than for other tissues.[31] Even with increasing doses of vitamin E (400 to 4,000 IU/day) for 5 months in Parkinson's patients, there was no enrichment of the ventrical cerebrospinal fluid in spite of major increases in the plasma.[107] For this reason, if antioxidants have a role in reducing the risk or delaying the onset of the disease they would be potentially more effective if administered before or at the early stages of pathogenesis. It is also essential to consider the intracellular location of oxidative stress in specific disease states and the potential to target antioxidants to those locations (such as the mitochondrial respiratory chain). It is very unlikely that antioxidants would reverse nerve damage and their role at the clinical stage may be very limited with the exception of an apparently significant effect in reducing the severity of tardive dyskinesia caused by neuroleptic drugs.

REFERENCES

1. Evans H, Burr G. Development of paralysis in the suckling young of mothers deprived of vitamin E. J Biol Chem 1928;76:273-97.
2. Goettsch M, Pappenheimer M. Nutritional muscular dystrophy in the guinea pig and rabbit. J Exp Med 1931;54:145-65.
3. Pappenheimer AM, Goettsch M. A cerebellar disorder in chicks, apparently of nutritional origin. J Exp Med 1931;54:145-65.
4. Kayden HJ, Silber R. The role of vitamin E deficiency in the abnormal autohemolysis of acanthocytosis. Trans. Assoc. Am. Phys. 1965;78:334-341.
5. Sokol RJ. Vitamin E deficiency and neurologic disease. Annu. Rev. Nutr. 1988;8:351-373.
6. Sokol RJ, Heubi JE, Iannaccone ST, Bove KE, Balistreri WF. Vitamin E deficiency with normal serum vitamin E concentrations in children with chronic cholestasis. N. Engl. J. Med. 1984;310:1209-1212.
7. Argao EA, Heubi JE. Fat-soluble vitamin deficiency in infants and children. Curr Opin Pediatr 1993;5:562-6.
8. Leo MA, Ahmed S, Aleynik SI, Siegel JH, Kasmin F, Lieber CS. Carotenoids and tocopherols in various hepatobiliary conditions. J Hepatol 1995;23:550-6.

9. Lepage G, Champagne J, Ronco N, *et al.* Supplementation with carotenoids corrects increased lipid peroxidation in children with cystic fibrosis [published erratum appears in Am J Clin Nutr 1997 Feb;65(2):578]. Am J Clin Nutr 1996;64:87-93.
10. Winklhofer-Roob BM, van't Hof MA, Shmerling DH. Response to oral beta-carotene supplementation in patients with cystic fibrosis: a 16-month follow-up study. Acta Paediatr 1995;84:1132-6.
11. Winklhofer-Roob BM, Tuchschmid PE, Molinari L, Shmerling DH. Response to a single oral dose of all-rac-alpha-tocopheryl acetate in patients with cystic fibrosis and in healthy individuals. Am J Clin Nutr 1996;63:717-21.
12. Papas AM. Determinants of antioxidant status in humans. Lipids 1996;31:S77-82.
13. Brown RK, Kelly FJ. Evidence for increased oxidative damage in patients with cystic fibrosis. Pediatr Res 1994;36:487-93.
14. Brown RK, Wyatt H, Price JF, Kelly FJ. Pulmonary dysfunction in cystic fibrosis is associated with oxidative stress. Eur Respir J 1996;9:334-9.
15. Langley SC, Brown RK, Kelly FJ. Reduced free-radical-trapping capacity and altered plasma antioxidant status in cystic fibrosis. Pediatr Res 1993;33:247-50.
16. Singh S, Shackleton G, Ah-Sing E, Chakraborty J, Bailey ME. Antioxidant defenses in the bile duct-ligated rat. Gastroenterology 1992;103:1625-9.
17. Sokol RJ. Fat-soluble vitamins and their importance in patients with cholestatic liver diseases. Gastroenterol Clin North Am 1994;23:673-705.
18. Borlongan CV, Kanning K, Poulos SG, Freeman TB, Cahill DW, Sanberg PR. Free radical damage and oxidative stress in Huntington's disease. J Fla Med Assoc 1996;83:335-41.
19. Ebadi M, Srinivasan SK, Baxi MD. Oxidative stress and antioxidant therapy in Parkinson's disease. Prog Neurobiol 1996;48:1-19.
20. Jenner P. Oxidative stress in Parkinson's disease and other neurodegenerative disorders. Pathol Biol (Paris) 1996;44:57-64.
21. Jenner P, Olanow CW. Oxidative stress and the pathogenesis of Parkinson's disease. Neurology 1996;47:S161-70.
22. Lyras L, Cairns NJ, Jenner A, Jenner P, Halliwell B. An assessment of oxidative damage to proteins, lipids, and DNA in brain from patients with Alzheimer's disease. J Neurochem 1997;68:2061-9.
23. Owen AD, Schapira AH, Jenner P, Marsden CD. Oxidative stress and Parkinson's disease. Ann NY Acad Sci 1996;786:217-23.
24. Simonian NA, Coyle JT. Oxidative stress in neurodegenerative diseases. Annu Rev Pharmacol Toxicol 1996;36:83-106.
25. Knight JA. Reactive oxygen species and the neurodegenerative disorders. Ann Clin Lab Sci 1997;27:11-25.
26. Lai CT, Yu PH. Dopamine- and L-beta-3,4-dihydroxyphenylalanine hydrochloride (L-Dopa)-induced cytotoxicity towards catecholaminergic neuroblastoma SH-SY5Y cells. Effects of oxidative stress and antioxidative factors. Biochem Pharmacol 1997;53:363-72.
27. Lai CT, Yu PH. R(-)-deprenyl potentiates dopamine-induced cytotoxicity toward catecholaminergic neuroblastoma SH-SY5Y cells. Toxicol Appl Pharmacol 1997;142:186-91.
28. Group TsS. Effects of tocopherol and deprenyl on the progression of disability in early Parkinson's disease. The Parkinson Study Group. N Engl J Med 1993;328:176-83.
29. Sano M, Ernesto C, Thomas RG, *et al.* A controlled trial of selegiline, alpha-tocopherol, or both as treatment for Alzheimer's disease. The Alzheimer's Disease Cooperative Study. N Engl J Med 1997;336:1216-22.
30. de Rijk MC, Breteler MM, den Breeijen JH, *et al.* Dietary antioxidants and Parkinson disease. The Rotterdam Study. Arch Neurol 1997;54:762-5.

31. Kayden HJ, Traber MG. Absorption, lipoprotein transport and regulation of plasma concentrations of vitamin E in humans. J. Lipid Res. 1993;34:343-358.
32. Muller DPR, Harries JT, Lloyd JK. The relative importance of the factors involved in the absorption of vitamin E in children. Gut 1974;15:966-971.
33. Sokol RJ, Kayden HJ, Bettis DB, *et al.* Isolated vitamin E deficiency in the absence of fat malabsorption - familial and sporadic cases: Characterization and investigation of causes. J. Lab. Clin. Med. 1988;111:548-559.
34. Kayden HJ, Sokol RJ, Traber MG. Familial vitamin E deficiency in the absence of lipid malabsorption. In: Hayaishi O, Mino M, Eds. *Clinical and Nutritional Aspects of Vitamin E.* Amsterdam, Netherlands: Elsevier Sci. Publ., 1987:193-197.
35. Muller DP. Antioxidant therapy in neurological disorders. Adv Exp Med Biol 1990;264:475-84.
36. Sokol RJ. Vitamin E and neurologic function in man. Free Rad. Biol. Med. 1988;6:189-207.
37. Kayden HJ, Hatam LJ, Traber MG. The measurement of nanograms of tocopherol from needle aspiration biopsies of adipose tissue: normal and abetalipoproteinemic subjects. J. Lipid Res 1983; 24:652-656.
38. Azizi E, Zaidman J, Eschchar J. Abetalipoproteinemia treated with parental and oral vitamins A and E, and with medium chain triglycerides. Acta Paediatr Scand 1978;67:797-801.
39. Bishara S, Merin S, Cooper M, Aziz E, Delpre G, Deckelbaum RJ. Combined vitamin A and E therapy prevents retinal electrophysiological deterioration in abetalipoproteinaemia. Brit. J. Ophthal. 1982;12:767-770.
40. Traber MG, Sokol RJ, Ringel SP, Neville HE, Thellman CA, Kayden HJ. Lack of tocopherol in peripheral nerves of vitamin E-deficient patients with peripheral neuropathy. N. Engl. J. Med. 1987;317:262-265.
41. Anderson C, Townley R, Freeman J. Unusual causes of steatorrhea in infancy and childhood. Med J Aust 1961;11:617-21.
42. Sokol RJ, Heubi JE, Iannaccone S, Bove KE, Harris RE, Balistreri WF. The mechanism causing vitamin E deficiency during chronic childhood cholestasis. Gastroenterology 1983;85:1172-1182.
43. Sokol R, Ballistreri W, Hoolnagle J, Jones E. Vitamin E deficiency in adults with chronic liver disease. Am J Clin Nutr 1985;41.
44. Sokol RJ, Guggenheim M, Iannaccone ST, *et al.* Improved neurologic function after long-term correction of vitamin E deficiency in children with chronic cholestasis. N. Engl. J. Med. 1985;313:1580-1586.
45. Rosenblum JL, Keating JP, Prensky AL, Nelson JS. A progressive neurologic syndrome in children with chronic liver disease. N. Engl. J. Med. 1981;304:503-508.
46. Jeffrey GP, Muller DPR, Burroughs AK, *et al.* Vitamin E deficiency and its clinical significance in adults with primary biliary cirrhosis and other forms of chronic liver disease. J Hepatol 1987;4:307-317.
47. Sokol RJ, Kim YS, Hoofnagle JH, Heubi JE, Jones EA, Balistreri WF. Intestinal malabsorption of vitamin E in primary biliary cirrhosis. Gastroenterology 1989;96:479-486.
48. Guggenheim M, Ringel S, Silverman A, Grabert B. Progressive neuromuscular disease in chidren with chronic cholestasis and vitamin E deficiency: Diagnosis and treatment with alpha tocopherol. J Ped 1982;100:51-58.
49. Tomasi L. Reversibility of human myopathy caused by vitamin E deficiency. Neurology 1979;29:1182-6.
50. Sokol RJ, Butler-Simon N, Conner C, *et al.* Multicenter trial of d-α-tocopheryl polyethylene glycol 1000 succinate for treatment of vitamin E deficiency in children with chronic cholestasis. Gastroenterology 1993;104:1727-1735.

51. Burton GW, Traber MG, Acuff RV, *et al.* Human plasma and tissue alpha-tocopherol concentrations in response to supplementation with dueterated natural and synthetic vitamin E. Am J Clin Nutr (submitted) 1997.
52. Acuff RV, Thedford SS, Hidiroglou NN, Papas AM, Odom TA, Jr. Relative bioavailability of RRR- and all-rac-alpha-tocopheryl acetate in humans: studies using deuterated compounds. Am J Clin Nutr 1994;60:397-402.
53. Alvarez F, Landrieu P, Lemonnier F, Bernard O, Alagille D. Vitamin E deficiency is responsible for neurologic abnormalities in cholestatic children. J Pediatr Scand 1985;107:422-5.
54. Sokol RJ, Butler-Simon NA, Bettis D, Smith DJ, Silverman A. Tocopheryl polyethylene glycol 1000 succinate therapy for vitamin E deficiency during chronic childhood cholestasis: neurologic outcome. J. Pediatr. 1987;111:830-836.
55. Socha P, Koletzko B, Pawlowska J, Proszynska K, Socha J. Treatment of cholestatic children with water-soluble vitamin E (alpha-tocopheryl polyethylene glycol succinate): effects on serum vitamin E, lipid peroxides, and polyunsaturated fatty acids. J Pediatr Gastroenterol Nutr 1997;24:189-93.
56. Sokol RJ, Johnson KE, Karrer FM, Narkewicz MR, Smith D, Kam I. Improvement of cyclosporin absorption in children after liver transplantation by means of water-soluble vitamin E. Lancet 1991;338:212-214.
57. Farrell PM. Deficiency states, pharmacological effects, and nutrient requirements. In: Machlin L, Ed. *Vitamin E: A Comprehensive Treatise*. New York, NY: Marcel Dekker, 1980:520-620.
58. Winklhofer-Roob BM, Puhl H, Khoschsorur G, van't Hof MA, Esterbauer H, Shmerling DH. Enhanced resistance to oxidation of low density lipoproteins and decreased lipid peroxide formation during beta-carotene supplementation in cystic fibrosis. Free Radic Biol Med 1995;18:849-59.
59. Peters SA, Kelly FJ. Vitamin E supplementation in cystic fibrosis. J Pediatr Gastroenterol Nutr 1996;22:341-5.
60. Winklhofer-Roob BM, Ellemunter H, Fruhwirth M, *et al.* Plasma vitamin C concentrations in patients with cystic fibrosis: evidence of associations with lung inflammation. Am J Clin Nutr 1997;65:1858-66.
61. Laplante P, Vanasse M, Michaud J, Geoffroy G, Brochu P. A progressive neurological syndrome associated with an isolated vitamin E deficiency. Can. J. Neurol. Sci. 1984;11:561-564.
62. Yokota T, Tsuchiya K, Furukawa T, Tsukagoshi H, Miyakawa H, Hasumura Y. Vitamin E deficiency in acquired fat malabsorption. J Neurol 1990;237:103-6.
63. Krendel DA, Gilchrest JM, Johnson AO, Bossen EH. Isolated deficiency of vitamin E with progressive neurologic deterioration. Neurology 1987;37:538-540.
64. Stumpf DA, Sokol R, Bettis D, *et al.* Friedreich's disease: V. Variant form with vitamin E deficiency and normal fat absorption. Neurology 1987;37:68-74.
65. Gutmann L, Shockcor W, Gutmann L, Kien V. Vitamin E-deficient spinocerebellar syndrome due to intestinal lymphangiectasia. Neurology 1986;36:554-6.
66. Acherman Z, Eliashiv S, Reches A, Zimmerman J. Neurological manifestations in celiac disease and vitamin E deficiency. J Clin Gastroenterol 1989;11:603-5.
67. Braunstein H. Tocopherol deficiency in adults with chronic pancreatitis. Gastroenterology 1961;40:224-31.
68. Traber MG, Schiano TD, Steephen AC, Kayden HJ, Shike M. Efficacy of water soluble vitamin E in the treatment of vitamin E malabsorption in the short bowel syndrome. Am. J. Clin. Nutr. 1994;59:1270-1274.
69. Amiel J, Maziere J, Beucler I, *et al.* Familial isolated vitamin E deficiency. Extensive study of a large family with a 5-year therapeutic follow-up. J. Inherit. Metab. Dis. 1995;18:333-40.

70. Behl C, Skutella T, Lezoualc'h F, *et al.* Neuroprotection against oxidative stress by estrogens: structure- activity relationship. Mol Pharmacol 1997;51:535-41.
71. Harding AE, Matthews S, Jones S, Ellis CJK, Booth IW, Muller DPR. Spinocerebellar degeneration associated with a selective defect of vitamin E absorption. N. Engl. J. Med. 1985;313:32-35.
72. Traber MG, Sokol RJ, Burton GW, *et al.* Impaired ability of patients with familial isolated vitamin E deficiency to incorporate alpha-tocopherol into lipoproteins. J Clin Invest 1990;85:397-407.
73. Arita M, Sato Y, Miyata A, *et al.* Human alpha-tocopherol transfer protein: cDNA cloning, expression and chromosomal localization. Biochem. J. 1995;306:437-443.
74. Hentati A, Deng H-X, Hung W-Y, *et al.* Human α-tocopherol transfer protein: gene organziation and identification of mutations in patients with familial vitamin E deficiency. Am. J. Human Genetics. 1995;57 suppl. 4:A214.
75. Hosomi A, Arita M, Sato Y, *et al.* Affinity for alpha-tocopherol transfer protein as a determinant of the biological activities of vitamin E analogs. FEBS Lett 1997;409:105-8.
76. Hentati A, Deng H-X, Hung W-Y, *et al.* Gene structure and mutations in familial vitamin E deficiency. Ann. Neurol. 1996;39:295-300.
77. Doerflinger N, Linder C, Ouahchi K, *et al.* Ataxia with vitamin E deficiency: refinement of genetic localization and analysis of linkage disequilibrium by using new markers in 14 families. Am J Hum Genet 1995;56:1116-24.
78. Ouahchi K, Arita M, Kayden H, *et al.* Ataxia with isolated vitamin E deficiency is caused by mutations in the alpha-tocopherol transfer protein. Nat Genet 1995;9:141-5.
79. Ben Hamida C, Doerflinger N, Belal S, *et al.* Localization of Friedreich ataxia phenotype with selective vitamin E deficiency to chromosome 8q by homozygosity mapping. Nature Genetics 1993;5:195-200.
80. Ben Hamida M, Belal S, Sirugo G, *et al.* Friedreich's ataxia phenotype not linked to chromosome 9 and associated with selective autosomal recessive vitamin E deficiency in two inbred Tunisian families. Neurology 1993;43:2179-2183.
81. Lendon CL, Ashall F, Goate AM. Exploring the etiology of Alzheimer disease using molecular genetics. JAMA 1997;277:825-31.
82. Lopera F, Ardilla A, Martinez A, *et al.* Clinical features of early-onset Alzheimer disease in a large kindred with an E280A presenilin-1 mutation. JAMA 1997;277:793-9.
83. Davis JN 2nd, Parker WD Jr. Evidence that two reports of mtDNA cytochrome c oxidase "mutations" in Alzheimer's disease are based on nDNA pseudogenes of recent evolutionary origin. Biochem Biophys Res Commun 1998:244:877-83.
84. Adams JD, Jr., Klaidman LK, Odunze IN, Shen HC, Miller CA. Alzheimer's and Parkinson's Disease, brain levels of glutathione disulfide, and vitamin E. Mol. Chem. Neuropath. 1991;14:213-226.
85. Famulari AL, Marschoff ER, Llesuy SF, *et al.* The antioxidant enzymatic blood profile in Alzheimer's and vascular diseases. Their association and a possible assay to differentiate demented subjects and controls. J Neurol Sci 1996;141:69-78.
86. Zaman Z, Roche S, Fielden P, Frost PG, Niriella DC, Cayley AC. Plasma concentrations of vitamins A and E and carotenoids in Alzheimer's disease. Age Ageing 1992;21:91-94.
87. Metcalfe T, Bowen DM, Muller DP. Vitamin E concentrations in human brain of patients with Alzheimer's disease, fetuses with Down's syndrome, centenarians, and controls. Neurochem Res 1989;14:1209-12.
88. Polymeropoulos MH, Lavedan C, Leroy E, *et al.* Mutation in the alpha-synuclein gene identified in families with Parkinson's disease. Science 1997;276:2045-7.

89. Olanow CW. Oxidation reactions in Parkinson's disease. Neurology 1990;40:suppl 32-7.
90. Spencer JP, Jenner A, Butler J, *et al.* Evaluation of the pro-oxidant and antioxidant actions of L-DOPA and dopamine *in vitro*: implications for Parkinson's disease. Free Radic Res 1996;24:95-105.
91. Tohgi H, Abe T, Saheki M, Hamato F, Sasaki K, Takahashi S. Reduced and oxidized forms of glutathione and alpha-tocopherol in the cerebrospinal fluid of parkinsonian patients: comparison between before and after L-dopa treatment. Neurosci Lett 1995;184:21-4.
92. Fahn S. A pilot trial of high-dose alpha-tocopherol and ascorbate in early Parkinson's disease. Ann Neurol 1992;32:S128-32.
93. Morens DM, Grandinetti A, Waslien CI, Park CB, Ross GW, White LR. Case-control study of idiopathic Parkinson's disease and dietary vitamin E intake. Neurology 1996;46:1270-4.
94. Scheider WL, Hershey LA, Vena JE, Holmlund T, Marshall JR, Freudenheim. Dietary antioxidants and other dietary factors in the etiology of Parkinson's disease. Mov Disord 1997;12:190-6.
95. Cadet JL, Lohr JB. Possible involvement of free radicals in neuroleptic-induced movement disorders: Evidence from treatment of tardive dyskinesia with vitamin E. Ann. N.Y. Acad. Sci. 1989;450:176-185.
96. Adler LA, Peselow E, Rotrosen J, *et al.* Vitamin E treatment of tardive dyskinesia. Am J Psychiatry 1993;150:1405-7.
97. Akhtar S, Jajor TR, Kumar S. Vitamin E in the treatment of tardive dyskinesia. J Postgrad Med 1993;39:124-6.
98. Dabiri LM, Pasta D, Darby JK, Mosbacher D. Effectiveness of vitamin E for treatment of long-term tardive dyskinesia. Am J Psychiatry 1994;151:925-6.
99. Dorevitch A, Kalian M, Shlafman M, Lerner V. Treatment of long-term tardive dyskinesia with vitamin E. Biol Psychiatry 1997;41:114-6.
100. Elkashef AM, Ruskin PE, Bacher N, Barrett D. Vitamin E in the treatment of tardive dyskinesia. Am J Psychiatry 1990;147:505-6.
101. Lohr JB, Caligiuri MP. A double-blind placebo-controlled study of vitamin E treatment of tardive dyskinesia. J. Clin. Psychiat. 1996;57:167-173.
102. Tracy K, Adler LA, Rotrosen J, Edson R, Lavori P. Interrater reliability issues in multicenter trials, Part I: Theoretical concepts and operational procedures used in Department of Veterans Affairs Cooperative Study #394. Psychopharmacol Bull 1997;33:53-7.
103. Rosen DR, Bowling AC, Patterson D, *et al.* A frequent ala 4 to val superoxide dismutase-1 mutation is associated with a rapidly progressive familial amyotrophic lateral sclerosis. Hum Mol Genet 1994;3:981-7.
104. Peyser CE, Folstein M, Chase GA, *et al.* Trial of d-alpha-tocopherol in Huntington's disease. Am J Psychiatry 1995;152:1771-5.
105. Scherzinger E, Lurz R, Turmaine M, *et al.* Huntingtin-Encoded Polyglutamine Expansions Form Amyloid-like Protein Aggregates *In Vitro* and *In Vivo*. Cell 1997;90:549-58.
106. Koroshetz WJ, Jenkins BG, Rosen BR, Beal MF. Energy metabolism defects in Huntington's disease and effects of coenzyme Q10. Ann Neurol 1997;41:160-5.
107. Pappert EJ, Tangney CC, Goetz CG, *et al.* Alpha-tocopherol in the ventricular cerebrospinal fluid of Parkinson's disease patients: dose-response study and correlations with plasma levels. Neurology 1996;47:1037-42.

26

Alpha-Lipoic Acid in Health and Disease

Sharon V. Landvik, M.S., R.D.
Vitamin E Research and Information Service, La Grange, Illinois, USA

Lester Packer, Ph.D.
Department of Molecular and Cell Biology
University of California, Berkeley, California, USA

INTRODUCTION

The metabolic role of alpha-lipoic acid (thioctic acid) has been known for many years. Alpha-lipoic acid has also recently received considerable attention as an effective antioxidant. Antioxidants are believed to have an important role in prevention of free radical-mediated chronic and degenerative diseases. Alpha-lipoic acid is currently under active investigation in prevention and treatment of a number of conditions that involve oxidative stress.[1,2] The present chapter is concerned with the functions of alpha-lipoic acid and the current research status of preventive and therapeutic applications of alpha-lipoic acid in a number of free radical-mediated conditions.

0-8493-8009-X/98/$0.00+$.50

FUNCTIONS

Alpha-lipoic acid functions as an essential cofactor in metabolic reactions involved in energy utilization.[3] Research in muscle and fat cells has demonstrated that alpha-lipoic acid stimulates glucose transport and has a positive effect on insulin-stimulated glucose uptake.[4] Alpha-lipoic acid and its reduced form, dihydrolipoic acid, may also have effects on genes and regulatory proteins involved in normal growth and metabolism.[1]

Alpha-lipoic acid and dihydrolipoic acid are effective as both fat-soluble and water-soluble antioxidants. Alpha-lipoic acid is readily absorbed, transported and taken up by cells and is reduced to dihydrolipoic acid in various tissues, including the brain.[5] Dihydrolipoic acid is also transported from cells and can provide antioxidant protection to the extracellular compartment (Table 1).

Table 1
Reactive Oxygen Species Scavenged by Alpha-Lipoic Acid and Dihydrolipoic Acid

	Scavenged by	
Oxidant	**Alpha-Lipoic Acid**	**Dihydrolipoic Acid**
Hydrogen peroxide	Yes	Yes
Singlet oxygen	Yes	No
Hydroxyl radical	Yes	Yes
Nitric oxide radical	Yes	Yes
Superoxide radical	No	Yes
Hypochlorous acid	Yes	Yes
Peroxynitrite	Yes	Yes
Peroxyl radical	No	Yes

Alpha-lipoic acid scavenges hydroxyl radicals, singlet oxygen, hydrogen peroxide, hypochlorous acid, peroxynitrite and nitric oxide. In addition to the reactive oxygen species scavenged by alpha-lipoic acid, dihydrolipoic acid scavenges peroxyl radicals and superoxide radical.[1,2] Alpha-lipoic acid and dihydrolipoic acid may also exert an antioxidant effect through chelation of copper, iron, and other transition metals.[1,6]

Dihydrolipoic acid reduces other antioxidants from their oxidized or radical forms, thus regenerating them (including glutathione and vitamin C directly and vitamin E indirectly).[2] In animal studies, alpha-lipoic acid supplementation prevented symptoms of vitamin C and vitamin E deficiency, indicating a synergy between alpha-lipoic acid and other antioxidants.[7,8] Alpha-lipoic acid supplementation has been shown to increase intracellular levels of the antioxidant enzyme glutathione by 30-70%.[9]

Based on the demonstrated functions of alpha-lipoic acid, it would be expected to be effective against conditions in which oxidative stress has a role.[3] A number of experimental and clinical studies have evaluated the beneficial effects of alpha-lipoic acid in such conditions as ischemia-reperfusion injury, heavy metal poisoning, radiation injury, cataracts, and complications of diabetes.[1]

ALPHA-LIPOIC ACID IN HEALTH AND DISEASE

Ischemia-Reperfusion Injury

In a cell culture model of hypoxia, alpha-lipoic acid protected neurons from damage if added 24 hours before hypoxia but did not have a protective effect if added only one hour before hypoxia.[10] Studies in mice demonstrated a protective effect of dihydrolipoic acid, but not alpha-lipoic acid, against ischemia-reperfusion injury in the brain.[11,12] However, alpha-lipoic acid was protective against ischemia-reperfusion injury in a gerbil animal model. Animals treated with alpha-lipoic acid for seven days prior to ischemia-reperfusion injury had less change in locomotor activity and less damage to brain cells than control animals.[13] In rats, pretreatment with alpha-lipoic acid before brain ischemia reduced mortality from 78% to 26% in the 24-hour period following reperfusion. Alpha-lipoic acid pretreatment almost completely abolished the ischemia-reperfusion-induced losses of glutathione in the brain and significantly reduced the elevation in lipid peroxidation associated with ischemia.[5]

In another study, hearts from rats fed alpha-lipoic acid were protected against ischemia-reperfusion injury in an isolated system. Alpha-lipoic acid preserved vitamin E in heart tissue, decreased lipid peroxidation, and improved recovery of left ventricular function following ischemia.[14] The addition of dihydrolipoic acid to the reperfusion buffer in a working heart system accelerated the recovery of aortic blood flow during reperfusion.[15]

Heavy Metal Poisoning

Research in animal models has shown beneficial effects of alpha-lipoic acid in the treatment of heavy metal poisoning. Alpha-lipoic acid completely protected mice and dogs from arsenite poisoning at ratios of alpha-lipoic acid to arsenite of at least 8:1. Complete protection from mercury poisoning was also observed in mice treated with high doses of alpha-lipoic acid but alpha-lipoic acid was ineffective against lead and gold poisoning.[16] In a rat model, alpha-lipoic acid treatment completely prevented cadmium-induced lipid peroxidation in heart, brain, and testes and restored activities of ATPase and catalase. Brain glutathione concentrations decreased 63% in rats treated with cadmium but increased only 4% in rats treated with alpha-lipoic acid and cadmium.[17]

Radiation Injury

Studies have also evaluated the effects of alpha-lipoic acid on radiation injury in animals and humans. In mice, alpha-lipoic acid, but not dihydrolipoic acid, protected against radiation injury to cells involved in blood cell formation.[18] Alpha-lipoic acid administration increased survival rates of irradiated mice from 35% in untreated animals to 90% in alpha-lipoic acid-treated animals.[9] In children living in areas affected by the Chernobyl accident, alpha-lipoic acid treatment lowered levels of chemiluminescence (a marker for lipid peroxidation) to levels of children who were not exposed to radiation. Combined treatment with alpha-lipoic acid and vitamin E further decreased chemiluminescence to below normal levels. Kidney and liver functions were also normalized by alpha-lipoic acid treatment.[19]

Cataracts

Administration of L-buthionine (S,R)-sulfoximine (BSO) to preweanling mice produces cataracts. In a study in newborn mice, all animals treated with BSO alone developed cataracts. Supplementation with alpha-lipoic acid decreased the incidence of cataracts to 40%. Lens concentrations of glutathione, vitamin C, and vitamin E, which decreased after BSO treatment, were restored to levels similar to controls. The researchers noted that the protective effect of alpha-lipoic acid on cataract development could have major therapeutic value.[20] Cataract development in rat lens cultures exposed to high concentrations of glucose was prevented by alpha-lipoic acid.[21]

Diabetes

Insulin resistance is a major characteristic in type II (non-insulin-dependent) diabetes. Therapeutic agents that enhance glucose uptake by skeletal muscle are potentially useful in type II diabetes. Animal research suggests that alpha-lipoic acid enhances insulin-stimulated glucose transport activity, non-oxidative glucose disposal, and glucose oxidation in peripheral tissues.[22] Using the obese Zucker rat as an animal model of obesity in insulin resistance, intravenous administration of alpha-lipoic acid markedly increased glucose uptake in the presence or absence of insulin. Alpha-lipoic acid treatment was also associated with significantly lower plasma levels of insulin and free fatty acids.[23] Alpha-lipoic acid lowered glucose levels during an oral glucose tolerance test.[24] Plasma glucose levels were also decreased after chronic and acute intraperitoneal administration of alpha-lipoic acid to diabetic rats.[25]

The effects of alpha-lipoic acid on glucose disposal have also been investigated in patients with diabetes (Table 2). In patients with type II diabetes, intravenous administration of 1000 mg alpha-lipoic acid enhanced insulin-stimulated glucose disposal by approximately 50%.[26] In another study of patients with type II diabetes, baseline insulin-stimulated glucose disposal was markedly impaired compared to healthy controls. Daily intravenous infusion of 500 mg alpha-lipoic acid for 10 days increased insulin-stimulated glucose disposal by approximately 30%.[22]

Studies have also demonstrated beneficial effects of alpha-lipoic acid on neuropathy, a common long-term complication of diabetes. In a study in rats, development of streptozotocin-induced diabetes resulted in a 100% increase in nerve vascular resistance and a 50% decrease in nerve blood flow. Intravenous administration of alpha-lipoic acid reversed these changes in a dose-dependent manner. Glutathione levels in sciatic nerve were significantly decreased in diabetic animals compared to controls but were restored to normal values by alpha-lipoic acid.[27]

A number of studies have also evaluated the effects of alpha-lipoic acid administration in treatment of neuropathy in patients with diabetes (Table 2). Alpha-lipoic acid appears to have very low toxicity and is used in Germany in treatment of patients with diabetic neuropathy. Results of a study of type I and type II diabetes showed clinical improvement in neurological symptoms in patients orally supplemented with alpha-lipoic acid, vitamin E, or selenium for 12 weeks but no improvement was observed in the control group. Blood levels of malondialdehyde (MDA-an index of lipid peroxidation) decreased in the supplemented groups but not in the control group.[28]

In a double-blind study, intravenous administration of alpha-lipoic acid (200 mg per day for 21 days) alleviated symptoms in a number of patients. Prior to treatment, six patients had moderate pain and four had severe pain. Following treatment, five patients had no pain, four had moderate pain, and one had severe pain. However, there were no changes in vibration sense or nerve conduction velocity over the three-week period.[29]

In a multicenter, double-blind study of patients with type II diabetes, clinical measures of neuropathy (pain, numbness, paresthesia, and burning sensation) improved significantly after intravenous treatment with alpha-lipoic acid (600 mg or 1200 mg five times per week for three weeks). Vibration sense and nerve conduction velocity did not change during the short-term study but the researchers noted that longer periods are usually required for significant changes to occur in these parameters.[30]

Research currently in progress is also evaluating effects of oral administration of alpha-lipoic acid on insulin resistance and symptoms of complications in patients with diabetes.

Table 2
Human Studies of Efficacy of Alpha-Lipoic Acid in Diabetes

Dosage	Study Finding	Ref.
1000 mg alpha-lipoic acid	50% increase in insulin-stimulated glucose disposal	26
500 mg alpha-lipoic acid per day for 10 days	30% increase in insulin-stimulated glucose disposal	22
600 mg alpha-lipoic acid per day for 2 weeks, then 300 mg per day for 10 weeks, or 1575 I.U. vitamin E or 100 μg selenium per day	Improvement in neurological symptoms, decrease in blood MDA levels	28
200 mg alpha-lipoic acid per day for 21 days	Decrease in pain in most subjects, no change in vibration sense or nerve conduction velocity	29
600 mg or 1200 mg alpha-lipoic acid 5 times per week for 3 weeks	Improvement in clinical measures of neuropathy, no change in vibration sense or nerve conduction velocity	30

SUMMARY

Alpha-lipoic acid and its reduced form, dihydrolipoic acid, are effective lipid-soluble and water-soluble antioxidants and also regenerate other antioxidants. Alpha-lipoic acid also has an important role in metabolic reactions. The results of animal and human studies have demonstrated beneficial effects of alpha-lipoic acid treatment in a number of conditions associated with oxidative stress, including ischemia-reperfusion injury, heavy metal poisoning, radiation injury, cataracts, and complications of diabetes. Research is continuing on the specific protective effects of alpha-lipoic acid in these conditions, as well as in other conditions in which oxidative stress has a role.

REFERENCES

1. Packer, L. and Witt, E. H., Alpha-lipoic acid as a biological antioxidant, *Free Rad. Biol. Med.,* 19, 227, 1995.
2. Packer, L., Tritschler, H. J., and Klaus, W., Neuroprotection by the metabolic antioxidant alpha-lipoic acid, *Free Rad. Biol. Med.,* 22, 359, 1997.
3. Packer, L. and Tritschler, H. J., Alpha-lipoic acid: the metabolic antioxidant. *Free Rad. Biol. Med.,* 20, 625, 1996.
4. Estrada, D. E., Ewart, H. S., Tsakiridis, T., Volchuk, A., Ramial, T., Tritschler, H. J., and Kilp, A., Stimulation of glucose uptake by the natural coenzyme alpha-lipoic acid/thioctic acid. Participation of elements of the insulin signaling pathway, *Diabetes,* 45, 1798, 1996.
5. Panigrahi, M., Sadguna, Y., Shivakumar, B. R., Sastry, V. R. K., Roy, S., Packer, L, and Ravindranath, V., Alpha-lipoic acid protects against reperfusion injury following cerebral ischemia in rats, *Brain Res.,* 717, 184, 1996.
6. Scott, B. C., Aruoma, O. I., Evans, P. J., O'Neill, C., van der Vliet, A., Cross, C. E., Tritschler, H. J., and Halliwell, B., Lipoic and dihydrolipoic acids as antioxidants: a critical evaluation, *Free Rad. Res.,* 20, 119, 1994.
7. Rosenberg, H. R. and Culik, R., Effect of alpha-lipoic acid on vitamin C and vitamin E deficiencies, *Arch. Biochem. Biophys.,* 80, 86, 1959.
8. Podda, M., Tritschler, H. J., Ulrich, H., and Packer, L., Alpha-lipoic acid supplementation prevents symptoms of vitamin E deficiency, *Biochem. Biophys. Res. Comm.,* 204, 98, 1994.
9. Busse, E., Zimmer, G., Schopohl, B., and Kornhuber, B., Influence of alpha-lipoic acid on intracellular glutathione *in vitro* and *in vivo*, *Arzneim.-Forsch.,* 42, 829, 1992.
10. Muller, U. and Krieglstein, J., Prolonged treatment with alpha-lipoic acid protects cultured neurons against hypoxic, glutamate- or iron-induced injury, *J. Cereb. Blood Flow Metab.,*15, 624, 1995.
11. Prehn, J. H. M., Karkoutly, C., Nuglisch, J., Pdruche, B., and Krieglstein, J., Dihydrolipoic acid protects neurons against ischemic/hypoxic damage, in *Pharmacology of Cerebral Ischemia,* Krieglstein, J. and Oberpichler, H., Eds., Wissenschaftliche Verlagsgesellscheaft mbH, 1990, pp. 357-362.
12. Backhaus, C., Karkoutly, C., Welsch, M., and Krieglstein, J., A mouse model of focal cerebral ischemia for screening neuroprotective drug effects, *J. Pharmacol. Methods,* 27, 27, 1992.
13. Cao, X. and Phillis, J. W., The free radical scavenger, alpha-lipoic acid, protects against cerebral ischemia-reperfusion injury in gerbils, *Free Rad. Res.,* 23, 365, 1995.

14. Serbinova, E., Khwaja, S., Reznick, A. A., and Packer, L., Thioctic acid protects against ischemia-reperfusion injury in the isolated perfused Langendorff heart, *Free Rad. Res. Comm.* 17, 49, 1992.
15. Assadnazari, H., Zimmer, G., Freisleben, H. J., Werk, W., and Leibfritz, D., Cardioprotective efficiency of dihydrolipoic acid in working rat hearts during hypoxia and reoxygenation, *Arzneim.-Forsch.*, 43, 425, 1993.
16. Grunert, R. R., The effect of dl-alpha-lipoic acid on heavy metal intoxication in mice and dogs, *Arch. Biochem. Biophys.* 86, 190, 1960.
17. Sumathi, R., Devi, V. K., and Varalakshmi, P., DL-alpha-lipoic acid protection against cadmium-induced tissue lipid peroxidation, *Med. Sci. Res.*, 22, 23, 1994.
18. Ramakrishnan, N., Wolfe, W. W., and Catravas, G. N., Radioprotection of hematopoietic tissues in mice by lipoic acid, *Radiation Res.*, 130, 360, 1992.
19. Korkina, L. G., Afanas'ef, I. B., and Diplock, A T., Antioxidant therapy in children affected by irradiation from the Chernobyl nuclear accident, *Biochem. Soc. Trans.*, 21, 314S, 1993.
20. Maitra, I., Serbinova, E., Tritschler, H., and Packer, L., Alpha-lipoic acid prevents buthionine sulfoximine-induced cataract formation in newborn rats, *Free Rad. Biol. Med.*, 18, 823, 1995.
21. Kilic, F., Packer, L., and Trevithick, J. R., Modeling cortical cataractogenesis 17: *In vitro* effect of alpha-lipoic acid on glucose-induced lens membrane damage, a model of diabetic cataractogenesis, *Biochem. Molec. Biol. Intl.*, 37, 361, 1995.
22. Jacob, S., Henriksen, E. J., Tritschler, H. J., Augustin, H. J., and Dietze, G. J., Improvement of insulin-stimulated glucose disposal in type 2 diabetes after repeated parenteral administration of thioctic acid, *Exp. Clin. Endocrinol. Diabetes*, 104, 284, 1996.
23. Jacob, S., Streeper, R. S., Fogt, D. L., Hokama, J Y., Tritschler, H. J., Dietze, G. J., and Henriksen, E. J., The antioxidant alpha-lipoic acid enhances insulin-stimulated glucose metabolism in insulin-resistant rat skeletal muscle, *Diabetes*, 45, 1024, 1996.
24. Natraj, C. V., Gandhi, V M., and Menon, K. K., Lipoic acid and diabetes: Effect of dihydrolipoic acid administration in diabetic rats and rabbits, *J. Biosc.* 6, 37, 1984.
25. Bashan, N., Khamisi, M., Vaknin, U., and Potashnik, R., Effect of lipoic acid on glucose homeostasis and muscle glucose transporters in diabetic rats (abstract), *Diabetologia*, 37, A60, 1994.
26. Jacob, S., Henriksen, E J., Schiemann, A. L., Simon, I., Clancy, D. E., Tritschler, H. J., Jung, W. I., Augustin, H. J., and Dietze, G. J., Enhancement of glucose disposal in patients with type 2 diabetes by alpha-lipoic acid, *Arzneim.-Forsch.*, 45, 872, 1995.
27. Nagamatsu, M., Nickander, K. K., Schmelzer, J. D., Raya, A., Wittrock, D. A., Tritschler, H. J., and Low, P. A., Lipoic acid improves nerve blood flow, reduces oxidative stress, and improves distal nerve conduction in experimental diabetic neuropathy, *Diabetes Care*, 18, 1160, 1995.
28. Kahler, W., Kuklinski, B., Ruhlmann, C., and Plotz, C., Diabetes mellitus - a free radical-associated disease: Effects of adjuvant supplementation of antioxidants, in *The Role of Antioxidants in Diabetes Mellitus: Oxygen Radicals and Antioxidants in Diabetes*, Gries, F. A. and Wessel, K., Eds., Verl. Gruppe, 1993, pp. 33-53.
29. Sachse, G. and Wilms, B., Efficacy of thioctic acid in the therapy of peripheral diabetic neuropathy, in *Aspects of Autonomic Neuropathy in Diabetes*, Gries, F. A., Freund, H. J., Rabe, F., and Berger, H., Eds., G. Thieme, 1980, pp. 105-108.
30. Ziegler, D., Hanefeld, M., Ruhnau, K. J., Meibner, H. P., Lobisch, M., Schutte, K., Gries, F.A., and The ALADIN Study Group, Treatment of symptomatic diabetic peripheral neuropathy with the antioxidant alpha-lipoic acid, *Diabetologia*, 38, 1425, 1995.

Part 7

Current Issues and Emerging Research

27

Current Issues and Emerging Research

Andreas M. Papas, Ph.D.
Health and Nutrition
Eastman Chemical Company, Kingsport, Tennessee, USA

INTRODUCTION

Research focus on the role of antioxidants in nutrition and health is fairly recent. For this reason, many findings from *in vitro*, animal studies, and small clinical studies have yet to be confirmed. The example of β-carotene, which appeared very promising from epidemiological studies but failed to reduce the incidence of lung cancer or heart disease in three major intervention trials, fueled a major scientific and public policy debate. The issues in this debate range from safety and optimum intake to the methodology for establishing efficacy and making public policy recommendations.

The strong scientific and public interest in the role of antioxidants expanded the focus of research from reducing the risk of chronic diseases to improving the general feeling of wellness, mental function, and expanding the life-span. This chapter will review some of the major current issues in the scientific and public debate and the emerging new areas of research.

0-8493-8009-X/98/$0.00+$.50

CURRENT ISSUES

Optimum Intake

Our knowledge of the optimum intake of antioxidants is limited for very few and completely absent for the great majority of them. Some antioxidants such as vitamins A, C, and E, and selenium are essential nutrients with established Recommended Dietary Allowances (RDAs). Almost all antioxidant phytochemicals, however, such as carotenoids, flavonoids, and tocotrienols are not considered essential nutrients and, for this reason, no RDAs have been established. The scientific debate on how to determine the optimum intake of antioxidants has been complicated by a continuing paradigm shift of our view of the role of nutrients and phytochemicals in nutrition and health (Figure 1).

The RDAs were defined as the levels of intake of essential nutrients that, on the basis of scientific knowledge, were judged by the Food and Nutrition Board (of the United States National Research Council) to be adequate to meet the nutrient needs of practically all healthy persons.[1] The United States Department of Agriculture developed Recommended Daily Allowances (USRDAs) which are slightly different than the RDAs. Similar guidelines have been developed by European countries and Japan.

RDAs – A New Paradigm?

The two principal methods used to establish the current RDAs focused on the levels of nutrients needed to prevent deficiency and the average intake of apparently healthy people from the food supply.[1] In contrast, the new paradigm focuses on the levels needed to improve wellness and reduce the risk of disease. While these levels are not known, there are strong suggestions that, for some nutrients, they are significantly higher than the RDAs. The examples of vitamin E and C illustrate this point very well.

For vitamin E, the RDA is 12-15 IU and the USRDA is 30 IU. European recommendations range from 2.3–18 IU with an upper limit of 45 IU. Intake from our diet is less than 11 IU/day and is apparently sufficient to prevent clinical deficiency. Epidemiological data and limited clinical intervention studies indicate that levels in excess of 100 IU are needed for prevention of disease. For example, the Health Professionals Study suggested that the risk of heart disease was lower in those receiving more than 100 IU/day.[2,3] Other studies (reviewed in Chapter 16 and by Weber *et al.*[4]) measuring oxidation of LDL and immune responses suggested that levels higher than the RDA are needed for optimum response.[5,6] A very recent study with elderly[7] evaluated doses of 60, 200, or 800 mg/d of vitamin E for 235 days. Vitamin E improved delayed-type hypersensitivity skin response (DTH) and antibody response to hepatitis B and tetanus. From the doses tested, the most effective was 200 mg/day which is significantly higher than the RDA. Several major clinical studies have or are evaluating daily doses of 50-2000 IU/day. These studies are reviewed in Chapters 21-26. The most popular doses for consumers taking vitamin E are 400, 800, 100, and 200 IU.

Similarly, for vitamin C the RDA is 60 mg and European countries recommend levels of 45-80 mg. A recent study reviewed in Chapter 9 suggested, on the basis of several criteria such as steady-state concentration, urinary excretion, cell concentration, bioavailability, and toxic effects, that the RDA should be increased to 200 mg.[8] The most popular doses for consumers taking vitamin C supplements are 500, 1000, and 250 mg.

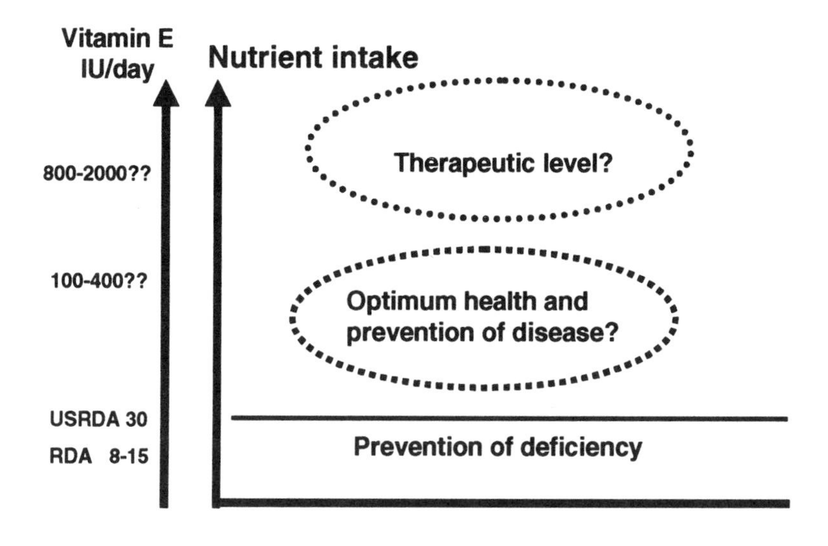

Figure 1. The proposed new paradigm in determining the optimum intake of nutrients. For vitamin E 100-400 IU are being evaluated in major intervention trials for reducing the risk of disease. Higher levels, up to 2000 IU/day have been used in some studies in the elderly.

This proposed new paradigm has affected our view of the role of phytochemicals for which there are no RDAs. The levels tested are generally severalfold higher than what is consumed in common diets.

This paradigm, however, remains quite controversial and is the subject of major debate in the scientific and public health communities[9,10] and in industry.[11] It is very unlikely that the RDAs will be revised soon in accordance with this paradigm. It is very likely, however, that for some nutrients the

RDAs will be revised for individual groups (elderly, athletes, women of reproductive age, etc.) even without wide acceptance of the paradigm. The recent consensus is that calcium intake higher than the RDA may be beneficial for some groups and recommends that women at the reproductive stage consume 400 mg folic acid daily.

The two major arguments against consuming antioxidant vitamins at levels higher than the RDAs are:

- The safety of long-term intake of high levels is not known. In addition, at high levels, antioxidants may function as prooxidants (see below).
- There is no conclusive evidence from clinical double blind, placebo/control intervention studies that higher levels are helpful for prevention of disease.

Safety

Vitamins A, C, and E

Safety is of paramount importance in making recommendations for antioxidant intake. Some antioxidants like vitamin A and Se are extremely toxic at high levels.[1,11] At doses 10 times higher than the RDA, vitamin A causes toxic symptoms including headaches, vomiting, bone abnormalities, and liver damage. Selenium causes nail and hair abnormalities and other toxic effects at doses of over 6 times the RDAs. For hormone antioxidants like melatonin, there is concern for their long-term effects even if short-term studies indicate that they are safe.

Vitamins C and E appear safe even at levels many times higher than the RDAs.[12,13] For vitamin E, side effects have been rare,[14,15] even with doses of 2000 IU/day for two years in two studies, one with patients in early stages of Parkinson's disease and in a very recent study with Alzheimer's patients.[16,17] Major ongoing clinical studies evaluate levels of vitamin E above 100 IU. Vitamin C up to 1000 mg/day had no adverse clinical effects including calculi, but excretion of oxalate and uric acid in the urine increased significantly.[8] Some ongoing clinical trials evaluate doses up to 500 mg.

Even though vitamins E and C are considered safe, they can be harmful in certain conditions. For example, vitamin E can exacerbate problems with blood coagulation for persons with vitamin K deficiency[14,15] and may increase the effect of anticoagulant medications because it reduces adhesion of platelets. Vitamin C accentuates Fe toxicity in conditions of impaired iron metabolism such as hemochromatosis or transfusion therapy because it enhances the absorption of Fe and reduces the Fe^{3+} form to the more prooxidant Fe^{2+}. There are also interactions of these vitamins with other nutrients and drugs which must be considered especially at high dose levels.[18,19]

β-Carotene

β-Carotene provides a good example of the safety issues in evaluating antioxidant phytochemicals and determining their effective safe use levels. β-Carotene has been used widely as food colorant and as a source of vitamin A. β-Carotene was considered safe even at high levels because its absorption and conversion to vitamin A in the intestine, liver, and other organs is low. This perception of safety was shaken recently after two major clinical intervention studies, the α-tocopherol, β-carotene (ATBC)[20] Study and β-carotene and retinol efficacy trial (CARET), discussed in Chapters 8 and 23 suggested that β-carotene increased the risk of lung cancer in current smokers. In the ATBC study, 50 to 69-year-old smokers received 20 mg/day synthetic for 5-8 years; in the CARET study, smokers, former smokers, and asbestos workers received 30 mg/day synthetic β-carotene and 25,000 IU of vitamin A as retinyl palmitate.[21] In another major study (Physicians, see chapter by Hennekens), healthy male physicians received 50 mg synthetic β-carotene on alternate days for about 12 years that did not appear to increase the risk of lung cancer in smokers or cause any other adverse effects.[22]

Although an adverse effect of β-carotene is not conclusive,[11] there has been significant debate as to the reasons for the results of the ATBC and CARET studies. In evaluating these findings, it is also important to understand that the *effective* dose in the ATBC study was 60 times and in the CARET 90 times higher than the *effective* dose from foods. The term *effective* describes the actual amount absorbed. Due to formulation in a water-dispersible microencapsulated form, the absorption of the β-carotene used in these two studies was probably 10-fold higher than from food. Among the mechanisms proposed were interaction with alcohol (ATBC) and/or additive effect with vitamin A (CARET). The most commonly proposed mechanism, however, is based on a prooxidant effect not only of β-carotene but all antioxidants at high doses.

Other Antioxidants

A number of antioxidant phytochemicals, such as lycopene, lutein, tocotrienols, and isoflavones have been introduced commercially as nutritional supplements. While there have been no safety concerns for these natural compounds, it is very important that their safety is carefully evaluated especially prior to their use at high levels. It is often assumed that natural phytochemicals and plant extracts are inherently safe. Of course this is incorrect as evidenced by adverse effects of ephedra.

Prooxidant Effects

It has been known for some time that antioxidants, at high levels and under some conditions *in vitro* and in foods, act as prooxidants. For this reason, food antioxidants are used within a relatively narrow range in order to reduce the probability of prooxidant effects. Whether antioxidants from our diet, and especially high levels from nutritional supplements, have prooxidant effects in humans remains a matter of scientific debate and controversy.

α-Tocopherol

Stocker and his workers studied the prooxidant effects of α-tocopherol on human low-density lipoproteins (LDL).[23] When challenged with free radicals *in vitro* in a system devoid of other antioxidants, LDL oxidized faster when enriched with α-tocopherol either by dosing the donor of the blood or by addition to extracted LDL. It was proposed that α-tocopherol, as the most reactive molecule in LDL, acts as radical sink, pulling radicals from the aqueous phase into the LDL particle. The tocopheryl radical in LDL is fairly immobile because its lipophilic tail anchors it to the particle. This radical can be reduced to tocopherol by other antioxidants such as ascorbic acid, coenzyme Q_{10}, etc.[24-26] In the absence of such agents, other radicals react with, and destroy the tocopherol in LDL leaving it very vulnerable to further free radical damage. Other antioxidants, which the researchers describe as co-antioxidants of α-tocopherol, reduce the tocopheryl radical and prevent its prooxidant effects. They proposed that small amphiphilic antioxidants are particularly efficient because they can shuttle free radicals out from the lipophilic LDL. The same researchers showed *in vitro*, that ascorbic acid and coenzyme Q_{10} prevented the prooxidant effect α-tocopherol. They suggested that other antioxidants such as bilirubin, aminophenol, and catechins have a similar effect.

Several studies evaluated in healthy volunteers the effects of a large range of doses of α-tocopherol (25-1200 IU/day) for 4-12 weeks on Cu-catalyzed LDL oxidation.[6,27] The overall conclusion from these studies was that α-tocopherol increased resistance of LDL to oxidation in a dose dependent manner. No prooxidant effects were apparent even at 1200 IU. Similar results were obtained in two studies with diabetics. In the first study with 21 insulin-dependent-diabetes males, 1600 IU/day for 10 weeks of α-tocopherol increased resistance of LDL to oxidation.[28] In the second, 1200 IU for 8 weeks increased LDL resistance to oxidation in both insulin-dependent and non-insulin-dependent diabetics.[29]

Recently, there has been one report of prooxidant effects of α-tocopherol in humans.[30] This study was conducted with 100 Scottish males (50 smokers and 50 nonsmokers) from a population with habitually low vitamin E and vitamin C intakes. Supplementation for 20 weeks with 70, 140, 560, and 1050 mg d-α-tocopherol/day (equivalent to 104, 209, 834, and 1565 IU) was associated with a significant decrease in susceptibility of erythrocytes to peroxidation. However, red cells of nonsmokers receiving 1050 mg had increased susceptibility to peroxidation and reduced plasma ascorbate concentration. Thus, it would appear that high and prolonged vitamin E intake has prooxidant activity in nonsmokers. This observation for vitamin E seems opposite to the hypothesis proposed by some for a prooxidant effect of β-carotene in smokers and apparently no similar effect in nonsmokers or former smokers. This hypothesis has not been confirmed and the potential prooxidant mechanisms, if they actually occur, are not understood.

These data and the long history of use of α-tocopherol at daily doses of 100-800 IU, without adverse effects, would suggest that prooxidant effects observed *in-vitro*, may not occur in healthy people except in rare special conditions. There are several reasons supporting this hypothesis:

- Antioxidants do not function in isolation but as a part of a complex system. As discussed above, the prooxidant effect of α-tocopherol on LDL *in vitro* is prevented by other antioxidants such as ascorbic acid and coenzyme Q_{10}. It would be practically impossible to create a situation *in vivo* where only one antioxidant is present. It is more likely, however, to alter significantly the relative abundance of antioxidants by supplementation with large doses of individual antioxidants. As discussed in several chapters, large doses of single antioxidants not only increase their level in blood and tissues but may also interfere with the absorption, transport, and tissue uptake of others.
- Our body has strong mechanisms, that regulate the metabolism of antioxidants and prevent excessive accumulation in blood and tissues. For example, α-tocopherol concentration in the blood appears to increase with supplementation in a quadratic manner with essentially linear increases up to approximately 400 IU/day and small increases thereafter.[31,32] Similarly, blood levels of ascorbic acid reach a plateau at doses above 200 mg/day. Mechanisms may exist for regulation of other antioxidants, although for many of them, and especially for phytochemicals, these mechanisms have not been studied. These mechanisms do not prevent large changes in the blood and tissue levels of antioxidants especially with large doses.

Vitamin C

People suffering from the hereditary diseases idiopathic hemochromatosis and thalassemia (hemoglobin is defective) have excess unbound Fe, which acts as a strong prooxidant. Vitamin C can accentuate this prooxidant effect by reducing Fe^{3+} to Fe^{2+}.[18,19,33] Also vitamin C and other antioxidants, such as flavonoids may increase unbound Fe overload by reducing Fe^{3+} in the gut to the more soluble Fe^{2+} thus increasing absorption.[34]

Other Antioxidants

We know little about prooxidant effects of many antioxidants especially of phytochemicals. It has been suggested, but not confirmed, that β-carotene may act as prooxidant in current smokers. Flavonoids have polyphenolic structure and are susceptible to autoxidation.[34] Free radicals are probably formed during their redox cycling. Ubisemiquinone, the intermediate of ubiquinone redox cycling, can undergo autoxidation to produce superoxide radicals. Another proposed mechanism for the flavonoid prooxidant effects, originally proposed for quercetin and later for gossypol, is the formation of ternary complexes of DNA, Cu, and flavonoids. Some flavonoids show mutagenic effects *in vitro*[35] but there are no such reports for similar effects *in vivo*. Actually many of them are studied for reducing the risk of cancer.

The Continuing Debate

While prooxidant effects, like that of vitamin C in hematochromatosis, are very plausible, there is little conclusive clinical evidence that does actually occur. There is also very little, and sometimes conflicting, information of other prooxidant effects *in vivo*. For example, α-tocopherol, applied topically, appeared to promote initiated skin tumors in mice suggesting a strong prooxidant effect.[36] Yet in another study in humans, α-tocopherol applied topically was very effective in reducing the severity of musositis caused by chemotherapy.[37] Furthermore, vitamin E has been used extensively for many years in cosmetics and for other skin and wound treatments without reported adverse clinical effects.

The debate on the prooxidant effects of antioxidants, and especially their significance in human nutrition and health, will continue for some time until additional research resolves the many remaining questions. The limited research available todate suggests:

- Prooxidant effects do occur *in vitro* and in foods and the mechanisms involved are reasonably well understood. In contrast, there is very limited evidence of prooxidant effects *in vivo* and the mechanisms involved, especially the interactions of the many components of the antioxidant system, are not understood as well.
- Some common threads emerge from research to date and merit further study. It appears that prooxidant effects *in vitro* are stronger when other

antioxidants are absent or are present proportionately in very small amounts. This would suggest that other antioxidants can prevent prooxidant effects because they scavenge the free radical form of antioxidants. As discussed above, it would be practically impossible to create a situation *in vivo* where only one antioxidant is present and this may explain the rare occurrence of prooxidant effects *in vivo*.

- It is also possible that antioxidants may have quite opposite effects in normal and precancerous or cancerous tissues. As discussed above, α-tocopherol is a promoter of induced skin tumors in mice but it seems to reverse mucositis in humans caused by chemotherapy.
- Finally, antioxidants have major nonantioxidant effects including signal transduction, enzyme inhibition and others. It would be important to understand these effects and determine whether they reduce or contribute to prooxidant effects.

Nutritional Supplements

There is practical unanimity that a balanced diet is the preferred source of nutrients and antioxidants. For this reason, it is recommended that we consume at least 5-9 servings per day of fruits and vegetables, which are rich sources of antioxidants. This unanimity, however, is replaced by heated debate regarding the use of nutritional supplements in general including antioxidants.

Arguments Against Nutritional Supplements

- We know very little about the safety of long-term use of many antioxidants, especially at levels severalfold higher than available from the diet. This is particularly true for antioxidant phytochemicals, which are now introduced as nutritional supplements.
- For many antioxidants there is no conclusive evidence of efficacy. Data from epidemiological studies cannot substitute for intervention studies as shown by the ATBC and CARET studies for β-carotene.
- Antioxidants may have prooxidant effects, especially when provided as single entities at large doses (see discussion above).
- Nutritional supplements provide a false sense of health security, which causes people to reduce their vigilance regarding their diet, exercise, and healthier lifestyles.

Arguments in Favor of Using Nutritional Supplements

- While there has been significant increase in consumption of fruits and vegetables, the average is still 4.3 servings per day, which is below the 5-

9 servings recommended. In addition, there are segments of the population consuming significantly less.[38,39]

- Even with a well-balanced diet, it is very difficult to meet the RDA for some antioxidants. Vitamin E provides a good example. Studies indicate that average daily intake is below 11 IU.[40] To achieve intake of 30 IU (USRDA), it is necessary to consume a well-balanced diet containing 30% or more of calories from carefully chosen fat sources. Individuals on a fat-restricted diet or with conditions that limit the digestion of dietary fats may require a supplement to reach even the USRDA levels.
- The strongest argument in favor of supplements is the new proposed paradigm, namely, that intakes higher than the RDAs may be required for optimum health and for reducing the risk of disease. Some antioxidants can be obtained from foods even at quantities severalfold higher than the RDAs. For example, 3-4 oranges can supply 200 mg vitamin C, the level suggested recently as optimum. For vitamin E, several studies reviewed above, suggest that intake of 100 IU or higher is needed. It would be extremely difficult to obtain this amount of vitamin E from the diet. For example, 474 g corn oil, 1.5 kg raw peanuts, or 5.3 kg raw spinach are needed to supply 100 IU.

The Continuing Debate

There are valid arguments on both sides of this debate. Especially valid is the argument that efficacy and safety data for long-term use of high levels of some antioxidants are absent or incomplete. Unfortunately, it will take decades before all necessary research is completed. This raises a serious dilemma. As discussed above, a recent study showed that Alzheimer's patients benefit from very large doses of vitamin E (2000 IU),[17] which could not be obtained from the diet. Ideally, these results should be confirmed in other intervention studies, including titration studies, to determine the optimum level before public health recommendations are made. This work will take at least several years and possibly decades and will be of little help to current patients. Less serious, yet important decisions face the elderly. Several nutrients and antioxidants show significant promise for boosting the immune system and reducing the risk of chronic disease and infection. Yet, the evidence is not conclusive. Thus, use of nutritional supplements becomes a decision of potential benefit versus risk and, for some antioxidants such as vitamins E and C, the potential benefits outweigh the risk. There are also other groups such as AIDS patients, athletes, and pregnant women with special nutritional needs which may not be met easily in the diet.

The main argument, however, is whether healthy people benefit from intakes of nutrients higher than the RDAs. This argument will be resolved only when scientists reach a consensus on two other underlying issues. The first is the proposed new paradigm that levels severalfold higher than the RDAs are needed for optimum health and for reducing the risk of disease as discussed above. The second is whether it is reasonable to expect that the great majority of the population will consume balanced diets. Since it is very unlikely that these issues will be resolved soon, the use of nutritional supplement will continue to be a matter of personal decision based on the perception of benefit and risk.

Antioxidant Status of the Digesta

Currently antioxidant status is almost exclusively considered in the context of blood and other tissues. It may be appropriate, however, to consider the digesta as a major component.[41] From the time of ingestion of food to excretion of fecal material, digesta undergoes major physical and chemical changes including acidification, complex enzymatic and other reactions, emulsification of lipids with bile salts, etc. In addition, the microflora in the gut is an integral part of the digestion and may influence absorption and may produce free radicals or antioxidants. Microflora is affected by diet composition, disease, medication, and other factors. The many complex reactions occurring in the gut could lead to production of free radicals and other metabolites which may have a direct effect in the development of digestive cancers, intestinal inflammation, and possibly other diseases. In addition, harmful end-products are absorbed and can cause tissue damage. Current concepts of absorption and bioavailability may not fully reflect the utility of various compounds and formulations. The role of the antioxidant status of the digesta using as an example the role of tocopherols in colon cancer was discussed in an earlier chapter.

Antioxidant Status: What is Optimal?

Scientists agree that a significant imbalance in the antioxidant status favoring prooxidants is harmful. Would tipping the balance in favor of prooxidants, however, be beneficial? The answer is probably no for several reasons.

- We derive our energy from oxidation, which requires at least slightly prooxidant conditions.
- It is not desirable to eliminate production of reactive oxygen species and free radicals because, at least some, are essential components of our body's defense mechanism against invading microorganisms.
- Finally, it is not known whether it is possible under practical conditions, even with significant diet modification and supplementation, to achieve such significant change in the metabolic environment of the body.
- Some researchers suggest that boosting the antioxidant status has no

benefits and can be harmful because it creates the conditions for antioxidants to become prooxidants[19] (discussed above). Fortunately, a large number of intervention clinical studies are now in progress and will help enhance our understanding of the antioxidant status in health and disease.

EMERGING RESEARCH

Brain Function

The role of antioxidants for improving brain function and delaying the onset of degenerative diseases appears very promising and is becoming a major and exciting area of research. This optimism is based on the emerging unified concept, which suggests that free radicals, resulting mostly from impaired glucose metabolism, contribute to the development of degenerative brain diseases.[42-44] There are two very distinct and equally important areas of interest.

1. Delay of the onset and progression of diseases such as Alzheimer's, Parkinson's, Huntington's, amyotrophic lateral sclerosis (ALS), and others. In addition, antioxidants may help with the management of these diseases by reducing the severity of their symptoms and the side effects of drugs.
2. Improving brain function of healthy people. Consumers have very strong interest in maintaining and even strengthening their memory, their mental alertness, their ability to think and focus, and other mental capabilities. This is apparent from the strong demand for products that promise to enhance brain function (ginseng, Ginkgo biloba and dehydroepiandrosterone (DHEA)) even in the absence of conclusive evidence.

Antioxidants and Diseases of the Brain

Two studies point to the large potential of this research. The first, a double-blind, placebo-controlled, randomized, multicenter trial in patients with Alzheimer's disease of moderate severity, very high levels of α-tocopherol (2000 IU day) delayed progression of this debilitating disease by approximately 7 months.[17] The implications for other diseases such as Parkinson's are extremely important. A major placebo-controlled, multicenter trial with patients in the early stages of Parkinson's disease showed no benefits from high vitamin E supplementation (2000 IU day).[16] Other studies, however, suggested that vitamin E reduces the severity of the symptoms of the disease and side effects of the powerful neuroleptic drugs used in these patients.[45]

It would be extremely interesting to find out whether α-tocopherol and other antioxidants, taken from a young age, would delay significantly the onset of these major and other degenerative diseases of the brain such as ALS and Huntington's. A unified hypothesis has been suggested for the development of these degenerative brain diseases. Specifically, it has been suggested that a common characteristic of these diseases is impaired energy metabolism in the mitochondria of brain cells, which disrupts the normal oxidation of glucose and causes electrons to be diverted and produce free radicals. Mitochondrial defects in the first and last steps of glucose oxidation have been suggested for Parkinson's and Alzheimer's disease, respectively. Similar defects are being suggested for ALS and in Huntington's. The reported genetic link of Alzheimer's disease to mutations in the genes encoding two mitochondrial cytochrome c oxidase subunits (CO1 and CO2), however, has been attributed to an artifact (discussed in Chapter 25). For this reason, this hypothesis may be applicable to some, but not all these diseases.

Improving Memory and Brain Function

A particular extract of Ginkgo biloba, EGb 761, has been used in Europe to treat cognitive disorders. In the United States and other countries, Ginkgo biloba has been marketed as an aid to improve memory and brain function. Evifence of its efficacy has been very limited. A recent intervention study evaluated the effect of EGb 761 with over 200 Alzheimer patients for one year.[46] The results indicated that one-third of the Alzheimer's patients taking the ginkgo extracts improved in tasks involving memory. Approximately half of the group did not show improved memory, but showed no signs of increased memory loss. These improvements are equivalent to a six-month delay in the progression of dementia.

These preliminary results suggest that phytochemicals may improve memory and brain function. The researchers suggested that the effect of the Ginkgo extract may be due to its antioxidant properties. The effectiveness of vitamin E in delaying the progression of Alzheimer's disease supports the hypothesis that antioxidant mechanisms may be partially responsible for the observed effects. While these effects were observed in Alzheimer's patients, it is very intriguing to determine the effects of these and other antioxidants in healthy people, especially the elderly.

Aging and Extending the Life-Span

In the past, scientists were very apprehensive of publicly discussing the potential for significantly expanding the life span lest they would be ridiculed. For this reason, research on aging focused on reducing the risk of chronic disease and improving the quality of life (Figure 2). (The productive research on the role of antioxidant status in aging has been reviewed in Chapters 13 and 17.) The scope of research on aging is now changing and there is open scientific debate and preliminary research suggesting that life span can be extended for years and even decades.

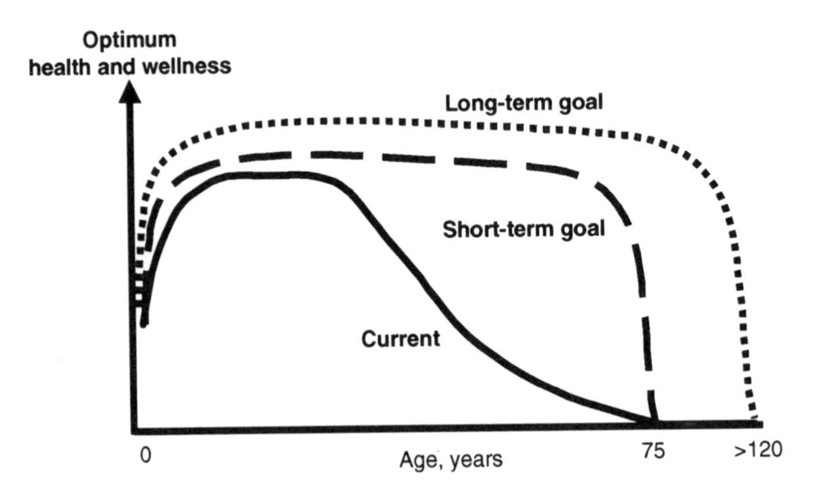

Figure 2. The changing paradigm of research on aging. The long-term focus includes extention of the life span in addition to reducing the risk of disease and improving wellness.

There is good basis for optimism. It has been known for some time that reducing by 30% the caloric intake of rats increased their life span by 30-40%. Caloric restriction reduced their body temperature by 1°C probably as a result of slower metabolic rate.[47] Another important development has been the discovery of telomeres, sequences of DNA at the end of the DNA strands, which protect the integrity of the genetic material. With repeated replications, telomeres become very short and possibly ineffective. An enzyme named telomerase preserves and possibly repairs telomeres thus opening the potential for using genetic engineering.[48] Is caloric restriction reducing cell division and thus delaying the damage to telomeres?

Another mechanism, proposed recently, suggests that glycosylation causes complexes of proteins with carbohydrates which trigger further accumulation of proteins leading to stiffening of joints, development of cataracts, and other chronic diseases.[49-51] Glycosylation occurs rapidly in diabetics, which are more prone to these diseases. It is believed that excessive production of free radicals in diabetics contributes to the higher incidence for these chronic diseases. Higher metabolic rate from high caloric intake may lead to increased production of free radicals which, in turn, may damage proteins and increase the production of factors facilitating glycosylation[52] and adherence of platelets.

A recent study at the University of Arizona[53] points to a potentially large role for free radicals and antioxidants. This study with rats investigated the effects of high vitamin E and/or high beta-carotene diets on band 3 proteins, which function as anion transporters, acid base regulators, CO_2 transporters, and structural proteins that provide a framework for membrane lipids that link the plasma membrane to the cytoskeleton. Senescent cell antigen (SCA), which terminates the life of cells, is a degradation product of band 3. Vitamin E prevented the observed age-related decline in anion transport by lymphocytes and the generation of aged band 3 leading to SCA formation. β-Carotene had no significant effect. Since increased aged band 3 and decreased anion transport are initial steps in band 3 aging, which leads to generation of SCA and death of the cell, vitamin E prevents or delays aging of band 3-related proteins in lymphocytes and brain. These very preliminary findings point to a new and potentially very exciting area of research for extending the life span. This will be a significant expansion to the ongoing research for improving the quality in the elderly.

Quality of Life

This term, for the purpose of this discussion, is used to describe a rather elusive feeling of wellness, which is strongly desired and actively pursued. Different people have varying expectations from a feeling of wellness. Some common expectations include:

- Feeling of high energy and absence of fatigue.
- High mental alertness, strong memory, and ability to focus and handle complex mental tasks.
- Increased resistance to infectious and chronic diseases. In the past, research focused primarily on life-threatening diseases such as heart disease and cancer. Future research will most likely be expanded to diseases such as the common cold that, while not life threatening, interfere with the quality of life.

Infectious Diseases

Important preliminary research, reviewed in Chapter 17, indicated that vitamin E increased delayed-type hypersensitivity skin response and antibody response to hepatitis B and tetanus in elderly humans.[7] This work suggests that there may be potential for reducing infection. Other researchers reported that a cloned and sequenced amyocarditic coxsackievirus B3 (CVB3/0), which caused little or no pathology in the hearts of vitamin E-supplemented mice, induced extensive cardiac pathology in vitamin E-deficient mice suggesting that this virus changed to a virulent phenotype.[54]

Similar observations were made in selenium-deficient mice.[55] The authors suggested that the nutritional antioxidant status of the host determines the severity of certain viral infections. There are many implications of these findings for other viruses and infectious diseases.

Management of Existing Chronic Diseases Such as Arthritis and Diabetes

There is substantial research, reviewed in other chapters, suggesting that antioxidants and particularly vitamin E, help reduce arthritic inflammation and improve glucose and lipid profile in diabetics. Because diabetes increases the risk of other chronic diseases, such as cataracts, arthritis, and heart disease, the role of antioxidants merits further research.

Depression

A number of clinical studies indicated that extracts of the plant Hypericum perforatum (St. John's wort) are effective for the treatment of mild to moderately severe depression.[56,57] The mechanisms involved are not understood but some researchers suggested that antioxidant compounds in the extract may be responsible in part for this effect. This research is insufficient for suggesting a role of antioxidants in the management or treatment of depression. It is, however, an area of significant interest due to prevalence of this disease and the side effects of some antidepressant drugs.

Beyond Antioxidant Function: Other Biological Effects

Recent research indicates that antioxidants have significant and sometimes quite different metabolic effects, which may be independent or only partially related to their function as antioxidants. The following are major examples of such effects:

- Signal transduction. Drs. Őzer and Azzi discussed in Chapter 20 the effects of tocopherols, tocotrienols, and other antioxidants on protein kinase C (PKC) and other important events in cell growth and communication. Quercetin has been suggested to enhance the transforming growth factor β_1 ($TGF\beta_1$) to post-transcriptional levels.[58] Lycopene and other antioxidants may play a role in cell communication.[59]
- Blocking estrogen-binding sites. It is believed that some flavonoids such as genistein, diadzein, and quercetin may help reduce the risk of breast, ovarian, and some other cancers by reducing the number of receptor sites available to estrogens.
- Inhibition of interleukin 1β (IL-1β) and monocyte-cell adhesion, a cru-

cial event in atherogenesis. These effects seem to be mediated by inhibition of PKC and NFκB.

- Post-transcriptional suppression of 3-hydroxy-3-methylglutaryl-coenzyme A (HMG-CoA) reductase. This enzyme is important for the synthesis of cholesterol. Tocotrienols inhibit its activity.[60]
- Control of extracellular fluids. LLU-α, a proposed metabolite of γ-tocopherol, may inhibit the 70 pS K^+ channel in the apical membrane in the kidney. LLU-α is considered an endogenous natriuretic factor.[61]
- Inhibition of modification of brain and lymphocyte band 3 proteins.[53] We discussed above the potential role of this modification by vitamin E and possibly other antioxidants on cell life span.
- Enhancing the action of drugs. Vitamin E and another antioxidant compound attenuated the effect of cancer drug 5-fluorouracil on tumors of human colon cancer cells transplanted into mice. The researchers suggested that vitamin E enhanced the action of the drug by turning on the gene p21 in cancer cells thus inducing death of the cells by apoptosis.

Future research will help us understand these mechanisms better and identify other mechanisms of action of antioxidants. Such information will be extremely useful in understanding the biological effects and safety issues. In addition, it may provide important biological markers for selective active compounds for further study.

CONCLUSION

Research on antioxidants has substantially increased our understanding of their function and their role in nutrition and health. As often happens with research in a new field, answers in some studies were partial or contradictory and the new knowledge generated more questions.

The debate on the issues of optimum intake, long-term safety, and pro-oxidant effects of antioxidants will continue for at least several years. It is possible that ongoing major intervention clinical trials like the Women's Health study, the HOPE study, and others (discussed in earlier chapters) will help answer these questions for vitamin E and provide some indication regarding the proposed new paradigm of health and prevention of disease versus prevention of deficiency.

Future research will expand in the fields of brain function, wellness, resistance to infectious diseases, and increasing the life span. The impetus and funding for these areas of research will be affected by results of the ongoing major clinical intervention trials.

REFERENCES

1. NRC. Recommended Dietary Allowances. 10 ed. Washington, D.C.: National Academy Press, 1989.
2. Stampfer MJ, Hennekens CH, Manson JE, Colditz GA, Rosner B, Willett WC. Vitamin E consumption and the risk of coronary disease in women. N Engl J Med 1993;328:1444-9.
3. Rimm EB, Stampfer MJ, Ascherio A, Giovannucci E, Colditz GA, Willett WC. Vitamin E consumption and the risk of coronary heart disease in men. N. Engl. J. Med. 1993;328:1450-1456.
4. Weber P, Bendich A, Machlin LJ. Vitamin E and human health: rationale for determining recommended intake levels. Nutrition 1997;13:450-60.
5. Meydani SN, Wu D, Santos MS, Hayek MG. Antioxidants and immune response in aged persons: overview of present evidence. Am J Clin Nutr 1995;62:1462S-1476S.
6. Jialal I, Fuller CJ, Huet BA. The effect of α-tocopherol supplementation on LDL oxidation. A dose-response study. Arterioscler. Thromb. Vasc. Biol. 1995;15:190-198.
7. Meydani SN, Meydani M, Blumberg JB, *et al.* Vitamin E supplementation and *in vivo* immune response in healthy elderly subjects. A randomized controlled trial. JAMA 1997;277:1380-6.
8. Levine M, Conry-Cantilena C, Wang Y, *et al.* Vitamin C pharmacokinetics in healthy volunteers: evidence for a recommended dietary allowance. Proc Natl Acad Sci USA 1996;93:3704-9.
9. Lachance P, Langseth L. The RDA concept: time for a change? Nutr Rev 1994;52:266-70.
10. Russell RM. New views on the RDAs for older adults. J Am Diet Assoc 1997;97:515-8.
11. Hathcock JN. Vitamins and minerals: efficacy and safety. Am J Clin Nutr 1997;66:427-37.
12. Meyers DG, Maloley PA, Weeks D. Safety of antioxidant vitamins. Arch Intern Med 1996;156:925-35.
13. Diplock AT. Safety of antioxidant vitamins and beta-carotene. Am J Clin Nutr 1995;62:1510S-1516S.
14. Bendich A, Machlin LJ. The safety of oral intake of vitamin E: data from clinical studies from 1986 to 1991. In: Packer L, Fuchs J, Eds. *Vitamin E in Health and Disease*. New York, NY: Marcel Dekker, Inc., 1993:411-416.
15. Kappus H, Diplock A. Tolerance and safety of vitamin E: a toxicological position report. Free Rad. Biol. Med. 1992;13:55-74.
16. Group TPS. Effects of tocopherol and deprenyl on the progression of disability in early Parkinson's disease. N. Engl. J. Med. 1993;328:176-183.
17. Sano M, Ernesto C, Thomas RG, *et al.* A controlled trial of selegiline, alpha-tocopherol, or both as treatment for Alzheimer's disease. The Alzheimer's Disease Cooperative Study. N Engl J Med 1997;336:1216-22.
18. Herbert V, Shaw SJ, E., Stopler-Kasdan T. Most free-radical injury is iron related: It is promoted by iron, hemin, holoferritin, and vitamin C, and inhibited by desferrioxamine and apoferritin. Stem Cells 12, 1994: 289-303.
19. Herbert V. The antioxidant supplement myth. Am. J. Clin. Nutr, 1994:157-158.
20. The Alpha-Tocopherol B-CCPSG. The effect of vitamin E and beta carotene on the incidence of lung cancer and other cancers in male smokers. The Alpha-Tocopherol, Beta Carotene Cancer Prevention Study Group. N Engl J Med 1994;330:1029-35.
21. Omenn GS, Goodman GE, Thornquist MD, *et al.* Effects of a combination of beta carotene and vitamin A on lung cancer and cardiovascular disease. N Engl J Med 1996;334:1150-5.

22. Hennekens CH, Buring JE, Manson JE, *et al.* Lack of effect of long-term supplementation with beta carotene on the incidence of malignant neoplasms and cardiovascular disease. N Engl J Med 1996;334:1145-9.
23. Bowry VW, Stocker R. Tocopherol-mediated peroxidation. The prooxidant effect of vitamin E on the radical-initiated oxidation of human low-density lipoprotein. J. Am. Chem. Soc. 115 1993: 6029-6044.
24. Kontush A, Finckh B, Karten B, Kohlschutter A, Beisiegel U. Antioxidant and prooxidant activity of alpha-tocopherol in human plasma and low density lipoprotein. J Lipid Res 1996;37:1436-48.
25. Stocker R, Frei B. Endogenous antioxidant defences in human blood plasma. In: Sies H, ed. *Oxidative Stress. Oxidants and Antioxidants.* London: Academic Press, 1991:213-243.
26. Thomas SR, Neuzil J, Stocker R. Cosupplementation with coenzyme Q prevents the prooxidant effect of alpha-tocopherol and increases the resistance of LDL to transition metal-dependent oxidation initiation. Arterio. Thromb. Vasc. Biol. 1996;16:687-696.
27. Princen HM, van Duyvenvoorde W, Buytenhek R, *et al.* Supplementation with low doses of vitamin E protects LDL from lipid peroxidation in men and women. Arterioscler Thromb Vasc Biol 1995;15:325-33.
28. Reaven PD, Herold DA, Barnett J, Edelman S. Effects of Vitamin E on susceptibility of low-density lipoprotein and low-density lipoprotein subfractions to oxidation and on protein glycation in NIDDM. Diabetes Care 1995;18:807-16.
29. Fuller CJ, Chandalia M, Garg A, Grundy SM, Jialal I. RRR-alpha-tocopheryl acetate supplementation at pharmacologic doses decreases low-density-lipoprotein oxidative susceptibility but not protein glycation in patients with diabetes mellitus. Am J Clin Nutr 1996;63:753-9.
30. Brown KM, Morrice PC, Duthie GG. Erythrocyte vitamin E and plasma ascorbate concentrations in relation to erythrocyte peroxidation in smokers and nonsmokers: dose response to vitamin E supplementation. Am J Clin Nutr 1997;65:496-502.
31. Dimitrov MV, Meyer C, Gilliland D, Ruppenthal M, Chenowith W, Malone W. Plasma tocopherol concentrations in response to supplemental vitamin E. Am. J. Clin. Nutr. 1991;53:723-729.
32. Traber MG. Regulation of human plasma vitamin E. In: Sies H, Ed. *Antioxidants in Disease Mechanisms and Therapeutic Strategies.* San Diego, CA: Academic Press, 1996:49-63.
33. Young IS, Trouton TG, Torney JJ, McMaster D, Callender ME, Trimble ER. Antioxidant status and lipid peroxidation in hereditary haemochromatosis. Free Radic Biol Med 1994;16:393-7.
34. Cao G, Sofic E, Prior RL. Antioxidant and prooxidant behavior of flavonoids: structure-activity relationships. Free Radic Biol Med 1997;22:749-60.
35. Stich HF. The beneficial and hazardous effects of simple phenolic compounds. Mutat Res 1991;259:307-24.
36. Mitchell REJ, McCann R. Vitamin E is a complete tumor promoter in mouse skin. Carcinogenesis, 1993: 659-662.
37. Wadleigh RG, Redman RS, Graham ML, Krasnow SH, Anderson A, Cohen MH. Vitamin E in the treatment of chemotherapy-induced mucositis. Am J Med 1992;92:481-4.
38. Krebs-Smith SM, Cook A, Subar AF, Cleveland L, Friday J. U.S. adults' fruit and vegetable intakes, 1989 to 1991: a revised baseline for the Healthy People 2000 objective. Am J Public Health 1995;85:1623-9.
39. Cleveland LE, Cook DA, Krebs-Smith SM, Friday J. Method for assessing food intakes in terms of servings based on food guidance. Am J Clin Nutr 1997;65:1254S-1263S.
40. Murphy SP, Subar AF, Block G. Vitamin E intakes and sources in the United States. Am J Clin Nutr 1990;52:361-7.

41. Stone WL, Papas AM. Tocopherols and the etiology of colon cancer. J Natl Cancer Inst 1997;89:1006-14.
42. Jenner P. Oxidative stress in Parkinson's disease and other neurodegenerative disorders. Pathol Biol (Paris) 1996;44:57-64.
43. Knight JA. Reactive oxygen species and the neurodegenerative disorders. Ann Clin Lab Sci 1997;27:11-25.
44. Simonian NA, Coyle JT. Oxidative stress in neurodegenerative diseases. Annu Rev Pharmacol Toxicol 1996;36:83-106.
45. Lohr JB, Caligiuri MP. A double-blind placebo-controlled study of vitamin E treatment of tardive dyskinesia. J Clin Psychiatry 1996;57:167-73.
46. Le Bars PL, Katz MM, Berman N, Itil TM, Freedman AM, Schatzberg AF. A placebo-controlled, double-blind, randomized trial of an extract of ginkgo biloba for dementia. JAMA 1997;278:1327-1332.
47. McCarter RJ. Role of caloric restriction in the prolongation of life. Clin Geriatr Med 1995;11:553-65.
48. Counter CM. The roles of telomeres and telomerase in cell life span. Mutat Res 1996;366:45-63.
49. Sullivan R. Contributions to senescence: non-enzymatic glycosylation of proteins. Arch Physiol Biochem 1996;104:797-806.
50. Bruel A, Oxlund H. Changes in biomechanical properties, composition of collagen and elastin, and advanced glycation endproducts of the rat aorta in relation to age. Atherosclerosis 1996;127:155-65.
51. Deguine V, Labat-Robert J, Ferrari P, Pouliquen Y, Menasche M, Robert L. Aging of the vitreous body. Role of glycation and free radicals. Pathol Biol (Paris) 1997;45:321-30.
52. Spencer RP. Life prolongation with dietary restriction: protection of genome and core metabolism and the role of glycosylation. Med Hypotheses 1993;40:102-4.
53. Poulin JE, Cover C, Gustafson MR, Kay MB. Vitamin E prevents oxidative modification of brain and lymphocyte band 3 proteins during aging. Proc Natl Acad Sci USA 1996;93:5600-3.
54. Beck MA, Kolbeck PC, Rohr LH, Shi Q, Morris VC, Levander OA. Vitamin E deficiency intensifies the myocardial injury of coxsackievirus B3 infection of mice. J. Nutr. 1994;124: 345-358.
55. Beck MA, Kolbeck S, Q., P.C., Rohr LH, Morris VC, Levander OA. Increased virulence of a human enterovirus (coxsackievirus B3) in selenium-deficient mice. J. Infect. Dis 1994;10: 351-357.
56. Linde K, Ramirez G, Mulrow CD, Pauls A, Weidenhammer W, Melchart D. St John's wort for depression - an overview and meta-analysis of randomised clinical trials. BMJ 1996;313:253-8.
57. Volz HP. Controlled clinical trials of hypericum extracts in depressed patients - an overview. Pharmacopsychiatry 1997;2:72-6.
58. Scambia G, Panici PB, Ranelletti FO, *et al.* Quercetin enhances transforming growth factor beta 1 secretion by human ovarian cancer cells. Int J Cancer 1994;57:211-5.
59. Stahl W, Sies H. Lycopene: a biologically important carotenoid for humans? Arch Biochem Biophys 1996;336:1-9.
60. Parker RA, Pearce BC, Clark RW, Gordon DA, Wright JJ. Tocotrienols regulate cholesterol production in mammalian cells by post-transcriptional suppression of 3-hydroxy-3-methylglutaryl-coenzyme A reductase. J Biol Chem 1993;268:11230-8.
61. Wechter WJ, Kantoci D, Murray ED, Jr., D'Amico DC, Jung ME, Wang WH. A new endogenous natriuretic factor: LLU-alpha. Proc Natl Acad Sci USA 1996;93:6002-7.

Epilogue

The current stage of our knowledge of the antioxidant status in humans, especially in relation to diet and physiological stage and its impact on nutrition and health, was reflected in a recent workshop organized by the Panel on Dietary Antioxidants. The Food and Nutrition Board of the Institute of Medicine, National Academy of Sciences appointed this panel to develop dietary reference intakes.

The decision of the National Academy of Sciences to undertake this study is indicative of the major research advances made and the strong scientific and public health interest to evaluate and apply this knowledge. In the first workshop organized by this panel, top experts in the field debated, without reaching a consensus, the definition of antioxidants and whether major classes of phytochemicals should be considered as antioxidants. Yet the same experts described our excellent understanding of the mechanisms of oxidation and antioxidant function. Thus, despite great advances, major gaps remain in our knowledge especially in measuring the antioxidant status in humans and in determining the role of antioxidants in health and prevention of disease.

Fortunately, research in this field has been increasing very substantially and will fill many of the existing knowledge gaps. The additional knowledge will contribute to the development of practical recommendations for nutrition and health. This process, however, is likely to be long and arduous. Until then, individual decisions will be made on the basis of the available scientific information. I hope this book will contribute in our understanding and effective use of the knowledge gained to date.

Index

B

D

E

F

G

H

I

J

K

L

M

N

O

Q

R

S

U

V

Also by Edvard Radzinsky

The Last Tsar:

The Life and Death

of Nicholas II

THE FIRST IN-DEPTH BIOGRAPHY BASED ON EXPLOSIVE NEW DOCUMENTS FROM RUSSIA'S SECRET ARCHIVES

EDVARD RADZINSKY

TRANSLATED BY

H. T. WILLETTS

DOUBLEDAY

New York London Toronto Sydney Auckland

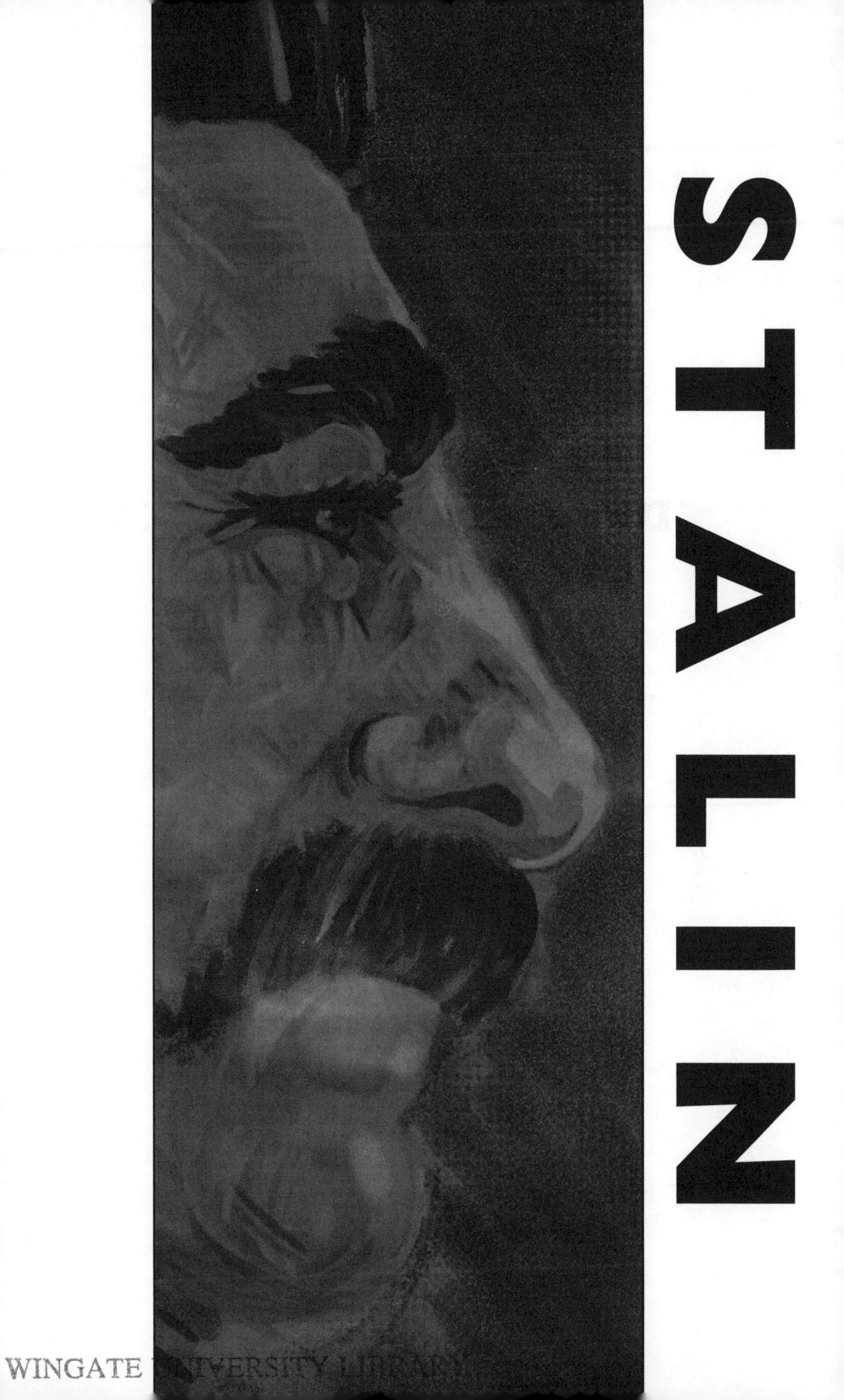
STALIN

PUBLISHED BY DOUBLEDAY
a division of Bantam Doubleday Dell Publishing Group, Inc.
1540 Broadway, New York, New York 10036

DOUBLEDAY and the portrayal of an anchor with a
dolphin are trademarks of Doubleday, a division of Bantam Doubleday
Dell Publishing Group, Inc.

Book design by Jennifer Ann Daddio
Frontispiece by Hal Brigish

Library of Congress Cataloging-in-Publication Data
Radzinskiĭ, Ėdvard.
Stalin: the first in-depth biography based on explosive new
documents from Russia's secret archives / Edvard Radzinsky;
translated by H. T. Willetts. — 1st ed.
p. cm.
Includes bibliographical references and index.
1. Stalin, Joseph, 1878–1953—Sources. 2. Heads of state—Soviet
Union—Biography—Sources. 3. Soviet Union—History—1925–1953—
Sources. I. Title.
DK268.S8R29 1996
947.084′2—dc20 95-4495
CIP

ISBN 0-385-47397-4

Translated from the Russian by H. T. Willetts

Printed in the United States of America
April 1996

1 3 5 7 9 10 8 6 4 2

First Edition

CONTENTS

NOTE

The dates used in this book up to February 1918 follow the old-style Julian calendar, which was in use in Russia until that month. In the nineteenth century the Julian calendar lagged twelve days behind the Gregorian calendar used in the West; in the twentieth century, the Julian calendar lagged thirteen days behind.

PREFACE

I have been thinking about this book all my life. My father dreamt of it till the day of his death. It is to him that I dedicate it.

I can still see that antediluvian day in March 1953 when the improbable happened: the event which it would have been a crime even to think of in our country.

I can see the unbearably bright March sunshine and the endless line of those eager to make their farewells to him. I see myself in the crowd of mourners. How lonely I felt among all those grief-crazed people. Because I myself hated him.

I had suffered a revulsion of feeling toward Stalin as an upperclassman at school: a transition from mindless adoration to a no-less ardent hatred, such as only the very young experience and only after mindless love.

This change of heart was brought about by my father and by his dangerous stories about Stalin. The real Stalin. Whenever my father spoke of him, he ended with the same words: *Perhaps someday you will write about him.*

My father was an intellectual with a passionate love of European democracy. He often repeated a saying which he attributed to President Masaryk of Czechoslovakia: "What is happiness? It is having the right to go out onto the main square and to shout at the top of your voice, 'Lord, what a bad government we have!'" My father came from a well-to-do Jewish family. He was a rising young lawyer, twenty-eight years old, when the February Revolution brought down the monarchy. He enthusiastically welcomed the bourgeois Provisional Government. This was *his* revolution. This was *his* government.

But the few months of freedom were soon at an end, and the Bolsheviks came to power.

Why did he—a highly educated man fluent in English, German, and French—not go abroad? It is the old, old story: he was always devoted to that great and tragic country.

In the early twenties, while some vestige of freedom survived, my father edited an Odessan magazine called *Shkvall* (Squall) and wrote screenplays for early Soviet films. His close friends at the time were the writer Yuri Olesha, the theorist of the avant-garde

Viktor Shklovsky, and also the film director Sergei Eisenstein. After my father's death I discovered, miraculously preserved between the pages of one of his books, a letter from Eisenstein complete with a number of brilliant indent drawings—relics of their youthful amusements.

But the epoch of thought control arrived, and the country became a great prison. My father did not grumble but went on living, or rather existing, quietly, inconspicuously.

He gave up journalism and began writing for the theater. He dramatized novels by one of the writers most esteemed by Stalin, Peter Andreevich Pavlenko, author of the scenarios for two famous films, *The Oath* and *The Fall of Berlin*, in which Stalin is among the dramatis personae. Pavlenko's ultrapatriotic screenplay *Alexander Nevsky*, about the thirteenth-century Russian warrior who defeated the Teutonic Knights, was filmed by the great director Eisenstein.

Pavlenko also wrote novels. Stalin conferred on him the highest of literary awards, the Stalin Prize, four times. Pavlenko had seen the Leader on a number of occasions. He had the entrée to the magic circle surrounding the God-Man.

Pavlenko's name saved my father. Many of his friends vanished in the camps, but he himself was not touched. According to the logic of the time, my father's arrest would have cast a shadow on the famous Pavlenko himself.

My father realized, however, that this protection might end at any moment. He expected, and was prepared for, something horrible. Yet in spite of living under the ax, in spite of his thwarted career, he never stopped smiling. His favorite hero was the skeptical philosopher in Anatole France's novel *Les Dieux ont soif*, a man who observed the horrors of the French Revolution with mournful irony. My father observed the dreadful life of Stalin's Russia with the same sort of smile. Irony and compassion were his watchwords.

In my memory he always wears that smile.

My father died in 1969. That is when I began writing this book. I have written it with no feeling of hatred for the Boss. I wanted only to understand the man himself and the horror through which we lived: I wrote surrounded by ghosts of those whom I saw in my childhood. I have included their stories about the Boss in this book, stories which my father loved to retell, always ending with the same refrain: *Perhaps someday you will write about him.*

STALIN

PROLOGUE: THE NAME

And authority was given it over every tribe and people and tongue and nation . . . and it was allowed to give breath to the image of the beast, so that the image of the beast should even speak, and to cause those who would not worship the image of the beast to be slain.
—Revelation 13:7, 15

Then a mighty angel took up a stone . . . and threw it into the sea, saying: "So shall Babylon the great city be thrown down with violence, and shall be found no more . . . for . . . all nations were deceived by thy sorcery. And in her was found the blood of prophets and of saints and of all who have been slain on earth."
—Revelation 18:21–24

Every day the largest country in the world woke up with his name on its lips. All day long that name rang out in the voices of actors, resounded in song, stared out from the pages of every newspaper. That name was conferred, as the highest of honors, on factories, collective farms, streets, and towns. During the most terrible of all wars, soldiers went to their deaths intoning his name. During that war the city of Stalingrad bled almost to death; it lost all of its inhabitants, the ground became one great scab bristling with shells, but the city that bore his name was not surrendered to the enemy. During the political trials organized by him, his victims glorified his name as they died. Even in the camps, his portrait looked down on millions of people who, corralled behind barbed wire at his behest, turned rivers back in their course, raised cities beyond the Arctic Circle, and perished in their hundreds of thousands. Statues of this man in granite and bronze towered over the immense country.

A gigantic statue of Stalin stood beside the Volga-Don canal—one of several built by his prisoners. One event in the history of that statue seems comically symbolic of the Stalin era: the custodian who looked after the statue was horrified to discover one day that migrating birds had taken to resting on its head. Birds cannot be punished. But people can. So the mortally terrified oblast authorities found a solution. They ran a high-tension electric current through the gigantic head. So now the statue stood there surrounded by a carpet of dead birds. Every morning the custodian plowed the little corpses under, and, thus manured, the ground brought forth flowers. While the statue, cleansed of bird droppings, gazed out on the great expanse beyond the Volga, fertilized by the bodies not of birds but of human beings, by the unmarked graves of those who had built the great canal.

To think how much he meant to us! Yuri Borisov, an important industrial manager in Stalin's time, used to tell this story in the sixties:

> Comrade Stalin sent for me. I had been in conversation with him before. I went there with a mist before my eyes. I rapped out the answer to his question looking him straight in the eye and trying not to blink. We all knew that saying of his: "If a man's eyes wander his conscience isn't clear." He listened to my answer, then held out his hand and said, "Thank you, comrade." When I felt his handshake it was like being struck by lightning. I hid my hand inside my coat cuff, got into my car, and rushed home. Without stopping to answer my worried wife's questions I went to the cot where my small son was sleeping, stretched out my hand, and rubbed his head with it, so that he too would feel the warmth of Stalin's touch.

Winston Churchill recalled, "Stalin made a very great impression on us. . . . When he entered the conference room at Yalta everybody stood up as if at a word of command. And, strange to tell, for some reason stood with their hands along the seams of their trousers." Churchill also said that on one occasion he was determined not to stand up, but when Stalin entered it was as if some extraterrestrial force lifted him from his seat.

During the war President Roosevelt used to speak warmly of Stalin—"good old Uncle Joe."

Even in 1959, when the whole world had heard of good old Uncle Joe's crimes, Churchill, speaking in the House of Commons on the eightieth anniversary of Stalin's birth, said, "It was Russia's great good luck that in the years of its greatest tribulations the country had at its head a genius and an unyielding military leader like Stalin." If only Churchill had known what the "unyielding military leader" had been planning in the distant days of March 1953.

But on March 1, 1953, Stalin lay on the floor of his room, felled by a stroke. In the capital of his empire, an empire replete with his glory, in which he had made himself a god in his own lifetime, he lay helpless in an empty room, in a pool of his own urine.

At different times he was called a paranoiac, a monster, or just a common gangster.

But his character and the motives for his actions remain just as mysterious now as they were on the sunny March day of his death. Stalin stole away into the shadows of history in his soft Caucasian boots. But now after the fall of the Soviet empire, his own menacing shadow looms again on the horizon. The fallen empire, once the greatest of the twentieth century, remembers its founder more and more frequently, and "the Boss," "Our Father and Teacher," is returning to his country in a cloud of new and menacing myths.

The Secret

He had succeeded in plunging the story of his life and the whole history of his country into impenetrable darkness. Systematically destroying his comrades-in-arms, he at once obliterated every trace of them in history. He personally directed the constant and relentless purging of the archives. He surrounded with the deepest secrecy everything even remotely relevant to the sources of his power. He converted the archives into closely guarded fortresses. Even now, if you are given access to the documents which used to be so jealously guarded, you find yourself confronting yet another mystery.

He had foreseen this too.

Here are a few excerpts from the secret minutes of Politburo meetings, preserved in the President's Archive:

> 1920. "Decisions of the Politburo on particularly serious matters must not be recorded in the official minutes."

> 1923. ". . . in confirmation of a previous decision of the Politburo nothing except the final resolutions should be noted in the minutes of the Politburo."

1924. "The work of all employees of the Secretariat of the Central Committee is to be treated as a Party secret."

1927. Adoption of measures "to ensure maximum secrecy."

This secrecy was not his invention. It was traditional in the Order of Sword Bearers, as its leader, Stalin, once called the Communist Party.

Stalin made the tradition absolute.

So that the moment we set about writing his life, we set foot in that great darkness.

The President's Archive

As a student at the Institute of Historical-Archival Studies, I already knew about this most secret of all archives. It contained, my professor said, a wealth of secrets with which only those of the Vatican could compete.

This archive was directly controlled by the leadership of the Communist Party and located in a secret department of its own. This was where documents originating in all those higher Party organs which governed the country for seven decades were preserved, together with Stalin's *personal* archive. This was only right, since by then the history of the Party, and that of the country, had become Stalin's history. This collection subsequently formed the basis of the "President's Archive," which was put together under Gorbachev. It was where the new president, Boris Yeltsin, discovered the secret agreements that Stalin made with Hitler's Germany.

I was given the unique opportunity to work in the President's Archive.

Documents from two other archives are also used in this book. First, there is the former Central Party Archive, the holy of holies of the Communist Party, previously inaccessible to historians. This is where the history of the underground group of revolutionaries who, in 1917, seized power over one-sixth of the world is preserved—in steel safes behind special doors. Documents in this archive are more often than not marked "Strictly Secret." Now that the Party itself has collapsed, the Party Archive has bashfully changed its name and is now called the Russian Center for the Preservation and Study of Documents Relating to Modern History (RTsKhIDNI). But to me it will always be the Party Archive, and that is what I shall call it in this book. I yearned for so long to enter the Party Archive and have set foot in it only now that the reign of that incorrigibly conspiratorial party of which our hero was the head has ended.

There are also, of course, what used to be the secret holdings of the State Archive of the October Revolution. After the collapse of the USSR, it swiftly changed its name to State Archive of the Russian Federation. This too I shall call by its former name—Archive of the October Revolution, a more accurate description. It contains documents relating to the Revolution and to famous Bolsheviks—Stalin's murdered comrades-in-arms—as well as Stalin's Special Files (secret reports to the Leader).

These are the three main archives in which I carried out my search for Stalin. The secret Stalin. The Stalin hidden from us for half a century.

I shall also make use of documents from another archive that is inaccessible even now. This is the archive of the former KGB. That is where we find the biggest "blood bank" in the world—the case records of those who were shot. Hundreds of thousands of them. I have been able with the help of "third parties" to consult certain documents of interest to me in that archive.

It should be noted that the KGB Archive itself has begun lavishly publishing its documents since perestroika. But I never forget the words of a former KGB officer: "Just remember that this is sometimes one of the KGB's little games—'fabrication with a view to publication.'" Putting it more simply—"Beware of Greeks bearing gifts." This applies particularly to the memoirs of former KGB officers. Those of Ivan Sudoplatov, one of Stalin's spies, may serve as an example. *Special Assignments* is their splendid title. Special assignments meant directing the enemy along a false trail, smearing Western idols, covering agents in the field, and naming nonexistent agents. Sudoplatov was still carrying on the struggle with one foot in the grave. Could the final "special assignment" for such people have been deathbed disinformation?

After giving interviews in which I said that I was writing a book about "Stalin, the First Revolutionary Tsar," I started receiving a lot of letters.

I was amused by this repetition of what happened with my previous book, about the last Russian tsar, Nicholas II.

These letters contain no sensational information, but they convey invaluable details about a vanished age, which has left behind a multitude of falsifications and the most mendacious literature in the world. For the most part, these letters were written by elderly people who had long ago withdrawn from active life and wished before departing this world to record what they had witnessed. They rarely say anything about themselves. As a rule, I know only a name and address (in some cases only the city from which the letter has come). This is not the result of carelessness, but of fear. That fear, inculcated in the people from their childhood by their Father and Teacher, will die only when they die. In my book I simply indicate the names of each of these unselfish coauthors and the town from which he or she wrote to me. I thank all of my voluntary helpers, inhabitants of the vanished empire called the USSR, yet another Russian Atlantis.

INTRODUCTION: AN ENIGMATIC STORY

I often recall a conversation which took place in the latter half of the sixties. I was young, but already the author of two fashionable plays, when I got to know Elena Sergeevna Bulgakova, the widow of the most mystical writer of the Stalin era. In Stalin's lifetime, Mikhail Bulgakov was famous for several forbidden plays and for one which was staged, *The Days of the Turbins*. Stalin had a strange, barely comprehensible love for this play and went to see it at the Moscow Arts Theater on innumerable occasions.

In the sixties most of Bulgakov's works were banned, as before, and many fantastic stories were told about his life. The one that interested me was the story of his play about Stalin, and I asked Elena Sergeevna about it. The conversation that resulted seemed to me so remarkable that I wrote it down in my diary.

> *Myself:* I have heard that in 1939 there was some suggestion that Mikhail Sergeevich should write a play about Stalin.
>
> *Elena Sergeevna:* Perfectly true. It was indeed *suggested*. The director of the Moscow Arts Theater came to see us. He was the one who suggested writing such a play for Stalin's jubilee. Misha was undecided at first but finally agreed—he had a special attitude to Stalin. He wrote an interesting romantic play about the young Koba [the young Stalin's Party pseudonym]. At first everything went well. The theater accepted the play. Even the bureaucrats in charge of cultural matters were delighted. [Later I checked Elena Sergeevna's story against her published diary. On May 11, 1939, she had written, "B. (Bulgakov) reads his story at the Committee for the Arts. They liked the play very much."] The theater intended to stage the play in December 1939, in honor of its hero's sixtieth birthday. But then they submitted it to Stalin, and he vetoed it. That's about all there is to be said.

If I had not been a Soviet playwright myself at the time, I should have left it at that. As it was I recognized at once the bizarre nature of what I had been told.

It was 1939, remember—at the height of the Stalinist terror. The whole country is in the grip of fear. Any ideological error is denounced as a hostile act. Who would have dared at such a time to commission from Bulgakov, the author of several forbidden plays, a play for the anniversary of the Leader himself? Commission it, what's more, for the country's premier theater? Those responsible for the arts at the time were already frightened out of their wits: who among them would have dared take such a responsibility upon himself? No one, of course, except . . . except the hero of the projected play himself, the unlikely devotee of *Days of the Turbins.*

So then, it can obviously only have been Stalin who commissioned the play. Another question then arises.

As a playwright myself, I knew very well that bureaucrats lived in constant fear. Even in the relatively safe sixties the cultural administrators did their best to avoid making decisions. Surely in the dreadful year 1939 bureaucrats half dead with fear would not suddenly have found the courage to enthuse over a play by Bulgakov, who had made several mistakes in the past. It seems improbable! Or, rather, it becomes probable on one assumption: that the customer had approved it himself.

Why then did he subsequently ban it? I continued my conversation with Elena Sergeevna:

Myself: When was the play discussed?

Elena Sergeevna: In the summer . . . it was July.

Myself: And when was it banned?

Elena Sergeevna: In August.

Myself: Something must have happened between those two events?

Elena Sergeevna (smiling; she could have read my thoughts): Misha arranged with the theater to go to Georgia. He was anxious to talk to eyewitnesses of events there, who remembered Koba in his youth. There were not many left by then, Koba had destroyed them all. . . . We set off, the designer, the producer, I myself, and Misha . . . Misha dreamt of working in Georgian archives.

Myself: In the archives?

Elena Sergeevna: Yes, well, he'd been writing without any documents. When he asked the theater to help him consult documents about Stalin's youth, the answer was that no such documents existed. So he decided to look for himself. We set out in perfect comfort, in an international carriage. We were getting ready to enjoy a banquet in our compartment when a telegram caught up with us: "Journey no longer necessary. Return to Moscow." In Moscow Misha was informed that the play had been read in Stalin's secretariat, and the verdict was that no one must try to turn Stalin into a literary image and put invented words into his mouth. Stalin himself was supposed to have said, "All young people are alike, why write a play about the young Stalin?"

Stalin's explanation was a strange one. Many works about the young Stalin were published in those years. But they were written just as the play had been—*without* documents. Their authors made use of official information about the life of the great revolutionary Koba. Of course!

Bulgakov's fatal mistake, obviously, was wanting to consult archival documents. The moment he tried to go beyond the limits of that official information, the play was doomed. The episode rebounded on the author with fatal results. Bulgakov fell sick and died.

I remembered myself as a child, sitting in my room; in the adjoining room my father was talking to the writer Pavlenko, one of the most highly regarded writers of the Stalin era. My father was earning our livelihood by adapting Pavlenko's novels for the stage. Pavlenko had written screenplays for films in which Stalin himself was portrayed. That day Pavlenko and my father were discussing future plans. The door was ajar, and I heard my father calmly asking, "Why don't you write about the youth of Joseph Vissarionovich? . . . Nobody has done it properly. You lived in the Caucasus for a long time . . ."

Pavlenko interrupted so harshly that I didn't recognize his voice: "It's no good trying to describe the sun before it has risen."

More Riddles: The Vanishing Birthdays

"Stalin (Dzhugashvili), Joseph Vissarionovich, was born on December 21 (December 9, Old Style), 1879." That is the birth date you will find in many of the world's encyclopedias. It is a date I remember well. I committed the one and only crime of my life because of that date. In one of the lower forms at school we sent him birthday greetings every year. In a reverent silence I described my love for him. Like all my classmates I was a believer, and I trembled as I imagined him reading our letters. But back home, as I was telling my father what I had written, I realized with horror that I had made a grammatical mistake. And he, Stalin, would learn that I was illiterate. It was more than I could bear. As soon as it got light I went to school, broke a window, and crept into the staff room. I found the pile of compositions. What a stroke of luck: they hadn't been checked yet. So I corrected my mistake.

Now, ages later, I am sitting in the famous Central Party Archive. I have before me a photocopy of the entry in the records of the Cathedral of the Assumption at Gori registering the birth of Joseph Dzhugashvili.

> 1878. Born December 6. Christened December 17, parents Vissarion Ivanovich Dzhugashvili, peasant, and his lawful wedded wife, Ekaterina Georgievna, residents of the township of Gori. Godfather—Tsikhitatrishvili, peasant, resident of Gori.

The sacrament was performed by Archpriest Khakalov, assisted by Subdeacon Kvinikidze.

Was he then born a whole year and three days earlier than his official date of birth? The date which the whole country had celebrated solemnly for so many years? Had it been celebrating the wrong date all those years? The date given here is no mistake. The same archive contains young Joseph Dzhugashvili's school-leaving certificate, issued by the Gori Junior Seminary. It reads: "Born on the sixth day of the month of December 1878." Here too we find a curriculum vitae written by Stalin himself in 1920. The year 1878 is given in his own handwriting.

The official date of birth is indeed fictitious. But when was it invented? And why?

The first question is easily answered: the fictitious date first appears immediately after Stalin's official elevation. In April 1922 Lenin made him Secretary General—head of the Party. And as early as December 1922, Stalin's secretary Tovstukha makes out a new CV for him, in which he alters the year of his birth to 1879, and the day to December 21. From then onward, our hero avoided writing his own CV. His secretaries did it for him. The fictitious date was entered in their handwriting. As always, it had nothing to do with him. The false date became official. But again—*why?*

I am sitting in the former Party Archive with Tovstukha's papers before me. He was Stalin's confidential assistant until 1935. He died in that year, luckily for him, inasmuch as after that date Stalin would destroy most of his entourage.

I peruse Tovstukha's papers, trying to find some sort of clue, but he left no diaries, no personal records of any kind. For that matter, those whom he served behaved likewise. On principle. Neither Stalin nor Lenin nor any of their associates kept diaries. For the revolutionary, nothing personal is supposed to exist. Only the Party and its cause. This useful principle enabled them to take their Party's secrets to the grave.

During a break from my work, an old man comes up to me in the corridor—one of those Party ancients who while away their leisure hours in the archives. He does not introduce himself, and I do not ask his name. I know from experience that it pays not to be inquisitive if you hope to obtain interesting information. This is what he says:

> I see you're interested in Tovstukha. I used to meet him at one time, in fact I even worked with him. He was a tall, thin man, typical intellectual. Died of tuberculosis. I visited him in the government sanatorium, the Pines, when he lay dying. He asked me to play the revolutionary songs of his youth on my guitar. He wept. He didn't want to die. Stalin had him buried in the Kremlin wall. He appreciated Tovstukha's services. Tovstukha had been his secretary. But, no less important, he was effectively in charge of the Party Archive. He collected all the Lenin documents. Stalin used those documents to destroy his opponents. One of his secretaries, Bazhanov, escaped abroad. He had a lot to say about Tovstukha in his book. But he didn't realize what Tovstukha's most important service to Stalin was. It happened when Stalin was already the country's Boss. In 1929 it was decided to make Stalin's fiftieth birthday the occasion for nationwide celebrations. Tovstukha began removing from the archives all documents concerning Stalin, particularly his prerevolutionary career, ostensibly in order to write a full biography. But no full biography appeared. The mountain brought forth a mouse: the result was the misbegotten *Short Biography*. He collected the documents to make sure that they were never published. Putting it more precisely, he *suppressed* documents. But I don't think it was his own idea. We were all *his* servants. We all did whatever Stalin, the Boss, wanted. As soon as he got hold of documents, Tovstukha referred them to the Boss. And they of-

> ten didn't return. The explanation given to people like me, who worked with Tovstukha, was Stalin's modesty: he didn't like superfluous mentions of his past. And the superfluous included all documents about his life before October 1917. People quoted a remark of his: "I did nothing worth mentioning compared with other revolutionaries."

I often remembered the old man's words as I looked through Tovstukha's papers. Take his correspondence with the accredited historian of the Party, Emelyan Yaroslavsky. In 1935 Yaroslavsky contemplated writing a biography of the Leader. He wrote to Tovstukha saying that he would like to consult sources for Stalin's life before October 1917 and asked what Tovstukha thought about his idea of writing a detailed biography of the Leader. Tovstukha replied, "I feel skeptical . . . the materials for this purpose are practically nonexistent. The archival sources are poor, they get you nowhere." Yaroslavsky was experienced enough to know who was dictating Tovstukha's answer, and there was an immediate change of plan. He wrote his biography of Stalin—but without using new documents.

There is a widely known story that the reason Stalin cooled toward Gorky was the great proletarian writer's stubborn reluctance to write the Leader's biography. But Tovstukha's archive points to a different explanation. Gorky evidently asked Tovstukha for materials to write the biography. And Tovstukha replied: "I am sending you, rather late in the day, some materials relevant to the Stalin biography. As I warned you, the materials are pretty meager."

This delay in answering the great proletarian writer, in such a context, could mean only one thing: that the biography should not be written. Gorky promptly dropped the idea.

All these stories show that Stalin did not want to recall the life of the revolutionary Koba and was perhaps so eager to distance himself from it that he even changed the date of his birth.

What was it in Koba's career that inspired such obvious unease in Stalin?

ONE

SOSO: HIS LIFE AND DEATH

1 THE LITTLE ANGEL

"Look at the map. You will see that the Caucasus is the center of the world."
—An English traveler

Soso's Town

It is 1878. The little Georgian town of Gori, birthplace of Joseph (Iosif) Dzhugashvili, slumbers against a background of distant mountains.

Soso, his mother called him, Georgian fashion.

Maxim Gorky, who was to be Stalin's favorite writer, wandering around the Caucasus at the end of the nineteenth century, described Gori as follows:

> Gori, a town at the mouth of the river Kura, quite small, no bigger than a fair-sized village. There is a high hill in the middle of it. On the hill stands a fortress. The whole place has a picturesque wildness all its own. The sultry sky over the town, the noisy, turbulent waters of the Kura, mountains in the near distance, with their "City of Caves," and farther away the Caucasus range, with its sprinkling of snow that never melts.

This sets the scene in which our hero's life begins. An ominous note is introduced into this idyllic landscape by the grim ruins looking down on the town from a steep cliff—the ruins of the castle from which Georgian feudal princes once ruled that region and waged bloody war on the Georgian kings.

We cross the bridge over the Kura into the little town. Gori wakes at sunrise, before the burning heat sets in. Herdsmen go from yard to yard to collect the cows. Sleepy people sit on little balconies. Church doors are unlocked and old women in black hurry to the morning service. Rafts speed down the boisterous Kura. Listless water carriers follow the movements of the daring raftsmen as they fill the leather bottles which they will then carry from house to house on the backs of their skinny nags.

The long main street bisects the town. It used to be called Tsarskaya Street, because Tsar Nicholas I once visited Gori. Later, of course, it became Stalin Street. Little shops and two-storied houses hide among trees. This is the lower part of the town, in which the rich live. From Gori, Armenian, Azerbaijani, and Jewish merchants once traded with the whole world. As you would expect in an Eastern town, the center of its life was the market—a typical oriental bazaar. Along its dark aisles innumerable little shops sold everything imaginable, from matches to precious stones. Tailors measured their clients outside in the street: the tailor sprinkled soot on the ground, the client lay down, and the tailor sat on him, pressing him into the soot. Nearby, barbers would give haircuts and shampoos, or draw teeth with pliers. Shopkeepers drank wine and played *nardy* (a board game like chess). The town madman might turn up in the market, followed by a crowd of teasing boys.

> Little Soso often came to bazaar. His mother did the laundry for a Jewish merchant who traded there. Soso never teased the madman. Soso defended him. The Jewish merchant was softhearted. He pitied the madman and often gave Soso presents for being kind to him. Soso shared the money with us to buy sweets. Although Soso's family was poor, he despised money. (Letter from N. Goglidze, Kiev)

Life was quite different in the upper town, where the future Leader's father, the cobbler Vissarion (Beso) Dzhugashvili, lived. He had set up house in a hovel after marrying Ekaterina (Keke) Georgievna Geladze, who had been born into the family of a serf. Her father died early, but although money was short her mother somehow saw to it that Keke learned to read and write. She was not yet sixteen when she met Dzhugashvili, who had only recently arrived in Gori from his family's little village of Didi Lilo.

A Dangerous Great-Grandfather

There is a story attached to the family's arrival in Didi Lilo. Beso's forebears had previously lived in a mountain hamlet in the Liakhvis Ravine. Like Keke's, they were serfs. Their masters were Georgian warrior princes—the princely Asatiani family. Soso's great-grandfather Zaza Dzhugashvili took part in a bloody peasant revolt. He was seized, cruelly flogged, and thrown into jail. He escaped, rebelled again, was arrested again, and again escaped. That was when he settled in the village of Didi Lilo, near Tiflis (now Tbilisi), got married, and at last found peace.

The old rebel's son Vano took no part in peasant risings, but lived a life of peace and quiet. He, however, left two sons, Beso and Georgi. Their grandfather's spirit was reborn in them. The wild Georgi was knifed in a drunken brawl, and Beso, no mean brawler and drunkard himself, left the quiet village for Tiflis. It was there that the semiliterate Beso became a shoemaker, working in the big Adelkhanov leather factory, which supplied boots to the troops in the Caucasus.

Beso once visited friends of his in Gori, also shoemakers. Their guild was the largest in the town, ninety-two strong. There he first set eyes on the sixteen-year-old Keke. Girls mature early in Georgia. A sixteen-year-old has been an adult woman for some time. Did she fall in love with Beso? Among people so poor, struggling to exist, common sense will pass for love. She had no dowry, and he was a shoemaker—in other words, he would never be short of a crust. It was a good match.

Excerpt from the register of marriages for 1874:

> Joined in wedlock on May 17, Vissarion Dzhugashvili, peasant, temporarily resident in Gori, Orthodox Christian, age of bridegroom 24, and Ekaterina, daughter of Glakh Geladze, peasant, formerly resident in Gori, deceased. Orthodox Christian, her first marriage, aged 16.

This was how Beso Dzhugashvili became a Gori resident.

Wedding feasts go on for a long time in Georgia. The guests drink to the music of pipers for days on end. So she was able to learn a great deal about her chosen one before the celebrations were over. Drinking in Georgia is an occasion for jollity and for endless toasts. But Beso was a morose and frightening drinker. He got drunk quickly. And instead of delivering the eulogies customary at a Georgian feast, he was soon looking for a fight. He was a man consumed by anger. He was dark, of medium height, lean, low-browed, with mustache and beard. Koba would look very much like him. Keke was pretty, with a light complexion and freckles. She was religious and literate. She loved music.

In the early years of her marriage Keke gave birth regularly, but her children died one after another. In 1876 Mikhail died in his cradle, and Georgi died soon after birth. Nature seemed to be against the birth of a child to the morose bootmaker.

THE DEVIL AMIRAN

Near the ruined castle of Gori there is a strangely shaped boulder. A huge, perfectly spherical ball of stone. According to popular legend, the giant Amiran had played ball with it. Amiran was a Caucasian variant of Prometheus, but he was an evil Prometheus, a demon of destruction chained up somewhere on the summit of the Caucasus range. There was an ancient custom in Gori: once a year all the blacksmiths hammered on their anvils in the night so that this terrible spirit of destruction would not descend from his cliff.

BUT THE BLACKSMITHS HAMMERED IN VAIN

On December 6, 1878, a third boy was born to Keke. Keke prayed hard for God to grant the child life. And her prayer was answered: the infant lived. He was christened on December 17. This boy would play with the terrestrial globe as Amiran had played with his stone ball.

The shoemaker Beso's little home survives to this day. In the years of Stalin's greatness a marble pavilion was erected over his hovel. Stalin, the ex-seminarist, remembered that this had been done with the stable in which the Savior was born.

A little single-story brick house. . . . The morose Beso sat outside cutting the leather for his boots. Father, mother, and son shared the one and only room. There was also a dark, smoke-blackened basement.

The scant light through the basement window illuminates a wooden cradle. His cradle, in which two infants before him—his dead brothers—had once wept and wailed.

Soso, then, survived. And Keke, in gratitude for the life vouchsafed him, resolved to dedicate the infant to God's service.

Soselo ("Little Soso"), as she tenderly called him, must become a priest.

The part of the town in which Beso's house stood was known as the Russian quarter, because Russian soldiers were stationed in a barracks nearby. So other children often called Soso "the Russian." This would lodge in his subconscious, with strange results. He would never feel the stirring of Georgian nationalist sentiment. Only his first revolutionary pseudonym—almost a childish nickname—had any connection with Georgia. As a professional revolutionary, he used only Russian names when living underground. He would later describe his homeland sarcastically as "that small area of Russia which calls itself Georgia."

His Mother: Shameful Rumors

Our hero's childhood is dimly lit. The marble pavilion covering Beso's little house conceals many secrets.

"My parents were simple people, but they treated me not so badly," Stalin said in conversation with the German writer Emil Ludwig. A very different story was sometimes told in Georgia.

> I lived in Tiflis up to the age of seventeen, and one close acquaintance of mine was an old woman who had previously lived in Gori. She told me that he invariably referred to his mother as "the prostitute." In Georgia even the most desperate criminals respect their mothers. After the age of seventeen Stalin visited his mother perhaps twice. He did not come to her funeral. (Marina Khachaturova, Russian journalist, in conversation with author)

> His mother never went to see him in Moscow. Can you imagine a Georgian becoming Tsar and not sending for his mother? He never wrote to her. He didn't come to her funeral. . . . They say that he openly referred to her as "the old prostitute," or something of the sort. The fact is that Beso lived in Tiflis, and never sent them money. That drunkard spent it all on drink. Keke had to work for her living and to pay for her son's education, so she went round the houses of the rich, laundering and sewing. She was quite young. You can imagine the rest. Even in his lifetime, when everybody was afraid of everything, people said, "Stalin was not the son of that illiterate Beso." One name mentioned was that of Przhevalsky. (Letter from N. Goglidze, Kiev)

The Russian explorer Przhevalsky did indeed visit Gori. His mustachioed face, in encyclopedias published in Stalin's time, is suspiciously like that of Stalin.

> After Stalin's death, when terror disappeared, people started naming several supposititious fathers. There was even one Jew, a merchant, among them. But the name most often mentioned was that of Yakov Egnatashvili. He was a wealthy wine merchant, a boxing enthusiast, and one of those Keke worked for.

> Yakov Egnatashvili must have had some reason for funding Soso's seminary education. People said that Stalin called his first son Yakov in honor of Egnatashvili. . . . I have seen a portrait of this Georgian hero . . . he was certainly nothing like the puny Soso. . . . But, obviously, whenever Beso came back from Tiflis he would hear all these rumors. Perhaps that is why he used to beat little Soso like he did. He would beat his wife half to death as well. Mother and son used to take refuge with neighbors. So when Stalin grew up, he could not help despising his fallen mother, as any Georgian would. That was why he never invited her to Moscow, and never wrote to her. (Letter from N. Goglidze, Kiev)

> Even in his lifetime, when people vanished for a single wrong word about him, he was openly spoken of as the illegitimate son of the great Przhevalsky. These stories could go unpunished only because they had approval from on high. It wasn't just his hatred for his drunken father, but a matter of political importance. The point is that he had, by then, become Tsar of all Russia. So instead of the illiterate Georgian drunkard, he wanted an eminent Russian for his daddy. But in Georgia a married woman who goes astray is a fallen woman. This was the origin of the dirty legends about his mother. (Letter from I. Nodia, Tbilisi)

The Truth About His Mother

In the summer of 1993 I was given permission to work in the President's Archive. I enter the Kremlin through the Spassky Gate—which used to see the entrance of a long cortege of identical automobiles, with the Leader's car concealed somewhere among them. A panorama opens out before me: golden domes, the Tsar Cannon (the biggest cannon in the world in the seventeenth century, which proved incapable of firing) and nearby another giant, the Tsar Bell, which cracked as soon as it was cast and never rang. Stalin saw these two derisory symbols of old Russia every day.

I turn right, just as his car would have done, because in 1993 the President's Archive was in Stalin's former quarters in the Kremlin. The apartment has been converted, but the high doors, with glass knobs which once felt the warmth of his hands, are still there. As is the old mirror which seems still to hold his reflection. I sit under Stalin's ceiling and look through his personal papers.

"Medical History of J. V. Stalin, Patient of the Kremlin Polyclinic". . . similar medical records for his wife, who died in mysterious circumstances . . . his correspondence with his wife, affectionate words, put on paper by a terrible man . . . his correspondence with his children . . . and . . . *his letters to his mother.*

Yes, it was all false—the story of his hatred for his mother, of his calling her "the prostitute." He had loved her and written to her as any son should all those years, right up to her death. Little yellowing pages, covered with bold handwriting in the Georgian script. (His mother never succeeded in learning Russian.)

After the Revolution, he installed the former laundress and housemaid in a palace, formerly that of the tsar's viceroy in the Caucasus. But she occupied only one tiny room, like her little room in their old hovel. She sat there with her friends, other lonely old women clad all in black, like so many crows.

His letters to her were brief. As his wife would explain later, he hated long personal letters. "16 April 1922: Dear mama. Greetings, keep well, don't let sorrow enter your heart. Remember the saying 'while I live I will live joyously, when I die the graveyard worms will rejoice.' " He ends almost every letter with good wishes in traditional Georgian form: "Live ten thousand years, mama dear."

The sort of letters a loving son usually writes. He sends her photographs of his wife, money, medicines, begs her not to be downhearted in spite of her many ailments. And sees to it that his wife accompanies his short letters with long ones of her own.

From one of his wife's letters to his mother: "Everything is fine with us. We . . . were expecting you here, but it seems you couldn't manage it." Yes, it was the other way round: they invite his mother, they ask her to come and see them. But she will not come. Yet his mother never overlooks the slightest sign of neglect on the part of her busy son. He has to make excuses: "Greetings, Mama dear. . . . It's a long time since I got a letter from you. I must have offended you, but what can I do, God knows how busy I am." . . . "Greetings, Mama dear. Of course I owe you an apology for not writing recently. But what can I do—I'm snowed under with work and couldn't take time out to write."

They continually invited his mother to Moscow. And she continually refused to come. In one of her last letters, his wife writes despairingly: "Still, summer is not that far off, maybe we shall see each other. But why don't you come to us sometime? It's very embarrassing the way you spoil us with presents." So then—she spoiled them by sending presents but would not go to see them, however much they begged her. They had installed her in a palace, but she persisted in living in one room.

Yes, but he spent his holidays in the Caucasus, not very far away, and wouldn't go to see her. Or was he afraid to? Whatever the truth may be, it was not until 1935, when he knew that she was very ill and that he might never see her again, that he went there. Stalinist propaganda converted their meeting into a Christmas story. But two snippets of truth slipped through the net (remembered by N. Kipshidze, a doctor who treated Keke in her old age).

"Why did you beat me so hard?" he asked his mother. "That's why you turned out so well," Keke answered.

And: "Joseph—who exactly are you now?" his mother asked him.

It was difficult not to know who her son had become, when his portrait was displayed on every street. She was simply inviting him to boast a bit. And he did. "Remember the tsar? Well, I'm like a tsar." To which she said something so naive that the whole country laughed heartily: "You'd have done better to have become a priest."

But this reply, from a pious woman, sums up his tragedy, and the whole secret of her relations with her son.

His Childhood: Beat Him!

Drunken Beso was, of course, Soso's real father—you have only to compare pictures of father and son. It could not have been otherwise: Keke was a chaste and deeply religious girl. And anyway, husband and wife were never apart in the year of Soso's birth. Beso lived in Gori at that time, making boots to order for the Adelkhanov factory in Tiflis. And drinking. There were dreadful scenes. N. Kipshidze remembered stories she told him: "One day when his father was drunk he picked him up and threw him violently to the floor. There was blood in the boy's urine for days afterwards." The big fistfights with no holds barred—that was what little Soso saw from the day he was born.

In the early years, when these drunken horrors occurred, the hapless Keke would grab the terrified child and run off to the neighbors. But a more mature Keke, toughened by heavy work, resisted her husband more stubbornly from year to year, while drunken Beso grew weaker. The time came when she fearlessly exchanged blow for blow, and Beso began feeling more and more uncomfortable at home, where he was no longer lord and master. It was more than the morose Beso could bear. That, evidently, was why he took it into his head to leave for

Tiflis and the Adelkhanov factory. Mother and son were left to themselves.

It was not only in his features that the boy resembled his father. "His harsh home life left him embittered. He was an embittered, insolent, rude, stubborn child with an intolerable character." Thus was he described by 112-year-old Hana Moshiashvili, a Georgian Jewish woman, once a friend of Keke, who emigrated to Israel in 1972. "His mother was head of the family now, and the fist which had subdued his father was now applied to the upbringing of their son. She beat him unmercifully for disobedience."

The verb *to beat* lodged forever in his subconscious. *To beat* also means "to educate." It was to be his favorite word in the fight with political opponents.

ANTI-SEMITISM

The seeds of another cruel feeling were planted in his childhood.

Anti-Semitism is not a Caucasian characteristic. From ancient times innumerable peoples have lived in the Caucasus, side by side. The Georgian Prince A. Sumbatov writes, "Persecution of the Jews was unknown in Georgia. Significantly, there is no Georgian equivalent of the insulting Russian word *zhid.* The only word used is *uria,* corresponding to the Russian *evrei* [Hebrew]." The Jews had been in Georgia since time immemorial, as small tailors, moneylenders, shoemakers. Jewish cobblers were expert at making Georgian boots to suit any taste: because they were well-to-do and consummate masters of their craft, they were hated by the drunken ne'er-do-well Beso. As a small child Soso was given his first lessons in malice toward the Jews by his father.

When Beso left, Keke did not go back on her vow: little Soso must become a priest. Needing money for his education, she would take on any job that was offered—helping with housework, sewing, laundering. Keke knew that the boy had an unusual memory and was capable of learning. He was also musical, like his mother—and that was important if he was to officiate in church.

Keke often worked now in the houses of rich Jewish traders. Her friend Hana recommended her to them. And her skinny little boy went with her. While she did the chores, the bright boy amused the householders. They liked this clever child. David Pismamedov, a Gori Jew, was one of them: "I often gave him money and bought books for him. I loved him like my own son, and he reciprocated." Had he but known how proud and touchy that boy was! How Soso hated every kopeck he accepted!

Many years later, in 1924, David went to Moscow and decided to look up the boy Soso, who had by then become General Secretary of the ruling party: "They wouldn't let me in at first, but when he was told who wanted to see him he came out himself, embraced me, and said 'My grandpa's come, my father.' "

Perhaps this meeting gave rise to the rumor about a rich Jewish father. . . . But Stalin simply wanted David, once a very rich man, to see what the miserable beggar Soso had become. To the end of his days he went on naively settling accounts with his poverty-stricken childhood. It was then, in his childhood, that his beloved mother's humiliation, their everlasting hunger, their poverty, sowed hatred and resentment in the morbidly touchy boy's mind. Hatred above all for them—those rich Jewish traders.

> Little Joseph got used to our family and was like a son to us. . . . They argued a lot, the little Joseph and the big one (my husband). When he got a bit older, Soso often said to big Joseph: "I respect you greatly, but look out: if you don't give up trade I shan't spare you." As for Russian Jews, he disliked the lot of them. (Hana Moshiashvili)

(This was not something she had imagined. His son Yakov would express exactly the same sentiments years later, as a POW in the Second World War. He told an interrogator, "I have only one thing to say about the Jews. They don't know how to work. As they see it, trade is what really matters.")

Soso's feelings were reinforced by jealousy and resentment. Insulting gossip about his mother and her visits to the homes of rich Jews made its furtive appearance at this time. This is how anti-Semitic feelings, so alien to the Caucasus, developed in little Soso. His friend Davrishevi remembered his grandmother reading the New Testament to them—the story of Judas's kiss of betrayal. " 'But why didn't Jesus draw his saber?' little Soso asked indignantly. 'He couldn't do that,' Grandma answered. 'He had to sacrifice himself for our salvation.' " That was something little Soso was incapable of understanding. All through his childhood he had been taught to answer blow with blow. He resolved to do what seemed to him the obvious thing: to take vengeance on the Jews! Even in those days he was a good organizer, but he himself remained behind the scenes for fear of his mother's heavy hand. One typical plan was carried out by little friends—they let a pig into the synagogue. They were found out but did not give Soso away. Shortly afterward an Orthodox priest told his parishioners in church, "There are those among us, some lost sheep, who a few days ago committed a sacrilege in one of God's houses." That was quite beyond Soso's understanding. How could anyone defend people of another faith?!

"Angelic Voices"

In 1888 Keke's dream came true. Soso entered the Gori Church School. His mother had seen to it that he was as good as the rest of them. Keke decided to change her clientele: from then on she laundered and cleaned in his teachers' houses.

The Gori Church School was a big, two-story building. It had its own chapel in the upper story. It was there that another pupil, David Suliashvili, first saw him.

> It was a church fast, and three singers sang the penitential prayers. Those with the best voices were always selected and Soso was always one of these. . . . At vespers three boys in surplices chanted the prayers on their knees . . . the angelic voices of the three children . . . the golden chancel gates were open . . . the priest lifted up his hands to heaven, and we prostrated ourselves, filled with an ecstasy not of this world.

Like Soso, David Suliashvili would complete his studies for the priesthood only to become a professional revolutionary instead. Subsequently, their paths parted: Suliashvili's successful rival went on to become the country's Leader and dispatch him to a prison camp, together with other old Bolsheviks.

But for the moment they were kneeling in their little church. Who could have known that this angelic little boy would become the man who would destroy more people than all the wars in history?

2

The Three Musketeers

Mikhail Peradze (who also attended the Gori Church School) tells us:

> Soso's favorite game was *krivi* (a sort of collective boxing match between children). There were two teams of boxers: one drawn from those who lived in the upper town, the other representing the lower town. We pummeled each other unmercifully, and weedy little Soso was one of the craftiest scrappers. He had the knack of popping up unexpectedly behind a stronger opponent. But the well-fed children from the lower town were always stronger.

Peradze—the most powerful boxer in the town—invited Soso to change sides ("our team is the stronger"), but he refused. Of course he did—on the other team he was number one. He never lost his love of "beating."

Soso also had the knack of dominating others. He organized an elite group from among the strongest boys. He called them the "Three Musketeers." Petya Kapanadze, Grisha Glurdzhidze, and Peradze were the three strongest boys and carried out the orders of the pocket d'Artagnan, Soso, without a murmur. After he had become Stalin and annihilated the revolutionary Koba's comrades-in-arms, he still preserved a sentimental attachment (unusual for him) to little Soso's friends. In the hungry years of the war he sent all three of them what were, for that time, considerable sums of money. "Please accept a small gift from me. Yours, Soso," the sixty-eight-year-old writes to the septuagenarian Petya Kapanadze, little Soso's friend. This and other, similar notes are still to be found in his archives.

The course at the Gori Church School lasted four years, and throughout his time there Soso was the star pupil. Students were not allowed to leave the building in the evening. A boyhood friend of his recalls that "the people who were sent to check up always found Soso indoors and busy with his lessons." While his mother was doing other people's housework he studied diligently. And she was happy: he *would* be a priest.

One of the teachers, Dmitri Khakhutashvili, would be remembered by his pupils for the rest of their lives. He introduced the discipline of the rod, in the fullest sense, into the classroom. The boys had to sit stock-still, with their hands on the desk in front of them, and look their fearsome teacher straight in the eye. If one of them showed signs of life and looked away, he would be rapped on his knuckles immediately. "If your eyes wander it means you're up to something nasty" was the teacher's favorite saying. Little Soso learned, and never forgot, the power of a steady gaze and the terror felt by a man who does not dare to look away.

Teachers in the Church School gave their pupils a rough time. There were exceptions: Belyaev, the supervisor, was kind and gentle. But because the pupils were not afraid of him, they did not respect him. That was another lesson for Soso to remember. One day Belyaev took the boys to the City of Caves—those mysterious caverns in the mountains. On the way there they had to cross a wide and turbulent stream. Soso and the other boys jumped over, but tubby Belyaev couldn't manage it. One of his pupils stepped into the water and "made a back" for the teacher. That was his only hope of crossing the stream. They all heard Soso's quiet voice saying, "What are you then, a donkey? I wouldn't make a back for the Lord God himself." He was morbidly proud, like many people who have been humiliated too often.

The Devil's Hoof

He was also defiantly rude, as children with physical defects often are. As if it wasn't enough to be small and weedy, his face was pockmarked, the legacy of an illness at the age of six. "Pocky" was his nickname in police reports. But that wasn't all.

> He was an excellent swimmer but shy about swimming in the Kura. His foot was deformed in some way, and my great-grandfather, who was in the upper classes at school with him, once twitted him with having "the devil's hoof in his shoe." It cost him dear. Soso said nothing. But the school strongman, Peradze, used to follow Soso around like a dog on a leash in those days. My great-grandfather had forgotten all about it when Peradze gave him a savage beating. (Letter from K. Dzhivilegov)

In the President's Archive, reading the "Medical History of J. V. Stalin," I turned a page and found this written about our hero: "Webbed toes on left foot."

The Mysterious Arm

In innumerable pictures Stalin is portrayed with the fingers of his left hand curled around a pipe. This famous pipe, which became part of his image, was really intended to conceal the deformity of his left hand. He told his second wife, Nadezhda, in 1917 that a phaeton, a horse and cart, had run into him when he was a child and that because there was no money for a doctor his arm had not mended properly. The contusion had turned septic and as a result the arm had become crooked. This coincides with the version, dictated by him, which I found in his "Medical History": "Atrophy of the shoulder and elbow joints of the left arm. Result of a contusion at the age of six, followed by a prolonged septic condition in the region of the elbow joint." S. Goglitsidze, Soso's contemporary, remembers the incident as follows:

> At Epiphany a great crowd of people gathered near the bridge over the Kura. Nobody noticed the phaeton charging downhill out of control . . . it crashed into the crowd and ran into Soso. The shaft struck his cheek and knocked him off his feet, but fortunately the wheels only passed *over the boy's legs.* People crowded round, and Soso was carried home. When she saw her crippled son his mother could not suppress a shriek, but the doctor said that his internal organs were undamaged . . . and he returned to his studies a few weeks later.

Another witness also tells us that the phaeton injured a leg. It obviously could not have run over his arm without crushing his "internal organs." So it *must* have run over his leg. And he was treated by a doctor and made well again quickly. Not a word here about an injury to his arm. Evidently, the crippled arm did not date from his childhood.

The story of the deformed arm belongs to a later and darker period in our hero's life, and to later chapters in this book.

Yet Another Mystery

But we are forgetting Beso. He came home occasionally and, as before, his wife's willfulness infuriated him.

> Beso often said to her: "Want your son to become a bishop, do you? You'll never live to see it. I'm a cobbler, and that's what he's going to be." Afterwards he just carried the boy off to Tiflis and got him a job in the Adelkhanov factory. Soso helped the other workers, did odd jobs for the older hands. But Keke was no longer afraid of her husband. She turned up in Tiflis and carried her son away. (From S. Goglitsidze's reminiscences)

She had defeated her husband yet again. And humiliated him. He never returned to Gori after that (perhaps 1888 or 1889). He vanished. Contemporaries of Soso, and his biographers, say that Beso later "died in a drunken brawl."

What did Soso himself have to say about it?

In 1909, many years after his father's death "in a drunken brawl," Soso was arrested, not for the first time, for revolutionary activity and sent to Vologda. Among the "Reports on Person under Surveillance" which have survived we find the following:

> Case No. 136, Vologda Gendarme Administration. Joseph Vissarionov Dzhugashvili, born in peasant family. Father, Vissarion Ivanov, aged 55, and mother, Ekaterina, . . . place of residence: mother in Gori, father, no fixed abode.

Not until 1912 did Soso give a different account for police records: "Father dead, mother living in Gori."

How can we explain this? By his passion for confusing the police? Or is there something else?

Was his father in fact still alive? Remember that Beso's brother had been killed, all those years ago, in a drunken brawl. Was the story of his death simply transferred to the missing Beso?

This is a letter I received from N. Korkiya, of Tver.

> In 1931 I met an old man in Sukhumi. He was standing by a meat pie shop on the seafront, begging. I didn't give him anything, he was very drunk. Suddenly he yelled at me—"D'you know who you've just refused money to?"—with a lot of obscene language to follow. The place I was staying at was a few steps away from the pie shop, and my landlady saw the whole scene through the window. When I got in she said in a whisper:

"When he's really drunk he says he fathered Joseph Vissarionovich. Yells at the top of his voice, 'I made him, with this ——— of mine!' The lunatic will shout himself into his grave one of these days." When I got back the following year, the old man wasn't there, of course. He used to live in a cellar next door to the pie shop, and people had seen him picked up and driven away in the night.

This, of course, is just one legend among others. But one thing is clear: his father vanished.

Life in Gori is drab and monotonous. Nothing that ever happened there made a greater impression than the public execution of two criminals. It was February 13, 1892. A thousand people crowded round the foot of the scaffold. The Church School pupils formed a separate group in the crowd. The idea was that "the spectacle of an execution should instill a feeling of the inevitability of retribution, a dread of transgression," Peter Kapanadze wrote in his memoirs. "We were terribly depressed by the execution. The commandment 'thou shalt not kill' did not square with the execution of two peasants. During the execution the rope broke, but the men were hanged a second time."

Among the crowd at the scaffold were two future acquaintances: Gorky and Soso. Gorky described the execution, Soso stored it up in his memory. He had learned that commandments can be broken. Was that when it first occurred to him that the Church School might be deceiving its pupils?

Once he began to suspect it, he could never stop.

Soso left school in 1894 with top marks and entered the first form of the Tiflis Seminary.

Tiflis at the end of the century: a beautiful, merry, drunken, sunwashed city. A world that little Soso saw for the first time. Pick up the *Photographic Catalog* of Caucasian scenes and types, published at the beginning of the century, and you will see the milling throng: the dignified Georgian in his *cherkesska,* the chattering artisans in workshops along the narrow streets, the raucous sellers of Georgian bread, the street musicians with their ancient Eastern instrument the *zurnach,* the brazen hucksters, never quite sober.

The students lived in the seminary building, on full board, walled in from that southern city brimful of temptations. A bleak asceticism brooded over the seminary, preparing its pupils for a life in the Lord's service. In the early morning when they longed to lie in, they had to rise for prayers. Then, a hurried light breakfast followed by long hours in the classroom, more prayers, a meager dinner, a brief walk around the city, and it was time for the seminary gates to close. By ten in the evening, when the Southern city was just coming to life, the seminarists had said their prayers and were on their way to bed. This was how Soso's adolescence progressed. Soso's fellow student I. Iremashvili wrote in his memoirs, "We felt like prisoners, forced to spend our young lives in this place although innocent."

Many of those hot-blooded, early-ripening Southern youths were not at all ready for this life of service. They longed for a different sort of education, one that would allow them to enjoy life's pleasures while satisfying the thirst for sacrifice, for some higher purpose, which the reading of the holy books and the noble dreams of youth had implanted in them.

And they found such a creed. The older boys spoke of certain illicit organizations, whose proclaimed purpose was that of the first Christians—service, martyrdom even, for the good of all mankind.

A Little Revolutionary History: "A Land of Slaves"

The Russian Empire was a land of peasants, with an age-old tradition of serfdom. The "serf right" was abolished only in the second half of the nineteenth century—in 1861. Until then, the great majority of peasants were the property of their masters, the landowners. From time to time the empire was shaken by bloody peasant revolts, but these were just as bloodily repressed, and arbitrary rule and meek submission again prevailed throughout that immense country: "A nation of slaves. All slaves, from the lowest to the highest," in the words of one of the initiators of the revolutionary movement in Russia, Nikolai Chernyshevsky. The antiquated form of land tenure that prevailed in the countryside partly explained the slavish submissiveness of the peasants. This was the peasant commune *(obshchina)*, an institution abolished long ago in Western Europe. The individual peasant had no right to own land; instead, land was held in common by all members of the commune. The commune made all its decisions collectively. Any rebellious individual dissolved in this meek, downtrodden mass. That was why Russian tsars cherished the commune. It was valued not only by them but also by the first revolutionaries. Whereas the tsar saw in it a way of preserving the great past, what the first Russian radicals, Alexander Herzen and Chernyshevsky, saw in it was the great future. Collective property and collective decision making—these were the socialist instincts which would enable Russia to bypass heartless capitalism and enter socialism directly. All that was required was the revolutionizing of the illiterate *muzhik*. For this, agitators—latter-day apostles—were needed. "Summon Russia to the Axe," urged Chernyshevsky, author of the famous novel *What Is to Be Done?*, the Russian revolutionaries' Revelation.

This was the origin of "populism," the creed of those who put their faith in the common people, in the subconscious socialism of the downtrodden Russian peasant.

Both the tsar and the revolutionaries were right. But for the "commune" mentality neither the three centuries of the Romanov monarchy nor the subsequent victory of the Bolsheviks in Russia would have been possible. Yet their first encounters with the people, as they really were, were not happy experiences for the revolutionaries. In 1874 hundreds of young people (most from well-to-do families) adopted false names, acquired forged passports, and set out to incite the Russian peasant to revolt. But this "going to the people" merely alarmed the peasants. Most of the luckless apostles were seized by the police or by the peasants themselves.

Meanwhile the development of revolutionary ideas went on apace among the intelligentsia. One of the dominant influences on the Russian Populist movement was the publicist Peter Tkachev. He joined the revolutionary movement at the age of seventeen as a student and was arrested and imprisoned in the Peter and Paul Fortress. He later succeeded in escaping abroad and became the acknowledged leader of the Russian Jacobins. He published abroad an antigovernment journal called *Nabat* (The Tocsin). He never returned to Russia, but died abroad in a home for the insane at the age of forty-one.

Tkachev's original contribution to Russian revolutionary thought was the idea that a popular uprising is not necessary for the success of a revolution. Revolution can be successfully carried out by a narrow conspiratorial group of revolutionary leaders. They must seize power first and then transform a country accustomed to slavish submission. They would speed the Russian people, full steam ahead, along the route to socialism into the bright future. But the expectation was that for the sake of that bright future *the majority of the population must be exterminated*. Otherwise, because of its backwardness, it would only hinder entry into the socialist paradise.

Precepts of the Latter-Day Apostles

One of the pillars of revolutionary socialism was Mikhail Bakunin, the father of Russian anarchism. Bakunin's ideas provided the basis for the *Revolutionary's Catechism,* written by Sergei Nechaev, the founder of a secret society which styled itself "People's Vengeance." The *Catechism* prescribed that the revolutionary should break with the laws of the civilized world: "Our task is terrible, universal destruction." He must be merciless, expect no mercy for himself, and be ready to die. To carry out his work of destroying the system, he must infiltrate all social formations . . . including the *police.* He must exploit rich and influential people, subordinating them to himself. He must aggravate the miseries of the common people, so as to exhaust their patience and incite them to rebel. And, finally, he must ally himself with criminals, "unite with the savage world of the violent criminal, the only true revolutionary in Russia. . . . Every fully initiated revolutionary must control several revolutionaries of the second or third category (not fully initiated), whom he must look upon as *part of the common capital, placed completely at his disposal."* Many Russian revolutionaries, forbidden to live in St. Petersburg, chose to reside in blissful Tiflis. Clever boys from the seminary often came into contact with them. Soso was one of those who met them and was given a copy of the *Catechism.*

He read the new commandments after lights out with the help of a candle end.

Without Tkachev and the *Revolutionary's Catechism,* we shall never understand either our hero or the history of Russia in the twentieth century.

What particularly attracted the seminarists was the idea, at once alarming and thrilling, of revolutionary terror. Fearing the advance of capitalism in Russia and its destructive effect on the commune, that bulwark of socialism in the future, the revolutionaries resolved to hasten the collapse of the system. They would overthrow tsarism by an unremitting campaign of terrorism against the most important official personages—and by assassinating the tsar himself. They did succeed in murdering Tsar Alexander II, but instead of a popular explosion, what followed was the benighted reign of Alexander III. It was during this period that the Marxists hived off from the Populist movement.

The Revolutionary Messiah

Symbolically, the first leaders were Georgi Plekhanov, son of a Russian landowner, and Pavel Axelrod, a poor Jew. They adopted Marxism, Russian-fashion, as a bible which foretold the future. And, in accordance with the Great Teaching, Marx's Russian followers sat down to await results as capitalism developed in their country. For, according to Marx capitalism begets its own murderer, the proletariat—while the proletariat inevitably fathers socialist revolution. The long wait ahead was, of course, rather embarrassing. For the dread murderer of capitalism (like capitalism itself) was in the early embryonic stage in Russia. But the Russian Marxists were resolved to lead it forward from early infancy to revolution and, for this purpose, to create a proletarian party.

Marxism quickly conquered the Tiflis Seminary. Many of its alumni would become revolutionaries. The seminarists readily absorbed Marxist teaching. Self-sacrifice in the service of the poor and the oppressed, the protest against an unjust society, the promise of a Kingdom of Righteousness and the enthronement of a new Messiah (the World Proletariat)—all these ideas seemed to coincide with those implanted by their religious upbringing. Only God was superseded. But by way of compensation they could now live in the real world and enjoy its consolations. Also abolished was the injunction—so strange to young ears—to "return good for evil"; instead, these young savages, sons of a warlike people, were granted the right to be ruthless to the enemies of the new Messiah. Little Soso's question "Why didn't Jesus draw his saber?" was resolved. Most important of all, their lowly social position was declared unjust, and they acquired the right to change it themselves. Soso now became a regular listener to Marxist debates.

Revolution was slowly ripening. And the poor but proud boy found the revolution's great promise—"He that was nothing shall be all"—more seductive all the time. Later, he would write, "I joined the revolutionary movement at fifteen."

The Poet

His character changed—jollity and love of games were no more.

"He became pensive, seemed gloomy and introspective, was never without a book," wrote one of his contemporaries later. Never without a new book, to be precise. In this phase of his life he was already in possession of the secret.

"There is no God, they are deceiving us," he told a classmate, and showed the frightened boy Darwin's book. This was when he learned to hide his thoughts. A secret unbeliever, he answered his teacher's questions as brilliantly as ever, even when the content and purpose of the lesson were religious. Duplicity became the staple of his existence.

His break with the past and his loneliness found expression—as it so often does with adolescents—in verse. He sent his verses to the newspaper *Iveria.* This was not just another newspaper. It was edited and published by the king of Georgian poets, Prince Ilya Chavchavadze. *Iveria* printed Soso's poems: the usual sentimental, adolescent musings about the moon, about flowers. Altogether the poet Soso had seven poems published in *Iveria* in 1895–96. The first was a bravura piece, with this felicitous beginning:

> Blossom, my native Iveria!
> Exult, O land of my birth!

The last of them struck a tragic note:

> Where once the strings of his lyre resounded
> The mob has set a vial filled with poison
> Before the hounded man,
> Crying "Drink, accursed one, such is
> Thy lot, the reward for thy songs.
> We have no need of your truth
> And your heavenly strains!"

Yes, he is preparing himself for a martyr's career. He remembers the words of the *Catechism:* "The revolutionary is a doomed man." Legend has it that Chavchavadze himself believed in the poet's future and cheered him on his way: "This is the road for you to follow, my son." It is rather more than a legend. One of Soso's poems was reprinted in 1907 in the *Georgian Chrestomathy: A Collection of the Finest Examples of Georgian Poetry.*

But by 1907 our poet's compositions were of quite a different order.

The Parricide's Gift: His Revolutionary Name

Those verses were his final farewell to little Soso. His new name would shortly be born. As befit a poet, he was under the spell of a literary character, Koba, the hero of his favorite book in his youth, *The Parricide,* the work of the Georgian author Kazbegi. Koba was a Georgian Robin Hood, fearlessly robbing the rich. Yet again the same old Bakuninist maxim: "Let us unite with the savage world of the violent criminal—the only revolutionary in Russia."

The title of this favorite work of his is significant. It all fit. He had rebelled against the Father. And just at this time he had killed the Father in himself. The erstwhile brilliant seminarist was now the revolutionary Koba. Koba was to be the revolutionary pseudonym by which he was most often known for many years to come.

His Future Teacher

Another revolutionary was living at this time in Siberian exile. He was only eight years older than Koba but was destined to play an extraordinary role in his life. His name was Vladimir Ulyanov. The twentieth century remembers him by his revolutionary pseudonym: Lenin.

How unlike the two of them were. The son of an actual state counsellor (the civil rank corresponding to the military rank of general in tsarist Russia) and a member of the gentry class by birth, Lenin grew up in an intellectual Russian family. His parents idolized their children. His father devoted his life to education as a district school inspector. In his boyhood Lenin roamed the paths of his grandfather's country estate.

The son of a drunken cobbler, Koba had got nothing from his father but beatings, and nothing from life but poverty.

And yet . . . they were also strangely alike.

In his childhood Lenin was rude and arrogant. Like Koba. Lenin was quick-tempered, yet he could be surprisingly patient, secretive, and cold. Like Koba.

Both had poetic natures. The young Lenin walked the avenues of his grandfather's estate absorbed in Turgenev's love story *A Nest of Gentlefolk*. Young Koba wrote sentimental verses. Both were small and both fanatically, almost insanely, determined always to come out on top, even in boyhood games. Both lost their fathers early; both were idolized by their mothers.

Neither of them at first intended to become a revolutionary. Lenin did so after suffering an indescribable shock: the tragic death of his older brother, hanged for his part in a plot to assassinate Alexander III. His mother's suffering and the sudden change in their social position were enough to make him hate life's injustice. His executed brother's favorite reading, Chernyshevsky's novel *What Is to Be Done?*, in Lenin's own words, "replowed" him.

Just as *The Parricide* replowed Koba. The crude romantic trash which was Koba's reading and the famous philosopher-revolutionary's book had something in common: both were about the elimination of injustice by violence.

And both young men, as they embraced revolution, took the same lesson to heart: the true revolutionary must be merciless, and not be afraid of blood. Both had devoted supporters, and both possessed "charisma"—the mysterious ability to dominate people by exerting a hypnotic influence over them.

3

Expulsion

He succeeded in making contact with the revolutionary underground. Versifying was at an end forever. During his absences from the seminary he now ran Marxist discussion groups for workers. He joined the Social Democratic organization called Mesame Dasi.

In 1898 his name is one of the most prominent in the seminary's record of student misdemeanors: "On the reading of forbidden books by J. Dzhugashvili . . . On the publication of an illegal manuscript journal by J. Dzhugashvili . . ." And so on. He has taught himself to answer his teachers' remonstrances with a contemptuous smile. He despises these deceivers, these servants of a nonexistent God.

He no longer studies. He is not prepared to waste time on it. Yet, interestingly, he becomes one of the most important figures in the life of the seminary. The whole establishment divides into friends and enemies of Koba. Even his enemies fear his secretive, vengeful character, his subtle sarcasm, his rough outbursts of anger. And the vengeance of his friends. The strongest boys for some reason slavishly submit to this puny seminarist with the little eyes, which blaze with a menacing yellow light when he is furious.

Friendship between men is highly prized in Georgia. He has many friends. To be more precise, there are those who believe in him, and they count as "friends." In reality, he is alone now, as he will be in the future. It is just that some young men are made to feel sure of his friendship and are then used in his struggle with those whom he regards as enemies. There was Soso Iremashvili, who would write so much in his memoirs about their friendship; there was the perfervid Misha Davitashvili, at one time his faithful shadow . . . there were, and would be, so many who believed in his friendship.

His name continued to appear in the conduct register: "Reading forbidden books, answering the inspector rudely . . . Joseph Dzhugashvili's room searched" (they were looking for "forbidden books"). He seemed to be challenging the administration to expel him from the seminary. Why didn't he just leave? Because he still had not lost his fear of his mother. At this period he no longer went home for vacations. He was avoiding a showdown.

In 1899 it finally happened: he was expelled. "Chucked out of the seminary for Marxist propaganda" is his own explanation. But the truth is different. Koba actually preferred to make a much less dangerous exit from the seminary.

I have before me an excerpt from the minutes of a general meeting of the seminary's governing body: "On the dismissal of Joseph Dzhugashvili from the Seminary for *failure to sit an examination.*"

As always, he was behaving cautiously.

In the last year of the dying century he had decided where his future lay: he would play a major part in the history of the coming century.

His mother heard the news—he had renounced the service of God. Her sacrifices had been in vain. It was a dreadful blow for pious Keke. She feared that God would abandon Soso, and that the Devil would move in.

At Christmas Koba started work. It was the first, and last, ordinary job in his life. The relevant entry in the records of the Tiflis Main Physical Observatory—"On the engagement of Joseph Dzhugashvili, December 26, 1899"—has survived.

He arrived at the observatory after Christmas, as the century neared its end. A certain A. Dombrovsky, who worked beside him, has described his duties there: "Joseph worked as an observer-calculator. There was no automatic recording apparatus, so all the meteorological data were recorded, round the clock, by human observers. Day and night. The daytime observer worked until 9 P.M., when the man on night duty relieved him."

On New Year's Eve Koba was on night duty in an empty observatory. The others had all gone to celebrate the end of a century.

A magical night: the transition from one millennium to another. The twentieth century, of which nothing yet was known, had arrived, and the man destined to determine its course was peering into the depths of the universe.

Work in the observatory was a blind. His little room there was a hiding place for illegal literature, including the leaflets of the Tiflis committee of the recently founded Russian Social Democratic Workers Party (RSDRP).

Foundation of His Party

In the dying days of the century, Russian Marxist émigrés passed from words to deeds. Plekhanov and Axelrod insisted on the establishment of a Marxist workers' party. The new party was founded with the participation of the General Union of Jewish Workers in Lithuania, Poland, and Russia (the Bund), a mass movement uniting more than twenty thousand Jews. These Jewish Social Democrats were Marxists and anti-Zionists—they believed that only socialism would put an end to anti-Semitism.

In 1898, with the active participation of the Bund, a clandestine congress held in Minsk marked the solemn inauguration of the Russian Social Democratic Workers Party. The Congress chose a Central Committee and called for the establishment of local committees. The majority of the Central Committee were arrested immediately after the Congress, but local committees multiplied. One of them appeared in Tiflis, with Koba among its members.

The Spark

At this time Lenin was a political exile in Siberia. As soon as he had served his sentence, he emigrated. Once abroad, he won over Plekhanov, Axelrod and other Marxist émigrés to his idea of creating an out-of-the-ordinary newspaper. It would have its agents all over Russia. The duty of these agents would be to dig themselves in to the newly founded RSDRP committees and give a militant lead. They would pave the way for a new congress to create a truly militant party. "Give us such an organization of revolutionaries and we will turn Russia upside down," wrote Lenin. The newspaper was called *Iskra* (The Spark). Its epigraph—"From the spark a flame will be kindled"—summed up its program. Lenin and his associates were determined to put old Russia to the torch.

They would succeed. Most of *Iskra*'s agents would see the revolution victorious, only to perish after it in Stalin's camps.

In 1900 an agent of Lenin's *Iskra,* Viktor Kurnatovsky, appeared in Tiflis introducing Lenin's central ideas to the city. Above all: the party must be organized on the strictest conspiratorial principles. There could be no broad discussion, no freedom of opinion in the party. It was a militant organization, with revolution as its aim and, hence, implicit discipline to orders from the center and rigid discipline. Marxism was the holy of holies to the new party. Any attempt to revise any Marxist tenet must be condemned as the work of enemies of the working class. Koba was quick to appreciate the power of this ironclad Marxism and promptly became a Leninist.

First Blood

The strength of these new ideas was tested in action. The Tiflis committee began preparing a workers' demonstration, which was meant to end bloodily. Koba and Kurnatovsky both had high hopes of this bloodshed. I. Iremashvili, an acquaintance of Koba's from the seminary, remembered Koba "frequently repeating that a bloody struggle must bring the quickest results." What Iremashvili did not know was that Koba was only repeating the Leninist slogans which Kurnatovsky had brought with him.

At about this time Koba's mother visited him at the observatory and stayed for a while. Keke evidently tried to make Soso return to the seminary. She had not yet given up hope. She did not know that her Soso was dead and that Koba had taken over. As yet only his new brothers, the revolutionaries, knew him by that name. But the poor woman soon realized her impotence. God had departed from Soso's heart, and the man talking to her was a stranger, the terrifying Koba. His mother went home to Gori.

The arrests began a month before the demonstration was due. Kurnatovsky was arrested, but Koba managed to disappear. He handed in a request for release from his employment on the eve of the demonstration. He was discharged from the observatory at the end of March but was allowed to retain for the time being the little room.

1901. On May 1 people in warm overcoats and sheepskin caps appeared in the center of the city. They were workers, steeling themselves for a clash with Cossacks carrying whips. Two thousand demonstrators assembled in the city center. Cries of "Down with autocracy!" rang out as the police began dispersing the turbulent crowd. And blood began to flow: that of wounded and arrested demonstrators. All this was a novelty in that gay, lighthearted Southern city. "The revolutionary movement can be said to have come out into the open for the first time in the Caucasus," *Iskra* noted with satisfaction.

There were arrests and house searches in the city. The little room in the observatory was searched, but Koba himself was long gone. He would often show this impressive ability to vanish at decisive and dangerous moments. "Koba, one of the ringleaders wanted by the police, managed to escape . . . he ran away to Gori . . . where he made a clandestine visit to my apartment at dead of night," remembered I. Iremashvili. The argument with his mother must have continued in Gori. Still, a mother had to help her son hide. And she did. But could she love this Koba, now that the flame of hatred burned in his heart? She who had deified her little Soso and dreamed of seeing him a priest?

Koba was uncomfortable in his mother's house. He returned to Tiflis, in spite of the danger, at the first opportunity.

TWO

KOBA

4

ENIGMATIC KOBA

"LENIN'S LEFT LEG"

In Tiflis, Koba melted into the revolutionary underground. His life now was that of a professional revolutionary, an "illegal" in revolutionary terminology. Forged documents, endless "safe houses," underground print shops concealed in cellars. A secret association of young people called the Tiflis Committee of the RSDRP. As Trotsky wrote in his book on Stalin, "Those were the days of the eighteen-to-thirty-year-olds. Revolutionaries older than that were few and far between. The words 'committee' and 'party' still had an aura of novelty. They charmed young ears like a seductive melody. Anyone who joined the organization knew that prison and exile awaited him in a few months' time. It was a matter of honor to hold out as long as possible before being arrested, and to remain firm in the face of the gendarmes." Those few months went by, and Koba was still at liberty.

Iremashvili remembered: "I visited Koba several times in his wretched little room. He would be wearing a black Russian blouse with the red tie so typical of Social Democrats. You never saw him in anything but that dirty blouse and unpolished shoes. He hated everything reminiscent of the bourgeois." Trotsky wrote sarcastically that "a dirty blouse and unpolished footwear were the general recognition signs of revolutionaries, especially in the provinces." Yes, a naive young Koba was trying hard to look like a real revolutionary. It was all just as it should be: wearing a dirty blouse, frequenting workers' groups to explain the teaching of Karl Marx. There he developed that threadbare style of his, which was so easy for a semiliterate audience to understand. The style which would later bring him victory over the orator Trotsky.

The East cannot do without a cult. And the "Asiatic," as the Bolshevik Krasin called him, found his god in Lenin. "He worshiped Lenin, he deified Lenin. He lived on Lenin's thoughts, copied him so closely that we jokingly called him 'Lenin's left leg,'" remembered the revolutionary R. Arsenidze.

Koba's god did not let him down. Lenin's *What Is To Be Done?*, which came out in 1902, was a bombshell. Before that, Marxists had despondently told each other that until capitalism was fully developed in Russia not a single hair would fall from the head of the autocracy. Revolution was relegated to the dim and distant future, and revolutionaries had to work for future generations. In his book Lenin gave them fresh hope. He announced that a powerful conspiratorial organization of professional revolutionaries could accomplish the revolution by means of a coup. Theirs was a country of age-old submissiveness. In Russia it was necessary only to seize power—and society would submit. A secret organization of heroes would be able to overthrow the autocracy. How congenial all this was to Koba!

More Bloodshed

Staying on in Tiflis would aggravate the danger of arrest. Being arrested, however, was, according to Trotsky, an obligatory item on the revolutionary's agenda, since it offered him a chance of that greatest of thrills—the *defendant's address to the court.* True revolutionaries were eager to be arrested so that they could convert the court into a platform for propaganda. But Koba was an ineffective speaker, with a muffled voice, slow speech, and a Georgian accent. He felt sure of himself only at liberty, and in the conspiratorial shadows. So Koba was dispatched by the committee to Batum.

A Southern port. Narrow streets, a wind from the sea, cool little courtyards where drying linen is forever flapping in the breeze like the sails of ships. A town made for love and for mirth. Here his clandestine work continues. His contemporaries fall in love, marry, take the first steps in a career. But Koba flits from one "illegal" apartment to another like a man possessed. A workers' demonstration is planned, on such a scale that it is almost an uprising. Much blood will be spilled. He knows the awesome secret: in great bloodshed great revolutions are born.

The unknown youth now had a meticulous chronicler—the police. Seventeen years of his life in the new century would be written up in police records. Policemen would leave accurate portraits of him. Together with photographs, full face and profile. The police are my strange coauthors. I am looking through the files of the Tiflis Gendarme Administration. Reports by policemen on the activities of the Tiflis organization of the RSDRP, on workers' meetings conducted by J. Dzhugashvili.

According to I. Iremashvili, Koba becomes more and more "the leader of a small group of Lenin's supporters in Georgia." Yes. Right from the start he was the leader. And a despot. In one police report we read that "the Batum organization is headed by Dzhugashvili. Dzhugashvili's despotism has aroused the indignation of many members, and there is a schism within the organization."

But look at the results of his despotism. Quiet Batum is shaken by a workers' demonstration on an unprecedented scale. There are clashes with the police, in which fifteen or so are killed and many injured. Blood and fury . . . another success!

The police made arrests in the town, but he had disappeared yet again. He fled to the mountains. The revolutionary Kato Bachidze tells us that "when he was forced to go into hiding after the demonstration Koba passed through the mountain hamlet of Krom. A peasant woman sheltered him, let him wash and rest up."

Mountains, sunlight, little white houses, old men lazily drinking wine in the shade of trees. Time stood still. This was where his forebears had lived for centuries. No, this was not the life for him. But it would be dangerous to return to Tiflis; he had been on the wanted list there for a long time, and going back to Gori was equally impossible—they would be looking for him there. He decided to take an unexpected step: return to the scene of his crime, to Batum. The police did not anticipate such impudence. He managed to remain at large for a whole month.

This was when he took another step up in the Party hierarchy: he was elected to the All-Caucasian Committee of the RSDRP.

First Arrest

It was a Southern spring night, and the revolutionaries were meeting secretly. But there was a provocateur among them, and the building was surrounded by the police. The police now supplemented his biography with the "report of the Inspector-in-charge, Fourth Precinct, City of Batum, on the arrest at 12:00 P.M. on April 5, 1902, of J. Dzhugashvili at a workers' meeting in the apartment of M. Darivelidze." Koba was carried off to jail through the happy city at the hour when his carefree contemporaries were pouring out of the taverns. Locked up for the first time, and in the dreaded Batum jail. This was the beginning of his prison Odyssey: Batum to Kutaisi.

We Learn, Bit by Bit, We Learn

An Asiatic jail. Physical abuse, beatings from the warders, filth, total deprivation of rights. Criminals beat up political prisoners. He was completely lost.

In desperation he tossed an unsigned letter out of a prison window, with a message for his mother: "If you are asked when your son left Gori, tell them he was in Gori all the time." The warders of course intercepted his mail. His naive impulse was followed by helpless despair.

But it didn't take him long to get used to prison. " 'We learn, bit by bit, we learn.' Joseph Vissarionovich liked repeating those words. With his soft accent and his light laugh," Peter Pavlenko narrated to my father.

"We learn, bit by bit, we learn." One discovery was that in prison the power of the warders was paralleled by the invisible power of the criminals. It was not difficult for this pauper son of a drunkard to find a common language with them. He soon became "one of us." He honored the commandment of the *Revolutionary's Catechism:* "Ally yourself with the criminal world." He realized their potential, the contribution that criminals could make to revolution.

Lenin always appreciated this ability of Koba's to find a common language with criminals. When units comprising former jailbirds and drunken soldiers mutinied during the Civil War, Lenin's immediate suggestion was "let's send Comrade Stalin—he knows how to talk to people like that."

Power

His new acquaintances respected physical strength. That was something he lacked. But inured as he was from childhood to beatings, he showed his fellow prisoners something different: contempt for physical force. The prison authorities had decided to teach the political prisoners a lesson. "The day after Easter the first company was lined up in two ranks. The political prisoners were made to run the gauntlet. Koba passed between the ranks book in hand, refusing to bow his head under the rain of blows from the rifle butts," wrote the revolutionary N. Vereshchak in his reminiscences.

Before long Koba had seized power in the prison, just as he had at school, in the seminary, and in the committee. The criminals were subdued by the strange power emanating from this swarthy little man with the angry yellow eyes.

In prison he adopted a rigid routine: every morning began with physical exercises, followed by an attempt to learn some German (true revolutionaries had to read Marx in the original). He never learned the language properly. His achievements in prison were of a different kind. Anyone who refused to recognize his authority became the victim of cruel beatings, administered by his new criminal friends.

And now the small, pockmarked Georgian with a shock of black hair was about to go into exile for the first time. "Koba was handcuffed to a companion. When he caught sight of me he smiled. He had a strange smile which sometimes sent a shiver down your spine," Vereshchak recalled.

Happy, Happy Day!

He was transported by stages to the rim of the world—the Siberian village of Nizhnyaya Uda in the province of Irkutsk. The Southerner found himself in the Siberian cold wearing his one and only overcoat, the black *demi-saison*. In his own country, snow rested only on the mountain heights, but now he was surrounded by it on every side. A flat land of cruel frosts.

But there, in exile, he received a letter from the god Lenin. In his book *Stalin,* Trotsky laughingly explained that this was just an ordinary circular, that Krupskaya, Lenin's wife, had distributed copies of a letter signed by Lenin to all his provincial supporters. But the naive Koba did not know that. His god had taken notice of him! He always remembered that day, and included it in all his biographies.

Born in a Stable

In exile he learned the details of a great event which no newspaper reported. On July 30, 1903, in Brussels, Lenin's dream became reality. Some forty revolutionaries gathered in a small barn. A scrap of paper pinned to the barn door bore the inscription "Congress of the Russian Social Democratic Workers Party." That barn was to see the birth of the atheists' Messiah—the Party which was meant to make all mankind happy.

The Congress in the barn was presided over by Plekhanov. From its very first sessions Lenin set about splitting the Party even before it came into being. With a group of young supporters he came out in opposition to Plekhanov and all the established authorities of Russian socialism. He insisted on a rigidly centralized organization resembling a religious order. Plekhanov and Martov stood out for some semblance of freedom of discussion, something more like European social democratic practice. But Lenin was immovable. He succeeded in splitting the Congress and uniting his supporters in a breakaway group. In the vote on one item under discussion his opponents found themselves in the minority, and Lenin adroitly labeled them Mensheviks ("minority men"), the name by which they have gone down in history. He assumed the proud name of Bolshevik ("majority man"). How Koba must have laughed when he learned that those fools (Mensheviks) had accepted such a demeaning name! How could such people hope to lead the Party? The Congress was followed by an unrelenting struggle between Bolsheviks and Mensheviks, a struggle for power over the Party, in all the provincial committees. They would fight each other, raucously and ruthlessly, at every Congress, for the best part of two decades.

Koba would finally put an end to this struggle in the thirties by exterminating the last revolutionary Mensheviks in the prison camps.

Escapes: So Successful, So Strange

It was November and the Siberian winter had set in, with blizzards one day and cruel frost the next. In this pitilessly cold land he pined for the warmth and the mountains of home. According to Sergei Alliluyev, Stalin's future father-in-law, Koba made his first attempt to escape in November 1903, but frostbite in his ears and nose forced him to return to Uda. Police records tell us, however, that "the political exile Dzhugashvili" was on the run again by January 5, 1904.

He traveled across Russia all the way to Tiflis, using forged documents in the name of a Russian peasant. A Russian peasant? With Georgian features and a Georgian accent! Right across Russia! And nobody stopped him.

Now he is living in Tiflis. And this is another strange thing. Trotsky wrote that "a prominent revolutionary rarely returned to his native place; he would be too conspicuous." If he did return to his hometown, an illegal was at once caught in the net of police surveillance. Statistics show that he would be under arrest within six months at the latest. But Koba would remain at large as an illegal from January 1904 to March 1908—four years—without ever once being detained. The Tiflis Okhrana, which was responsible for security throughout the Caucasus, failed to locate him in four whole years. That is what we read in his official biography. But there are other sources of information: "In 1905 he was arrested and escaped from prison" (from a report on J. Dzhugashvili compiled in 1911 by the head of the Tiflis Department of State Security, I. Pastryulin). "28. 01. 1906 I. Dzhugashvili was arrested in Mikha Bocharidze's apartment" (police records). He was, then, arrested, and more than once? And as before succeeded in escaping? And was not afraid to return to the dangerous Caucasus? Why?

In Tiflis Koba got to know Sergei Alliluyev.

"We first met in 1904—he had just escaped from exile," wrote Alliluyev in his memoirs. Alliluyev had been in the Party from the day it was founded and had worked in the railroad workshops where Koba had preached Marxism to workers' groups. Alliluyev's wife was a madly romantic beauty. She was not yet fourteen when she tied her clothes up in a bundle, slung it over her shoulder, and eloped with him. She was now thirty—and as capable as ever of romantic infatuations. But every new romance ended in her returning to the good-natured Sergei. There is a horrid legend that this passionate woman was not unmoved by Koba's arrival on the scene and that the birth of her younger daughter, Nadya, who was to be Koba's second wife, may have been the result of this infatuation. It is only a legend. The infant Nadya had made her appearance before Koba met Alliluyev.

More Riddles, More Questions

Nineteen hundred five had arrived, and the hitherto unshakable empire was rocked by the first Russian Revolution, which took Bolsheviks and Mensheviks alike by surprise. They were still arguing about revolution when, suddenly, it began. Mass disorders, attacks on the police, mutinies in the army, barricades . . . revolution is always theater. Enter the *jeunes premiers*—the dazzling orators. In this time of the orators Koba was effaced, withdrew into the shadows. That, at least, is what Trotsky wrote about him later.

But there was something strange, something mysterious about those "shadows." We know that he was editing a minuscule newspaper—the *Caucasian Workers' News Sheet*—in Tiflis. And also writing a theoretical work paraphrasing Lenin's ideas. But was this all that the ever-active Koba could find to do in the days of revolution?

No, of course not. There was something else. And that "something" the great conspirator has concealed from us. Most skillfully. It is significant that the mysterious arrests which he ignores in his biography occurred in those years. It is significant that this was when Lenin first took notice of Koba, and Koba made his way to Tammerfors for the first Bolshevik conference.

Using once again a passport belonging to someone with a Russian surname, this Georgian had no difficulty in crossing the frontier. And this in the days of revolution, when trains for Finland teemed with secret agents looking for revolutionaries in hiding there. But Koba escaped arrest. Yet again, his luck held.

Meeting His God

At Tammerfors he saw Lenin for the first time. The naiveté, the primitive uncouthness of Koba as he then was shows clearly in his account of this meeting with his idol:

> In my imagination I pictured Lenin as a giant. How disappointed I was to see a very ordinary human being. . . . It is generally accepted that a great man must arrive late at meetings . . . so that participants will await his appearance with reverent awe. . . . [But to his amazement Lenin arrived on time] . . . and chatted with rank-and-file delegates.

His surprise was genuine, because Koba himself—as a woman revolutionary, F. Knunyants, writes—"was always late for meetings—not very late, but regularly late."

He did not address the Congress. Nor—as Trotsky quite fairly noted later—did he make his mark on this occasion outside the conference room. Yet Lenin again summoned him to take part in the Fourth Congress, in Stockholm, and, although he had still done nothing to distinguish himself, invited him to yet another Congress, this time in London.

Let us note in passing that these visits to foreign capitals made no impression on the ex-poet. He never subsequently mentioned them. What Trotsky tells us about his own first encounter with Paris will serve as an explanation for Koba too: "To take in Paris you have to expend too much of yourself. I had my own sphere of activity which brooked no rival: revolution." In this respect they were all alike. The revolutionary Maria Essen describes a walk with Lenin in the Swiss mountains. Lenin and this young woman are standing on a mountaintop: "The view is boundless . . . the glare from the snow is intolerably bright. . . . I am in the mood for high poetry . . . about to recite Shakespeare and Byron . . . when I look at Vladimir Ilyich. He sits there deep in thought, and suddenly raps out 'Say what you like, the Mensheviks are really shitting on us!' " Koba was just the same. He didn't visit museums, didn't wander the streets. To them, all these bourgeois cities were just bivouacs on the road to revolution.

Lenin, then, summons him to conferences, though, as before, he "does nothing in particular to distinguish himself." It would be more accurate to say that he sometimes revealed a characteristic which Lenin, as a rule, found particularly odious. In the narrow revolutionary milieu, some of Koba's shocking utterances must surely have reached Lenin's ears. This one, for instance: "Lenin is indignant because God has given him comrades like the Mensheviks. What sort of people are they, in fact, these Martovs, Dans, and Axelrods? Circumcised Yids, the lot of them. Then there's that old bag Vera Zasulich. You can neither march into battle with them nor make merry with them." Or this: "They don't like fighting, these treacherous shopkeepers. The Jewish people have produced only traitors, people useless in battle" (quoted from I. David's *History of the Jews in the Caucasus*).

These are the very words spoken by the young, still wild Koba. If there were any doubt about it we could point to an article written by Koba himself and published in the underground newspaper *Bakinsky Rabochii* (Baku Worker) in 1907. This is Koba's own account of his participation in the London Congress of the RSDRP, at which he expressed the same thoughts in the same lighthearted fashion, describing the Mensheviks as a "completely Jewish group" and concluding that "it would not be a bad idea for us Bolsheviks to organize a pogrom in the Party."

Why, then, did Lenin, surrounded as he was by Jewish revolutionaries, and himself with Jewish blood in his family, excuse such a display of the anti-Semitism which all genuine intellectuals detested? It can be explained only by the requirement of the *Revolutionary's Catechism* that "comrades are to be valued only in accordance with their usefulness to the cause." If Lenin could overlook such utterances, Koba must have been needed by "the cause." Very much needed. He must in fact have distinguished himself in some important way.

Koba's Secret

Koba and Trotsky first met at the London Congress. Trotsky arrived at the Congress in a blaze of glory, eclipsing the god Lenin. In contrast to the émigré theorists, who spent all their time arguing about revolution, Trotsky had been in the thick of it back in Russia. In the last days of the legendary Petersburg Soviet he had been a leader, and crowds had listened to him with rapt attention. He had been arrested and had stood trial fearlessly. Sentenced to exile for life, he had escaped from Siberia, traveling more than four hundred miles on reindeer sledges. Trotsky simply failed to notice the tongue-tied provincial with a Georgian accent and—for some reason—the ridiculous Russian Party pseudonym Ivanovich. Trotsky did notice someone else, and later wrote about him. One brilliant young orator, hitherto unknown, made such an impression that he was immediately elected to the Central Committee of the RSDRP. The orator's name was Zinoviev. This was the Party pseudonym under which the young Bolshevik Grigori Radomyslsky became overnight a Party notable.

Imagine the ambitious Koba's feelings when he witnessed the sudden elevation of this blabbermouth—a Jew into the bargain—and the glorification of that other self-infatuated Jew Trotsky, realizing all the time that the Party would never hear of his own services to it. One person, though, did know of them—Lenin.

Immediately after the London Congress Lenin made for Berlin, and Koba went to meet him there. He mentioned this in the interview he gave many years later to the German writer Emil Ludwig. But on the content of Lenin's discussions with him in Berlin he would say nothing.

After that he was on the train again, returning safely to Tiflis. Another fantastic piece of luck.

Shortly after Koba's return to Tiflis the subject of his discussion with Lenin in Berlin would become clear.

Gold

It happened on June 26, 1907—a hot summer's day. Erevan Square in Tiflis was crowded as always. A colorful, cheerful crowd. Two carriages with a Cossack escort turned into the square. They were carrying a large sum of money for the state bank. Almost simultaneously two phaetons drove into the square. One of them held a man in officer's uniform; the other carried two ladies. At a command from the "officer," a band of something like fifty people seemed to rise out of the ground, barring the way to the carriages with the money. Bombs rained on the Cossacks and on bystanders. Amidst the smoke and the uproar the bandits threw themselves into the carriages. One policeman's deposition reported that "the criminals seized a sack containing money under cover of the smoke and suffocating fumes. . . . They opened fire from revolvers at several points in the square and made their escape."

Several people lay dead in the square—Cossacks, policemen, and soldiers, torn to pieces by bombs. Passersby lay mutilated among the wreckage of the shattered carriages. According to Trotsky, "There was no doubt in Party circles that Koba had personally participated in this bloody operation." There was blood, always a great deal of blood, wherever the small, dark man turned up.

The Criminal Wing of the Party

After Stalin's death, Nikita Khrushchev, in his famous speech on the cult of Stalin's person, expressed outrage that Stalin had downgraded the role of the Politburo by creating working parties within the Central Committee—the "fives" and "sixes," vested with plenary powers—"card-players' terminology," Khrushchev indignantly called it. But Khrushchev belonged to the post-Lenin generation of the Party and did not know (or pretended not to know) that he was assailing one of the oldest traditions of the conspiratorial organization which called itself the Communist Party. "Threes," "fives," and other such "narrow formations" set up by the leader within the directorate, and known only to the participants and the Leader himself, first appeared in Lenin's time. One of these Leninist "threes" was directly connected to the raid on Erevan Square.

"Poison, the Knife, and the Noose"

At the end of the nineteenth century, the ideas of revolutionary terrorism held sway over the minds of many young people. Murder in the name of the revolution was considered "an act of revolutionary retribution." Robbing banks or rich people's homes to raise funds for the revolution was called "expropriation." The militants and fighting squads who carried out these murders and expropriations were seen as so many romantic Robin Hoods. "We met with love and sympathy on every side . . . we had helpers in every stratum of society," the terrorist Vera Figner wrote.

When he was planning a sequel to *The Brothers Karamazov,* Fyodor Dostoevsky thought of making the meek little monk Alyosha Karamazov a terrorist. Lenin's brother Alexander *was* a terrorist. Under Stalin the official ideology stubbornly insisted that Bolshevism had eschewed terrorism from the very beginning. All the textbooks cited Lenin's (apocryphal) words after his brother's execution: "We shall take a different path." This was just another official fiction. The revolutionary Nechaev, of whom the young Lenin thought so highly (and who became the hero of Dostoevsky's *Devils*), said that "poison, the knife, and the noose are sanctified by the revolution." And an admirer of Jacobinism like the young Lenin would never think of renouncing terrorism.

During the 1905 Revolution Lenin called for the "schooling of young fighters" by participation in "the murder of policemen and in ar-son" and in the development of a whole program of terrorism. But he knew that as soon as a revolutionary party engaged in direct action, the police too were activated and provocateurs were implanted in the Party.

THE WORLD OF THE PROVOCATEUR

The famous terrorist organization called the People's Will was for a time headed by the provocateur Degaev, and the fighting squad of the Socialist Revolutionary Party by the provocateur Azef. Lenin, therefore, ran his own militant organization on rigidly conspiratorial lines right from the start. This was very helpful when he needed to conceal the militant groups not only from the police but from his own Party.

When the 1905 Revolution ended in defeat, more and more fighting squads turned into gangs of common thieves. There were many examples of "expropriated" money being spent on drink, women, and cocaine. The Mensheviks called for the disbandment of fighting squads.

Lenin and the revolutionaries in emigration were in a difficult situation. As Trotsky wrote, "Before the 1905 Revolution the revolutionary movement was financed either by the bourgeoisie or by the radical intelligentsia." But in the bloody year 1905 the Russian intelligentsia took its first look at the true face of revolution, at the ruthless face of a Russian popular rising. And was horrified by what it saw. The money stopped flowing.

But the comfortable lifestyle of the émigrés, the debates on revolution in Parisian cafés, the activities of revolutionaries underground in Russia—all these things required a very great deal of money. "In the circumstances, the seizure of money by force seemed to be the only means possible," Trotsky wrote. At the Stockholm Congress of the Party, Lenin tried to defend the fighting squads. But there were too many instances of mere brigandage, and the Mensheviks were afraid that they would bring the movement into disrepute. The London Congress, therefore, categorically forbade expropriations and decreed the dissolution of the fighting squads.

By then, however, Lenin had already formed a secret group within the Party, of which the Party as a whole knew nothing. The police were better informed. "The main inspiration for and general direction of direct action was Lenin himself," wrote the gendarme General Spiridovich. And the former Bolshevik Alexinsky, who was very close to Lenin in those days, tells us that "a 'Threesome,' the existence of which was concealed not only from the police but from Party members, was set up within the Central Committee." Trotsky gives us the composition of this "threesome": Bogdanov, Lenin, and Krasin.

A Party Secret: The Great Terrorists

In the notes to Lenin's works there is an opaque reference to Krasin which reads: "Directed the technical bureau attached to the Central Committee." Even after the Revolution Krupskaya would write evasively that "Party members now know of the work which Krasin carried out in arming the fighting squads. . . . All this was done conspiratorially. Vladimir Ilyich was more aware than anybody of this work of Krasin's."

The great terrorist Leonid Krasin, member of the Central Committee of the RSDRP, studied at the Petersburg Technological Institute, was expelled for revolutionary activity, and served a prison sentence. He was a brilliant engineer and a handsome man famous for his success with women. But bombs were his true passion. Bombs for the revolution. "His dream was to create a bomb the size of a walnut," Trotsky declared. Bombs required a lot of money. And Krasin found a great variety of ways of obtaining it.

In May 1905, a certain Savva Morozov took up residence in a villa at Nice. Famous for his wealth and his generosity to needy causes, Morozov had been a great help to the revolutionaries. He was in a state of deep depression. After a visit from Krasin, he made a will leaving his insurance policy to the actress Maria Yurkovskaya Andreeva. She was not just an actress, she was also an agent of the Bolshevik Central Committee. Shortly afterward Morozov was found with a bullet in his heart. Had he shot himself? Or had he been shot by someone else? Only Krasin knew the answer.

The story of the Morozov money does not end there. Nikolai Shmit, Morozov's nephew, was the owner of a large furniture factory—and secretly a member of the RSDRP. During the 1905 Revolution he had organized a workers' rising in his own factory, and he had gone to prison for it. He had often announced for all to hear that the whole of his enormous estate was willed to his beloved Party. In 1907 he committed suicide, in prison, in strange circumstances. And no will was ever found. His heirs were his two sisters. But Krasin had his own way of dealing with the situation. To begin with, the Bolshevik Nikolai Andrikanis was deployed against the older sister, with instructions to marry her. He did so, but, alas, did not hand over the money to the Party. Next, the young Bolshevik Vasili Lozinski (Party nickname "Taratuta") was dispatched to deal with the younger sister, Elizaveta. He made her his mistress and ensured that she would testify in court in favor of the Bolsheviks.

"Could you have done it? . . . Neither could I. . . . The good thing about Taratuta is that he stops at nothing. . . . He's irreplaceable," Lenin told Nikolai Rozhkov, a member of the Central Committee. The irreplaceable person is the one who stops at nothing—that was another lesson Koba would learn in the Leninist universities. "We learn, bit by bit, we learn."

The Bolsheviks won the civil action over the Shmit inheritance and received an enormous sum. The Morozov and Shmit fortunes went toward the manufacture of Krasin's bombs, and the organization of raids and robberies. And this outlay was returned with interest. Bomb factories, Krasin's creation, were now set up in the provinces.

"Krasin's alchemy was greatly democratized" was Trotsky's joke. That was why there was much more bloodshed in those years, although the Revolution was waning. In 1905 the terrorists killed 233 people. In 1907 the toll rose to 1,231. The more money the revolutionary parties needed, the more murders and expropriations there were.

The taciturn Koba was one of those who operated with Krasin's bombs at this time.

We can only guess when it first occurred to Lenin to use the devoted Georgian for "bomb work." Lenin had given him full credit for the organizing talent he had shown in the bloody demonstrations in Georgia. And for his conspiratorial abilities. And his skill in making contact with dangerous criminal elements. Lenin now created a partnership between the wily Koba and the legendary Kamo.

Bewitched by Soso

Kamo was the Party pseudonym of the Armenian Simon Ter-Petrosyan. His daring and physical strength were legendary in the Party. He had to his credit the seizure of shipments in Batum, in Tiflis. Not many people knew that Kamo was no longer alone. He had a friend of long standing at his side—a friend who gave him orders. Because not many knew about their common past.

Simon, like Koba, was born in Gori. His father's opulent home was not far from Koba's hovel. From their childhood days little Simon was the masterful Soso's obedient shadow. Kamo's sister Dzhavaira remembers how "our father used to get furious: 'What do you see in that ragamuffin Soso? Aren't there any worthwhile people in Gori? He'll get you into trouble.' But it was no good. Soso had a magnetic influence on us. As for my brother—he was simply bewitched by him."

Simon was a typical golem: diabolically cunning, strong, cruel, and with the brain of a child. The fearless and fantastically proud Simon, always flustered in Stalin's presence, became strangely dependent. His Party pseudonym itself originated in one of Stalin's sarcastic jokes. Stalin once asked him to deliver a parcel. "Kamo?" (for "Komu?"—"To whom?") asked Simon in his usual mangled Russian. Stalin laughed and started calling him "Kamo" from then on. Making fun of Simon would have cost anyone else his life. But he tolerated this—and much more—from Koba. The master went further and made this joke-name Simon's Party pseudonym, but the golem could not be angry with him. Simon was content to become Kamo. And so Koba, as Trotsky says, gave birth to a name which passed into history.

But the Erevan Square raid surpassed all Kamo's other exploits. This magnificent theatrical event was, from start to finish, Koba's composition. Kamo meticulously followed the score he was given. This was the first show Koba put on for all Europe to see.

"The Swiss burghers were frightened to death . . . they could talk of nothing except the Russian 'exes,'" Krupskaya wrote ecstatically to Lenin from Switzerland. "The Devil alone knows how this uniquely audacious robbery was carried out," wrote the Tiflis *New Times.* Koba evidently couldn't contain himself. His previous terrorist feats had been performed anonymously, which was his preference, but the whole Party soon knew about his participation in the Erevan Square robbery.

Several Bolsheviks were jailed after this affair. Even the experienced Kamo was arrested as soon as he arrived in Berlin. But Koba, yet again, was strangely invulnerable. The robbery on Erevan Square was only one of his terrorist exploits. I. Iremashvili writes that "before this he had taken part in the assassination of General Gryaznov, the military dictator of Georgia in 1906. The general was to have been killed by Menshevik terrorists, but they were too slow about it. So Koba organized his assassination, and was greatly amused when the Mensheviks claimed responsibility."

Pavlenko told my father that "Stalin injured his arm during one of the 'exes.' He was skillful and brave. When the money was snatched in Tiflis he was one of those who attacked the carriage." But Koba never forgot that the Party had prohibited terrorist acts. It was not fitting for the Party and the country to have as their Leader a reckless bandit—even one who had robbed for the good of the cause. This was why, when he became Stalin, he would take pains to conceal Koba's terrorist activity. It was, however, only too well known. In 1918 the Menshevik Martov declared that Stalin had no right to occupy leading positions in the Party, since he "had, in his time, been expelled for his involvement in expropriations." Koba asked for a Party tribunal. "Never in my life," he said, "was I either tried by a Party organization or expelled. This is a vile slander." But in spite of his indignation Koba did not speak of not participating in terror. Martov insisted that witnesses should be called. He produced fresh evidence of Koba's participation in the expropriation of the steamship *Nikolai I*. But he could not summon witnesses from the Caucasus, which was cut off by the war. The matter petered out.

"Just as His Comrades Persuaded Him to Write His Memoirs . . ."

But his past as Koba always worried Stalin. Many of Koba's comrades-in-brigandage would end their days with a bullet in the head in Stalin's camps.

Inevitably Koba's main comrade-in-arms in reckless exploits, Kamo, would be the first to depart this life. This happened immediately after Stalin's elevation to the post of General Secretary of the Party. On July 15, 1922, Kamo was riding a bicycle in Tiflis, when an automobile, one of the very few in the city at the time, bore down on him. There was a dreadful collision. According to a Tiflis newspaper, "Comrade Kamo was hit so hard that he was thrown off his cycle, his head struck the pavement, and he lost consciousness. He died in hospital without coming to." At his funeral, Mamia Orkhelashvili lamented that "Comrade Kamo perished just as his comrades had persuaded him to work on his memoirs and provided him with a stenographer for this purpose. The irony of fate!" Was it Fate's little joke? Or one of his erstwhile friend's?

Fate Turns Its Back on Koba

But in the distant days of 1907, as the Palestinian revolutionary Asad-Bey writes, "He was straight and honest and content with little. All the rest he sent to Lenin."

Throughout those dark years he was living, or rather hiding, in Baku, in the oil fields. This was evidently Lenin's decision. He would henceforward always take care of faithful Koba. "At the wish of the Party I was transferred to Baku. Two years of revolutionary work among the oil workers toughened me," Koba wrote.

He did indeed carry on "revolutionary work in the oil fields." Together with his fighting squad he exacted protection money from the oil magnates by threatening to fire their wells. Sometimes the revolutionaries carried out the threat, and an angry red glow, together with clouds of smoke, hung over the oil fields for weeks on end. They also organized strikes, though these were profitable rather than otherwise to the owners. They raised the price of oil and made an additional payment. Yet Koba himself lived more or less the life of a tramp. All the proceeds were sent in full and promptly to Lenin. This was not easy for him now that he was married, and his wife had borne him a son.

Love

He had met the revolutionary Alexander Svanidze (Party pseudonym "Alyosha") in safe houses in Tiflis. Alyosha introduced Koba to his sister. Like Koba's mother, she was called Ekaterina. Her forebears were from Didi Lilo, the hamlet where Koba's father had been born. She was very handsome. And very gentle and docile. Not like those free and easy, garrulous women revolutionaries. But nonetheless—a revolutionary's sister. David Suliashvili, another former seminarist who had become a revolutionary, regularly visited the Svanidze house at the time and considered himself engaged to her. The handsome Suliashvili versus Koba. The revolutionary Faina Knunyants paints a pitiless picture of Koba in those years. He was "small, weak, with some sort of deformity, wearing a Russian blouse too big for him, and a ridiculous Turkish fez on his head." But Ekaterina saw him differently. He had the glamour of Georgia's favorite romantic brigand who robs the rich for the sake of the poor. Then again, his awareness of his power over others was itself fascinating. Molotov recollected in his old age that Stalin had "always been attractive to women."

It was love, of course! She was as religious as his mother. They married secretly, and in church. The wedding was not kept secret only from the police. A church wedding meant disgrace for a revolutionary.

"There was hardly a single case of a revolutionary intellectual marrying a believer," Trotsky wrote contemptuously. Koba killed people. Koba lived a life of near destitution, but it was his dream to have a real family, the family of which he had been deprived in childhood. He could found such a family only with an innocent and pious girl. Freethinking women revolutionaries, forever on the move from one illegal apartment to the next and from one male comrade's bed to another, were no good to him. Now he had found her. "Hunted by the tsarist Okhrana he could find love only on the humble hearth of his own family," noted Iremashvili.

They rented a room on the oil field—a squat adobe cottage, with a Turk for a landlord. Ekaterina (Kato) worked as a seamstress. Everything in their beggarly dwelling was sparkling clean, everything was covered with embroideries and lace of her making. His home, his hearth—a traditional family. But in spite of all this he remained the same ferocious revolutionary as before. According to Iremashvili, "He was terrifying in political argument. If he had been able to, he would have exterminated his opponent with fire and sword."

She tried hard to make a home of the house to which he so rarely came, for fear of arrest. When he did come it was only at dead of night, to vanish again at first light. She bore him a son, Yakov. With a babe in arms to look after, she had difficulty making ends meet. As always, they had no money. The enormous sums which he obtained went immediately to Lenin. And in any case this near pauper despised money. To him, it was part of the system which he had set out to destroy. When money came his way he unhesitatingly distributed it among his friends. Sergei Alliluyev writes that "I was supposed to go to Petersburg at the end of July 1907, and had no money, so on the advice of comrades I went to see Koba." Koba immediately offered him money, but Alliluyev could see how poor he was and of course refused to take it. Koba was adamant. He kept trying to force the money on Alliluyev, saying "Take it, take it, you may need it," until Alliluyev finally gave in and took it. The Alliluyevs owed him a lot. It was Koba who had saved Sergei's little girl from drowning. That same little Nadya.

His wife sat at home with no money and a wailing infant, and Koba had vanished into the night. After a while she fell ill, and Koba had no money to pay for treatment. Nor could he show himself very often at the little house. It was too dangerous. She was near death. In the autumn he was forced to move her to Tiflis. Her family lived there. The Svanidzes could look after her. But it was too late. "Kato died in his arms," wrote Iremashvili. A photograph preserved by the Svanidze family shows Koba, looking frightened and disheveled, standing over her coffin, unhappy and bewildered. That was how he killed his first wife.

Another Riddle

Yakov was born shortly before his mother's death, and the year of his birth is given in all official documents as 1908. But I found in the Party Archive a photocopy of a newspaper report that "the death of Ekaterina Svanidze occurred on November 25, 1907."

Was Yakov, then, born after his mother's death? One explanation given for this discrepancy is that Yakov was indeed born in 1907, but to delay his call-up to the tsarist army for a year, the local priest agreed to record the date as 1908. This appears to be the truth of the matter. But the question remains: when Yakov was given his passport after the October Revolution, why did the all-powerful Stalin not correct the date?

He did not correct it because everything to do with the life of the mysterious Koba was later painstakingly complicated by Joseph Stalin.

The newborn child was left in the care of the dead woman's sister. The Revolution found Yakov living in his aunt's family home and he would not move out until 1922. Only then did Koba—now Stalin and in Moscow—send for his son.

"After his wife's death Koba showed great zeal in organizing the assassination of princes, priests, and the bourgeois," wrote Iremashvili. But this was the time when strange rumors also made their appearance—dreadful rumors since their subject was a revolutionary. Koba, fortune's favorite, who managed to elude all his pursuers, Koba the fearless, was in reality a provocateur insinuated by the police into the revolutionary movement.

Koba's arrest put a stop to these rumors for the time being.

More Big Surprises

Koba was now in prison. Documents found in his possession when he was arrested proved his membership of the banned Baku Committee of the RSDRP: this gave the police the right to bring a further charge against him, which could result in a sentence to imprisonment with hard labor. But the Baku Gendarme Administration for some reason closed its eyes to these documents and recommended only that Koba should be returned to exile, this time in Solvychegodsk, for a term of three years. There followed another surprising decision: the Special Conference of the Ministry of the Interior banished Koba for a mere two years.

The exiles' route to the godforsaken little town of Solvychegodsk lay through Vyatka. In Vyatka jail Koba fell sick with typhus. He was transferred from his cell to the provincial hospital.

At Solvychegodsk he rented a room in the house of a certain Grigorov. At that time the tiny township was one of the centers of revolutionary life: a population of 2,000 was increased by 450 political exiles. All these socialists, living at the expense of the state which had banished them, spent their days arguing about the coming revolution.

Under Stalin, life in exile would be quite different.

He made a complete recovery in Solvychegodsk and by early summer he was on the run. According to police reports he escaped on June 24, 1909. As before, he was not afraid to make the Caucasus his refuge.

He was at large there for nine months, was arrested on March 22, 1910, and under investigation for three months. The deputy director of the Baku Gendarme Administration, N. Gelibatovsky, drafted the following recommendation: "In view of his persistent participation in the activities of revolutionary parties, in which he has occupied a very prominent position, and in view of his two escapes, . . . the highest penalty, banishment to the remotest regions of Siberia for five years, is appropriate." And once again the improbable happened. The recommendation was ignored. The decision adopted instead was a mild one: the incorrigible Koba was deported all the way back to—Solvychegodsk! That was how his third period of banishment began.

A Riddle, This Time a Romantic One

On October 29, 1910, he took up residence again in the otherwise unknown Grigorov's house. But this time it was not for long. It can hardly have been because conditions were bad there; if they had been bad, he would not have moved in again. Some other factor was possibly at work.

On January 10, 1911, Koba moved to the house of a young widow, Maria Prokopievna Kuzakova. She herself has described their first meeting:

> In the winter of 1910 a middle-aged man called on me and asked, "Did my friend Asiatani lodge with you?" The visitor's name was Joseph Vissarionovich Dzhugashvili. He wasn't dressed for winter—he wore a thin black overcoat and a felt hat. He had come looking for a room to rent. "How old are you?" "How old would you say?" "Somewhere around forty." He burst out laughing. "I'm only twenty-nine."

Kuzakova described her house as follows: "There wasn't much room in the house, the children slept on the floor, and sometimes they got very noisy, so it was no good trying to read." It obviously cannot have been the domestic amenities that attracted Koba and made him change his address.

The Mysterious Kuzakov

In 1978 the seventieth birthday of one of the television bosses, Constantin Stepanovich Kuzakov, was marked by a special program. He was the son of that same Maria Kuzakova.

Everybody in television knew that he was also Stalin's son. They were remarkably alike. Moreover, Constantin Stepanovich's life story was full of mystery. Someone highly placed in television told me that "soon after Joseph Vissarionovich's elevation the widow was summoned to the capital and given an apartment in a new government building. The young Kuzakov got a higher education and occupied high positions, on the vice-ministerial level. All his life he never saw Stalin. But during the cruel Stalinist repressions when people in important positions were being annihilated, Kuzakov's turn came. He was expelled from the Party, and it looked as though his days were numbered. He immediately appealed to Stalin directly. I have seen his appeal myself, in his personal file, with the decision taken by Stalin in person: 'Not to be touched.' And Kuzakov was immediately left in peace." In Kuzakov's curriculum vitae the date of his birth is given as 1908. But according to the same document his father died in 1905. Work that one out! Of course, the year 1908 is given for reasons of tact. Just as in the widow's story of her acquaintance with Stalin, published in *Pravda,* the date of their meeting is given as 1910.

Koba must, of course, have met her early in 1909, during his first period of banishment in Solvychegodsk, since his friend, the Georgian revolutionary Asatiani, was lodging with her at the time. Koba was feeling the loss of his wife acutely. The good widow evidently helped him to forget. That was why when Koba turned up in Solvychegodsk again he moved in with her noisy household. So Constantin Stepanovich was most probably born a year later. I saw him on a number of occasions. The resemblance became more and more marked as he aged. He knew it, and played on it to some extent: he grew a mustache like Stalin's, was slow and deliberate in manner, laconic. Svetlana Alliluyeva wrote that according to her aunts Koba had lived with a peasant woman during one of his spells of Siberian exile, "and there must be a son somewhere."

Here, as elsewhere in Koba's life story, the facts were successfully muddled by Stalin: a rumor would be put around that the son in question had been born in Turukhansk.

(At the very end of September 1995, when this book was about to be printed, I was pleased to be able to inform my publishers of the latest Moscow sensation: the newspaper *Arguments and Facts* printed an interview with Kuzakov himself, titled "Kuzakov: Son of Stalin." The suppositions turned out to be true: approaching his ninetieth year Kuzakov decided to disclose that which he had kept silent about throughout his long life. "I was still a child when I learned that I was Stalin's son," he told the correspondent.)

Another Enigmatic Story

Koba's exile came to an end, and so did his life in Kuzakova's boisterous quarters with its rambunctious children, all of them, so spiteful tongues asserted, greatly resembling exiles who had formerly lodged there.

Denied the right to leave for the capital, Koba chose to reside in Vologda. All this time Lenin had been thinking of the dark, audacious Georgian. He sent him impatient invitations. Koba himself writes about this in a letter intercepted by the police: "Ilyich & Co. keep urging me to go to one of the two centers [i.e., Moscow or Petersburg] before I finish my sentence. I should like to finish it so as to have more scope for my work on a legal footing, but if the need is urgent I will of course take off."

Another oddity. Why was this great conspirator so strangely trusting? How could he forget that the police opened and read letters?

The Police Department shortly afterward received from its agent the news that, "as might be expected, the Caucasian [that was what the police called Koba] will leave shortly for Petersburg or Moscow to see representatives of the organization there, and will be under surveillance all the way. It might be better to carry out a search and arrest him right now in Vologda."

But there was no arrest. Those in charge of the department seemed not to hear, and did not react at all. Shortly afterward, Lenin gave the order, and Koba took off for Petersburg. According to a detective's report: "3.45: The Caucasian arrived at the station with his baggage and got into a third class carriage on the train for St. Petersburg. . . . The Caucasian left on the aforementioned train for St. Petersburg." And no attempt was made to stop him. Why?

To aid an escape, revolutionaries used two kinds of documents. There were false documents made from expired passports, stolen from local government offices, chemically processed, and filled in with new particulars. There were also "iron" passports—genuine documents, sold by local residents, who then waited a while before reporting their "loss" to the police.

Sure enough, after Koba's departure an "application from P. A. Chizhikov, domiciled in Vologda, in connection with loss of his passport" appears in the records of the Gendarme Administration. The passport had, however, already been found. A certain "Chizhikov" was arrested in a Petersburg guesthouse, and turned out to be the fugitive J. Dzhugashvili.

Another puzzle. It was clear from the start that flight to Petersburg was pointless. Prime Minister Stolypin had just been killed by a revolver shot in Kiev, and the whole police force was on the alert. Petersburg was flooded with police agents. How could anyone with the Russian name Chizhikov in his passport, and Georgian features, hope to survive? Especially someone who behaved as strangely as Koba now did in Petersburg?

He was cautious to begin with. In his memoirs, Sergei Alliluyev tells us that Koba "left the Nikolaevsky Station and decided to walk around the city for a while . . . in the hope of meeting somebody in the street. That was less risky than looking for people at addresses he knew. He spent the whole day walking round in the rain. The crowd on the Nevsky Prospect was thinning out, the lights of advertisements were going out, when he caught sight of Todria. The whole police force was out and about after Stolypin's assassination. The two men decided to rent a furnished room. The doorman handled his passport dubiously—his name was given there as Pavel Chizhikov. Next morning Todria brought him to our place."

At this point the story again becomes difficult to understand. Alliluyev looks through the window and sees plainclothes men. The apartment was obviously being watched. But Koba, suspicious Koba, makes a joke of it, and seems strangely unconcerned. Later, accompanied by the worker Zabelin, he eludes observation with remarkable ease and spends the night at Zabelin's place, after which he returns to the very same furnished room, knowing that he is under surveillance.

"From what Stalin himself told us," wrote Anna Alliluyeva, Sergei's oldest daughter, "he was arrested on his return to the lodging house, late at night after he had gone to sleep."

That he was arrested is not at all surprising. The surprising thing is that he behaved so carelessly.

And so his three days in Petersburg ended in mystery. Examination of his case went on until mid-December. Once again, Koba was given a light sentence: he was exiled for three years, and with the right to choose his place of residence. Yet again he chose Vologda.

Historical Personages Gather

In the investigators' files on Dzhugashvili we catch a glimpse of someone else who was to be famous: Vyacheslav Skryabin. The revolutionary Skryabin's Party pseudonym was "Molotov." That was the name under which the future Minister of Foreign Affairs would partition Europe and go down in history.

Looking through his meager files in the Party Archive I find the curriculum vitae which he wrote on being arrested at the age of nineteen. The future minister, I find, is another who did not complete his education. He had founded a secret revolutionary organization in the Kazan Modern School and, as a result, was expelled and sent to live under police surveillance in Solvychegodsk.

So the two of them had lived in the same place—though not at the same time. Fate had chosen to postpone their meeting. When Dzhugashvili fled to Petersburg, his future loyal henchman had only just turned up in Solvychegodsk. Living, to begin with, in the very same hospitable household, that of Kuzakova.

The romantic lives of young people in exile. How young they were, how full of hope, on the threshold of the second decade of a young century. Their century. One which would bring these unknown youths power and glory. Followed—for most of them—by their destruction.

Placed on the Central Committee by Lenin Himself

He arrived in Vologda at the end of December 1911. It was Christmas, and the town was joyfully celebrating the great holiday.

"We," wrote Koba's old classmate I. Iremashvili in his memoirs, "felt like convicts, condemned to spend the years of our youth in this place although guilty of nothing."

In the new year Koba's fortunes took an immediate turn for the better. Sergo Ordzhonikidze, an old friend of his and an important Party functionary, came to Vologda to see him. Grigori Ordzhonikidze, whose Party alias was "Sergo," was younger than Koba. He was born in 1886 in a Georgian gentry family. He joined the revolutionary movement at seventeen, was imprisoned, emigrated, and lived for some time in France. He was famous in the Party for his quick temper and his habit of arguing furiously and yelling at his opponents. It was because of this that delegates to one Congress were reluctant to elect him to the Central Committee. Lenin, however, greatly valued Sergo's loyalty, and craftily claimed that he shouted so loudly at his opponents because he was deaf in one ear. Now, in 1912, Ordzhonikidze had been sent back to Russia by Lenin, to work underground.

It was Ordzhonikidze who told Koba about surprising happenings in the Party. The indefatigable Lenin had carried out a coup!

After the defeat of the 1905 Revolution, rank and file members of the Party, Mensheviks and Bolsheviks alike, had striven to repair the breach. This became a matter of urgency when the Mensheviks found themselves short of funds. They tried to arrange a discussion of the Shmit legacy: the money, willed to the RSDRP as a whole, had been seized by the Bolsheviks. The two sides agreed to hold an All-Russian Conference of the RSDRP, with a view to reuniting the warring factions once and for all. Few of them believed it possible.

"Needless to say at any such conference a bunch of brawlers living outside Russia would try to outshout each other . . . and it was the purest self-deception to expect anything sensible from these fighting-cocks," the famous revolutionary Rosa Luxemburg sarcastically remarked.

She did not know her Lenin. All *he* wanted was to show the Party that "we have done everything we could to restore unity." After which he accused the Mensheviks of unwillingness to cooperate and in January 1912 carried out a blatant coup. He convened a conference of Bolsheviks in Prague. They proclaimed themselves sole representatives of the RSDRP and elected a Central Committee consisting only of Bolsheviks. Lenin, Zinoviev, and Ordzhonikidze himself, who had taken a most active part in preparations for the Prague Conference, were among those elected to the Central Committee. Koba was not.

Koba was brought into the Central Committee later, by Lenin in person.

There were indignant letters from Plekhanov, from Trotsky, from the Menshevik leaders, from the German socialists—but Lenin simply ignored them.

This was when Koba began to master a crucial lesson in the art of leadership in the new century: complete disregard of public opinion.

Ordzhonikidze conveyed the leader's will: Koba must escape. On

February 28, 1912, a few days after his meeting with Ordzhonikidze, he ran away yet again.

Once he was clear of his place of exile, the new Central Committee member became frantically active. Pining for the sun in the vast Siberian wilderness, he began with a trip back to Tiflis. Then he made for Petersburg, inspecting provincial Party committees en route. The police painstakingly touched up his portrait: "face pockmarked, eyes hazel, mustache black, nose unremarkable. Special distinguishing marks: wart over right eyebrow, left arm does not bend at elbow." The revolutionary Vera Shveitser adds to the portrait: "On the way back to Petersburg he called at Rostov. He left me instructions for the work of the Don Committee. Almost the whole Central Committee was imprisoned at the time. We walked all the way to the station, and to disguise the purpose of our meeting drank a cup of coffee and spent two hours there waiting for the train. He was wearing a black autumn overcoat . . . his hat was dark gray, almost black." The same old overcoat, the same old hat. The man in black.

As Nadezhda Krupskaya told it, "Lenin was greatly exercised by the elections to the State Duma (parliament). For the sake of that institution he had already sacrificed some of those closest to him, dispatching Inessa Armand and Georgi Safarov to take part in the electoral campaign. [Armand was Lenin's mistress—Krupskaya had to reconcile herself to her existence—while Safarov was then acting as secretary to the Leader.] Inessa and Safarov, whom Lenin pumped full of instructions, were immediately arrested in Petersburg." That was when Lenin had made Koba escape. He arrived in Petersburg without incident.

After the Revolution Safarov would be one of the leaders in the Red Urals, and would sign the warrant for the execution of the imperial family. Only to be executed himself on Stalin's orders some twenty years later.

Another Fantastic Journey

In Petersburg Koba now took charge of the electoral campaign. This was when he met Skryabin (Molotov), who was also living illegally in the capital. They were joined by another revolutionary, Sverdlov. On this occasion Koba was uncharacteristically circumspect. Arrests were usually made at night, so this time Koba did not go home at night. After a get-together with workers to discuss electoral tactics, he would spend the whole night wandering from one cabman's tearoom or tavern to another.

Koba sat waiting for morning in a choking haze of tobacco smoke among cabbies and homeless drunks, dozing at their tables. Sleepless nights left him so weary that he could hardly stand on his feet.

In spite of all this, spring in Petersburg ended with his arrest. But whereas in September 1911 he had been at liberty for exactly three days, this time it was several weeks. He was arrested on April 22 and sent—instead of to Vologda—to the harsh Narym region. But he had no intention of staying around for the icy Narym winter, and in September he escaped with no difficulty whatsoever. For the fifth time. There is a telegram in the Police Department's files which reads: "Dzhugashvili escaped Narym region . . . intends go to Lenin for consultation . . . in event of discovery request not arrest immediately . . . better as he attempts to cross frontier."

But in spite of these orders, in spite of police surveillance, he manages in some mysterious manner to cross the frontier safely.

He travels first to Cracow, to see Lenin, and in November coolly returns to Petersburg. Then at the end of December he makes his way back, with no difficulty at all, to Lenin in Cracow to take part in the February conference of the Central Committee. And all this without an external passport. How was it possible?

What follows is his own explanation, as retold by Anna Alliluyeva. It seems that "Koba did not have the address of his dispatcher [the person who was to help him across the frontier] . . . but he met a Polish shoemaker in the market . . . and when the Pole learned that Koba's father had also been a shoemaker, in Georgia, which was also oppressed, like Poland . . . he immediately agreed to guide him over the frontier. The Pole wouldn't take any money, and his parting words were . . . 'We sons of oppressed nations must help each other.' . . . I heard this story many years after the Revolution. . . . He laughed as he told it to us."

It was indeed a story for naive little girls, to be told with a laugh. The question remains: how *did* he manage to get abroad twice, without an external passport, and when the police had been alerted?

Bloody Marxism

Once abroad, he was able to observe the free and easy life of the Bolshevik émigrés, debating in cafés over coffee. Some of them had their wives and children with them and lived a normal life, paid for with money earned by illegals like himself, working in inhuman conditions in Russia. Here, at last, was his opportunity to talk to Lenin. What did they talk about? Probably the same things that Lenin discussed with Valentinov and other congenial revolutionaries. Valentinov has reproduced these conversations for us.

The number one subject was "bloody Marxism": "Being a Marxist [Lenin told Valentinov] doesn't just mean learning Marxist formulas off by heart . . . a parrot can do that. . . . To be a Marxist you need the right psychology . . . what people call Jacobinism. . . . Jacobinism means fighting for your objective with no fear whatsoever of resolute actions, not fighting in white gloves . . . not fearing to resort to the guillotine. . . . A difference in attitudes to Jacobinism is precisely what divides the world socialist movement into two camps—the revolutionary and the reformist." Valentinov added that "Lenin spoke so passionately that there were red spots over his cheekbones and his eyes became pinpoints." Jacobinism and the guillotine were lessons which Koba would remember well.

Following Lenin, he moved on to Austria.

In his eternal black overcoat and dark hat he turns up next in Vienna.

Trotsky was in Vienna in 1913, staying with one Skobelev (the son of a rich citizen of Baku) who was a faithful disciple of his at the time, but later an opponent and a minister in the Provisional Government. "Suddenly," wrote Trotsky, "the door opened without a knock and . . . a strange figure appeared on the threshold: a very thin man, rather short, his face swarthy with a grayish tinge and clearly visible pockmarks. He looked anything but friendly. This stranger emitted a guttural sound, which might have been taken for a greeting, silently poured himself a glass of tea, and just as silently left the room. 'That's the Caucasian, Dzhugashvili,' Skobelev explained. 'He's just got into the Bolshevik Central Committee and is obviously beginning to play an important part there.' The impression he made was difficult to describe, but no ordinary one . . . the a priori hostility, the grim concentration."

Trotsky, then, had finally taken notice of him.

The Marvelous Georgian of Steel

Meanwhile, Stalin went back with his cup of tea to the work he had interrupted.

Lenin had invited the non-Russian Koba to come out against the "Bundist bastards," Jewish socialists so incapable of forgetting their Jewishness that they were demanding national-cultural autonomy. Did

Lenin perhaps want to take advantage of Koba's anti-Semitism—much as he himself hated such sentiments—for the good of the cause?

Koba worked away diligently. He wrote about the world of the future, in which the great ideal of internationalism would triumph, and there would be no miserable little nations, but the one world of the victorious proletariat. Lenin painstakingly edited the work. "We have here a marvelous Georgian, who has sat down to write a big article", he wrote to Gorky. (The eminent writer Maxim Gorky had enjoyed great popularity from the beginning of the twentieth century. To the Russian intelligentsia his name symbolized revolutionary ideas. The younger generation called him "The Stormy Petrel of the Coming Revolution." He was a friend of Tolstoy, Chekhov . . . and also of Lenin.)

Koba signed this article "Stalin"—"Man of Steel." He was following the fashion. Skryabin, for example, had become Molotov, the man who smites the enemy like a hammer *(molot)*. There was a Bolshevik called Bronevoi—as hard as armor plating *(bronya)*. And so on. But Koba did not become Stalinov, on the analogy of Molotov. He chose Stalin, to sound like Lenin. These naive sobriquets made the intellectual Trotsky smile.

From Vienna, Koba wrote a letter to Lenin's favorite, Malinovsky, who led the Bolshevik group in the Duma. Malinovsky was a brilliant orator, and the organizer of a metalworkers' union. As in Koba's case, Lenin himself had procured Malinovsky's election to the Central Committee of the Party. But in addition to his important Party responsibility Malinovsky carried out other duties as an informer on the payroll of the police department.

To judge from the letter, Koba and his addressee in Petersburg were close acquaintances. They were both illegals, both belonged to the category of Party leaders who worked inside Russia instead of sitting it out abroad. In his frank letter Koba complained to Malinovsky that the theoretical work he is engaged on is rubbish, poppycock. That was how he defined his own theoretical pursuits. He was bored. He could never be number one at this—he could only repeat Lenin's thoughts. But Lenin was now sending him to Russia.

Arrested Again

Koba, then, returned to Petersburg, to supervise the work of the Duma group. Once again he behaved with extreme caution. But to no avail. The writer Yuri Trifonov told this story:

> My Bolshevik grandmother T. Slovatinskaya lived in a "safe house" with her daughter, my future mother. Hiding in one of the rooms was A. Solts, a Bolshevik with terms of exile and imprisonment behind him. He lived in a tiny room meant for a servant. One day Solts told my grandmother that he would be bringing along a comrade, the "Caucasian," whom he wished to introduce to her. It turned out that this Caucasian had been sharing with Solts for some days, without ever leaving the room. I don't know how they made room for the two of them on that narrow iron bed. Evidently, my grandmother said, the usual unwritten rules of conspiracy did not allow them to confide even in me. . . . That was how I met Stalin. At first I found him too serious, too reserved and shy. He seemed to be afraid above all of giving trouble or inconveniencing anybody. I had difficulty in persuading him to sleep in the large room, where he would be more comfortable. When I left for work I always asked him to have dinner with the children, . . . but he shut himself up in his room all day and lived on beer and bread. . . . He was arrested in the spring of 1913, at a charity concert. We often organized concerts jointly with some student "friends-from-home" society, ostensibly for charity, but in reality to collect money for the Party. . . . I remember it as if it were today. . . . He was sitting at a little table, chatting with Malinovsky, the deputy, when he noticed that he was being watched. . . . He went out to the artists' dressing room for a minute and sent someone to fetch me. . . . He said that the police had turned up, that he could not get away, and would shortly be arrested. He asked me to let it be known that he had been with Malinovsky before the concert. . . . Sure enough, as soon as Stalin went back in, two plainclothes men approached his table and asked him to leave with them. Nobody knew as yet that Malinovsky was a provocateur.

Over the Edge of the World

This time the punishment was harsh. Koba was banished to the Turukhan region for four years.

It was a long journey in a barred rail truck, across the Urals and Siberia to Krasnoyarsk. And from there to the rim of the world—the Turukhan region. He was taken by boat up the turbulent Yenisei to the village of Monastyrskoe. And on from there beyond the end of the world to a settlement called Kostino. Then beyond the Arctic Circle to the settlement of Kureika. The scenes that awaited him were enough to fill any inhabitant of his sunny homeland with despair—endless icebound winter, a short, wet summer with clouds of midges and troubled white nights. A place where time stood still. A limitless icy sky, and under it a mere speck of humanity. This was where the Bolshevik Joseph Dubrovinsky, Lenin's comrade-in-arms, had committed suicide; this was where another well-known Bolshevik, Spandaryan, would die of tuberculosis.

It was 1913, and the country was celebrating the tricentenary of the Romanov dynasty, solemnly observing the holiday of its tsars. The regime looked unshakable, and Lenin sadly acknowledged that there would be no revolution in his lifetime.

Koba wrote pathetic, self-pitying letters right and left.

"I don't think I've ever had to endure such a dreadful situation," he wrote to the Bolshevik group in the Duma. "My money's all gone, I've started getting a worrying cough of some sort now that the cold is intensifying (37 degrees below). I've got no provisions, neither bread nor sugar, everything here is dear, I must have milk, I must have firewood . . . but there's no money. I have no well-off friends or acquaintances, I have absolutely no one to turn to. What I'm asking is that if the group still has its fund for the repressed let it allot me say sixty rubles."

And this to the editors of *Prosveshchenie*: "I don't have a single penny, and I'm right out of provisions. . . . I did have some money but it all went on warm clothing . . . couldn't you stir up people you know and raise say twenty or thirty rubles. That would be a real life-saver."

He wrote to the Alliluyev family as well. They sent him money as soon as they heard that he was destitute. He responded: "I ask only one thing: don't waste money on me, you need it yourself, you have a large family. . . . I shall be quite happy if you just send me the occasional postcard with a view. . . . In this accursed land nature is hideously bare, and I have fretted myself stupid longing for a landscape to look at, if only on paper." In later years he hated writing long letters. But in those days, and in that terrible place, letters were the only possible means of talking to friends and relatives, and this lonely man had no one nearer than a family whom he half-knew.

The Party Archive has preserved a story called "Into the Blizzard," dictated by him to Alliluyev's son Fyodor. Evidently, when he was courting Nadya Alliluyeva, Koba, like Shakespeare's Othello, told stories about his "tormented past," how he would go out into the Arctic night to catch the fish which were "his only food" and how on one occasion he had nearly perished: "The frost was getting harder all the time, the snow and the shadows from ice hummocks were bluish in the moonlight . . . the icy wilderness . . . a north wind sprang up, the snow whirled, the stars were hidden. . . . He had wandered into a blizzard. . . . The landmarks disappeared in the blizzard. At each gust of the icy wind his face grew number until it turned into an icy mask. The pain was excruciating. His steaming breath froze as it left his mouth. His head and breast were encrusted with ice, it was impossible to breathe, his eyelids were stuck together by hoarfrost. His body was losing heat fast. But . . . on and on he went. And he made it."

While all this was happening Lenin more than once discussed ways of helping Koba to escape. But Koba's "boots" (that was what they called the passports necessary for an escape) somehow never arrived. Why did he himself make no attempt to escape? He, who had escaped from places of banishment so often, would surely escape from the most dreadful of them all. But he suffered, and continued tamely living in this hell. Why? The answer to this question may be connected with the main enigma about Koba.

The Thirteenth Provocateur

When I was a young student at the Historical-Archival Institute doing my practical work in the Central Party Archive in Moscow, I saw there the (top-secret) card index of the Moscow Security Police Department. It was a listing of revolutionaries: blue cards for Bolsheviks, white for Kadets, pink for Socialist Revolutionaries (SRs). On the backs of cards were the pseudonyms of provocateurs who had supplied information to the police. Recruiting a valuable provocateur could open the way to promotion for a Police Department official. They took good care of their protégés. The head of the Security Police, V. Zubatov, often said, "You must regard your collaborator as a married woman with whom you are having an affair. One careless step and you will ruin her."

After the February Revolution the Provisional Government set up several commissions of inquiry, and many important provocateurs were exposed. But with the advent of the Bolsheviks to power, a remarkable change took place. The Special Commission attached to the Archive of Revolutionary History in Petrograd worked on exposing provocateurs for just one more year, then, in 1919, it was abolished. Its work resulted in the exposure of twelve provocateurs who had operated among the Bolsheviks. A thirteenth, whose pseudonym was "Vasili," was never exposed.

Koba: The Riddle of Riddles

Rumors that Koba was a provocateur began to appear at the very beginning of his career. When I started writing this book, Olga Shatunovskaya, a member of the Party since 1916 and at one time the personal secretary of Stepan Shaumyan, the chairman of the Baku Commune, was living on the Kutuzov Prospect. She had, of course, been imprisoned by Stalin in the thirties, but was rehabilitated in Khrushchev's time, and afterward occupied an important post as a member of the Party Control Commission. Shatunovskaya stated publicly on a number of occasions that Shaumyan had been absolutely convinced that Stalin was a provocateur. He used to talk about his own arrest in 1905 at a safe house known to one person only—Koba. An underground print shop existed for three years in a Tiflis suburb, until in spring 1906 it was raided by the police. Once again, rumor insistently pointed to Koba.

We know of Shaumyan's suspicions not only from Shatunovskaya's account, but from documents recently published. The following document was preserved in the secret section of the Archive of the October Revolution:

> To the Baku Division of the State Security Police. The Baku Committee of the RSDRP met yesterday. Those present—Dzhugashvili—Stalin, who had come from the Party center, committee member "Kuzma" [S. Shaumyan's Party pseudonym], and others. Members confronted Dzhugashvili-Stalin with the accusation that he was a provocateur and an agent of the Security Police. And that he had embezzled Party funds. Dzhugashvili-Stalin reciprocated with charges of his own. *Fikus* [fig tree].

"Fikus" was the pseudonym by which Nikolai Erikov was known to the police. This revolutionary, who lived underground, was a secret collaborator of the Security Police from 1909 to 1917. He had been a Party member from the day it was founded.

The agent Fikus passed on another very curious piece of information: "The 150 rubles sent by the Central Committee to set up . . . [a printing press] are in Kuzma's possession, and he at present refuses to hand them over to Koba. . . . Koba has asked him about it several times, but he stubbornly refuses, openly showing his distrust of Koba."

It was at that moment of maximum tension that Koba was arrested by the police. His arrest and exile put a stop to the awful rumors for the time being. We now find Shaumyan writing sympathetically that "we were told the other day that Koba is being sent to the Far North, and he hasn't a single kopeck, he has no overcoat, and nothing at all to wear."

The first edition of Stalin's *Short Biography* says that he was "arrested eight times, and escaped from exile seven times." A text of the biography with Stalin's emendations is preserved in the Party Archive. For the second edition in 1947, Stalin made a very interesting emendation. The old text reads, "between 1902 and 1913 Stalin was arrested eight times"; Stalin corrects this to "seven." The old text says, "Stalin escaped from places of banishment six times"; he corrects this to "five." One of his periods of detention evidently worried him, and he decided to remove it. In Shatunovskaya's opinion, it was the one during which he became a provocateur.

When I heard Shatunovskaya's stories, Khrushchev's Thaw was coming to an end. She bombarded me with the names of old Bolsheviks who had known about Stalin's role as a provocateur: V. Sheboldayev, Secretary of the Rostov obkom (regional chapter of the party); Politburo member S. Kosior; Marshal Yakir. A letter from L. G. Korin from Tomsk says: "The rumor that Stalin had been a provocateur was well known in the Communist International. My father, an old Bolshevik, told me that at some Comintern meeting Radek read out the Police Department's secret instructions on the recruitment of provocateurs. This was done to teach Communist parties how to combat provocateurs and how to recruit agents of their own. And Radek read it out with Stalin's unmistakable slight accent."

Amusingly, I stumbled on these secret instructions when I was looking into the secret Comintern files. Here are a few extracts:

> Secret agents are most useful to the Security Department if they are at the top of the Party. . . . If it is unable to recruit an agent of this sort, the Security Division tries to help its agent to rise from the lower levels to the summit of the party. . . .
>
> The most suitable people to work on are those who return from exile without authorization, those detained when trying to cross the frontier, those arrested with incriminating objects in-

> tended for dispatch. . . . If a secret agent is in danger of exposure he is arrested together with other members of his party, including the one by whom they were told that he was a provocateur.

So we can easily imagine that, as Korin says, "Radek's reading was a great success with the initiated among his listeners."

Shatunovskaya told me that the materials on Stalin's career as a provocateur were shown to Khrushchev, but when people asked for further investigation Khrushchev threw up his hands and said, "It's impossible. It would mean that our country was ruled for thirty years by an agent of the tsarist Secret Police."

Was Our Country Ruled for Thirty Years by an Agent of the Tsarist Secret Police?

Consider all his fantastic escapes, his trips abroad, the strange complaisance of the police, the endless list of futile coded telegrams asking for Koba to be intercepted, arrested, and never for some reason taking effect.

Consider one of those coded telegrams in the Archive, from the head of the Moscow Okhrana Division A. Martynov to the Petersburg Division: "November 1, 1912 . . . Koba Dzhugashvili on his way to Petersburg should be detained before he leaves for abroad." But Koba went on his way via Petersburg and across the frontier. Yet again. And would take part together with Lenin in the Bolsheviks' Prague Conference. At which, incidentally, the provocateur Malinovsky would also be present. Can he really have been an Okhrana agent?

The Mirror

To understand it we must recall the strange story of his close acquaintance and correspondent Roman Malinovsky. Malinovsky was the head of the Metalworkers Trade Union. As early as 1911 some members of the Party harbored serious suspicions of him. He had been elected to the State Duma by a Moscow constituency and became leader of the Bolshevik group in that body. When the president of the Duma learned of his service in the police, Malinovsky was invited to leave without fuss. He disappeared from the capital.

The Bolsheviks were alarmed by his inexplicable disappearance. Rumors of his double-dealing were recalled, an investigation was ordered, and a commission set up. Malinovsky agreed to appear before the commission. It gave all his accusers a hearing. But Lenin stoutly defended Malinovsky, and the commission declared the accusations against him unproven. At the same time, the commission decided not to make public a personal matter which Malinovsky offered in explanation of his withdrawal from the Duma. Lenin continued defending his favorite with all his might. When the young Bukharin, already an influential member of the RSDRP, savagely attacked Malinovsky, Lenin wrote him a letter on Central Committee paper: if he went on slandering Malinovsky, he would be expelled from the Party himself. Rehabilitated, Malinovsky continued working for the Party. During the war he volunteered for army service, with secret instructions to surrender to the Germans and become a POW. In the Party Archive is a solicitous letter, dated 1915, from Lenin telling Malinovsky that warm clothes had been sent to the POW camp for him. After the February Revolution in 1917, Malinovsky's role as provocateur was proved beyond doubt. But Lenin fought on to the end: he flatly informed the Provisional Government's commission that he did not believe that Malinovsky was a provocateur. The documentary evidence mounted up, however, and in the end the Bolsheviks had to give in. Malinovsky's name became a synonym for double-dealing, alongside those of Azef and Degaev. Yet shortly after the victory of the October Revolution Malinovsky came back from Germany to Petrograd. He was immediately arrested and sent on to Moscow, and stood trial on November 5. He made a curious statement in court, which is mentioned by Louis Fischer in his biography of Lenin: "Lenin must know about my connection with the police." He asked for a confrontation, but the Investigating Commission of the Supreme Tribunal had him shot in a hurry. Those are the facts. The question which naturally arises is why did Malinovsky return?

In his testimony to the Provisional Government's commission Lenin said, "I do not believe that Malinovsky was a provocateur, because . . . if Malinovsky had been a provocateur the Security Police would have gained less from it than our party did." Lenin's answer, perhaps, holds the key to a surprising situation. Malinovsky did indeed do the Party much more good than harm. The Security Police, under pressure to preserve Malinovsky's cover, made the authorities tolerate his inflammatory speeches in the Duma and the existence of *Pravda,* the Bolshevik newspaper in which subversive articles were published. Vissarionov, one of the top men in the Security Police, says much the same: "When I started reading his speeches in the Duma I came to the conclusion that we could not go on working with him." In this statement we hear the voice of a disappointed man.

Thinking over the Malinovsky story, I remembered something that happened when I was a young man studying at the Historical-Archival Institute. It was a year devoted to practical work on the card indexes, one of provocateurs and one of revolutionaries, referred to earlier. In those days this archive often received requests from old Bolsheviks applying for a pension in recognition of their services to the Revolution. These services were checked against the card index of revolutionaries and at the same time against the card index of provocateurs. Sometimes the same names occurred in both indexes. The meritorious revolutionary was found to be neither more nor less than a provocateur.

During my time in the archive I witnessed the following incident. One of these old Bolsheviks asked for evidence of his revolutionary activity. A woman archivist found his name on both indexes. He arrived at the archive, suspecting nothing, to collect his certificate. The woman in charge of our practical course had a soft spot for me and allowed me to sit in on the interview. I still remember him—a tall old man with exquisitely groomed snow-white hair. And I shall never forget how he laughed when they told him about their discovery. I reproduce from memory the extraordinary conversation that followed.

He: Yes, I was on the force as an agent, but never was one.
Archivist: I don't understand you.
He: I was working with the Party's consent. That was how we obtained information. Unfortunately, those who planted me on the police were shot long ago by Stalin. You'll have to take my word for it.
Archivist: But you betrayed . . . [she named various revolutionaries].
He: That was done by agreement.
Archivist: With whom?
He: With those who planted me. But I can assure you that if those I betrayed had known about it they would have approved of my actions. Our lives belonged to the Party. For the good of the Party we were ready to sacrifice our freedom and our lives.
Archivist: But you didn't ask your victims first?
He: That's a pretty bourgeois way of thinking. Still, I suppose it's difficult to understand nowadays. The revolutionaries are all

> dead, and the bourgeois are still with us. *Thermidor* has conquered.

I can see him now rising from his chair and walking out without saying goodbye.

Let us remember Bakunin's *Catechism:* infiltrate all social groupings, including the police. The well-known socialist Angelica Balabanova recorded how surprised she was when Lenin expressed his readiness to make use of provocateurs for the good of the cause: "When will you begin to understand life? Provocateurs? If I could I would station them in Kornilov's encampment [referring to the general who was the leader of the Russian Army]."

My Version

First—my version of Malinovsky. When the police got to know about his dark past (which included rape and robbery, among other things) they began blackmailing him, and invited him to become an agent. He evidently decided to tell Lenin about it. He had studied Lenin closely, and as he expected the Leader made light of his past crimes. They had not been committed against the Party, and from the point of view of the *Catechism,* which called for collaboration with violent criminals, Malinovsky was blameless. The police, however, had him cornered. They could not be allowed to blacken him, since that would blacken the Party. Not surprisingly, Lenin had an idea absolutely in the spirit of the *Catechism*: Malinovsky must agree to become a provocateur, so that he could use the police for his own purposes. As the relationship between Malinovsky and the police developed, "a few comrades" had to be sacrificed. But only those least needed were turned in, while Malinovsky became incomparably more useful to the cause. It was thanks to the police that Malinovsky got into the Duma, where he fulminated against the autocracy unhindered. He was also very helpful to the Bolshevik newspaper *Pravda.* His activities as a provocateur were conducted in the strictest secrecy, as always, and it seems most likely that no one except the Leader knew about them. That was why Malinovsky returned to Russia once the Revolution was over. But he had forgotten the *Catechism:* the good of the cause was what mattered most. Lenin could not admit the existence of his Party's criminal wing. So the tribunal had the forgetful Malinovsky shot.

This was hardly a unique case. In a party which had always acknowledged that "all things are permitted for the good of the revolutionary cause," the practice of using double agents was not uncommon. The wily Koba was better suited than anyone to this role. It may be that Koba was given permission to establish contact with the police so that he could carry on the "bomb business" more effectively. That would explain why escape was so easy for him, and why he showed so little concern for his own safety. And also why Lenin was untroubled by his strangely successful escape attempts and his suspiciously easy trips abroad. Here too, of course, others had to be sacrificed. But Koba, in all probability, did not give away only "unwanted" comrades. He could simultaneously use the police to settle accounts with his personal enemies. The money which the police paid him Koba would, of course, hand over to the Party.

"When parting company with a secret collaborator, be careful not to strain relations with him, but take care at the same time not to put him in a position in which he could subsequently exploit the person in charge of the investigation," reads one of the Secret Police Department instructions. But, as happened with Malinovsky, the police began to suspect that Koba was playing a double game. When he lost their patronage he was compelled to behave more cautiously. He had to give up his part in the "exes" (expropriations) and concentrate on work with the Duma group. He was valuable to Lenin as an organizer capable of conducting an election campaign, but once the Duma elections were over he was much less useful to the Party. Others could oversee the routine work of the Bolshevik group in the Duma—in other words, carry out Lenin's instructions from abroad. It seems possible that Malinovsky was allowed to turn Koba in. When he heard of Malinovsky's flight, Koba would draw his own conclusions. He had been betrayed. They had sacrificed him.

He did not, however, realize it immediately. He wrote to Lenin from exile in Turukhan. He felt sure that they would save him, help him to escape. Now that he had no help from the police he could not manage it alone.

"Koba sends greetings, and reports that he is in good health," Lenin wrote to V. Karpinsky in August 1915. But there were no letters for Koba. Lenin had other things on his mind. While Koba was rotting at Turukhansk, the First World War had broken out. And with it a great squabble among socialists. The majority supported their own governments. But Lenin proclaimed that "the defeat of tsarism" would now be the lesser evil. Defeat in war, soldiers' blood—that was now the way to revolution. A few months later, when Lenin decided to revive the Russian Bureau of the Central Committee, he began showing an interest in Koba again. "Important request," he wrote to Karpinsky. "Find out Koba's surname (Joseph Dzh—? We've forgotten. Most important!!!)."

Yes—Lenin could no longer recall the faithful Koba's surname. Then he changed his mind, and faithful Koba is not mentioned again. Koba himself kept trying to remind people of his existence. He wrote an article on the "national question": Lenin had once much enjoyed seeing his own thoughts copied down by the non-Russian Koba. Koba sent the article to him. Lenin did not answer.

Reinforcements arrived in Siberia. Obeying Lenin's wish, the Bolsheviks in the Duma had voted against war credits. The deputies toured Russia, agitating against the war. The whole Duma group was arrested.

SUMMING UP

His conversations with the deputies can have left Koba in no doubt about Malinovsky's role. And the miserable role assigned to himself. For the second time in his life Koba suffered a terrible spiritual upheaval. The first time he had lost his belief in God. Now he lost his belief in the god Lenin. And in his comrades.

He started hating everybody.

He may have reviewed his career to date. He was thirty-seven. His life was more than half over. And what was he? A member of the Central Committee of a party of windbags, most of them in jail, the rest blackguarding each other in foreign parts. His life was a failure. He spent whole days lying with his face to the wall. He stopped tidying his room and washing the dishes after meals. Sverdlov, who shared his lodging, described how Koba thought it funny to put plates with scraps of food sticking to them on the floor and watch the dogs lick them. Sverdlov gave a sigh of relief when he moved to a different house.

Meanwhile, the authorities had begun calling up political exiles for military service. They didn't trust Sverdlov enough to draft him, but they decided to take Koba, which tells us that he was still looked upon favorably.

Once more the Georgian was carried half-frozen over the tundra and down an icebound river. Six weeks later, at the end of 1916, exhausted by the journey, he was delivered at last to the medical examiner in Krasnoyarsk. But luck was with him: his withered left arm earned the future Supreme Commander exemption from military service.

His term of exile was due to end on June 7, 1917, but again the powers that be showed their goodwill: on February 20, three and a half months early, he was given permission to leave for the township of Achinsk. One of Lenin's close associates, Lev Kamenev, was living in exile there at the time. Kamenev, editor of *Pravda* and a member of the State Duma, had been put on trial with the other Bolshevik deputies in 1915. But his behavior in court had been strange, or, to put it more precisely, cowardly: unlike the other Duma Bolsheviks, he had refused to condemn the war. In spite of this he was exiled to the Turukhan region.

As soon as he arrived Kamenev was called before a comrades' court made up of other exiled Bolsheviks. Only members of the Central Committee took part in it. And Kamenev found it strangely easy to vindicate himself. He passed on some message which resulted in the adoption of a resolution approving the conduct of all the deputies tried by the tsarist court.

After the February Revolution some of the younger Bolshevik leaders in Petrograd attempted to put Kamenev on trial again. His august reply was that "for party-political reasons he could not offer explanations of his conduct in court pending prior discussion with Comrade Lenin." In other words, he made it clear to the young Petrograd Bolsheviks that there were things which only the leaders of the Party were allowed to know. Sure enough, when Lenin arrived in Petrograd the "coward" Kamenev became a member of the Central Committee with Lenin's approval. Evidently, this was another instance of the "double game" which Koba knew so well. Kamenev had been instructed by Lenin to belie his convictions in court. Lenin had tried to preserve the freedom of a Duma deputy devoted to him, but the police had seen through the maneuver, and Kamenev was exiled.

In Achinsk Koba visited Kamenev quite frequently. Kamenev, with his professorial beard, would hold forth, educating the uncouth Georgian, while Koba listened, said nothing, and puffed away at his pipe. He was learning. If Kamenev had only known what an inferno there was in the Georgian's soul. How much he now understood. And how he had changed.

The Year 17

"The year 17, whoever that may be," the great, mad poet V. Khlebnikov called it in his visions of the future. Defeats in battle, the shortage of food, and a cold winter awakened the hopes of the revolutionaries.

"Something is happening in the world. I am afraid to open the newspaper in the morning," wrote the poet Blok.

In a sketch written for the newspaper *Russian Word,* the poet Teffi listed the words most often heard in crowded places: "They're selling the fatherland. . . . The cost of living goes up all the time. . . . The government isn't doing a thing." And the great producer Meyerhold put on a play called *Masquerade,* where, against a background of fantastically luxurious scenery, "someone" minced and flitted—this "someone" being Death.

And then—it happened. Suddenly. As always in Russia. That which no one could have thought possible a year earlier: revolution in Petrograd! "The whole edifice crumbled, without so much as a cloud of dust, and very quickly," wrote A. Shchusev, the architect who was to build the Lenin Mausoleum. The writer Bunin recorded something a cabbie said to him: "We're an ignorant people. Make one of us get up and the rest all follow."

The jails were thrown open, local Security Police headquarters set on fire. Somebody had incited the crowd. And among other things destroyed in this revolutionary conflagration were lists of secret collaborators with the Security Police. The stupendous news soon reached Achinsk: the tsar had abdicated, and a Provisional Government formed by the Duma had assumed power. Koba's fortunes were transformed in a split second. His former energy was reawakened. But this was a different Koba.

Kamenev and Koba hurried back to the revolutionary capital. A large group of Siberian exiles traveled in the same train. It was cold in the carriage. Koba was frozen, in agony, and Kamenev sacrificed his own warm socks. The exiles, including the unknown failure Koba, were given an enthusiastic welcome at stations along the line. They were now "victims of the accursed tsarist regime." As always happens in Russia when rulers fall, society at large woke up to its hatred of everything connected with their reign.

On March 12 the Trans-Siberian express set him down in Petrograd. He was in good time—one of the first exiled Bolsheviks to arrive in the capital. Koba at once made his way to the home of Sergei Alliluyev. "He was still wearing the same suit, the same Russian blouse and felt boots, but his face looked considerably older. He amused us with his impersonations of the orators who had organized receptions at the stations," wrote Anna Alliluyeva in her memoirs.

He had cheered up.

Koba in the Atmosphere of the "Gentle Revolution"

A March of sunny days. The soldiers who had carried out the revolution were still sitting peacefully in the cafés of Petrograd, whose proprietors fed them gratis. They belonged to units of the Petrograd garrison stationed in the city; those which on various excuses had managed to dodge service at the front and stay on in the capital. The army in the field contemptuously called the Petrograd garrison the "Sprinter Battalions" because those of them who were sent to the front ran away from their very first battle. They hated the war, and had quickly become an easy target for revolutionary propaganda. Now they felt like heroes, because they had refused to fire on the people.

The intelligentsia were happy: censorship had been abolished, there was freedom of speech for the first time ever. Political parties mushroomed. At the theater famous actresses came out front and sang the "Marseillaise" before the show began, rattling chains from the prop room, broken to symbolize Russia's liberation. Freedom, freedom! In the streets of Petrograd there was red everywhere—red flags, the red ribbons of never-ending demonstrations. It was all uncannily reminiscent of blood. The only black in sight was that of burnt-out police stations. And the sun seemed to shine more brightly than ever that spring. Even the deposed empress said so in a letter she wrote to the tsar after his abdication—"such brilliant sunshine." Yet the killings had already begun: officers were murdered by soldiers, policemen were beaten to death by all who felt like joining in. The press shortly reported the assassination of the governor general of Tver. The same newspapers, however, explained that he was "a well-known reactionary."

Yesterday's exile, of course, followed these events with great interest. He could understand the revolutionary mood of the capital, with its intelligentsia and a garrison unwilling to go to the front. But the rest of Russia, Holy Russia, all those millions of peasants who only yesterday were praying for the tsar, God's anointed, what would they say? Well, they spoke.

"How easily the countryside renounced the tsar. It's incredible—as if they were blowing a hair from their sleeve," an astonished journalist wrote in *Russian Word* that March. So those who had said that revolution from above was a possibility had been right? It was true then: in a country of slaves people fear strength and will submit to it. "We learn, bit by bit, we learn."

The Turukhan exiles went into action almost as soon as they alighted from the train. Lenin, Zinoviev, and other Bolshevik leaders were still abroad. As in 1905 they had neither planned the revolution nor taken part in it and they now found themselves cut off from Russia. As Russian subjects they did not have the right to travel across a Germany at war with their country. The exiles feverishly discussed what to do next. The Bolshevik organizations in Petrograd were controlled by youngsters: Vyacheslav Skryabin—Molotov, whom we met earlier—and two working-class comrades of his own age, Shlyapnikov and Zalutsky. In early March they had already made arrangements for the publication of *Pravda,* the official Bolshevik newspaper. Molotov and certain young Party functionaries of the second rank were the senior editors. Not so long ago they had met in garrets, but now the Bolsheviks had requisitioned the luxurious house of the ballerina Ksheshinskaya, once the mistress of the tsar and his brothers. There was a sort of cruel irony in it: this notorious "love nest" now housed the roughest of all radical parties.

Koba and Kamenev at once made their way to the ex-favorite's house. Workers in black jackets and soldiers in gray greatcoats scurried up and down a once elegant staircase, littered now with cigarette butts. Underwood typewriters chattered away in the chamber which was now the workroom of the Party secretariat.

The young Petrograd comrades were less than delighted to see these influential new arrivals. But the comrades from Turukhan took a firm line. "In 1917 Stalin and Kamenev cleverly shoved me off the *Pravda* editorial team. Without unnecessary fuss, quite delicately," Molotov recollected at the age of ninety.

The days of raging crowds, of street action and of oratory had returned. But our former poet spent the whole of this period in the editorial office of *Pravda.*

6

Opening Move: Encounter with Power

His *Pravda* articles, so strangely forgetful of his teacher Lenin's views, would astound historians. Koba evidently liked this bourgeois revolution, which had so successfully transformed his life. While Shlyapnikov and the young Petrograd comrades invoked Leninist slogans—fraternization at the front and an immediate end to the war—Koba was writing in *Pravda* that "the slogan 'Down with the War' is completely useless for practical purposes at the present time." Kamenev went further and called on the soldiers to answer the Germans bullet for bullet.

But Koba was not merely writing. Together with Kamenev he turned the policy of the Petrograd Bolsheviks upside down. He extolled the Russian Social Democratic Party and launched a campaign which, for a follower of Lenin, could only be called criminal: to unite the Bolsheviks with their foes, the left-wing Mensheviks.

Trotsky would later write of Koba losing his head, following Kamenev's lead, and promoting Menshevik ideas. Trotsky was right. But he did not understand *why* this happened.

A second center of power had been established in Petrograd side by side with the Provisional Government at the very beginning of the Revolution: the Soviets of Workers' and Soldiers' Deputies. The word "Soviet" itself was a felicitous creation of the 1905 Revolution. The word in its time-honored sense implied communal deliberation in an assembly of equals. It was deeply rooted in the peasant mentality and the Russian tradition of "conciliarity."

While the Duma, swept along on a revolutionary tide, strove to prevent chaos, two revolutionary parties, the Socialist Revolutionaries and the Mensheviks, quickly held "flying elections" (by a simple show of hands) in barracks and in factories. And as early as February 27 they announced the creation of a Petrograd Soviet. The Soviet comprised delegates from the workers and, most important, from military units. It was controlled, of course, by those who had so skillfully orchestrated the elections—the SRs and Menshevik revolutionary intellectuals. Thus, another claimant to power now existed in the Tavrida Palace, where the Duma held its sessions. One whose power relied on the support of the mob.

With the help of the soldiers' deputies, the Soviet could control the garrison. It issued the famous "order number 1": henceforward army units were to be governed by soldiers' committees, and officers were to be supervised by rankers. This spelled an end to discipline. The persecution of officers began immediately. The president of the Soviet, the Socialist Revolutionary A. Kerensky, was immediately co-opted to the Provisional Government.

A new custom, suggested by the Soviet, was introduced: troops presented themselves at the Tavrida Palace while the Duma was in session, supposedly to show support for the Duma. But as early as March 3 the president of the Duma, M. Rodzyanko, narrowly escaped being shot by sailors who had come along. Koba could now observe the same scene from day to day: the approaches to the palace packed with crowds of gray-clad soldiers and black-clad workers. Trucks overloaded with soldiers and workers barged their way through the crowd. The streets bristled with bayonets and there was never a break in the yelling of the crowds, the red flags, the inflammatory oratory. People flooded out from the palace's vestibule. If you wanted to move at all you had to join this human torrent. The might of the Soviet grew and grew. Koba knew that the soldiers searching the apartments of former tsarist dignitaries were acting on the orders from the Soviet. They were rather shy about it at first: after the search they would look embarrassed and ask the gentleman victim of the search for a tip. That's Russia for you! But arrests were already being made. "Lickspittles of the old regime" were arrested and brought before the Soviet. One of those hauled in was old Shcheglovitov, a former minister in the tsar's government. Kerensky narrowly saved him from summary execution by the soldiers. They were already tearing off the old man's epaulettes when Kerensky confronted the mob, shouting, "Over my dead body!" On the eve of Koba's arrival the Soviet had compelled the Provisional Government to arrest the tsar, in spite of his abdication, and to consign tsarist ministers to the cells of the Peter and Paul Fortress.

For the time being, the Soviet could not supplant the Provisional Government, since in Russia's eyes the Duma and the government were the authors of the Revolution. But the Soviet quite openly asserted its overriding authority. The ominous formula "so far and no farther" made its appearance. The government could rule insofar as the Soviet supported it. The Soviet was a mighty power, and now Koba, the chronic failure, was part of that mighty force. The Soviet was headed by old acquaintances from Koba's Caucasian days—Georgian revolutionaries like the Menshevik Nikolai Chkheidze, its president. Another very influential figure, Irakli Tsereteli, was also a Georgian Menshevik. And they, of course, wanted to see their Georgian acquaintance Koba among the Bolshevik delegates to the Soviet. Yesterday's forgotten man shortly became a member of the Executive Committee of the Soviet, the real ruler of Petrograd.

Koba knew what those in power required of him. He knew what he was doing when he suddenly forgot Lenin's ideas, began echoing those of the Mensheviks, and gave his support to Kamenev. Intoxicated by the air of revolutionary Petrograd, like so many intellectuals, Kamenev was now preaching the "unification of democratic forces."

It became more serious as time went by. In one of his articles Koba was in favor of the idea of preserving a unitary Russian state. "He seemed to have forgotten his previous ideas on the nationalities question, written down on Lenin's instructions," Trotsky said sarcastically.

Once again, Trotsky was right. And once again, he failed to see the reason.

These ideas of sovereignty, of the preservation of empire, naturally pleased people in the Provisional Government. And they naturally took notice of Koba, the influential radical who nonetheless held such comfortable views. The new Koba began attacking on several fronts at once in this first but dazzling game of chess.

"Koba Stalin" was the name with which he signed his articles. The old Koba, the pathetic loyal fool who had been so ruthlessly exploited and so easily forgotten, had been left behind in Turukhansk. He would no longer be pulling the chestnuts out of the fire for anyone. From now on he served only himself. Himself and the Revolution, insofar as the Revolution could be of service to him.

Results of His Opening Moves

After only two weeks in Petrograd Koba had already seized control of a newspaper, become one of the main figures among the city's Bolsheviks, and joined the leadership of the Soviet, the effective holder of power. Yet in the Soviet he was strangely self-effacing. "When he was playing his modest part in the work of the Soviet the impression he made on me—and not only on me—was that of a gray blob, now dimly visible, now fading without trace. There is really nothing more to be said of him," observed the Menshevik Sukhanov. But Koba Stalin was no gray blob.

A New Piece on the Chessboard

In mid-March a woman no longer young, but still something of a beauty, turned up in *Pravda*'s editorial office. This was the famous ultra-Bolshevik Alexandra Kollontai, daughter of a tsarist general. She handed the editors two letters from Lenin, for publication. In these "Letters from Afar" Lenin's fury knew no bounds. He stigmatized both the Menshevik leaders of the Soviet and the Provisional Government. He ordered "no support for the bourgeois government." Lenin was announcing a change of course—toward a second revolution, a socialist revolution.

To Kamenev, all of this looked like the ravings of an émigré long divorced from Russia. But—Marx or no Marx—Lenin did not want to wait for the completion of democratic changes in backward Russia: that Asiatic peasant country, lacking as it did a strong proletariat, must nonetheless be steered toward proletarian revolution in a hurry. Trotsky had put forward similar ideas during the first Russian revolution, and Lenin had ridiculed him at the time. Yet now . . . the Leader's letters could not be left unpublished. It was evidently Kamenev's idea to publish the first, deleting the harshest words about the government and the Mensheviks, and then pretend to forget the second. Koba consented, knowing that in retrospect Kamenev would bear the main responsibility. Kamenev was the Party's leading journalist and he, Koba, was a mere "practical worker."

Koba was thinking more and more carefully about his future.

He had already sized up the freedom-loving windbags in the Soviet—eternally bickering democrats, scared by the steadily rising waves of mindless Russian rebellion. Chkheidze, Tsereteli, Jewish idealists like Dan, Nakhamkis, and the rest of them—how could they cope with this elemental force? True, the Bolsheviks were only just emerging from underground, but Koba knew the full strength of that ruthless "mothballed" organization. Accustomed as it was to rigid discipline, to unquestioning obedience, it was nothing without a Leader. But with a Leader . . .

Its Leader was due to arrive shortly. Koba did not doubt that the Germans would agree to let Lenin and his comrades-in-arms pass unhindered. He had, of course, heard by then of the firm ties which had unexpectedly linked the Bolsheviks with the kaiser's Germany. He knew that Lenin would return to Russia with lots of money.

This was money the Bolsheviks had been receiving since the beginning of the war. There was nothing strange about it. Lenin was agitating for the defeat of tsarist Russia, for the conversion of the war with Germany into a civil war inside Russia, with the workers and peasants in soldiers' greatcoats, turning their weapons against "their own" bourgeoisie.

Koba could easily deduce the scale of German support from the large subsidies received by his newspaper, *Pravda*. And from the generous funds for arms which went to the military organization set up within the Party. With this money the Party was, with feverish haste, establishing a Red Guard with units throughout Russia.

German Gold

Koba had not gone to live with the hospitable Alliluyevs, although they had told him that there "was always a room waiting for him." Instead, he moved into a large flat shared by the young leaders of the Petrograd Bolsheviks.

"Stalin and I lived in the same apartment at that time," Molotov wrote. "He was a bachelor, and so was I. It was a large apartment on the Petrograd side. I shared a room with Zalutsky, then there was Smilga (the Bolshevik Smilga) with his wife, and Stalin joined us. It was a sort of commune we had there." And that was where Koba could have heard a great deal of talk about German gold. Possibly from a frequent visitor to the apartment, a colleague in the leadership of the Petersburg Bolsheviks, Shlyapnikov. German money had paid for Shlyapnikov's travels between the European capitals during the war, and for the printing and dispatch to Russia of masses of defeatist propaganda—and German gold. This was one of Bolshevism's shameful secrets, and many attempts would be made to prove it untrue. But documents from the secret German archives published after the fall of Nazi Germany revealed that the Bolsheviks continued to receive German money even after the October Revolution. "It is in our best interests that the Bolsheviks should remain in power. . . . If you need more money telegraph the amount"—so wrote Kuhlmann, the German minister of foreign affairs, to the German ambassador in Moscow, Baron Mirbach.

Did the Bolsheviks take money from the Germans? Certainly. Were they, then, German agents? Certainly not. They were simply obeying their *Catechism:* "Make use of the Devil himself if the Revolution requires it." Lenin could have no scruples about taking the money. Yet again, Koba realized that all things were permitted for the good of the cause. "We learn, bit by bit, we learn."

Koba's Expectations Realized

A Russian rebellion: once it starts there's no restraining it. During the first days of the Revolution, while the intelligentsia were joyfully hailing the "dawn of Russian freedom," the famous artist Somov noted in his diary that "so far the crowd is good-humored, but I believe that there will be a great bloodletting." Nothing is more dangerous than eternal Russia with the bit between her teeth.

The man who was eager to fan the spreading flames into a conflagration was on his way. Koba judged correctly what the advent of his Jacobin Leader, furnished with German gold, would mean. In Russia he would find waiting for him an organization battle-hardened in the underground, and the army in a state of collapse and unwilling to fight. Koba knew instinctively to whom the future belonged. That was why he was so cautious in the Soviet: from mid-March onward he was waiting for the new master. Kamenev would answer for *Pravda*'s sins, but he, Koba, would have to answer for his stance in the Soviet. He adopted his favorite tactic—impenetrable silence. He was present in the Soviet, yet absent. A gray blob. He realized that the time for speeches was over, and the time for action at hand. His time.

The train on which Lenin and thirty or so other Russian revolutionary émigrés were passengers crossed the Russian frontier on April 3. It had traveled unhindered through a Germany at war with Russia. As General Hoffman later wrote, "We had the idea of using these Russians to speed up the demoralization of the Russian army." And Ludendorff, in his memoirs, observed that "this journey was justified from a military point of view."

What these German generals would subsequently write was obvious enough to the general public at the time. Krupskaya recalled how apprehensive Lenin was at the prospect of "the savage outcry from the chauvinists" upon their return, and even thought that it might end with him being put on trial and "carted off to the Peter and Paul [Fortress]." They were also worried about the practicalities. It was Easter Day, and they were afraid that they would arrive late and have difficulty finding a cab.

Instead of which a Bolshevik delegation was waiting for Lenin at the

Finnish frontier. Koba was not among them. He had preferred to let Ilyich vent his wrath on Kamenev. It went just as he expected. A member of the delegation, Fyodor Raskolnikov, who represented the pro-Bolshevik sailors in their mutiny against their officers at the beginning of the Revolution, described the scene as follows in his memoirs. The welcoming party came in and sat down on a sofa, and Lenin immediately attacked Kamenev. (Koba would later improve on history. Hundreds of paintings showed the joyous meeting between the great leaders Stalin and Lenin.) Then it was night, and an enormous crowd had gathered at the Finland Station. What awaited Lenin was not a cell in the Peter and Paul Fortress, but a reception committee from the mighty Soviet, led by its president, Chkheidze, whom Lenin had so unmercifully vilified in his letters. A guard of honor and an armored car had been provided for the small, bald-headed man who had never addressed more than a handful of émigrés. At last Lenin saw the great crowds he had always longed for. From the armored car he called on his listeners to realize the insane utopian dream, to ensure the victory of socialist revolution. Only a year ago all this had been delirium, pure fantasy. And now . . . the crowds, the floodlights, the armored car.

Winning Moves

Who had organized Chkheidze's arrival at the station? He was president of the Soviet, which was the real master of the situation in Petrograd, and his appearance legalized the scandalous circumstances in which Lenin and his henchmen had returned. Who had worked to persuade Chkheidze that the rumors about German money only served the right-wing forces and that his presence at the station would put an end to this reactionary talk?

Lenin was bound to appreciate the service which Koba and Kamenev, both old members of the Bolshevik Party, had performed for him.

Late that evening Lenin laid his "April Theses" before an audience. His address was a bombshell. No support for the bourgeois Provisional Government! No more "up to a point," no more "insofar as." All power must belong to the Soviets. But what must have struck Koba most forcibly was the ease with which Lenin had discarded the most familiar Marxist dogmas. Marx had written about the inevitable accession to power of the bourgeoisie after a democratic revolution. And here was Lenin declaring that the bourgeoisie had come to power in Russia as the result of a mistake on the part of the proletariat and calling for immediate transition to a socialist revolution. The astonished audience heard a man who used to represent Marxism as gospel truth calmly reject one of its main postulates. Koba realized yet again that all things are permitted to the Leader.

He immediately adjusted his own views by 180 degrees. Koba Stalin now wrote article after article for *Pravda* in which he slavishly expounded Lenin's ideas. The Boss was back.

The Bolsheviks met in conference on April 29. In the great hall of which the ballerina Ksheshinskaya had been so fond, Lenin repeated the message of his "April Theses." Kamenev chose to defend his own beliefs and railed against Lenin. Whereupon Lenin unleashed Koba. Koba spoke in his new style—without systematic argument, crudely and brazenly garbling Kamenev's views. He lambasted his friend of yesterday unmercifully. This was a new Koba—a Koba who from now on had no friends. His line prevailed. The delegates turned on Kamenev, reminding themselves of all his past sins.

Then came the election of the Central Committee, and Lenin personally proposed Koba. "We have known 'Comrade Koba' for very many years," Lenin asserted. "He is a good worker in any responsible position." The audience took its Leader's point: Koba's earlier articles were not to be held against him. The "good worker" collected ninety-seven votes, more than anyone except Lenin and Zinoviev. This was a great victory. Koba was finally playing a leading role. What he had failed to win by devotion he had won at once by dirty tricks. Lenin nonetheless had to support Kamenev as well: Lev Borisovich knew too much, and had indeed done a great deal for Lenin. To the amazement of his audience Lenin, usually so unforgiving, suppressed the story of Kamenev's behavior on trial: "The incident is closed." And that was that. He recommended Kamenev too for the Central Committee, and the conference duly elected him.

Koba was not mistaken in Lenin. They began working to seize power there and then, at the conference. They decided to enmesh the whole country in a network of Bolshevik cells and detachments of the Red Guard. For this purpose Lenin selected an organizer of genius, Koba's onetime roommate in exile in Turukhan, Yakov Sverdlov. Party functionaries were quickly on their way to the provinces, to prepare a new revolution, with German money in their pockets. Russia would soon be ablaze.

After the conference a narrow inner leadership called the Bureau of the Central Committee was elected. It would later be known as the

Politburo and would become the official ruling body of one-sixth of the earth's land surface for many decades. The first Bureau had four members: Lenin, his faithful assistant Zinoviev, Kamenev, and Koba Stalin. In May 1917 Koba was already a member of the Party's four-man leadership.

They had set their course toward a new revolution. Lenin the Jacobin called his policy "peaceful," but he was preparing to shed blood. He had need now of that wily terrorist who had proved his worth in the Party's most dubious deeds. Lenin knew too that Koba would always voice *his* thoughts. Koba's instant capitulation had given him fresh assurance of it.

Koba, however, soon had to make room for someone else. As did the other members of the Bureau. May saw the return of Trotsky to Russia.

The Second Queen

He had been a Menshevik, and vehemently denounced the Bolsheviks, then distanced himself from the Mensheviks in turn. This "freelance revolutionary," a brilliant journalist and outstanding orator, had fought against Lenin throughout, calling him the "Dictator," the "future Robespierre," while Lenin called Trotsky "Yudushka" (after a character in one of Lenin's favorite novels, *The Golovlyov Family,* by Shchedrin; Yudushka was a monster of greed, cunning, cruelty, and hypocrisy). These were the mildest of the insults they exchanged. But now, since February, the gap between the views of these old enemies had surprisingly narrowed. Lenin was now the spokesman for Trotsky's old dream of "permanent revolution," and they uttered in a single voice the battle calls to rebellion: "All power to the Soviets" and "Down with the Provisional Government." There was a third slogan, the most fearful of all, calling for the defeat of Russia and the conversion of war with Germany into civil war. The foes had traveled in opposite directions for so many years—and finally met.

Trotsky's very first speech, at the station, electrified the crowd. A great actor in the drama of revolution had taken the stage again. Lenin sorely needed such an ally, but he knew that Trotsky, fame's spoiled darling, would never be the first to seek reconciliation. So, after all those years of vilification, he took the initiative himself and traveled "the road to Canossa" just a few days after Trotsky's return. He made Zinoviev and Kamenev assist in the negotiations—or rather the suasions. Trotsky's former enemies urged him to join the Bolshevik Party together with his supporters. Trotsky was stubborn: he demanded the abandonment of the name Bolsheviks. Lenin refused, but continued his efforts at persuasion. Kamenev and Zinoviev jealously watched Lenin humiliating himself, and Trotsky behaving as though he was the Party's leader even before he had joined it.

A Useful Piece on the Board

Trotsky began cooperating with Lenin. But Koba was not worried.

Trotsky was later convinced that Koba had always envied and hated him. He was mistaken. Koba's feelings were dictated by the game of chess he was playing. And, strange as it may seem, Trotsky's arrival was very helpful to him. He could see into other men's souls, or at least read their baser emotions. He knew that the advent of the new favorite would bind the three of them—he, Kamenev, and Zinoviev, the three faithful old servants—more closely together. Henceforth they would be as one. What is more, he knew that Lenin would never forgive Trotsky for the long years of struggle against him, would never regard him as "one of us." He would always be wondering anxiously about the next move of this unmanageable revolutionary, who felt himself to be co-Leader and Lenin's equal.

Koba realized that Lenin would appreciate hatred for Trotsky. To outdo others in your devotion to Lenin you must exhibit a particular hatred of Trotsky.

A Complicated Maneuver

The first All-Russian Congress of Soviets opened on June 3. One episode in the proceedings would find a place in all books about the Revolution. The Menshevik Tsereteli declared that "there is at present no party in Russia which would say 'just put power in our hands and go away, we will take your place.' There is no such party in Russia." At which Lenin shouted from the body of the hall, "There is such a Party!" It seemed preposterous: a miserable nine percent of the delegates at the Congress were Bolsheviks.

But at a joint meeting of the Bolshevik military organization and the Central Committee on June 6, Lenin proposed that they should organize a demonstration and show how strong the Party was, in spite of its small numbers.

"All power to the Soviets!" and "Down with the ten capitalist ministers!" were the belligerent slogans of this allegedly peaceful demonstration. I. Smilga told the Central Committee, of which he was a member, in so many words that "if events lead to a clash those taking part must seize the post office and telegraph buildings and the arsenal." M. Latsis echoed this: "With the support of the machine gun regiment we must occupy the station, the banks, the arsenal, and the post and telegraph buildings." Yes, the impatient Lenin was getting ready for a first attempt at a Bolshevik coup. How could he fail to make use of Koba, who had organized bloody demonstrations in Georgia? Koba was, of course, at the center of events. He it was who drafted the appeal to "all toilers and to all the workers and soldiers of Petrograd." But his participation was a matter of the utmost secrecy; he was, after all, an influential member of the Executive Committee of the Soviet, and he had to be kept there in case the demonstration was a failure. Hence his rejoinders in the course of the Central Committee session: "We must neither force the pace, nor let any opportunity slip. . . . Our duty is to organize a demonstration . . . but [there must be] no attempt to seize the telegraph office."

As early as June 9 rumors of an impending Bolshevik demonstration against the government were spread at the Congress of Soviets. The Menshevik Gechkori read out to the Congress a leaflet with Koba's appeal, which he had picked up in the street.

Taken in conjunction with Lenin's declaration, the demonstration acquired a sinister significance. Tsereteli, speaking from the rostrum, said that "what we have here is a Bolshevik conspiracy to seize power." A storm of indignation swept through the hall, and Chkheidze said that "tomorrow may prove a fateful day."

Kamenev, Koba, and the other members of the Bolshevik group feigned astonishment and voted with the Congress as a whole against the demonstration. The Provisional Government warned that any resort to violence would be met with the full force of the state power, and Lenin decided to back down. It was decided overnight to cancel the demonstration. This decision prompted Koba to make an amusing move. He gave notice of his resignation from the Central Committee, arguing that the decision to cancel the demonstration was a mistake. He knew very well that this was not a dangerous move, that he would be invited to withdraw his resignation. That indeed was what happened. But his declaration had revealed to the Party as a whole what until then had been a secret—his part in organizing the demonstration. It showed too what a bold and uncompromising fellow Koba was. Koba the chess player.

An "In-Depth" Language

While I was working in the Party Archive, one of my anonymous informants told me: "Bolshevik documents are peculiar in that wherever they say 'peaceful demonstration' they most probably mean 'armed uprising.' The general rule is that 'yes' almost invariably means 'no.' Somebody has called this an 'in-depth' language—a false-bottomed language, in which words have two or three meanings. Add to this that Stalin was a grand master. To understand the reasons for his moves you must look at the result. Only then will certain things become clear." I often recall these words. Koba really *did* want an armed demonstration. We shall not understand why until much later.

The Congress of Soviets, then, reacted indignantly to news that preparations for a demonstration were under way. A storm blew up. It looked for a while as if the Bolsheviks would be torn limb from limb. The harshest measures were proposed, and then it all petered out. Instead, the Congress resolved to "organize a demonstration" of its own. A peaceful one, of course, with "Trust the Congress and the Government" as its slogan. But it cost a great deal of intrigue behind the scenes to jockey the delegates into adopting this idiotic resolution, which instead of condemning the Bolsheviks in effect authorized them to carry on with the demonstration they had organized. Who foisted this stupid motion on the Congress? It was the handiwork of a genius at intrigue. Koba's scheme is taking its course, though for the present its purpose remains unclear.

A spectacular demonstration, with Bolshevik slogans, took place on June 18. It was a triumph. Two articles about the demonstration appeared in *Pravda,* by Lenin and by Koba. One by each of the two organizers. "A bright, sunny day," Koba wrote. "The procession to the Field of Mars went on from morning till evening. . . . An endless forest of banners. . . . There was a steady roar from the crowd. . . . Every now and then cries of 'All power to the Soviet. . . . Down with the capitalist ministers' rang out."

No more than two hours after this success, Lenin, in consultation with other members of the Central Committee, decided that it was time for the proletarian masses to show just how strong they were.

The ailing Provisional Government was going through one of its regular crises. Russia's wrangling democrats had created a favorable situation for an attempt to seize power. Lenin resolved to take advantage of it.

Not Necessary, Yet Necessary

The hand that would someday write Stalin's masterpieces can be clearly seen in the organization of the July action. Rumors that it was about to be sent to the front were circulated in the First Machine Gun Regiment, which teemed with Bolshevik agitators. Soldiers who preferred to do their fighting at political meetings were furious, and called for armed resistance. The Bolsheviks, of course, urged them to cancel the demonstration. One of the leaders of the military organization, V. Nevsky, described how they went about it: "I gave my advice in such a way that only a fool could conclude from my speech that the demonstration should not take place." The regiment naturally had no wish to look like fools. They had mastered the "in-depth" language of the agitators: when they said "Don't act," they meant "Act."

A regimental meeting on July 2 called for an uprising. The regiment sent delegates to other army units, to factories, and to Kronstadt. Soldiers came out onto the streets fully armed. Lenin was reported ill; he disappeared from active life.

In the Kronstadt Fortress the sailors were in permanent session. The rebels among them had distinguished themselves at the very beginning of the Revolution. During those first, "bloodless" days, sailors on vessels of the Baltic fleet had shot 120 officers. They tore off Admiral Viren's epaulettes, dragged him to Anchor Square, and killed him. Admiral Butakov and 36 other senior officers were shot on the same day. The naval fortress became a stronghold of piratical freedom. The newly organized Bolshevik Committee assumed the leadership of the mutinous sailors. Kronstadt had become a Leninist citadel. When representatives of the Machine Gun Regiment appeared there, the comedy continued as before: the Bolsheviks urged the sailors to disobey the machine gunners' call to arms, but urged them in such a way that they obeyed it. The Bolshevik midshipman Raskolnikov, one of the leaders of Red Kronstadt, wrote, "We had very nice custom according to which I telephoned Petrograd daily and asked for Lenin, Zinoviev, or Kamenev . . . to get my instructions."

The Kronstadters received instructions from one other leader. The poet Demyan Biedny described how he was once sitting in *Pravda*'s editorial office when the phone on Koba's desk rang. An inquiry from Kronstadt—should the sailors turn up in Petrograd for a demonstration with or without their weapons? Koba took a puff or two on his pipe and answered, "Well, hacks like me always carry our own weapons—our pencils—with us . . . what do you do with yours?"

As ever, he was at the center of the action, yet uninvolved. That very same day, as Tsereteli related in his *Reminiscences of the February Revolution,* Koba stated at a session of the Soviet that armed soldiers and workers were eager to take to the streets, but that the Bolsheviks had dispatched agitators to restrain them. Koba asked for this statement to be recorded, then he took his leave. Chkheidze told Tsereteli with a wry smile that "men of peace have no need to put their peaceful intentions on record."

Koba did not, of course, expect to be believed. It was simply the latest move in his game: he had chosen the convenient role of peace-loving intermediary between the Soviets and the Bolsheviks. He may possibly have persuaded Lenin to allot him that role. A Georgian would obviously find it easier to reach an accommodation with other Georgians if the demonstration was a failure.

On July 4, armed Kronstadters set sail to take control of Petrograd. They disembarked on Vasilievsky Island, with "their weapons." An endless procession of armed sailors made for Ksheshinskaya's mansion. Naturally, the peace-loving Koba was not at Bolshevik headquarters. Lunacharsky and Sverdlov, Bolsheviks of secondary importance, came out on the balcony to address the crowd, but the sailors demanded Lenin, and they were told that he was ill. The sailors began to feel uneasy. Knowing that Lenin was in the building, the exhausted Raskolnikov tracked him down to his hiding place, and the "sick man" had to make a (very cautious) speech. Then the demonstrators went on to the Tavrida Palace, to insist that the Soviet take power. Once there, the sailors arrested Chernov, leader of the Socialist Revolutionary Party, who came out to meet them. They were about to drive away with him and shoot him, when Trotsky, realizing that there would be a heavy price to pay for this, jumped onto the hood of the car. From that platform, he began extolling the sailors, "the fine flower and the pride of the Russian Revolution," but concluded his panegyric with the words "Citizen Chernov, you are free."

Disorderly demonstrations continued throughout the day. Crowds of workers and armed sailors roamed the streets. Lenin had by now moved to the Tavrida Palace. But this was the moment at which troops loyal to the government arrived from the front. The fate of the action was decided. Midshipman Raskolnikov prepared to stand siege in Ksheshinskaya's mansion.

The Endgame Begun

The attempted coup was crushed. Lenin had lost. The question arises—what about Koba? True, in the event of victory he would have come to power with the Party. But even in the event of defeat he was on his way to power. Power *within* the Party. That explains his torturous maneuvers.

The Provisional Government was carrying out a secret investigation at the time. Evgeny Yermolenko, who had returned from across the German lines, testified that he had been recruited by the Germans to agitate in favor of peace with Germany, and that Lenin likewise had been commissioned by the Germans to do everything in his power to undermine confidence in the Provisional Government. These activities were funded by the German general staff. Yermolenko also indicated the channels by which the money reached Lenin. The Directorate of Military Intelligence at Supreme Headquarters latched onto the investigation, and from that moment Lenin was under surveillance. Intercepted telegrams showed that the Bolsheviks were receiving large sums of money from abroad.

Kerensky personally took charge of the inquiry into Lenin's involvement in these activities. Only a very narrow circle knew about it. But the Socialist Revolutionary Kerensky realized that proof of Bolshevik guilt could be used by the army, the monarchists, and reactionaries generally, against the forces of the left. How could he fail to inform his party brethren, the SR leadership, and his Menshevik collaborators in the Soviet, of this investigation? Rumors of a secret inquiry soon reached the general public. Obviously, they could not have been unknown to Koba, a Georgian member of the Soviet Executive Committee. Koba calculated that any Bolshevik demonstration would prompt the government to make use of this investigation, and that the accusations leveled at them would exclude the Bolshevik leadership and Trotsky from legal activity. They were all, in one way or another, connected with German money. Only one leader of the first rank was not tarred with this brush—Koba himself. Nor had he stepped into the limelight during the July rebellion. He would be the only one left at liberty.

Yet again it happened just as he expected. Toward evening on July 4, P. Pererzev, the Minister of Justice, made known some of the findings of the inquiry (still in progress) into the connections between Lenin and the Bolsheviks on the one hand and the Germans on the other. That night the Bolsheviks hastily called off the demonstration, but it was too late. Proceedings against "the spies" were already under way. The genie was out of the bottle. Lenin, of course, also knew about this delayed-action bomb. Was this perhaps why he had been in such a hurry, and risked the July action?

Lenin turned to Koba. He was the only immaculate member of the leadership. The Georgian Koba went to see the Georgian Chkheidze and asked him to "nip the slanders in the bud" and forbid the publication of materials relating to the case before the investigation was completed. Koba got his way. Chkheidze promised. But Koba, an experienced journalist himself, could easily see that it would be impossible to prevent publication of such sensational material by one newspaper or another. A defiant newspaper came forward immediately: the bold *Living Word* published letters from two revolutionaries, N. Pankratov, who had been imprisoned for many years in the Schlusselburg Fortress, and a former associate of Lenin's, Aleksinsky. Both denounced Lenin and his comrades as spies. The endgame had begun.

The Endgame: Koba's Victory

Troops newly arrived from the front surrounded Ksheshinskaya's former residence. The government ordered the organization of a task force to storm the building. Sailors under Raskolnikov's command prepared to defend it. But this was a gesture of despair. The grim-faced, unshaven front-line soldiers hated and longed to avenge themselves on these sailors who had always skulked in the rear.

Once again Koba saved the situation by parleying with the Soviet. No blood was shed, and the building was surrendered without a fight. Koba made his way next to the Peter and Paul Fortress. The Kronstadters installed there were determined to defend themselves. Soldiers had surrounded the fortress and were about to fire on the "German spies." But Koba talked the sailors round with an unhurried speech and a few Georgian jokes. They agreed to surrender their weapons and returned peacefully to Kronstadt. The peacemaker had twice succeeded in preventing bloodshed.

On July 6, the Provisional Government signed a warrant for the arrest of the Bolshevik leaders. The names of Lenin, Trotsky, Zinoviev, Kamenev, and Lunacharsky were on the list. Lunacharsky and Trotsky were plucked from their beds and taken straight to jail. But Lenin and his faithful aide Zinoviev managed to vanish underground. It was Koba again who helped them do it.

Lenin hid at first in the apartment of a Bolshevik called Kayurov.

But Krupskaya wrote, "Kayurov's son was an anarchist, and the young people were always fiddling with bombs, which was not altogether appropriate in a conspiratorial apartment."

Sergo Ordzhonikidze said in his memoirs that "many prominent Bolsheviks took the view that since such a grave accusation had been leveled at the Leader of the Party he should stand trial and clear himself and the Party." And Lenin told Krupskaya that "Grigori [Zinoviev] and I have decided to stand trial. . . . Let us say goodbye. We may never see each other again." He was very anxious not to go to jail. And, of course, Koba came to his aid yet again. He thought up another of his comedies with a predetermined ending. He sent Ordzhonikidze to the Soviet to ask about the conditions Ilyich could expect in jail. When told, Koba immediately declared the conditions unacceptable. He made the statement which Lenin so wanted to hear: "The Junkers will never get Lenin as far as the jail—they'll kill him on the way." Meaning that Lenin must *not* go to jail at all. The Central Committee followed this with a ruling that "in view of the danger to his life Lenin must not stand trial."

Lenin himself had no wish to remain in Petrograd. He was naturally afraid of standing trial. Once more the faithful Koba came to his aid. He found Lenin and Zinoviev another refuge, in the house of a worker called Yemelyanov, not far from Sestroretsk. Faithful Koba even escorted Lenin to the railway station. Koba, his savior.

Yemelyanov hid the fugitives in a shack out in the hay fields on the lake shore. Lenin and Zinoviev would remain there until autumn. So for the present the Party was left in the charge of Koba Stalin.

His lengthy game of chess had ended in victory.

Trying on the Leader's Clothes

Kerensky, the head of the Provisional Government, was afraid that the "espionage" affair would strengthen the forces of the right. The arrest of Trotsky and the disappearance of Lenin gave him all that he wanted. He did not believe that they would return to politics after such a scandal.

The espionage case was postponed indefinitely. What is more, the Red Guard was not disarmed, Bolshevik newspapers continued to publish, and the Bolsheviks prepared for their next Congress unhindered. The Congress was semilegal, and Kerensky's government studiously averted its eyes from the assembly of three hundred Bolshevik delegates. The proceedings were presided over by Koba Stalin, trying himself out for the first time in the role of Leader.

Lenin, however, remained in control of the Party from his shack, and submitted to the Congress what would have been the key points in his report. These were read aloud by Koba, who made the two main speeches at the Congress: the Central Committee's wartime report and a statement on the political situation. He also made the closing speech.

Stalin would later designate Lenin's shack one of the shrines of the Communist religion. Thousands of pictures by Soviet artists show Lenin all alone there, busily writing his immortal works, or Lenin welcoming to the shack his friend Koba. The shack's other occupant, Zinoviev, would later vanish from the far-famed shack, destroyed by Stalin. Yemelyanov would be expelled from the Party and banished, and his two sons would both perish in Stalin's camps.

The shack itself was always kept in good repair, and Stalin decided in 1947, its thirtieth anniversary, to have it enclosed in marble. Then, on his orders, a live exhibit was introduced to the shack—the aged Yemelyanov. The old man, having lost his children, and by now half-blind, would tell visitors all about the immortal friendship between Koba and Lenin. And about their meetings in 1917—when "one of my sons used to bring Stalin to the shack by boat."

They did in fact meet there on a number of occasions. It was there that Lenin passed on to Koba the Party's new and somewhat alarming slogans. Kerensky's government was called "an organ of counterrevolution," while the Soviets were a "fig leaf" to cover the government's nakedness. Lenin canceled the slogan "All power to the Soviets," and called on the Party to prepare for an armed uprising.

After Lenin's departure, Stalin left the bachelor apartment where he had lived so contentedly and moved in with the Alliluyevs, taking over the room which had recently hidden Lenin and Zinoviev. As always, Koba tried not to put his hosts to any trouble. "What he did about his meals, and where, apart from his early morning tea, I don't know," wrote Fyodor Alliluyev in his memoirs. "I sometimes saw him devouring bread, sausage, and smoked sea carp at a stall opposite our building. That was obviously his dinner—and perhaps his lunch too."

The move coincided with his hour of destiny—the Sixth Congress. But Koba possessed only one cotton shirt and a jacket that had seen better days. The Alliluyevs decided, Fyodor recounted, that "the Leader could not direct the work of the Congress looking like that. So we bought him a new suit. He didn't like ties. Mother sewed on a high collar so that it was like a military tunic." That form of dress would be known to history as the typical costume of a Bolshevik Leader. It was really, of course, Koba's own invention. His semimilitary appearance symbolized his secret pursuit of the Great Dream—the world revolution which the Bolsheviks were initiating. That was why they were about to seize power in Russia. Later on, Lenin too would wear the semimilitary tunic.

Love

Every day he went home from the Congress to the Alliluyev apartment. He enjoyed the company of those innocent girls, and their admiration for him. That was probably his reason for moving in. Nadezhda was still at high school. She looked Georgian, with her swarthy complexion and mild brown eyes.

In that little apartment it was the old, old story: Othello, no longer young, told the youthful Desdemona stories of his ordeals and his exploits. Fyodor Alliluyev dutifully recorded Koba's account of terrible nights in exile at Turukhan. And Nadya's sister Anna remembered his moving stories about the dog Tishka, with whom he talked the lonely Turukhan evenings away. On one occasion Koba brought Kamo along, that same Kamo who was the subject of legends in the Alliluyev household, and the girls noted the legendary hero's slavish devotion to their lodger. It is not hard to imagine the impression Koba made on a high school girl, while the lonely, middle-aged Georgian himself was captivated by the charm of youthful innocence and, above all, by the girl's rapt idolization of him.

Anna Alliluyeva remembered it all, and conscientiously described what Koba was like in those days. When she brought out a volume of reminiscences in 1947, neither she nor her publishers realized that Joseph Stalin was not at all fond of recalling his life as Koba. Poor Anna was packed off to a prison cell. She emerged from solitary confinement only after Koba's death, by then half-insane.

The Provisional Government Grows Weaker

Russian democracy was expiring in never-ending harangues and altercations.

The Romanovs had ruled, and Russia had remained silent, for three hundred years. It now seemed likely to go on talking for the next three hundred. It was as if the country had gone mad: workers were not working, peasants were not sowing, soldiers were not fighting. The whole country was engaged in one interminable political meeting. Innumerable parties held innumerable sessions. Demagogy reigned triumphant.

The army was too tired to fight. The Galician offensive launched by Kerensky ended in disaster—that desperately tired army lost a hundred thousand soldiers. The army wanted to go home. But instead of making peace, the obtuse government called for another offensive. As in the past, no attempt was made to address the crucial issue of land reform. Lenin meanwhile promised it all: land for the peasants and peace for Russia. Bolshevik newspapers and agitators were busy subverting the army at the front. The Germans had not wasted their money. The bacillus of Bolshevism was now killing the Provisional Government. As General Krasnov wrote, "We saw the very same picture almost everywhere—along the railroads, in trucks, or in the saddle . . . dragoons sitting or standing round some slick character in an army greatcoat." By autumn Kerensky's government resembled that of the dethroned tsar. It was supported by no one. In spite of the espionage affair, the influence of the Bolsheviks had risen steeply.

Kerensky knew that his authority was declining rapidly. A firm hand was needed to prevent the collapse of the regime. Lenin's latest ideas, on the itinerary toward armed uprising, were now filtering into the press. The commander in chief, General Kornilov, demanded action to forestall a Bolshevik coup. He asked Kerensky for plenary powers to restore order at the front and in the rear, and dispatched General Krymov's cavalry corps to Petrograd. Kerensky, who had been in favor of this to begin with, took fright at the last moment. He was afraid that once order was restored, he himself might be discarded. He declared General Kornilov's advance mutinous. The poet Zinaida Gippius noted at that time that "a Bolshevik rising is expected from day to day, and this made it necessary to send in troops from the front. I am almost certain that the divisions were marching for Kerensky, with his full knowledge . . . and in response to an informal order from him." (Many decades later, in 1991, Gorbachev would behave exactly as Kerensky did.)

Kerensky replaced Kornilov, and called "all democratic forces," including the Bolsheviks, to help him. Lenin's decision was instantaneous: he would ally himself with the government against Kornilov. Kerensky accepted this dangerous gift, and the Bolsheviks were summoned by Kerensky to defend the Winter Palace.

Another of history's little jokes. Just a few months later one of the *Aurora*'s guns would open fire on the palace and announce to all the world the end of Kerensky's government.

Lenin made splendid use of his contact with the government. He armed his supporters in every urban center. Once the "Kornilov mutiny" was put down, Bolsheviks were gradually released from prison. The leaders—Kamenev, Trotsky, and the others—returned. But Lenin did not show himself in Petrograd. He remained in the Finnish hiding place to which Koba had solicitously transferred him from the shack as soon as the autumn rains set in.

Trotsky would write that "the return to work of Central Committee members who had been forcibly removed from it for a time ousted [Stalin] from the eminence which he had occupied at the time of the Congress. His work went on in a sealed vessel unknown to the masses and unnoticed by the enemy." Yet again he had failed to understand Koba. Koba did indeed withdraw into the shadows, but gladly so. For a truly anxious time was at hand. On September 12 and 14 two extremely dangerous letters were delivered from Lenin, still in Finland: the time for the uprising was now!

September proved fatal to the Provisional Government. The Germans seized islands in the Baltic, and an assault on Kronstadt and Petrograd was expected. The government prepared to evacuate the capital. There was an outbreak of looting in the city. The palaces of Grand Dukes Alexander Mikhailovich and Andrei Vladimirovich were sacked. Gold, silver, diamonds, coin collections, and porcelain vanished. The imperial family's favorite home, the Alexander Palace, was also plundered. The loot was sold on the open market. The newspapers were dotted with advertisements such as "I buy *objets d'art* at the highest prices."

Meanwhile the Bolsheviks were beginning to seize power in Soviets all over the country. In Petrograd people spoke openly of an imminent Bolshevik uprising. In a letter to Gorky, the artist Benoit observed that "our terrified public is horrified by the specter of Bolshevism. . . . Everything we believed in is doomed, Petersburg is doomed. The plot against Petersburg is nearing realization."

This was the moment when, at his request, Lenin's first letter calling for a Bolshevik seizure of power was delivered to Koba, who read it to other members of the Central Committee: "If we seize power at once in Moscow and Petersburg we shall undoubtedly conquer."

In the course of this discussion, Koba proposed that these letters should be distributed to the most important Party organizations for consideration. He avoided expressing any opinion himself. But the majority supported the idea of an uprising, and Koba voted with them. These were dangerous moments.

Russia in Flames

The Bolsheviks seized control of the Petrograd Soviet and Trotsky became its chairman. Then, on October 9, something which Lenin had eagerly awaited happened: conflict erupted between the disintegrating garrison and the government. The government attempted to pull back reliable troops from the front, and the Soviet immediately came out in defense of the garrison. Trotsky set up a committee of the Soviet to "provide for the defense of Petrograd against the Germans and secure it from attack by reactionaries—Kornilovites military and civilian." Trotsky would convert this committee into the legitimate general staff of the Bolshevik uprising.

The Central Committee's most famous session took place on October 10. All the leaders were present. For the first time Lenin and his recent shack-mate Zinoviev put in an appearance, clean-shaven by way of disguise. Lenin spoke on the current situation: "Armed uprising is inevitable, and the time for it is ripe." Nor would they be alone. Commenting on news of unrest in the German navy, Lenin saw it as evidence of the "ripening of world revolution throughout Europe." He sensed the dubiety of his associates, but was able to infect them with his own faith. Lenin's outstanding characteristic was freedom from doubt about his message of the moment, although the very next instant he might be saying the opposite with the same absolute certainty. This was another characteristic of the true leader which Koba would adopt.

Koba voted with the majority for the uprising, but did not speak. A Political Bureau was set up for the political direction of the uprising and Lenin saw to it that Koba was included.

Zinoviev and Kamenev spoke against the uprising, predicting that it would fail. Neither man could forget the terrible July days. Defeated in the Central Committee, Kamenev took a rash step. On October 18, in a statement to Gorky's newspaper *New Life,* he made clear his own and Zinoviev's position: the uprising was doomed to defeat, it would have disastrous consequences for the Party and for the prospects of the Revolution. Lenin was furious. He wrote to the Central Committee demanding the expulsion of these "strikebreakers of the Revolution" from the Party. They had betrayed the secret decision to organize an uprising, said Lenin, although in fact there was nothing secret about it. "Rumors are circulating in the city that the Bolsheviks intend to take action on October 20," the schoolgirl Nadezhda Alliluyeva wrote, in her bold hand, to friends.

Thinking better of it, Zinoviev sent off a craven letter to *Workers' Path* (the name assumed by *Pravda* after it was banned in July). He was at pains to prove that there were and could be "no serious differences of opinion" between Lenin and himself. He had simply been "misunderstood." And something strange happened. The editor of the newspaper, Koba, not only published the letter, but added a note supporting Zinoviev, and even ventured some slight criticism of Lenin's intransigence.

Why Was He So Bold?

The Central Committee met to discuss Zinoviev's and Kamenev's misdemeanor, and Trotsky demanded their expulsion from the Central Committee. Koba's proposal was quite different: these two comrades should be required to submit to the will of the Central Committee, but should be kept in it. Trotsky's proposal prevailed, whereupon Koba announced his own resignation from *Workers' Path*. He knew—as he had known when he threatened to resign on other occasions—that he would emerge unscathed. Sure enough, the Central Committee refused to accept his resignation. There would be many such "resignations" in times to come. But why did he support Zinoviev and Kamenev?

For one thing, by attaching to himself two of the most important members of the Party he hoped to form a cabal of his own. Second, if the uprising ended in failure, his line would be that he had stood up for those who were against it. We shall see his third reason more clearly later.

For the present, he left it to Trotsky and others to prepare for the risky uprising. Koba himself was busy preparing the agenda for the Second All-Russian Congress of Soviets.

The Man Who Missed the Revolution

"On Trotsky's initiative the Bolsheviks launched the uprising on October 24," an eyewitness reported. "Another of fate's ironies: the command center of the uprising was set up in the Smolny Palace, in the famous Young Ladies' Institute, where the daughters of the Russian aristocracy had learned how to behave. Machine guns and cannon stood at the palace doors. Inside there was a scene of feverish activity: councils of war in the schoolrooms, mass meetings without a break in the great hall, soldiers, workers, sailors everywhere." One person missing from the epicenter of the uprising was Koba.

The editor-in-chief of the Bolshevik newspapers was at his post—in his office. On October 24 *Workers' Path* published an "Appeal to the

Population—to the Workers and Sailors" written by Koba: "If you all act together and steadfastly no one will dare to oppose the will of the people. The old government will make way for a new one, and the stronger, the more disciplined, the more powerful your show of force the more peaceful the old government's departure will be." *Peaceful.* He was sticking to his old line.

The government had tried to act first. A detachment of government troops had burst into the print shop early that morning, confiscated copies of the newspaper, and sealed the entrance. Koba sent the printers to look for support. A participant in these events tells us that "the Volhynian Regiment immediately sent a company. And the very fact that the government had closed the print shop, and that our company had come to stand guard on it, openly emboldened the whole district." But Koba knew that those who came off best in the first exchange of fire often went on to lose the battle.

He had put things to rights in the print shop before the morning was out. And then? Can he really have remained in the editorial office throughout that historic day, while the coup was carried out?

In the Smolny Palace, a hastily organized, extraordinary meeting of the Central Committee had been in session since early morning. It had adopted Kamenev's proposal that "no member of the Central Committee shall leave the Smolny today without a special ruling from the Committee." Old disputes were forgotten: yesterday's panickers, Kamenev and Zinoviev, were there among the leaders of the uprising. Final orders for the seizure of power in the capital were given out. Trotsky directed the whole operation. Party functionaries drove off to their battle stations. The whole leadership of the Party took part in the uprising.

With two exceptions. The Party was keeping its Leader hidden in an "illegal" apartment. In case of failure. But where was Koba? Trotsky described him as "The Man Who Missed the Revolution." According to Trotsky, "When roles in this drama were distributed among the actors, no one mentioned Stalin's name. No one suggested any assignment for him. He had simply dropped out of the game."

Had they forgotten him? Forgotten the man who only yesterday had taken charge of the Congress? One of the Party's leaders? And what of Lenin? How could Lenin fail to make use of such an experienced organizer and successful terrorist in the decisive hour of the Revolution? Can he have given Koba permission to sit out the October Revolution in a newspaper office? Naive questions. Did he then simply avoid committing himself, disappear, using his editorial work as an excuse? But if that was so, would not Lenin have noticed his cautious behavior? Or rather his cowardice? If he did, why would he make this coward a member of his first government on the day after the coup? Why did Koba spend several days after the coup closeted with Lenin? If cowardice was not the explanation—what was?

Koba's Most Secret Chess Game

Koba had not, of course, "dropped out of the game." It was just that he was playing a game of his own, one of which Trotsky should have known. Anna Alliluyeva wrote, "Immediately before the October Revolution Lenin came to our house. One afternoon the doorbell rang. 'Whom are you looking for?' A man I didn't know was standing on the threshold. 'Is Stalin at home?' I recognized Lenin by his voice. Mother offered him something to eat. Lenin refused. After a short discussion he and Stalin left the house together."

Obviously, editing a newspaper was very far from being Koba's main job at that time. His main job was liaison with Lenin, who was lying low in a clandestine apartment.

Anna Alliluyeva's memoirs were written at the time of the Stalin cult, and we must treat them with caution. But Trotsky himself declared that "contact with Lenin was mainly through Stalin," then added, pointedly, "as he was the person of least interest to the police." But let me suggest that Lenin's contact was mainly through Stalin because he was the person who had already saved Lenin in the dangerous July days. Lenin was very cautious. His timidity, his dread of physical punishment, evidently stemmed from the shock he had suffered as an adolescent when his brother died on the gallows. In the manuscript of Sergei Alliluyev's *Memoirs* there is an amusing description of Lenin on the eve of his departure for Yemelyanov's shack, studying his route to the station on a map. Alliluyev assured him that he knew the route perfectly, and that it was safe, but in the middle of the night Lenin insisted on checking everything meticulously.

Lenin knew that, should the uprising fail, his punishment would be merciless. So he entrusted himself to the tried and tested Koba, who had demonstrated his competence during the July days. For the sake of Lenin's safety, Koba now had to make himself as uninteresting to the police as possible. It was, then, for Lenin's sake that he absented himself from the Smolny. We see now that the Party had found a task for Koba while the coup was in progress, and Koba had worked hard to be given this assignment. It made it possible for him to take the new Koba's favorite position: one in which he could exploit the fruits of victory, but remain safe in the event of defeat.

Because he had "dropped out of the game" for Lenin's sake, it was very easy for him to rejoin it immediately after the coup.

"The headquarters of the uprising were in the Smolny," wrote Pavlovsky, one of the organizers of the uprising. "But in case the Smolny was successfully stormed, there was an alternative headquarters, in the Peter and Paul Fortress, and there were front-line command posts, one in the Pavlovsk Regiment's barracks, another in the barracks of the Baltic fleet, a third on the cruiser *Aurora*."

Lenin's safety was evidently ensured in the same organized fashion. Koba arranged alternative apartments, and, in case the insurrection failed, he charted a route for the immediate removal of Lenin from Petrograd, most probably along the well-trod road to Finland. This duty would have devolved upon him as the person "of least interest to the police." Such was his important, if quite unheroic, assignment. He himself, and the other Party leaders, subsequently preferred to keep silent about it. But official Stalinist historiography would put Koba in the seething Smolny, directing the insurrection jointly with Lenin, and surrounded by figures without names. Almost all those who *had* played a part in the insurrection he would send to their deaths.

The Day of the Coup

All day Koba kept up his game of "peaceful intentions." He was officially attached to the Second Congress of Soviets, and around midday he turned up together with Trotsky at a preliminary conference of delegates. The Congress proper was due to open on the following day. One of the Socialist Revolutionary delegates asked, "What is the purpose of the Military-Revolutionary Committee—insurrection or the preservation of order?" And Koba unhesitatingly replied that it was "preservation of order." Koba paid fleeting visits to these gatherings and made peaceful declarations, but of course kept in close touch with his charge. The memoirs of V. Fofanova, the occupant of the apartment in which Lenin was hiding, are held in the former Party Archive. We read there that "when the 24th arrived, there was a public meeting at the Polytechnic Institute, at which Stalin was to speak, and we had to hand him a note from V. I. [Vladimir Ilyich Lenin]."

Lenin was evidently kept constantly informed by Koba and learned from him that the coup was proceeding successfully. The story of the February Revolution was obviously repeating itself—the uprising was meeting no resistance. That must have been why late that evening Lenin broke his arrangement to remain hidden in the apartment until victory was complete. His Finnish bodyguard, Raichia, would write later that "Ilyich asked for Stalin to be fetched," but realizing that this would "mean a great waste of time" he disguised himself and set off for the Smolny without Koba. He did not remove his disguise while there in spite of all the reports of victory. Trotsky recalled that "Vladimir Ilyich and I sat together. With a handkerchief tied round his face, as if he was suffering from toothache, and wearing enormous spectacles, he was rather a strange sight. The Menshevik Dan scrutinized this strange character as he passed by. Lenin nudged me and said, 'The rotters have recognized me.' "

Member of the Government

In the course of the night Lenin called a meeting of the Central Committee. The Bolshevik S. Ravich remembered that it took place "in a tiny room, round a badly lit table, with overcoats thrown down on the floor. People were continually knocking at the door, bringing news of the uprising's latest successes. Among those present were Lenin, Trotsky, Zinoviev, Kamenev . . . and Stalin."

Koba had hurried to the Smolny on his charge's heels, so obviously they were in continuous contact. This meeting was held to discuss the composition of the new Bolshevik government. Trotsky, whose mind was always on the French Revolution, proposed that the new ministers should call themselves People's Commissars. Lenin liked the idea. They then went on to discuss the composition of the government. Lenin, naturally, proposed that Trotsky, the organizer of the coup, should be president of the Council of People's Commissars. Trotsky would not hear of it, mentioning, among other reasons, his Jewishness. Lenin showed some embarrassment but nonetheless assumed that position himself and offered Trotsky "foreign affairs." He did not, of course, forget faithful Koba. The Georgian became head of the Commissariat for Nationalities. Now he was a minister.

The new head of government spent the rest of the night in the same little room, bedding down on a pile of newspapers. But there was no sleep for the new commissar. He was drafting an "Appeal to the People," announcing the overthrow of the Provisional Government. The overthrown government was, however, just where it had been, in the Winter Palace.

At 2:35 in the afternoon there was an emergency meeting of the Petrograd Soviet in what had once been the Assembly Hall of the Smolny. An eyewitness recalls the scene: "Two rows of massive white columns, lit by crystal chandeliers, the Presidium at a table on a dais, in the background an empty gilt frame from which a portrait of the emperor had been torn out. . . . Trotsky wore a black suit, as if dressed for a ball, with a soldier's greatcoat draped over it. In the name of the Soviet he announced that the Provisional Government no longer existed. . . . Trotsky's immortal speech is engraved on my memory. . . . It was like molten metal. . . . People listened with bated breath, resolved to follow him unquestioningly wherever he might lead them!" Lenin spoke next, announcing the victory of the workers' and peasants' Revolution. Molotov recalled, "I was in the Presidium, directly behind the rostrum. Lenin addressed the hall with one foot slightly raised. That was a habit he had when he spoke in public. I could see the sole of his shoe. And I noticed that it was worn right through."

The mighty Bolshevik regime began with a hole in its shoe. Koba would later produce an edited version of the proceedings. His historians omitted everything except Lenin's speech.

Even in the Smolny, Koba was yet to emerge from the shadows. The Provisional Government was still in the Winter Palace. For the time being the Bolsheviks were still mere mutineers. Lenin raged, "The Provisional Government must be finished off at whatever cost." Meanwhile, the Soviets began their Second Congress. Koba was not one of the many elected to the Presidium. Lenin was evidently still afraid; he still hadn't left off his disguise. And Koba, as before, had to remain in concealment somewhere in the Smolny, so that he could help the Leader of the Revolution disappear at any moment. Victory was, in fact, still not altogether certain. Kerensky had escaped from the encircled Winter Palace, and set off for the front in search of reinforcements. The Winter Palace itself was still holding out, with the Provisional Government still inside it. Podvoisky, one of the organizers of the armed uprising, wrote in his memoirs, "We should have taken the Winter Palace by the morning of the 25th. Zero hour was moved to noon, then to 6:00 P.M., after which no new time was fixed. Lenin paced the little room restlessly. He did not leave it for the opening of the Congress of Soviets. V.I. was swearing and shouting, he was ready to shoot us."

A New World

At 6:00 P.M. all approaches to the Winter Palace were blocked by insurgent troops. The defenders began to leave the palace. By midnight only a Women's Battalion and a handful of cadets remained. It was time to begin. Blank shells were fired from the cruiser *Aurora* and the Peter and Paul Fortress. The whole city heard them. After this came a live shell from a gun near the General Staff Archway. The pediment of the palace was damaged.

The February Revolution was nearing its end. The poet Zinaida Gippius recorded her impressions of that historic night: "It began in sunny springtime and ended on that dreadful gloomy autumn day . . . no one on the streets, the electricity lamps are out . . . big guns firing, I can hear them from here, the fighting drags on . . . From our balcony I can see shellbursts like flashes of lightning in the sky."

The shelling was followed by an assault on the palace. As Maria Bocharnikova, a top sergeant in the Women's Battalion, put it, "The Bolshevik victory that night was a victory over women."

The palace was finally taken at 1:50 A.M. on October 26. Foreign books in luxurious bindings were snatched from the Last Tsar's quarters. Precious objects were looted. Those searching the courtyard came upon the palace's wine cellars, and flung themselves upon the stocks of food and drink, dragging cases of wine and hams out into the square and off to the barracks. Meanwhile the arrested ministers were led across the courtyard and over the barricades, on their way to the Peter and Paul Fortress. Bocharnikova described the scene: "The women were arrested, and it was only thanks to the Grenadier Regiment that we were not raped. Our weapons were taken from us. . . . Only one woman was killed. But many of our number met their end when we separated and set off home without our weapons. Tipsy soldiers and sailors hunted women down, raped them, and threw them from the upper stories of houses down into the street." Bocharnikova survived on this occasion, only to be shot during the Civil War.

While this was going on, a pale and distraught Menshevik, Abramovich, was shouting himself hoarse, struggling to make himself heard over the uproar in the hall, telling the delegates that the *Aurora* was bombarding the palace, and demanding that the siege be called off immediately. His words were drowned in the storm of applause that greeted a sailor from the *Aurora,* who announced that the palace had been taken. "Only then," according to Trotsky, "did Lenin take off his wig and wash off his makeup."

The session went on until 5:00 A.M., after which the weary victors slept briefly. "Somebody spread blankets on the floor and put pillows down," Trotsky wrote, "and Vladimir Ilyich and I took a rest, lying side by side. . . . [Later that morning Lenin said,] 'The transition from the underground to power has been too sudden,' adding, 'my head is spinning,' for some reason in German." This touching scene, we may be sure, was witnessed by the loyal Koba. He knew very well what the friendship between the two leaders was worth.

How unutterably happy the organizers of the coup were as they went to sleep toward morning in the Smolny's numerous rooms. In one of them a small, pockmarked Georgian had fallen asleep with a cold pipe in his hand. The man who would one day exterminate all those happy souls.

The next day was cold and misty. Wet snow was falling. Groups of curious spectators crowded round the Winter Palace, staring at the overturned street lamps and the scattered woodpiles.

That morning a new world was born. Koba's world.

7

THE GREAT UTOPIA

The new society was like a child newly taken from the womb. It was covered with blood—but it had been born!
—R. Rolland

THE DREAMERS IN THE YOUNG LADIES' INSTITUTE

"After the victory Stalin moved into the Smolny," Fyodor Alliluyev tells us. And Molotov recalled that "for the first three days we did not leave the Smolny—I myself, Zinoviev, and Trotsky. Opposite were Stalin and Kamenev. We tried by fits and starts to picture the new life. Lenin, for instance, thought that, to begin with, the oppressive power of money, of capital, would be abolished in our country. We should do away with money altogether sometime in the twenties."

Mirages swirled in that smoke-filled room of the former school for young ladies. Something fantastic had happened: an armchair utopia had become reality. They had not simply seized power. They were determined to build the new world of their dreams: a classless society, money abolished, the state withering away. And to build it quickly. Now that the coup had succeeded, they must, Lenin thought, advance full speed ahead toward socialism. "Socialism is already staring us in the face through the windows of modern capitalism," he wrote jubilantly.

It all looked so easy: everything is monopolized in the interests of the victorious people, a single State Bank is established, a Leviathan to dominate the whole country. Everybody would take a turn governing everybody else. Literally the whole population would be involved in government: cooks would learn how to administer the state. And people would gradually reach the point at which nobody governed anybody else. The hateful state, which had enslaved mankind for centuries, would die away.

This was the dream which would lead them to create the most monstrous state of all.

The fair redivision of all land, proclaimed by Lenin on the

night of the coup, was a confidence trick. The Bolshevik dream was to create, in the future, collective farms in which no one could say "This is mine," and everything would be held in common. The "mine" must die. "Mine" always pointed the way to oppression. According to Peter Pavlenko, Stalin liked telling this story:

> Saint Francis taught men to live without property. One monk asked him: "Can I at least have a Bible of my own?" St. Francis answered: "If today you have your own Bible, tomorrow you'll start giving orders—telling somebody, 'Go and fetch my Bible.' "

They decided to replace "loathsome trading—that seedbed of capitalism" with universal distribution of foodstuffs by the state. In that way their main objective would be achieved: the power of money would be at an end. Gold they would use to pave the streets, gold would be the material of which lavatory pans were made. They referred to money contemptuously as "monetary tokens," and planned to print unconscionable quantities of it, to render the accursed stuff valueless. Christ's disciples expected the Second Coming to happen immediately, and the Bolsheviks believed that world revolution was imminent. It would create a completely new world. Scientific foresight had already brought revolution to Russia. Now it gave assurance of world revolution. Russia's great example was bound to attract others. Workers and peasants in soldiers' uniforms had grown utterly weary of war. Why should they be massacred in the interests of their bosses? Inspired by Russia's example, they would of course turn their bayonets against their oppressors. Give us world revolution! That was all they talked about during those days in the Smolny.

People's Commissar Koba issued decrees. Yesterday's political exile now signed, jointly with Lenin, a "Declaration of the Rights of the Peoples of Russia." All Russia's nationalities were guaranteed the right of self-determination. The empire of the Romanovs was coming apart at the seams: Poland, Finland, the Baltic countries, Ukraine, and the Caucasus all broke away. This would inevitably push the peoples of other empires even farther along the road to world revolution. From one day to another they expected to hear the awesome tramp of workers' battalions. For the present all they had to do was hold out in this fortress conquered by the proletariat, and surrounded by its enemies.

Steal What Was Stolen

The great revolutionary redistribution was already under way. The spoils were shared out in accordance with the new government's decrees: the land to the peasants, factories and mills to the workers. Peasant communes were seizing land, workers' committees were taking mills and factories into their own hands. Owners who did not run away in time were "taken out into an open field" and never seen again. Soldiers at the front distributed the contents of army stores. Then, weighed down with looted ammunition, they deserted the front and headed homeward, shooting officers as they went. "Steal what was stolen from you" is a slogan beloved of all revolutions. Looting sealed the support of the people for their new rulers. Throughout Russia's great expanses the story was the same.

But in Petrograd the Bolsheviks were still fighting for their lives. For the first two weeks they appeared to be doomed.

"We knew that the army might intervene at any moment and that the Bolsheviks would be done for," an old émigré told me in Bulgaria. The intelligentsia sat in apartments without light, waiting for their liberators. Nobody believed that the Bolsheviks would last long.

Kerensky himself moved on the capital immediately after the coup. Trotsky and Lenin organized the city's defenses and Koba was at Lenin's side throughout, his inseparable shadow. Z. Gippius wrote: "The Cossacks and Kerensky were already at Tsarskoe Selo, where the garrison surrendered to them . . . but his soldiers had been got at by agitators . . . they were surrounded by a great crowd, and fraternization began." The "mutiny" (as the Bolsheviks called the toppled premier's offensive) was crushed.

Retreat

> My grandfather used to tell me how they drove Kerensky's Cossacks out of Tsarskoe Selo. Plekhanov was living in Tsarskoe at the time. . . . They searched old Plekhanov's home several times—not because they did not know who he was. Ilyich had obviously never forgiven him for that famous utterance of his—that "Russia's history has not yet milled the flour from which the pie of socialism might be baked." Also in Tsarskoe, some soldiers came up to my grandfather in the street: "Want to buy an officer, daddy?" "What would I do with him?" "Shoot him,"

> they said, and roared with laughter. (Letter from B. Nelidov, Moscow)

Did the father of Russian Marxism, I wonder, get a good look at the triumph of his ideas? Plekhanov left Russia, and died in the following year.

Lenin's Shadow

One of Lenin's first decrees called for peace with Germany. At General Headquarters (GHQ) the commander-in-chief, Dukhonin, refused to negotiate an armistice. Lenin went to the radio station in person. With him, as always at that time, went his faithful shadow, Koba. Koba himself has described what happened next: "Lenin transmitted the order for Dukhonin's removal. He called on the soldiers to 'surround the generals and suspend military operations.' " Lenin appointed Ensign N. Krylenko, a Bolshevik, commander-in-chief. The new commander-in-chief immediately drove to GHQ with a detachment. He made a speech, after which the soldiers "surrounded" Dukhonin and savagely murdered him.

In Petrograd the civil servants repeatedly came out on strike. "The civil servants won't serve, the ministers aren't working, the banks don't open, the telephone doesn't ring," Gippius noted in her diary.

The commissars appointed by Lenin found no one in their ministries except cleaners and messengers.

One of those spending his days in a room at the Smolny was the Bolshevik Menzhinsky. His brother was a well-known banker, which was perhaps why Lenin had appointed him Minister of Finance. This aesthete, this sybarite in a luxurious fur coat, escorted by a detachment of Red Guards, paid a frustrating visit to the State Bank. The striking bank officials would not hand over the ten million rubles for which Lenin was asking. The man in charge of the country's finances, reduced to safebreaking, made off with five million rubles like a common thief.

As for Koba's "People's Commissariat," it existed at first only in Lenin's decree. But a few days later he acquired his first collaborator, an energetic one at that. A certain S. Peskovsky, who had taken part in the coup, now turned up in the Smolny to take part in the division of power. He wrote in his memoirs: "I decided to go to Trotsky and submit my application for a post in the Commissariat of Foreign Affairs. But Trotsky explained that it 'would be a pity to use an old Party member in such an unimportant capacity,' . . . [after which] I entered a room facing Ilyich's office. There I found Menzhinsky lolling on a couch, looking exhausted." Hearing that Peskovsky had studied at London University, Menzhinsky immediately offered him the directorship of the State Bank. But Peskovsky knew about the bank officials' strike, and preferred to go on looking. He went into the next office. This was Ilyich's office, which Stalin used on and off because he had no office of his own. Peskovsky obviously felt that this was where the power was, because he decided right away to work for Stalin. He asked Stalin if he had a commissariat. No, replied Stalin. "Well, I'll make you a commissariat," said Peskovsky. "I dashed around the Smolny, looking for a suitable place for a People's Commissariat," he recalled. "It was a complicated business. There was no room anywhere." In the end, he found a friend of his, there to represent some commission or other, in one of the rooms, and talked him into joining forces, complete with desk and part of a room. Peskovsky triumphantly planted a card with the title "Commissariat of Nationalities" on his desk and went to report to Stalin. The "imperturbable Stalin" silently inspected his "commissariat," was satisfied, and "returned to Lenin's office."

So, while he was in Smolny he used Lenin's office. Lenin evidently chose to keep Koba at his side. Who knew what Kerensky would do next? Or the generals, the army? He might have to run for it at a moment's notice. He wanted Koba near him, just in case.

Panic reigned among Lenin's closest associates throughout the first few weeks. Kamenev, who headed the Central Executive Committee elected at the Second Congress of Soviets, trembled, and Zinoviev was terrified. They saw their prophecies coming true: they wouldn't succeed in holding on to power unless they shared it with parties supported by the majority of the population. Otherwise there would be civil war. The People's Commissars appointed by Lenin were also losing their nerve. They too demanded the creation of a "multiparty government drawn from the socialist parties." The leadership of the Railmen's Union, Vizkhel, threatened to bring traffic on the railroads to a halt. With famine and an icy winter at the door (there was no fuel in the city) the Central Committee discussed the situation. Lenin and Trotsky were fully occupied with the defense of the capital against Kerensky, and in their absence the Central Committee agreed to create a multiparty government. Lenin was enraged. He had not seized power in order to share it with the Socialist Revolutionaries and the hated Mensheviks. Lenin never wavered in his support of one-party government. Kamenev demonstratively abandoned his post at the head of the Central Executive Committee, and some other Bolsheviks left the government.

An Office Which Only Two Could Enter

Meanwhile, what of Koba? While so many of those closest to Lenin were wavering, Koba remained faithful. But did it really matter? Who cared what he thought?

My father recalled that, arriving in Petrograd at the time, he saw enormous portraits of the leaders at the station: Lenin, Trotsky, Zinoviev. But there were no portraits of Stalin. Nor was his name known to the people. At that time he played only supporting roles. That is the unshakable view of many historians.

Imagine, then, my amazement when I saw in the former Party Archive a document headed "Instructions to the Guard on Lenin's Office," signed by Lenin himself in the early months of the new regime, on January 22, 1918. In accordance with these instructions only two people had the right to enter Lenin's office without prior notification and at any time—Trotsky and Stalin. Trotsky was the acknowledged joint leader of the October coup. Lenin was obliged to acknowledge it. But why Koba?

Because Koba was his shadow and the person he trusted above all others in the Party. Lenin was the Ruler. Koba was the Ruler's trusted aide. The others, of course, enjoyed much of the glory. But much glory does not always mean much power.

Koba would shortly prove it.

The "Punitive Sword"

Lenin and Trotsky were now putting the finishing touches to their program. Trotsky formulated it as follows: "All this petit bourgeois riffraff . . . once it realizes that our regime is strong will be with us. . . . When we crushed Krasnov's Cossacks on the outskirts of Petrograd a mass of sympathizers emerged on the following day. The petit bourgeois mass looks for the power to which it must submit. Whoever fails to understand that understands *nothing.*"

The ruthless, uncompromising exercise of power—that was the path they must follow. They shut down all opposition newspapers, and workers' squads wrecked the print shops.

Shortly afterward, in December 1917, they established the Cheka—the "Extraordinary Commission for Combating Counterrevolution and

Sabotage by Officials." The Cheka was the "punitive sword of the Revolution" (the new leaders loved rhetoric in the style of the French Revolution).

Gippius noted in her diary: "There are only two newspapers left—*Pravda* and *New Life* [Gorky's paper]. Horrifying stories are told about the torture chamber of the Peter and Paul Fortress." The Cheka, with the Polish professional revolutionary Dzherzhinsky at its head, filled the cells with aristocrats, officers, and striking civil servants. In the women's cells the wives and daughters of yesterday's bigwigs met prostitutes and thieves. It was announced in the city that in the night hours dangerous criminals could buy their way into the women's cells and enjoy their fun.

Civil servants, frightened by horrific rumors of torture chambers, hurried back to the new people's commissariats, while the mutinous Kamenev and the undisciplined commissars quickly submitted to the Leader's will. Kamenev repeated, as so often before, that "as time goes by I am more and more convinced that Ilyich does not make mistakes." But Lenin chose to install the docile Sverdlov in Kamenev's place, as head of the Central Executive Committee. The mighty organ of the Soviets was finally converted into an ornamental facade for the government. The Soviets were finished. The Party would rule. And the Party's Leader. Koba saw once again that *force majeure* worked very well in that country.

THE CONSTITUENT ASSEMBLY

Lenin's government also described itself as "provisional" and undertook to provide for immediate elections to a Constituent Assembly. Lenin promised at the victorious Second Congress to abide by the results of the imminent elections—the "will of the popular masses."

Koba was now given a splendid lesson in Leninist tactics. Lenin was in no doubt that the results of the elections would be unfavorable. But since he had no intention of surrendering power, the dismissal of the first freely elected Russian parliament was a prospect already dimly visible.

Lenin needed a revolutionary ally for this most unrevolutionary enterprise. He therefore offered the Left Socialist Revolutionaries seats in the government. They accepted, subject to a number of conditions—restoration of the freedom of the press and the suppression of the Cheka among them. Newspapers were allowed to appear, but the Cheka was not suppressed. Instead, a number of people on the extreme left of the Socialist Revolutionary Party were brought into it, but only in less important posts. SRs were also given seats in the government, but these were relatively unimportant. Elections to the Constituent Assembly followed. As Lenin had expected, the Bolsheviks and the Left Socialist Revolutionaries were the losers. But he was unperturbed—the Bolsheviks were victorious among the garrison troops in both capitals. The soldiers liked this new regime, under which they did not have to fight and could shoot their officers and break into rich Petersburg apartments and hold drunken public meetings. For the time being it was they who decided, these armed assemblies of soldiers' greatcoats and sailors' reefers. Lenin had the means of dispersing the Constituent Assembly. He could act.

Koba was behind the scenes. But in the dismissal of the Assembly we can see the hand of an expert organizer of mass demonstrations. Latvian snipers, other soldiers, and sailors surrounded the Tavrida Palace. Every street was packed with troops loyal to the Bolsheviks. Demonstrators supporting the Assembly were fired upon, as in tsarist times. The first session opened only after the dispersal of the demonstrators. In the hall, soldiers and sailors acted the part of spectators. The stenographic record shows that this, the one and only session, was accompanied throughout by shouting and whistling from the body of the hall. An amusing detail: when he put on his overcoat, Lenin found that his Browning was no longer in the pocket—someone had stolen it while the meeting was in progress. This tells you something about the invited audience. At 5:00 A.M., when he judged that the orators had been teased enough, the bearded giant Dybenko, who had served in the tsar's navy and now commanded the republic's naval forces, ordered the sailors on guard to terminate the session. The guard commander, the sailor Zheleznyakov, tapped the chairman on the shoulder and spoke his "historic words": "The guard is tired. It is time to go home."

Reactions to the dissolution of the Constituent Assembly were muted. Koba realized yet again how quickly the spirit of the intelligentsia could be broken by stern measures. "Lackeys of the imperialists," "slaves of the American dollar," "stabbers in the back"—such were the epithets with which *Pravda* escorted the first freely elected Russian parliament to its grave.

Twenty years later, in the same newspaper, Koba would escort to their graves Dybenko and the other old Bolsheviks who had so cheerfully dispersed the helpless Russian Assembly.

Peace with Germany

Once they helped to secure approval for the dismissal of the parliament at the next session of the Congress, the Left SRs had served their purpose. Lenin's government could rid itself of the prefix "provisional." Next to go would be the Left SRs. The clash would inevitably come, Lenin expected, during the peace negotiations with the Germans.

Lenin urgently needed peace. He had to have breathing space, to put an end to the power of the street meeting, to demobilize the unruly soldiery and create an army of his own. And, of course, the Germans were insisting on peace and he had to meet his obligations to his creditors.

The Germans had signed an armistice with the Bolsheviks in January. A highly representative delegation, headed by Trotsky, the second leader of the Revolution, had set off for Brest-Litovsk. Koba was not a member of the delegation. He had already chosen his role—that of Trotsky's enemy. It enabled him to stand aside in this dubious "German affair."

As they approached Brest, that most cynical of Bolsheviks, Karl Radek, made an eccentric display of idealism, feverishly throwing from the window of the train leaflets urging German soldiers to stop the war with their Russian brother-workers. In Brest, Trotsky continued Radek's ideological fun and games. He turned the negotiations into an interminable lecture in condemnation of imperialism. The German generals heard him out, and then presented him with the harsh conditions under which they would make peace: the Baltic states, the Ukraine, the Caucasus etc., would be lost to Russia.

Trotsky broke off the peace talks and returned to the capital for consultation. An endless dispute broke out within the Party. Lenin explained that breathing space was essential: "If we don't conclude peace—peace will be concluded by a different government." But the "left opposition," led by one of the Party's most talented theoreticians, the young Bukharin, demanded the rejection of the German conditions. "Lenin's mistake," Bukharin declared, "is that he looks at this matter from the Russian, not the international point of view. The international viewpoint calls not for a shameful peace but for revolutionary war, a war of self-sacrifice. The struggle of the first workers' and peasants' state in the world must rouse the European proletariat to rally to its defense immediately." In short, it must spark off the longed-for world revolution.

Lenin explained that there *would be* a world revolution, without fail—but there already *was* a Russian Revolution, the one they should be thinking about. Besides, there was no one to do the fighting. The army had disintegrated: "The Russian trenches are almost empty." Lenin insisted on peace at any price. Koba supported the Leader, and noted that "there is no revolutionary movement in the West. There is only potential—and we can't bank on potential." Lenin, of course, protested against this lack of faith. And Koba, also of course, meekly held his tongue.

He did, however, see clearly, as he listened to all these furious arguments about world revolution, that it was all superstitious nonsense. Marx's dogmas were now the Old Testament. Lenin served the New Testament, the one and only idea of which was to hang on to the power you have seized in *this* country. Koba had mastered the teaching of those who served the New Testament—you could ally yourself with the devil himself if it was necessary in order to win and keep power. He understood too what an enormous concentration of power there was in this broad-browed little man wearing an old suit and a shirt with a dirty collar. It was not hard to understand. He was just the same himself.

Lenin obtained the Central Committee's support. But agreed tactics were to drag out negotiations in expectation of world revolution. Only if faced with an ultimatum would they conclude a humiliating peace. Trotsky set off for Brest again. Once again the German generals had to listen to his impassioned outpourings. In the end, the Germans presented an ultimatum. But instead of concluding peace Trotsky uttered a paradoxical call for "neither peace nor war," and took his leave.

The Germans, inevitably, launched an attack. How eagerly people in Petrograd awaited them! "You'll see, when the Germans come they'll restore order" was a statement often heard on the city streets at the time.

But the Bolsheviks knew very well that the Germans would not come.

Lenin begged for peace. The attacking Germans put forward new, much more onerous conditions. Again Lenin summoned the Central Committee. He urged them to make peace at any price. Koba again supported Lenin. After endless discussion Lenin won. The shameful peace would be concluded.

Stalin's historians would never stop cursing Trotsky for his inexplicable move. But Lenin quickly forgave his crazy behavior. Why? Let Trotsky speak for himself: "I thought that before we signed the peace treaty it was essential at all costs to give the workers of Europe clear proof of the hostility between ourselves and the rulers of Germany." That was why he had provoked the Germans into starting military operations. It was all done to show the workers of Europe that "we signed the peace at bayonet point." Yes, it was all just a show. Like the proclamations scattered by Radek. The object was the same: cleanse the Bolsheviks of the "German agents" smear before making peace.

This game suited the Germans very well. It gave them the right to attack and help themselves to extra slices of the Russian cake. But they knew too that the offensive must be a limited one. If they bent the stick too far, if they didn't halt in time, the Bolsheviks would simply fall. And wounded national pride might give Russia fresh strength to resist. Instead of the loyal Bolsheviks they might get a government of war. And Lenin, of course, realized that the Germans would call a halt.

Both sides, then, knew that peace would be made. The simple truth was that both Bolshevik leaders put on the Brest show for the eyes of their uncomprehending Party and allowed the Germans to "pinch a bit off the Russian cake." Both sides needed this German offensive along the whole front: it enabled the Bolsheviks to explain Brest to the proletariat, while the Germans were repaid in territory for their gold. Lenin was, in fact, paying not only for past support, but for that which the Germans went on generously providing.

After the signing of the Brest-Litovsk Treaty, Baron Mirbach became German ambassador to Russia. In his secret dispatches to the kaiser he described the aid which the Germans were now giving to the Bolsheviks. He did not believe that the Bolsheviks would last long: "I should be grateful for instructions on the following questions. Is the use of large sums in our own interests? What tendency should we support if the Bolsheviks do not hold on?" Berlin replied that "it is in our own best interests for the Bolsheviks to remain in power."

The peace treaty was discussed at the Seventh Congress of the Party. The nerve-racking struggle between Lenin and the "leftists" was resumed. Bukharin, Kollontai, and even Lenin's lover, Inessa Armand, were among the young intellectuals opposed to the treaty. Opposition was fashionable. The treaty cast too ambiguous a shadow. But what of Koba? To begin with, he took up his favorite position, midway between the disputants: drag out the negotiations, don't sign the treaty. But after one rebuke from Lenin, he immediately voted with his Leader, for peace. Still, his main aim had been achieved: he had more or less dissociated himself from this shameful peace.

After a long struggle Lenin won the Party's support for the Brest peace.

The Seventh Congress, at which the Brest treaty was approved, also changed the Party's name. It was now the "Communist Party." Another of history's little ironies, since this was the Congress at which the Party said farewell to communist idealism.

The shameful peace treaty consolidated the position of the new regime.

"I cannot picture the signature of Emperor Hohenzollern side by side with the signature of Bronstein-Trotsky," wrote the well-known journalist Yablonovsky. But he was obliged to picture it.

Now, with the help of the treaty, the next step was to get rid of the Left SRs.

"Wake Up, Old Fellow, We Aren't in the Smolny Now"

This was a feat which Lenin preferred to perform in a more convenient setting. He decided to transfer the capital to Moscow.

The move was meant partly as further proof that there was no secret understanding with the Germans: the Bolsheviks were so distrustful of the German imperialists, so afraid of a sudden attack, that they were transferring the capital to the heartland of Russia. In reality they had decided to exchange Petrograd with its hostile intelligentsia and its SR militants for quiet, patriarchal Moscow.

Lenin and the other senior leaders installed themselves in the Kremlin. Trotsky remarked on the strangeness of it—the Kremlin with its medieval walls and gilded domes as the citadel of the Revolution. It was in fact symbolic. Removal to the capital of the tsars signified the beginning of a new reign. Revolution and utopia would gradually die.

The senior leaders moved into the Cavalry Block opposite the Poteshny Palace. The previous occupants were evicted, or passed on to the Cheka. The chimes from the Spassky Tower were adjusted: the "Internationale" replaced "God Save the Tsar." The new potentates' cars drove into the Kremlin through the Spassky Gate, under an icon with an extinguished lamp behind shattered glass.

Trotsky wrote: "The furniture in my room was of Karelian birch, there was a clock with Cupid and Psyche on the mantel shelf. . . . We ironically asked the Cupids and Psyches whether they'd been expecting us." Trotsky tells a funny story about a certain Stupishin, an old Kremlin retainer, who one dinnertime served buckwheat gruel in plates decorated with imperial eagles, and carefully turned the plates so that the eagles looked the eaters straight in the eye. Trotsky shouldn't have found it so funny. The old servant Stupishin, the Cupids and Psyches sensed at once that their new masters had arrived. Lenin's favorite words of reproach to his fellow warriors then were: "Wake up, old fellow, we aren't in the Smolny now."

Lenin of course saw to it that another new resident would be right beside him in the Kremlin—faithful Koba. Koba too was given a Kremlin apartment with Cupids and Psyches and mirrors. Koba knew, though, that the Party rank and file looked askance at the rapid rise of their leaders to this lordly lifestyle. When he first set foot in his Kremlin apartment, Koba said, "Why all this upper-class luxury?" and smashed an antique mirror with a kick. The bourgeois Cupids and Psyches soon winged their way to the scrap heap.

Another Lesson from the Leader

Once settled in Moscow, Lenin got to work on the Left SRs. The Fourth Congress of Soviets—the first held in Moscow—met in the Hall of Columns of the House of Unions. The Congress was held to ratify the Brest treaty. Lenin was in no doubt that there would be a fierce fight, ending in the restoration of undivided power to his Party. The Congress opened with the reading of a message from President Woodrow Wilson, expressing his sympathy with the Russian people, which had cast off the yoke of autocracy. The Congress adopted a reply in which it promised Wilson speedy liberation from the yoke of capital and the establishment of socialism throughout the world. They had their fun with Wilson, and then joined battle. After a statement from Lenin, B. Kamkov, a Left SR ideologist never seen without a revolver dangling at his side, declared that his party did not want to share responsibility for the disgraceful Brest treaty. He condemned the Bolsheviks' ties with the Germans, calling Lenin's party "counterhands for German imperialism." Lenin gave as good as he got. He called the Left SRs "soap bubbles" and "accomplices of the bourgeoisie." The docile Congress (there were nearly 800 Bolsheviks present to 284 Left SRs) of course passed a resolution approving the peace, and the Left SRs had to withdraw from the government.

The settlement of accounts by installments—using one enemy to destroy another—was almost over. Koba would take to heart all that he learned in Lenin's universities. "We learn, bit by bit, we learn."

Once again the Bolshevik leaders were jubilant, this time because they had knocked the stupid SRs out of the game. (Twenty years later, most of those rejoicing would be sitting in the Hall of Columns again. That was the place in which Koba would stage his trials of Old Bolsheviks, the place from which they would be taken under sentence of death by shooting. But for the present they were jubilant.)

Lenin, though, knew that the SR militants would not leave it at that. He had to hurry, before the enraged countryside exploded. He knew that the peasant world would shortly become his enemy. For hunger was advancing on Petrograd and Moscow. And with it—civil war.

In the Fiery Cage

The prophecy of those who had urged Lenin not to take power had come true. The breathing space turned out to be a short one. Civil War broke out over the great expanses of Russia. Or rather a multitude of wars. One of them was the war with foreign interventionists: all the powers that had fought each other in the World War began helping themselves to pieces of the dying Romanov empire.

In spring 1918 the Germans occupied the newly independent Ukraine. German troops also headed southward to the Caucasus, where they controlled part of the territory of the Georgian, Armenian, and Azerbaijani republics.

The Turks also invaded Transcaucasia and seized a number of Black Sea ports, including Batum, the city in which Koba had begun his revolutionary career.

Four hundred thousand square miles of the dismembered empire's territory, and sixty million of its subjects, were now in the hands of the Germans and their allies.

The Entente countries, still at war with the Germans, naturally could not remain mere observers of these events. In March 1918 British and French troops landed at Murmansk in northern Russia.

Lenin and Koba contacted the chairman of the Murmansk Soviet, Alexeyev (Yuryev) on the direct line. (A transcript of this conversation can be found in volume 1 of the collection *Documents on the Foreign Policy of the USSR.)* Alexeyev explained that the Soviet had reached an agreement with the British, who had undertaken to defend the North from German incursions and to provision the hungry city of Murmansk.

Koba's reply to Alexeyev was that "the British never give their help gratis, nor do the French. . . . It seems to us that you have to some extent let yourself be taken in." He recommended annulling the agreement, but the hungry people of Murmansk refused to budge. (Koba did not forget this exchange with Alexeyev, who was shot once the war was over.)

As early as July 1, four thousand British, French, American, Italian, and Serbian soldiers disembarked at Murmansk and began to spread out over northern Russia. Archangel was occupied in August 1918.

The Americans, as Louis Fischer correctly writes in his *Lenin,* were extremely reluctant to take part in the intervention. The "Russian question" tormented President Wilson for almost a year before he wrote to Colonel House that "I have been sweating over the question of what is right and feasible to do in Russia."

But in the end Wilson had to agree, and not only because the Bolshevik usurpers had allied themselves with the Entente's German enemies. He was also alarmed by the prospect of a universal conflagration, of that world revolution for which Lenin was tirelessly calling, the persistent Bolshevik threat to plunge a war-ruined world into chaos.

Luckily for the Allies, there were at the time some fifty thousand well-armed and well-trained foreign soldiers in Siberia—Czechs and Slovaks taken prisoner by the tsar's army. The Czech lands and Slovakia had been part of the Austro-Hungarian Empire, which had fought on the German side against Russia. But Czechs and Slovaks, unwilling to fight against brother Slavs, had surrendered to the Russians in their thousands. They had been released immediately after the February Revolution. France, which was running short of manpower, rearmed the Czechoslovak Legion and was preparing to transfer it to the western front when the October Revolution took place. The allies now found a different use for the Czechs and Slovaks. The Legion troops were traveling along the Trans-Siberian Railway at the time. The Bolsheviks demanded that they should surrender their arms. On May 14, the Legion mutinied. The troops refused to disarm, and made their way across Siberia toward the Urals, sweeping away Soviet authorities as they went. They were joined by Cossacks also in revolt against the Bolsheviks, and tsarist officers who had taken refuge in Siberia.

Ekaterinburg, the capital of the Red Urals, fell to the Legion on July 25. (The Bolsheviks had shot the tsar and his family on the eve of the city's surrender.) The Czechs and Slovaks crossed the Urals and seized Samara and Simbirsk (Lenin's birthplace) and occupied Kazan.

In July of that same summer, a terrible one for the Bolsheviks, an invasion force landed from British and Japanese vessels at anchor at Vladivostok, capital of the Russian Far East. Japanese troops entered the city on August 3. Under an agreement between the United States and Japan, seven thousand soldiers from each country were to take part in the Far Eastern operation, but by August there were no fewer than seventy thousand Japanese on Russian soil.

Foreign intervention was the background to the most terrible, ruthless, and bestial of wars within Russia itself—a war fought by Russians against Russians.

Brother Against Brother

On the eve of the October Revolution the Russian army had been plunged into chaos. The White general Denikin described the situation in his memoirs: "Armed robbery and looting is rife on all the railroads and waterways." Reports from the front said in so many words that "we no longer have the strength to fight with people who have neither conscience nor sense of honor. The units passing through sweep everything away, destroy crops, cattle, and poultry, break into government warehouses, drink themselves unconscious, set fire to houses. . . ."

The armed rabble of ex-soldiers, intoxicated with their new freedom and brutalized by drink, and the anarchic mass of rebellious peasants were the main props of the Bolsheviks after their seizure of power.

"There is nothing more terrible than a Russian peasant rebellion. It is mindless and ruthless." That is how Russia's greatest poet, Alexander Pushkin, described it. "Mindless and ruthless"—his words were echoed by many writers describing the Civil War. After centuries of slavery and brutal treatment by their masters, the pent-up brute force of the Russian people found its outlet in hideous atrocities. In the 1920s, the famous Russian writer Alexei Tolstoy, then living in Berlin, liked to show people a photograph taken during the Civil War. A giant of a man, armed to the teeth, reclined picturesquely in an armchair. At his side, on a little table, stood a severed human head. This was the pose chosen by Ataman Angel, leader of one of the innumerable gangs that raped and robbed peaceful citizens in the years of the Civil War.

Revolts broke out in southern Russia immediately after the seizure of power by the Bolsheviks. The Cossacks—a privileged military caste which had always been regarded as the main prop of tsardom—were up in arms. (Before the Revolution there had been eleven Cossack "armies"—those of the Don, the Kuban, Orenburg, the Urals, and Siberia among them.) As early as November 1917 the tsarist general Kaledin, ataman of the Don Cossacks, had raised a rebellion against the Bolsheviks. In the same month in the southern Urals, the Orenburg Cossacks had revolted under the leadership of General Dutov. Kaledin was crushed in January 1918, and Dutov in April, by the revolutionary armies.

General Kaledin, reporting his defeat to the "government" on the

Don, uttered ominous words: "Our situation is hopeless. The population denies us its support." He interrupted those who tried to argue: "Gentlemen, keep it short. Idle talk is what has destroyed Russia." Kaledin shot himself that same day, January 29.

These Cossack revolts were only the beginning. Officers from all over Russia fled to the Don and the Kuban.

On November 2, 1917, coincidentally with the Kaledin rebellion, General Alexeyev, a former chief of staff, began recruiting in southern Russia a "volunteer army" to fight the Bolsheviks. This event is regarded as the beginning of the White movement. The Bolsheviks, who fought under the Red Flag, were henceforward referred to as "the Reds," and those who rose against them called themselves "the Whites," or "White Guard." "Whiteness" was thought of as a symbol of spiritual purity, of freedom from blood-guilt.

In January 1918 General Anton Denikin announced the creation of the Armed Forces of South Russia, with which the volunteer army and the Don army shortly merged, under Denikin as commander-in-chief.

Another group of White forces began to take shape in the northwest. The anti-Bolshevik movement there was headed by Nikolai Yudenich, a front-line general in the First World War. For exceptional valor he had been decorated with the most prestigious of Russian military awards, the Order of St. George First Class. (Only one other White Guard commander, General N. Ivanov, shared this distinction.) Yudenich's army was joined by White officers who had fled to newly independent Estonia, and by some Estonians.

The White armies absorbed many of the finest officers schooled by the First World War. But outstanding former tsarist officers and generals were also found in the Red army. In some cases brothers found themselves on opposite sides. Thus, General Y. Plyushchik-Plyushchevsky served with the Whites, and his brother Grigori, also a general, with the Reds. General P. Makhrov was in the volunteer army, while his brother Major-General N. Makhrov fought for the Bolsheviks. M. Berens was a White admiral under General Wrangel, while his brother Evgeny Berens commanded all the Bolshevik naval forces in April 1919.

Brother made war on brother. The capture and execution of brother by brother, father by son would be unremarkable events in the years of Civil War.

Having lost three-quarters of the country's territory, Lenin and the

Bolsheviks were trapped in a cage of fire, with the Germans to the west and south, the Entente powers to the east, Denikin's forces to the south, and Yudenich's army to the northwest.

The Bolsheviks were left with only a small area around Moscow and Petrograd. But both capitals remained in their hands and from this vantage point they could continue proudly representing themselves as the legitimate government, fighting against mutineers and foreign invaders.

From March 1918 Trotsky commanded the republic's armed forces. Inside the cage of fire his armored train sped from one forward position to another. Until October 1917 the Bolsheviks had supported those anarchic elements which threatened to reduce the army to a rabble of looters. Now they had turned full circle. Trotsky began hastily reconstituting the regular army which revolutionaries had so hated and the destruction of which was part of the utopian dream.

Trotsky realized that such an army could not be created without military experts. So, to the amazement and fury of revolutionary soldiers, former tsarist officers who agreed to cooperate with the Bolsheviks reappeared in the Red army, insisting, as before, on the discipline which the rank and file detested. Trotsky did not entirely trust these military experts—*voenspetsy,* as the Reds called them for short. Their families became in effect hostages. But Trotsky's most important innovation was the institution of "military commissars." Every decision made by a *voenspets* was subject to the approval of a military commissar, who also assisted in reinforcing what was now called "revolutionary discipline."

Trotsky tirelessly harangued the troops to raise morale. My father heard him speak on a number of occasions. He looked like a typical intellectual, but when he began to speak his face became almost Mephistophelian, and the crowd was spellbound.

Magnetic as he was, Trotsky's rhetoric would have been less effective if his speeches had not been accompanied by the sound of rifle fire. For desertion, for indiscipline, for cowardice—the penalty was execution by shooting. "One of the most important principles in the training of our army," said Trotsky, "is that no offense should go unpunished. The penalty must follow immediately."

Koba could not help being impressed by the results. Within a very short time, Trotsky converted an exhausted rabble of barrack-room lawyers into a Bolshevik army.

But Trotsky was following an example set by someone else. Koba remembered that after the October coup Kamenev, trying to curry favor with the soldiers, had proposed that the new regime's first decree should abolish capital punishment in the army. Trotsky had agreed. But when Lenin arrived in the Smolny and heard about the proposed decree he was indignant: "What nonsense! How can you carry out a revolution without shooting people?" The decree was buried. Another lesson learned.

8 THE CRISIS MANAGER

The sufferings of war were compounded by a cruel famine. The countryside refused to surrender its grain to the Bolsheviks for nothing. Kulaks, as the wealthier—that is, the ablest—peasants were called, began hiding the grain they had produced by the sweat of their brows. Lenin organized his Committees of the Village Poor. The "poor"—the laziest, most resentful peasants—were given power in the villages. Armed squads of workers were dispatched from the towns to the countryside. Together with the village poor they were to confiscate the grain held by kulaks. In the event, "food squads" did not collect very much grain, but quickly turned into gangs of drunken marauders.

Petrograd and Moscow were dying of hunger. Lenin had posted Trotsky to the front, and now he dispatched his second hope, Koba, to bring in the grain. On May 24, Koba was put in charge of food stocks. In southern Russia he set off for Tsaritsyn, the most important Bolshevik outpost in the south, through which a thin trickle of grain from the northern Caucasus was still reaching the center. It was Koba's job to turn the trickle into a flood.

NIGHTS IN AN OVERHEATED RAILCAR

"In 1918 Comrade Stalin said, 'Come and work with me, as secretary in the People's Commissariat,' " Fyodor Alliluyev wrote in his memoirs. "Comrade Stalin's staff consisted at the time of one secretary—myself—and one typist—my sister." And so, at the end of May 1918, the People's Commissariat was deserted: the whole trio was getting ready for its journey. "Comrade Stalin only gave me a couple of days' notice that we were about to leave," Alliluyev continued. "I was used to obeying him without argument."

The Kazan station was packed with "bag people" (speculators, usually peasants, who carried sacks of fresh food to hungry towns or sold it at railroad stations) and half-starved homeless children when this trio turned up—a girl not yet sixteen, a tall young man, and a short, middle-aged Georgian, with a squad of Red army men to see them off.

In spite of "instructions from the Council of People's Commissars" and Koba's awesome credentials, a train was found for them only after a lengthy altercation between Koba and the stationmaster. Not many people knew as yet who this Georgian was.

"The train hesitantly set off in the direction of Kislovodsk, stopping at every signal," Alliluyev wrote. The three of them assembled in the lounge car. This had previously belonged to the gypsy songstress Valtseva and was upholstered with a jolly, light blue silk.

In May 1918 the whole of the south was gripped by madness. The travelers can hardly have been sure that they would ever see Tsaritsyn. The Germans were keeping up their slow advance southward, and mutinous bands of General Krasnov's Cossacks were active on the approaches to the city. There were also anarchist groups, showing the black flag under the walls of Tsaritsyn, fighting the Germans at one moment and turning against Soviet forces the next. The mountain tribes too were in a continual state of high excitement. There was no knowing how it would all end. The train might be seized by the Germans, by the Cossacks, by the anarchists, by almost anybody.

Stalin slept in the lounge car, the brother and sister in a separate compartment. "Only one track ran to the south, and that was jammed with convoys of troops," Alliluyev noted. "Our train scarcely moved, and at every station we heard complaints that 'the Cossacks took up the track yesterday.' "

Koba realized that he had to hurry. Every delay increased the time wasted in traveling, and also the likelihood of an attack. At night the train was blacked out and slipped through stations in a hurry or hid on sidetracks. Stations were dark and dirty. There were drunken shouts from soldiers on the platforms, and the sound of accordions, or more frequently of rifle fire. Old Russia on the spree. But the train could defend itself. Koba's armed task force was four hundred strong. Among them the elite guard of the Revolution, the Latvian riflemen, battle-hardened in the execution squads.

Lenin had dispatched Koba to the south with the widest discretionary powers. "A telegram from Ordzhonikidze reached us en route: 'the anarchist Petrenko has revolted in Tsaritsyn,' " Alliluyev recalled.

The authorities there had attempted to evacuate the gold reserves and valuables taken from the safes of the bourgeoisie, and Petrenko's force had ambushed the train carrying this gold, launching empty wagons in its path. Men were killed in the collision. The groans of the wounded were deafening. The bandits lying beside the track forced their way onto the train, seized the money, and, obeying what was then the general rule, held a political meeting. Fiery speeches were delivered among the corpses and the burning railcars. The meeting ruled that the money belonged to the people, so they started sharing out gold coins, hiding them inside their dirty footcloths. For good measure they stripped the dead of their boots, and shot those still living. They were caught at it by Ordzhonikidze's armored train, and immediately surrendered. But that night two surviving columns of bandits led by Petrenko and the famous woman Cossack Chieftain Marusya burst into the city. Marusya—Maria Nikiforovna—was an alumna of the Smolny Institute for Daughters of the Gentry. A cocaine addict, insanely lustful and cruel, she was surrounded not by her languid school friends but by drunken riffraff. Ataman Marusya was executed in the open street, wearing her white Cossack frock coat and her shaggy fur hat. A little later Koba received another telegram from Sergo: Petrenko had been caught and shot.

"This was the situation in Tsaritsyn on the eve of Koba's arrival," Alliluyev went on. "Toward morning on June 6 we found ourselves in the endless maze of tracks round Tsaritsyn, all of them jammed by trains. . . . Tsaritsyn's dirty-white station building loomed before us. At dinner in the hotel I saw ample evidence that the city was well-off for food. It was only three days since Stalin had treated us to a Sovnarkom [i.e., government] dinner: vobla soup with a small piece of black bread. Here you could get a first-class meal for a ruble and a half." The country round about was choking on its grain surplus. But how could it be brought from the back of beyond to Tsaritsyn? And sent on from there to Moscow?

Koba embarked on a revolutionary solution of the problem with a round of executions, just to inspire respect for his decisions. He shot everybody involved in black marketeering or counterrevolutionary activity. Or anybody who might become involved.

"Not a day passed without executions by shooting in the local Cheka HQ," wrote Henri Barbusse, Stalin's enthusiastic admirer. The city was a crazy quilt of all the political groupings produced by the Revolution. They had all congregated in this proving ground—Socialist Revolutionaries, anarchists, monarchists. So there was no shortage of people to shoot.

Trucks kept their engines running at night, to drown out the noise of shots and the screams. Bodies were stuffed into sacks and buried by moonlight. When day dawned, relatives of the dead swarmed round the communal graves, digging up the fresh earth to find their loved ones for reburial.

This was when Koba ordered the execution of the engineer Alexeyev, on suspicion of conspiring against the Bolsheviks. Alexeyev's mother was a well-known Populist revolutionary. Lenin was told of his arrest and gave orders by telegraph that he should be brought to Moscow. Koba, however, was not one to change his decisions. His word must be law. Alexeyev's two sons, boys of sixteen and fourteen, were shot with their father. N. Valentinov wrote that "Stalin informed the soldiers, who did not want to shoot them, that these were the children of the White Guard General Alexeyev," and that sufficed.

Shortly afterward Koba sent a telegram to Lenin: "In spite of all the muddle in every area of the local economy it is possible to restore order . . . In a week's time we shall be sending about a million poods [18,000 tons] to Moscow." All this time he was living and working in a railcar. "For two and a half months the railcar was our operational HQ," Alliluyev wrote. "The temperature was around 40 [104°F], and the railcar got as hot as a brazier. The roof remained just as hot at night. Inside the car you forgot what it was like to be cool."

That was where it all happened: after the shootings by night, in the overheated railcar. From then on Koba's young secretary, Nadya Alliluyeva, was his wife. In time of revolution no formal ceremony was needed. They simply declared themselves man and wife.

The Riddle of Fyodor's Madness

In that same year, 1918, Fyodor Alliluyev, the author of the notes from which I have been quoting, suddenly and mysteriously lost his mind. He suffered a shock of some sort, as a result of which for the rest of his life bouts of insanity alternated with rare intervals of lucidity, during which he could work and write. Svetlana Alliluyeva (Stalin's daughter by Nadya) offers an explanation of his mental breakdown in her memoirs. Her story is that Kamo's men decided to play a trick on Fyodor. The whole squad pretended that they had been killed, smearing themselves with bullock's blood to make it more convincing. Fedya saw this spectacle and went mad. Svetlana evidently heard this account from relatives when she was adult. But it looks very odd indeed if we remember that this was a time when killing confronted you at every turn, when bodies were stacked out in the streets of Tsaritsyn, and bloody murder was part of everyday life.

I myself am reminded of a version without documentary support which is sometimes cited even in serious scholarly literature. According to this, Nadya was raped by Koba during the journey to Tsaritsyn. Her brother heard her screams and burst into the compartment. And Koba was forced at gunpoint to marry her.

This stupid and sordid fabrication perhaps preserves the distant echo of a true tragedy. Nadya was, of course, in love with the revolutionary hero. Perhaps what happened was what had to happen in that overheated railcar, when her morose idol returned from an insane orgy of executions. The cry in the night, which brought her unfortunate brother Fedya running to the rescue, was one of passion. He rushed into the unlocked carriage and saw his adored sister with the elderly Georgian—though only fortyish, this Georgian whom he idolized must have seemed an old man to Fedya. Violation of chastity seems a terrible thing to an adolescent. Idealistic Russian youths cannot always live with it. But all this is impermissible conjecture. All we know for sure is that it was night, that there was a railcar, and that these were three people—in the maddening heat under the stars of 1918.

Undermining Trotsky

Authority in a front-line town belongs in the first place to the military. Koba, who had never seen battle, tried now to take over from the military authorities. The North Caucasian Military District was under the command of A. Snesarev, a tsarist general who had changed sides. Several other former tsarist officers were working with him. They had all been assigned to Tsaritsyn by Trotsky. So Koba began playing a game which was sure to please Lenin: he wrote an endless string of complaints against Trotsky. Single combat with Trotsky was, however, dangerous. Koba needed a comrade-in-arms to act for him when risks had to be taken. Troops which had fought their way through from the Don were just then arriving in Tsaritsyn. They entered the city with Klim Voroshilov, originally a turner and fitter, then a professional revolutionary, and now a Red army commander, at their head. Koba knew how to win over such people, and Voroshilov, who was not very bright, became his devoted comrade. In any battle you need an ideological banner. So if Trotsky favored the employment of ex-tsarist officers as "military experts," Voroshilov and Koba were naturally against it. They joined in attacking Trotsky's people, accusing them of treason.

JULY FRENZY

On July 4, the Fifth Congress of Soviets opened in Moscow. Koba must have followed the surprising course of events there with great interest.

At first it was all straightforward: Trotsky arrived from the front to deliver a fiery speech threatening with execution all those who broke the agreements reached at Brest. This provoked the expected reaction from the Left Socialist Revolutionaries. Kamkov, the same Kamkov with the revolver at his side, waving his fists wildly, pitched into the German ambassador, Baron Mirbach, and "Bolshevik lackeys." The SRs loved the village as a parent loves a favorite child. Kamkov varied his insults about Bolshevik toadying to the "German imperialists" with promises to "sling your requisitioning squads and your committees of the poor out of the village by the scruff of their necks."

Delegates of the two parties sprang up from their seats shaking their fists at each other.

But Lenin was calm. And amused.

The Left SRs went into action on July 6. Two of them, Y. Blyumkin, who was in charge of the Cheka's counterespionage section, and N. Andreev arrived at the German embassy. Blyumkin was a typical product of that ruthless period. Nadezhda Mandelstam described him sitting, drunk, in a café, swearing vilely and adding names at random to the list of those to be executed. The poet Mandelstam plucked the list from his hands and tore it up. Dzherzhinsky heard about this incident and promised to have Blyumkin shot immediately, but the following day Blyumkin was at liberty and painting the town as before. Bolsheviks had a weakness for the Socialist Revolutionary Blyumkin.

Once inside the embassy Blyumkin asked to see Mirbach. He and Andreev were taken to the ambassador's study, where Blyumkin whipped out a revolver and fired. Mirbach rushed toward an adjoining room, but Blyumkin threw a grenade after him. Mirbach was killed. Andreev and Blyumkin then jumped from a window into the street, where a car was awaiting them. Blyumkin landed awkwardly, broke a leg, and had to crawl to the car. Nonetheless they succeeded in making their escape, thanks to the surprisingly slow reflexes of the Latvian riflemen on guard.

The Central Committee of the SR Party had decided to assassinate the German ambassador in order to nullify the Brest treaty. But what happened next was not easy to understand.

Members of the SR Central Committee gathered at the headquarters of a well-armed Cheka squad under the command of an SR called Popov. Blyumkin joined them. The mutinous squad was quite close to the Kremlin, but no attempt was made to seize it.

Dzherzhinsky turned up to demand Blyumkin's arrest. The SRs arrested Dzherzhinsky instead. But still they made no move. They were waiting for something. Toward evening they seized the telegraph office, but only to tell Russia and the world that Mirbach's assassination was not the signal for a rising against the Bolsheviks. It had been carried out only to wreck the treasonable peace agreement. The mutinous squad was not, it seemed, contemplating an attack on the regime. It meant only to demonstrate its disagreement with the Bolsheviks. It was difficult to imagine anything more stupid.

Lenin had been given the right to act ruthlessly. The headquarters of the eccentric mutineers were stormed and wrecked by Latvian riflemen, and the Left SR delegates to the Congress of Soviets were arrested. Lenin's dearest wish had been granted. The Left SRs had ceased to exist as a political force. As had the man who knew too much—Ambassador Mirbach.

How could the SRs have followed such a stupidly suicidal course, one which so admirably suited and in no way threatened the Bolsheviks? It was a miracle, pure and simple!

Koba, though, did not believe in miracles. The great chess player inevitably sensed that there was some hidden factor at work: someone had induced the SRs to behave so irrationally.

The Bolsheviks and the tsar's security service had fought each other for years. Planting provocateurs on each other was an old habit of theirs. Not surprisingly, the Cheka had from the moment it came into existence added this tried and proven method of the tsarist secret police, provocation, to its arsenal. The Cheka's most brilliant operations in those early years—the arrest of the famous terrorist Savinkov, or the arrest of the British diplomat Lockhart—were the result of provocations, the planting of a double agent in the enemy camp. Koba was bound to see the fingerprints of a provocateur on the affair of the SR mutiny. Sure enough, something strange happened to Blyumkin, Mirbach's assassin. When the Bolsheviks occupied the Cheka section's headquarters, he was left there with his broken leg. He was one of the leaders of that division of the Cheka, the one whom Dzherzhinsky had come in person to arrest—but nobody recognized him. He was taken, unrecognized, to a city hospital, from which he escaped to present himself, a voluntary penitent, to the Cheka. Sentenced to three years' imprisonment, he received amnesty soon after, and immediately joined the Bolsheviks. Blyumkin then worked in Trotsky's secretariat, and after that in the Cheka and the GPU (State Political Administration).

Koba, then, was given a chance to appreciate the present power, and the potential, of this recently established but mighty Cheka. He did appreciate it. Nor did he forget Blyumkin.

After Trotsky's fall and his banishment abroad, the GPU sent Blyumkin to Tibet, Damascus, and Constantinople in the guise of a pilgrim. He called on his former chief, Trotsky, en route. This was, beyond any doubt, his main assignment—to find out the exile's plans—and at the same time feel out his former supporters.

On his return, Blyumkin delivered a letter from Trotsky to a former close associate of his, Karl Radek. But that cleverest of cynics knew only too well how things worked, and immediately told Koba.

Blyumkin had to be shot immediately.

After the engineered "Left SR mutiny," Koba may well have reminded himself of Lenin's rule: "If the end is important enough, the means by which it is attained are unimportant." A banal aphorism, terrifying to the petit bourgeois, yet so obvious to the true revolutionary. Lenin wrote: "Let us suppose that Kalyaev [who assassinated Nicholas II's uncle] in order to kill the tyrant gets hold of a revolver from the vilest of men promising him money and vodka. Can we condemn Kalyaev for doing a deal with a criminal? Any sensible person will say no."

Our Hand Will Not Tremble

Lenin's objective had been achieved: the roundup of the Left SRs was under way, and it was legal. On July 7 Koba, in Tsaritsyn, received a telegram from Lenin: "Essential crush these wretched hysterical adventurers wherever. Show no mercy to Left SRs, and keep us informed regularly." Koba replied: "Rest assured our hand will not tremble. Our enemies will learn what enemies are . . . the track south of Tsaritsyn has not yet been repaired. I am chasing them up and bawling them out. . . . You may be sure we shall spare nobody, neither ourselves nor anyone else, and will give you the grain whatever happens."

He did indeed "spare no one." And as early as July 18, five wagonloads of grain left for Moscow. He was producing the grain. And other things besides.

BLACK GOLD

"Sent letter by special messenger to Baku," he informed Lenin cryptically. As soon as he arrived in Tsaritsyn, Koba had made contact with the city of his youth, and with the remarkable man who would be his associate for the rest of his life. The Soviet regime had quickly asserted its authority in Baku. The Baku Soviet was controlled by one of Koba's old enemies, Shaumyan. But the new regime collapsed just as quickly as it had been established, under pressure from Turkish and British troops, and the Baku commissars, with Shaumyan at their head, were shot. Only one of the twenty-six miraculously survived—the Armenian Anastas Mikoyan.

Mikoyan had joined the Party in 1915 at the age of twenty. He had been one of the most active members of the Baku commune. After its destruction Mikoyan remained in the Baku underground.

Baku meant oil, and without oil, war was impossible. So the cunning Mikoyan, the Bolshevik, under instructions from Koba in Tsaritsyn, made contact with the Baku capitalists. Mikoyan paid generously, in gold, and they shut their eyes to the fact that the oil was going to Lenin. Very, very soon the Bolsheviks would be in Baku, and oil would be the death of those who owned it.

For the time being Koba was busy reinforcing Mikoyan's fleet with vessels of his own, while continuing to bombard Lenin with telegrams about the struggle with Trotsky: "Get it into his head that . . . there is plenty of grain in the south but that to seize it I NEED FULL MILITARY AUTHORITY. I have written about this before, but have received no answer. Very well. If that is the situation, I shall demote those commanders and commissars who are ruining the operation . . . and the absence of a scrap of paper from Trotsky will not stop me."

Lenin chided him for this continual in-fighting, but Koba sensed that he had his Leader's approval, and kept it up. Acting on Koba's orders, Voroshilov forcibly took command of the Third and Fifth Armies. He and Koba jointly organized an offensive. Koba took part in it himself, from an armored train. The attack misfired, but this defeat had an unexpected result: Trotsky's protégé Snesarev was recalled to Moscow. A military council for the northern Caucasus was set up, headed by . . . Koba! Lenin loved Koba. And appreciated his struggle with Trotsky.

Koba now had a free hand, and Lenin was told in a telegram that "the military council has inherited a run-down estate. Have had to start all over again." The ruinous condition of the "estate" was said to be due to a "conspiracy" on the part of the "military experts." And on August 22, in the night, a barge put out into the middle of the Volga. On board were the "military experts" brought in by Trotsky and Snesarev, and arrested by Koba. All were shot.

The offensive had failed, but Koba stoutly defended Tsaritsyn. The city was never surrendered. Grain and oil got through to Moscow.

News from Moscow: A Shot

At the end of August 1918 Lenin was wounded after addressing workers at the Mikhelson factory. He ended his speech with the slogan "Freedom or death!" and walked down the steps from the platform and across the yard toward a waiting car. Then came three revolver shots, and Lenin fell beside the car, struck by two bullets.

Many legends have grown up around the attempt on Lenin's life. The official files are in the former Central Archive of the KGB, and in 1995 I was able to consult them. Among them is the testimony of Lenin's driver, K. Gill, who was waiting for him in the car and saw the whole thing. Lenin left the building, Gill tells us, "surrounded by women and men. . . . He was only three steps away from the car . . . when I saw, not more than three paces to his left, a woman's hand holding a Browning revolver protruding from a group of several people. Three shots were fired."

Photographs attached to the file illustrate the details of the attack: the would-be assassin was standing by the front left wheel of the car, Lenin by the back wheel, facing her at a distance of three paces.

"I rushed toward the spot where the shots were coming from," Gill testified. "The woman threw the revolver down at my feet and vanished in the crowd. . . . A woman medical assistant who happened to be in the crowd and two other persons [obviously Lenin's bodyguard] helped me to put Lenin in the car and the four of us drove off to the Kremlin."

Gill carried the Leader home at breakneck speed. Lenin was able to go upstairs to his Kremlin apartment unaided. According to the official communiqué: "One bullet entered below the left shoulder blade and lodged in the right side of his neck . . . the other penetrated his left shoulder. The patient is fully conscious. The best surgeons have been called in to treat him." Doctor Rozanov wrote later that "Lenin's life was not in danger."

The Leader's wound would shortly release rivers of blood.

A young woman in a black dress was detained just a few blocks away from the site of the attempted assassination. This was Fanny Kaplan, a revolutionary who had been imprisoned under the tsar for taking part in the preparation of a terrorist act.

In her depositions she stated: "I shot Lenin because I believe that he is delaying the realization of the socialist ideal by decades. . . . I decided to take this step back in February. . . . The Bolsheviks are conspirators. They have seized power without the people's consent." Asked about her accomplices and her party allegiance, Kaplan said, "I made the attempt entirely by myself."

The investigation was carried out quickly, although historians find that many questions remain unanswered. How, for instance, did the half-blind Kaplan manage to hit Lenin? Was there, perhaps, another assassin, who managed to escape? The Russian historian Volkogonov writes in his *Lenin*: "It was not Kaplan who fired the shots. She was merely the one prepared to accept responsibility." In my view, everything about the event is perfectly logical: it was precisely because she was half-blind that Kaplan failed to wound Lenin fatally at a distance of three paces. A much more interesting question is whether she did have accomplices, and whether she in fact belonged to a political party or "acted independently" as she claimed.

On September 3 the Kremlin commandant, Malkov, led Kaplan out into the yard and shot her in the back of the neck, with the Bolshevik poet Demyan Biedny as an interested spectator. The Cheka put out the rumor that Lenin personally had pardoned the revolutionary Kaplan. The rumor lingered for decades.

Trotsky and his army were near Kazan, fighting the attacking Czechs. The moment he heard about the attempt on Lenin, Trotsky left the front and rushed to Moscow. He felt himself to be Lenin's heir.

Koba, however, remained in place at Tsaritsyn. What could he have achieved in a Moscow without Lenin? He was, after all, a member of the ruling group only on Lenin's authority.

At about this time a student, L. Kenigisser, killed Trotsky's friend Uritsky, the chairman of the Cheka in Petrograd. Kenigisser's explanation was that he had killed Uritsky to avenge executed officers and the death of a friend of his.

Trotsky made a fiery speech on the need for retribution, and on September 2, after a stormy debate in the Central Committee, the Bolsheviks launched their campaign of Red Terror.

Koba heard about it in Tsaritsyn.

Russia Awash with Blood

The Terror had, in fact, been in progress throughout 1918, without prior warning. It had been there in the summer, when the whole imperial family was shot in a dirty cellar at Ekaterinburg. When Koba was busy shooting officers at Tsaritsyn. When Jews with their bellies ripped open littered the streets of Ukrainian towns. When Lenin, shortly before the attempt on his life, was told of a peasant revolt in Penza and telegraphed: "Terror against kulaks, priests, and White Guardists. Imprison suspicious persons in concentration camps outside city."

Throughout that year people were tortured and murdered all over the country. Both sides killed people: the bloody cellars of the Bolshevik Cheka sections were no different from the blood-washed cellars of White Guard counterespionage units. In both, people were swathed in barbed wire, eyes were gouged out, gloves were made of human skin, people were impaled. Denikin's government was horrified by the bestial savagery of its warriors, while on the other side, punishment where no crime had been committed was officially acknowledged policy. The decision on Red Terror was made public on September 5, 1918.

After the assassination of Alexander II in 1881, tsarist ministers had debated whether or not to declare "each and every member of a revolutionary party responsible for any further crime, however small, and outside the law." They could not bring themselves to do it. The Bolsheviks could and did.

A hostage system was introduced. Five hundred "representatives of the overthrown classes"—if we rely only on official figures—were shot immediately after Uritsky's assassination. In Kronstadt, four hundred former officers were lined up in front of three deep trenches and shot.

Revenge of course had nothing to do with it. It would have been strange to wreak vengeance on former tsarist ministers and to kill senators and clergymen because Kaplan had shot Lenin. The terror had a much broader purpose, which Trotsky partly revealed when discussing reasons for the murder of the imperial family. It was necessary, he said, "to give our own ranks a jolt, show them that there is no going back. Ahead of us lies total victory, or total disaster." Complicity in crime brings people together, makes them realize that it is victory, or retribution. It was, moreover, as Trotsky also wrote, necessary to "horrify and terrify the enemy." But not only the enemy. The population at large had to be terrified. The Red Terror meant that the regime had the right to punish where there was no crime, it meant that the common man lived in a state of constant Kafkaesque dread, a feeling that, confronted with authority, he had no rights. This was the ultimate meaning of the Terror. And Koba took the lesson to heart.

That was the point at which "the living spirit of the Revolution finally took wing, and flew away," as M. Spiridonova wrote in prison.

Dress Rehearsal for Stalinist Terror

Whoever takes captives, to captivity he goes. Whoever slays with the sword, he must be slain.
—Revelation 13:10

The Red Terror escalated. G. Petrovsky, People's Commissar for Internal Affairs, signed an "Order Concerning Hostages," according to which "all right-wing Socialist Revolutionaries known to local Soviets are to be arrested immediately. A significant number of hostages must be taken from among the bourgeoisie and the officer class. The slightest attempt to resist should be met by wholesale shooting."

A campaign of mass murder developed throughout the country. In the *Cheka Weekly* we read:

Executions Reported by Provincial Cheka Sections:	
Novgorod Cheka	38 persons
Pskov Cheka	31
Yaroslavl	38
Poshekhon	31

Terror was becoming a nationwide competition. Lists of people who could expect to die were pasted up all over the country. A typical announcement would read: "At the least sign of counterrevolutionary activity these persons will be shot immediately"—followed by the names of dozens of hostages. It became common practice to take a husband hostage and wait for his hapless wife to come and purchase his life with her body. Chekists invited the wives of arrested officers to join in their drinking bouts. This was part of the routine training for new Cheka personnel.

All of them would later serve Koba, only to perish later in his camps.

Kamenev, Zinoviev, and Trotsky all extolled the Terror in public. Even the humane Bukharin stated that "proletarian coercion in all forms, beginning with execution, is the method by which communist man is fashioned from the human material of the capitalist epoch."

As for Koba, he did not care to discuss the subject. He simply acted. And horror gripped Tsaritsyn.

As the Chekists warmed to their task they called for "a deepening of the Terror." We read in the *Cheka Weekly* that "in many towns mass executions of hostages have already been carried out. And that is good. In such matters half-measures are worst of all. They exacerbate the enemy without weakening him." The author of this article wanted to go further, and called for the authorization of torture. It was time to get rid of petit bourgeois ideology.

But the bloodthirsty omnipotence of the Cheka was beginning to provoke murmurs of dissent in the Party itself. In a letter to *Pravda* one Communist wrote, "We are turning the slogan 'all power to the Soviets' into 'all power to the Cheka.'" After this a commission was set up "to acquaint the public with the activity of" the Cheka. Koba was among its members, and the executioner of Tsaritsyn now emerged as a restraining force, an opponent of extreme measures. In general, the center, the halfway point between contestants, was becoming more and more frequently his favorite position. He made one exception: where Trotsky was concerned he was always passionately ready to do battle. He knew that Lenin appreciated this ardor of his.

The commission ruled that the call for the use of torture was a mistake, the young hotheads in the Cheka were told what could be said and what must never be mentioned, even if it had to be done.

These ideas about the need to use torture *he* would put into practice in twenty years' time. And the cruel idiots who had called for it in 1918 would learn on their own skins what torture means.

Ha-ha

When Stalin died he left behind thousands of books in his Kremlin apartment and at his dacha in Kuntsevo. There was émigré, White Guard literature, and there were works by old acquaintances whom he had killed: Trotsky, Zinoviev, Kamenev, Bukharin. Their books, confiscated everywhere else in the country, lived on in his library. In the Khrushchev period the library was broken up, and only books annotated by Stalin were left behind. The laconic Koba had left a great number of marginal notes in his books, and these jottings offer a curious way in to the Great Conspirator's private thoughts.

In the Party Archive, I leafed through two of his books, both about terror. The first was Trotsky's *Terror and Communism* (1920). Wherever Trotsky extolled terror and revolutionary violence Koba made an enthusiastic note: "Right!" "Well said!" "Yes!" We can see him, alone with himself, expressing his real opinion of his enemy, who, as we shall shortly see, was always his teacher! A teacher second only to Lenin.

The second book was *Terrorism and Communism,* by the German Social Democrat Karl Kautsky. "The leaders of the proletariat," Kautsky wrote, "have begun to resort to extreme measures, bloody measures—to terror." Koba has ringed these words, and written "ha-ha" in the margin. The Civil War leader, who had witnessed massacres from day to day, who had waded through a sea of blood, finds it funny, this "bourgeois fear of blood." He writes "nota bene" beside this passage in Marx: "There is only one way to shorten and ease the convulsions of the old society and the bloody birth pangs of the new—revolutionary terror." Koba took the lesson to heart.

N.B.: Terror is the quickest way to the new society.

"All Power to the Cheka!"

Koba was bound to cast a sympathetic and curious eye on the Cheka, this new power born of terror. Its credo appeared in *Red Sword,* the organ of the Special Corps of the Cheka: "All things are permitted us, because we were the first in the world to take up the sword . . . in the name of the liberation and emancipation of all men from slavery! Who is to reproach us, armed as we are with this sacred sword, who is to reproach us for the manner of our struggle?" This was a thought which Koba would realize fully two decades later. And its authors would learn in full what it meant in practice.

Trotsky Mightier Still

In early September the Red army, under Trotsky's leadership, struck a number of powerful blows. In a space of three days they took Kazan, Samara, and Lenin's hometown, Simbirsk.

Lenin, who had only just recovered from his wound, telegraphed his congratulations to Trotsky.

In the second half of September Koba arrived in Moscow to visit Lenin now that he was well again. And Lenin, of course, at Koba's request, sent a congratulatory telegram to the commander on the southern front, Voroshilov. Trotsky took this as a snub to himself: yet again Lenin was conniving at Koba's self-promotion. He reacted boldly, sending P. Sytin, a former tsarist general, to Tsaritsyn as front commander.

Koba and Voroshilov refused to accept his authority. As usual, they sent a coded telegram to Lenin: "Sytin is a man . . . who does not deserve our trust. . . . Necessary to discuss in Central Committee behavior of Trotsky who shows disrespect for senior Party members in favor of traitors in ranks of military experts." Trotsky replied immediately: "Categorically insist on recall of Stalin. Things are going badly on Tsaritsyn front, in spite of our superior forces. Voroshilov able to command a regiment, but not an army of 50,000 men." Lenin could not contradict Trotsky just then, and in October 1918 Koba was recalled to Moscow.

In Moscow he realized at once that he would have to capitulate. Trotsky was too powerful. He informed Voroshilov that he had "just been sent to see Lenin. He is furious and insists we rethink."

Koba's contrariness disappeared immediately. "I think we can settle this matter quietly," he told Lenin pacifically, and beat a hasty retreat. In his *Pravda* article on the first anniversary of the Bolshevik regime he sang the praises of Trotsky: "All the work in connection with the practical organization of the uprising was carried out under the immediate direction of . . . Comrade Trotsky. . . . For the garrison's speedy decision to side with the Soviets, and the skillful organization of the Military Revolutionary Committee's work, the Party is indebted primarily and chiefly to Comrade Trotsky." To keep Koba at the front, Lenin himself undertook the task of reconciliation. He informed Trotsky that "on his arrival Stalin persuaded Voroshilov to submit completely to orders from the Center." Koba also knew when to retreat.

Life in Utopia

In Moscow the Bolsheviks were getting ready to celebrate the first anniversary of the October Revolution. They were entitled to celebrate—they had been governing the country for a whole year. Who would ever have believed it! The artist Annenkov remembered how he helped to decorate the capital for this occasion. Although there was no cloth to be had in Moscow, thousands of red streamers and thousands of red banners fluttered over the city. A hungry city, but a beautiful red city! They discovered late in the day that they had forgotten the most important thing of all—to erect the platform from which Lenin, now recovered from his bullet wounds, was to deliver a speech at 9:00 next morning. Annenkov made a rough sketch, fires were lit on the square, and work went on all night. The job was done by "a brigade of professors and intellectuals," forced to carry it out by way of "compulsory labor education." By 8:00 A.M. the platform was up, and Lenin was able to make his speech from it. Trotsky stood at the front of the rostrum as Lenin's heir.

Koba saw the platform, and must have appreciated its significance. It was a public declaration of the order of precedence. What had been going on behind the scenes of the regime would now be advertised from that platform for all to see. On the very spot from which Lenin was now holding forth, Koba would erect his Mausoleum. It would become the new Rostrum, on which Koba would line up his own associates in order of precedence.

The vital concerns of ordinary people living in that beflagged capital were quite different. When could they get bread? Where could they get firewood? Bread was brought in from the provinces by "bag people." The militia would arrest them and confiscate their bread. But still they infiltrated the hungry city. There were hundreds of them in houses and courtyards around the stations. People passed on their addresses. In our household a scrap of paper with one such address survived for several years: "First building after the station, there's a fence in the yard, the second board is loose, go through and there's another yard. There's a rubbish dump in that yard and somebody will be waiting behind that rubbish dump with bread." The starving intelligentsia crept from one such address to another, trying to exchange family treasures for bread.

Front doorways and basements were full of *besprizorniki*—homeless children of vanished parents. Homeless little girls were sold for bread.

There is a story by Zamyatin called "The Cave," about an intellectual dying of cold and hunger in a big, unheated apartment, which has become a primitive cave. Like any primitive man, he goes hunting—in his case to steal his neighbor's firewood. But most "gentry apartments" had by now been "filled in" by quartering proletarians on the former occupants. A huge increase in the incidence of savage assaults and murders, together with constant hunger, changed people. Yesterday's humanist was today's robber with violence; ordinary, good-natured people became cruel animals. Three and a half years of war and nearly two years of revolution had stripped away the veneer of civilization. The poet Blok, dying of revulsion from life as it had become, said, "I am suffocating. . . . We are all suffocating. World revolution is turning into universal angina pectoris."

Long Live World Revolution!

Throughout this time of hunger and bloodshed Lenin conjured his party to stand fast: "The workers of all countries look to us with hope. You can hear their voice saying, 'Hold out just a little longer and we will come to your aid, and by our joint efforts we will cast the imperialist predators into the abyss.' " In the same vein, an article of Koba's suggested stockpiling grain for these hungry republics of the future. Nevertheless, he knew already that the regime would hold out whether world revolution came or not. The terror had taught him once and for all how it would be done.

But . . . it came to pass! Just when it seemed that they were near the end of their resistance, their hopes were realized!

There was no sleep in the Kremlin on the night of November 9–10: revolution had broken out in Germany. First the defeat of the Czechs, then this second miracle!

The Hohenzollern monarchy had collapsed, and Karl Liebknecht had proclaimed from the balcony of the royal palace the creation of a new Soviet republic.

Germany was now ruled by German Soviets. A second great empire had disappeared from the map of Europe.

The Bolshevik envoy in Berlin began secretly purchasing arms for the German revolutionaries. A little while ago the Germans had been assisting revolution in Russia. Now Lenin was reciprocating. Just as secretly. The Bolshevik embassy became the headquarters of the German revolution.

On November 12 came another revolution, this time in Austria. Yet another monarchy was replaced by a republic. All doubt was now dispelled: exactly one year after the October Revolution, world revolution had arrived! Koba was amazed to see yet another of Lenin's prophecies become reality. Crowds of joyful revolutionaries paraded all day in front of the Moscow Soviet's building. But it all ended in victory for moderate socialists, and the creation of more of those bourgeois republics which Lenin so loathed. Hope flared again at the beginning of 1919, when left-wing Social Democrats—the Spartacus League, to which Liebknecht and Rosa Luxemburg belonged—rose in revolt. Soldiers and sailors seized the Reichskanzlerei in Berlin. But the rising was suppressed. Luxemburg and Liebknecht were murdered by extremists, their bodies thrown in a canal. In accordance with the doctrine of Red Terror, the reply to these murders was the execution of four Romanovs, uncles of the Last Tsar. One of them, Grand Duke Nikolai Mikhailovich, was a liberal and a historian of note. Gorky interceded for him, and Lenin, of course, promised to consider the illustrious writer's petition. He simultaneously ordered Zinoviev not to let the grand duke get away, and to hurry it up. The image of Lenin the intellectual remained untarnished. And the grand dukes were shot.

Koba admired this procedure. It was something else that he would take over from the Leader.

The German armies now hurriedly abandoned the Ukraine and Transcaucasia. But this made the situation no easier.

In the Ukraine, German rule was replaced by that of Simon Petlyura, a nationalist enemy of the Bolsheviks; the British made their appearance in the Caucasus, while the Don Cossacks, who had been encouraged and armed by the Germans, put themselves under Anton Denikin's command and henceforward implicitly obeyed his orders. But the Bolsheviks were to face their worst ordeal in the east.

In November 1918, while the Bolsheviks were rejoicing in the German revolution, something terrible happened in Siberia: over the vast expanse from the Pacific Ocean to the Volga basin power passed into the hands of one of the ablest Russian commanders—Alexander Kolchak.

The son of a humble artillery officer, he had reached the climax of a brilliant career as a rear admiral, and on the eve of the Revolution was commanding the Black Sea fleet. After the February Revolution he had tried to check the spread of anarchy by ordering the decommissioning of the most rebellious ships. Mutinies had broken out, and the Provisional Government, hoping to curry favor with the sailors, sacrificed the admiral. Kolchak was relieved of his post and sent to the United States as head of a naval mission.

In October 1918, Kolchak arrived in Omsk and a month later a right-wing government of Kadets and monarchists was set up under his leadership. The enormous human resources of Siberia were in Kolchak's hands. He also held the gold reserves of the Russian Empire, seized by the Czechoslovak Legion in Kazan.

Kolchak's army began its victorious march across Siberia.

We're All Only Human

Lenin decided to send Stalin to the front again. But Koba would first have to make his peace with Trotsky. When all other attempts at a reconciliation failed, Lenin took matters into his own hands. At the end of November he sent a telegram to Trotsky: "Are you willing to try to reach an understanding with Stalin? He is ready to come to see you about it. Do you think it possible, on certain conditions, to put aside previous frictions and arrange to work together, which is what Stalin so much wants? As far as I personally am concerned I think it is essential to make every effort to arrange things so that you and Stalin can work together."

Voroshilov had already been banished from Tsaritsyn. He had been given the post of People's Commissar for Internal Affairs in the Ukrainian government, with a proviso that he would not be allowed to interfere in military matters. Trotsky could consider himself satisfied. And shortly afterward Lenin was writing, "There are several reports from the Perm area about the catastrophic condition of the army. . . . I am thinking of sending Stalin there. . . . I'm afraid Smilga may be too soft." Catastrophe had already occurred in the Urals. Drunkenness and looting were rife in the army outside Perm. After its defeats at the hands of Kolchak the army was in its death agony. Koba was dispatched to Perm together with the head of the Cheka, Dzherzhinsky. He lived up to Lenin's hopes: a round of merciless executions speedily rendered the army fighting fit.

But Kolchak seemed to be irresistible. By the spring of 1919 his 400,000-strong army had crossed the Urals, and he was now advancing on Samara. From there the road to Moscow lay open to the White Guard.

Yet again—the mirage of world revolution: in March 1919 Communists, led by Bela Kun, a Hungarian prisoner of war in Russia who had joined the Bolsheviks, set up a Hungarian republic. Trotsky proposed in the Central Committee that they should go to the aid of Hungary without delay. Koba took no part in such futile discussions. This was no time to be worrying about Hungary. Kolchak had gone over to the offensive, and General Yudenich was outside Petrograd. Passionate speeches were made about Hungary in the Central Committee, and that was the end of it. An International Division was formed in Kiev to help Hungary, but funds for it for some reason never arrived. The Hungarian republic shortly collapsed. For some time to come, the history of Bolshevism would be the history of Russia itself. The great dream of world revolution remained just a dream.

That spring, at the Eighth Congress of the Party, Koba resumed his favorite game, and mounted another attack on Trotsky. What came to be called the "military" opposition united a number of Party members with military ambitions of their own. They openly opposed Trotsky's policy of reliance on "military experts"—former tsarist officers who had gone over to the Bolsheviks. The opposition denounced them as secret enemies and traitors.

Lenin happily permitted these attacks on Trotsky, and then, of course, came out in support of him. It was perfectly clear that without the tsarist officers the army would degenerate into a rabble of irregulars. Lenin mercilessly castigated the "partisan mentality." And who should rally to his support but Koba! He had been the real organizer of the opposition behind the scenes. He now came out against them—at Lenin's side. Lenin was grateful to Koba—he had given Trotsky another slap in the face—and admired him for his ingenuity. He appointed Koba to a special commission, whose task it was to reconcile Trotsky with the opposition. He did not forget to defend Koba's executions at Tsaritsyn: "When Comrade Stalin was shooting people at Tsaritsyn I thought it a mistake, and sent a telegram urging him to be cautious. I was in error. We're all only human." Koba had to be spotlessly clean. Because Lenin was getting the faithful Georgian ready for a new job.

A Thousand Posts

Early in 1919 Sverdlov, the man of iron through whom all of Lenin's decisions were transmitted, died. Lenin looked around for someone to take over his role. Who better than Koba? A brilliant organizer. He could always put the squeeze on and get a result. A will of steel. Not afraid to dabble in blood. And he hated Trotsky. Lenin needed in a high position someone able to deal with the self-infatuated Trotsky and his fondness for wild schemes.

As we remember, fate had thrown Sverdlov and Koba together on a number of occasions. They had shared a room in exile at Turukhansk and had jointly organized a Duma electoral campaign. This little man with the little black beard, the black leather jacket, and eyes inflamed by constant insomnia was simultaneously chairman of the Central Executive Committee, the country's highest legislative organ, and secretary of the Party's Central Committee, as if to symbolize the fusion of Party and state. Sverdlov concentrated in his own hands all bureaucratic and organizational work, and was always in possession of the Party's biggest secrets. It was from Sverdlov that Trotsky heard about the shooting of the royal family. After the publication of my book about Nicholas II I received an unsigned letter, which read in part as follows: "Do you know that N. Krestinsky [People's Commissar for Finance in 1918] had the valuables taken from the bodies of the dead Romanovs brought to Moscow, and that Sverdlov added them to what was called 'the Party's emergency fund'? This fund, consisting of jewels, was established by the Bolsheviks in case the Party lost power, and was kept by Sverdlov in a secret safe."

I viewed this information with skepticism, but shortly afterward I succeeded in examining a transcript of a speech made by Yurovsky, who organized the execution of the royal family. In this speech, to an audience of Old Bolsheviks, he mentions that "valuables taken from the tsar and his family after their execution were taken by N. N. Krestinsky to Moscow." Further, Bazhanov, Stalin's onetime secretary who defected to the West, mentions in his book that after Sverdlov's death his widow, with Stalin's blessing, went on keeping these valuables "in case the Party lost power."

On March 25, 1919, a Politburo (Political Bureau) was elected from among the members of the Central Committee. The prototypes of the Politburo created by Lenin before the Revolution had been qualitatively different. They had operated within the Party and expired in due course. But now the Party embraced the whole country. Lenin's intention was that henceforward the history of the country would be the history of the Party. The "million-handed" Party would penetrate every area of the country's life, and the Politburo would be the nerve center of the Party. Once a week, on "Lenin's Thursdays," members of the Politburo met in strictest secrecy to act as the real government of the country. Ill-educated revolutionaries in the Politburo made decisions on the multifarious problems of the country's economic life. *They* were the initiated, armed with the gift of prophetic foresight, thanks to the scriptures according to the great theorist Marx. From among the major leaders of the Party Lenin brought Kamenev and Trotsky into the Politburo. And also Koba. This was the nerve center. Zinoviev and Bukharin he made only associate members. Lenin also set up an Organization Bureau, to supervise the current work of the Party, and made Koba a member of this body too. Even this was not enough. He appointed Koba to two People's Commissariats—Nationalities and the very important Workers' and Peasants' Inspectorate. It was still not enough. Throughout this period a great number of commissions came into being to manage the day-to-day life of the country under the Politburo's guidance. Lenin appointed Koba to all the particularly important commissions, usually steering Trotsky in the same direction. Koba never forgot that he was there to do battle with the great Lev, giving Lenin the opportunity to act as impartial arbiter. Lenin often authorized Koba to conduct meetings of the government in his absence. . . . This, then, was the new Koba—member of the Politburo and the Orgburo, People's Commissar twice over, representative of the Central Committee and the Revolutionary Military Council on the Petrograd, western, and southern fronts. Add to this all those commissions. . . .

At the Eleventh Congress in 1922 one prominent Bolshevik, E. Preobrazhensky, would note with astonishment the vast authority which Lenin had concentrated in Koba's hands: "Take Stalin, for instance. . . . Is it conceivable that one man can take responsibility for the work of two commissariats, while simultaneously working in the Politburo, the Orgburo, and a dozen commissions?" But Lenin would not surrender his favorite: "We need a man whom any representative of any national group can approach, a man to whom he can speak in detail. Where can we find such a man? I don't think Comrade Preobrazhensky could name any candidate other than Comrade Stalin. . . . We have to have a man with authority at the head of it . . . otherwise we shall drown in a sea of petty intrigue."

In May, when he was already within a short distance of Samara, Kolchak suffered a crushing defeat. This was no temporary setback. Still in May, Lenin telegraphed the Revolutionary Military Council as follows: "Can you guarantee that rumors about the disintegration of Kolchak's forces and mass desertions to us are not exaggerated?" The rumors were confirmed. Yet again the Bolsheviks had stood their ground. Ironically, just when Kolchak's power was waning, the long-awaited unification of the White forces finally took place: Yudenich in the northwest and Denikin in the south recognized Kolchak as "Supreme Ruler of Russia."

Taking advantage of the fact that the main Bolshevik forces had been drawn eastward, Yudenich suddenly broke through the Bolshevik lines in the northwest and advanced on Petrograd. His force was very small—a single corps. But his agents had infiltrated the garrisons around Petrograd and were trying to provoke a mutiny, which the daring breakthrough was meant to support. Yudenich advanced rapidly on Petrograd. Zinoviev, chairman of the Petrograd Soviet, panicked. "Zinoviev knew no intermediate states. He was either in the seventh heaven or lying on his couch heaving sighs," wrote Trotsky.

Lenin could not rely on Zinoviev. He sent Koba to Petrograd, with ominous instructions to "take whatever extraordinary measures are necessary."

Petrograd was expecting Yudenich to arrive at any moment. Koba reached the city on May 19. He acted in the usual way: electricity was cut off. The apartments of "former persons" were searched by candlelight. Hostages—aristocrats, officers, tsarist bureaucrats, priests—were shot. The city was frightened out of its wits. Resistance within the city was broken, but on June 12 the garrisons of two forts outside Petrograd, the Red Hill and the Gray Horse, mutinied.

Koba realized that if the mutiny was not put down immediately the fire would spread to other forts. Some ships of the Baltic fleet went over to the mutineers. But by June 15 simultaneous attacks by land and sea had quelled the mutiny.

Koba proudly telegraphed Lenin: "The speedy capture of Red Hill is due to the roughest intervention on my part in operational matters, to the extent of canceling orders and imposing my own. I consider it my duty to state that I shall continue to act in this way."

The White offensive had misfired, and Yudenich retreated.

In October 1919 Yudenich launched another menacing attack on Petrograd, this time with a whole army. Lenin was ready to abandon the former capital, but Trotsky successfully defended it. Koba was elsewhere—on the southern front—at the time. Stalinist historians subsequently remedied the situation by merging Yudenich's two offensives, so that Koba became the sole savior of revolutionary Petrograd.

In the second half of 1919 General Denikin led the "Armed Forces of South Russia" against Moscow, threatening to join with Kolchak's armies, and at the beginning of September Lenin sent Koba, the acknowledged expert in crisis management, to the southern front. Denikin took Kursk at the end of that month, and Orel in October. The Whites were drawing near the capital. Posters bearing the slogan "Everything for the struggle against Denikin" were pasted up all over Moscow.

Denikin was halted, as Kolchak had been, on his way to Moscow. October proved fatal to the general. Before the month was out he had lost Orel.

The White army began to retreat. Koba had performed his role. A Red cavalry army, commanded by a former cavalry sergeant major in the tsar's army, smashed the elite Cossack troops of the tsarist generals Mamontov and Shkuro. Koba informed Lenin by telegraph that "the spoils captured include all the enemy's armored trains" and that the "halo of invincibility around the names of General Mamontov and Shkuro had been dispelled."

Budenny's cavalry mercilessly harassed Denikin's units as they fell back toward the Black Sea.

By the beginning of 1920 the Civil War had been won by the Bolsheviks. After a series of defeats Kolchak had also retreated, into Siberia. His shattered army melted away. As a favor from the Czechoslovak Legion, the former Supreme Ruler of Russia was given a railroad car, in which he got as far as Irkutsk. The Bolsheviks were there before him, and in return for permission to leave Russia without hindrance the Czechoslovak Legion had to hand over the luckless admiral to them. Kolchak listened calmly as he was sentenced to death by shooting, and asked permission to smoke one last pipe. A platoon of Red army soldiers executed the admiral at dawn, and his body was pushed through a hole in the ice on the river Angara.

Meanwhile, after withdrawing into the Crimea, Denikin had resigned and had been replaced as commander-in-chief by Baron Wrangel, who continued the struggle to hold on to the peninsula. The Crimea was the last stronghold of a vanishing Russia. The Bolsheviks had already occupied the Ukraine.

The incredible had happened: the Reds, half-starved, wretchedly uniformed, many of them without boots, had defeated the best tsarist officers, a magnificently equipped regular army, and elite Cossack units. How can we explain this miracle? Why were both Kolchak and Denikin suddenly pulled up short and routed on their victorious progress toward Moscow?

Roman Gul, a White Guard officer, wrote in his book *Campaign on the Ice,* "The people did not want to join the Whites . . . after all, they were the former masters. . . . The peasant did not trust us. That was disastrous for the peasant and for Russia as a whole." The same class hatred of peasants for their former masters helped the Bolsheviks. As soon as the "masters" reappeared, the peasants forgot Bolshevik oppression completely. The masters made this easier for them—they tried to reintroduce tsarist laws and took land away from the peasants to restore it to the landowners. As a result, the might of Denikin's and Kolchak's armies was destroyed by the merciless peasant war that flared up in their wake.

In addition to this, the White armies were fatally weakened by an age-old Russian ill: thievery. At the beginning of the nineteenth century the Russian writer and historian Karamazin was asked for a succinct description of his country. He summed it up in a single word (in Russian): "They steal."

General Denikin complained in his memoirs that "after the glorious victories at Kursk and Kharkov . . . the area to the rear of the White army was clogged with trains which the regiments had loaded with goods of all kinds." "Goods and chattels," we may add, "taken from the population." Brutality and looting helped to demoralize the White movement and to alienate peaceful civilians. "A wave of violence and pillage swept over the whole theater of the Civil War," Denikin wrote sadly, "often effacing the differences between the savior and the enemy."

Add to all this another typically Russian failing: the jealous hostility between Generals Wrangel and Denikin, the endless squabbling between generals on Kolchak's and on Yudenich's staff. A good deal has been written about this.

One other factor was disastrous for the Whites: killing fellow countrymen, brothers, their "own people," inspired in them a horror which they could not suppress. The Bolsheviks, Koba, Lenin, the political commissars in the Red army had no such feeling: their "people" was the world revolution, and they were at war not with fellow countrymen but with "exploiters," whom they were killing to bring happiness to the dispossessed everywhere on earth. This was what the political commissars taught Red soldiers. In one of the most popular Red army songs of the day, "Granada," the singer gives as his reason for leaving a little cottage and going to war his desire to endow the Spanish peasant with land.

The country, bled dry by fratricidal strife, lay in ruins.

But "the worse, the better." The dream of which the Bolsheviks sang in their anthem, the "Internationale," had come true. The old Russia had been "razed to its foundations" in total war. The tsar and his family had perished, the most illustrious families of old Russia had either been wiped out or had fled abroad, the old order had been completely destroyed. Nothing but "naked human beings on naked earth" remained.

It was possible now to resume building a Bolshevik world.

Victory forced Lenin to think about relations with other countries. He had to rescue his country from a universal boycott. But the regime was compromised by the Red Terror. Nor were Western socialists overjoyed with it. The beginning of 1920 saw the abandonment of capital punishment by order of the Cheka. This was an action intended for Western eyes. The night on which the decision came into force was uniquely horrible. The regime had no intention of letting its enemies go free, and that night many "former persons" were shot in the country's jails. The Cheka's day of clemency had become a day of blood. This was another lesson for Koba: you can forgive your enemy, but you must destroy him first.

The Expert on Catastrophes Offers to Resign

From autumn 1919 onward, Koba sent one stinging missive after another to the Central Committee asking to be recalled from the front. Such as:

> To begin with I am a little overtired, and should like permission to detach myself for a certain time from the hectic work at the most dangerous points in the front line, where rest is out of the question, and to concentrate for a little while on "quiet work" in the rear (I'm not asking a lot, I don't want a holiday in a dacha somewhere, I just want a change of work—that would be holiday enough).

And a telegram to Lenin:

> May I remind you again of my request to you to recall me and send someone else worthy of the Central Committee's trust. In the event of obstinacy on your part I shall be compelled to leave without authorization.

He refuses to back down, grumbles all the time, shows how offended he is by the Central Committee's refusal to retire his enemy Trotsky, and says that because of this he no longer wants to be "the expert at mucking out the war department's stables."

In reality, he was making a new move before anyone else could. He had been quick to realize that the war was won. Tomorrow all those bemedaled cavalrymen would count for nothing, and so would Trotsky with his Commissariat of War. It was high time to hurry back to the home front. That was where the power lay now—in the rear.

He was mistaken. The war was not yet over. At the end of April Poland attacked Soviet Russia. It had failed to do so earlier, when the Bolsheviks were on the brink of the abyss and the blow might have been fatal. The Poles had been too afraid that the tsarist generals might win and that their country, robbed of its independence so often in the past, would revert to the Russian Empire.

The death penalty was reintroduced immediately.

"Any scoundrel who urges retreat will be shot. Any soldier who abandons his post will be shot," read a directive from Trotsky.

The Poles got as far as Kiev and were driven back.

Then in the spring of 1920 a military putsch in Berlin was crushed and Lenin decided that events were repeating themselves: after the suppression of "Germany's General Kornilov," its October Revolution was next on the agenda. Lenin announced to the Ninth Party Congress that "the time is not far off when we shall be walking hand in hand with a German Soviet government." That was why after the Red army had driven the Poles out of the Ukraine Lenin was in favor of attacking Poland. The Red army would march across that country to aid a Soviet Germany.

Koba, who was eager to return to Moscow, spoke out against "certain comrades who not content just to defend our republic . . . declare that they can make peace only in a Red Soviet Warsaw." Trotsky, knowing how weary the army was, also opposed the war. But Lenin was adamant, and at the beginning of July an army 150,000 strong under the command of the twenty-seven-year-old Tukhachevsky advanced from the Smolensk region. "Give us Warsaw" was the favorite slogan at the time. Covering twelve miles a day, they marched in quest of the world revolution. Wearing dirty foot rags and broken boots or bast clogs, many of them without uniform, they reached the Vistula. The buildings of Warsaw could already be seen from the nearest hill. But the peasants whose grain they confiscated were for some reason less than delighted by their presence. Nor did the Germans raise the expected revolt. Meanwhile the Polish army had pulled itself together and began spilling a great deal of blood in self-defense.

Koba fought against the Poles in the South. He was the commissar responsible for the southern army group jointly with army commander Yegorov. Budenny's First Cavalry Army was their main striking force. In an attempt to reinforce Tukhachevsky's attack, Trotsky ordered the southern front to transfer Budenny's cavalry to him. Koba refused. He had long ago lost all enthusiasm for "pulling chestnuts out of the fire for other people," and he had grandiose plans of his own. He had decided that while Tukhachevsky was trying to take Warsaw he himself would take Lvov, strike at Warsaw from there, and then, in a lightning move through Austria, break through into Germany to support the revolution. In the end, both armies—that of Tukhachevsky and that of Koba and Yegorov—would be repulsed and driven back into Russia.

Lenin, however, forgave Koba even this and decided to send him against the Crimea. While the fighting was going on in Poland, Wrangel had emerged from the Crimea to occupy adjacent regions. In August 1920 it was decided to unite the two armies operating against Poland on the western front under Tukhachevsky's command and at the same time to open up a southern front against Wrangel. Lenin instructed Koba to set up his headquarters on the southern front as a matter of urgency: "We have just put the separation of fronts through the Politburo. You are to concern yourself solely with Wrangel. The Wrangel danger is becoming enormous and there is a growing inclination in the Central Committee to make peace with bourgeois Poland. I beg you to consider the Wrangel situation carefully and let us know your conclusion."

Koba, however, was in such a hurry to get to Moscow that he replied almost rudely: "I got your note about the separation of fronts. The Politburo ought not to occupy itself with trivialities. I can go on working at the front here for two weeks at the maximum. Look for a replacement." The familiar tone of the brave slave to duty offended by the unrelenting intrigues of his enemies. Lenin took pity on him. We hear echoes of his compassion in a letter to A. Joffe: "Take Stalin, for instance. . . . Fate has not once in the last three years permitted him to be People's Commissar either of the Workers' and Peasants' Inspectorate or of the Commissariat for Nationalities." Lenin corrected fate's error. In September 1920 he recalled faithful Koba to Moscow.

If Koba was eager to get back to the home front it was not just to be closer to the center of power. He was forty years old, and it was time he had a home of his own. His young wife was expecting a child. And it was high time to summon from Georgia that other child, the half-forgotten son born in that other life which had vanished forever. Back in Moscow, Koba heard that the Crimea had fallen. A line of unassailable trenches and the marshes of the sluggish river Sivash had barred the entry to the Crimea, but an avalanche of Red soldiers, using mountains of their own dead for cover, had launched a frontal attack and poured into the peninsula. Koba again learned the important lesson: Trotsky knew how to use people ruthlessly, and that was how he won his victories.

Someday I will describe in full the exodus from the Crimea: the milling crowds in the ports, the embarkment on ships bound for Constantinople, the despair of those left behind, and my father, there on the quayside, deciding after all not to leave Russia. And how he managed to survive afterward. Because afterward came the massacre. Bela Kun, the leader of the Hungarian Revolution, who had taken refuge in Russia, wrote that "the Crimea is a bottle from which not a single counterrevolutionary will escape. The Crimea is three years behind in its revolutionary development, but we will quickly bring it up to date." Koba saw how they managed it. Machine guns chattered for months on end and tens of thousands perished. Many of those executed were thrown into old wells dug long ago by the Genoese. Some victims-in-waiting were forced to dig their own graves. The stench of corpses hung over the Crimea. But the Crimea was purged of Whites.

At the end of the year Koba had to endure yet another of Trotsky's triumphs—the celebrations on the third anniversary of the October Revolution. They celebrated extravagantly, because this event coincided with victory in the Civil War and the final conquest of the country. A grandiose pageant was organized, with "The Night the Winter Palace Was Taken" as its theme. Ballet dancers, circus artists, machine gunners and other soldiers all had parts in it. The *Aurora* was to open the proceedings with a historic single round, but unfortunately it began firing shot after shot without a break: the cease-fire signal could not be given, because the telephone was out of order. It required a messenger on a bicycle to put an end to this farce. While the *Aurora* boomed away, soldiers of the Red army stormed the palace, over a barricade behind which ballerinas cast as members of the Women's Battalion and circus artists impersonating the kadets were sheltering. At that point the palace was suddenly illuminated. Shadows appeared behind the white-curtained windows to produce the effect of fighting. A battle of silhouettes! By way of finale all the searchlights were beamed onto the banner, now red, fluttering over the Winter Palace.

Those who had played a major part in the coup were all invited to the show. Koba was not among them. Next came a succession of formal meetings, and the newspapers published the reminiscences of heroes of the coup. Koba's name was nowhere to be found. But he was unperturbed. He knew that the past had died along with the great utopia. All that was left was a ballet-and-circus extravaganza, with the *Aurora*'s cannon going mad. And shadows.

The Leader's Love

The Leader knew how unfair it was. Lenin loved Koba. He knew that Trotsky and all the petty intellectuals of the Party only *tried* to be cruel. Their harshness was unnatural, hysterical, like their love for the Revolution. Had not Zinoviev said, "Revolution? The International? These are great events, but if they touch Paris I shall cry my eyes out."

But Koba was genuinely cruel, like the Revolution itself. He was as rough, as bloodthirsty, as treacherous as revolution itself, and as single-minded and primitive. For the sake of the Revolution he would set fire not just to Paris but to the whole world. Such was the picture of Koba drawn for Lenin by Koba himself. And there was something else just as important. The true revolutionary Koba never missed a chance to show his contempt for that caricature of a revolutionary Trotsky, forever Lenin's brother and Lenin's foe.

No sooner had he returned from the front than Lenin's favorite fell dangerously ill. For a time, Koba seemed likely to die. He was laid low by an acute attack of septic appendicitis. His exhausted organism had no resistance. He had spent his whole life languishing in exile, on the run, stumbling from jail to jail, and then on the front line. And always—work, work, work.

Dr. V. Rozanov, who attended Koba, recalled that "the operation was a very serious one. As well as removing the appendix we had to carry out a major resection of the blind gut. It was difficult to guarantee the result of the operation." Fyodor Alliluyev tells us that "the patient was so weak that they decided to operate on him under local anesthetic. But he was in so much pain that they were compelled to suspend the operation and give him chloroform. After that he lay there as gaunt and pale as death, almost transparent, bearing the imprint of a terrible weakness." Dr. Rozanov adds, "Vladimir Ilyich rang me at the local hospital twice a day—morning and evening. He did not merely inquire about Stalin's health, he asked for the most thorough report possible." After the operation, when the danger was past, Lenin himself consulted Rozanov about Koba's convalescence. He insisted on sending him to the mountains of his homeland, the Caucasus, "somewhere so remote that no one can bother him."

By 1921 Koba's native Caucasus had been reconquered by the Bolsheviks. Armenia and Azerbaijan fell first, then came the end of independent Georgia. Koba's old acquaintances Chkeidze and Tsereteli emigrated. Toward the end of May Koba, newly risen from his sickbed, flew to Nalchik, a town in the mountains of the northern Caucasus, to recuperate in a sanatorium.

After nearly a month breathing the mountain air, he was his old self again. At the beginning of July he finally set out for Tiflis, at the request of Ordzhonikidze, the Bolshevik leader in the Caucasus. A turbulent plenary meeting of the Caucasian Bureau of the Party was in progress when he arrived. Koba supported Ordzhonikidze, who was devoted to him. While in Tiflis he saw his mother, for the first time in many years. And also his older son.

Lenin, always solicitous, sent an angry telegram to Ordzhonikidze on July 4, inquiring by what right Stalin's convalescence had been interrupted and asking to be sent the doctors' report on his state of health. On August 8, Koba left for Moscow after making a full recovery.

Throughout 1921 Lenin was tireless in his concern for Koba. Now that he had a newborn son, Vasily, in Moscow, Koba asked for a quieter apartment without explaining the situation. Lenin himself joined in his search for a new home:

> To Comrade Belenki, Guard Commander: Stalin's present apartment in the Kremlin is one in which he can get no sleep. . . . I'm told that you have undertaken to move him to a quieter apartment. Please do this quickly.

But the Kremlin was overpopulated by the new lords and masters, and Lenin decided to install Koba in the Great Kremlin Palace, in the historic state rooms. Nothing was too good for Koba. This was too much for Trotsky. His wife, who was in charge of the Kremlin museums, also protested. Lenin wrote her a placatory letter and suggested moving valuable furniture out of the rooms in question. In the end, Lenin's obliging friend Serebryakov gave up his own apartment to Koba. In his tender concern for Koba Lenin had the Politburo adopt a special resolution "obliging Comrade Stalin to spend three days a week at his dacha." It was in this period of tender affection that Lenin—half-joking, half in earnest—offered to marry Koba to his sister Maria. He was very surprised to learn that Koba was already married.

Lenin was not sentimental. The reason for his love, his touching solicitude for Koba was of course strictly practical. Koba's death would have been a tremendous blow to him, just when he had planned his latest dizzy somersault. And Koba had been assigned a special role.

Farewell to Utopia

The end of the Civil War did not bring peace to Russia. While the war raged Lenin had consolidated the state, bugbear of all revolutionaries, and buried the Great Utopia. With the economy it was the other way around. Using the Civil War as his excuse, Lenin had realized a number of Marx's fantasies. He called them "war communism." Industry was nationalized and private trade was prohibited. From 1919 a tax in kind was imposed on the peasant. This meant that all of his grain, except that needed to feed his family, was confiscated. The peasant had no right to trade in grain. Now that the Civil War was over the peasants expected changes. But the Party rank and file believed that having won the war they would go on from war communism to peace communism. Onward, along the road to the Great Utopia! Only the peasant now refused to surrender his grain.

Ever since the "mutiny" of 1918, the peasants' well-wishers, the Socialist Revolutionaries, had been in Butyrki Prison—in the "socialist wing," as their part of the prison was jestingly called. But news of the peasant unrest which had begun to flare up reached them even there. They learned too that the revolutionary Lenin, only yesterday their ally, was suppressing these revolts with a cruelty of which the dethroned tsar would never have dreamed. Lenin ordered: "The revolt of five kulak cantons must be mercilessly suppressed. An example must be made by (1) hanging—execution must be by hanging, so that the people can see it—at least 100 known kulaks, (2) publishing their names, (3) confiscating all their grain, (4) naming hostages—and doing all this in such a way that people for hundreds of versts around can see it and tremble." Molotov complacently recalled in his old age how "Lenin gave orders to suppress the Tambov rising by setting fire to everything."

In May 1921 Tukhachevsky, no less, was appointed commander of the "Tambov army to combat banditry." An order issued by him on June 12, 1921, reads: "remnants of the defeated gangs are gathering in the woods. . . . I hereby order you to clear these woods using poison gas in such a way that it will spread and destroy anything hiding in there." The commander was sent 250 barrels of chlorine. By then thousands of rebels were already held in the concentration camps which had been hastily set up around Tambov. Tukhachevsky had 45,000 soldiers, 706 machine guns, 5 armored trains, and 18 airplanes. He laid waste with poison gas and fire a large part of the Tambov region. (My nanny, Masha, fled from her Tambov village to Moscow. Her father and brothers were shot before her eyes. Masha woke up screaming every night of her life. She could never forget the heroic feats of the illustrious commander.)

But these were peasants—counterrevolutionaries through the ages. "The Vendée"—a word familiar to the revolutionary ear—explained it all. Soon afterward, though, the sailors—"the pride and joy of the Russian Revolution"—were up in arms. On the last day of February 1921, exactly four years after the February Revolution, Kronstadt rebelled yet again.

Trotsky in person went to put down the mutiny, with the famous Tukhachevsky lending a hand. Koba gave no sign of life. He realized that the Party looked on with mixed feelings as the former tsarist officer Tukhachevsky and the Bolshevik leader Trotsky dealt with the sailors. Kronstadt held out. The rebels' newspaper described how "Marshal Trotsky, up to his knees in blood, opened fire on revolutionary Kronstadt, which has risen against the Communist autocracy to reestablish real Soviet power."

Lenin made the Party as such help shed the blood of the disloyal. At the Tenth Party Congress, in March, three hundred of the delegates were mobilized and sent out over the icebound Gulf of Finland to storm Kronstadt. The rising was suppressed, but some of the Kronstadt rebels escaped over the ice to Finland.

Koba forgot nothing. After the defeat of Hitler, the People's Commissariat of Internal Affairs would bring the hapless Kronstadters, old men by now, back from Finland, and dispatch them to Stalin's camps.

"The cuckoo has cuckooed its last" was Trotsky's verdict on the sailors' revolt. The country was weary of privations. The last rebels had once been the bulwark of the regime. Lenin now performed a fantastic *salto mortale.* He buried utopia and the dreams of Karl Marx, and announced to a stunned audience at the Tenth Congress the transition to the New Economic Policy (NEP).

The Secret of NEP

The October coup had created deep divisions in the Russian intelligentsia. Some of its most brilliant representatives emigrated, or were exiled, to the West, while many of those who remained in Russia hated the Bolsheviks. My father was a journalist who used the English word "Waiting" as his nom de plume. He was waiting for *that regime* to fall. But, like many other intellectuals, he had faith in NEP. They decided that the Bolsheviks had finally come to their senses. N. Valentinov described how a group of brilliant economists wrote a secret paper entitled "The Fate of the Main Ideas of the October Revolution." They came to the conclusion that as a result of Lenin's proclamation of NEP nothing was left of the ideas with which the Bolsheviks had come to power four years earlier. Instead of the state withering away, they were constructing a new and mighty state. Instead of the disappearance of money, NEP called for the reinforcement of the ruble. Lenin had abolished the forcible confiscation of grain, replaced it with an ordinary tax in kind, and—horror of horrors!—permitted the peasant to sell his surplus grain. The free market, that once-detested mainstay of capitalism, was reappearing. Gone was the dream of collective farms, which the peasants would be compelled to join. Instead the peasants were set free. True, lip service to the dream of world revolution was still obligatory, but that was all. The Bolsheviks were already trading with capitalist countries. Their minds were on the prosperity of their own country, not on a universal conflagration. This was how a group of clever intellectuals understood NEP. While in the West the émigré professor Ustryalov welcomed this "new wave of common sense set rolling by the breath of the vast peasant country," and joyfully exclaimed that "Lenin is one of us. Lenin is a true son of Russia. Lenin is a national hero."

Many people believed Lenin when he said that NEP was meant to be "serious and for a long time." My father and other nonparty intellectuals may be forgiven for this, but how could N. Valentinov forget the traditions of the Party at whose headwaters he had once stood? How could he forget Rule Number 1—that statements by the Party's leaders were only the product of tactical considerations, whereas the real, long-term plans, the Party's strategy, had to remain hidden, to be revealed at some future time? A certain person, for instance, assured everyone in 1924 that class warfare was on the wane. He made mock of those who exaggerated the kulak danger. He insisted that the Party should show the greatest tolerance toward those who had gone astray. That certain person was Stalin, who just a few years later would herd the peasants into collective farms, extirpate the kulaks, and present the slogan "Intensify class warfare" as the country's be-all and end-all. This, it seemed, was strategy. Yesterday's lie was tactics.

So when Lenin declared that NEP was "serious and for a long time," it meant only that he wanted people to think so. At the very same time, he was writing the Commissar for Foreign Trade, the ex-terrorist Krasin, that "it's a very great mistake to think that NEP means the end of terror. We shall resort to terror again, and to economic terror. Foreigners are now buying up our officials with bribes. . . . My dears, when the moment comes I shall hang you for it." In a secret note he offered Kursky, the Commissar for Justice, his own draft version of a clause to be added to the criminal code, defining the nature of terror and the situations which justified its use. Even as he introduced NEP Lenin was already thinking about the retribution to be meted out when the Bolsheviks abandoned it and reverted to the Great Utopia. This is why during NEP the land itself, major industries, foreign trade, the banks, and transport all remained in the hands of the Bolshevik state. Lenin's creed remained what it had always been: the dictatorship of the proletariat, which meant "power relying on force, with no limitations, unrestricted by any laws." Could power of this kind coexist with a NEP that was meant seriously and meant to last? To Lenin, NEP was just a breathing space, like the Brest peace. When Trotsky called NEP a maneuver, that was the truth of it. But it was not a truth that the Party could be told, because Lenin was eager to obtain funds from the West. Capitalism must come to his aid, so that he could destroy it later.

But for this to happen the West had to believe that Jacobinism was finished—seriously and for a long time—now that NEP had arrived!

A tragedy was in the making. Lenin would have to do battle with an indignant Party ignorant of this truth. A Party which now believed that what had to be taken seriously was the death of the Great Utopia. Lenin knew that the opposition would take advantage of this situation. He tells us that "NEP gave rise to panic, grumbling, despondency, and indignation in the Party."

NEP. Smart hansom cabs and private cars on the streets, carrying the hated "unculled bourgeois" as the Party called them, beautiful women in mink coats, and casinos reappeared. Moscow plunged into a life of feverish enjoyment. Foodstuffs surfaced from underground. New restaurants opened.

It was all so reminiscent of Thermidor, the month in which the French Revolution died—a memory hateful to the Bolsheviks.

It reminds us, too, of Moscow in 1992.

There were murmurs of discontent from ordinary Party members, who sensed the possibility of dissent within the leadership.

"We have conjured up the devil of the market," warned Trotsky.

9 THE BIRTH OF STALIN

LENIN'S NEW ROLE FOR KOBA

Lenin had allowed for the explosion of indignation within the Party that NEP would cause. While liberating the economy, he now imposed the strictest discipline on the Party. On his initiative the Tenth Congress adopted a resolution forbidding the formation of factions within the Party. Factionalism became punishable by expulsion. Lenin sought to stifle the very possibility of opposition. The wording of this resolution, unthinkable in a democratic party, grated on the ear, and it was therefore kept secret from the public.

In the spring of the following year, 1922, Lenin introduced a new post—General Secretary of the Party—and in April, on his proposal, Koba was elected to the post. Some suppose that it was meant to be a purely executive position and that only Koba's malign genius made it so influential in the Party. This is to misunderstand both the situation and Lenin himself. The post of General Secretary was the latest in a series of measures adopted by Lenin against dissidence in the Party. He knew that discontent would grow as NEP took its course and that the eternally rebellious Trotsky would inevitably make a move. Lenin, with all his experience, knew that although factionalism was now banned he had to be wary of open rebellion on the part of the old guard. By 1922 he had begun to feel very tired, exhausted by the constant struggle at Congress after Congress with opposition groups—the "Workers' Opposition" and all the rest. He was also tormented by inexplicable headaches, which were becoming more and more painful. He decided to create a machine capable of organizing more businesslike and pacific Congresses. This was the Secretariat, headed by faithful Koba. The tried and trusty Koba was to ensure that Congresses behaved themselves. He must learn how to control the Party. Put more simply, he must tame it. That was the meaning of the new post. No wonder that Lenin defined the functions of the Secretariat in disingenuously vague terms. The Politburo had been set up to decide the most important questions of policy, the Orgburo to deal with major organizational questions. The implication was that the Secretariat would deal with less important questions.

But with this went a dangerous proviso: any decision by the Secretariat which went unchallenged by members of the Orgburo automatically became a decision of the Orgburo. Any decision of the Secretariat unchallenged by members of the Politburo became a Politburo decision. So that from its inception it was possible for the Secretariat to decide matters of the greatest importance. On Koba's proposal, his old acquaintance Molotov became Second Secretary. (Lenin had affectionately nicknamed him "Stone Arse" because of his diligence and his ability to work twenty-four hours a day.) The Secretariat and the Orgburo annexed by Koba (and run by the loyal Molotov) began to control all appointments within the Party.

A Silent Coup Within the Leadership

Still in 1922, Lenin said at a Politburo meeting that "we [he meant Trotsky and himself] are in our fifties, you [the rest] are all in your forties. We must prepare the thirty- and twenty-year-old comrades who will replace us—select them and train them for leadership." So it was not Koba's but Lenin's idea to replace the leading cadres. The leader was tired of the old guard, his brilliant and eternally carping associates. So he gave Koba the job of preparing replacements. Brilliance must be replaced by efficiency. Koba saw the possibilities and carried out his task enthusiastically. This, for instance, explains the emergence of thirty-year-old Lazar Kaganovich, a shoemaker by trade, like Koba's father. Born in a Jewish shtetl, he was semiliterate but extremely hardworking. Molotov discovered him and introduced him to Koba, who put him in charge of the Central Committee's organizational department. Kaganovich had under him a team of Central Committee "instructors," who were sent to the provinces to check the work of local Party organizations. The future of a local leader depended on their reports. Kaganovich's department was shortly given the right to appoint local Party officials on the spot. Provincial Party organizations were now entirely in Koba's hands. Kaganovich set about the gigantic task of installing the right people, checking up on their loyalty, generally shaking up Party officialdom. In less than a year forty-three secretaries of *guberniya* Party organizations (the plenipotentiary rulers in the provinces) were checked and confirmed. These Party mandarins were endowed with power beyond the dreams of the tsar's governor-general.

In the General Secretary's copy of Trotsky's *Terrorism and Communism,* beside a sentence of Trotsky's about the Party's leadership in the state apparatus, Koba's marginal comment is a single word: *indivisible.*

The power to appoint congenial provincial party leaders and inspect their work—this was the simple lever which enabled Koba to subordinate the Party to himself within a very short time. Trotsky understood what was happening, was dismayed, but it was, alas, too late. Local leaders acceptable to Koba and dependent on the Secretariat were in place everywhere. They were ready to constitute a new, manipulated majority at Congresses. And if any of the Kremlin boyars made bold to defy this majority, he would be hounded out of the Party, in accordance with Lenin's prohibition of factionalism. Koba had carried out his task successfully. A docile Party had been created, in a very short time.

But Lenin was not destined to take advantage of it.

The GPU Knows Everything

In February 1922, after inventing the post of General Secretary, Lenin reformed the Cheka. Its new name was the State Political Administration attached to the People's Commissariat of Internal Affairs—GPU for short. But before 1923 was out, it was renamed Unified State Political Administration (OGPU). (In common usage it was the GPU as before, and its staff were still GPU men. So GPU is the name which will often be used in our narrative.) The GPU was detached from the People's Commissariat for Internal Affairs and officially answerable to the Council of People's Commissars, but in reality to Lenin and the Politburo. All this was advertised as the end of the "bloody Cheka." It was announced that the GPU's only tasks now were the struggle against serious crimes which endangered the state and intelligence gathering. In reality the ill-defined functions of the old Cheka remained sacrosanct. The collegium of the GPU retained the right to shoot any Russian citizen without exception, and with no questions asked. A triumvirate consisting of the chairman of the GPU, his assistant, and the investigator in charge of the case also had powers of summary execution. The threesome took its decision without calling the accused or his defending lawyer, and the accused was not informed of the verdict until shortly before his execution. Koba immediately involved the newly formed GPU in his offensive against the opposition. For the reorganization of the Cheka was really just another part of Lenin's plan to tame the Party. To begin with, the GPU was used in the fight against rival revolutionary parties. It was permitted to employ former officials of the tsarist secret police against SRs and Mensheviks: they had so much experience in hunting down those other revolutionaries. The GPU also set its sights on its own Party's heretics. A new order from the Central

Committee obliged all Party members to inform the GPU of all "anti-Party" talk and all opposition groups within the Party. Lenin and Koba had thereby thrust the GPU into the intra-Party struggle. Members of the Party had a duty to inform against their Party comrades. Members of the collegium of the GPU were listed as employees of the Central Committee, so their appointment too was in Koba's gift. The semiliterate sailors with bombs and the Bolshevik hotheads soon disappeared from the GPU.

Koba involved the GPU more and more in the life of the Party. After the privations of the prerevolutionary period, high Party functionaries were greedily enjoying life. The GPU now kept the General Secretary regularly informed of fun and games among the bigwigs: the adventures of such high Party functionaries as Kalinin and Yenukidze with ballerinas; the visits of the commissar of education, Lunacharsky, to the Actors' Club, from which the cultural supremo was carried to his car, to the accompaniment of loud female laughter, as the lights were dimmed at dawn; and the scandalous exploits of Kamenev's young son Lyutik. For that matter, Kamenev himself had taken a mistress. All this was known to the GPU and to Koba. Files were now kept on Party officials.

Let Us Clean Russia and Keep It Clean

An operation which shocked the Russian intelligentsia at large was carried out at this time. An operation devised by Lenin. In the last days of 1922 a steamship from Russia put into the port of Stettin in Poland. There was no one waiting to welcome the new arrivals. They found a few horse-drawn wagons, loaded their luggage onto them, and walked behind in the roadway, husbands and wives arm in arm. "They" were the fine flower and pride of Russian philosophy and social thought, all those who had shaped Russia's social awareness in the early years of the twentieth century: Lossky, Berdyaev, Frank, Kizevetter, Prince Trubetskoy, Ilyin . . . 160 of them, eminent professors, philosophers, poets, and writers, the whole intellectual potential of Russia cast out at a stroke.

Pravda published an article about the expulsion under the headline "First Warning." It was just that. Throughout 1922, while he was implementing the New Economic Policy, Lenin was also systematically purging the country of dissidents. With the General Secretary, faithful Koba, at his side. In a dispatch to Koba, he said, "With reference to the expulsion of Mensheviks, Kadets etc. from Russia . . . several hundred such gentlemen should be mercilessly expelled. Let us make Russia clean for a long time to come." A special commission attached to the Politburo worked tirelessly. List after list of expellees was drawn up. And Koba's rough handiwork can be seen in the systematic and unwavering implementation of Lenin's scheme.

Leaving Russia was a grotesque tragedy for these people.

"We thought we should be returning in a year's time. . . . That was all we lived for," wrote the daughter of the eminent agricultural scientist Professor A. Ugrimov. In Prague in the seventies I met a very old woman, the daughter of the eminent historian Professor Kizevetter. She had lived with her suitcase ready, packed, since 1922. She was still waiting.

Lenin's illness interrupted the gigantic purge which was getting under way. But the General Secretary had mastered its slogan: "Let us make Russia clean for a long time to come."

THE NEW TOWER OF BABEL

Lenin also steered General Secretary Koba in the direction of the Comintern (Communist International), which had close links with the GPU. The third Communist International had been set up in 1919, when the dream of world revolution still lived. It was joined by Communist parties obedient to Moscow. When they founded the Comintern, Lenin and Trotsky had written candidly in its manifesto that "the international proletariat will not sheathe its sword until we have created a world Federation of Soviet Republics. . . . The Comintern is the party of the revolutionary rising of the international proletariat."

The Comintern offices were on Manège Square. There were several "sections" on each floor, representing, in toto, the whole world. Three Communist universities trained the cadres who should someday set the world on fire. Radek, Zinoviev, Bukharin, and Kamenev all gave lectures there. Koba now began to speak there quite frequently. An old Comintern member, V. Saveliev, wrote me: "I am nearing the end of my ninth decade. . . . I had some connection with the Comintern. For that I was given an eighteen-year rest cure in Stalin's camps. The Comintern was a great organization. Stalin utilized it brilliantly. I was just a boy. I remember the head of Comintern, Zinoviev—red-faced, plump. . . . We taught Western Communists to operate underground, to manage illegal organizations, to organize disorders, etc. The heads of the GPU often came to our meetings. Zinoviev, paraphrasing Trotsky, called the GPU 'the glory and the pride of our Party.' The GPU acted in conjunction with the Comintern. In 1920, when we were thinking of helping the

German revolution, the GPU blew up an arsenal in Poland, just in case we had to go to the aid of the Germans via Poland. . . . If Stalin took something on he 'squeezed hard,' 'got a stranglehold' on it. . . . Zinoviev didn't like work, and after Stalin was appointed Gensek [General Secretary] all the most secret business of the Comintern was done through him."

The gigantic resources of the country, seized by the Bolsheviks who so hated money, were lavished on the preparation of world revolution. In March 1922, for instance, 4 million lire were allocated to the Italian Communist Party, 47 million marks to the Germans, 640,000 francs to the French. The list was endless. Starving Moscow was feeding the Communist Parties of the whole world. People were swollen with hunger, but never mind, the world revolution was at hand. The Comintern spent money without counting, squandered it recklessly. Money often disappeared together with Comintern agents. When Koba became Gensek he set about introducing some system of auditing expenditures. A report from G. Safarov informed Koba that 200,000 gold rubles had disappeared in Korea. Koba also looked into the millions spent on Germany, and tried to make Zinoviev account for them. In 1921 alone, 62 million marks had been paid out to fund a revolution. The payment was made partly in currency, partly in jewelry, some of it taken from the imperial family when they were executed. It included, for instance, a pearl necklace belonging to Russia's last empress. All those millions of marks had been kept in the apartment of a Comintern agent, stuffed into files, cupboards, suitcases, boxes. The commission of inquiry set up by Koba uncovered total chaos and a complete absence of accountability. Koba now began to oversee not only the expenditures but the whole life of the Comintern.

Studying the (invariably top-secret) documents of the Comintern Commission for Illegal Work in the Party Archive, I saw how Koba's shadow hangs over all subversive activity the commission organized in Germany, Italy, Hungary, Czechoslovakia, the United States, Lithuania, and Latvia. Safe houses, clandestine printing presses, sabotage—the former terrorist knew all about such things. He tied in Comintern activities more and more closely with those of the secret police. Terrorists were to be planted in every country of the world. The Comintern's most secret business was now referred to the Gensek.

THE COMRADES HAMMER

At the beginning of the nineties I managed to obtain a photocopy of what was still a secret document, held by the Party Archive. Penciled on the document were the words "Strictly Secret—from Lenin to Comrade Stalin." This was a "report from Boris Reinstein" on Comrade Dr. Julius Hammer and the American company run by him and his son Dr. Armand Hammer, which had obtained concessions in Soviet asbestos workings, among other things. (Boris Reinstein, a Russian Jew, had emigrated to the United States at the end of the nineteenth century and returned to Russia in 1917 to take part in the Revolution. He became an influential Comintern official and, needless to say, later disappeared in Stalin's camps.) Reinstein's note reads:

> Dear Vladimir Ilyich
>
> Herewith some information on Comrade Julius Hammer and his company, but I beg you to ensure that this report does not fall into the hands of people who are not entirely reliable, since if a copy falls into the hands of the American government it could have a disastrous effect on Julius Hammer's situation, which is already very difficult. Having worked for 25 years (1892–1917) in the American Socialist Workers Party I know Comrade Julius Hammer intimately as a sincere and self-sacrificing Marxist. . . . Having built up a profitable medical practice he has always given generous financial help to the socialist movement. . . . After America's entry into the war it was impossible for him to make a dash for Russia so he decided instead to play the bourgeoisie at their own game, i.e., to make a lot of money but use it to support revolution. He succeeded brilliantly. . . . He and his family are said to have amassed a great deal of money. At the beginning of 1919 Narkomindel [the People's Commissariat for Foreign Affairs] sent money to Comrade Martens. [Martens, a New York resident, had been appointed Soviet Russia's first ambassador to the United States, although that country refused to recognize the Soviet government at the time.] When Martens's funds ran out, Comrade Hammer saved his office from liquidation with a loan amounting in total to $50,000. Later . . . when Russia needed to obtain machinery for the oil fields, he loaned $11,000 for that purpose. . . . After the foundation of Comintern he broke with the Socialist Workers

Party because of its ambiguous attitude to the International. . . . In September 1919, with [John] Reed and others, he initiated the Communist movement in America. Besides actively participating in the Communist Congress he gave the Party generous financial support, advancing more than $250,000 for that purpose. The American government suspected that Comrade Hammer was subsidizing Martens's Soviet bureau and the Communist movement, and tried to find an excuse to get rid of him. Deporting an American citizen occupying a prominent social position was, however, impossible. . . . An excuse finally presented itself . . . a woman patient of his, on whom he had been forced for clinical reasons to perform an abortion, died. The government seized on this, induced the dead woman's husband to prosecute, and forced the jury to bring in a verdict of guilty at all costs. As a result, he was sentenced to imprisonment with hard labor for a term of from 31/2 to 15 years. This means that he could be released after a little over a year (he has been in Sing Sing jail, near New York, for over two years now) but even after that the government could make his political behavior the excuse for throwing him in jail again and keeping him there for the full 15 years. . . . He and his sons are the main shareholders in a big firm . . . and are now set to work from behind bars to induce his company to support Soviet Russia. In summer 1921 he sent his son Armand, who had recently qualified as a doctor, to Moscow. Armand is their company secretary. Armand Hammer brought with him as a present from his father a full set of surgical instruments, large enough to equip a whole hospital, and worth a great deal of money. Following in his father's footsteps, the young man—on learning that there was a scheme to set up in Moscow a model American hospital, with funds furnished by friends of the Soviet Union, . . . gave $25,000 toward it. Making a tour of enterprises in the Urals last year he saw that well-equipped factories were at a standstill because the workers were short of food, and offered—after consulting his father—to provide one million poods [18,000 tons] of grain in return for Russian goods. The contract was made through Vneshtorg [the Soviet Foreign Trade Agency], and one shipment of grain (about 150,000 poods) arrived, but then there was a holdup, partly because our caviar, for which there was a brisk sale at $10 a pound, was found on analysis to contain chemical preservatives

> in quantities not permitted by American law. . . . Since the Russian goods were threatened with confiscation the ship had to be diverted first to a Canadian port. A safe way has now been found to deliver the caviar directly to the more profitable United States market. . . . A large joint American company, with several financial bigwigs, has now been set up on young Dr. Hammer's initiative specially to develop Russian enterprises. . . . It is clear from all that has been said here that we have in the two Comrades Hammer and their company a connection of great value to us, and that it is in our interest to remove all obstacles from their path.

In a secret report (the original was in English) the GPU noted that "on his return journey, at the request of Comintern, Hammer carried $34,000 in cash, which he delivered to the Communist Party in the USA. During this period the USA had placed an embargo on all exports to Russia, and Hammer's success in getting grain and machines through was unprecedented."

The Leader's Illness

Throughout 1921 Lenin was plagued by the same excruciating headaches and by neurasthenia. Koba advised a trip to the sunny Caucasus. But to Lenin, just thinking about the fatigues of travel was daunting, as it might be to anyone approaching his end. Lenin wrote to Ordzhonikidze, "I'm afraid a long journey might result in exhaustion by all the nonsensical fuss and bustle rather than a cure for my nerves."

Lenin spent less and less time in the Kremlin, and more and more in Nizhny Novgorod, near Moscow, on the estate of that enigmatic person, the late Savva Morozov. He was persuaded to call in the doctors, although he had little confidence in Bolshevik "Doctor-comrades." As he once wrote to Maxim Gorky, "Ninety-nine out of a hundred of our doctor-comrades are asses." In the old Russia which Lenin had destroyed, German doctors were regarded as the best. And sure enough, doctors were summoned from capitalist Germany to diagnose the Leader's strange condition. Professor F. Klemperer and his colleagues found nothing particularly alarming, just a slight neurasthenia. They explained his headaches by the bullets left in his head after the assassination attempt. They removed the bullets. But . . .

Morozov's country home brought him no luck.

At Gorky, on May 26, Lenin suffered a stroke. His right-side extremities were partly paralyzed and his speech was affected. As he confided to Trotsky later, "I could neither speak nor write. I had to learn all over again."

This was the beginning of the tragic period in Lenin's life, his losing battle with sickness which ended with his death two and a half years later.

The communiqué on "The Illness and Death of V. I. Ulyanov (Lenin)," published in *Pravda,* lists the eminent Russian and German doctors and the junior medical personnel, some forty names in all, who treated Lenin, or were called in for consultation, in the course of his illness. Among them we find F. Klemperer, O. Förster, V. Kramer, V. Osipov, F. Gautier, S. Dobrogayev, all of whom subsequently published reminiscences, and Dr. Kramer, whose unpublished notes on Lenin's illness are in the President's Archive.

There is a well-known story that Koba's immediate reaction to the stroke was "Lenin's kaput." That is a lie—he could never have said that. Not faithful Koba. Cautious Koba. He was never in a hurry, never rash.

But he did, of course, realize that the Leader was walking with death. It could happen at any minute. A few years before it would have spelled the end for Koba. But now . . . now he would remain just where he was, with the terrifying power which he had amassed. He had done what neither Sverdlov nor Lenin himself had managed to do—made the Party manageable. Add to that a docile GPU . . .

While Lenin was learning to talk the doctors argued over the precise diagnosis. They even mentioned the possibility of hereditary syphilis. They journeyed to Astrakhan, where Lenin's forebears had lived, to make inquiries, but discovered nothing definite. In the meantime Lenin began to show signs of recovery. He was forbidden to read the newspapers, he still had attacks, he could not receive visitors. But he was already asking for faithful Koba. Throughout July, August, and September Koba regularly visited Lenin at Gorky. Lenin was feeling better all the time, and he decided to escape from the doctors' tutelage. He appealed to Koba—as was only right; the Gensek, faithful Koba, was monitoring the Leader's treatment. Lenin wrote to him in July 1922: "The doctors are evidently creating a legend which cannot go unrefuted. They lost their heads completely after my severe attack on Friday, and did something utterly stupid—tried to forbid political discussion. . . . I got extremely angry and sent them packing. . . . I want you here most urgently to tell you in time what to do if my illness gets worse. I can say it all in 15 minutes. . . . Only fools can blame 'talking politics.' If I ever get agitated it is for lack of sensible conversation. I hope you'll understand that, and send the doctors packing."

On July 13 Koba was at Gorky with the Leader. In *Pravda,* he himself would give a humorous description of this idyllic meeting: " 'I'm not allowed to read newspapers,' Lenin remarked ironically. 'I'm not allowed to talk politics. I steer clear of any scrap of paper lying around on the desk, for fear it might be a newspaper.' I laughed and praised Comrade Lenin's self-discipline to the skies. Then we both laughed at the doctors, who cannot understand that when professional politicians meet they can't help talking politics." This article was part of an ideological stunt thought up by the resourceful Koba: a special issue of *Pravda* to tell the world that the Leader had recovered. There were several photographs of Lenin, and among them one of Lenin and Stalin sitting side by side on a bench.

Koba also described their conversations on that sunlit bench. Lenin "complained that he was out of touch with events . . . he was interested in everything: the harvest prospects, the trial of the SRs." (Thirty-five right-wing Socialist Revolutionaries, including eleven prominent members of the Party's Central Committee, who had distinguished themselves in the struggle against the Last Tsar, were standing trial at the time. The trial had been extremely well prepared, and Koba's hand, with which we are familiar from the Stalinist trials of the future, is clearly visible in this one.

(The records of the case, still held by the Central Archive of the KGB, run to several volumes. I was able to consult some of them.

(The "star" of the trial was a certain G. Semyonov, who had commanded the SR "fighting squad." He had been arrested by the Cheka back in 1919, and would have been sentenced to death had he not "honestly repented," "sincerely broken with his past," and joined the Bolshevik Party while in jail. Semyonov had then been planted in the SR Party as an informer. Later he was given still more serious tasks. The records contain a letter from Trotsky testifying to Semyonov's "devotion to the revolution," as evinced by his work as a Soviet agent in Polish territory in 1920.

(In 1922 Semyonov carried out a new assignment: he appeared as one of the accused in the trial of right-wing Socialist Revolutionaries. He made statements on a number of subversive actions secretly planned by the Right SR Party's Central Committee and on their links with foreign agencies. He claimed that Fanny Kaplan had been briefed for her attempt on Lenin's life by the Right SR Central Committee and was a member of its terrorist group. However, his statement that he regarded Kaplan as the "best person to carry out the attack on Lenin" showed that he can never even have seen that half-deaf, half-blind woman.

(Nikolai Krylenko, who had exchanged the post of commander-in-chief for that of public prosecutor of the republic, demanded the death penalty for the SR leaders.

(Bukharin and Radek spoiled everything. Eager to be seen as "civilized socialists" at the Third International, they promised that the Socialist Revolutionaries would not be executed. This misreading of the situation of course infuriated Lenin. The pacification of the Party and the country was proceeding. That was why rebellious intellectuals had been deported. Why Lenin had made Koba General Secretary. And why the SRs had to be executed.)

This was something Lenin and Koba must have discussed on that sunlit bench. In any case, as soon as he rose from his sickbed Lenin published in *Pravda* an article calling for the blood of the SRs. Twelve of them were sentenced to death. But Bukharin's promises had to be taken into account, and the sentence specified that the execution of the SRs was to "take place only after the first terrorist act against the Bolsheviks."

The SRs, spared for the time being, Krylenko, who had condemned them, and the provocateur Semyonov would all perish together in the days of Stalinist terror.

Meanwhile, a Lenin full of energy, the old Lenin, was ready for work again. But, as Lunacharsky wrote, "Everyone was aware of a worrying impediment in his speech. It was particularly frightening when he just stopped short in the middle of a statement, turned pale, and could only continue with a terrible effort."

It was Koba's official duty to supervise Lenin's treatment and he was kept reliably informed by the doctors. The illness was expected to recur. A second stroke might follow at any time. Koba, the great chess player who could always see several moves ahead, drew his conclusion.

Lenin himself realized his condition. It was time to turn once more to faithful Koba.

Koba and the Poison

Trotsky wrote: "During Lenin's second illness, in February 1923, Stalin told a meeting of the Politburo that Lenin had unexpectedly sent for him and asked to be supplied with poison, since he . . . foresaw that another stroke was imminent. He did not believe the doctors, because it had not been difficult to catch them out in contradictions . . . and he was suffering unbearable agonies. . . . I remember how strange, how inappropriate to the circumstances, Stalin's looks seemed to me. The request he was passing on had a tragic character, but his face was frozen in a half-smile, as if it were a mask. 'There can, of course, be no question of carrying out that request,' I exclaimed. 'I told him all that,' Stalin retorted, rather irritably, 'but he just dismissed it. The old man is suffering, says he wants to have poison handy. He will do it only if he becomes convinced that his situation is hopeless. . . . The old man is suffering,' Stalin repeated, 'he's obviously got something in mind.' "

Trotsky went on to ask: "Why was Stalin the one Lenin turned to at such a time? . . . The answer is simple: Lenin saw in Stalin the only man who would [i.e., the only man cruel enough to] carry out his tragic request."

Maria Ulyanova also wrote about Lenin's request for poison. But the circumstances as she described them were quite different. Shortly before her death Lenin's sister wrote a note which was found among her private papers, immediately landed in the secret section of the Party Archive, and was made available to historians only half a century later. It was a penitential act on her part. Feeling that death was near, she wrote:

> I consider it my duty to say something, however briefly, about Ilyich's real attitude to Stalin in the last period of his life [since in previous statements] I did not tell the whole truth.
>
> In the winter of 1921–1922 V.I. fell ill. Around that time, I don't know exactly when, he told Stalin that he would probably end up paralyzed, and made him promise to help him get and to administer potassium cyanide if that should happen. Stalin promised. . . . The reason why he chose to ask Stalin was that he knew him to be a hard man, a man of steel, devoid of sentimentality. There was no one else whom he could ask to do such a thing. V.I. made the same request to Stalin in May 1922, after his first stroke. V.I. had decided that he was finished, and asked for Stalin to be fetched. He was so insistent that they dared not refuse him. Stalin spent a little time with V.I., really not more than five minutes, and when he came out of the room he told me and Bukharin that V.I. had asked him to get him the poison,

> since the time had come to carry out his promise. Stalin promised, he and V.I. embraced, and Stalin left the room. But after talking it over together we decided that we should try to reassure V.I., so Stalin went back into his room and said that after talking to the doctors he was convinced that all was not yet lost, and that the time to carry out V.I.'s request had not yet come. V.I. cheered up considerably although he said to Stalin, "Are you fooling me?" "When did I ever try to fool you?" Stalin said. They parted, and didn't see each other again until V.I. started getting better. . . . In those days Stalin was with him more often than the others.

So Trotsky was right about one thing—there was a request for poison. But Trotsky placed it in 1923, by which time Lenin and Koba were enemies. Maria Ulyanova places it in 1922, when they were the best of friends. Lenin's request to Koba was an expression of implicit trust in him, at a time when, so Maria Ulyanova tells us, "Stalin was with him more often than any of the others."

I used to think that Trotsky had made a mistake, perhaps a deliberate mistake, to make his readers believe that Stalin was already Lenin's enemy when he carried out his request. Imagine my amazement when, working in the President's Archive, I learned that Stalin had indeed been asked again, in 1923, to obtain poison for Lenin. But this time the request came, as we shall see, not from Lenin himself. By then, Lenin could not "summon Stalin . . . and request," as Trotsky says he did. He could not even speak.

But first we must return to 1922.

What did they talk about when Koba visited him? Maria Ulyanova says, "On that occasion, and during subsequent visits, they talked about Trotsky." In the intervals of his illness Lenin saw many things clearly. While he was ill, his suspicious nature had made him form an alliance against Trotsky. He now knew that the danger came from a different quarter. He evidently received alarming news from Kamenev, Zinoviev, and even Trotsky: that the Party was now completely controlled by Koba. He himself, of course, had made Koba General Secretary, to create an apparatus to manage the Party. And Koba had carried out his wishes. But times had changed. Lenin was now a sick man, his illness might become acute at any moment, and if it did . . . who could tell how Koba, with the Party apparatus at his command, might behave? He had evidently succeeded in undermining Lenin's authority.

Lenin took fright and decided to remove Koba from the post of General Secretary. An excuse was needed. Lenin found one.

THE DISAPPEARANCE OF KOBA, THE EMERGENCE OF STALIN

In 1922 Lenin decided to regularize the position of the republics. Parts of the old tsarist empire—Ukraine, Belorussia, and the Transcaucasian Federation—were now formally independent of Russia, but in fact governed by protégés of Moscow. Lenin was planning the next step—unification.

In Lenin's absence Koba had proposed abandoning secrecy in favor of frankness: the "independent" republics should all enter into a Russian federation, retaining only local autonomy. This caused grumblings in the republics, especially in Georgia, which had only recently lost its independence. The Georgian leader, Budu Mdivani, realized how difficult it would be to tell the Georgians that the clock was being turned back to tsarist times. He asked to be given a fig leaf: let Georgia enjoy independence, at least on paper. Lenin supported him, and put forward his own concept of a Union of Soviet Socialist Republics (USSR). The republics were to enjoy equal rights, on paper, and even the right to leave the future union. This was enough to satisfy the "independents" in Georgia, and at the same time it allowed Lenin to open his campaign against Koba. Koba—and another non-Russian who favored federation, the leader of the Transcaucasian Bolsheviks, Ordzhonikidze—knew how deep-seated nationalist sentiment was in the republics, and how dangerous even formal independence might become tomorrow. In the heat of debate the temperamental Ordzhonikidze struck the "independent" Mdivani. This gave Lenin a splendid excuse. He denounced Koba's and Ordzhonikidze's policy as "Great Russian chauvinism," and promoted Ordzhonikidze's punch to the status of a crime.

Kamenev, who realized that Lenin would not last much longer and lived in mortal fear that Trotsky might become supreme, decided to honor his alliance with Koba, and immediately reported to him that "Ilyich is ready for war in defense of independence."

Koba realized that Lenin no longer felt the same toward him, and of course knew why. He invited Kamenev to join him in rebellion, and wrote in reply to his note that "in my view we must show firmness against Ilyich." In other words, he was no longer afraid. The doctors made their reports to the Gensek, and Koba had been informed that another stroke was inevitable. Lenin, however, took effective action. He dispatched a special commission to Georgia, and drew Koba's enemy

Trotsky into the struggle against him. A Lenin-Trotsky combination meant that the result was a foregone conclusion. No one could stand up to both leaders.

Lenin now resolved to destroy Koba at the next (Twelfth) Party Congress and, according to Trotsky, he had a bombshell ready.

Kamenev got cold feet, and wrote to Koba, "If V.I. insists, resistance will get more difficult." Koba replied gloomily, "I don't know—let him do what he thinks best." Koba meant to wait. He was good at that. He began drafting a declaration on the formation of a Union of Republics, just as Ilyich wished. But Lenin did not accept his surrender. At the beginning of October, he wrote to Kamenev, "I am declaring war on Great Russian chauvinism." Kamenev saw that there was no way of stopping Ilyich.

Lenin was in constant contact with Trotsky on the Caucasian problem through his secretary Fotieva:

> *Trotsky:* So he isn't looking for a compromise with Stalin, even if the line is the correct one?
> *Fotieva:* Right. He doesn't trust Stalin, and wants to attack him openly before the whole Party. He's preparing a bombshell. . . . Ilyich's condition is deteriorating from one hour to the next. He has difficulty speaking, and he's afraid he'll collapse completely before he can act. When he handed me the note he told me: "If I don't want to be too late I must speak out sooner than I meant to."

Trotsky, however, was not the only one who heard this from Fotieva. She also kept Koba informed about everything that happened in Lenin's office. She knew from Ilyich's worsening condition that a new master was on the threshold. (Lidia Fotieva was one of the few close associates of Lenin whom Koba would not touch. In 1938 he would send her to work in the Lenin museum. Lavishly decorated and rewarded, she died in 1975, in her nineties, outliving Koba, and indeed almost outliving the Soviet era.)

Kamenev turned up in Trotsky's office. Trotsky wrote, "He was a sufficiently experienced politician to realize that it was not just a question of Georgia, but of the whole role of Stalin in the Party." Fainthearted Kamenev had deserted Koba.

The downfall of Ilyich's one-time favorite seemed imminent. But . . .

Koba's information proved accurate. The struggle and his hard feelings proved too much for Lenin.

The doctors demanded complete rest for Lenin. Koba clarified their demands: In mid-December he carried a resolution at a plenary meeting of the Central Committee placing "personal responsibility for the *isolation* of Comrade Lenin—in respect both of his personal dealings with officials and of his correspondence" on the Gensek. Meetings with Lenin were forbidden. Neither friends nor members of his household were allowed to tell Ilyich anything about political events, in case it overexcited him.

The Leader himself was not informed of the Party's decision. But what sort of leader was he now? The Leader had vanished, leaving only a sick man in his place. Koba too had vanished, and Joseph Stalin had appeared on the scene. A graduate of Lenin's university, summa cum laude.

THREE

STALIN: HIS LIFE, HIS DEATH

10

The tyrant grows from a root called popular representation. To begin with he smiles at and embraces all whom he meets. . . . He promises much. . . . But having become a tyrant and realizing that the citizens who made possible his elevation now condemn him the tyrant will be forced willy-nilly to destroy those who condemn him, until he has neither friends nor enemies left.
—Plato

Meeting with Stalin

The Central Committee plenum adopted a decision recommended by Lenin before his illness: the monopoly of foreign trade was to remain in the hands of the state. Trotsky took the lead in supporting this decision. He was obviously now playing what used to be Koba's role vis-à-vis Lenin. Krupskaya informed Lenin that his proposal had prevailed and the moment he recovered from his stroke he dictated a letter to Trotsky: "We seem to have taken the position without firing a single shot. . . . I suggest we do not stop there but continue the offensive." By "offensive" Lenin meant the attack on Koba. Lenin was a skillful fighter. Next day, Kamenev, alarmed by the obvious rapprochement between Trotsky and Lenin, informed Stalin in a note that the two leaders were in contact: "Joseph, Trotsky rang me tonight to say he had received a note in which the Old Man expresses his satisfaction with the resolution on foreign trade." Stalin replied: "Comrade Kamenev, how was the Old Man able to organize correspondence when Dr. Ferster has absolutely forbidden it?" The tone of this note is new. He is no longer just "Joseph"; he is the Gensek, who allows no one to act in breach of a Party decision.

Stalin then rang Krupskaya and rudely berated her.

Krupskaya was in a state of shock. According to Maria Ulyanova, when she got home she "was quite unlike her usual self.

She rolled about the floor, sobbing." This was evidently when Krupskaya lost her self-control and told Lenin how she had been insulted. Lenin was in a rage, and wrote to Stalin breaking off relations. At the same time, Krupskaya wrote a furious letter to Kamenev: "Stalin has taken it upon himself to treat me in the rudest possible way. . . . Never in all these thirty years have I heard a single rude word from any comrade, and the interests of the Party and of Ilyich are no less dear to me than to Comrade Stalin. At present I need all the self-control I can muster. I know better than any doctor what may and what may not be talked about. . . . And certainly better than Stalin does. I am appealing to you, and to Grigori, as V.I.'s closest comrades, and I beg you to protect me from rude interference in my private life, from vulgar abuse and threats. I too am a living person, and my nerves are strained to the utmost." She did not understand what had happened. Lenin's wife had, for the first time in her life, seen Stalin. Until then she had known only faithful Koba.

But once she had recovered her composure Krupskaya began to appreciate the new situation and to realize how helpless she was. She must have immediately begged Lenin's secretary not to send his letter to Stalin just yet. Meanwhile, Kamenev had realized when he received Krupskaya's letter that hostilities with Stalin had been resumed. He sought Trotsky out at once. They discussed what the situation in the Party would be in the wake of this note. And both decided to leave Stalin where he was. Trotsky subsequently described this scene: "I am in favor of preserving the status quo," he told Kamenev. "If Lenin gets on his feet for the Congress, which is not very likely, we will discuss the matter further. I am against liquidating Stalin, but agree with Lenin on the essential point. Stalin's resolution on the nationalities question is no good at all. . . . That apart, Stalin must immediately write Krupskaya a letter of apology."

In the middle of the night Kamenev informed Trotsky that Stalin had accepted all their conditions and that Krupskaya would receive a written apology. That was evidently when she persuaded Lenin not to send the letter. According to Maria Ulyanova's memoirs, "she told V.I. that she and Stalin had already made their peace."

Lenin consented. He was always able to control his impulses. He decided to prepare for another attack before sending the letter. But Stalin was evidently informed of everything that happened in Lenin's household. Maria Ulyanova recalled, "One morning Stalin called me into his office. He looked distraught. 'I didn't sleep at all last night,' he told me. 'What does Ilyich think I am, treating me as some sort of traitor, when I love him with all my heart? Try and let him know what I've said.' "

Stalin had decided to act the part of Koba one last time. But he had learned a very important lesson: Trotsky and Kamenev hated each other so much, and each so much feared the other's elevation, that they would both support him, even against Lenin's will.

The Indefatigable V.I.

Lenin had been living in the Kremlin. He should have left for Nizhny Novgorod but a heavy snowfall had blocked the road. He wasted no time. As soon as he felt a little better he resumed his offensive. At the end of December he began dictating his "Letter to the Congress"—a document which has gone down in history as "Lenin's Testament" because Lenin himself stipulated that it should be read out at the first Congress after his death, and not before. In this letter, he gave character sketches of his closest comrades-in-arms, noting the significant faults of each of them. He got to Stalin last, juxtaposing him with Trotsky.

> Relations between Stalin and Trotsky account for more than half the danger of the schism . . . which could be avoided . . . by increasing the membership of the Central Committee. . . . Since becoming Gensek Comrade Stalin has concentrated immense power in his own hands, and I am not sure that he will always succeed in using that power with the requisite caution. On the other hand, Comrade Trotsky is perhaps the ablest person in present Central Committee, but is too boastfully sure of himself and too carried away by the strictly administrative side of things.

The document was typed by a secretary, and the original drafts were burned. Copies were placed in envelopes marked "Strictly Secret," and sent to Krupskaya, to be opened only after Lenin's death.

But one copy, sealed with wax, remained in the Secretariat.

Why did the Leader, who was obsessively secretive, suddenly behave so naively? Did he truly believe that a copy passed to his Secretariat would remain unknown to his comrades-in-arms? Had he no inkling of the rule that servants do not carry out the wishes of former masters? Or of the fact that secretaries might not carry out the requests of their former chief?

Fotieva Takes Care of It

Fotieva's letter to Kamenev is still there in the Party Archive: "Comrade Stalin was given V.I.'s letter to the Congress on Saturday, December 23. . . . However, it transpired after this that V.I. wanted the letter to be kept strictly secret in Archives, and to be opened only by himself or by Krupskaya. . . . I asked those comrades who know the contents of this letter to . . . regard it as a record of V.I.'s personal opinion, which no one else was meant to know." Fotieva's letter is marked: "Read by Stalin. To Trotsky only." Trotsky said later, "Naturally, I told nobody about V.I.'s letter."

We see then that Fotieva failed to understand Lenin's instructions and "happened" to pass the letter immediately to Stalin. Stalin in turn passed it on to Trotsky and Kamenev. Why? Because it contained quite unflattering character sketches of both of them. Which meant that both of them were extremely anxious that no one else got wind of it. In this way Stalin made certain that he had allies in his effort to conceal the letter.

But at the beginning of January the indefatigable Lenin added a supplement to his text:

> Stalin is too rude. This is a fault which can easily be tolerated in our own circle, in dealings between fellow Communists, but it becomes intolerable in the office of Gensek. I therefore propose that some way be found of *transferring* Stalin from that post and appointing to it someone else who would differ from Stalin in one respect only, that he was more tolerant, more loyal, more polite, and more considerate, less capricious etc., in his dealings with comrades.

Lenin didn't leave it at that. He began writing a series of articles, one of which was sharply critical of Rabkrin, Stalin's former Commissariat.

Koba evidently heard about it immediately, and in February 1923 the doctor told Lenin that he was "categorically forbidden newspapers, visits, and political information." Fotieva plucked up her courage immediately after Stalin's death and recalled that "Lenin at once saw that these prohibitions were not simply doctor's orders. . . . He began to feel worse. They had upset him so much that his lips trembled. . . . V.I. obviously got the impression that it was not the doctors who were advising the Central Committee, but the Central Committee giving instructions to the doctors."

Lenin nonetheless thought of a way of escaping from Stalin's tutelage. On March 5 he suddenly sent Stalin a furious letter about the incident with Krupskaya (which had supposedly been laid to rest):

> Dear Comrade Stalin! You were so rude as to call my wife to the telephone and abuse her. Although she told you that she agreed to forget what had been said . . . I do not intend to forget so easily what was done against me, and needless to say I regard anything done against my wife as done against me. I ask you, therefore, to consider whether you are willing to take back what was said, or whether you prefer to break off relations between us.
>
> Respectfully yours,
> Lenin
> Copies to Comrades Kamenev and Zinoviev

This was Lenin's attempt to break out of jail. Surely a man with whom he had broken off relations could not continue keeping watch over him? Even if Stalin did apologize, he would find a way of prolonging the quarrel, so that the Central Committee would have to do something. Lenin did not know that Stalin had anticipated this move too. Already on February 1 he had asked the Politburo to relieve him of responsibility for looking after the sick Lenin. But Koba knew that Zinoviev and Kamenev were frightened by the dying leader's attempts to ally himself with their enemy Trotsky, and would not want Lenin to escape from his supervision. His expectations were realized. The Politburo turned down his request. So he was now, at the Party's request, Lenin's jailer forever.

"Help! . . . the Devil . . . Oh, the Devil . . ."

Stalin received Lenin's letter next morning. But he was unperturbed. He had heard what had happened the previous night. Lenin's rage had cost him dearly, and during the night he had lost the gift of speech. He kept whispering disconnected phrases and inarticulate sounds, which the doctors recorded: "Help—oh . . . the devil . . . devil . . . evi helped, if it . . . evi. . . ." "Evi" was obviously "the devil" again. And although the former Leader recovered his speech toward morning, Stalin was in no doubt: the devil could be of no more help to him. It would be soon!

Stalin promptly wrote his reply. That letter would be kept hidden for decades in a secret archive. I am now reading it—the last letter from the former Koba to the former Leader.

> Comrade Lenin! Five weeks ago I had a conversation with Comrade Nadezhda Konstantinovna [Krupskaya]. . . . I spoke to her by telephone approximately as follows: "The doctors have forbidden anyone to give Ilyich political information. . . . You, however, seem to be disrupting this regimen. You must not play with Ilyich's life," and so on. I do not think that anyone could find anything rude in these words . . . anything aimed "against you." However, if you think that in order to preserve relations between us I ought to take back the words mentioned above I can take them back, though unable to understand what it is all about, where I am to blame, and what exactly is wanted of me.

A stiff letter. Time for this semicorpse to realize that Koba was dead, and that Stalin did not stand on ceremony. Lenin, however, never read it.

On March 10 Stalin heard that a stroke had deprived Lenin of the ability to read and write, and of speech.

A Wife Asks for Poison

Stalin received a request which he immediately reported in writing to members of the Politburo. On March 17 Krupskaya, "in the strictest secrecy, . . . communicated to me V. I. Ilyich's request to obtain and pass on to him a quantity of potassium cyanide. . . . N.K. said that V. I. Ilyich's suffering was beyond belief. . . . I must declare that I lack the strength to carry out the request and I am compelled to refuse this mission . . . and hereby inform the Politburo accordingly." The unfortunate Leader was by now scarcely able to think at all. Krupskaya herself was trying to carry out his former wish and spare him from further suffering. In fact, Stalin informed his friends in the triumvirate, Zinoviev and Kamenev, that "Nadezhda Konstantinovna said . . . she had 'tried to give him cyanide' but 'couldn't go through with it,' and so was 'asking for Stalin's support.' " But Stalin was a connoisseur of character. He knew that his partners would subsequently accuse him. No, Ilyich must oblige by dying unaided. The members of the Politburo naturally approved his decision. So now his hands were clean.

THE CLAIMANTS

The struggle in the Kremlin now began in earnest. It was a fight not merely for power, but for life. Each of the claimants knew how to make political enemies pay in blood. These were leaders molded by the Civil War and the Red Terror and in Lenin's academies. They thought of the country as a "fortress under siege," and in such conditions ruthlessness was the supreme virtue. Trotsky, neatly summing up their common creed, spoke of "priestly—or quakerish—driveling about the sanctity of human life." So each of them knew what the price of defeat might be. Stalin alone was extremely cautious in calling for blood. He seemed more moderate than the others. His record included no bloody words. Only bloody deeds. And, as a rule, secret deeds.

How did the claimants compare? Stalin, incontestably, came first. He did not, of course, have Trotsky's fame. He had little fame, but a great deal of power. Lenin had concentrated power over the Party in *his* hands, and power over the country in the Party's hands. He controlled the whole central Party machine and the local Party committees—the 15,000 Party functionaries with dictatorial power over the country's political and economic life were his protégés.

After Stalin came the Kamenev-Zinoviev duo. Kamenev was chairman of the Moscow Soviet and Lenin's deputy in the Council of People's Commissars, "an exceptionally capable and willing workhorse," one who could "pull two carts at once," Lenin said of him. Zinoviev was head man in Petrograd and also presided over Comintern.

Finally there was Trotsky. He was in charge of the republic's armed forces. But the army had been scaled down by demobilization. Thanks to Lenin's efforts his "brother-enemy" was now the least influential of the claimants, the farthest removed from all key posts. Nonetheless, Trotsky was still the glamorous Second Leader of the Revolution.

One last name—Bukharin, editor of *Pravda,* and the Party's leading theoretician. He was not himself a contender. But it was very important whom he chose to support.

Trotsky was first off the mark. On March 13 the newspapers published a guarded bulletin on "the deterioration in Lenin's health." Next day an article by one of Trotsky's closest associates, Karl Radek, appeared in *Pravda*: "Lev Trotsky: Organizer of Our Victories." To the man in the street, and to ordinary Party members, this must have looked like a signal: Trotsky was to be the Leader's successor. Trotsky was now in a hurry for the Congress.

The Twelfth Party Congress—the last not completely orchestrated by Stalin—was held in April. At the Congress Trotsky's supporters spread rumors of some sort of will in which Lenin named Trotsky as his successor. Trotsky delivered a brilliant speech on the state of industry. It was greeted with thunderous applause. "Indecent—Lenin never got a reception like that," Voroshilov commented. It enraged the envious Zinoviev and frightened Kamenev. Fear of Trotsky finally forced Kamenev, Zinoviev, and Bukharin to ally themselves with the Gensek. Stalin was the force which could stand up to the very dangerous Lev.

In May the publication of bulletins on Lenin's health ceased. The country was told that the threat to his life had passed, and began to believe that he had indeed returned to work. This was Stalin's idea. Armed with a special decision of the Central Committee, he introduced a "check on all information concerning Ilyich's health." Trotsky was obliged to obtain information from Dr. F. Gautier, his own doctor as well as one of Lenin's. Stalin had Gautier removed.

In May Lenin was moved to Nizhny Novgorod. He was carried to the car on a stretcher. The unfortunate Leader wore a mindless smile.

By order of the Gensek, several photographs of Lenin were taken around this time, and the artist Annenkov was called in to paint a final portrait. "Semirecumbent in a chaise longue, wrapped up in a blanket, and staring past us with the blank stare of a man in second childhood, Lenin could serve as a model only for an illustration of his own illness," Annenkov noted. But Stalin wanted documentary proof that in the last phase of his life Lenin had been imbecile, so that his last jottings might look like a product of feeble-mindedness. Krupskaya, however, vetoed the portrait. On May 6, 1923, she wrote to Inessa Armand, the daughter of Lenin's mistress (also Inessa), who had died in 1920. "You reproach me for not writing to you, but you cannot possibly imagine what things are like here . . . there are no words for what is going on at present. . . . Everybody has left us—they express sympathy but are afraid to call on us. The only thing that keeps me going is that Volodya is glad to see me in the morning, he takes my hand, and sometimes we exchange a few words about things for which however there are no words."

Lenin Improves

Lenin not only survived—he began to improve. Stalin no longer visited Nizhny Novgorod and he allowed no one else to do so, alleging that this was the sick man's own wish. Lenin still could not speak, but he was hard at work. Exercise books which Krupskaya used to teach the Leader to speak are preserved in the Party Archive: "This is our dog. Its name is Jack. It is playing. . . ." The words which Lenin repeated most successfully were *proletariat, people, revolution, bourgeois, Congress,* etc. Words and phrases disappeared from his memory as fast as he mastered them, but his understanding of what others were saying was restored. And he no longer had difficulty in analyzing what was happening. For instance, because he liked picking mushrooms they "used to collect a few in advance and plant them beside the path along which he was usually taken in his wheelchair," recalled Dr. V. Osipov, one of his doctors. "On one occasion, he touched a mushroom with his cane and it fell over. This underestimation of his intellectual capacity greatly annoyed him."

The doctors' case notes were always read carefully by the Gensek. He was kept informed, among other things, of the dangerous fits of anger which alarmed those present. Lenin was in a hurry to get well. Krupskaya recalled that "I used to say 'see—your speech is coming back, but slowly. Think of it as a temporary stay in jail.' " Lenin knew that he was in jail, and was evidently thinking furiously of ways to break out.

Tovstukha was now working furiously, collecting Lenin's documents. I found in the Party Archive a warrant authorizing Tovstukha to remove documents originating with Lenin from the archives of his comrades-in-arms. Stalin was planning another game of chess. One in which these documents would be invaluable.

Meanwhile anonymous brochures with such titles as "Small Biography of a Big Man" were beginning to find their way round Moscow. They set out to prove, using quotations from Lenin himself, that Trotsky had always been against him. This "bathroom literature," as Trotsky contemptuously called it, was disseminated in the provinces too. Tovstukha was doing his job.

"You've Got It Too Good, My Friends"

In summer 1923 most of the leaders went on holiday. Zinoviev and Bukharin made for Kislovodsk, leaving Kamenev in Moscow.

The Gensek, needless to say, stayed put in sweltering Moscow. He had no time for holidays. It was work, endless work. Besides, the strange improvement in the Leader's health troubled him.

During the summer intermission in their fight with Trotsky, Zinoviev and Bukharin resolved to put pressure on Stalin, and make him share power with them. The holiday-makers wrote to him in a humorous vein: "29.07.23 . . . Two ordinary citizens propose the introduction of Zinoviev, Trotsky, and Stalin into the secretariat, to consolidate it."

The purpose of the letter was not, however, humorous. Their idea was to level the odds. If they succeeded, he would be compelled to ally himself with Zinoviev in order to defeat Trotsky—in other words, to carry out their decisions. Stalin must indeed have been amused. They seemed to take him for an idiot.

At the same time Zinoviev wrote to Kamenev: ". . . and you allow Stalin to treat us with undisguised contempt. [He mentions innumerable examples of Stalin's highhanded behavior while they were away on vacation.] We are not going to put up with it any longer." The Gensek, of course, knew about their correspondence. The trusty GPU was already keeping an eye on each of them. But he knew the way to calm them down. He wrote to Bukharin and Zinoviev, telling them that he did not "know what to do to stop you abusing me. It would have been better if you had written me a little note in clear and precise terms. Always supposing, of course, that you think it possible for us to go working together in future (for . . . I have begun to realize that you are half-inclined to hasten the breach which you think unavoidable). . . . Do what you think best. In 8–10 days time I am going on leave (I'm tired, worn out). All the best. PS. How lucky you people are. You have the leisure to think up all sorts of crazy things, . . . while I'm here doing the heavy work, miserable as a dog on a chain. Which is all my own fault. This is enough to get anybody down. You've got it too good, my friends! J. St."

This ploy never failed. The hint that he might resign terrified them: if he went, Trotsky might step in. He could use the same trick on Trotsky—who also knew that if he went, Zinoviev and Kamenev would move in. They were indeed afraid of the "rough, primitive Georgian." But they were much more frightened of each other. Their hatred of each other ensured that Stalin would win the endgame.

Zinoviev and Kamenev wrote back immediately: "All this talk about a breach is, of course, just the result of your tiredness. It is out of the question. Where are you thinking of going on vacation? Regards."

He had made a close study of these gentlemen. They weren't afraid only of Trotsky. They were afraid of work. They did not like the hard grind. They preferred representational roles. Let *him* get on with the work. Well, so he would. He wrote to them at once about Lenin's "Letter to the Congress." He of course knew all about the letter. He wanted to find out how much they knew.

On August 10, 1923, they responded: "Yes, there is a letter from V.I. in which he advises the Congress not to elect you Secretary. We—Bukharin, Kamenev and I [Zinoviev]—decided not to tell you about it for the time being . . . for the obvious reason that . . . we did not want to upset you. But these are all small matters. The essential point is that *there is no Ilyich now.* The Secretariat of the Central Committee (with no disrespect to you) in practice *decides everything.* Collaboration on an equal footing is impossible with our present setup. Hence our efforts to find a better form of collaboration. We do not doubt for a minute that we shall come to an arrangement."

They still lived in hope that he would voluntarily give up the machine he had created. How this must have amused him.

But one thing may have worried him. *They* thought that "there is no Ilyich now": *he* was horrified to see Lenin recovering!

Krupskaya observed, "From July he started recovering rapidly, he was soon able not only to sit up but even to walk, with the aid of a cane . . . and his speech began to come back to him—in October, as it happened."

Another event in October must have come as a great shock to Stalin: Lenin put in an appearance in Moscow. But as soon as he returned to Nizhny Novgorod the nightmare began again. His recovery was cut short, and Lenin began to die. Can something have happened during his visit to Moscow?

A Kremlin Mystery

"One fine morning," Krupskaya wrote, "he went to the garage unaided, got into the car and insisted on being driven to Moscow. . . . When he got there he went round all the rooms, called at his office, looked in on Sovnarkom, sorted out his copybooks, collected three volumes of Hegel, . . . and then decided to go for a ride round the city. Next day he was in a hurry to get back to Nizhny Novgorod. Moscow wasn't mentioned again."

But there was someone else in the car with him besides his faithful wife. Maria Ulyanova accompanied them. Krupskaya's failure to mention it is not due to mere forgetfulness.

N. Valentinov, of whom we have heard before, has published a story attributed to Maria Ulyanova: "All the way from Nizhny Novgorod Lenin kept hurrying the driver up. . . . After looking in at his office in Sovnarkom Lenin went to his apartment. He spent a long time searching for something there. He got extremely annoyed about it, and went into convulsions. . . . Maria told the doctor about it when she arrived. . . . Krupskaya called the doctor in afterward and said: 'V.I. is sick. He may have a somewhat distorted view of things. I don't want the rumor to get around that letters or documents have been stolen from him. A rumor of that sort can only cause great unpleasantness. Please forget everything that Maria Ilyinishna said to you . . . she joins me in this request.' " But what was it Lenin was looking for in his office?

Lenin's "Letter to the Congress" leaves us with a distinct impression that something is left unsaid. For instance, Lenin writes to the Congress about Stalin's "immense power," and expresses his apprehension that he will not always "use it cautiously enough." Should Stalin, then, be relieved of his post? Lenin makes no such suggestion. What is more, as if to demonstrate that there is no one to replace Stalin, he gives unflattering character sketches of other Party leaders. So he is not to be removed? What then should be done? All that is needed, apparently, is to enlarge the membership of the Central Committee by bringing in more workers. Are these workers supposed to curb the lust for power of Stalin and the other Party bosses? Can Lenin really have been so naive? After Stalin's rudeness to Krupskaya Lenin added another paragraph in which he now demanded Stalin's "transfer from the post of Gensek." Did he leave it at that, with no recommendation for a replacement? No name mentioned? That could cause chaos. A Leader cannot leave his Party without precise instructions. They must have been there. But where are they now?

With all his political experience Lenin was bound to realize that a letter containing such demeaning descriptions of all his heirs might simply never reach the Party. It would unite them in the wish to suppress it. (That, incidentally, is what actually happened. When the American Communist Max Eastman once mentioned it, Trotsky promptly declared that no such letter existed.)

Another strange thing: of all those mentioned in the letter Stalin appears in the most favorable light. He is the one Lenin accuses of rudeness and intolerance, but that was never regarded as a fault in the proletarian party. And the postscript calling for Stalin's transfer could be regarded as an emotional outburst, the result of Stalin's clash with Krupskaya. Surely a brilliant journalist like Lenin could not fail to realize all this if he had been eager to remove Stalin. So where does that leave us?

The most likely explanation is that the text that has come down to us is only part of the letter and that the expert conspirator Lenin deliberately left this variant in the Secretariat, allowing for the unreliability of the office staff, and for Koba's hyperactivity. This text was meant for Koba-Stalin.

Was there then, another, fuller, text? If so, he might have kept it in a secret place in his Kremlin office. Possibly his proposals to the Congress were also there. Was there a recommendation, for example, to replace the Gensek with a triumvirate of secretaries—Trotsky, Zinoviev, and Stalin? A proposal which would reduce Stalin's influence to nothing?

It may be that a story told by Annenkov, the artist, shows traces of this full text. After Lenin's death the artist, working in the Lenin Institute, saw there a jar containing the Leader's brain. He was astonished to find that one of the cerebral hemispheres was healthy, and of normal weight, while the other seemed to be hanging by a thread and was shriveled, no bigger than a walnut. He also saw in the institute rough drafts of Lenin's last writings, which utterly amazed him. These were Lenin's recommendations on ways of deceiving "deaf-mutes"—the name used here for Western European capitalists. Annenkov reproduces them in his own words: "In their pursuit of profit the capitalists of the whole world will want to conquer the Soviet market. Blinded by their greed for gain they will be ready to close their eyes to our activities, to turn themselves into deaf-mutes. As a result we shall obtain from them the goods and the money to create an army. Their capital will raise it to the level of perfection. For a future victorious attack on our own creditors. We will make the deaf-mutes work for their own destruction, but to do so we must first do a thorough job of turning them into deaf-mutes." This was followed by a plan in outline: NEP, the fictitious separation of Party and government, reestablishment of relations with all countries, do everything possible to make the deaf-mutes believe, etc.

Lenin's intention in visiting his Kremlin office was to check the full text of his "Letter to the Congress." But the Gensek too was an experienced conspirator. He had anticipated something of the sort, and had already checked the office himself. The text had vanished. Hence, obviously, the unhappy Leader's seizure. The last lines of a note written by

Maria Ulyanova shortly before she died read as follows: "V.I. valued Stalin as a practical worker, but thought it essential to find some means of restraining his idiosyncrasies and his oddities, on account of which he thought that Stalin should be removed from the post of Gensek. He said so specifically in his political testament, which never reached the Party, but I will deal with that on another occasion."

There was no other occasion. Maria died soon after. Or was there? Did she write later about the missing testament? And did Ulyanova pay for the "other occasion" with her life?

11

THE END OF THE OCTOBER LEADERS

Trotsky Attacks

Trotsky realized the full horror of the dying Leader's legacy. The secret resolution forbidding factionalism, ordered by Lenin and adopted at the Tenth Party Congress in 1921, made it possible for Trotsky's enemies to shut his mouth at any time. All they needed was a simple majority, and that was provided for: the Gensek had organized it in advance. In a letter to the Central Committee, yesterday's champion of the toughest methods possible now called for Party democracy. At the same time, a letter repeating Trotsky's demands for democracy and signed by forty-six prominent Party members was sent to the Central Committee. Among these latter-day supporters of democracy was Alexander Beloborodov, former Party boss of the Red Urals, who had organized the execution of the tsar and his family at Ekaterinburg, and was now Dzherzhinsky's deputy in the bloody Cheka. Other equally ruthless Bolsheviks had also signed the letter. In his reply the Gensek ridiculed them: "In the ranks of the opposition we find such comrades as Comrade Beloborodov, whose democratism lingers on in the memories of Russian workers, Rozengoltz, whose democratism did little for the health of workers on our waterways and railroads, Pyatakov, whose democratism had the Donbas not just crying out but howling." He went through the whole list of signatories, recalling the bloody deeds of which they had so recently been guilty.

But his allies in the triumvirate were frightened and unsure of themselves. Knowing how they feared Trotsky, he met them halfway, and at the same time took the wind out of Trotsky's sails, with promises to follow the Party's electoral traditions, and other fine words. He had, however, studied Lev closely enough to know that concessions would only whet his appetite. Sure enough, the "permanently inflamed Lev Davidovich," as his enemies laughingly called him, sent *Pravda* an article entitled "A New Course," repeating his denunciation: "Leadership is degenerating into mere command. We must put an end to this old course and adopt a New Course. The degeneration of our old guard (i.e., Stalin, Zinoviev, Kamenev, etc.) is not precluded. We must look to the young." Trotsky had thereby compelled Stalin's timorous comrades-in-arms to join the fight.

Kamenev and Zinoviev were not long in replying. Bukharin also spoke out: "Bolshevism always did, and still does, value the apparat." Heated discussion followed. "The Party was in a fever. Debates went on night after night, all night long," Zinoviev wrote later. The country read the newspapers with astonishment: the Party which had constantly stressed its unity was torn by controversy over the need for democracy in the Party, while a country crushed by terror looked on. (My father and his friends, as he often told me, were sure that all these debates were a cunning farce, to be followed by new calamities for the intelligentsia.)

To the delight of his allies, Stalin demonstrated for the first time the strength of the apparat he had created. A Party conference, the first organized by him, was held in January 1924. It was unsparing in its condemnation of Trotsky and the opposition, and it decided that the secret resolution (Lenin's resolution) "on expulsion from the Party for factional activity" should be made public for the first time. Trotsky had always acted alone: in 1917 he had been able to make use of an organization created by Lenin. His calculation now was that he could take the conference by storm. But this was the twentieth century: the age of individuals was over.

Death and Deification: The Imperishable God

By October the previous year Lenin had given up the struggle and was rapidly sinking. The Leader who had once been such a brilliant seminarist devised an unprecedented propaganda campaign which might have been called "Departure of the Messiah." Stalin had taken the measure of this country long ago. Under the Romanovs, during the Revolution, in the past and in the future, it was forever looking for a god and tsar. (We shall hear his own formulation of this idea later.) He decided to present it with a new god, in place of the one overthrown by the Bolsheviks. An atheist Messiah, the God Lenin.

In the autumn months he was already planning the "Ascension." He sent delegations to Nizhny Novgorod. Ritual farewells to the Messiah were instituted: representatives of the toiling masses vowed to the departing God that they would continue his immortal work. Representatives of the heroic Red army made their farewells. Lenin was enrolled for all eternity as an honorary Red army man, and presented with a bundle containing his uniform. In November the half-dead Lenin had to receive the proletariat as represented by a delegation from the Glukhov factory. An old workman delivered greetings which were also an epitaph: "I am a blacksmith. . . . We shall forge all that you have designed."

Lenin still had several months to live when the Gensek first spoke about his funeral in the Politburo: "I learn that this question is also a matter of great concern to some of our provincial comrades." He went on to report a surprising request made by those comrades: "Do not bury Vladimir Ilyich. It is essential that Ilyich remains physically with us." Trotsky, who was present, realized that Stalin intended to transform the atheist Ulyanov into a sacred relic to be worshiped by the faithful. Molotov recalls that "Krupskaya was against it, but we did it by decision of the Central Committee. Stalin insisted." He had his way and produced an imperishable Marxist god.

He had thought of everything. When the death of the God was imminent, doctors advised the ailing Trotsky to take a cure at Sukhumi. After Lev's departure Stalin saw to it that none of the remaining leaders visited Lenin, in case one of them turned up at the Messiah's bedside at the very moment when he began withdrawing into eternity, and turned the dying man's mumblings into "last words" to suit himself.

But it happened just as he feared. Bukharin, who was receiving medical treatment right there in Nizhny Novgorod, appeared at Lenin's bedside. He described that "when I rushed into Ilyich's room . . . he heaved one last sigh. His head fell backward, his face was terribly pale, I could hear a hoarse gurgle, his arms went slack."

Stalin corrected Bukharin's mistake, simply wiped him out of the deathbed scene, transferred him from Nizhny Novgorod to Moscow. As a result, Zinoviev was shortly writing in an article that "Ilyich had died. . . . An hour later we were on our way to Nizhny Novgorod where Ilyich was already lying dead—Bukharin, Tomsky, Kalinin, Stalin, Kamenev, and I."

Trotsky would later speak of "Stalin's poison." But this is irrelevant. Professor V. Shklovsky, son of the eminent physician M. Shklovsky, found in his father's records the testimony (originally meant to be destroyed) of V. Osipov, one of the senior doctors attending Lenin, and the speech therapist S. Dobrogayev. We read in particular that "the final diagnosis dismisses the stories of the syphilitic character of Lenin's disease, or of arsenic poisoning. It was atherosclerosis, mainly affecting the cerebral blood vessels. The calcium deposit was so thick that during dissection the tweezers made a noise as if they were rapping on stone. Lenin's parents also died of this disease." But the story that Lenin had been poisoned would never die. Stalin killed too many others for anyone to believe that he had not also sent his most dangerous enemy to the grave.

While preparations were being made for Lenin's funeral, a telegram was sent to Trotsky: "Funeral takes place on Saturday, you cannot get here in time. The Politburo thinks that the state of your health makes it essential for you to go to Sukhumi. Stalin."

In fact the funeral had been postponed until Sunday. But Stalin was not simply lying. Where there is a god there are loyal and disloyal disciples. The disloyal, who have insulted the Messiah in his lifetime, must not be present at his obsequies.

Stalin devised a grandiose plan for the God's funeral. The arrival of the Body by train was a solemn ceremony in itself (the compartment which held the sacred remains and the locomotive which pulled it would be stationed forever in a building clad in granite and marble). The loyal disciples devotedly bore the precious Body from the station across Moscow to the Hall of Columns of the House of Unions. Few of those helping to carry the Lord's coffin would survive.

At 7:00 P.M. the public were admitted to the Hall of Columns. The God Lenin lay there in his khaki tunic. And Stalin, also wearing a tunic, kept vigil over him. People filed past all night long. The frost was incredible, and bonfires were lit. There was a frozen mist; people were wreathed in the steam of their own breath.

The Body had been embalmed on the morning of January 22. It was a temporary job, done so that the Messiah could lie in state in the Hall of Columns for several days. But Stalin had thought up a fantastic scheme: he would show that the Bolsheviks could conquer even death. The God would be imperishable. Thousands of telegrams from workers called for postponement of the funeral. In response to the wishes of them and millions of others, the Kremlin announced: "It has been decided to preserve the coffin with Lenin's body in a special Mausoleum on Red Square near the Kremlin wall." Simultaneously, "at the request of the workers of Petrograd" the capital of the Romanov empire was renamed Leningrad.

By the end of January a wooden mausoleum designed by A. Shchusev had been erected over the coffin. Stalin meanwhile was working out the details of the new cult. "Red corners" in honor of Lenin would be set up all over the country. At one time the "red corner" was where the icons were hung in a peasant hut. Now portraits of the God Lenin would hang there.

Behind the closed doors of the Mausoleum Stalin's unprecedented idea was already being realized. When experts declared that contemporary science lacked the means of preserving a body for any considerable length of time, other experts were found. The anatomist Vladimir Vorobyov and the young biochemist Boris Zbarsky undertook to embalm the body as required.

The scientists worked day and night, and Stalin himself went down into the Mausoleum several times. He obtained a result in time for the Thirteenth Congress in May. Kamenev, presiding, announced on the second day that after the morning session delegates would be able to see Lenin in his new immortal guise. They were stunned. Asked by Zbarsky whether "the likeness has been preserved," Lenin's brother said, "I can't say anything, I'm overcome. He's lying there looking just as he did when I saw him after he died." Thus, Stalin's present to the first Congress held without Lenin was—Lenin.

When he had created an empire, he would rebuild the wretched little wooden Mausoleum in marble, porphyry, and labradorite, with columns of different kinds of granite. Such would be made the dwelling place of the imperishable God, his holiest shrine in the atheist empire. Krupskaya, when she lived in the Kremlin complex, often went down into the Mausoleum. Zbarsky tells us that "six months or so before she died she visited the Mausoleum. She stared for a long time, and then said 'he's just the same, and I'm getting so old.' "

In the West, not everybody believed in the "ever-living" Lenin. They alleged that the figure lying in the Mausoleum was a wax doll. So Stalin arranged in the thirties for a group of Western journalists to be shown the relics worshiped by Bolsheviks. Lenin's biographer, Louis Fischer, was one of their number. He has described how "Zbarsky opened the glass case containing the remains, and pinched Lenin's nose. Then he turned his head to right and left. That was no wax doll. It was Lenin. The iconoclast had become a relic."

Stalin had given them their imperishable God. Next he must give them a tsar.

GENERAL SECRETARY, NOW AND FOREVER

The Thirteenth Party Congress had arrived. Lenin's "Letter to the Congress" was to be read there. On the eve of the Congress Krupskaya solemnly presented the Central Committee with certain sealed packets.

Emelyan Yaroslavsky recalled that "when these few pages written by Lenin were read to the members of the Central Committee the reaction was one of incomprehension and alarm." It was true. The members of the Central Committee could not understand what Lenin wanted. Why was he abusing all the leaders, without suggesting any replacement? Why should Stalin be driven out of the Secretariat if all he could be reproached with was rudeness? Besides, they all knew that it was Lenin, not Stalin himself, who had "concentrated power" in the Gensek's hands. It was all rather embarrassing because it seemed that the only reason for these attacks was that Ilyich's wife had been offended. That Stalin was terrified of this letter, that he was saved by Kamenev, and so on, is mere legend. Kamenev spoke for everyone when he said that "our dear Ilyich's sickness prevented him at times from being fair. And since Stalin has already confessed to the character faults noted by Lenin and will, of course, correct them, we should begin by accepting the possibility of leaving Stalin in the post of Secretary General." And so, out of concern for Lenin's reputation, it was resolved that these "sickbed documents" should not be reproduced. They would be read to each delegation separately.

Stalin's hand-picked Congress, with support from Kamenev and Zinoviev, swallowed the letter without difficulty. Trotsky remained silent. The Congress was followed by a plenary meeting of the Central Committee, to elect its General Secretary. This was where Stalin made one of his favorite moves. He offered his resignation: that was what the Messiah had wanted, and for him the will of the God Lenin was sacred. It happened exactly as he expected: they all—Trotsky, Kamenev, and Zinoviev, because they hated each other—voted unanimously that he should remain. So now he had become Gensek at their wish. From now on he could tell them all that "you got what you asked for!"

On January 31, 1924, he had announced the "Leninist draft"—a mass recruiting drive to enlarge the Party. It was as if the God Lenin was appealing to his people from the grave. The Party gained 240,000 new members. By 1930 almost 70 percent of Party members had joined during Stalin's tenure as Gensek. He was preparing the Party for the game he meant to play.

TROTSKY OUTMANEUVERED

"Lessons of October," Trotsky titled his crucial new article. In it he disingenuously lauded the departed God Lenin for resurrecting *his,* Trotsky's, theory of permanent revolution, harnessing an inert Party, and—together with Trotsky—leading it to victory, despite the craven behavior of Zinoviev and Kamenev. This was yet another reminder that he, Trotsky, was the October leader, that Zinoviev and Kamenev were cowards, that Stalin was simply irrelevant, and further that the Party had always been inert. The implication was obvious: why should anyone submit to the Party majority?

This was suicide. Zinoviev and Kamenev immediately fell upon the weakened Trotsky, and Stalin joined in the chorus of outrage. Forgetting his previous utterances, Stalin coolly asserted that "Comrade Trotsky did not, and could not, play any special part either in the Party or in the October Revolution." He had learned it from Lenin, of course: to the Leader, all things are permitted. This was the beginning of a campaign to separate Lev from the Messiah. Trotsky's disagreements with the God Lenin were harped on endlessly. Trotsky agreed that he had come to Lenin struggling, but asserted that ultimately he had come over to him fully and completely. He was the former sinner who had become the apostle Paul. The others had now to show that his conversion was not genuine. Stalin drew the chief ideologist, Bukharin, into the fight, and he found new and deadly ammunition in Lenin's last articles.

Lenin had in the past often asserted that a socialist society could not be constructed in a single country, and Trotsky, following his lead, had often repeated this "elementary Marxist truth." Now here was Bukharin triumphantly quoting Lenin's last article, "On Cooperation," in which he said, "All the conditions for building socialism already exist in Russia." This was by no means all that Bukharin found in Lenin's last articles. Lenin, he also pointed out, spoke of an alliance with the peasants, whereas Trotsky was still repeating Lenin's earlier belief that clashes with this hostile class were inevitable. Trotsky could not argue that Lenin's last articles were merely a maneuver, that they were written in the context of the temporary New Economic Policy, to deceive the "deaf-mutes." The God could not, of course, be guilty of low cunning. Thus, the "ever-living" Ilyich reached out from his Mausoleum to finish off his eternal friend-and-enemy.

Zinoviev and Kamenev moved at a plenary meeting of the Central Committee that Trotsky should be expelled from the Party—only to be opposed by Stalin. To the amazement of his allies, who wanted blood, Stalin persuaded the Central Committee not to expel Trotsky, nor even to remove him from the Politburo. They did not realize that the game was still in its opening stage. It was not yet time to remove a once powerful piece from the board. On the contrary, it would soon be their turn to leave the board, while Trotsky, who hated them, might prove useful to the Gensek in dealing with the "victors"—for that was how these foolish fellows now thought of themselves. But while leaving Lev in the Politburo he clipped his claws. Trotsky lost his post as chairman of the Revolutionary Military Council: the founder of the Red army was removed from the army. A letter from P. A. Koloskov reads in part:

> Bazhanov, Stalin's secretary at the time, who later escaped to the West, correctly describes Trotsky's finale. My father told the same story. . . . Trotsky made a thunderous speech. And rushed towards the exit. He intended to slam the door as he left. But the session was taking place in the Throne Room of the Kremlin Palace. The door was, as it happened, too heavy. Some doors can't be slammed. The wretched fellow ended up wrestling with the door handle. . . . But it wasn't all one big joke. The day before, Trotsky's supporters had put it to him that while he was still in charge of the army he should have Stalin, Zinoviev, etc. arrested as traitors to the Revolution. This was in the evening. Night fell, and there was still no answer from Trotsky. By then the other camp knew all about it. It was a night of acute anxiety. Koba sat in a corner sucking his pipe, then suddenly vanished. Zinoviev, in hysterics, sent people to look for him. He was nowhere to be found. At dawn Trotsky told his associates that he would not do it. He could not let the Party accuse him of that most terrible of sins for a revolutionary—Bonapartism. The Party's major dogma was that all political activity outside the Party was counterrevolutionary. An appeal to the people or the army would lead to the creation of a new Napoleon and ruin the Party. The freedom-loving Trotsky was also the supreme dogmatist. He was like the wolf who would sooner face a bullet than run past the red flags. Koba reappeared next morning as suddenly as he had vanished.

His next moves were made quickly. M. Frunze was put in charge of the army. A prominent Civil War commander, Frunze was not Stalin's man, which was why Zinoviev and Kamenev supported his appointment. Frunze was given the task of reorganizing the army. Of the old unruly army only the officers and NCOs were retained. The new army was drawn from the peasant youth called up in the autumn. Once that was done, Frunze developed an ulcer, and when his condition became acute a dubious operation was performed on him, by order of the Politburo. He died on the operating table, and his wife, convinced that he had been murdered, committed suicide. Stalin's loyal servant Klim Voroshilov was now put in charge of the Red army. The maneuver paid off. Voroshilov, who looked like a florid counter-jumper, hated the brilliant Tukhachevsky, whom some people, greatly daring, called Napoleon. War between them was inevitable, but then again, Voroshilov also hated Trotsky and was not likely to forget his humiliation at Tsaritsyn. So what lay ahead was a ruthless purge of Trotskyists in the army. Stalin had appointed the right man.

The Right Is Right . . . for the Moment

It was now Zinoviev's and Kamenev's turn. Stalin made the last remaining leader, Bukharin, his ally. Bukharin was now at the head of a faction known in the Party as "rightist." He and his associates, the Trades Union chief Tomsky and the chairman of the Council of People's Commissars, Rykov, were in favor of prolonging NEP and of the alliance with the middle peasantry, and against collectivization, against superindustrialization, against war on the kulak. In short, they favored unhurried, peaceful development. Bukharin quoted copiously from Lenin's last articles: everything now had to be reinforced with quotations from the God. Bukharin's enemies, however, could produce plenty of quotations contradicting him, also from the God.

On April 14, 1925, *Pravda* published an article by Bukharin with a slogan addressed to the peasants: "Enrich yourselves, develop your holdings. And don't worry that they may be taken away from you." The country sighed with relief. With Trotsky's fall things were obviously beginning to change for the better.

Old Party members were flabbergasted by Bukharin's slogan. A rich peasant! This was a knockout blow to utopia. Kamenev asked Stalin for an explanation. Stalin puffed at his pipe enigmatically and said nothing. Zinoviev and Kamenev decided that it was time to call Bukharin to order. By destroying Bukharin they would give Stalin a bit of a scare. He had lured this foolish pair out into the open: they now spent all their time sniping at Bukharin, while Stalin remained silent. Waiting. The decisive battle was joined at the Fourteenth Congress in December 1925. Zinoviev declared, "There exists within the Party a most dangerous right deviation. It lies in the underestimation of the danger from the kulak—the rural capitalist. The kulak, uniting with the urban capitalists, the NEP men, and the bourgeois intelligentsia will devour the Party and the Revolution."

Stalin would reproduce Zinoviev's thoughts almost word for word some years later, when he himself was ready to destroy Bukharin and the other right-wingers. But now it was the turn of Zinoviev and Kamenev. For the time being he passionately defended Bukharin: "You want Bukharin's blood? We shall not let you have his blood."

Bukharin would recall these words as he went to his death thirteen years later. But one of Stalin's rejoinders augured ill for the rightists: "But if you ask Communists what the Party most wants, I think 99 Communists out of 100 would say that the Party wants above all to hear the slogan 'Beat the kulak.' " Although he was defending Bukharin, he knew very well that the Party was eager to continue the revolution and to have done with the hated capitalists and the hated NEP—that betrayal of the Great Utopia. Even then, as he thought over his future moves, he had no doubt that the Party would applaud him when the time came to deal with the rightists. Meanwhile, history was repeating itself in a most amusing way: the ruthless sanctions which Zinoviev and Kamenev had tried to invoke against Trotsky were now invoked against them by the hyperintellectual Bukharin.

From start to finish the proceedings of the Fourteenth Congress had a surprising accompaniment. When Lenin had dismissed the Constituent Assembly organized uproar had been one of his ploys. Stalin now made use of this example. Kamenev tried in vain to shout above the noise of a frenzied audience: "You will not force me to be silent, however loudly a small group of comrades may shout. . . . Stalin cannot play the part of unifier of the Bolshevik general staff. We are against one-man rule, against the creation of a Leader!" To which the whole hall yelled in reply: "Untrue! Rubbish! We want Stalin! Stalin!" The stenographic record is one continuous "voice from the hall," supposedly personifying the people, identified here with the lower levels of the Party.

Koba's handpicked Congress was not merely obedient. The delegates no longer believed in the sincerity of those arguing on the platform. Yesterday Zinoviev and Kamenev had joined Stalin in attacking Trotsky, today Zinoviev and Kamenev sided with Trotsky against Stalin. The Leningrad dictator, bloodstained Zinoviev, now demanding democracy, made just as strange a spectacle as the dictator Trotsky calling for democracy. The shrewd Mikoyan summed it up neatly: "When Zinoviev has a majority he is in favor of iron discipline, when he hasn't he is against it." The delegates knew by now that this was all merely a struggle for power. Ideas no longer mattered. So they eagerly demonstrated their support of Koba: there might at least be some career advantage in it.

Krupskaya, however, tried to retain her independence, and came out in support of Zinoviev and Kamenev. The majority, she said, was not always in the right, witness Lenin's defeat at the Stockholm Congress. Stalin politely contradicted her on the platform—and less politely in the lobbies. Molotov remembered Stalin saying about her that "she may use the same lavatory as Lenin, but that doesn't mean she knows anything about Leninism."

On the platform, however, he was the embodiment of peaceableness and moderation: "Methods such as amputation and bloodletting are infectious. If we chop off one person today, another tomorrow . . . what will be left of our Party?" kindly, tolerant Stalin asked the Fourteenth Party Congress. He cited the resolution drafted by Lenin for the Tenth Congress, which spoke of measures against splitters up to and including expulsion, and his furious audience demanded their immediate application. His reply was, "Wait a while, comrades, don't be in such a hurry." He had staged this spectacle, and for the present the role he had chosen for himself was to pacify his audience, to play the wise, calm, anything but bloodthirsty leader.

Zinoviev and Kamenev were condemned by the Congress. It was total defeat—559 votes against them, 65 for, to the novel accompaniment of approving shouts, as Stalin's tame Congress drew to its close. His new-fangled system of selecting delegates had worked splendidly.

Bukharin and his rightist sympathizers, happy that they had defeated their enemies, all praised this system. Just as Kamenev and Zinoviev had recently praised it after defeating their enemy Trotsky at the previous Congress.

The rightists did not realize what lay ahead, nor did Kamenev and Zinoviev. Only later the rules of the game would become clear: one of them was that Stalin shared power with different people and factions each time. But only from one Congress to the next. For one move at a time. Trotsky had taken no part in these latest polemics. He looked on sardonically while Stalin deftly rammed the fool's cap marked "oppositionist" on the heads of his allies of yesterday.

Trotsky now sat through Party meetings pointedly reading French novels.

"Knock Their Teeth Out"

At this Congress Stalin was singled out for the first time from the other members of the Politburo. His name no longer appeared in alphabetical order. He had removed Kamenev from his post as chairman of the Council of Labor and Defense. He now had a stable majority in the Politburo. The new members—Voroshilov, Molotov, and Kalinin—were his obedient servants. He mercifully left Zinoviev in place for the time being, but took the precaution of drawing his teeth: Zinoviev lost control of the dangerous city of Leningrad, and his supporters were ruthlessly expelled from the local leadership. The purge was directed by the new Leningrad boss, Sergei Kirov (Party pseudonym of the worker Kostrikov). Kirov was an effective organizer, with no experience of intrigue, a modest, efficient provincial. And efficient people were what the times called for. Kirov had won back the Caucasus for the Bolsheviks, and had tracked down Stalin's son Yakov in Georgia. Stalin was friends with Kirov. (I have seen only one affectionate inscription in Stalin's hand, and that was in a book presented to Kirov: "To my friend and favorite brother from the author." He wrote to no one else in such terms.)

He also left Trotsky in the Politburo. He still had to accustom the Party to the new position of yesterday's leaders. To this end the dread epithet "factionalist" would soon be regularly attached to their names.

For the present he appointed Trotsky to a relatively unimportant post in the Supreme Economic Council. The rumor current in Moscow was that he intended to make Lev head of the council in the near future. Trotsky let himself be influenced by this rumor, and bided his time. But nothing happened, and he finally realized that Stalin had made a fool of him. Throughout 1926 he was ill. It was a nervous disorder. His friend Joffe, formerly ambassador to Germany, made use of his connections to arrange medical treatment for Trotsky in that country. He left Moscow.

Stalin had also departed, for a holiday in Sochi, leaving Moscow in Molotov's hands. It was during this period that Molotov became his faithful shadow, as Koba had once been to Lenin. "Stone Arse" now wrote to him in Sochi almost every day. Every step the demoted leaders took was monitored by the GPU, and reported immediately in Molotov's letters.

He was a strange figure as he walked around Sochi in a white cotton suit, with his white trousers tucked into black jackboots. He explained to the loyal henchmen on holiday with him that the boots were "very convenient. That way you can give certain comrades a kick in their ugly mugs that'll knock their teeth out." This wasn't just a stupid joke.

One day he received startling news. And he prepared to knock out each and every tooth his enemies had left.

It turned out that Trotsky had returned from his cure in much better health and eager to "dispel the political shadows." Zinoviev and Kamenev had got to know of it, and approached him, offering an alliance. With the man they had so often betrayed, so often traduced! Like many others born in Russia, they suffered from the peculiarly Russian disease of naive romanticism. They believed that the three of them had only to appear together and the Party would immediately remember the heroic past and fall in behind its former leaders. They refused to see that the membership had long been eating out of the new potentate's hand, that the overwhelming majority of the bureaucrats who now managed the Party had been installed by Stalin, and that in any case the country had no wish at all to see the bloodstained ideas of the Revolution resurrected. Realistically, they could command the support of a mere handful of idealistic young Party fanatics. To attack with such forces would be suicide. Stalin was nonetheless certain that they would attack. The injured aristocratic pride of these ex-leaders would prevail.

While he waited he planned the "kicks to the face" in a series of letters:

> June 25. To Molotov, Rykov, Bukharin, and other friends . . . Zinoviev's group is now the inspiration of all schismatics. . . . This role has devolved upon their group because (a) it is more familiar with our methods than any other group. [As they might well be, since they had only recently joined in his effort to destroy Trotsky.] And (b) their group is on the whole stronger than others because it has in its hands the Comintern, which is a serious force. Our blow must be aimed specifically at this group. To unite Zinoviev and Trotsky in the same camp would be premature and at present strategically unsound. It is better to defeat them separately.

> August 30, 1926. Greetings, Molotov. The way things are going we cannot avoid . . . removing Grigori [Zinoviev] from Com-

intern. . . . Is the People's Commissariat of Foreign Affairs working to find a post for Kamenev?

And so the fate of Zinoviev and Kamenev was decided. Kamenev would be packed off with an ambassadorship. Eminent Bolsheviks who had once been Lenin's comrades-in-arms and were now "oppositionists" were dispatched to the overfed bourgeois world; in effect, into exile. To Berlin, N. Krestinsky, former secretary of the Central Committee and member of the Politburo; to Prague, the Trotskyist Antonov-Ovseenko, who in his day had announced the overthrow of the Provisional Government; to Paris, K. Rakovsky, onetime head of the Ukrainian government, accompanied by other influential members of Lenin's Central Committee, the Trotskyists Pyatakov and Preobrazhensky. Vienna, Argentina, Sweden, Persia . . . he scattered his enemies over the face of the earth. Let them rest a while and enjoy life. Just for a little while.

Meanwhile Krupskaya made another attempt to support Lenin's former comrades-in-arms.

On September 16, 1926, Stalin wrote Molotov: "Discussion with Krupskaya is at present not only inappropriate, but politically damaging. Krupskaya is a schismatic."

Back in Moscow, he warned Krupskaya jokingly that "if you carry on splitting the Party we'll find Lenin a different widow." And the man who would give the Party a new history, in which all the founding members of the Bolshevik Party would be depicted as its most vicious enemies, might have done just that. Krupskaya took fright, and remained frightened to the end of her life. Stalin would send her along to sit in on meetings of the Central Control Commission, where she would confirm the wildest fabrications against her husband's former associates.

A Desperate, Doomed Battle

That autumn, while he was still in the Caucasus, he learned that his wishes had been realized: the opposition was preparing for a desperate effort. On September 23, 1926, he wrote Molotov that if Trotsky had "gone raving mad" and meant to "stake everything on one last throw," so much the worse for him. In October oppositionists spoke out in Party cells at factories, calling for a debate. But they lost their nerve almost immediately, and acknowledged that their action had been "a breach of discipline." It was too late—Stalin was already hounding all those "October leaders" out of the Politburo. Zinoviev also ceased to manage the Comintern.

From that moment the opposition had nothing to lose. Battle was joined. A savage battle in which they were doomed.

And so a year later, on the eve of the Fifteenth Party Congress, on the tenth anniversary of the October coup which he had organized, and in the state which he had founded, Trotsky was obliged to set up an underground press to print his program. He knew he would not be able to read it out at the Congress—the audience, obeying Stalin, would shout him down. The GPU, needless to say, knew what was afoot, and this was just what Stalin had been waiting for. The underground press became the excuse for the immediate expulsion of Trotsky's supporters from the Party, and the arrest of many of them. Trotsky delivered his speech at a routine plenum of the Central Committee. His words were barely audible; he was interrupted by oaths and abuse, and the speech was accompanied throughout by cries of "Down with him!" "Get him out of here!" The same shouts drove Zinoviev from the platform. Stalin could be proud of himself. The system he had created was functioning with greater precision from one day to the next.

The opposition then organized demonstrations in Moscow and Leningrad on November 7. These were the last two open demonstrations against the Stalinist regime. The GPU, of course, knew about them in advance but allowed them to take place. In Lenin's Party submitting Party differences to the judgment of the crowd was considered the greatest of crimes. The opposition had signed their own sentence. And Stalin, of course, a brilliant organizer of demonstrations himself, was well prepared.

On the morning of November 7 a small crowd, most of them students, moved toward Red Square, carrying banners with opposition slogans: "Let us direct our fire to the right—at the kulak and the NEP man," "Long live the leaders of the World Revolution, Trotsky and Zinoviev." The GPU did its work, and a handpicked "public" soon attached itself to the column. The procession reached Okhotny Ryad, not far from the Kremlin. Here the criminal appeal to the non-Party masses was to be made, from the balcony of the former Paris hotel. Stalin let them get on with it. Smilga and Preobrazhensky, both members of Lenin's Central Committee, draped a streamer with the slogan "Back to Lenin" over the balcony. Those marching in support of the opposition shouted "Hurrah!" The "toilers" immediately "acted in protest," blowing whistles supplied in advance, throwing tomatoes they just happened to be carrying. A group headed by the secretary of the district Party Committee, Ryutin, arrived by car and tried to break in through the locked door. At the same time a Red army soldier climbed the sheer wall to the balcony and tore down the slogan, to the laughter of the mob. Ryutin and his companions found a way into the building and began assaulting the oppositionists. Ultimately they would all perish: the beaten—Smilga and Preobrazhensky—and the beater—Ryutin—alike.

Meanwhile loud shouts of "Bash the oppositionists" were heard from the crowd, and, more loudly still, "Down with the Yid oppositionists." Those demonstrating in favor of the opposition were first beaten up and then arrested.

While all this was going on preparations were being made for a solemn meeting in the Bolshoi Theater to mark the tenth anniversary of the October Revolution. After the ceremonies the famous director Eisenstein was supposed to show his film *October.* He was not ready in time. G. Alexandrov, who was then Eisenstein's assistant director, remembered: "At four Stalin came into the cutting room. He greeted us and said, 'Is Trotsky in your picture?' Eisenstein said, 'Yes.' After viewing it Stalin said categorically that the picture must not be shown with Trotsky in it." So the great director Eisenstein set to work excising from the film *October* the man who had been the father of October.

On November 14 Trotsky and Zinoviev were expelled from the Party. A little later one hundred cinemas were simultaneously screening the revolutionary blockbuster *October*—minus Trotsky. Krupskaya warmly approved of it, and wrote in *Pravda:* "You feel that a new art has emerged and is already taking shape in our country. That art has a colossal future." She was right. A new art had emerged. And Stalin would harness Eisenstein, and all the other geniuses of the medium, to its service.

At the Fifteenth Congress in December, to the usual accompaniment from the hall of approval for himself and indignation with the opposition, he said: "We make one condition: the opposition must renounce its views openly and honestly before the whole world. It must stigmatize the errors which it has committed . . . it must deliver up its cells to us, and make it possible for the Party to disband them completely. Either that, or let them quit the Party. If they won't go quietly—we'll chuck them out." This triggered shouts of "Right!" and prolonged applause.

He knew, of course, that all these former leaders were not yet ready to scourge themselves "before all the world" and "openly and honestly" hand over their supporters (the "cells") to the GPU. But in this way he obtained the right to "chuck them out." The Congress confirmed the expulsion of Trotsky, Zinoviev, and seventy or so other oppositionists from the Party, including such notables as Pyatakov, Radek, and Smilga. Kamenev was expelled from the Central Committee. In that anniversary year he calmly drove almost all of the God Lenin's henchmen out of the Party. Nor did he leave it at that. In speeches made by his allies, the oppositionists' former comrades, there were interesting hints of further action. A. Rykov, for instance, proclaimed that "in the situation which the opposition was endeavoring to create . . . we cannot, in my opinion, guarantee that in the very near future we shall not have to enlarge our prison population somewhat."

Shouting and clapping, his audience was preparing its own future.

Speeches like that of Rykov enabled Stalin to go further and to do something which the former Kremlin boyars could never have expected. All those ex-members of the Central Committee—Radek, Smilga, Beloborodov, Muralov, Preobrazhensky, I. Smirnov—were banished, as in tsarist times. And as the above-mentioned Bolsheviks themselves had banished their former fellow revolutionaries, the SRs.

The living symbol of world revolution, Lev Trotsky, was also banished. After the November demonstration he was evicted from his apartment in the Kremlin. While he looked for another, he stayed with his friend A. Beloborodov, the imperial family's murderer. Trotsky's banishment was carried out in the best tradition. First, Bukharin informed Trotsky by telephone of the decision to banish him. Trotsky, naturally, thought of organizing a demonstration for the day of his banishment. But Stalin had plans of his own. He instructed Bukharin to tell Lev that his departure had been postponed for two days. Then, the very next day, an "escort" arrived to take Lev to the station. Trotsky locked himself in his room, but, as Molotov described it, "Trotsky was carried out of his department. Two men carried him. One was my chief bodyguard Pogudil. He was a mighty boozer."

"They're carrying Trotsky out!" his son was shouting, and ringing the doorbells of all the other apartments. None of those living in the building opened up. Stalin had them trained by now. They carried Trotsky downstairs to a waiting car without interference. On the station platform his son still kept shouting, appealing to the railroad employees: "Look! Look how they're carrying Trotsky!" But the station was empty, and the railroad staff were unmoved. Trotsky had had his day.

All those benighted semiliterate workers, introduced into the Party by the "Lenin draft," sighed happily. No longer could it be said of their Party that "the Jews rule." They were grateful to Stalin. Radek made a sour joke: "Moses led the Jews out of Egypt, Stalin led them out of the Politburo."

Zinoviev and Kamenev again took fright, and immediately recanted, publicly condemning their views as anti-Leninist. Zinoviev was reinstated in 1929.

The Best Pupil

During the days of mourning for Lenin, Stalin, among others, made a speech. The former seminarist had not forgotten his homiletics. He spoke of the commandments bequeathed by the God Lenin, and vowed to carry them out. As indeed he did, in the shortest possible time. Lenin had intended to tame the rebellious old guard: Stalin made this an imperative. Lenin had adopted a menacing resolution on Party unity: Stalin made it an iron law. Indeed, he had every right to say: "I declare that the present regime in the Party is the exact expression of the regime which was established in the Party under Lenin at the time of the Tenth and Eleventh Congresses."

What now lay ahead was the abandonment of NEP and the final pacification of the country. Russia was about to meet its new tsar.

His mind turned to the future of a state that now belonged to him. Among his first steps were his attempts to lure back the great émigrés. Approaches were made to Gorky. The eminent "Bard of the Proletariat" and "Stormy Petrel of the Revolution" had not accepted the October coup. He had branded his friend of yesterday, Lenin, as "an adventurer, prepared to betray the interests of the proletariat in the most shameful fashion." Throughout 1918 his newspaper *New Life* had condemned Bolshevik terrorism. Koba had said of him that "the Russian Revolution has overthrown quite a few authorities, and we fear that the lost laurels of these great ones give Gorky sleepless nights, we fear that Gorky feels a fatal urge to join the has-beens—well, it's up to him. The Revolution neither pities nor buries its dead."

But Gorky had been equally uncompromising, and written a play about the sordid aspects of the new regime. Zinoviev, as boss of Petrograd, repeated the treatment meted out to the writer by "accursed tsarism": the play was banned, and Gorky's apartment was searched. Zinoviev added a new wrinkle: he threatened to arrest people close to Gorky. But Gorky would not be put off. In *New Life* he wrote, "This is just what we expect from a regime which fears the light of publicity, is antidemocratic, tramples on basic civic rights . . . and sends punitive expeditionary forces against peasants." Zinoviev closed the newspaper down, and Lenin had to advise the father of proletarian literature to remove himself from the first proletarian state. Gorky left Russia in 1922, ostensibly to seek medical treatment. But now that his archenemy Zinoviev had been driven out of Leningrad, Stalin's orders were that Gorky should be persuaded to return. The homecoming of the "Stormy Petrel of the Revolution" would sanctify the advent of a new Leader. Stalin made the new chief of the secret police, Genrikh Yagoda, responsible for bringing Gorky back.

Negotiations were going on simultaneously with another celebrity, one who had never belonged to the Party, the composer Sergei Prokofiev. The enticement of Prokofiev was also a GPU operation. In January 1927, after many changes of mind, Prokofiev decided to visit "Bolshevizia" with his wife.

As soon as Prokofiev arrived in the country from Paris "a certain Zucker" was attached to him as his "constant companion." This "employee of the Supreme Executive Committee" (as he described himself to Prokofiev) was, of course, a GPU agent.

Prokofiev was taken to the best hotel, the Metropole. In his diary, the "naive person with gray eyes" (as his friends called him) wrote: "An enormous room with a delightful view of the Bolshoi Theater, but no bath, the water for washing yourself was in jugs. . . . The crowd in the streets was good-natured—could these be the wild beasts who had so horrified the whole world? Hotel servants take tips, as they do everywhere, and are polite. . . . Zucker spent the whole journey enthusiastically explaining the beneficial activities of his Party. It proved to be very interesting, and on a planetary scale."

The processing continued. Prokofiev was taken to a "special restaurant," where the meal was "exceptionally tasty" and the service just as good. There were "grouse, marvelous whipped cream," and "in general a host of forgotten Russian things." When he entered the Conservatoire the orchestra welcomed him with a triumphal march. Back at the hotel he was handed a "letter of an erotic, and indeed demonic character . . . with telephone number enclosed" (the omniscient organization overlooked nothing). In the end, an old friend told him that " 'life here is impossible: you're watched and spied on the whole time, it's sheer torture . . . every sixth person is a spy.' "

Zucker finally decided to show his complete confidence in Prokofiev by taking him along "as a guest" to the Kremlin. The company chosen for this occasion was as "intellectual" as could be arranged: a friend of Kamenev's, Trotsky's sister, Kamenev's wife (Kamenev himself had by then been dispatched to Rome as ambassador).

The Kamenevs still had quarters in the Kremlin. "Soldiers with rifles and bayonets gleaming in the sunshine guard the Kremlin," Prokofiev noted. Zucker kept up a gushing commentary: the man who just passed us is a minister of something or other, this is where Lenin did this or that, look, the revolutionary poet Demyan Biedny lives here, " 'but living here can be very inconvenient,' Zucker told me, 'if you just want to invite somebody as a guest . . . there's a lot of bother with passes. . . .' We were taken to an enormous, comfortable room with magnificent armchairs and bookcases. We were shown in with a certain ceremony, there was an aura of deference, Olga Davidovna [Trotsky's sister] seemed lively and pleasant. . . . Later Litvinov (Deputy Commissar for Foreign Affairs) and his wife put in an appearance. They both announced that they loved music. Zucker tactfully hinted that it would be nice if I played something. . . . The new revolutionary forces took their ease to the strains of my compositions."

The visit dragged on till after midnight, when they walked through the darkness to the car. "Litvinov's wife carried her muddy shoes along the endless Kremlin corridors. . . . 'How I love this quiet Kremlin,' she exclaimed. It was amusing, if you knew how turbulently active that very same Kremlin was in the world."

Both Zucker and Kamenev's wife would be shot.

But Prokofiev liked what he saw. He paid several subsequent visits to the USSR and eventually resettled there. Yagoda had succeeded.

Return to Revolution

In those days many people still had the pre-Revolution habit of keeping diaries, most of which would vanish with their authors in the time of Terror. A few prudent people, my father among them, would burn their diaries for fear of arrest. So what little has trickled through time's cruel sieve is doubly precious.

This is from the diary of I. Schutz, a teacher of history: "In the provinces people spoke openly of famine. The peasants have instinctively devised a specific tactic which has spread everywhere. Their tactic is to keep their grain out of sight and they are such artists at concealment that look as he may no one will ever find it. . . . Hence the startling news that in Odessa scouts are posted to look out for bread, and in the Caucasus, the country's granary, restaurants offer 'dinner with bread' as if that was something miraculous."

He had set out to implement Bukharin's policy of "alliance with the peasantry," and the result was a shortage of bread. Once they felt themselves free the peasants simply refused to sell grain to the state at low prices. There was no food for the towns, and none for the army, which, although Europe was at peace, was steadily expanding.

Stalin would shut himself up in his study, and pace the floor, sucking his pipe. The power was in his hands. His rivals for the leadership had been laid low. Bukharin—"Bukhkashka," as the Party derisively called him—was, of course, not a rival. For Stalin what he should do next was no longer a question. Later, when he was thinking over his disagreements with Stalin, Bukharin would recall an "economic" discussion they had back in 1925. In the course of the discussion Stalin had said that if they gambled on NEP for long it would beget capitalism.

For him, the wager on NEP was of course only a maneuver in the fight with Trotsky and Zinoviev. And a breathing space, as Lenin had willed it, while the Party gathered strength. The essential question was when this pause for breath should end. It must not be left too late. Stalin agreed completely with the ousted leftists that "NEP for a long time" would mean the end of the Soviet regime.

Seventy years later the Gorbachev episode would prove yet again that a prison cannot be made self-financing. One-party rule cannot survive where someone has even minimal economic freedom.

As he paced his study nerving himself to *begin,* he saw already the mirage of a unique country. One that united the Marxist economic utopia of which they had dreamt in 1917 with a mighty state. There would be a single bank, a single economic plan, a peasantry organized in collective farms, and a pyramid of lesser leaders, all-powerful at their own level. At the top of the pyramid would be the Supreme Leader, his word instantly made flesh in the lesser leaders. There would be ruthless discipline, ruthless punishments. Gigantic resources would be concentrated in the hands of the state and the Leader. He would be able to create a huge industrial economy. And hence a huge army. . . . And then, and then . . . the Great Leninist Dream of World Revolution. "The head spins!"

The forces to execute the great turn were already in place. He announced at the Fifteenth Party Congress that "*guberniya* and oblast committees have taken over the business of economic management." The pyramid of leaders—provincial Party secretaries endowed with plenary powers—which he had created, his Order of Sword Bearers, controlled the whole life of the country. He could turn things whichever way he chose. He knew how eager the Party was for the turnaround. It viewed Bukharin's compliments to the petite bourgeoisie with contempt. The militants of the Party longed to hear again the favorite word of the Civil War—"Kill!" "Kill the kulak!" "Finish off the bourgeois!" The writer A. Vinogradov said in a letter to Gorky that "when the two children of a champion metalworker throw a schoolmate under a streetcar because he is a doctor's son and their class enemy—it means that utterly inhuman elemental forces have been unleashed and are running riot."

These were the elemental forces of the Russian Revolution, and Stalin would reawaken them. He would revive the romanticism of October, the slogans of the revolutionary upsurge: "No compromise!" "Class war to the death!" To build a society like none ever seen before, in which there would be neither peasants nor shopkeepers nor petit bourgeois.

In revolutionary battle dress he began building himself an empire. It gladdened him now to see the peasants withholding their grain. The specter of famine untied his hands. He uttered the call for which the Party was waiting. The bourgeois have forgotten the might of the Great Revolution. Very well, we'll remind them that the Revolution goes on!

Decrees on the forcible confiscation of grain, like those of years gone by, were drafted once more. Squads of factory workers and Cheka agents went once more from village to village. Stalin chased his comrades-in-arms out of their offices to extort grain. Molotov recalled, "We squeezed grain out of all those who had any. . . . On January 1, 1928, I was in the Ukraine, pumping grain, and Stalin said, 'I could give you a big kiss for the job you've done there,' and told me he felt an urge to go off to Siberia himself."

Stalin left for Siberia on January 15, 1928. He visited Novosibirsk, Barnaul, and Omsk. He returned from his trip in the foulest of tempers. According to a letter from N. Krotov, "Stalin went on from Omsk to some village or other. It was said that he spent his whole time there haranguing the peasants to make them hand over their grain. While he was at it one of them up and yelled at him, 'Dance us a *lezginka,* you Georgian so-and-so, and maybe we'll give you some grain!' He came back from Siberia with a decree already drafted: if the kulak did not surrender grain in the quantities required, punitive measures were to be used. He squeezed pretty hard. And he pumped out the grain."

They had dared to laugh at him. They wouldn't do it again. This people only understood strength.

In his copy of Lenin's *Materialism and Empiriocriticism,* which I examined in the archives, Stalin left an amusing inscription on the flyleaf: "(1) weakness (2) laziness (3) stupidity are the only things that can be called vices. All else, in the absence of the above-mentioned, is virtue."

All Else Is Virtue

Bukharin and his team were horrified: Stalin had simply reverted to war communism.

He had in fact gone further, and began to speak of collectivizing the peasantry. He had supposed that the mild Bukharin would meekly submit. But to his amazement Bukharin was furious, and a series of skirmishes developed. In spring 1928 Bukharin mobilized his supporters, Rykov, then head of government, and the Trades Union leader Tomsky, and they all wrote notes to the Politburo about the threat to the alliance between the proletariat and the peasantry, naturally invoking Lenin. Stalin did not intend to annihilate Bukharin just yet. He was making a

180-degree turn, and needed Bukharin to explain it from the standpoint of Marxism. He summoned a plenary meeting of the Central Committee and gave a simple account of the future in a formula heard for the first time: "The advance . . . toward socialism . . . inevitably leads to resistance on the part of the exploiting classes . . . [and to] the sharpening of the class struggle."

The population at large did not read boring political speeches, and so didn't realize that that sentence had been passed. His lackluster words concealed a sea of blood. As a near neighbor of ours, an old Party member, once explained to my father, "When class war is waged there has to be terror. If class war is intensified—the terror must also be intensified." My father did not believe him and merely laughed.

The plenary meetings were a grueling experience. Bukharin refused to give in. Rykov and Tomsky supported him. In the privacy of his study Stalin tried to coax Bukharin: "You and I are the Himalayas—all the others are nonentities. Let's reach an understanding." But Bukharin stood his ground. The expert on Leninism had simply failed to grasp what Lenin was about. Bukharin with his European education had not understood the main lesson which the ignorant Koba had mastered in the Leninist academies: NEP and a free peasantry spelled the doom of Bolshevik power. A single day without terror was dangerous; two days without terror meant death to the Party. At Politburo meetings he began raising his voice to Bukharin, who immediately quoted his remark about "nonentities" to the other members present, hoping to make them angry. This was foolish of him—they really were nonentities. All they felt was fear; they hated Bukharin for his humiliating candor. Stalin (so Bukharin told Kamenev later) grew furious; he shouted at Bukharin, "It's a lie, you've made that up." And so it went, with hysterical outbursts and ugly scenes at every meeting.

"Soft as wax" Bukharin kept fighting back. He even tried to enlist Kalinin and Voroshilov, promising to sweep Stalin away at some future Politburo meeting. Two other Politburo members, Rykov and Tomsky, were after all his allies. Kalinin was of two minds. A former peasant himself, he was of course against collectivization. The proletarian poet Demyan Biedny was given the job of bringing the old man to his senses. Biedny, the Party's pet poet, resided in the Kremlin, and his enormous apartment, his mahogany furniture, his children's governess, his chef, and his housekeeper were legendary among hungry writers. Demyan knew how to show gratitude for blessings received. At the beginning of

March an article of his in *Izvestia* (the government newspaper) assailed certain "older men in authority" who got involved with "young artistes from the world of light opera." Kalinin was having an affair at the time with a certain Tatyana Bakh, who had risen to stardom as his protégée. He saw at once that the drubbing would be ruthless, and shaming. For Stalin had a new weapon—the GPU dossier. Kalinin capitulated. The fun-loving playboy Voroshilov quickly took the hint from Kalinin's experience.

But Bukharin's activities were becoming more and more serious. Stalin learned that he had talked to the GPU chiefs, Yagoda and Trilisser, and then he called on his ousted enemy Kamenev. This was in July 1928. Kamenev wrote to Zinoviev that "Bukharin was in a state of terminal shock. His lips twitched violently with agitation." Trotsky had once been visited by his ferocious enemies Kamenev and Zinoviev, now Kamenev had been visited by *their* ferocious enemy Bukharin, also seeking an alliance and declaring that previous differences were immaterial. Let's ally ourselves against Koba!

Kamenev summarized Bukharin's part in the discussion as follows: "Stalin is a Genghis Khan, an unscrupulous intriguer, who sacrifices everything else to the preservation of his power. . . . He changes his theories according to whom he needs to get rid of next. . . . We quarreled so violently that we started calling each other 'liar,' etc. . . . The differences between us and Stalin are many times more serious than our former differences with you. . . . It would be much better for us to have Zinoviev and Kamenev in the Politburo rather than Stalin." He went on to explain Stalin's new concept, which was the reason for their disagreements. "Stalin's line was that capitalism grows at the expense of its colonies. We have no colonies, and no one will make us loans. We must therefore rely on tribute from our own peasantry. Stalin knows that there will be resistance. Hence his theory that as socialism grows so does resistance to it."

> *Kamenev:* What are your forces?
> *Bukharin:* Myself, Rykov, Tomsky, and Uglanov [leader of the Moscow Bolsheviks]. The Leningraders are mostly with us, but they are frightened. Voroshilov and Kalinin let us down at the last moment. It is becoming clear that the middle of the road Chekist [his name for most ordinary members of the Central Committee] would also be for Stalin.

Of those with power he for some reason identified Yagoda and Trilisser as his supporters. It may have been thanks to "supporter" Yagoda that news of this meeting with Kamenev reached Stalin immediately, together with a transcript of their discussion.

Kamenev realized that Bukharin and his friends were helpless. And as naive as he himself once had been. He remarked that the tone of Bukharin's statement showed a "total hatred for Stalin" and a "total breakdown of relations." He asked Bukharin, "What will become of us?" "He will try to buy us with important posts . . . so that we can help him to suffocate us," Bukharin replied.

The naive Bukharin was mistaken. Kamenev had long been awaiting an approach from Stalin. Stalin had, after all, now adopted Kamenev and Zinoviev's program. All that they had asked for he was now carrying out. Bukharin's story only poured oil on the flames. Bukharin was doomed: alliance with him would lead nowhere. Why should he, Kamenev, spare Bukharin, who not so long ago had been calling for *their* blood? The best thing for him to do was to inform Stalin of this visit as soon as Bukharin left.

Bukharin was, in any case, behind the times. Stalin needed no help from other former leaders—he could easily smother the rightists without it. Kamenev grew tired of waiting for Stalin's call, and went himself to see Voroshilov in December. He spent two hours "groveling and praising the Central Committee's policies to the skies." Voroshilov said not a single word in reply.

To close his account with the former leaders, Stalin exiled Trotsky from Russia in January 1929. As Zinoviev rightly remarked, there was "nobody left to protest to." Stalin showed that he had not lost his sense of humor: Trotsky, who regarded himself as a true Leninist, was deported from Russia on the steamship *Ilyich*. Why didn't Stalin kill him? Because he needed Trotsky alive. For future games. Trotsky would become a center of counterrevolutionary activity, and Stalin could accuse his enemies of being in contact with it. Trotsky was the bait with which he would catch his future victims. The chess player always thought several moves, very many moves ahead. Just now he had to settle accounts with Bukharin. He would set to work via Trotsky.

In 1938, on the eve of his execution, Bukharin would write a letter to Stalin: "When I was with you once in summer 1928 you said to me, 'Do you know why I am friends with you? It's because you are incapable of intrigue—aren't you?' I said yes. And that was at the very time when I was running to Kamenev." Poor Bukharin didn't understand a thing.

Stalin had received reports of Bukharin's conversation with Kamenev immediately, from several sources. He asked the hapless intellectual whether or not he was "capable of intrigue" to make him squirm. And when the other man, worried out of his mind, told a lie, Stalin felt entitled to feel a mortal hatred for the liar and traitor.

His GPU also arranged for a record of Bukharin's conversation with Kamenev to reach Trotsky. He knew that Trotsky hated Bukharin, and would not spare him; he would publish the information immediately. As always, his calculations proved correct. Once abroad, Lev published the transcript, and presented Stalin with a bombshell: the right to speak of a compact between the rightists and their predecessors in opposition.

At this point Stalin gained some new supporters. Radek and other Trotskyists could now surrender honorably. Stalin had, after all, "turned his fire to the right." Stalin must be supported, and the "left flank of the Party occupied, before it is occupied by others," as the exiles wrote to each other. In order to return, they had first to sacrifice Trotsky, their vanished leader. Radek appealed to the exiled Trotskyists, "We have brought ourselves to exile and imprisonment. I have broken with Trotsky, we are now political enemies."

"You Must Believe That White Is Black"

Why was it so easy for them to change their views and betray each other? Pyatakov, once a leading Trotskyist and subsequently a staunch Stalinist, startled Valentinov with this explanation: "For the Party's sake you can and *must* at 24 hours' notice change all your convictions and force yourself to believe that white is black." For the Party's sake! When the former seminarist Stalin called the Party the Order of Sword Bearers he had just that in mind: the sacred nature of the Party. Trotsky expressed the same thought in his dictum "the Party is always right." Like the church, their Party remained pure even if those who served it erred. For, like the church, the Party was founded on scripture, in its case the sacred Marxist texts, which would never allow the Party as a whole to err, or sinful individual members to change its sacred nature.

Hence the principle "everything for the Party," which allowed them to betray themselves and humble themselves before Stalin—the head of the Sacred Party.

Professions of repentance came pouring in, and Stalin graciously allowed the repentant "leftists" to return from exile. Pyatakov, Smilga, Rakovsky, Beloborodov, and other notables condemned Trotsky and came back into the Party. Their prestige and their energy were very helpful to Stalin in what historians would call the Year of the Great Turn.

Back in 1925, when Stalin, in alliance with the rightists, was attacking Kamenev and Zinoviev in Leningrad, the poet Sergei Yesenin had committed suicide in the Hotel Angleterre. In Russia poets are prophets. One of Yesenin's regular drunken hallucinations was a horrifying Black Man. The great peasant poet even then sensed Stalin's approach. Now the hour had come. The Black Man had readied himself to destroy the age-old Russian village as Yesenin had known it.

From April 1929 the turnaround was official. The Year of the Great Turn had begun. The greatest experiment of the twentieth century, which promised endless bloodshed. But what did blood matter, when ahead of them lay the great future? Stalin meant to attain it by revolutionary means, in the shortest possible time. Very soon the resistance of the village would be destroyed, as would a considerable section of the middle peasantry. The rest would be united in *kolkhozy,* collective farms. The unpaid labor of tillers of the soil gathered together thus would produce colossal funds for investment. He would build a huge industrial economy. This too in the shortest time imaginable. He would make the workers forget about wages. And holidays. Revolutionary enthusiasm—that was the thing! The country could look forward to unprecedented privations, industrial accidents resulting from unheard-of tempos which neither worn-out machinery nor half-starved workers could endure. He knew that people were unhappy when they did not understand the source of their agony, so, feeling charitable toward his fellow citizens, he decided in advance to provide the country with culprits for its future miseries. The blame must lie with "enemies"—this was the eternal Russian explanation for all the nation's woes. He remembered how during the First World War the tsar's government had quickly found a plausible explanation for the defeats incurred by their incompetent generals: spies were responsible! And the people were happy to believe it. He thought up a new variant: the modern equivalent of those spies would be the engineers. Wreckers! Experts trained in the days of the tsars who, naturally, hated the dictatorship of the proletariat and tried to sabotage it. He could count on the ignorant loathing of the semiliterate masses for the educated, the intelligentsia. And on what had as a result become the mob's favorite word: "Kill!"

As he approached the turning point, he had to plunge the country into an atmosphere of constant fear. Only fear could excuse possible excesses in advance and reduce the people to the level of subservience necessary for the Great Change. And to unmask the "wreckers," he called upon the GPU; now the secret police began to gain a powerful hold on the public mind.

The Gladiatorial Games

That was the origin of a unique spectacle: the show trials, first of their kind, in the late twenties.

As the decade neared its end, life was drab and hunger prevailed. Everywhere swarmed hoards of physically unclean people. Migrants from the countryside had taken possession of the towns: people who wiped their noses with their hands and were used to living, eating, and sleeping in a single room, often parents and children together. The huge apartments of the upper class had become communal dwellings, housing a dozen or so families. In the mornings members of different households, indecently half-clad, stood chatting in the queue for the lavatory or washbasin. And the regular subject of conversation was the trials of those wreckers whom the valiant GPU was constantly unmasking. The detective stories told in court, and the awesome sentences handed down, brought a little variety into the dreary lives of ordinary people. The trials were a peculiar variant of the Roman gladiatorial games.

A Talented Scoundrel

The GPU was headed by Vyacheslav Menzhinsky. A sybarite and snob, born in a wealthy family, he had joined the revolutionary movement at an early age. In 1909 he had described Lenin, in a Socialist Revolutionary newspaper, as a "political Jesuit." When Menzhinsky made friends with the Bolsheviks after the February Revolution Lenin had spoken just as warmly of him: "Our business will be extensive enough to find work for every scoundrel with talent."

After October he was made People's Commissar of Finance, but created such chaos that he was quickly removed. Then, in 1919, Lenin suddenly remembered that Menzhinsky was a lawyer and found a suitable place for him in the senior ranks of the Cheka. He had guessed correctly: the "scoundrel" proved invaluable in concocting bafflingly complicated provocations. It was a highly specialized intellectual game. Though Menzhinsky had a hand in all the dreadful deeds of the Red Terror, he fastidiously absented himself from the torture chamber and from executions. As soon as he was appointed Gensek, Stalin established a close relationship with this strange person. Since Dzherzhinsky, formally in charge of the Cheka, was also responsible for a multitude of other duties, Menzhinsky became the effective head of the Bolshevik secret service, and Stalin confirmed him in that post after Dzherzhinsky's death.

Menzhinsky was faithfully served by Genrikh Yagoda. Yagoda helped the maestro to improve on his methods, and provocation became the regular modus operandi of the Cheka (GPU). Menzhinsky was responsible for setting the dizzying confidence game in motion. With the help of a spurious anti-Bolshevik organization created by the Cheka, Menzhinsky lured an old acquaintance of his, the legendary SR terrorist Boris Savinkov, back to Russia. Savinkov, who had assassinated an uncle of the Last Tsar and certain of his ministers, had become an implacable enemy of the Bolsheviks. But after lengthy discussions with Menzhinsky, he announced that he "now recognized the Soviet regime and no other." For this sensational declaration Menzhinsky commuted his death sentence, and apparently promised a pardon at some time in the future. In 1926 it was announced that Savinkov had committed suicide—but shortly before this he had given this warning to his son: "If you hear that I have laid hands on myself, don't believe it." Menzhinsky knew the rule: you can forgive your enemy, but you must destroy him beforehand.

It was in Menzhinsky's time that a large number of well-educated and foppish young men arrived in the GPU. Their past was anything but proletarian. They were ruthless careerists. The genuine fanatics, with their fevered dreams of world revolution, went on working side by side with these people, and hating them.

In 1927 Stalin organized a grandiose jubilee—the Party and the whole country celebrated the tenth birthday of the Cheka, now the GPU, the "punitive sword of the Revolution." Most of those with whom Menzhinsky had shared the experience of October 1917, and who had helped to found his institution, had fallen from power. Now they themselves were under surveillance by the GPU. But Menzhinsky was still in place. Interminable speeches were delivered, earlier eulogies of the GPU were cited. Particularly pleasing were the words of the intellectuals' intellectual Nikolai Bukharin: "The GPU has accomplished the greatest miracle of all time. . . . It has succeeded in changing the very nature of Russian man."

He was right. For the first time in Russia informing on others was proclaimed a virtue, and the secret police became heroes. At the ceremonial meeting, instead of the speech expected of him, Menzhinsky spoke these few words: "The Cheka's greatest merit is that it knows how to keep silent." Then he laughed and left the stage.

But in 1928–1929, Menzhinsky sensed that the wind was changing. Not so long ago the official line was that all the main enemies had been eradicated, but now the Caucasian in the Kremlin was officially proclaiming that *not only are our enemies not eradicated—there are millions of them.* The Leader had obviously decided to resurrect the Red Terror, but the gigantic task ahead held no attraction for Menzhinsky. Since his wife's death he had been sick with boredom. Stalin sensed his weariness, and lost interest in him. When the show trials began, Menzhinsky was his collaborator, but from the end of 1930 he worked more and more closely with the vice commissar, Yagoda.

In 1930, yet another of Lenin's old comrades-in-arms was driven out of office by Stalin. This was Chicherin, People's Commissar for Foreign Affairs and a friend of Menzhinsky. At once a Bolshevik and a scion of the Naryshkin clan, who were related to the Romanovs, Chicherin was a solitary, a strange person who liked to shut himself up in his apartment and play his beloved Mozart for days at a time. Stalin replaced Chicherin with an enemy of his, the energetic Litvinov. Having a Jew at the head of his Foreign Office also helped Stalin to avoid accusations of anti-Semitism abroad. Besides, he was already thinking of repairing relations with America.

Menzhinsky occasionally called on Chicherin. Chicherin would play Mozart, while Menzhinsky listened in silence. He knew that his department had ears everywhere. He was by then only a fleeting visitor to his place of work. Mostly, he stayed at home studying Old Persian, so that he could read Omar Khayam in the original.

Stalin stopped summoning him to the Kremlin, but could not allow him to retire. He knew too much. Menzhinsky was nominally head of the GPU until 1934, when Yagoda, apparently, poisoned this strange relic of the Leninist epoch.

Stalin now began working intensively with Yagoda.

Genrikh Yagoda owed his rise to the Sverdlov family. The older Sverdlov, a rich Nizhny Novgorod merchant, had believed in the Revolution and had helped revolutionaries by making seals for forged documents. His son Yakov had naturally joined the revolutionaries himself, and had become the first nominal head of government in Bolshevik Russia.

As a boy Yagoda ran errands for the older Sverdlov. The old man helped him get an education. He was trained as a pharmacist, and would make good use of his skills at a later date.

After the October Revolution Yagoda found himself working for the

Cheka. He still clung to the powerful Sverdlov family: his wife was related to Yakov himself. In the twenties he was already one of the top men in the all-powerful GPU. It was Yagoda who enmeshed the country in a network of informers during those early years of the Soviet regime. Lenin's formula "every Party member must be a Chekist" was expanded under Yagoda: now every citizen had to become a Chekist. An invitation to become an informer was proof of the Party's confidence in you.

A Unique Spectacle: The Show Trials

In the year of the Cheka's glorious anniversary, several dozens of engineers were arrested in the Donbass mines and charged with "wrecking." The investigation, or rather the rehearsals for an incredible theatrical event, went on through 1927 and 1928. Yagoda's interrogators were extremely frank with the bewildered detainees. Bewildered because they had naturally begun by denying the charges, but had been told that no one would believe them and that what was required was not protestations of innocence but cooperation. The unfortunate engineers were told that the false charges against them had a lofty ideological purpose. The building of socialism now in progress had no precedents, and an admission from the accused that they were saboteurs was calculated to excite the wrath of the people against capitalism, heighten their vigilance against real enemies, and increase the productivity of labor. In return they were promised their lives.

The premiere took place in Moscow on May 20, 1928—the public trial of the "Shakhtintsy"—"wreckers" in the mines of the Donbass. Fifty-three engineers were called before the court. The diplomatic corps's box was full, newspaper reporters from all over the world were present. The show was a success: all the accused joined in enthusiastic self-flagellation, and even dissociated themselves from their overzealous defense counsel. They seemed to vie with the public prosecutor, N. Krylenko, in aggravating the charges against them. Worldly-wise intellectuals at once dubbed the trial of the Shakhtintsy "Prosecutor Krylenko's Fables." (I. A. Krylov (1769–1844) was the Russian Aesop.)

The public prosecutor called for twenty-two death sentences. But out of gratitude for the cooperation of the accused, only five executions were ordered. A mere five innocent people killed—what did they matter measured against the Party's planetary goals? Stalin was able to draw the necessary conclusion at a plenary meeting of the Central Committee: "We are confronted with an obvious escalation of class warfare. Needless to say, things of this kind will happen again." This was an order: in every factory the search for wreckers, for "our own Shakhtintsy," was on.

End of the Right

Battles with Bukharin and the rightists went on throughout 1929. One right-wing member of the Central Committee, Ryutin, subsequently gave this character sketch of his leader: "As a political leader Bukharin is beneath criticism . . . clever but shortsighted. Honest, but weak, he quickly lapses into lethargy, is incapable of long struggle with a serious enemy . . . panics easily, cannot provide leadership to the masses, needs to be led himself." Nonetheless, Bukharin took hold of himself and fought back. Stalin guessed the main reason for this stubbornness. The GPU had informed him that young Marxists from the Institute of Red Professors regularly met Bukharin in the apartment of Postyshev, a secretary of the Central Committee. These young people called themselves the "Bukharin school." While Postyshev himself was away from Moscow, his wife, who worked at the Marx-Engels Institute, put the apartment at their disposal. Bukharin went straight there after Politburo meetings to tell them about his daring deeds and speeches. Softhearted Bukharin reveled in the adoration of these young Marxists, particularly the young female Marxists. Let him carry on with it, Stalin decided. Bukharin's resistance was now grist for his mill: he aimed thunderbolt after thunderbolt at the right, intensifying an atmosphere of terror. At every plenum he set out to annihilate Bukharin. And, of course, it worked: Bukharin took fright. Attempts at a reconciliation followed. Bukharin and Tomsky, who just a little while ago had called him "Genghis Khan," now spoke of their friendship with Comrade Stalin. At a subsequent plenum Stalin recalled how Bukharin had gone to see Kamenev, and how that "irreproachable and loyal member of the Party" had suggested that the two of them should "change the composition of the Politburo."

In November 1929 the rightists publicly capitulated. Rykov spoke for all of them: they were now for the general line of the Party, for the destruction of the kulak, for the policy which Bukharin only yesterday had called "the military-feudal exploitation of the peasantry." Stalin "deemed their declaration unsatisfactory." They would have to go on crawling in public for a long time to come. Meanwhile he booted

Bukharin out of the Politburo. Rightists were pilloried all over the country, condemned at staff meetings in factories, in learned institutes, in kindergartens, and even at cemeteries.

Rightists and wreckers were anathematized by turns. From morning till evening the radio never paused in its imprecations. Trials now followed each other without a break. A group of people belonging to the old aristocracy were arrested at the Monastery of the Trinity and St. Sergius, the most important in Russia. Evicted from their homes and denied work elsewhere, they had sought refuge in the monastery, where they worked in the museum and taught in the seminary. Now they were denounced as wreckers and arrested.

The Fate of Religion

From the very beginning of the Bolshevik regime religion had been under attack. T. Samsonov, head of a secret department of the Cheka, wrote to Dzherzhinsky on December 4, 1920, that "communism and religion are mutually exclusive. . . . No machinery can destroy religion except that of the [Cheka]. In its plans to demoralize the church the Cheka has recently focused its attention on the rank and file of the priesthood. Only through them, by long, intensive, and painstaking work, shall we succeed in destroying and dismantling the church completely." In building a new society with a new religion the onetime seminarist followed the behests of Ilyich. He kept a careful eye on the personnel of the church. The GPU was always at the church's side. And Stalin was physically destroying church buildings, as Lenin had willed.

The famous seventeenth-century church of St. Paraskevi on Okhotny Ryad was destroyed. Curious crowds stared wild-eyed as the great bell, nine tons in weight, was hurled to the ground. Five thousand people joined enthusiastically in demolishing the Monastery of St. Simon. But the high point of the campaign was the collective destruction by a crowd many thousands strong of the Church of Christ the Savior, the largest place of worship in Moscow. As a symbol, Stalin decided to erect on the site of this Christian temple the greatest temple of the new regime—the Palace of the Soviets, to be crowned with a gigantic statue of the God Lenin.

Such churches as survived were converted into storehouses. Children were told at school to bring icons for a public bonfire, and were given posters of Lenin to hang in their place. Newspapers published letters to the editor announcing that some former priest had broken with religion forever. The slogan "religion is the opium of the people" was displayed everywhere and anywhere.

THE GREAT CHANGE BEGINS

Throughout 1929 the country was preparing for Stalin's fiftieth birthday, in December. Or, to be precise, for the fictitious birthday which he had chosen for himself. Thousands upon thousands of articles were written about the beloved Leader. In honor of the Great Jubilee mills and factories reported unprecedented successes. The radio blared frenzied congratulations. In a Moscow psychiatric hospital, A. Kochin, a fifty-three-year-old professor of mathematics who had lost his mind, shouted the praises of the Leader incessantly, interrupting them only to heap recherché imprecations on the wreckers.

On his fiftieth birthday he could pause to sum up his achievements. The last of Lenin's comrades-in-arms had been driven out of the leadership. It was now, during these birthday celebrations, that the absolute character of his power became obvious for all to see. His coronation was to come at the next Congress. I. Schutz noted in his diary that "everybody expects sensations at the Congress. . . . The Leader will dominate everything."

He composed a modest reply "to all the organizations and comrades who have congratulated me . . . I regard your greetings as addressed to the great Party of the working class which bore me and reared me in its own image and likeness."

The use of biblical language—"in its own image and likeness"—was deliberate. So was the statement that he was born not of woman, but of the Party. As he became tsar he resolved also to become a god. A Bolshevik Trinity, a triune godhead, was emerging. Marx, Lenin, and himself. Gods of the earth.

The shattered leaders of the right tried to make their peace with him. On the night of January 1, 1930, Bukharin and Tomsky arrived at Stalin's apartment with bottles of wine to see the New Year in. The reconciliation took place: he still needed "little Bukharin." He had no comparable theoretician of his own. And after all, they were both "Himalayas."

He chose his anniversary to initiate the Great Change.

While he was celebrating the New Year with his family, his humiliated foes, and his servile henchmen, preparations were being made out on the boundless frozen expanses of Russia. Special freight cars stood ready on the rail tracks. Previously used to transport cattle they were waiting now to transport human beings.

Toward the end of 1929, shortly before his birthday, he had published an article entitled "The Year of the Great Turn." In it he defined the task ahead as "the liquidation of the kulak as a class." A twentieth-century state was planning the organized destruction of fellow citizens who worked on the land. Together with the kulak, the old Russian village was to be destroyed. The Revolution had endowed the peasants with land. Now they were required to give it back, and to surrender their cattle for communal use. Instead of "my own"—so dear to the peasant heart—they must learn to say "ours." The better-off peasants, the kulaks, would naturally not want any of this and would be obstructive. Therefore, to economize on time, he decided to proceed in revolutionary fashion and simply destroy them. He put faithful Molotov at the head of a commission to finalize the solution. Molotov labored diligently. And bloodily.

In a very short time the commission had drawn up a plan for the total extermination of the kulak. Kulaks were deported to the far North, to the Urals, Kazakhstan, and Siberia. Kondratiev, Yurovsky, and Chayanov, economists of note in their day, suggested using kulaks—often the ablest and hardest-working peasants—to till the virgin lands. Let them have on long-term lease the uncultivated open spaces abandoned by Kazakh nomads. They did not realize that his present concern was not with economics. His objective was political: the complete and utter destruction of a class. The revolutionary Tkachev's formula—"We must ask ourselves how many people we need to keep"—had prevailed.

In February, Molotov and his commission divided the kulaks into groups. First, the counterrevolutionary kulak activists. They would be sent to the camps, or shot, and their families deported to the remotest regions. Second, whatever was left of the wealthiest kulaks. They would be deported to remote and infertile areas. Third, those with less prosperous holdings. They would be evicted and put down outside the boundaries of the collective farms.

Nobody knew exactly who belonged to which category. It was impossible to say definitely who was a "kulak," to distinguish "kulaks" from "middle peasants." The unfortunate prosperous peasant was completely at the mercy of the GPU, the Party authorities, and, above all, the malicious "village poor." Well-off peasants voluntarily surrendered their property to the kolkhoz, imploring those in charge not to class them as kulaks. But the idle and shiftless rural paupers took their revenge: the new masters were inexorable. I. Vareikis, a member of the Central Committee and of Molotov's commission, wrote with satisfaction that "dekulakization is being carried out with the active participation of the poor. The poor accompany the commissions in large groups and confiscate cattle and other property. On their own initiative they post a watch on the roads out of villages at night, with the object of detaining kulaks trying to escape."

All over the country, as women howled and sobbed, the unfortunates were loaded onto carts, which moved out of the village under the watchful eyes of the GPU. People gazed round at the empty houses which had been their family homes for centuries. They were leaving behind a life which they would never see again.

The Molotov commission deported fifty thousand kulak families to the far northern territory. The Northern Territorial Committee had reported that it could take only twenty thousand: the huts, without heat or light, were not yet ready. Stalin's telegraphed response to the problem was: "The Central Committee cannot agree to a decision which overturns the resettlement plans already adopted by the Party." And: "Novosibirsk. To Secretary of the Siberian Territorial Committee Eikhe: Take all necessary preparatory measures for reception in mid-April of not fewer than 15,000 kulak families." Telegrams such as these sped to every provincial committee. And Stalin's plans were carried out in full. Freight cars unloaded people out in the open steppe, into a hungry wilderness fenced with barbed wire. A whole class was being destroyed.

The commission did its work well. Its members were the new Stalin boyars, the obkom secretaries installed by Stalin, Party leaders all-important in their own provinces. Together, of course, with Yagoda, representing the GPU. The onetime head of the commission, Molotov, recalled at the age of ninety that "we made a pretty good job of collectivization. . . . I personally delineated the resettlement areas. . . . Around 400,000 were deported." S. Kosior, a new member of the Politburo, who was on the commission, told the commission that "we must inflict a really annihilating blow on the kulaks," while S. Kirov wrote picturesquely of "columns of tractors digging the kulaks' graves." If Kirov had only known it, graves were being dug for others besides the kulaks.

Kirov, Kosior, and Vareikis would all perish. Ninety percent of the commission's membership (nineteen out of twenty-one) would soon be lying in unmarked holes, victims of Stalin's purges. But for the present they worked with a will destroying others. Train after train after train transported peasants in cattle wagons. There were floodlights on the roofs of the wagons, and guards with dogs inside.

The poor peasants and those of the middle peasants who survived were united in collective farms. The kulaks' carefully tended herds, their well-built houses, goods and chattels accumulated over the centuries, money in the savings banks—all had to be handed over to the kolkhoz. The kolkhoz originated in the bloody misappropriation of other people's property.

All Party organizations raised their targets with feverish haste and undertook to complete collectivization in the shortest possible time. Naturally, lip service was paid to the principle of voluntary membership. Or, as the current joke went, "voluntary-compulsory membership." The GPU herded the peasants into the kolkhoz to the strains of music and singing. Local Party leaders knew that it was a case of either 100 percent collectivization or hand in your Party card. In his old age Molotov recalled a joke popular with the general public at the time: "How do you get rid of lice?" "Write 'kolkhoz' on your head and they'll all run away at once."

There were rebellions. A bloody riot, in which kolkhoz chairmen and GPU plenipotentiaries were killed, flared up in the Ryazan area. The rising was savagely suppressed. (That was when my nanny's sister, the tall and beautiful Pasha, turned up in the city. Half-asleep, I heard Pasha telling my mother in the next room how she had set fire to her cottage so that "those devils wouldn't get their hands on it.")

Putting down the risings was the Red army's job. But Stalin knew the effect all this might have on an army made up mainly of peasants' sons. He had not yet completely tamed the country; he still had to think of such things. Hence his article "Dizziness with Success." It seemed, he explained, that "certain comrades," dizzied by the headlong voluntary rush of the masses to join the kolkhoz, had become overzealous. These "certain comrades" had sometimes forcibly collectivized. Worst of all, they had confused middle peasants with kulaks. All these "comrades" would, of course, prove to be crypto-Trotskyists, deliberately trying to sabotage collectivization. *They* were responsible for the deviations from the correct line. A wave of trials swept over the country. Trials, this time, of the "malicious exaggerators." Stalin skillfully kept up the pressure of the Terror.

Pope Pius XI chose now to call for prayers for persecuted Christians in Russia. On the eve of the day appointed by the Pope for this universal prayer, Stalin published a decree "on the distortion of the Party line in the kolkhoz movement." Once again, it all was *their* fault: maliciously overzealous deviationists had, it seemed, forcibly closed down a number of churches.

And although priests and monks were not brought back from exile, although by the end of the year 80 percent of village churches were closed, people still enthused over the handful of churches reopened on Stalin's orders. He was skillfully reinventing a figure beloved of Russians: that of the good tsar with bad ministers.

Even after "Dizziness with Success," the extermination of better-off peasants continued to escalate. From all over the country convoys including children and old people were moved on "by stages" toward their places of exile. The trains were packed with people dying of cold and thirst. Children died on the journey, some of them killed by their mothers to spare them suffering. According to (understated) official figures, another 240,000 families had been deported by 1933. The gigantic revolutionary experiment was a success. The class which Lenin so hated, the prosperous Russian peasantry, no longer existed.

All this was accompanied by sensational trials. In the summer of 1930 cars raced around Moscow and throughout the surrounding countryside. The police were rounding up intellectuals. Yagoda had a new large-scale operation in hand. The flower of the intelligentsia—academicians, eminent scholars and scientists, technologists, professors, the economists Chayanov, Kondratiev, Yurovsky, etc.—were all arrested. Among the most important of those accused of "wrecking" was M. Ramzin, a famous specialist in boilermaking and director of the Moscow Thermo-Technical Institute. The GPU also announced the discovery of a powerful terrorist organization, with almost 200,000 underground members, and claimed that a clandestine Industrial Party had been plotting to seize power.

Those under arrest confessed to everything. Volumes have been written on the way in which the required testimony was obtained from them—how they were tortured by interrogation round the clock, denied sleep, and so on.

One thing unknown until the present was the extent of Stalin's involvement. Only now, after reading the new documents, can I say for sure that he personally staged the trials. And what a producer he was! How meticulously he worked out the details of this Grand Guignol. And even dictated the actors' lines.

AUTHOR! AUTHOR!

> July 2, 1930. Stalin to Menzhinsky. Strictly Personal. Ramzin's testimony is interesting. My suggestions—make one of the most important, crucial points of Ramzin's (future) depositions the question of intervention. And the dates of the planned intervention. Why was intervention postponed in 1930? Was it because Poland is not yet ready? Or perhaps Romania is not yet ready? Also—why did they postpone intervention until 1931? Could they postpone it till 1932?

In this concocted fantasy, the accused were being told that the imperialists were secretly preparing intervention in the Soviet republic. By admitting their involvement in the intervention scheme, the accused would automatically thwart it and save the country. They were invited to slander themselves out of true proportion, in return for which they were, of course, promised more lenient sentences. Ramzin agreed to admit in court that his "party" had welcomed the capitalists' plans to intervene against the USSR. But Stalin still needed to amplify Ramzin's "interesting testimony." The point was that there *was* no intervention. And he knew that there would be none. So now he suggested a variety of explanations as to why the intervention had not yet happened. And why it would not happen. Not all of the accused behaved as sensibly as Ramzin. In exasperation, Stalin demanded that "Messrs. Kondratiev, Yurovsky, Chayanov, etc., who are craftily trying to wriggle out of the intervention tendency should be made to run the gauntlet. We will make this material available to a section of Comintern. Then we shall conduct the broadest possible campaign against the interventionists, thereby frustrating and paralyzing attempts at intervention for the next year or two, which is not unimportant to us. Understand?" So it was all pure invention, devised by him to serve "not unimportant" ends. The fact that the "wriggling" Kondratievs were innocent *was* unimportant.

How exactly the intellectuals were "made to run the gauntlet" we can only guess. One way or another, his orders were carried out.

In a note to Molotov, Stalin wrote, "You must have received Kondratiev's *new testimony* by now. Yagoda brought it along to show me. I think that all these statements should be distributed to all members of the Central Committee." Capitalist plans for intervention and the atmosphere of a fortress under siege were required by the Terror. Stalin meant to keep the country in a permanent state of emergency.

At the very end of 1930 a grandiose new spectacle was mounted—the public trial of the "Industrial Party." The indefatigable Krylenko prosecuted, and once again the trial went splendidly. Workers' meetings all over the country demanded the execution of these "vile traitors," whereas in the courtroom spectators marveled at the extraordinary politeness shown to the accused by the judge: they were even allowed to smoke. The press was there in force, and the proceedings were filmed. The accused vied with one another in confessions of guilt. They readily supplied an amazing variety of information on their wrecking activities, and their links with hostile émigrés, foreign embassies, and even French President Poincaré himself. Still, things did not go absolutely smoothly. The "vile wrecker" Ramzin, for instance, asserted that his plans for intervention by foreign states included the formation of a government in waiting. His candidate for the post of Minister of Trade and Industry was the Russian capitalist Ryabrushinsky, with whom he had negotiated successfully. Unfortunately it transpired that Ryabrushinsky had managed to die before Ramzin could enter into "successful negotiations" with him.

Stalin was capable of gratitude. The main defendant, Ramzin, was sentenced to death by shooting, but this was commuted to imprisonment. The same Ramzin whose name had been anathema to the country at large was shortly released, and eventually became director of the very same Technological Institute, and a winner of the country's highest award, the Stalin Prize. Several other of the "inveterate wreckers" would be numbered among Stalin's pet scientists.

He still saw to it that blood was spilled abundantly. How can you have Terror without blood? The trials of intellectuals for sabotage in every branch of the economy went on without a break. Bacteriologists were tried on charges of spreading cattle plague and shot. Officials in the food industry were accused of organizing a famine, and forty-eight of them were shot. People, mostly professors and engineers, were sitting on the bare cement floors of the Butyrki Prison, sixty to eighty to a cell. Jails had long been known to the public as "Holiday Homes for Engineers and Technicians." Stalin tirelessly directed these "measures of no small importance."

> 13.9.30. Stalin to Molotov. All the testimony of wreckers in fish, meat, canned goods, and vegetables should be published imme-

> diately . . . followed in a week's time by the announcement that all these scoundrels have been shot. They must all be shot.

It seems fantastic. He himself organizes the trials, he declares innocent people to be criminals, yet he is genuinely indignant at their crimes. The actor has fully identified himself with his role.

But the damage done became more and more serious, and his commissars sounded the alarm. Skilled personnel had vanished completely. But here too he had a remedy to hand—to fill the gaps, to man the depopulated enterprises they began bringing engineers in from the jails! People who had sorely missed the jobs they had lost thought themselves lucky.

At the Sixteenth Congress in July 1930 he was truly crowned. In his report to the Congress he said frankly that NEP had been a maneuver. He had been building up his strength all the time, in the knowledge that "at the appropriate moment" he would destroy the old village and carry out industrialization:

> The Party chose the right moment to go over to the attack all along the front. What would have happened if we had listened to the right-wing opportunists of the Bukharin group, if we had refused to attack, had slowed down the development of industry, held back the development of collective and state farms, and based ourselves on individual peasant farming? We would surely have disrupted our industrial program . . . we would have found ourselves without bread . . . we would be sitting by a broken trough. What if we had listened to the left-wing opportunists grouped around Trotsky and Zinoviev, and launched an offensive in 1926–1927, when we had no way of replacing grain produced by kulaks with grain produced by collective and state farms? We should surely have come to grief that way . . . and found ourselves without bread . . . sitting beside a broken trough. [Applause] Advancing regardless dooms an offensive to failure. Our experience of the Civil War tells us that. . . . The basic orientation in the Party at the present moment is away from a socialist offensive limited to particular sectors of the economic front, and toward an offensive along the whole front.

But Whose Idea Was It?

In my memory, I am back in the seventies. In Moscow. It was early morning in the Lenin Library, as it was then called. As soon as the library opened, a little, thin-necked man appeared. The striking thing in his appearance was a pair of pince-nez of the sort once worn in tsarist Russia. But all those who frequented the library recognized that face and those pince-nez. They belonged to Vyacheslav Molotov.

One day I succeeded in introducing myself to him. It happened at the first night of some play or other at the Yermolova Theater. I had left my overcoat in the manager's office, and when I went to get it after the play I saw an old man in pince-nez outside the office door. I went in and the manager said, "Did you see Molotov? He left his coat here. I had to ask the old man to wait. We had an important guest tonight—our district Party secretary. I had to let him put his coat on and leave first, to avoid any embarrassment." The embarrassment was that Molotov had been expelled from the Party after his clash with Khrushchev. And now the man who had once controlled the destiny of postwar Europe had to wait while a district secretary got his overcoat on. *Sic transit gloria mundi.* I took Molotov's coat and galoshes, and the street clothes of his companion, and carried them out to him. His companion was an elderly lady, apparently his housekeeper. His wife was dead.

That was how we met.

He lived on Granovsky Street, quite near the theater. Which was why he valued his connection with it, and was concerned about embarrassing the manager.

I volunteered to see him home. It was a quiet winter night. I was stupid and impatient enough to start talking about Stalin right away. I sensed his uneasiness, and began with innocuous questions, such as "Why did Stalin wear boots even in summer? Many strange explanations have been given."

He answered me very politely. "Please tell me just one of them," he said. I suggested that the semimilitary tunic and the military boots hinted at war for world revolution.

He laughed dubiously. "Very poetic. Stalin, however, wrote poetry only in his early youth. As for the world revolution—we never did forget our obligation to the world proletariat. But unlike the Trotskyists who kept shouting about world revolution—we made one. Made one, and created a worldwide socialist camp. We didn't keep shouting about industrialization like the Trotskyists, but we did it. In just the same way, they talked about collectivization, but it was Stalin who brought the peasants into the kolkhoz. Although to begin with he seemed to be defending even kulaks. Incidentally, Lenin too only 'sort of believed' in NEP."

I remember to this day his flat voice and that sarcastic "sort of." But like an idiot I interrupted him. "You mean 'sort of' believed in NEP to appease the deaf-mutes?"

He was silent for a while, then said stiffly, "I don't know what you mean."

"I'm talking about Lenin's Testament. There was a rumor that there was a longer one somewhere."

"There was no longer Lenin Testament," he said in the same flat voice.

Later I read a little book by the poet Chuyev about his long conversations with Molotov. Chuyev asked him whether there were any secret agreements about the Baltic States. Molotov, who had drafted them himself, said that there were none.

I imagine that he answered in the same icy tone.

For the rest of the journey he remained silent. I rang him up occasionally after this but could never arrange another meeting. I had probably broken some sort of taboo.

But, invoking poetic license, let us suppose that there was a Testament. If so, when Stalin laid hands on it in Lenin's private office it would have been like finding a map of buried treasure. Kamenev once said of Lenin that "whenever I disagreed with him he always proved to be right." They all had faith in the God Lenin's compass. If Lenin's command in his Testament had been to regard NEP as "serious and here to stay" Koba, who as yet had little experience of leadership, would, just as energetically, have taken the country to the very end of that road. Ilyich, of course, had willed something different. To a radical like Lenin, NEP was merely the rocket designed to lift off his spacecraft and disappear. Was Stalin, at the Sixteenth Congress, putting into his own words the economic plan contained in Lenin's Testament?

The underlying idea of the plan was to squeeze a century of progress into ten years, by revolutionary means. This required industrialization, the collectivization of agriculture, and the creation of a manipulable Party, which would carry out the leader's injunctions to the letter instead of wasting time on discussion and opposition. Only such a Party could finally tame a country stirred up by revolution and create a united society. After that it could go on to make the Great Dream come true.

He allowed the rightist leaders to remain in the Central Committee, but slung Tomsky out of the Politburo. That body became once and for all a submissive tool in the hands of the Leader. True, the pathetic Rykov remained a member after acknowledging his errors, but he was often far from sober. In fact "vodka" was often called "rykovka" in Party circles. To teach him a lesson Stalin forced him to do penance over and over again.

The "Boss" Arrives

After the Congress Stalin set off for the South, as he always did in autumn. And as usual, he left Molotov in charge of "the business." "The business" was what the Party higher-ups more and more frequently called the Party and the country. And Stalin was more and more often referred to by the people and the Party alike as "the Boss."

Molotov was now number 2 in the country, the Boss's shadow. The Boss remembered that Molotov had once been the first to appreciate an unknown, pockmarked Georgian who arrived in Petrograd from nowhere, and had made way for him as editor of *Pravda* without a murmur.

When Koba was appointed to the new Secretariat of the Central Committee Molotov had been senior secretary for some time. The Central Committee machine was in his hands, but this too he surrendered to Stalin without a murmur.

The brilliant Trotsky thought Molotov a blockhead. Bukharin too complained to Kamenev of "that blockhead Molotov, who tries to teach me Marxism, and whom we call 'Stone Arse.'" Chuyev asked Molotov whether it was true that Lenin had called him "Stone Arse." Molotov answered with a laugh. "You ought to hear some of the things Lenin used to call other people. He was no blockhead."

Bazhanov, Stalin's former secretary, wrote about Molotov: "He is a very conscientious, not at all brilliant but extremely capable bureaucrat. . . . He is polite and good-natured." Molotov was essentially a good bureaucrat. An extremely hardworking machine, automatically carrying out the Boss's orders. After all, the Revolution had long ceased to be the green-eyed beloved mistress, and had become an aging wife. The time for brilliant people had gone, the time for businesslike management had arrived. And besides, against the background of Stalin's handpicked, proletarian Politburo, including such men as the cobbler Kaganovich and the metalworker Voroshilov, polite stone-bottomed Molotov with his pre-Revolution pince-nez looked like a genuine intellectual.

The age of "Unenlightened Absolutism" had arrived.

On vacation in the South, the Boss gave his shadow fresh instructions daily: "I think we need to solve the problem of the top people in the Soviets once and for all this autumn. First of all, Rykov must be dismissed . . . and their whole apparat must be disbanded. Second, you will have to take over from Rykov as chairman of the Council of People's Commissars and of the Council of Labor and Defense. All this is between ourselves; we'll talk about the details in the autumn. For the time being think it over together with a few very close friends. So long for now. Cordially yours, Stalin."

He was moving his pieces around the board quickly. The "business" was taking shape. In the last days of 1930 he removed Rykov from the Politburo. The Boss now made Molotov head of government.

"The Boss" was now in effect his official title. On June 12, 1932, Kaganovich wrote to Ordzhonikidze, "As before we are receiving regular and frequent directives from the Boss. . . . In practice he has to carry on working while he is on holiday. But there's no other way."

No, there would in the future be no other way. The Boss was in charge of everything. And the people, whose official history at the time stated that "the people overthrew all the bosses in 1917," now affectionately called him the Boss!

The Great Turn was a reality. The Bolshevik God lay in his Mausoleum, and a Bolshevik tsar known as "the Boss" had arrived.

Trouncing the rightists at the Sixteenth Congress, the Boss delighted his docile and eagerly attentive audience with an undemanding witticism: "Whenever there are difficulties, minor hitches, they immediately start worrying that something dreadful may happen. If they hear a cockroach rustling, they stagger back out of harm's way before it's more than halfway out of its lair, they're horror-struck and start howling that there's a catastrophe and the Soviet regime is doomed." The audience laughed, but he knew that they would soon be facing the famine of which the rightists had warned them.

A Welcome Famine

Collectivization and the destruction of kulaks—the most skillful cultivators—would inevitably lead to an unprecedented famine. Stalin and his GPU made their preparations. The endless trials of wreckers, the unremitting terror, excessive demands on workers, undernourishment, and living conditions fit only for animals had already broken the country's will. "Can these really be the people who made a revolution?"

asked a Western journalist, looking at the people meekly standing in line at a labor exchange.

In the winter of 1931–1932 the ex-midshipman Fyodor Raskolnikov, hero of revolutionary Kronstadt and subsequently a thriving diplomat, returned to his native land for a holiday. His wife described their impressions. All the food shops were empty. There was nothing to be seen except barrels of sauerkraut. Ration cards for bread had been introduced. The population was fed in canteens at factories and mills. But the most horrible sight of all confronted her in the street: "On one occasion . . . near the Nikitsky Gate, I suddenly saw a peasant who seemed to appear out of the ground, accompanied by a woman with a babe in arms. Two slightly older children clung to their mother's skirts. I was shocked by the expression of utter despair on these people's faces. The peasant doffed his cap and said in a breathless, imploring voice, 'For the love of Christ, give us something, only be quick about it, or they'll see and pick us up.' "

"What are you afraid of? Who will pick you up?" the famous revolutionary's wife asked in astonishment. She emptied her purse into his hand, and he disappeared, saying, "You don't know anything about what's going on here. Out in the country they're all starving to death." The Ukraine, the Volga region, the Caucasus, and Kazakhstan were in the grip of the severest of famines. Millions of starving people tried to escape to the towns, but bread was sold there only to townspeople holding ration cards. Emaciated peasants too weak to walk straight—wraithlike creatures, bearing little resemblance to human beings, with children transparent from hunger—arrived on the outskirts of towns begging for bread. The militia, or GPU agents in militia uniform, carted them away, while little boys pelted them with stones: they had been taught at school to hate the "accursed kulaks" and their children, "the kulak's brood." Teachers in every school told children the story of the kulak monsters who had murdered the Young Pioneer Pavlik Morozov. Morozov, a fourteen-year-old boy belonging to a village in the Sverdlov oblast, had denounced his father, a kulak, to the GPU. The son who had betrayed his father was murdered by kulaks in 1932, during the terrible famine. On the Boss's instructions, the son who had betrayed his father in Stalin's name, occupied an important place in all official propaganda. Stalin remembered what he had been taught in the seminary: "He who loves his father and mother more than he loves Me is unworthy of Me" (Matt. 4:37). Statues of Pavlik Morozov were erected all over the country.

He had achieved the impossible: he had silenced all talk of hunger. Any mention of "famine in the countryside" he condemned as "counter-revolutionary agitation." Millions were dying, but the nation hymned the praises of collectivization. Parades were organized on Red Square. There was never a line about the famine in the press or in works of literature. The village was dying in silence. At the height of the famine Yagoda and the GPU arranged a very successful tour for Bernard Shaw, who arrived with Lady Astor. Lady Astor was reputed to be an influential politician, and she was determined to ask Stalin about punitive measures, but in the end she just didn't dare. Shaw wrote that "Stalin received us like old friends and let us say all that we wanted to before modestly venturing to speak himself." He had simply seen through Shaw: this old man loved to talk. Stalin didn't hinder him. And old Shaw wrote about an "open-hearted, just, and honorable man . . . who owes his outstanding elevation to those very qualities, and not to anything dark and sinister." Shaw declared the USSR to be the country of the future. True, when he was asked why he did not remain in that country, the "Dear Liar," as Mrs. Patrick Campbell had called him, laughingly replied that "England is Hell, it's true, but it's my duty to remain in Hell." Those nice Western radicals—how they yearned to see utopia made reality.

Shaw wrote confidently that rumors of famine were pure invention.

No one knows how many people famine carried off. Estimates vary between five and eight million.

Stalin fought famine with his usual weapon—Terror. In August 1932 he personally drafted the famous law declaring that "persons misappropriating public property must be regarded as enemies of the people" and introduced savage penalties for any such offense. The people at large dubbed this the "five ears law," since it threatened any hungry person who stole a few ears of corn with execution by shooting or, at best, ten years' imprisonment. N. Krylenko, still People's Commissar for Justice, waxed indignant at a Central Committee meeting in January 1933: "We are sometimes up against flat refusal to apply this law rigidly. One People's Judge told me flatly that he could never bring himself to throw someone in jail for stealing four ears. What we're up against here is a deep prejudice, imbibed with their mothers' milk . . . a mistaken belief that people should be tried in accordance not with the Party's political guidelines but with considerations of 'higher justice.' "

Judges were told to base their decisions solely on the Party's guidelines. Very soon Krylenko would be given a practical demonstration of this principle on his own hide.

By January 1933, fifty-five thousand people had been convicted under the new law, and two thousand of them shot. People were dying of hunger, but dared not touch the kolkhoz grain. In spite of the famine, grain exports to Western Europe continued without interruption. He needed funds for the new factories under construction. In 1930 he sold 48 million poods (864,000 tons) of grain, in 1931, 51 million, in 1932, 18 million, and in the hungriest year of all, 1933, he still managed to sell 10 million poods. With the aid of fear, bloodshed, and hunger he led, or rather dragged, a broken-backed country along the road to industrialization.

He had foreseen the famine, and he needed it. The village, drained of its strength and near death from hunger, meekly succumbed to death by collectivization. The old revolutionary formula "the worse, the better" had proved its efficacy. But he still had work to do if he was to tame the country. Famine came to his aid once more. According to GPU estimates, more than one and a half million peasants had fled to the towns to escape from hunger and "de-kulakization." As if to defend the towns from the hungry, he bound the peasants to the land. Internal passports were introduced. But people living in rural areas were not allowed to hold their own passports, and anyone found in a town without one was arrested by the militia. The passport system deprived the peasants of freedom of movement, and gave the GPU and the militia an additional means of exercising tight control over all citizens. Another of history's ironies. Passports had existed in tsarist Russia, and their abolition was one of the main demands of the Revolution. Gone were October's dreams of the dismantling of the state: the monster state was now a reality.

While he was creating it, he paid unwearying attention to ideology.

Friend of the Arts

Here too the GPU became his main helper. Cudgeling confessions out of intellectuals was not Yagoda's only skill. He also did excellent work with intellectuals not yet in jail. His closest friends included some of the most eminent writers, and he invented an extraordinary way of showing his trust in them. Investigating officers would summon them to the GPU to listen in while suspects were interrogated. From an adjoining room the writers could hear the interrogator browbeating some unfortunate intellectual until, completely demoralized, he agreed to slander a friend. Among those who went along to the GPU and "listened in" were the brilliant Isaac Babel and Peter Pavlenko. Nadezhda Mandelstam wrote that "in 1934 Pavlenko's account of how he accepted an invitation from a GPU investigator out of curiosity and was present in hiding at a nocturnal interrogation, reached [the poet Anna] Akhmatova and myself. According to Pavlenko Osip Emilevich [Mandelstam] looked pitiful and confused during the interrogation. His trousers kept falling down, and he had to keep hitching them up. He gave irrelevant answers, talked all sorts of nonsense, and squirmed like a carp in a frying pan." The really horrifying thing was that Pavlenko did not realize how monstrous his story was. Time had already hardened most people's hearts. Yagoda was taming the writers, training them to collaborate with the GPU. Confiding the interrogators' secrets to them enabled him to ask for confidences in return—for their help and participation in the actual work of the secret police.

The wife of N. Yezhov, Stalin's most terrible torturer (and Yagoda's eventual successor), asked Nadezhda Mandelstam a naive question: "The writer Pilnyak visits us. Whom do you visit?" "Visiting" in this context meant enjoying the patronage of the mighty GPU.

Yagoda it was who had successfully carried out the Boss's order to bring Maxim Gorky back to the USSR. Beginning in 1928 Gorky, in Sorrento, was inundated with telegrams and letters from his homeland, in which workers' groups, prompted by the GPU, told him how they missed their bard.

In the same year, the Boss had organized celebrations in honor of Gorky's sixtieth birthday, the likes of which had never been seen. He knew how to do the honors. Portraits of the writer and articles about him filled all the newspapers. Through Yagoda's emissaries, the Boss offered Gorky the post of spiritual leader, second man in the state. The old, old story—"You and I are Himalayas."

Living abroad Gorky missed the matchless fame he had once enjoyed. He agreed to visit the USSR. Collectivization interested him. He had always hated the "half-savage, stupid, awkward people in Russian villages" (the peasantry). His hopes were raised by the fact that they would now be converted into a rural branch of the proletariat he so loved, as workers in state and collective farms.

When Gorky returned, Yagoda was his inseparable companion. "Yagodka" ("Little Berry") was Gorky's affectionate name for the secret police chief. "Little Berry" took him on a tour around the GPU's camps. Gorky was shown former thieves and prostitutes who had become shock workers (those who set new productivity standards). And all the time there was a constant, unbroken stream of flattery. The Boss knew people's weaknesses. In the camps Gorky was touched by the successes of reeducation. Moved to tears, he sang the praises of the GPU. He would return to the USSR to stay just as the trials of intellectuals were beginning, in the year of the Shakhtintsy affair. In an article for *Pravda,* the humanitarian Gorky supplied a formula which would become the motto of the Stalin era: "If the enemy refuses to surrender he must be destroyed."

The Boss was not mistaken in him. He had brought Gorky back to play a special part in the taming of the intelligentsia.

Taming the Intelligentsia

All this time, from 1929 on, a campaign against "ideological distortions" proceeded in parallel with the trials of wreckers. The intelligentsia was being taught caution in its use of the printed word. The slightest departure from the official view risked an accusation of perverting Marxism-Leninism, or worse.

Biologists, philosophers, educationists, and economists were all assailed. All branches of learning reported the discovery of "distortions." The "pseudo-academics," as they were now called, obediently did penance at public meetings.

Stalin was gradually eliminating shame. Fear is stronger than shame.

The cruel years that had gone before now looked like a reign of freedom. Quite recently, in 1926, the Moscow Arts Theater had been allowed to put on Mikhail Bulgakov's *Days of the Turbins.* It was a fantastic success. Spectators watched in amazement a play which portrayed White officers (the enemy) not as the usual monsters but as likable, decent people. The production infuriated writers who were members of the Party. But the play proved to have one seemingly inexplicable devotee and defender. The Boss went to see it time and time again. Was this really odd? Not at all. The play dramatized the wreckage of the old empire. And Stalin, as he settled accounts with the leaders of October, could already see the empire of the future.

Still, he did not believe in playing favorites. In 1929, while he was taming the intelligentsia, the Arts Theater accepted a new play from Bulgakov. *Flight* was about the end of the White army and its exodus from Russia. The heroes were the same, the ideas were the same as those of *Days of the Turbins.* But times had changed. The Boss had the play discussed in the Politburo. The body which governed the whole state was called on to examine a play which had not yet been shown. In his empire that sort of thing would be the norm. He knew that nothing was more important than ideology. He had taken to heart Lenin's dictum "the slightest relaxation in ideology will lead to loss of power by the Party." The Politburo accepted the recommendation of the commission it had set up that "staging of this play be deemed inexpedient." The verdict of P. Kerzhentsev, director of the Central Committee's Department of Agitation and Propaganda, is appended to the minutes: "The author's bias is quite clear: he is making excuses for people who are our enemies." As if at a word of command, the newspapers, each and every one, set about destroying Bulgakov. Agitprop did its job, and *The Days of the Turbins* was taken off. The experienced Kerzhentsev obviously intended to seek out the rightists in the arts.

The Boss, however, had other plans for Bulgakov.

My father was friends with Yuri Karlovich Olesha. They had both attended the Richelieu High School in Odessa. In the twenties and thirties Olesha was one of the most fashionable writers. But after that . . . well, he was never imprisoned; they merely stopped publishing him. He spent his time jotting down mundane aphorisms, drinking heavily, and, when truly drunk, throwing his scraps of paper into the wastebasket. In the fifties the whole street would turn round to look at the man with the disheveled mane of gray hair, the dirty scarf around his neck, and the aquiline nose. He often visited my father to ask for money, and they would talk for hours. On one such occasion he told my father how Bulgakov, driven into a corner, decided to write a letter to Stalin. The idea was put into his head by a dubious character widely believed to be an informer. Bulgakov had no money at all, and had tried in vain to find work with the Arts Theater. He nerved himself to write a desperate letter asking Stalin to let him go abroad. This was suicide when so many intellectuals were standing trial. As Olesha told the story: "It all happened in April. It was April 1 and we all played April fool jokes on each other. I knew about this letter, so I rang him up and said, with some sort of accent, 'Comrade Stalin wishes to speak to you.' He recognized my voice, told me to go to hell, and lay down (he always had a nap after dinner). But then the phone rang again. A voice at the other end said, 'Comrade Stalin will speak to you now.' He swore and hung up, thinking that I just wouldn't leave him alone. The phone rang again immediately, and he heard Stalin's secretary say sternly, 'Don't hang up. I hope you understand me.' Another voice, with a Georgian accent, cut in: 'What's the matter, are we getting on your nerves?' After Bulgakov had got over his embarrassment and greetings had been exchanged, Stalin said, 'I hear you're asking to be sent abroad.' Bulgakov, of course, answered as expected, that 'a Russian writer cannot work outside his Motherland,' and so on. 'You are right. I also believe that you want to work for the Arts Theater?' 'I should like to, yes, but . . . they've turned me down.' 'I think they'll agree.' With that he hung up. And almost immediately there was a call from the theater asking Bulgakov to start work there."

So Bulgakov wrote *Molière,* a play about a king who was Molière's only protector against a spiteful court camarilla. Kerzhentsev—who else?—instantly denounced the author to the Central Committee: "What is the author's political intention? Bulgakov . . . sets out to show the fate of a writer whose ideology is at odds with the political order, and whose plays are banned. Only the king stands up for Molière and defends him against his persecutors. . . . Molière has such lines as 'all my life I've been licking his (the king's) spurs with only one thought: don't trample on me. Maybe I haven't flattered you enough, maybe I haven't crawled enough?' The scene concludes with Molière exclaiming, 'I hate arbitrary tyranny' (we amended 'arbitrary' to 'the king's'). The idea around which the author builds his play is sufficiently clear." The Boss agreed with Kerzhentsev's recommendation to take the play out of the repertoire. But he remembered that only the king had helped Molière and took note of Molière's readiness, much as he hated tyranny, to serve his only protector, the king.

In 1936 the old Bolshevik Kerzhentsev would be shot. But Bulgakov survived.

Buried Alive

The Boss was gradually inculcating the idea that nothing escaped his attention. Everything of the slightest importance was reported to him. In 1931 a ticklish situation arose. The demolition of the Danilovsky Monastery was under discussion. The monastery's graveyard would also cease to exist. But this was where the remains of one of Russia's greatest writers, Gogol, had been laid to rest. The Boss decided that the writer's remains should be transferred from the Danilovsky to the Novodevichi cemetery. After this had been done, a strange, indeed terrifying rumor went around: when the grave was opened it was found that Gogol had been buried alive.

Historians of literature excitedly remembered the text of Gogol's will: "My body is not to be buried until unmistakable signs of decomposition appear. I mention this because in the course of my illness I have experienced moments of suspended animation, in which my heart and my pulse ceased to beat."

The Boss was informed. Yagoda gave him a detailed account of what had happened at the cemetery: the director of the Novodevichi cemetery, to which the remains were taken, invited a number of writers. Olesha, the novelist and short story writer Lidin, the poet Svetlov, and others duly arrived. Also present were certain friends of the director: he had distributed invitations freely as if they were complimentary theater tickets. And "comrades" from the department, who needed no invitation.

The coffin was opened and the astounded spectators saw lying there a skeleton with its skull twisted to one side.

While the remains were being transferred there was a certain amount of pilfering. Lidin took a small piece of Gogol's waistcoat. One of the director's friends helped himself to his boots, and even a bone.

These proceedings were not to the Boss's liking. Yagoda was given his instructions, and a few days later all the stolen articles were returned to the grave. Later the newspapers carried an official explanation of Gogol's posture: "There is nothing mysterious about the turning of the deceased's head. The sides of a coffin start to rot first, and the lid subsides under the weight of the soil above it, pressing down on the corpse's head, and causing it to turn gradually sideways. This is a quite frequent phenomenon." Stalin was satisfied. He did not want any awkward associations of ideas at a time when he was burying the art of the Revolution alive, burying the avant-garde and the Great Utopia together.

The beginning of the eighties. I am sitting on the beach at Pitsunda. Sitting next to me is Viktor Borisovich Shklovsky. The great theorist of left-wing art and friend of Mayakovsky. He is completely bald. His longish head gleams in the Pitsunda sunshine. He was, however, just as bald at the age of twenty. Throughout my childhood Viktor Borisovich was never out of my sight for long. He and my father worked on screenplays together. Only later did I learn that he was mainly responsible for the theories of the great avant-garde movement of the twenties. The shining sphere that was his head was glimpsed at all the famous debates of the decade. He is now ninety, and completely alone: the other participants in those controversies had gone to their graves long ago. Most of them to unmarked graves, shot in the days of Stalin's Terror. When he speaks, his thoughts are like the fallout of an atomic explosion. I write it all down as carefully as I can: "Gorky was one of the old school, he didn't know the first thing about the avant-garde, he thought it was all bogus. . . . Stalin did the right thing, sending for Gorky when he decided to do away with the art of the Revolution. Gorky didn't understand painting at all. All the main characters in the avant-garde were fully developed before the Revolution . . . Malevich, Meyerhold, Khlebnikov. . . . They hated the 'repositories'—their name for the palaces and galleries in which art languished. So after the Revolution they brought it out onto the streets. The great world of leftist art arrived. Tatlin, Malevich . . . Tatlin once came to see your father, do you remember? . . . No, of course not, you were only little. Tatlin was a poor creature by then, a broken man. In the twenties he'd been the Messiah. He hated Malevich. It was mutual. And also worshiped him. He put up that famous tent in his studio so that when Malevich called he couldn't steal his ideas. He was very serious, no sense of humor. After October he designed the Tower of the Third International—a symbol of the New Time. He thought of it as a modern Tower of Babel. The proletariat would reject God, and climb its spiral ramp to a new heaven. The heaven of the world revolution. Comintern was supposed to make the tower its headquarters. It was a synthesis of all that was new in architecture, sculpture, and painting. And of course nobody could possibly build it. It was just a dream. Later on he designed a costume for the proletariat which no tailor could make. Then he put on a play based on a poem by Khlebnikov, which no one could understand. Then he designed a flying machine which, needless to say, would not fly. As he saw it, art's only duty was to set the agenda for technology. All he did was done for the future."

He saw that Future. Vladimir Tatlin, the genius of the Great Utopia, lived in Moscow in obscurity and in constant fear until his death in 1956.

They argued about the new art. In the tiny rooms of communal flats urbanistic mirages were born in Asiatic Russia. And with them, countless literary movements. There was no furniture in these apartments—it had all been burned in the cold winter of 1918. Furniture was declared "petit bourgeois." Their women despised housework, and simply covered cigarette butts and remnants with a layer of newspaper. The floor was a little higher after every party. There, on this bed of newspaper, they made love to girls who, like them, believed in the new art.

Their mistresses' haunches reclined among reports of Party discussions and the battle cries of world revolution.

I ask Shklovsky why the left-wing intelligentsia sided with Stalin in his fight with Bukharin and the rightists. The rightists, he says, stood for "the world of the well-off, NEP, shopkeepers, prosperous peasant dimwits. We wanted something quite different. When Stalin sounded the call for industrialization we rejoiced. It meant—to us—that the time of urbanization and of the new art had arrived. Not for nothing was Tatlin awarded the title 'Honored Artist'—the highest distinction in those days."

Only to be denounced as a "bourgeois formalist" in 1932. As I listen to Shklovsky, I ask myself, Did they really believe? Or did they just think it wise to believe? After all, the country was already ruled by total terror. It forced Eisenstein to remake his *October.* And enabled the Boss to stifle the art of the Great Utopia calmly and without excuses.

One of the leaders of the avant-garde, Vladimir Mayakovsky, had dutifully performed the Russian poet's role of prophet. Like Yesenin before him, Mayakovsky had a feel for the future. On the threshold of the terrible thirties, with the end of left-wing art in sight, he ended his life with a bullet from a revolver. His best-known slogan in verse—"Life is good, and it's good to be alive!"—mocked the unfortunate man who lay on the floor with a bullet in his heart.

The avant-garde and the Great Utopia breathed their last beside him.

The avant-garde had wanted a revolution in art, but the new regime wanted art to serve the revolution. The first assault on leftist art was Lenin's idea. Immediately after establishing the post of General Secretary he had set up the RAPP—Russian Association of Proletarian Writers. RAPP, with its team of Party critics, undisguisedly sought to control art.

But many Trotskyists and Zinovievites had made themselves at home in RAPP. The Boss handled the situation neatly. When in 1932 he was about to abolish RAPP by decree, most of the writers interpreted this as a sign of relaxation, and were naturally delighted. The same decree, however, dissolved all other literary groupings. The avant-garde was simply decreed out of existence. He delayed publication of the decree so that the writers themselves could take the initiative in abolishing RAPP and suppressing the avant-garde.

THE GOODS WE NEED: PEOPLE'S SOULS

I was told about this famous meeting on various occasions by Peter Pavlenko and by two other writers, Evgeny Gabrilovich and Korneli Zelinsky.

On the eve of RAPP's dissolution the telephone rang in the homes of many well-known writers. They were asked to report to Gorky's residence, no reason given. The writers assembled as bidden.

Gorky, looking mysterious, met his guests on the stairway, and invited them into the drawing room. They sat there waiting for quite a while before the guests of honor finally appeared. Stalin, surrounded by his senior henchmen. Gabrilovich used to tell us how he could not take his eyes off the dictator: a small man in a dark green tunic of fine cloth, smelling of sweat and unwashed flesh. Gabrilovich remembered the thick black hair that tumbled over his narrow brow and the pockmarked face, the pallor of someone who worked indoors without a break. He moved quickly, as small people generally do, and laughed a lot in short bursts from under his mustache, looking for the moment sly and Georgian. But when he was silent his bushy brows rose at an angle and made him look harsh and grimly determined. He listened politely to the writers' statements. But from his responses everybody realized with amazement that he was supporting the non-Party writers against the mighty RAPP. Then he made a speech, in which he tore the former leaders of RAPP to pieces. He lavishly praised the writers there before him: "You produce goods that we need. Even more than machines and tanks and airplanes we need human souls." He went so far as to call writers "engineers of human souls." He liked that definition: people's souls interested him greatly. Chatting with the writers during a break in the proceedings, he repeated it, aiming a finger at the chest of one of them as he did so. The writer in question blurted out, "Me? Why me? I'm not arguing!" To which the artless Voroshilov retorted, "What's the good of just not arguing? You have to get on with it." The writer nodded vigorously. He wasn't sure exactly what "it" was, but he was eager to get on with it.

Among those present was Sholokhov, author of the celebrated novel *Quiet Flows the Don*. Rumors that Sholokhov had stolen his novel from a Cossack officer destroyed by the regime were already going around. People did not believe that a man so young and so unintellectual could have written a great book. Sholokhov was Stalin's writer, promoted by him. And he threatened to arrest those who said such things. The rumors nonetheless persisted, because nobody could understand why Sholokhov himself behaved so strangely and feebly, why he failed to defend himself. The authorship of *The Quiet Don* became one of the literary riddles of the century.

Yet it was all easily explicable. Poor Sholokhov didn't dare try to prove anything, because the man on whose life the novel was based had been arrested shortly before the first part appeared.

The Literary Riddle of the Age

> June 6, 1927. Case No. 45529 against Citizen Yermakov was heard by an OPU board. . . . Yermakov, Kharlampi Vasilievich was sentenced to death by shooting. (From a declassified case file)

The dossier includes a photograph of a young Cossack with a mustache, and a biography of Yermakov. His life story is that of Grigori Melikhov, hero of *The Quiet Don*. Yermakov, just like Melikhov, was called up for military service in 1913, fought in the First World War, was awarded four St. George Crosses, and promoted to the rank of ensign. Again like Melikhov, he had fought on the side of the Reds against Colonel Chernetsov's guerrillas, had behaved in the same way during the rebellion in the Cossack village of Veshenskaya, etc., etc.

It all becomes clear when you read the most intriguing document included in the dossier. This is a letter from the young Sholokhov, then a little-known writer, to Yermakov, in 1926: "Dear Comrade Yermakov, I need to obtain from you some additional information about the 1919 period. I hope that you will not refuse me the favor of supplying this information. . . . I plan to be with you in May-June this year. . . . Yours, Sholokhov."

Sholokhov, then, could not produce the simplest possible proof of his authorship—the name of his hero and informant. That would have meant killing the book, since Kharlampi Yermakov, hero of the best Soviet novel, was an enemy of the people, shot by the GPU. He was not rehabilitated until 1989, after Sholokhov's death. Sholokhov had to remain silent till the day he died. And carry on drinking.

In the Image of the Party

All writers—Party members and nonmembers alike—now had to unite in the Union of Writers, an organization modeled closely on Stalin's Party: it had secretaries, plenums, congresses—all just the same. He gave this Party-for-writers a leader of its own, the celebrated Gorky, with his aversion to left-wing art. This had been Stalin's reason for calling him home. It had all been planned in advance. Gorky's name was meant to blind European radicals to the suppression of the avant-garde.

Stalin had entrusted the organization of the Writers' Union to Bukharin. The work took him away from the day-to-day business of the Party, and a dependable overseer was attached to him—Ivan Gronsky, editor-in-chief of *Izvestia* and of the magazines *Novy Mir* and *Krasnaya Niva*.

The Seduction

Gronsky's reputation was that of a very nice if not very clever man. Here is a story told by that nice man in 1963, talking to staff members (including me) of the Gorky Archive: "I went to see Gorky once. A man of medium height was standing there. Gorky introduced him—His Highness Prince Svyatopolk-Mirsky. One of the most exalted names in tsarist Russia." They sat at the table. And Gronsky was struck by the fact that the more the prince drank, the more cautious he became. He did not like this, and when he got back he asked the GPU to look up whatever information they had on the prince. When he learned that Mirsky was an alumnus of the Corps of Pages, that he had known Denikin and Wrangel and had lived in England before returning to Russia, the vigilant Gronsky instantly "recognized the handiwork of the British Intelligence Service." He raised the matter with Yagoda and with Stalin personally. After which the hapless prince, who had been talked into moving to the USSR, vanished into the camps.

And here was Gronsky, who had spent a decade and a half in the hell of Stalin's camps himself, proudly telling us how vigilant he had been. So the very nice Gronsky had "belonged" in those crazy days. He may have been the first witness to tell the true story of the Boss's attitude to Gorky: "I heard Stalin on various occasions say things like 'Who does Alexei Maximovich think he is?' " Then he would start reeling off a long list of Gorky's attacks on the Bolsheviks. But he knew that Gorky was political capital. And immediately before the creation of the Writers' Union he bestowed Gorky's name on the city in which he was born, the main street in Moscow, and the famous Moscow Arts Theater.

Gronsky timidly questioned this last decision:

> *Gronsky:* Comrade Stalin, it's more Chekhov's theater.
> *Stalin:* That's of no importance. Gorky is a proud man, and we have to bind him to the Party with strong ropes.

Gronsky could not know that the Master was looking far ahead. In the bloody future of which Stalin was already thinking, Gorky would have to reconcile himself to many things. The Boss was winning him over in advance, binding him with the ropes of vainglory. Giving him something to lose. The Boss knew the power of vanity, that pathetic weakness of pathetic intellectuals, knew the bait to which they all rose with remarkable uniformity to become his lackeys. The French writer Henri Barbusse had been in Moscow for the Gorky jubilee. Shortly before, he had written an article in support of Trotsky, which had brought the wrath of the French Communist Party and Comintern down upon his head. "What fools. Barbusse is political capital and they're squandering it," Stalin said to Gronsky. He took over this capital himself—using the same old bait for Barbusse as for others.

During the Gorky celebrations at the Bolshoi Theater Barbusse was sitting modestly in the body of the hall. But then, in the middle of some ringing oration about Gorky, the Boss ordered Gronsky to extract him from the depths and invite him onto the platform. When the bewildered Barbusse, shepherded by Gronsky, appeared there, Stalin solemnly rose, interrupted the speaker, and began clapping. The Presidium, of course, followed the Boss's lead and sprang to their feet. The whole uncomprehending but obedient audience rose. Stalin surrendered his own seat to the thunderstruck Barbusse, and modestly retired to the third row. Barbusse was inspired to write this of him: "Whoever you are, all that is best in your destiny is in the hands of this man with the head of a scholar, the face of a worker, and the costume of an ordinary soldier."

"He was a great actor," Gronsky wrote. "He would be talking to somebody amicably, affectionately, all absolutely sincere. And as soon as he had seen that person to the door he'd say 'what a bastard.' "

The ideological reorganization continued. After the writers had been dealt with, uniformity was introduced in all cultural activity. The avant-garde in music and art was destroyed. Unions of Artists and Composers were created, and they too had secretaries, plenums, congresses. Two more mirror images of the Party. Henceforward there would be no unofficial groups in the arts. Gronsky assembled the artists in Moscow, and announced to a jeering audience: "Socialist Realism means making Rembrandt and Repin serve the working class."

The audience—all those innovators who had canceled bourgeois art—hissed him, but Gronsky told them, "You rage in vain, gentlemen. We want no more formalist junk." The Boss reinstated the old school—the artists of the empire. The hated realist Repin, who had painted a gigantic canvas showing the tsarist State Council in session, was proclaimed the model. The Academy of Arts was reestablished, former exhibits were restored to the Tretyakov Gallery, and the avant-garde was relegated to the tiniest of rooms.

Henceforward all those active in literature and the arts had to adopt a single creative method. They must follow the Party's example. Only those who accepted the prescribed method had the right to membership in the unions. Every departure from it had to be punished, like factionalism in the Party. The method, devised by Bukharin and Gorky, was called "Socialist Realism." Its essence was contained in the word *partiinost* ("Party spirit"). Only works which served the Party had the right to exist. Realism and accessibility, constituents of the method, precluded once and for all the beautiful delirium of the avant-garde.

The Boss took away their freedom but rewarded the members of the new unions. Artists were given magnificent rent-free studios and received extra rations in the hungry years. But the Boss was especially generous to writers. Separate apartments, out-of-town houses, rations well above the average, all went to emphasize the special ideological importance of these "engineers of souls." In exchange for their freedom, practitioners of the arts would become one of the most prestigious and highly paid groups in his kingdom.

At their meeting with the Boss in Gorky's house the writers, as yet unaware of the bounty to come, took advantage of a break in the discussion to beg favors. When the writer Leonov despondently hinted that his dacha did not suit him, the Boss made an unexpected and somber reply: "Kamenev's and Zinoviev's dachas are now vacant, you could move in there."

It was in fact a time when dachas became vacant in large numbers.

13

THE DREADFUL YEAR

THE ONLY GENUINE CONSPIRACY

He fought on without a pause throughout 1932 and ruthlessly demolished the Bukharin school. He had started the process a few years earlier. The genius Nikolai Ivanovich would soon have no one to show off to. In her memoirs, Anna Larina, Bukharin's wife, recalled Bukharin discovering as he came away from a Politburo meeting in 1929 that he had lost his favorite pencil. He went back to the committee room, bent down to pick up the pencil, and saw on the floor a scrap of paper with the words in Stalin's writing "Bukharin's pupils must be destroyed."

For a start, he made Bukharin not only renounce his beliefs but betray his faithful disciples, who were then banished from Moscow. But Stalin knew that young people would not submit. Just as he had expected, the GPU shortly informed him that Bukharin's pupils were holding meetings and carrying on "rightist" propaganda. In October 1932 some forty of Bukharin's followers were arrested.

That was how autumn 1932 began.

Molotov, reminiscing in old age, said, "It was all happening at once . . . famine, disturbances . . . no, you couldn't let your hand tremble, you couldn't go weak at the knees. If anybody did, it was watch it—you could get knocked off!" Never mind the hunger, never mind the corpses: Stalin would drag his helpless country along the road he had always envisioned for it.

Then, still in autumn 1932, the first genuine conspiracy against him arose within the Party.

On a sunny August morning in 1932 a group of obvious town dwellers turned up in Golovino, a village outside Moscow. The gathering included V. Kayurov, an old Bolshevik who had once hidden Lenin in 1917; Mikhail Ivanov, another of the old guard, a member of the Party since 1906; and Kayurov's son Vasili, a member of the Party since 1914.

The meeting had been called by Martemyan Ryutin. As recently as 1927 he had joined in beating up Trotskyist demonstrators. But Ryutin, who came of peasant stock and had been a village schoolteacher, could not reconcile himself to the rout of the rightists and the destruction of the village. The Boss had been compelled to have him "chucked out" of the district Party committee. In 1929 he was sent off to Siberia to play a leading part in the collectivization campaign. But Ryutin carried considerable weight in the Party, and the Boss decided to preserve him. He was recalled to Moscow and in February 1930 appointed to the Presidium of the Supreme Economic Council and put in charge of the film industry. In August 1930, while the Boss was on holiday in Sochi, Ryutin was also in the Caucasus. Stalin sent for him and suggested that he should recant in public and condemn the rightists. Nothing came of this conversation. Ryutin "wriggled out of it."

The Boss's response came in September 1930. It is clear from documents in the former State Archive of the October Revolution that an official of the People's Commissariat of the Defense Industry, one A. Nemov, also on holiday in the Caucasus, denounced Ryutin. When Nemov was confronted, he asserted that Ryutin had called Stalin a "trickster and political intriguer who will lead the country to ruin." Stalin thereupon wrote to Molotov on September 13 as follows: "It seems to me that in Ryutin's case we cannot limit ourselves to expulsion [from the Party]. He will have to be exiled to some remote place. These counterrevolutionary vermin must be disarmed completely."

He was expelled from the Party, and even arrested, but then released. He could not, of course, have been released without the approval of the Boss. Stalin had given the order, knowing that Ryutin would never give up and could therefore be used as bait for bigger fish.

It happened as he had expected. Once free, Ryutin immediately became active underground. He organized the League of True Marxists-Leninists to fight against the fake Marxist-Leninist Stalin. The GPU, of course, continued to keep him in its sights.

It was to put the League on a regular footing that Ryutin had called the meeting in Golovino. He made a speech on "the crisis of the Party and of the proletarian dictatorship." The gathering confirmed the program of the new league, adopted the text of an appeal, and elected a committee. Ryutin remained outside the committee for "conspiratorial reasons." They then dispersed and began distributing their documents. For the time being the Boss made no attempt to hinder them. Most of the documents ended up in the archives of the GPU, since almost all the recipients promptly notified that body.

Stalin knew that the documents had reached Bukharin.

One can picture him reading them, with their hair-raising indictments of the reckless pace of industrialization and collectivization, their insistence that "no change can be expected while Stalin is at the head of the Central Committee . . . [Stalin the] Great Agent-Provocateur, destroyer of the Party, gravedigger of revolution in Russia . . . the whole country has been muzzled . . . lack of rights, abuse of power, arbitrary use of force . . . progressive pauperization of the village . . . conversion of the countryside into a wilderness . . . naked coercion and repression . . . literature and art reduced to the level of handmaidens and props of the Stalinist leadership," and their conclusion that "we can either go on as we are, uncomplainingly awaiting the destruction of the dictatorship of the proletariat, or else we can remove this clique by force."

Zinoviev and Kamenev were also acquainted with the documents, but neither of them informed the GPU or the Central Committee. They had therefore failed in their duty as Party members to notify the Party and the GPU immediately of oppositional activity. They had fallen into Stalin's trap.

On September 15, 1932, the "counterrevolutionary" group was arrested by the GPU. Zinoviev and Kamenev were summoned by the Party Control Commission. They were charged with knowing about the group and failing to report it. The commission reminded Kamenev of his conversation with Bukharin and of his alliance with the Trotskyists. The October leaders were expelled from the Party and banished—Kamenev to Minusinsk, Zinoviev to Kustanai. Bukharin was not yet touched. The firm still had work for him to do. Meanwhile the evidence against him was piling up.

Stalin could now deal with Ryutin and his followers. On October 11 a GPU tribunal sentenced them to various terms of imprisonment. Ryutin got ten years and was sent to the GPU's maximum-security prison at Verkhne-Uralsk. So in 1932 the former village schoolteacher and former Party functionary celebrated the Revolution anniversary in a former tsarist jail.

While awaiting trial Ryutin wrote letters to his wife which remained unknown until recently. On November 7, 1932, he wrote, "I have now been here 24 hours. My nerves have more or less quieted down. I live now only in the hope that the Party and the Central Committee will in the end forgive their prodigal son."

Ryutin, who had so boldly described the horrors of Stalin's dictatorship, was now calling himself a "prodigal son" and yearning for forgiveness. In his appeal, he said, he had tried to be cautious, tactful, and polite. The Leninist taboo was still operative. Party members enjoyed immunity: only nonmembers were shot or beaten to death.

Famine, breakdowns in the factories, and peasant rebellions had all helped to stimulate opposition, but Yagoda and his network of informers nipped mutinous stirrings in the bud. For example, the Boss received a report of criminal remarks made on November 7 in the apartment of A. Eismont, an old Bolshevik and a Party official: "If you talk to members of the Central Committee individually, the majority of them are against Stalin, but when they come to vote, they vote unanimously 'in favor.' Suppose we go to see Alexander Petrovich Smirnov [another old Bolshevik] tomorrow—I know the first thing he'll say is 'Don't tell me there's nobody in this whole country incapable of removing him.' "

Eismont and Smirnov were arrested, but Stalin would shortly have other things on his mind. On the following night—November 8–9—during the main Bolshevik holiday, the anniversary of the October Revolution, while Ryutin was writing to his wife from the "isolator" and the trusting Eismont was enjoying a chat with a provocateur, a catastrophe occurred in Stalin's own household.

A Shot in the Night

The festival had, as always, been a busy time for him. On November 7, with his henchmen around him, he had reviewed a military parade on Red Square. November 8 was also a holiday, and the day on which all Party members made merry. Stalin and his wife were Voroshilov's guests. The whole of Soviet high society assembled in Voroshilov's Kremlin apartment that evening. Those present, of course, included Stalin's shadow, Molotov, accompanied by his wife. Stalin drank heavily that evening, trying to relax. He was very tired—it had been a terrible year. He knew that the people would not put up with another year of famine. Hungry bellies would overcome fear. His own docile henchmen would be the first to mutiny. Eismont and Ryutin were warning signals. But he let none of this show. He amused himself in his coarse fashion, lacing his conversation with foul language. His image as a rough soldier of the Party had become the reality.

The morning after this night of revelry, his wife was found with a bullet in her heart. A pistol—a little Walther, most convenient for a lady's handbag—lay beside her. It had been a present from her brother Pavel Alliluyev.

Nadezhda's Life and Mysterious Death

Kira Pavlovna Alliluyeva-Politkovskaya, Stalin's wife's niece, had graduated from a drama school. She was about to join the famous Maly Theater and to appear in a film when her mother's arrest in December 1948 (more later about the reasons for this), followed by her own arrest, cut short a very promising career. After her release, she appeared at various provincial theaters, worked as a television producer, and finally retired on a pension.

I went to see her in 1992 in her tiny apartment in a typical Moscow block in an out-of-the-way spot near the River Station.

She was still an attractive and charming woman, and in spite of the heavy blows fate had dealt her she was cheerful and remarkably sociable.

Theatrical people readily share each other's feelings. Perhaps that was why I found it so easy and enjoyable to talk to her.

She began with a little family history. . . . "The Alliluyev's great-grandmother was a gypsy and we are all dark, wild at times, hot-tempered. . . . They say Nadya was a merry girl, always laughing . . . but that was before my time. When they realized that he was courting her they all told her that he had a very difficult temperament. But she was in love with him, she thought that he was a romantic. He had a sort of Mephistophelian look about him, with his mane of jet black hair and his burning eyes. . . . In Petersburg she wasn't yet his wife—they were waiting till she was sixteen. When the government moved to Moscow, Nadya went with him to Tsaritsyn as his secretary, then became his wife."

Later she worked in Lenin's Secretariat, so it was not difficult for Koba to find out things through naive little Nadya. She had to leave this job when she was "in a certain condition." She was too embarrassed to say that she was pregnant, and pretended that her husband wanted her to leave. Lenin shrugged, and said something about "these Asiatics." He probably said it affectionately, since he was very fond of Koba in those days. In 1921, during one of the periodic purges, Nadya was expelled as "dead weight with no interest in the Party." She tried to excuse her inactivity by the birth of her child, but to no avail. Lenin, who was aiding Koba's rise at the time, would not allow anyone to injure his protégé. In December 1921 he wrote a letter about the services of the Alliluyev family to the Party, and Nadya was readmitted as a probationary member.

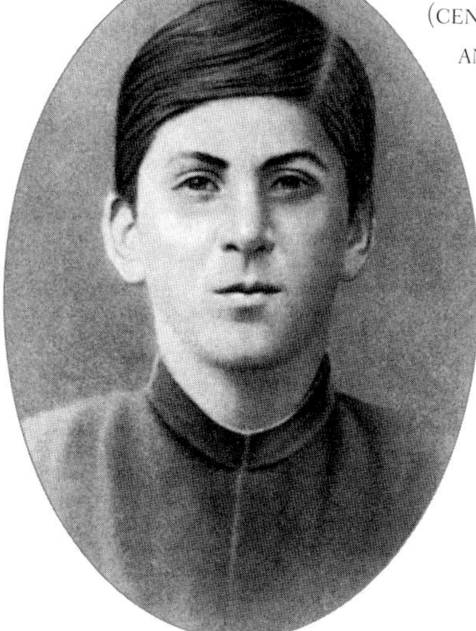

Stalin as a seminary student, Tiflis, 1894. (CENTRAL STATE ARCHIVES OF CINEMATOGRAPHIC AND PHOTO DOCUMENTS)

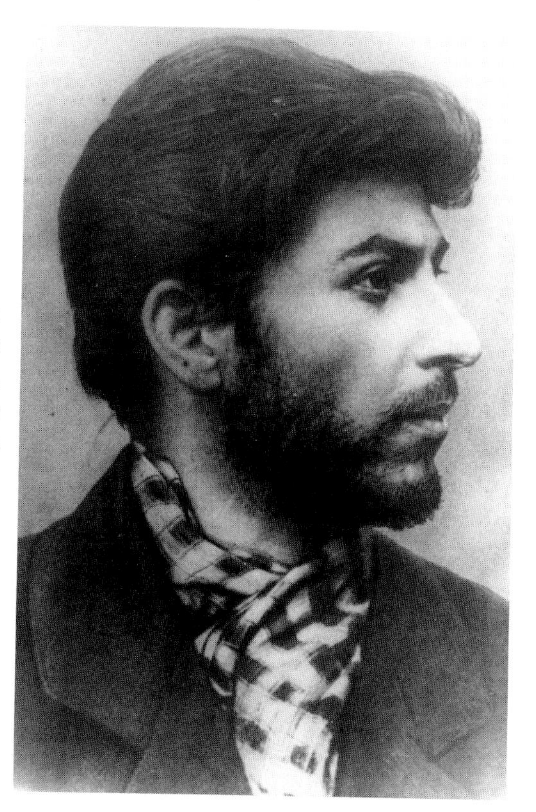

Stalin, the young revolutionary. Photo taken in 1902 by the Batum Regional Gendarme Administration. (PHOTO-NOVOSTI OF THE RUSSIAN INFORMATION AGENCY)

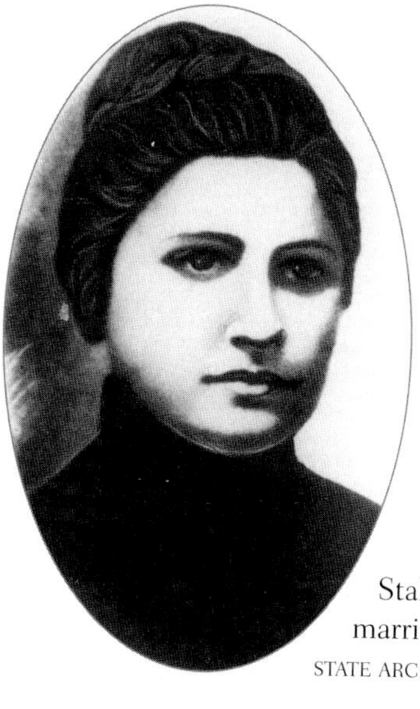

Stalin's first wife, Ekaterina Svanidze, whom he married in 1905. She died two years later. (CENTRAL STATE ARCHIVES OF CINEMATOGRAPHIC AND PHOTO DOCUMENTS)

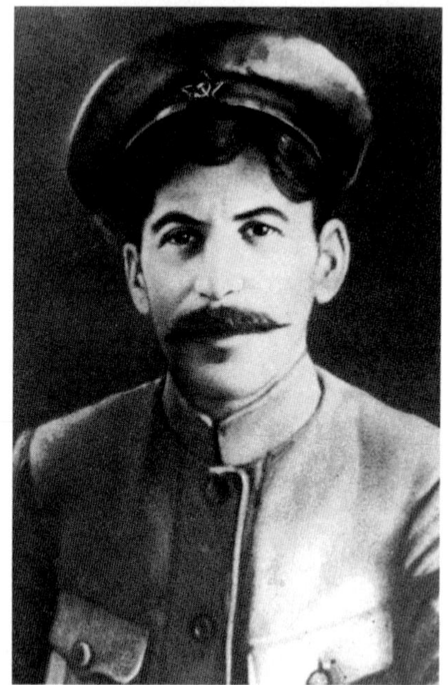

Stalin in his Civil War uniform, as a member of the Revolutionary Military Council of the Southern Front, 1918. (PHOTO-NOVOSTI OF THE RUSSIAN INFORMATION AGENCY)

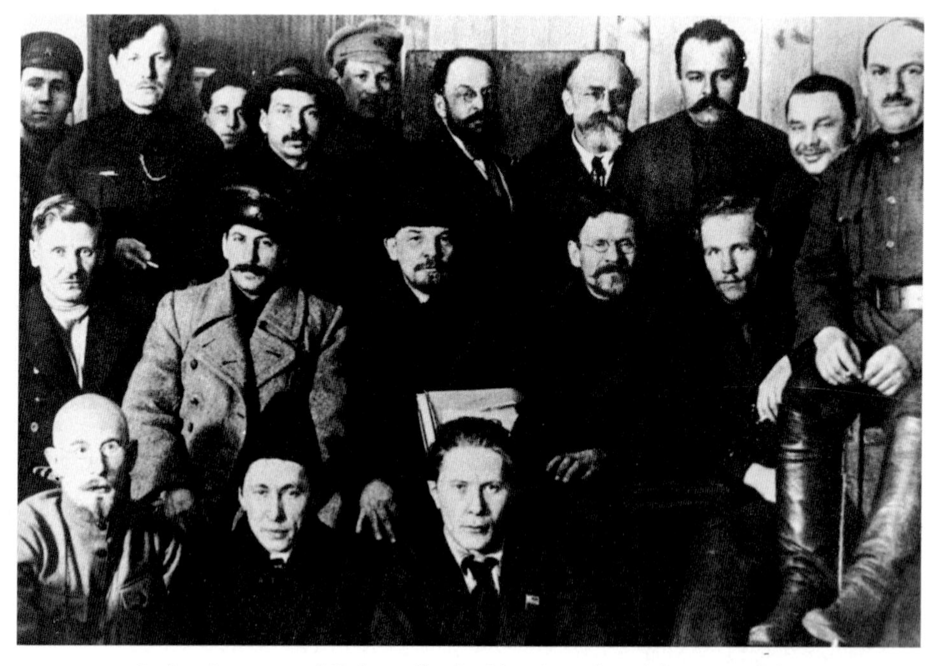

Stalin, Lenin, and Kalinin flanked by the other delegates of the Eighth Party Congress, the Kremlin, March 1919. (ARCHIVES OF THE INSTITUTE FOR MARXIST-LENINIST STUDIES)

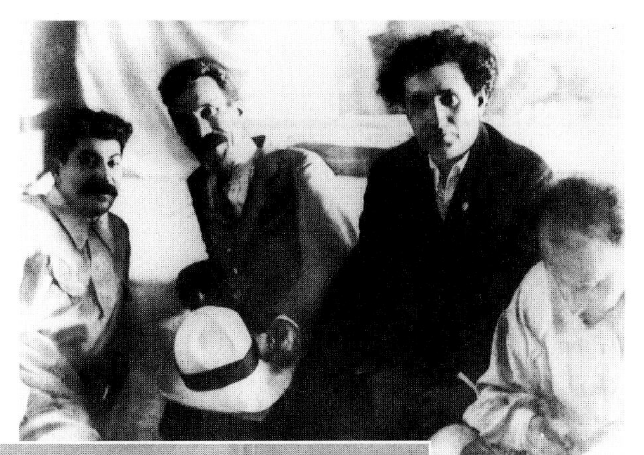

Stalin with three of his fellow Politburo members: Rykov, Zinoviev, Bukharin. Moscow, 1924. All three would later fall victim to Stalin's terror. (CENTRAL STATE ARCHIVES OF CINEMATOGRAPHIC AND PHOTO DOCUMENTS)

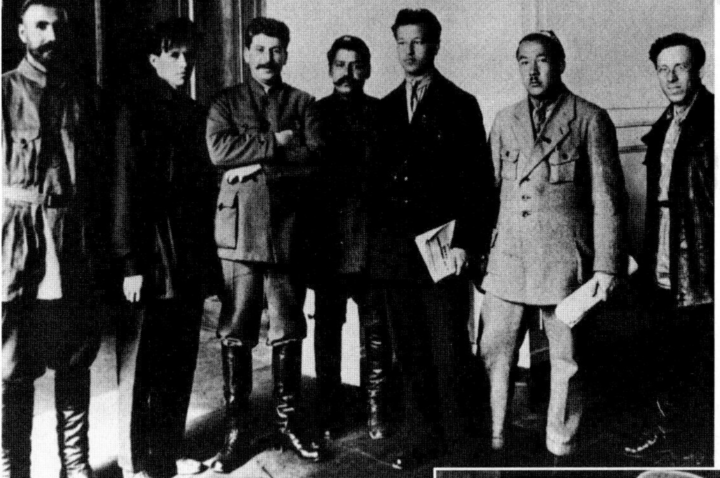

Stalin among delegates to the Fourteenth Party Congress, Moscow, 1925. (CENTRAL STATE ARCHIVES OF CINEMATOGRAPHIC AND PHOTO DOCUMENTS)

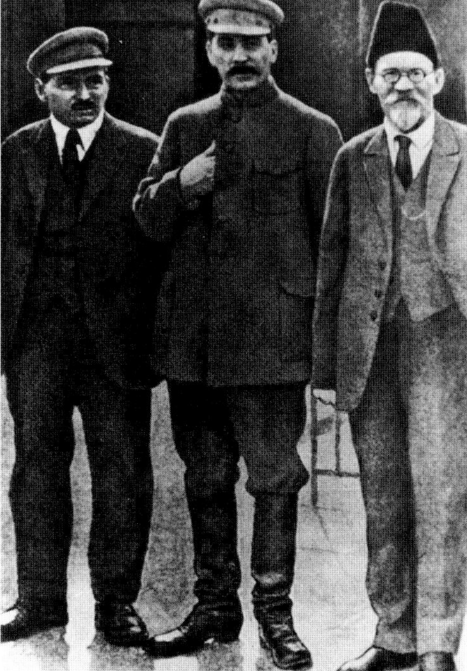

Stalin between Politburo colleagues Tomsky and Kalinin, Moscow, 1927. (CENTRAL STATE ARCHIVES OF CINEMATOGRAPHIC AND PHOTO DOCUMENTS)

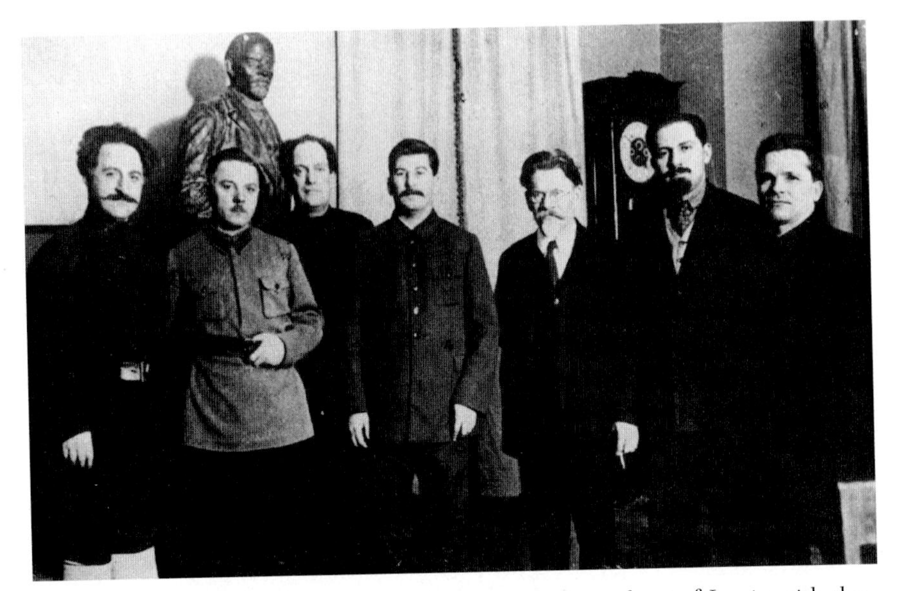

Stalin, having achieved supreme power, poses before a bust of Lenin with the party leaders most loyal to him, Moscow, 1929: from left, Ordzhonikidze, Voroshilov, Kuibyshev, Stalin, Kalinin, Kaganovich, Kirov.

(PHOTO-NOVOSTI OF THE RUSSIAN INFORMATION AGENCY)

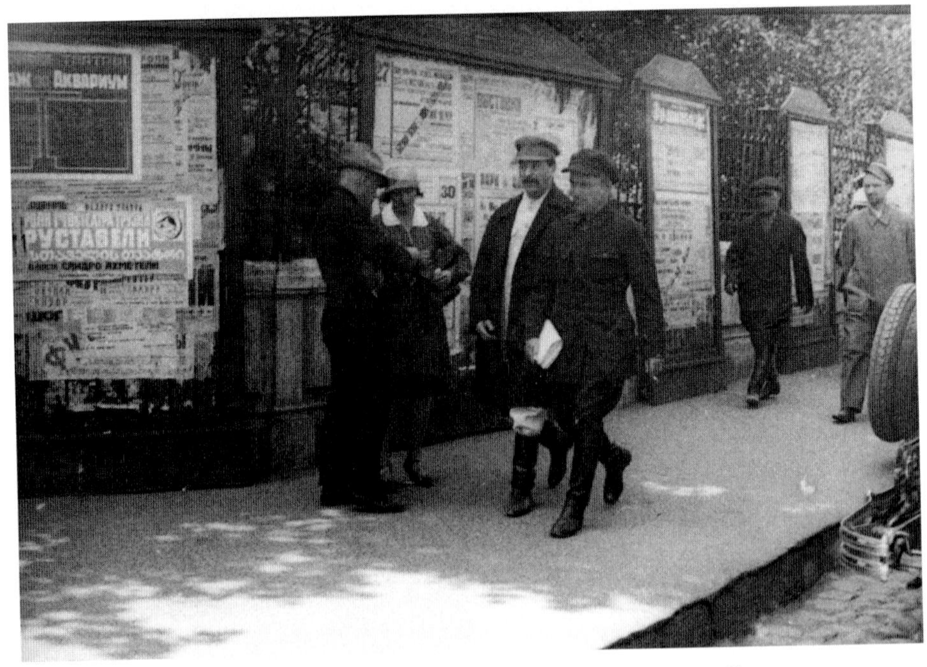

Stalin and Kirov making their way to the Sixteenth Party Congress, Moscow, June 1930.

(G. PETRUSOV/PHOTO-NOVOSTI OF THE RUSSIAN INFORMATION AGENCY)

Joking before the camera, 1930.
(CENTRAL STATE ARCHIVES OF CINEMATOGRAPHIC AND PHOTO DOCUMENTS)

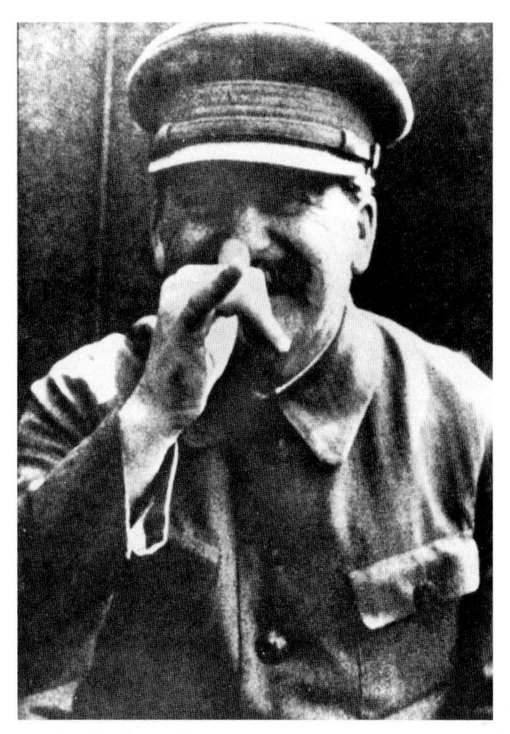

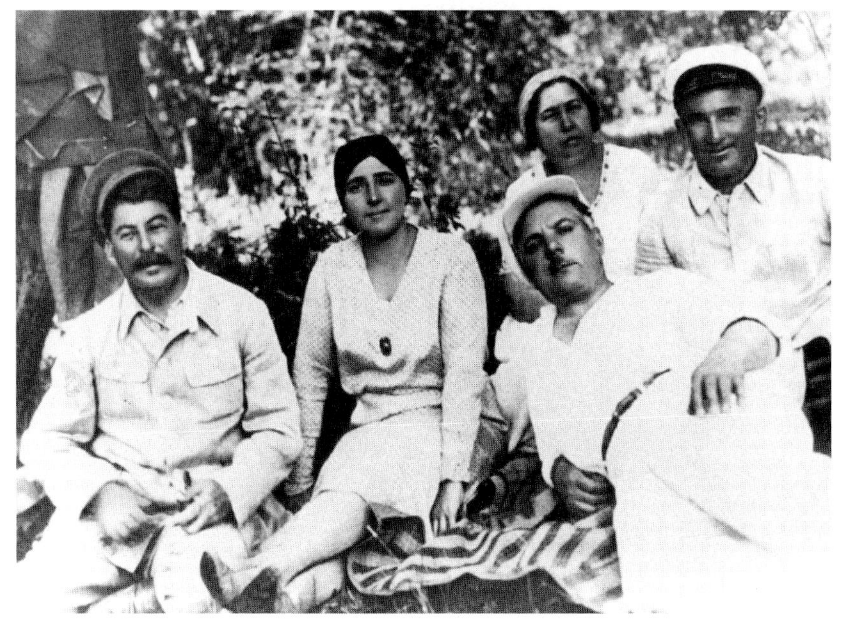

Stalin, Voroshilov, and their wives at Stalin's dacha, Zubalovo, c. 1930.
(Man at right is unidentified.)
(CENTRAL STATE ARCHIVES OF CINEMATOGRAPHIC AND PHOTO DOCUMENTS)

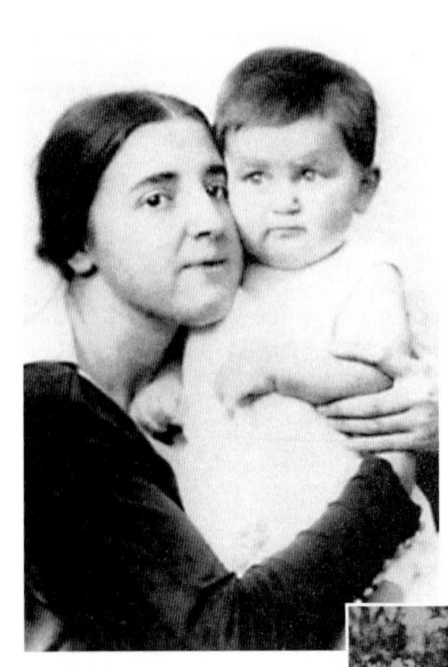

Nadezhda Alliluyeva, Stalin's second wife, with their son, Vasily, early 1920s. (CENTRAL STATE ARCHIVES OF CINEMATOGRAPHIC AND PHOTO DOCUMENTS)

Lavrenti Beria, then Caucasus party chief and later head of the Soviet secret police, with Stalin's daughter, Svetlana, c. 1935. Stalin is working in the background. (CENTRAL STATE ARCHIVES OF CINEMATOGRAPHIC AND PHOTO DOCUMENTS)

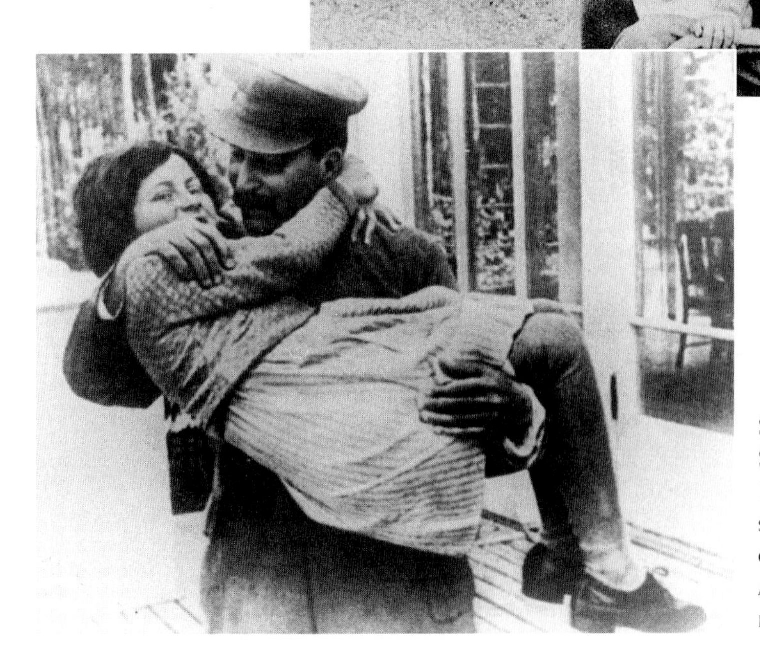

Stalin with Svetlana, mid-1930s. (CENTRAL STATE ARCHIVES OF CINEMATOGRAPHIC AND PHOTO DOCUMENTS)

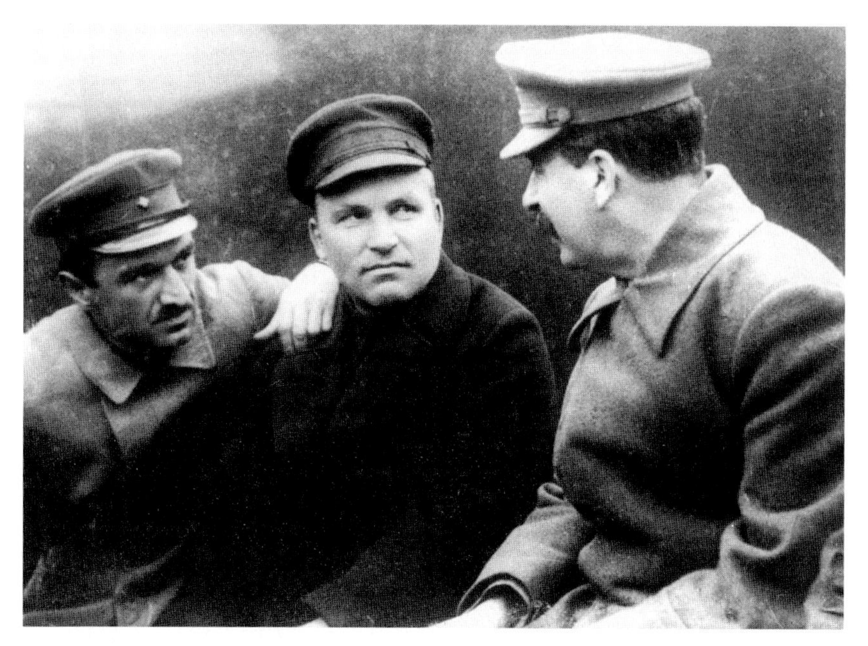

Mikoyan, Kirov, and Stalin, Moscow, 1932.
(CENTRAL STATE ARCHIVES OF CINEMATOGRAPHIC AND PHOTO DOCUMENTS)

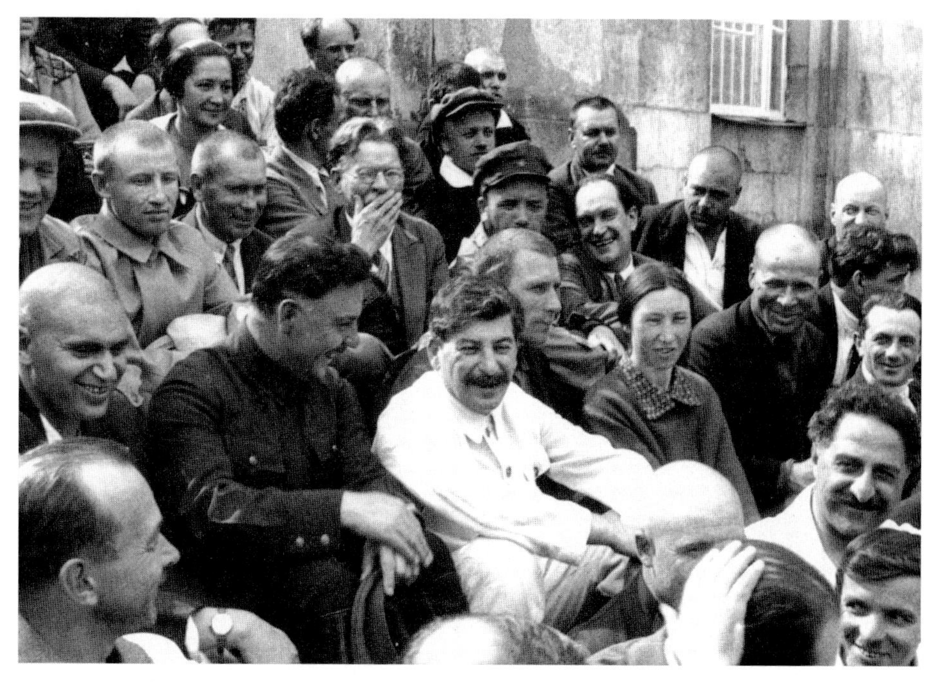

Stalin among delegates to the First Congress of Advanced Kolkhoz (Farmers' Collective) Workers, Moscow, 1933. Kalinin, behind Stalin, seems to be yawning. (G. PETRUSOV/PHOTO-NOVOSTI OF THE RUSSIAN INFORMATION AGENCY)

Stalin and Voroshilov wear national clothes presented to them by kolkhoz workers from Turkmenistan and Tadzhikistan. Moscow, 1935. (CENTRAL STATE ARCHIVES OF CINEMATOGRAPHIC AND PHOTO DOCUMENTS)

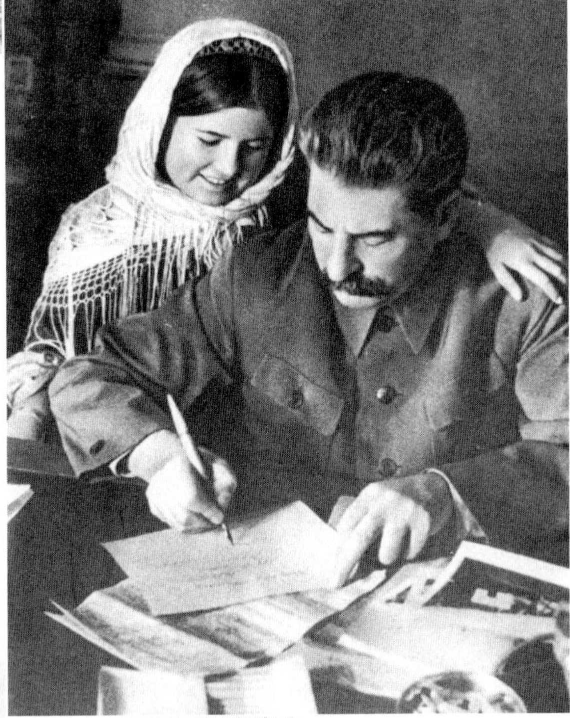

Stalin signing his autograph for Mamlakat Nakhangova, a Tadzhik girl who distinguished herself in picking cotton, 1935. (CENTRAL REVOLUTION MUSEUM ARCHIVE)

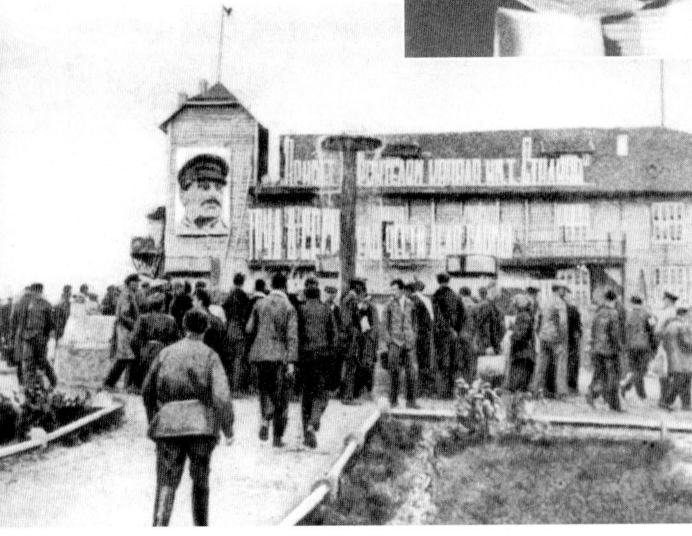

Prisoners in front of the "cultural barrack" at the forced labor camp on Stalin Channel, 1930s. (PHOTO-NOVOSTI OF THE RUSSIAN INFORMATION AGENCY)

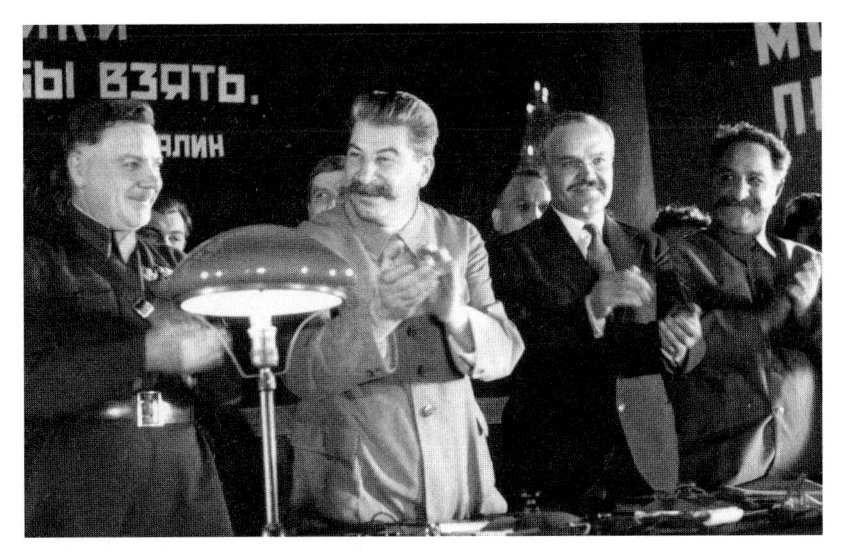

Voroshilov, Stalin, Molotov, and Ordzhonikidze, on the dais at the gala meeting in the Hall of Columns of the House of Unions to celebrate the opening of the Moscow Metro, 1935.
(G. PETRUSOV/PHOTO-NOVOSTI OF THE RUSSIAN INFORMATION AGENCY)

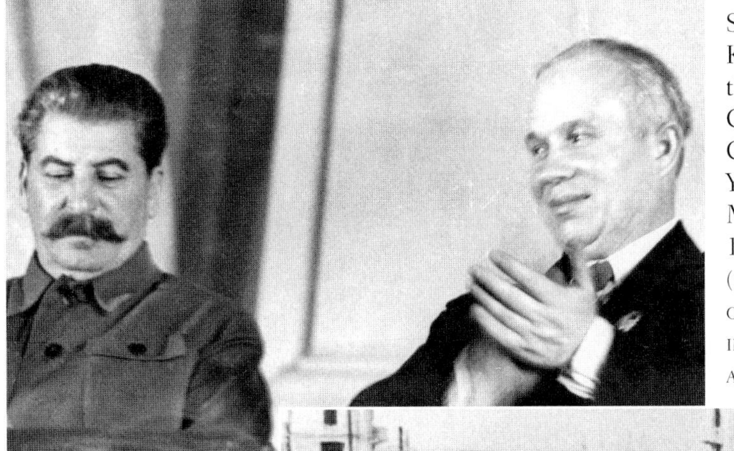

Stalin and Khrushchev at the Tenth Congress of the Communist Youth Movement, 1936.
(PHOTO-NOVOSTI OF THE RUSSIAN INFORMATION AGENCY)

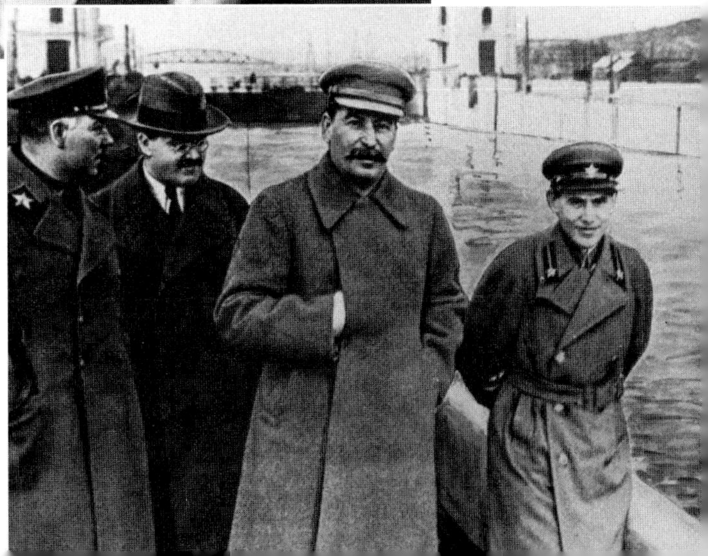

Voroshilov, Molotov, Stalin, and Yezhov at the opening of the Moscow-Volga Canal, 1937.
(CENTRAL STATE ARCHIVES OF CINEMATOGRAPHIC AND PHOTO DOCUMENTS)

Stalin in his office in the Kremlin, 1938.
(CENTRAL STATE ARCHIVES OF CINEMATOGRAPHIC AND PHOTO DOCUMENTS)

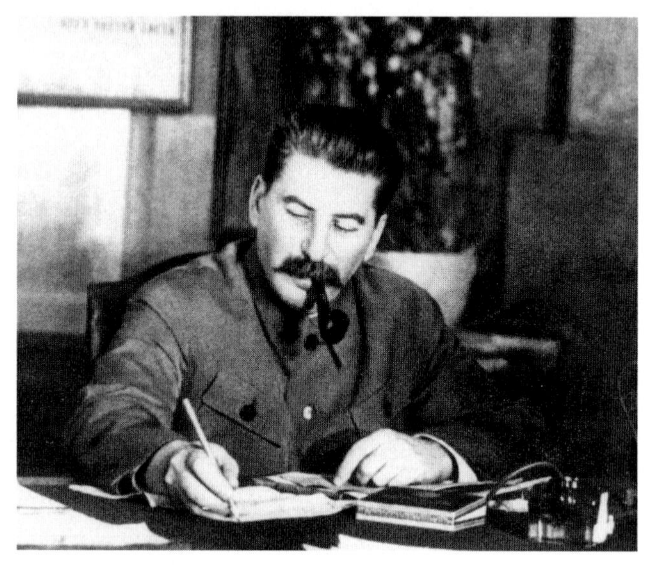

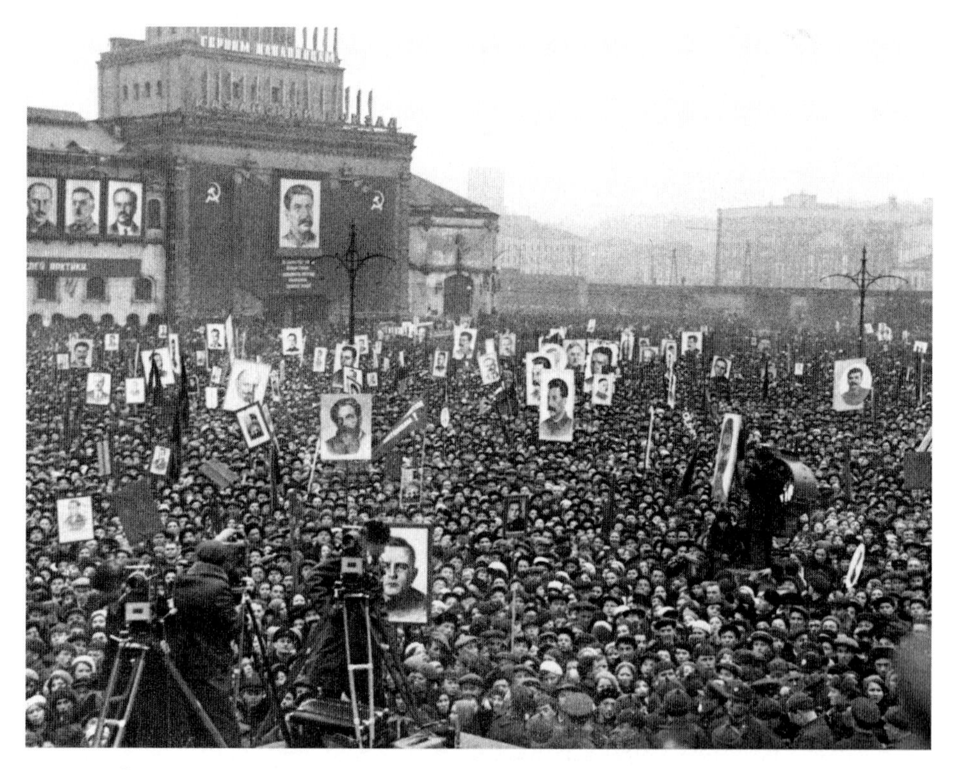

A demonstration to greet Soviet explorers returning from the North Pole, Belorussian Railway Station, Moscow, 1938.
(PRIVATE ARCHIVES)

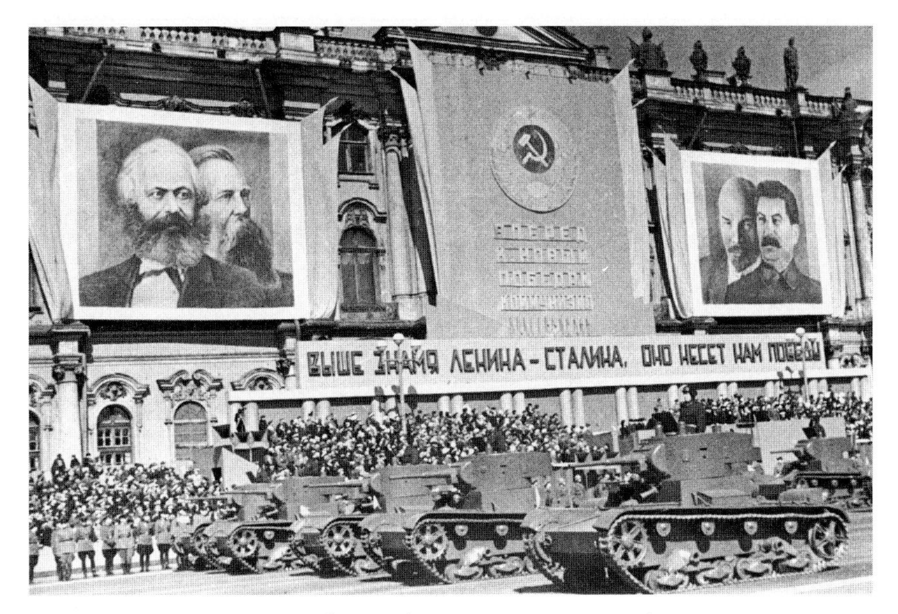

May Day parade in Palace Square, Leningrad, 1938.
(M. RADKIN/PHOTO-NOVOSTI OF THE RUSSIAN INFORMATION AGENCY)

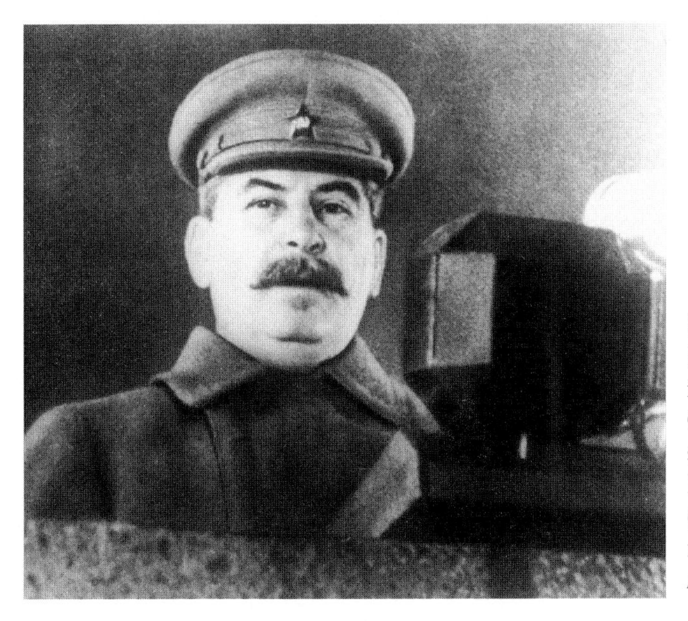

Stalin addressing Red army units in Red Square, while German troops surround Moscow, November 7, 1941.
(PHOTO-NOVOSTI OF THE RUSSIAN INFORMATION AGENCY)

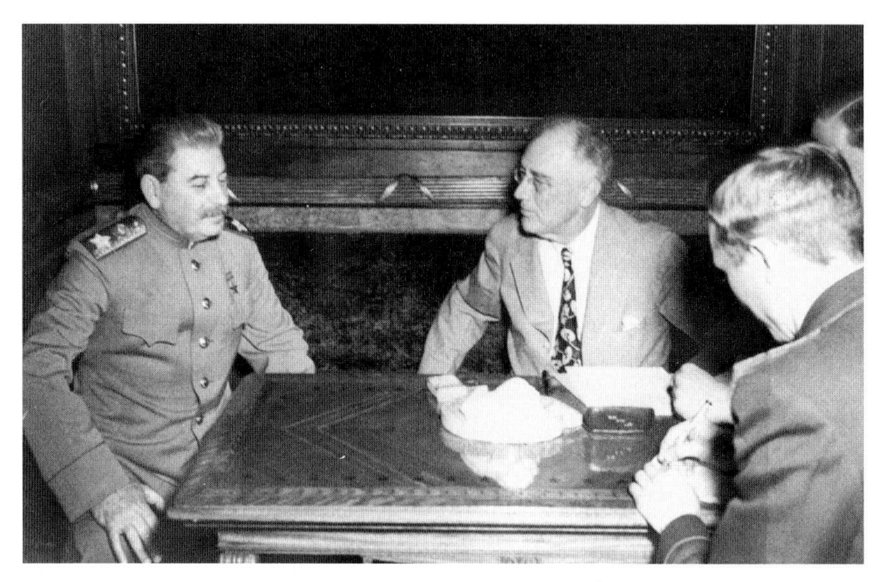

Stalin with Roosevelt at Yalta, February 1943.
(E. HADLEY/PHOTO-NOVOSTI OF THE RUSSIAN INFORMATION AGENCY)

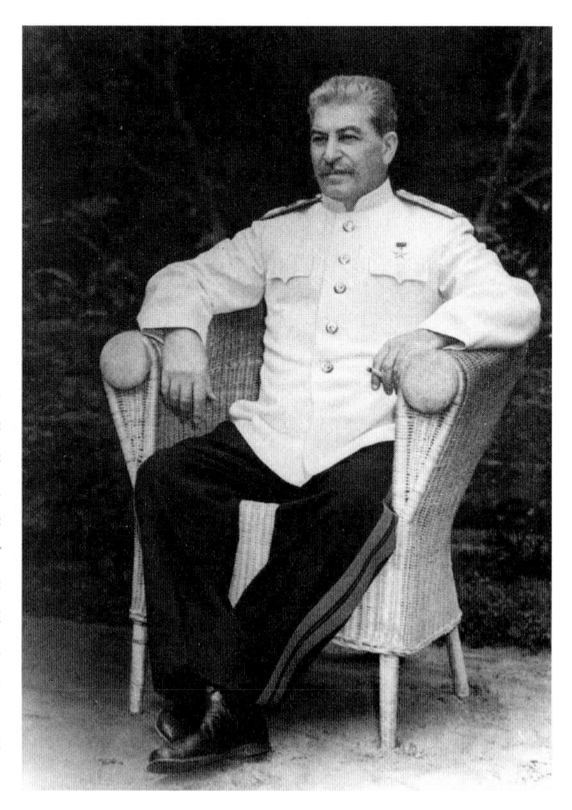

Stalin the victor, Potsdam, 1945. By this time his official titles were Generalissimus of the Soviet Union, Supreme Commander-in-Chief, Chairman of the State Committee for Defense, General Secretary of the Central Committee of the Bolshevik Communist Party, and Chairman of the Council of People's Commissars of the USSR.
(E. HADLEY/PHOTO-NOVOSTI OF THE RUSSIAN INFORMATION AGENCY)

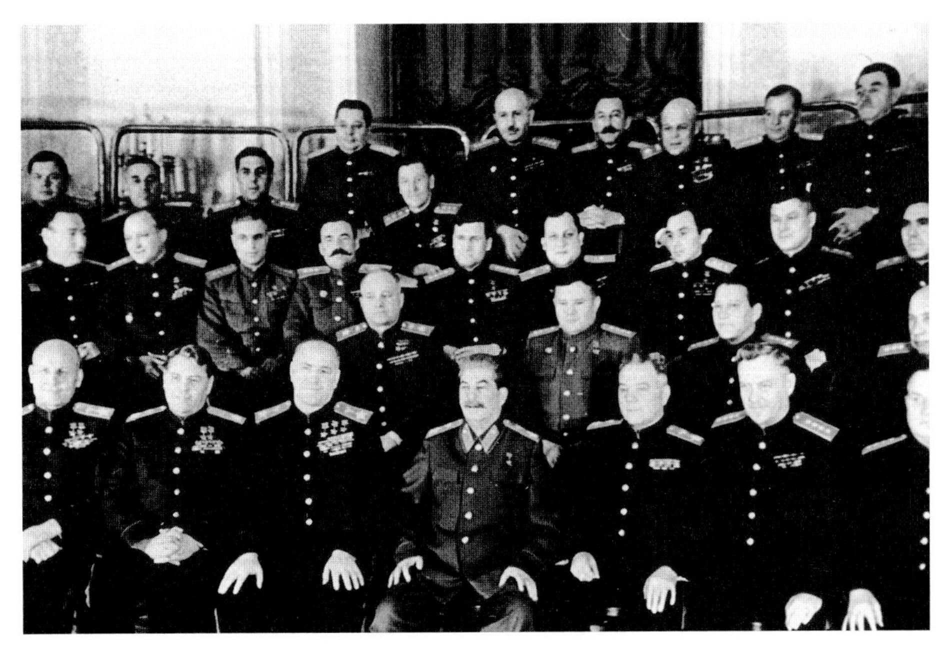

Stalin among his military leaders, Moscow, 1945.
(CENTRAL STATE ARCHIVES OF CINEMATOGRAPHIC AND PHOTO DOCUMENTS)

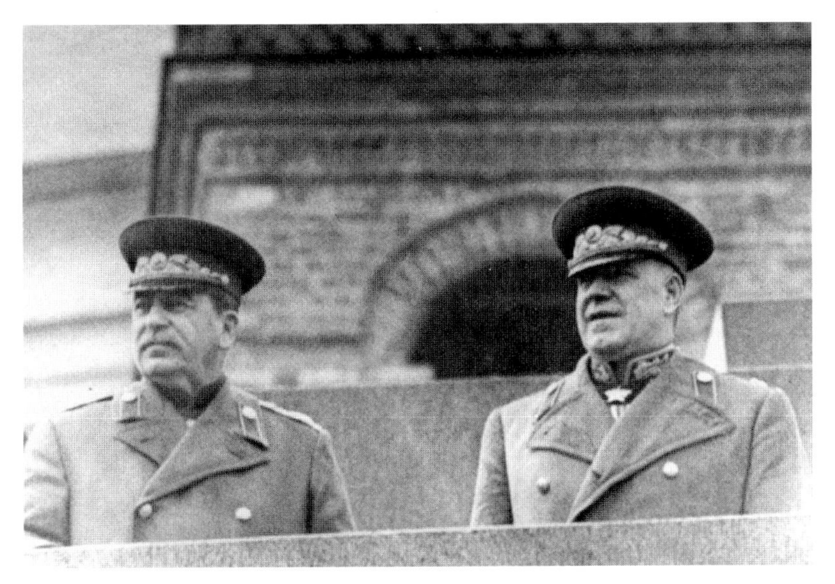

Stalin and Marshal Zhukov atop the Lenin Mausoleum, reviewing a victory parade in Red Square, June 24, 1945.
(E. HADLEY/PHOTO-NOVOSTI OF THE RUSSIAN INFORMATION AGENCY)

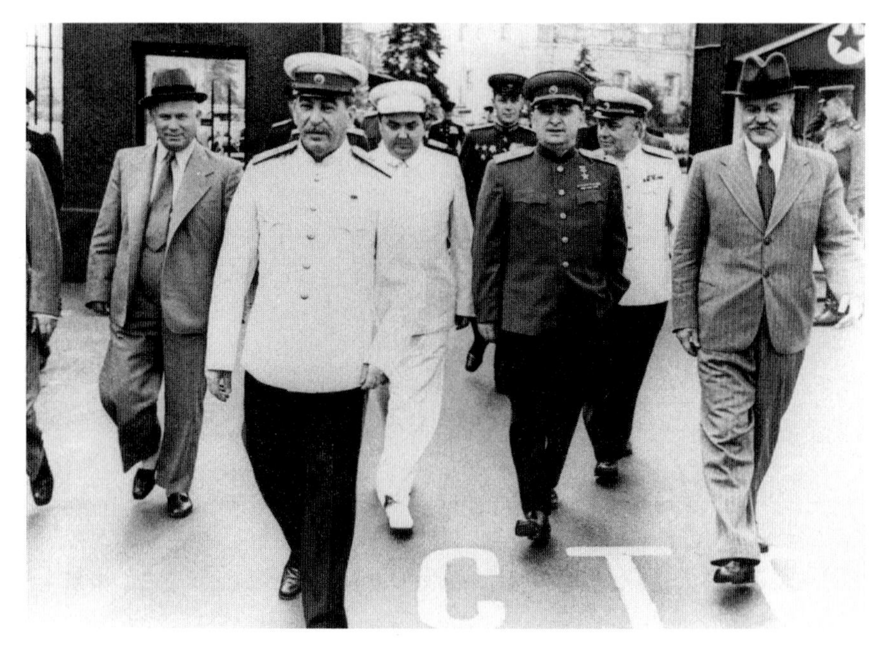

Stalin leads Khrushchev, Malenkov, Beria, and Molotov to Red Square for a sports parade, Moscow, July 1945.
(PHOTO-NOVOSTI OF THE RUSSIAN INFORMATION AGENCY)

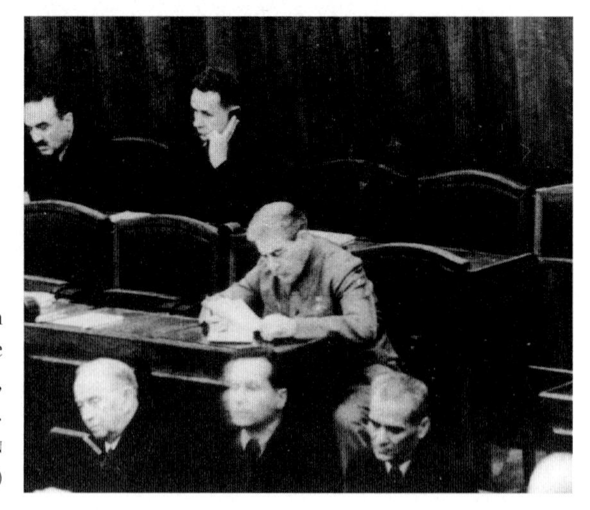

Stalin at the Nineteenth Party Congress, the last he would attend, Moscow, October 1952.
(PHOTO-NOVOSTI OF THE RUSSIAN INFORMATION AGENCY)

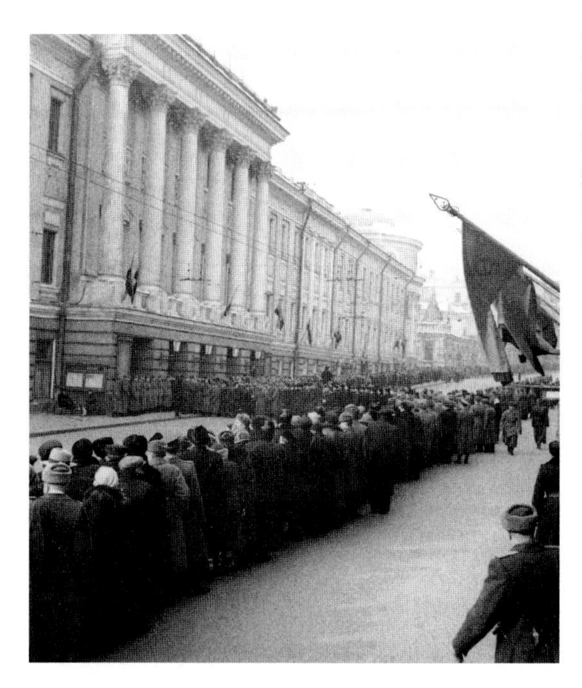

Following Stalin's death, people make their way to the Hall of Columns of the House of Unions, where Stalin's body lies in state. Moscow, March 1953.
(PHOTO-NOVOSTI OF THE RUSSIAN INFORMATION AGENCY)

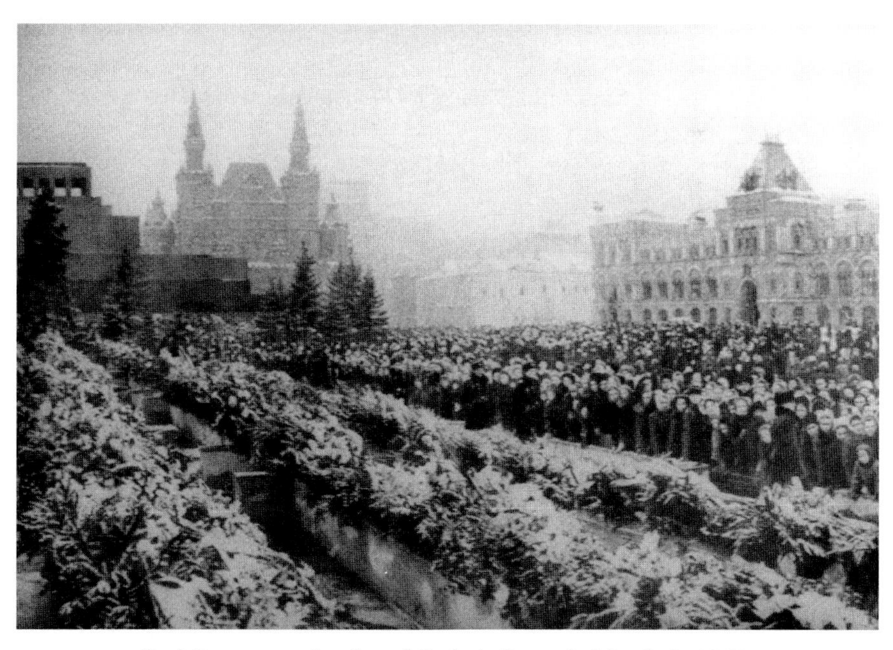

Red Square on the day of Stalin's funeral, March 9, 1953.
The crowds were so large that many were crushed to death.
(PHOTO-NOVOSTI OF THE RUSSIAN INFORMATION AGENCY)

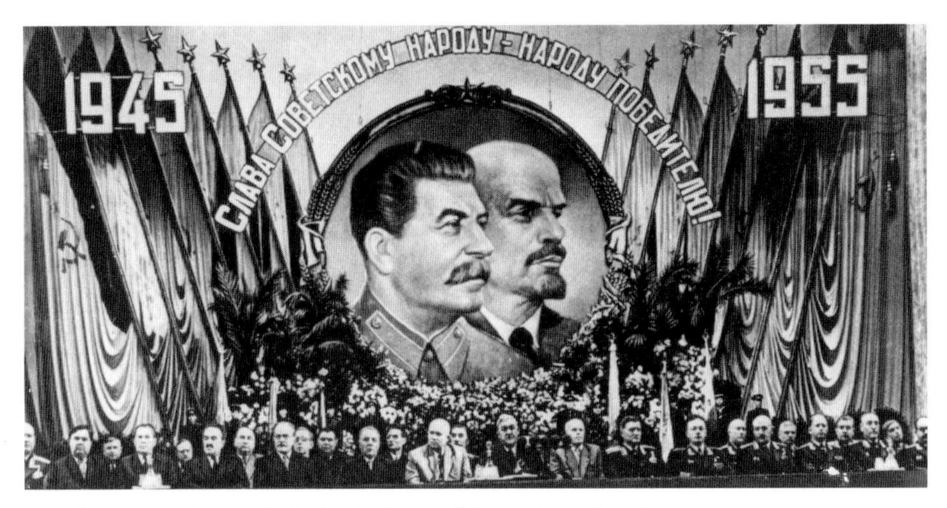

Two years after Stalin's death, his and Lenin's profiles loom over a meeting to commemorate the tenth anniversary of victory in World War II.
(PHOTO-NOVOSTI OF THE RUSSIAN INFORMATION AGENCY)

According to one witness, "she was beautiful at times, and very ugly at others—it depended on her mood." But another witness, Bazhanov, wrote in his book that "she was not beautiful, but she had a sweet, attractive face. At home Stalin was a tyrant, and Nadya sometimes told me with a sigh that 'he hasn't spoken for three days now, he won't talk to anyone, and he doesn't answer if anyone speaks to him; he's an extremely difficult man.' " She was obviously completely dominated by him at first, as his mother had once been by his father. But, like his mother, she soon started showing her independence and her hot temper. General Orlov, a defector once high up in the GPU, described in his memoirs how Pauker, commander of Stalin's bodyguard, once ridiculed him for calling Nadya "gentle," and said that she was in fact very hot-tempered.

It was a family characteristic. Alliluyeva-Politkovskaya told me a story about her father, Pavel, usually the kindest of men, breaking a billiard cue in half in a fit of uncontrollable anger. It was, she said with a charming little sigh, "his gypsy blood."

In their early years together, however, Stalin and Nadya were evidently happy. His vagabond days were over. For the first time in his life he had a home, the home she made for him in what had been the out-of-town mansion of the Zubalov family. The Zubalovs had owned refineries in Baku, in which he had once organized revolutionary study groups and strikes. It seemed especially fitting that he and that other Baku revolutionary, Mikoyan, should set up house in the former domain of the oil kings. The Zubalovs themselves had emigrated, leaving everything behind for the new occupants—Gobelins, marble statues, a park, a tennis court, a conservatory. That was a time when everything was going well for him, and he was rising rapidly. His old comrades lived nearby and they had so many memories to share—all those years of wandering, of imprisonment, of the sordid life underground, of terror and of blood.

She bore him a son. A son is a great happiness for a Georgian. Life was indeed kind to him. He wrote to Demyan Biedny in 1923, "I am glad you are feeling so cheerful. The American Whitman has neatly expressed our philosophy: 'We are alive, and our crimson blood seethes with the fire of unexpended strength.' "

There was, however, another boy in the house. A reminder of the other life that had vanished. In 1921 Kirov had brought back from the Caucasus the forgotten son Yakov. Bazhanov wrote, "In Stalin's apartment lived his older son, who was never called anything but 'Yasha.' He was a secretive youth, he looked cowed. He was always absorbed in his inner life. You could speak to him and he wouldn't hear, he always had a faraway look."

There are many stories about Nadya taking pity on Yasha, about what almost amounted to a love affair between them; there's no end to this nonsense. In fact she did not like her stepson, a painfully shy and rather obtuse boy. She wrote to his aunt Maria Svanidze that she had "given up all hope that he will ever start behaving sensibly. There is a complete absence of interest or purpose. I'm very sorry, and very upset for Joseph, he feels it keenly at times when he's talking to comrades."

V. Butochnikov, who made friends with this tongue-tied adolescent when they were both at the Kremlin Military School, tells us that "Yasha hardly ever joined in a lively conversation. He was exceptionally reserved, but also hot-tempered."

So there were three hot-tempered people under the same roof. The weakest of them was the first to give under the strain. Yasha could not indefinitely endure his father's unrelenting contempt. He was as sensual as all Georgians, and he decided to marry early. His father not only forbade it, he ridiculed him. Yasha attempted to shoot himself, but must have taken fright at the last moment and escaped with a flesh wound. After that he refused to stay at home, and made his escape to the Alliluyevs in Leningrad.

On April 9, 1928 Stalin wrote to Nadezhda, "Tell Yasha from me that he is behaving like a hooligan and a blackmailer, with whom I have, and can have, nothing in common. Let him live where and with whom he likes."

After the birth of her son Nadya gave up work and lived in seclusion. Stalin was always at work. He lived in a tight, all-male community of his own, forever surrounded by his comrades-in-arms. She tried to resume work as a secretary. Ordzhonikidze took her into his secretariat. But the work was boring and she loathed it. She gave up work again, but this time she had an excuse of sorts—she was carrying another child.

In those days the Svanidzes were fairly frequent visitors (Alyosha Svanidze was Joseph's first wife's brother). They had only recently returned to Moscow, and Alyosha's wife, a middle-aged singer from Tiflis, was drawn to Nadezhda by her own loneliness. Each complained to the other of her joyless and lonely existence, surrounded by aging female ex-revolutionaries, the wives of the Kremlin leaders.

Among Maria Svanidze's papers in the President's Archive I found this letter from Nadya:

> 11.1.26. I have absolutely nothing to do with anybody in Moscow. It seems strange at times to be without friends or close relations for so many years. But it obviously depends on one's character. It is strange, though, that I feel closer to non-Party people—women, of course. The obvious reason is that they're more easygoing. . . . There are a terrible lot of new prejudices. If you don't work you're just a "baba" (housewife), although your reason for not working may be that you don't consider unskilled labor worthwhile. . . . You can't imagine how unpleasant it is doing any old job just for the pay. You have to have some qualification, so that you needn't always be at someone's beck and call, which is what usually happens if you do secretarial work. . . . Joseph sends his greetings, he's very well disposed to you (says you're a "sensible baba"). Don't be angry—"baba" is his usual expression for people like us.

Rough masculine behavior characterized the family life of all real Bolsheviks. There was no bourgeois sentimentality. "Hard," "iron-hard," "steely"—this was the new complimentary language of the new order. What would you call a nonworking wife who could not be a Party comrade? A "baba" of course. Just a "baba."

As she became more adult, she began standing up to him more frequently, as his mother had stood up to his father. She no longer forgave his rudeness to her. There were rows, after which they might both sulk silently for days on end. She always addressed him politely as "You"; he called her "Thou." On one occasion he stopped talking to her and it was some days before she found out why. He had taken offense because she always called him "You." They were both good at taking offense and nursing grievances. Nonetheless, they loved each other. They were both strangely, indeed frighteningly, unsuited to family life. Left alone together for any length of time they drove each other mad with their sulks. Yet when they were parted they could not do without each other. Fortunately, they were never alone together for long except on holiday, in the South. In Moscow he was hardly ever at home; he would return in time to drink tea and go straight to bed.

Their second child was a daughter. She was light-haired, and he happily called her Svetlana. Russia's Leader had to have a fair-haired Russian daughter. He loved his daughter, but bitter quarrels between the two difficult characters continued. On one such occasion Nadya took her children and left him, forever, to live with the Alliluyevs in

Leningrad. It was strange how history had repeated itself. His mother had once fled from his father taking her children with her in exactly the same way.

But once again they made peace. She had decided to change her way of life. She would take up a profession and cease to be a "baba." He would no longer have to blush for her idleness. She knew how "morbidly proud" he was at all times. She decided to enroll at the Industrial Academy, acting on advice from Bukharin. He had been one of their closest family friends before civil war broke out within the Party. And since his capitulation he had started dropping in again. The children adored him. He had stocked his dacha with amusing animals—hedgehogs roamed the garden, and a tame fox lived up on the balcony.

(Svetlana later wrote that Bukharin's fox was still roaming around long after its master was shot.)

In 1929, while Nadya was taking the entrance examination for the academy, Stalin was taking his usual autumn holiday in the Caucasus. Previously they had always spent their vacation together. But this time she had gone away earlier, because of her studies at the academy. They wrote to each other, and he kept most of her letters to the end of his days. Her letters go only to 1931. Nothing for 1932, the year of her mysterious death. His own letters, predictably, are very short. As he had told Demyan Biedny, he loathed letter writing. Another feature of the Party mentality: letters and diaries, like all that was merely personal, belonged to the world which they had destroyed.

As I read these letters in the early nineties in the President's Archive—housed in what was once the Boss's own apartment—they seemed at first unrevealing. And yet, letters have this mysterious power: as you read them you begin to hear the voices of those who wrote them.

> 01.09.29. Greetings, Tatka! [He sometimes affectionately used her childhood nickname.] It seems I very nearly caught pneumonia in Nalchick. . . . I have a crepitus in both lungs, and my cough never stops. . . . It's all work, damn it.

> 02.09.29. Greetings, Joseph. [Without sentimental adjectives, Party fashion. "Dear Joseph" occurs now and then, but the endearments seldom go further.] I'm very glad to hear you're feeling better now you're in Sochi. You ask how I'm getting on at the Industrial Academy. I had to be there at 9 this morning. I left the house at 8:30, of course, but the tram broke down. I stood

> waiting for a bus—but it never came. I decided to take a taxi, so as not to be late—and what do you think happened, it stopped when it had gone about 200 meters. Another breakdown. I found it all terribly funny. When I finally got to the academy I had to wait two hours for my exam to begin.

Vestiges of the "Party norms" observed in the years immediately after the Revolution lived on: wives still traveled by tram.

> Tatka! How are things with you? It seems my first letter was mislaid and then delivered to your mother in the Kremlin. How stupid a person must be to accept and open other people's letters! I'm getting better gradually. A kiss. Yours, Joseph.

As soon as she got into the academy she attempted to interfere in Party matters. She wanted him to feel that she was no longer just a "baba." He was purging the leadership of rightists at the time, including, of course, those planted on *Pravda* by its former editor Bukharin.

> Dear Joseph! Molotov said that the Party section of *Pravda* was not following the Central Committee's line. [She goes on to plead for the head of the section, a certain Kovalev.] Sergo interrupted him, thumped the table in the traditional way, and said, "How long must this Kovalev nonsense on *Pravda* continue!" . . . I know that you greatly dislike me interfering, but I think you should intervene in this affair, which everyone knows is unjust. . . . Mama too you accused unfairly, it turns out that the letter was never delivered anyway.

As he saw it, the rightists were acting through her. There were many of them in the academy. Bukharin had known what he was doing when he influenced her choice. Stalin hit back.

> Tatka. I think you're right. If Kovalev really is guilty of anything the Bureau of the *Pravda* Editorial Board is guilty three times over, and they obviously want to make Kovalev their scapegoat. A great big kiss for my Tatka. [He wrote "great big" as his daughter, Svetlana, who could not pronounce her *r*'s would have said it.]

At first she was happy. She had helped him to understand the situation. Only later did she realize that as a result not only Kovalev had suffered—the whole editorial board had been ruthlessly purged.

But the crucial point is that she had intervened on behalf of the rightists. And he had made a note of it.

That the rightists had enormous influence in the Industrial Academy is not mere conjecture. Here is an excerpt from a penitent letter written by one of their leaders, N. Uglanov: "Throughout 1929 we endeavored to organize groups of supporters. We made a special effort to reinforce the right opposition in the Industrial Academy." It was true. She herself made a joke about their influence in a letter to him dated September 27, 1929: "Students here are graded as follows: kulak, middle peasant, poor peasant. There's any amount of laughter and argument every day. . . . They've put me down as a rightist." It is doubtful whether he approved of such jokes. When he fought, he felt only hatred.

In 1930 he sent her to Karlsbad. She needed treatment for a stomach complaint. It was obviously something fairly serious; otherwise he would never have sent her to German doctors. That was the year of his "coronation" at the Sixteenth Congress. As usual when they were parted, he was full of love and concern for her. Her illness alarmed him:

> 21.06.30. Tatka! What was the journey like, what did you see, have you been to the doctors, what do they say about your health, write and tell me. We start the Congress on the 26th. . . . Things aren't going too badly. I miss you very much, Tatka, I'm sitting at home, lonely and glum. . . . So long for now . . . come home soon. I kiss you.

> 02.07.30. Tatka! I got all three letters. I couldn't reply, I was very busy. Now at last I'm free. The Congress is over. I shall be expecting you. Don't be too long coming home. But stay a bit longer, if your health makes it necessary. . . . I kiss you.

Her health evidently did make it necessary. She did not get back to Moscow until the end of August. Meanwhile, she had seen a good deal of her brother Pavel.

Kira Alliluyeva-Politkovskaya told me: "She came to see us in Germany. I remember those days in Germany. . . . Papa [Pavel] was a buyer for some agency, Mama also worked in the Trade Mission."

Voroshilov had found Pavel a place in the Trade Mission so that he could report on the quality of German aviation equipment. He evidently had other assignments too, like all Bolsheviks abroad. General Orlov, the intelligence officer, said vaguely that he and Pavel worked together for two and a half years.

Kira continued, "It was Papa who gave her that little Walther revolver. She may have told him that she was having a hard time. I don't know, and never said anything about it either. . . . Anyway, it was Papa who gave her the revolver. Perhaps she complained to him. . . . When it all happened Stalin kept saying 'What a thing to give her.' Of course, Papa felt guilty afterward. It was a great shock to him. He loved her very much."

All that was still in the future. In 1930, when Nadya got back from Germany, Stalin was on vacation in the South. She joined him, but returned to Moscow shortly afterward.

> 10.09.30. . . . The Molotovs scolded me for leaving you alone. . . . I made my studies the excuse for leaving, but that of course was not the real reason. This summer I did not feel that you would like me if I prolonged my stay, quite the contrary. Last summer I felt very much that you would, but this time I didn't. It obviously made no sense to stay on in that frame of mind. I don't consider that I deserve reproaches, but as they see it, of course, I do. . . . You talk of coming back at the end of October. Surely you don't mean to stay so long? Write, if my letter doesn't make you cross—but please yourself. All the best. A kiss. Nadya.

It was jealousy. Simple jealousy.

> 24.09.30. Tell Molotov from me that they are wrong. As for your assumption that your presence in Sochi was not wanted, your reproaches to me are as unfair as Molotov's reproaches to you. Really, Tatka, I started the rumor that I might not return till October for reasons of secrecy. Only Tatka, Molotov, and maybe Sergo know the date of my arrival. Yours, Joseph.

She refused to change the subject. She was furious with him, but tried to conceal it with a joke.

> 6.10.30. I don't seem to have had news of you recently. I heard from an attractive young lady that you are looking extremely well, she saw you at dinner at Kalinin's place. She said that you were extremely jolly and made them all laugh, although they'd been shy in your august presence. I'm very glad.

She was jealous. He had become a potentate, and she could not resign herself to the fact that women now flirted with him. She imagined that he wanted to be with those women and that she was simply in his way. That was why she had left the South in such a hurry.

There was another series of furious quarrels that year.

In autumn 1931 they went on holiday together. But, as was now usual, she left early. She had classes at the academy. Her letters were calm and matter-of-fact. She had finally made up her mind to be his informant, "the eye of the sovereign," during his absence.

> Greetings, Joseph. I got back safely. . . . Moscow is looking better, but here and there it is like a woman trying to powder over her blemishes, especially when it rains and the paint runs down in streaks. . . . In the Kremlin everything is clean but the yard with the garage is ugly. The demolition of the church [of Christ the Savior] is going slowly. . . . Prices in the shops are very high, and stocks are very high as a result.

This was how she tried to powder over her grievances. With her new businesslike manner.

> 14.9.31. I'm glad you've learned how to write businesslike letters. . . . There's no news from Sochi. The Molotovs have left. . . . Keep me informed.

> 26.9.31. It's raining endlessly in Moscow. . . . It's damp and uncomfortable. The children of course have flu already, I evidently escape it by wrapping myself up warm. . . . By next post . . . I'm sending the book by Dmitrievsky (that defector) *On Stalin and Lenin*. . . . I read about it in the White press, where they say that it has very interesting material about you. Curious? That is why I asked them to get it for me.

At this time talk of the famine, the results of de-kulakization, and his inevitable fall echoed through the academy. She knew the state he was in, and had been pleased to find the book in which Dmitrievsky, once a Soviet diplomat, glorified him and annihilated Trotsky: "Stalin represents the national-socialist imperialism which aspires to destroy the West in its strongholds. . . . Stalin represents the new, nameless wave in the Party which did the dark and cruel work of the Revolution." (He had mentioned this "defector" contemptuously at the recent Congress, but had not ordered his liquidation. Unlike many other defectors, the wily Dmitrievsky stayed alive.)

This is his last answer to a letter of hers:

> 29.09.31. . . . There was a fantastic storm here. The gale howled for two days with the fury of an enraged beast. 18 large oaks were uprooted in our grounds. A great big kiss, Joseph.

They both knew what the fury of a wild beast was like.

In 1932 they went to Sochi together, taking the children. She returned to Moscow early, but her letters to him have disappeared.

There is, however, one letter written in this last year of her life. A letter to his mother.

> 12.03.32. You are very angry with me for not writing. I didn't write because I don't like writing letters. None of my family get letters from me, and they're all just as angry with me as you are. . . . I know you're very kind, and won't be angry with me for long. Things here seem to be all right, we're all well. The children are growing up, Vasya is 10 now and Svetlana is 5. . . . She and her father are great friends. . . . Altogether, we have terribly little free time, both Joseph and I. You've probably heard that I've gone back to school in my old age. I don't find studying difficult in itself. But it's pretty difficult trying to fit it in with my duties at home in the course of the day. Still, I'm not complaining, and so far I'm coping with it all quite successfully. Joseph has promised to write to you himself. As far as his health is concerned I can say that I marvel at his strength and his energy. Only a really healthy man could stand the amount of work he gets through. I wish you all the best, and kiss you many, many times, may you have a long, long life. . . . Yours, Nadya.

She herself had only a short time to live.

After Stalin's return to Moscow, tension in the household reached such a terrible point that, as Stalin's daughter Svetlana Alliluyeva (she took her mother's maiden name) wrote, "Mama thought more and more frequently of leaving my father." He was enjoying his new role as a lady-killer. It tickled his vanity. In retaliation, Nadya more and more frequently repeated at home the gossip about him that she heard at the academy, at the very time when the Ryutin documents were being passed around in the lecture rooms. He judged people by one criterion only: whether or not they were loyal to him, and he began to hate her. He was unfaithful more and more frequently, simply to hurt her. She would go mad and shout out to his face the insults which Orlov quotes in his book: "You're a torturer, that's what you are. You torture your own son, you torture your wife, you've tortured the whole people till they can take no more." It was a vicious circle.

And on November 8 the tragedy occurred. A mysterious tragedy.

Sixty years after the event I found myself trying to elucidate what exactly had happened on that terrible night. To this end, I interviewed Kira Alliluyeva-Politkovskaya, and also resolved to meet Nadezhda Stalin, the other Nadezhda's granddaughter and namesake.

She was the daughter of Stalin's son Vasily and his wife, Galina Burdonskaya. (Her French ancestor Bourdonnais arrived in Russia with Napoleon, was taken prisoner, and settled permanently in his new homeland.) Her French ancestry showed in the exceptional elegance of Nadezhda Stalin the younger, an enchanting woman.

She was born in 1943 at the height of the war with Hitler, and studied in drama school. (Incidentally, her brother Alexander also became a theatrical producer. Is it too whimsical to suppose that the genes of that great actor Joseph Stalin manifested themselves in this way?)

The younger Nadezhda, however, soon exchanged her career as an actress for family life. She married the son of the famous Stalinist writer Alexander Fadeyev, onetime head of the Writers' Union.

The younger Nadezhda allowed me to tape our conversation. I then combined it with my interview with Alliluyeva-Politkovskaya, with Molotov's reminiscences as recorded by the poet F. Chuyev, the memoirs of Bukharin's wife Anna Larina, the books by Svetlana, the daughter of Stalin and Nadezhda Alliluyeva, and, last but not least, the documents which I read in the President's Archive.

From all this material there gradually emerged the solution of the mysterious events of November 8, 1932.

Nadezhda had made particularly careful preparations for the anniversary party at the Voroshilovs' on November 8, her granddaughter Nadezhda recounted. "Anna Sergeevna Alliluyeva, grandmother's sister, used to tell us about the party. Nadya usually wore her hair in a severe bun. But on this occasion she chose a stylish hairdo. . . . Somebody had brought her a black dress with a rose pattern appliqué from Germany. It was November, but she ordered a tea rose to go with the dress, and she put it in her hair. She twirled around in front of Anna Sergeevna, showing off her dress, and asking what she thought of it." She had dressed up as if she was going to a ball. And, according to Nadezhda, "Somebody was paying far too much attention to her at the party, and Grandfather said something rude to her."

Molotov said that "the cause of Alliluyeva's death was, of course, jealousy. . . . There was a large gathering in Voroshilov's apartment. . . . Stalin rolled some bread into a ball and threw it at Yegorov's wife with everyone watching. . . . I saw it, and this seems to have had something to do with what happened."

These two contradictory versions can be reconciled. Nadya had gone to the party intending to show him how attractive she was. Obviously, when Yegorov's wife, who was famous for her amours, began flirting with him and he responded, Nadya also began making up to somebody. And was rudely rebuked for it. According to Svetlana, "He said to her 'Hey you' and she said 'My name isn't hey,' and left the table." Molotov said, "She [Nadya] was by then a bit of a psychopath. She left the party with my wife. They walked round the Kremlin grounds a bit, and she complained to my wife, 'He grumbles all the time . . . and why did he have to flirt like that?' But there was nothing to it: he'd had a little drink and was playing the fool, but it upset her."

Anna Larina, Bukharin's wife, also described the occasion: "On November 8 Nikolai Ivanovich [Bukharin] saw her at a banquet in the Kremlin. . . . According to Nikolai Ivanovich, Stalin, half-drunk, threw cigarette ends and orange peel in Nadezhda Sergeevna's face. She refused to put up with this rudeness, rose from the table, and left. They had been sitting opposite each other that evening, Stalin and Nadezhda. Nikolai Ivanovich was next to her. In the morning Nadezhda was found dead."

Kira Alliluyeva-Politkovskaya wrote: "Mama told me later that when Nadya got home she must have thought it all out in advance because she bolted her door. And nobody heard the shot. It was a little revolver, a lady's. . . . They say she left a letter, but nobody read it. The letter was for him, Stalin. . . . No doubt she poured her heart out in it." Nadya Stalin said: "In the morning they knocked on her door—and found her dead. . . . The rose she'd worn in her hair was lying on the floor by the door. She'd dropped it as she ran into the room. That is why the sculptor put a marble rose on her gravestone."

A Party member's life often ended with a pistol shot. If he disagreed with the Party, or the Party rejected him, only a bullet could resolve the problem satisfactorily.

Stalin knew how his enemies would explain Nadya's tragic end: they would say that she had chosen to die rather than remain married to him. He had lost not only his wife but his home. He was disgraced in the eyes of his comrades and of his enemies alike. He immediately made her suicide a state secret. Her obituary in *Pravda* stated, "A comrade dear to us, a person with a beautiful soul, is no more. A young woman still full of strength, a Bolshevik devoted to the Party and to the Revolution, has departed from us." The official communiqué said, "The Central Committee of the All-Union Communist Party with great sadness notifies comrades that on November 9, the death took place of an active and devoted member of the Party."

Nowhere was there a single word about the cause of death. The funeral was a hurried affair. On November 9 the coffin had already been transferred from the Kremlin apartment to the Great Hall in the building of the Central Executive Committee (now occupied by GUM) on Red Square.

There is a well-known legend that when she was lying in her coffin he went up to the coffin to pay his last respects—and pushed the coffin aside in a rage. Molotov recalled, "I had never seen Stalin weeping before, but as he stood there by the coffin tears ran down his cheeks. She loved Stalin very much—that is a fact. . . . He did not push the coffin: he went up to it and said, 'I didn't take enough care of you.' " We can be sure that he didn't push the coffin away. He never lost his self-control. Anna Larina, Bukharin's wife, described how "Nikolai Ivanovich was standing by the coffin. And Stalin thought fit at a moment like that to come up to Nikolai Ivanovich and say that after the banquet he had left for his dacha, and had been rung up in the morning and told what had happened." Kira Alliluyeva-Politkovskaya said, "She lay there looking very beautiful. . . . I remember that we walked to Novodevichi cemetery afterward . . . but Grandma [Nadya's mother] had lost the use of her legs after all that had happened and was taken by car."

Anna Larina, Bukharin's wife, wrote that "at the funeral Stalin asked them not to close the coffin. He raised Nadezhda Alliluyeva's head and began kissing it."

Then came the burial. Horses slowly drew the magnificent bier, draped with a dark red pall, right across the city from the Kremlin to the Novodevichi cemetery. Next day all Moscow was talking about the crowds of thousands, and how he had walked beside the bier without a hat and with his greatcoat unbuttoned.

His daughter Svetlana asserted that he did not join in the funeral procession. The fact remains that many people saw him walking behind the coffin. He was no coward, but he was inordinately afraid of an attempt on his life. His fear was that of an old terrorist, who knew how easy assassination is. Surely he would not have wanted to walk across Moscow?

As so often, he had outwitted everybody. He did, in fact, walk with the coffin, but only for the first ten minutes, as far as Manège Square—in other words, as far as the first inhabited buildings, where there might be some danger of a shot from a window. There he got into a car, while his first wife's brother, Alyosha Svanidze, also a shortish man with a black mustache, and wearing the same sort of greatcoat, walked on behind the coffin and was taken by the crowd for Stalin.

She was buried in a coffin and in the ground. The usual funeral rite of the Bolsheviks was cremation. Why was the custom not followed? Had he, perhaps, excommunicated her from the Party because of her suicide? Or was this the beginning of a new era? The Imperial Era. She had been the wife of the new tsar. He had chosen the cemetery of an ancient monastery in which the wives of Muscovite tsars lay buried.

After the funeral the country was unofficially informed that she had died of acute appendicitis. The GPU busily disseminated its account. Kira Alliluyeva-Politkovskaya said, "When Mama and Papa [Nadya's brother Pavel and his wife] arrived for the November celebrations they were overwhelmed with grief. They said that Nadezhda Alliluyeva had undergone an operation for appendicitis and died of heart failure in the course of it."

Only after Stalin's death did the Russian public discover that she had not died of natural causes. But at the time, other rumors soon circulated. He had too much blood on his hands. The intelligentsia immediately started saying that he had killed his wife.

Svetlana Alliluyeva, Stalin's daughter, said in her book that her nanny, shortly before she died, told her everything, saying she "wanted to confess." According to her nanny "My father usually slept in his study or in a little room with a telephone next to the dining room. He slept there that night, arriving home late from the anniversary banquet which Mama had left earlier. . . . These rooms were a long way from the servants' quarters—to get there you had to go along a little corridor past our bedrooms: Father's room was on the left, Mother's on the right. She was found dead in the morning by the housekeeper, Karolina Til, who had brought her her breakfast. She suddenly rushed into the nursery, trembling all over, and called nurse. . . . Mother was lying by the bed, covered with blood, with the little Walther pistol given to her by Pavlusha in her hand. They rushed to the telephone and called Avelya Enukidze, the chief bodyguard, and Molotov's wife, Polina, who was Mama's close friend. . . . Molotov and Voroshilov arrived."

We may doubt whether Polina Molotov was indeed such a close friend. We need only recall Nadya's letter, saying how incredibly lonely she felt among the Party wives. And Polina was just that—a haughty Party lady.

Molotov confirmed the nanny's story: "Stalin was at home and asleep at the time of the shot. He did not hear it. . . . Stalin always slept in his own room. When he finally went into the dining room he was told 'Joseph, Nadya is no longer with us.' " But, according to Nadya Stalin, who heard it from Anna Sergeevna Alliluyeva, "she came home and locked herself in . . . but Grandfather went off to the dacha."

Stalin, then, was not at his Kremlin apartment? Anna Larina, Bukharin's wife, as we know, said the same.

We see, then, that two witnesses, the nurse and Molotov, stated that he was in the house, while two others—at second hand—asserted that he was at the dacha. We also have the written testimony of another person, who saw Stalin in the Kremlin the morning after Nadya's death. This was Anna Korchagina, who worked as a cleaner in Stalin's apartment.

Did Stalin Shoot Her?

I leaf through a document consisting of several sheets covered with a semiliterate handwriting. This is a petition "To the head of the state, Comrade Kalinin," from Anna Gavrilovna Korchagina. She writes, in 1935, from a camp on the White Sea–Baltic Canal: "The charge against me was that in 1933 I was on vacation at the rest home of the Central Executive Committee. The workers from the CEC's library, Sinelobova and Burkova, were also on vacation. Sinelobova learned that I had worked for Comrade Stalin and questioned me about the death of

Nadezhda Sergeevna. I told her she died of heart trouble at the same time as acute appendicitis. That was all I ever said about it."

But in 1935 when the repressions began, Sinelobova's brother, who worked in the Kremlin commandant's office, was shot, and Sinelobova herself was arrested. "Sinelobov was in Comrade Stalin's apartment when Nadezhda Sergeevna died," Korchagina writes. "He was authorized to act for the Kremlin commandant. When they were arrested, as I learned during the investigation, Sinelobova gave evidence against me, that I had told her the cause of Nadezhda Sergeevna's death was Comrade Stalin, and that he had shot her. I could never have said it, it is impossible to think up such a vile lie about a man dear to me and all those for whom he has opened up a path to a bright life. I know very well that even you, Comrade Kalinin, know that Comrade Stalin was with Comrade Molotov out of town at his dacha that evening. I was not in Comrade Stalin's apartment at that time. We were doing the rooms in the other block, but we were rung up from the dacha and asked 'what has happened there?' . . . They rang Comrade Stalin from the Kremlin telling him to come home, and he made haste and left quickly . . . quite early. When I got to work at 9:00 A.M. I saw everybody was upset but they didn't tell us women workers anything until the coffin and flowers were brought, then they told us that Nadezhda Sergeevna was dead. They didn't tell us before so we wouldn't start howling and upsetting others. This is my faithful testimony to her natural death. On March 22, 1935, two comrades in army tunics came to see me. I thought it was to take me to work, but they took me to the Lubyanka [prison]. In the interrogation I told them everything as I'm telling you, but they shouted at me, 'She's lying, she's got eyes like a thief.' And they said a lot of insulting things. . . . I read the protocol, but I couldn't sign it, because what was there wasn't what I'd said, but when I started objecting they shouted at me ever so loud and one of the comrades came up to me and quietly laid his hand on my shoulder, then shouted, 'You'd better sign if you know what's good for you,' and I was so frightened I signed it all." After explaining what happened, Korchagina pleads for a pardon. Written on the petition are the words "referred to M.I. [Kalinin] personally," followed by his decision—"Reject. 8.3.35 Kalinin." So the hapless cleaner disappeared into the camps.

But let us remember these words: "Even you, Comrade Kalinin, know that Comrade Stalin was with Comrade Molotov out of town at his dacha that evening." That was the *official* version. The version given to the servants, which they were required to repeat. And which Stalin himself had "thought fit" to pass on to Bukharin as they stood beside the coffin. But what was the reality? Molotov and the nurse are of course right. They were both in the house and saw it all for themselves: the Boss was at home that night, but for some reason did not want anybody to know. Why? To understand it we must go back to Nadya's last evening.

She arrives for the party in a funereal dress with a rose on it. She is insulted. She flees from the party. Why was she so overwrought? Was it only jealousy? Was this a unique occasion? No, she had become "a bit of a psychopath," as Molotov put it.

Why? The answer turned out to be as horrifying as it was simple.

In the President's Archive I came across the "case history of Alliluyeva N.S.," compiled in the Kremlin Polyclinic. The Boss had kept it in his personal archive. I leafed through it. "Alliluyeva, Nadezhda Sergeevna, native of Baku, member of the Party from the age of 18."

At the end of the "case history" I was taken aback by an entry dated August 1932, which reads: "Acute pains in the abdominal region—return for further examination in 2–3 weeks' time." This was followed by one final alarming entry: "31.8.32. Examination to consider operation in 3–4 weeks." There are no further entries. So she committed suicide when she was due to have an operation. I had seen no previous mention of this in my reading!

There had evidently been a good reason for her journey to Karlsbad. She had been experiencing "acute pains in the abdominal region" for some time. Nothing concrete was said about the causes of her pains. But she was undergoing examinations and was being prepared for an operation of some sort. Yet a decision was taken not to record details of her illness. Which means that it must have been something very serious. Perhaps she had begun to suspect something when she was undergoing treatment in Karlsbad. Was that the reason for her heightened excitability all this time? And was that how the revolver, her brother Pavel's strange present, came into her possession? Did she ask him for it? A revolver was a Party member's loyal aid when life became unbearable. And the insult at the anniversary party could have been the last straw.

So she ran away from the party. Polina, Molotov's wife, caught up with her. They talked. Afterward, Polina herself would describe to Svetlana how they had walked around the Kremlin grounds and how she had calmed Nadya down. But Nadya had still insisted on going home. So the question arises, had Polina really succeeded in calming her down? Or had she even tried?

That was a terrible time full of terrible people. Polina Molotov was typical of the revolutionary women in that period. In 1949, when she was arrested on the Boss's orders, she told her life story under interrogation: "My name is Perl Semyonovna. Zhemchuzina was my Party pseudonym." "Did you work underground?" "Yes, in the Ukraine when Denikin's army was there. . . . While attending an international women's congress I met Molotov . . . and at the end of 1921 I became his wife." Polina, the underground revolutionary, Party activist, Commissar of the Food Industry, People's Commissar of the Fishing Industry. A victim of Stalin, this staunch revolutionary continued to deify him even after her release. Could she possibly have loved that "baba" Nadya, with her undisguised sympathy for Bukharin, who despised and hated Polina's husband? At a time when there was a fierce struggle for power and the presence of "that baba" at the Boss's side was so dangerous?

Nadya did genuinely sympathize with Bukharin. Anna Larina, Bukharin's wife, said, "She secretly shared his views on collectivization and found a convenient occasion to tell him so." And Molotov knew all about it. He told the poet Chuyev, "That she became Bukharin's follower is very unlikely. But she did, of course, allow herself to be influenced by him."

So if Polina ran after Nadya, it was more probably out of a sense of duty. The second lady in the land must comfort the first. If she tried to comfort her at all, she may have gone about it in a peculiar way. Polina may well have known a certain secret, any hint of which might be fatal for Nadya.

We find a trace of this secret in Maria Svanidze's diary, which I have read in the President's Archive.

"Now That I Know Everything"

This was the Maria who had confessed her loneliness to Nadya. Alyosha and Maria Svanidze were arrested in 1937, and Maria's papers were passed to Stalin. He kept them in his apartment, in his personal archive. With good reason.

Maria Svanidze had dared to make an entry in her diary which strangers could not possibly be allowed to read: "4.11.34. Saw J. [Joseph] again yesterday after a three-month interval. He got back from Sochi on the 29th. He looks fine, but has lost a lot of weight. We—I myself, Nyura [Anna, Nadya's sister], and Zhenya [Pavel Alliluyev's wife] . . . walked over to see him at 7:00 P.M., but he was not at home. . . . We spent some time with the children, and were sitting in Vasya's room when Joseph suddenly came down the corridor wearing a summer overcoat; in spite of the cold weather he never likes changing his clothes with the seasons and goes on wearing the summer clothes he is used to, and it's the same story in spring, when winter garments are left off and others have to be worn. . . . He invited us to a meal. He spoke to me kindly, asked after Alyosha, teased Zhenya about getting fat again. He treated her very affectionately. Now that I know everything I have watched them closely. They opened some champagne, and we drank toasts."

Zhenya, the wife of Nadya's brother, was a dream woman: a tall Russian beauty with light brown tresses and flushed cheeks. Her daughter, Kira Alliluyeva-Politkovskaya, said, "Mama's nickname was 'the rose of the Novgorod fields.' She was [five feet nine inches] tall. Just before she went into labor she split some logs—then she went off and gave birth to me."

Maria Svanidze's entry was made in 1934, long after Nadya's death. But the infatuation may have begun earlier. Here is another excerpt from my conversation with Alliluyeva-Politkovskaya:

> *Myself:* I've often read that Stalin sent all the Alliluyevs packing after his wife's death.
> *Alliluyeva-Politkovskaya:* On the contrary, he took us all to live in his dacha at Zubalovo. We lived there from 1932, Grandma, Grandpa, Seryozha [Alliluyeva-Politkovskaya's brother], and Mama and Papa, who came for weekends. . . . Stalin was generally stern and reserved, but he noticed when women dressed well. He used to say to Mama—"Zhenya, you ought to teach Soviet women how to dress."

Yes, he was under her spell before 1934. And if we remember how weary he had been of all those rows with his wife, of the eternal strife between them. . . .

Perhaps it is not too much to speculate that Zhemchuzina, when she was "calming" Nadya, only had to drop the slightest hint to make Nadya's gypsy blood boil. She ran, no, raced home and, most probably, sat waiting, ready for a furious argument with him, to avenge herself by pouring out her resentment. He arrived the worse for drink. There was an argument in her room, then he, inevitably, treated her to a few soldier's oaths and went off to bed. She threw her rose after him. In her rage and despair, she seized Pavel's present. The very thing! She had heard the rumors about Pavel's Zhenya, now she would seek help from Pavel's revolver.

When he heard the shot he knew at once what had happened. He saw her on the bed, covered with blood. . . . She was beyond help. So he decided to pretend that he was sleeping. Afterward, it all went as the nurse described it. The housekeeper went into her room. They woke him up. He realized that his enemies might say that he had killed her. It would be difficult to explain why he had not heard the shot in the silence of the night. It was then that he thought up the story, which everyone would have to repeat—the story which made poor Korchagina say, "Even you, Comrade Kalinin, know that Comrade Stalin was with Comrade Molotov out of town at his dacha that evening." The servants knew that he was in the apartment. And it was this strange divergence from the official version that gave rise to dreadful rumors.

After the funeral it was time for his usual occupation: looking for the culprits. He had no difficulty in finding them. His enemies. The ones who had poisoned her mind, whispered slanders in her ear. He had always suspected it. Now he knew he was right. Let us remember Molotov's previously quoted remark: "She [Nadya] did, of course, allow herself to be influenced by [Bukharin]." We can assume that he is echoing the Boss's words. Further, the commander of Stalin's bodyguard, N. Vlasik, told the historian Dr. N. Antipenko that Nadezhda once brought home and showed to Stalin a copy of Ryutin's appeal to the Party which had been slipped to her in a class at the Industrial Academy, and in which Stalin was called an "agent provocateur" and much else. Anna Larina, Bukharin's wife, wrote, "Nikolai Ivanovich remembered coming to the dacha at Zubalovo one day and walking in the grounds with Nadezhda Sergeevna. Stalin suddenly arrived, crept up to them, and looking straight at Nikolai Ivanovich said something terrible: 'I'll kill you.' Nikolai Ivanovich took it as a joke, but Nadezhda Sergeevna shuddered and turned pale." It was not, of course, jealousy. He was too sure of himself for that. And of her. It was the same old problem: Bukharin's influence on Nadya. He was of course afraid of what Bukharin and his wife might say to each other about famine in the countryside and about Ryutin's accusations. He was fed up to the teeth with *her* accusations, and could assume that many of them originated with Bukharin. So when he said "I'll kill you"—he meant it. We can easily reconstruct his grim logic: the rightists had brought her to her doom, deliberately destroyed his home life and his family. Significantly, Ryutin's conspiracy coincided with Nadezhda's death. He remembered more and more frequently the fate of Tsar Ivan the Terrible, and how the boyars in their struggle against him had poisoned his beloved wife. *They* had used poison, these others—poisoned words. Ivan, however, had taken a terrible revenge on them. His wrath too would be terrible. But he would not show his hand too soon. He was good at waiting.

Tsar Ivan the Terrible, as we shall see, would become his favorite historical character. It was he who commissioned the great Eisenstein to make a film about the terrible tsar. In the film, Ivan the Terrible, after losing his beloved wife as the result of the boyars' intrigues, plans a "great and merciless work"—the extermination of the rebellious boyars.

He made no public appearances for the rest of that terrible year. He shut himself up, trying to get over her death. Sucking his pipe. Thinking. And all the time his faithful shadow, Molotov, was at his side.

The fifteenth anniversary of the GPU was celebrated at the end of the year. He did not emerge even for that, but confined himself to sending greetings.

He left it after the New Year to convene a plenary meeting of the Central Committee, at which he summed up the results of the Great Turn and declared industrialization a success: "We had no iron and steel industry—now we do; we had no automobile industry—now we do; we had no tractor industry—now we do." He went on monotonously listing the new industries, to the inexhaustible applause of the audience: "We have moved into one of the top places in the production of electric power, oil products, and coal. . . . We have created a new iron and steel base in the East. Instead of an agrarian country we have become a mighty industrial country capable of producing all modern means of defense. . . . A country which was a hundred years behind had to be hurried up. The Party acted correctly in implementing a policy of accelerated growth."

Millions had perished in that terrifying dash forward. But he knew that the Reformer Tsar, Peter the Great, had also brought countless of his countrymen to their graves. Yes, millions had perished. But with their bodies he had paved the way to tomorrow, had brought the Great Dream closer to realization.

Now he needed a harvest. He sent seventeen thousand Party officials into the countryside to take the grain from the collective farms. And he got his harvest. The specter of famine receded. He had won.

A Warm Spell

After his wife's death he lived alone. From now on his was a male kingdom. Previously, leaders had sat with their wives in the government box at his favorite theater, the Bolshoi. After Nadya's death, wives were not invited. The Boss had no wife, so his servants had no wives. The whole Politburo now celebrated the New Year in the Kremlin with only men at the main table. Wives sat apart.

His mother, Keke, was told the official story, that Nadya had died of appendicitis. His mother believed in God and of course pondered over his second widowhood and God's anger. She sent him jam and fruit from his little homeland, as before. And as before, he never went to see her when he was in Sochi, but wrote her short letters regularly.

> Greetings, Mother dear. I got your letter. I also got the jam, the ginger, and the *churkhcheli* [Georgian sweets]. The children were very pleased and send you their thanks. I am well, don't worry about me, I can endure my lot. I don't know whether or not you need money. I'm sending you 500 rubles just in case. I'm also sending a photograph of me and the children. . . . Keep well, dear Mother, and keep your spirits up. A kiss. Your son Soso.

> 24.3.34. The children salute you. Since Nadya's death my personal life is hard. But never mind, a brave man must be brave at all times.

His period of seclusion was over. On June 12, 1933, he put in an appearance at a grandiose new show, a physical culture parade. Those perfect bodies, lightly clad, were supposed to testify to the might of the proletarian state. He knew that his henchmen had acquired bourgeois habits, and would be making their selection from the pretty girls on parade. Well, let them have their fun. While the warm spell lasted.

In 1933 the trials came to a full stop. There was even a rumor that his wife's death had changed him, that he had become much gentler.

He had succeeded in making the summer and autumn of 1933 a turning point. He deserved the credit for the excellent grain harvest. His cruel policies had forced people to work until they were exhausted. The collective farms obediently poured their grain into the state's bins. And it was proving to be a turning point in the attitude of party functionaries: now they could see he had been right all along. The revolutionary path, through blood and famine, was the one by which the people could be led into the bright future. "Stalin has conquered" was heard more and more frequently from people who only yesterday were reading Ryutin's program to each other.

His power would soon be absolute. The joke that follows dates from this time: "During the October holidays the Politburo is discussing what sort of present to give the Soviet people. One after another they suggest different concessions. Stalin speaks last: 'I propose that the day of the October anniversary be declared a day of collective flagellation.' His henchmen are horrified, but dare not object. On the October anniversary they assemble in the Kremlin fearing the worst. Shortly afterward they hear the buzz of a crowd. It gets nearer. By now the henchmen are cursing Stalin and hiding under the table. He is imperturbable. An excited security man rushes into the room. 'Comrade Stalin,' he says, 'a delegation of workers in the arts has broken into the grounds. They are demanding to be flogged first.' "

A warm spell. The trial of the young Party members who had supported Ryutin ended with light sentences. Ryutin himself wrote to his wife from prison in November 1933 that "only in the USSR, under the leadership of a great genius like our beloved Stalin, have such unprecedented successes in socialist construction been achieved." Ryutin had heard that Zinoviev and Kamenev had repented and been released, and he hoped for the same treatment.

Zinoviev and Kamenev had indeed been released, at the modest price of another recantation and a public glorification of the Boss. In a letter to *Pravda* in May 1933 Zinoviev acknowledged that he had deserved his punishment, and was ready to expiate his offense by working in any capacity. The Boss himself appealed to the Central Control Commission, humbly pleading for his enemies Kamenev and Zinoviev.

While he was thinking of the future, they had taken another step down the road to destruction. Their recent supporters now despised them. The Boss had them brought back to Moscow. The featherbrained coxcomb Zinoviev was given a job on the magazine *Bolshevik,* writing eulogies of the Leader in expectation of some senior Party post. The clever Kamenev, who had begun to understand the Boss's elaborate game plan, clearly suspected that this was only the first move. He distanced himself from politics, and told all the world that he had done so.

When Bukharin, convinced that Kamenev really had been forgiven, offered him a position as departmental editor on *Izvestia,* Kamenev's reply was "I want to lead a quiet, untroubled life. . . . I want people to forget me, and I hope Stalin won't even remember my name." The former head of state now worked quietly in the Institute of World Literature.

Ryutin, however, the Boss could not forgive. He was left in jail.

Trotsky's former court poet, Radek, was also given new posts. The Boss respected Radek's talent as a journalist: let him work while the sunny spell lasts, there's still plenty of time. The cynic Radek worked all out, condemning Trotsky and lauding the Boss. Now he was Stalin's bard. In 1933 he published a book called *The Architect of Soviet Society,* a hymn to Stalin, that "son of poverty who rebelled against the life of servitude in a seminary. . . . The waves of love, and of the people's trust lap against the serene, rocklike figure of our Leader." Yagoda, who had once personally arrested the oppositionist Radek, now respectfully quoted these panegyrics. Though some people thought that Radek was really ridiculing his subject.

Radek became one of the editors of *Izvestia,* working under Bukharin. The Boss had made Bukharin chief editor of that newspaper, the second most important in the country, and shortly afterward delegated to him the task of drafting a new constitution.

Not only his disarmed enemies but his faithful lackeys in the Politburo took it all seriously. He went to the Caucasus on vacation in autumn 1933, leaving Molotov, as usual, to look after "the business." During a Politburo meeting the new State Prosecutor, A. Vyshinsky, launched a routine attack on experts in industry. In reply, the Boss's friend Sergo Ordzhonikidze (People's Commissar for Heavy Industry) and Y. Yakoviev (People's Commissar for Agriculture) got the Politburo to censure Vyshinsky. The Boss wrote to Molotov immediately: "I consider Sergo's outburst in the Vyshinsky business the behavior of a hooligan. How could you give in to him? What does it all mean?"

The faithful servant took the point: the weather mustn't warm up too much too soon.

Throughout 1933 Stalin was busy organizing celebrations. The White Sea–Baltic Canal—constructed by convict labor and hymned by his writers—was completed. The country rejoiced. Together with his closest comrade-in-arms, Kirov, Stalin proceeded on board ship along the newly dug canal. His icebreakers were opening up the northern sea route. One old icebreaker, the *Chelyuskin,* got stuck in the ice, and Stalin turned the rescue of the crew into a magnificent piece of theater.

The eyes of the whole country were on these events. He organized a sumptuous reception in Moscow for the rescued sailors. All through 1933 loudspeakers pumped out deafening marches, and radio announcers extolled the Boss's latest victories. It was as if he was trying to forget his personal tragedy in the din of martial music and servile praise. A huge airplane was built, the *Maxim Gorky*, biggest in the world. Stalin approved the design for a Palace of the Soviets. It was meant to be a structure unlike any ever known. A building 1,300 feet high would be crowned with a 300-foot statue of Lenin. A grandiose hall would seat an audience of 21,000 for the Leader's speeches. Bolshevism's greatest shrine would rise on the site of the demolished Church of Christ the Savior.

That shrine, for all his orders and decrees, would never be built. The reason commonly given is shortage of funds. But in times when labor cost nothing and the Boss's will was law, this is no explanation. We are left with the explanation preferred by the people at large: "The Lord forbade it."

Stalin in Carpet Slippers

For years now the Boss had been fashioning a new lifestyle for Bolshevik leaders. Gone never to return were the democratic ways of the early years after the Revolution, when the families of Kremlin bigwigs traveled by public transport, stood in line with their fellow citizens, and were short of money. ("Joseph, send me 50 rubles or so if you can, they won't give me any money at the Industrial Academy until October 15 and right now I haven't a single kopeck," Nadya wrote to her husband in a postscript to a letter dated September 17, 1929.) The Boss's children were now taken to school in limousines, with bodyguards. Massive villas for the use of the rulers were erected outside Moscow, each in its own spacious grounds and with its own security guards. Academician E. Varga, an eminent economist and Comintern activist, noted sadly that "they have gardeners, cooks, maidservants, special doctors and nurses working for them—sometimes a staff of fifty or so—and all this at state expense. They have special trains, personal airplanes, personal guards, fleets of cars to service them and their families. . . . They get all their provisions and household goods for next to nothing. To live at this level in America you would have to be a multimillionaire." Varga, an old Comintern hand, could not help remembering Lenin's promise to create a society in which leaders would "receive the same salary as an average worker."

The former royal residences, and the palaces of the aristocracy, which Lenin in a special decree had generously presented to the toiling masses, soon passed into the hands of the new tsar and the new aristocracy. Stalin would be assigned the royal family's favorite palace, at Livadia in the Crimea; Molotov's holiday home would be the luxurious palace of Count Vorontsov. (In fact, the Boss made use of his palace only once: he preferred to take his holidays in one of the many government dachas in his native Caucasus.) Stalin was, however, careful to keep up appearances: all the luxuries with which he finally corrupted and demoralized the Party remained state property. Once he removed them from the Olympus of state power, former grandees and their families counted for nothing. The daughter of the once mighty Kaganovich told me that when her father was dismissed after Stalin's death the family was amazed to discover that they did not even possess any furniture of their own—everything belonged to the state. This system helped to make the Boss's henchmen zealous in his service.

In those years the Boss chose as his new main residence a government villa built at Kuntsevo, a suburb of Moscow, and called the "nearer dacha." He left his children, Vasya and Svetlana, at his former dacha in Zubalovo, where he used to spend the summer with Nadya. This was also the home of Nadya's parents, the Alliluyevs, and several of her relatives were regular visitors—her brother Pavel and his wife, Zhenya (whose relationship with Stalin was "observed" by Maria Svanidze), her half-crazy brother Fyodor, her sister Anna (pet name Nyura), who was married to a pillar of the secret police called Redens. Other visitors included the Svanidze couple, Maria and Alyosha, relatives of the Boss's first wife, and his older son Yakov.

After work the Boss always returned to his Kremlin apartment. But, as Svetlana would write later in her memoirs, he now always left to spend the night at the nearer dacha. The apartment evidently held too many memories of Nadezhda and of that fatal night.

ALYOSHA, MARIA, AND JOSEPH

His private life at this time seemed likely to remain a secret, and a source of legend. There was, however, one chronicler—a witness who enables us to catch a glimpse of this most secretive of human beings at home. Maria Svanidze.

Maria Svanidze was then in her forties (she was born in 1889). And she was more or less in love with Stalin.

Her husband, Alyosha Svanidze, was the brother of Stalin's first wife. Svetlana Alliluyeva describes "Uncle Alyosha" as "a handsome Georgian of the Svanetian type, a short fair-haired man with blue eyes and an aquiline nose. He had received a European education at German universities, paid for by the Party." Maria, a Jewish beauty, was a singer in the Tiflis opera company. She was already in her thirties when she divorced her first husband and married Alyosha. They had a son, to whom they gave the ultrarevolutionary name Dzhonrid (John Reed) in honor of the famous American Communist. Svanidze had worked in Georgia as head of the republic's Finance Ministry in Budu Mdivani's government.

In Moscow Maria saw a great deal of Nadya Stalin. Alyosha even wrote to his wife in care of Stalin's apartment. Maria was very fond of Nadya. A year after Nadya's death she wrote, "Now she's no longer with us, but her family and her home are dear to me. I went to see Nyura Redens [Nadya's sister Anna] yesterday. Pavel was there, and Zhenya . . . but it wasn't the same. I feel very lonely without Nadya."

She did, however, often visit the house which seemed so empty after Nadya's death. It was there that she "observed" Joseph and Zhenya. And all this time she kept up her diary. Many pages have been torn out. Did Maria destroy them herself in that terrible year 1937? Or did the diary's hero take the trouble to do it, when the diary came his way after Maria's arrest?

But all this was in the future. For the time being the Svanidzes belonged to the innermost circle of Stalin's friends. He called them Alyosha and Masha, they called him Joseph. Svetlana Alliluyeva described the Svanidzes as an ideal couple. But you need only read the diary to realize that the two Georgian revolutionaries had more in common than most friends. Alyosha's European veneer also concealed the fiery temperament of a barbarian. An entry in the diary, from 1923, the year in which the Svanidzes married, reads: "I cried bitterly after that wild scene of jealousy, and he sat on the edge of the bed beside me: 'It's all because we love each other, you know. . . . All the unpleasantness is over now' and he became so affectionate. When he makes jealous scenes it isn't so much because he's hurt and is suffering as because, according to him, I don't know how to behave . . . and my conduct is very bad when men are present." And an entry on March 30, 1934: "Why do I have to live with a man who hates and despises me, and why does he have to live with a woman who out of grief, despair, and resentment sometimes wishes him dead? But afterward, life together somehow becomes livable for a time, and you start clinging to it. . . . Of course, my age is more to blame . . . and the fear of poverty (absolutely beyond all reason in my case), and then again I want to say to hell with it all, I'm not going to sell myself . . . it's a vicious circle. . . . I'm badly wounded, my heart bleeds . . . I have to sort it out somehow . . . or it will all end tragically. I haven't been seeing anyone lately, except the Alliluyevs."

That was how things were between them. She sensed how much her adoration of Joseph upset Alyosha. But how severely she punished him by flaunting her adoration: "30.7.34. On July 28 J. [Joseph] left for Sochi. Because of Alyosha I couldn't see him before he left. I was vexed. For the last two months Alyosha has persistently deprived me of his company, which I find so interesting."

The Lady of the House

Maria described the strange family which Joseph established after Nadya's death. Little Svetlana was made "lady of the house" in place of her dead mother. From her he received at last what he had always wanted—unquestioning adoration. Her love expressed itself in a strange way. She used to give him written orders! The man to whom no one else dared give orders. It was a game which he took very seriously; he was a genuinely loving father. From Maria's diary:

> Svetlana hung around her father the whole time. He petted her, kissed her, admired her, lovingly gave her the choicest morsels from his plate. She wrote him "Order No. 4": he must allow her to spend holidays at Lipki—one of his dachas was there. . . . After dinner he was in a good humor. He went to the private intercity telephone, rang Kirov, and shared a joke with him. . . . He advised him to come to Moscow immediately, to defend Leningrad's interest. . . . Joseph loves Kirov, and . . . suddenly wanted to see him, so that they could steam themselves in a Russian bathhouse and play the fool together. Around 10 he got ready to go out of town with the children, complained that he was short of sleep, and obviously intended to catch up on his sleep when he got to the dacha. . . . We stayed on with Karolina Vasilievna (the housekeeper, she's been with them eight years), and talked about the children, about his son Vasya, he's doing badly at school, exploits his name and his father's position, is rude to all adults, including his teacher, it would, she said, be a blow to J. if he got to know all the details. He gets tired and wants peace and comfort at home. . . . Nadya made great efforts to bring up the children austerely, but since her death, every-

thing's gone to rack and ruin. . . . Joseph and I said goodbye for an indefinite period. . . . He is kind and warmhearted.

14.11.34. At 6:00 P.M. J[oseph] arrived with Vasya and Kirov. The little girls gave us a puppet show. J. said, "I've never seen anything so beautiful." He was smoking his pipe. He invited us to go with him to the nearer dacha, but as he had said earlier that he was going there to work, Zhenya and I didn't respond to his invitation. Sometimes he invites people simply out of courtesy. Svetlana wrote an order: "I order you to allow me to go to the theater or the cinema with you." And signed it "Svetlana, Mistress of the House." She handed it to him, and J. said: "Oh well. I must obey." They've been playing that game for a year now. Svetlana is the Mistress of the House, and she has several secretaries. Papa is No. 1 secretary, then come Molotov, Kaganovich, Ordzhonikidze, Kirov, and a few others. She is great friends with Kirov, because J. is on very good and close terms with him. Svetlana writes orders and pins them on the wall with drawing pins.

He was friends with Kirov. His friendship was genuine. And he was getting ready to murder him. Maria wrote: "He invited us (Alyosha and me) out to the nearer dacha. . . . He was a little irritable with the servants at supper. . . . We went home at 2:30, leaving him alone in that enormous house. My heart aches when I think of his loneliness."

Without Kirov he would be absolutely alone. But . . .

14

THE CONGRESS OF VICTORS

APOTHEOSIS

But there was no other way. That is what he must surely have said to himself early in 1934, after the famous Seventeenth Congress, which was to have marked the consummation of his triumph over his shattered foes.

It had all gone well to begin with. In his official report, accompanied by never-ending ovations from the hall, he had proudly declared that "whereas at the Fifteenth Congress we were still having to argue for the correctness of the Party line, and to do battle with certain anti-Leninist groups, and at the Sixteenth Congress finish off the last adherents of those groups, at this Congress . . . there is no one to fight. . . . Everybody sees that the Party line is victorious, the policy of industrialization is victorious . . . the policy of liquidation of the kulaks, and total collectivization is victorious. . . . Our country's experience has shown that the victory of socialism in a single country is perfectly possible."

After this, yesterday's oppositionists strove as never before to outdo each other in penitential eulogies. From Bukharin: "Stalin was entirely right when by brilliant deployment of Marxist-Leninist dialectic he utterly demolished several of the assumptions of the right deviationists, for which I was mainly responsible. . . . After the former leaders of the rightists had acknowledged their errors . . . resistance from the enemies of the Party found its expression in various small groups, which slipped with gathering speed headlong down the slope to counterrevolution. The remnants of the opposition within the Party were just the same—*among them several of my former pupils,* who were deservedly punished." And from Tomsky: "Comrade Stalin was the most consistent and the most brilliant of Lenin's pupils. . . . He saw farthest, and he most consistently led the Party along the correct Leninist path."

Such fulsome praise, all from the mouths of his former foes. Pyatakov, Sokolnikov, the list seems endless. And who first thought of the progressive combination "Marx-Engels-Lenin-Stalin"? Not Molotov, not Kaganovich. Zinoviev. The whole country heard the

October leaders acknowledge, one after another, their own nullity, and Stalin's superior wisdom.

His loyal henchmen were, of course, not to be outdone. "Brother Kirov" mentioned Stalin's name twenty-two times in his speech, showing an enviable ingenuity in his choice of epithets: "the helmsman of our great socialist construction," "the supreme strategist in the battle for the liberation of the toilers," and so on. From Kirov came a proposal without precedent in the history of Party Congresses, that "all the theses and conclusions contained in Comrade Stalin's report should be adopted as Party law and acted upon accordingly." Barely a year after the horrifying famine, the Congress declared that the "foundations of a socialist society" had already been laid. The country found that it was already living in the long-awaited age of socialism, the heart's desire of all revolutionaries.

"The Congress of Victors," Stalin decided to call it. Out of modesty, of course. It was really "the Congress of the Victor."

Behind the Scenes

And then it emerged that a bomb had been prepared for him. Yagoda's department had exerted itself, and Stalin learned what had been going on in the lobbies. Kirov also came and told him. Nikita Khrushchev, who took part in the Seventeenth Congress, and was then a young protégé of Kaganovich and a loyal Stalinist, later told the story: "At that time the secretary of the North Caucasian Territorial Party Committee, Sheboldayev, occupied a prominent position in the Party. This Sheboldayev, an old Bolshevik, came to Comrade Kirov during the Congress and said: 'The older comrades are talking about going back to Lenin's Testament and acting on it, in other words transferring Stalin to some other post, as Lenin recommended, and putting in his place someone who would show more tolerance to those around him. People are saying that it would be a good idea to promote you to the post of General Secretary.' . . . What Kirov's answer was I don't know, but it became known that Kirov had gone to Stalin and told him about his conversation with Sheboldayev. Stalin is supposed to have said, 'Thank you, I won't forget what I owe you.' "

There is also a deposition made by V. Verkhovykh, a delegate to the Congress, in 1960. He wrote that "S. Kosior, a candidate member of the Politburo, . . . told me that some people . . . had talked to Kirov, trying to get him to agree to be General Secretary. Kirov refused." Another delegate, Z. Nemtsova, told how Kirov gave the Leningrad delegation a dressing-down in their hotel for mentioning him as a possible General Secretary. This was the way people were talking in the lobbies while the Boss was being eulogized on the platform and wildly applauded from the hall. Another reminder that "however well you feed a wolf it hankers after the forest." The old Party would never fully accept him as its leader, never fully reconcile itself to him. The final proof of this came when the Congress which had glorified him came to cast its votes.

The Vote

The concluding item of business was the election by secret ballot of the Party's highest organ, the Central Committee. Only one candidate was nominated for each place to be filled. Every candidate obtaining more than fifty percent of the votes was considered elected. The Boss had deliberately arranged the mode of election so as to preclude choice.

Voting papers were distributed to the delegates and the election got under way. "Stalin," so Khrushchev recounted in his memoirs, "demonstratively walked up to the ballot box and dropped his papers in without looking."

This was an invitation to others to follow his example.

But then something unexpected happened. According to a widely known story, Zatonsky, the chairman of the Electoral Commission, anxiously informed Kaganovich, who was in charge of Congress arrangements, that 270 votes had been cast against Stalin.

In the note mentioned earlier, Verkhovykh wrote that "as a delegate to the Seventeenth Congress I was elected to the Tellers' Commission. The result of the voting was that . . . the largest number of votes 'against' went to Stalin, Molotov, and Kaganovich." O. Shatunovskaya, an old Party member, and also a teller at the Congress, wrote in a letter to the Central Committee in Khrushchev's time that 292 votes were cast against Stalin.

The biggest surprise is that the suppressed documentation of the tellers at the Seventeenth Congress survives in the Party Archive. During the Khrushchev Thaw the packets of voting papers were opened. It emerged that of 1,225 delegates who should have voted, only 1,059 appeared to have done so. Evidently, 166 "no" votes had been removed.

In spite of the 166 votes against him—and even if the number was in fact 292—Stalin would still have been duly elected to the Central Committee. Nonetheless, such a shocking number of "no" votes would have been a heavy blow to his prestige in the Party. As a result of the prompt remedial measures taken by Kaganovich, the official announcement of the Tellers' Commission showed that only three votes had been cast against Stalin, four against Kirov . . . and so on.

We see then that dozens of the delegates who had applauded Stalin voted against him in a secret ballot. "Cowardly double-dealers," he called them. There was not a single person in the ranks of the glorious Leninist guard brave enough to proclaim his beliefs out loud.

Of course everyone was afraid. Of course it could mean certain death. But even in the days of Nero's most terrible orgy of executions, some individuals spoke out openly against the emperor in the Roman Senate. They knew that it meant death, but they spoke out for all to hear.

The vote, then, was not just evidence of double-dealing. It showed that the system of terror Stalin had created was highly effective. And that he could now get to work without delay.

What they had voted for that day was their own destruction.

But for the present the warm spell continued. He gave them a little time to enjoy life under socialism, while he decided when to begin, and how many of them to remove.

Or rather (as Tkachev once put it) how many must be kept.

Of the 139 senior Party leaders present at the Congress, only 31 would die natural deaths.

Testing the Intelligentsia

In that same year, 1934, the poet Osip Mandelstam was arrested. This sent a shock wave through a Moscow enjoying the warm spell.

I am looking through the records of his case, which has been a legend for half a century: "Case No. 4108—Accused—Citizen Mandelstam, O., commenced 17.5.34." Then follows the report on the house search. That day in May, "letters, notes with telephone numbers and addresses, and manuscripts on separate sheets, forty-eight in number," were removed from his apartment. The unhappy poet was taken to the Lubyanka. Here is an excerpt from the record of his first interrogation on May 18: "Do you admit that you are guilty of writing works of a counterrevolutionary character?" "Yes, I am the author of the following verses:

"We don't live, we just nervously tiptoe through life
At ten paces our words are mere silence
And if an occasion for converse occurs
We remember the man from the Highlands

In the Kremlin, with chicken-necked chieftains all round
The rabble he mocks and relies on

. . . .

His whiskers droop, roachlike, from under his nose."

The transcript cites the complete text of this—one of the most famous works in twentieth-century Russian poetry—written against the Boss. "To whom did you give copies, or read this work?" "I gave no one copies, but I read it to my wife, my brother, the writer Khazin, the writer Anna Akhmatova and her son Lev Gumilev . . ." "What was their reaction?" Mandelstam answered this last question in detail. We see that the torture spoken of in contemporary legend was quite unnecessary. The poet spoke voluntarily, because he was demoralized, confused, a broken man. As so often, the intellectual capitulated. During a visit from his wife the unhappy poet, on the verge of madness because of his confession, told her whose names he had mentioned and begged her to warn them.

He was banished. In exile he became mentally ill. He used to wake his wife in the middle of the night and say he had seen Akhmatova arrested because of him, and had gone looking for Akhmatova's body in ravines.

Two eminent poets went into action. Anna Akhmatova succeeded in obtaining an interview with A. Enukidze, chairman of the Central Executive Committee, while Boris Pasternak sought Bukharin's aid. Bukharin in turn appealed to the Boss. I have read his letter in the President's Archive: "I thought I should write to you on a number of matters. . . . About the poet Mandelstam. He was recently arrested and banished. . . . I keep getting desperate telegrams from his wife telling me that he is mentally disturbed, that he has tried to jump out of the window, etc. My judgment of M. is that he is a first-class poet, but not at all a modern one, and that he is undoubtedly not quite normal. Since people keep appealing to me, and I don't know how he has gone wrong, I decided to write to you about this too. . . . P.S. Boris Pasternak is utterly flabbergasted by Mandelstam's arrest, and nobody else knows anything."

The Leader, who had been the butt of Mandelstam's verses, scrawled on Bukharin's letter. "Who authorized Mandelstam's arrest? Disgraceful." The proper response of an ex-poet to the arrest of another poet. Even one by whom he had been insulted. There followed one of those routine miracles: Mandelstam's sentence was immediately reviewed. And the Boss thought of a new move. He rang Pasternak.

Pasternak was taken aback. Petitioning Bukharin was one thing, talking to Stalin quite another.

> *Stalin:* Mandelstam's case is under review, everything will be all right. Why didn't you approach the writer's organization or me? [Stalin was no mere Bukharin, he was the poet's friend.] . . . If I were a poet and my friend got into trouble I would go to any length to help him.
> *Pasternak:* The writers' organization hasn't dealt with such matters since 1927, and if I hadn't made a fuss now you would probably never have known about it. [He questioned the word "friend," which was not strictly applicable to his relationship with Mandelstam.]
> *Stalin:* But he is a master of his craft, isn't he?
> *Pasternak:* Yes, but that's not really the point. [Pasternak was evasive, trying to understand what this terrible man was getting at.]
> *Stalin:* What is, then?
> *Pasternak:* It would be good if we could meet for a talk.
> *Stalin:* What about?
> *Pasternak:* About life and death.

Stalin replaced the receiver loudly.

Molotov described a postscript to the incident: "About Pasternak. Stalin rang and said he couldn't manage to defend his friend." Let us write in the missing words: rang and said with satisfaction.

Yet again, the talk was of the Boss's noble nature. Nobody dared wonder whether he, who had eyes for everything, could possibly have been unaware of the famous poet's arrest. Mandelstam's arrest and first conviction were, of course, ordered by him. This episode was for him a sort of test. It told him that the moment the intelligentsia started believing that the weather had changed for the better they had grown bolder. He still had not tamed them completely. But he would; that Pasternak, the boldest of them, was nonetheless afraid proved it. Did taming them completely mean teaching them not to notice the arrest of their friends? No—it meant teaching them to sing hymns of praise when friends were arrested.

Before the Offensive, a Breathing Space

The system he had created was working. The hierarchy of "party bosses," with the God-Boss at its summit, in a very short time had carried through industrialization and collectivization. The system's safety devices—the extrajudicial penal apparatus and the organs of agitation and propaganda—were operating effectively. The extrajudicial penal apparatus had been in complete control of the situation at that terrible moment in 1932. The ideological machine was not yet perfected, but a broad ideological front, on which the armies created by him (the cultural unions) would converge, had been opened. The population at large had also learned a great deal in the last few years: to look at starving people without noticing them, to work for a beggarly wage, to live in a house more like a hive, and to stand in line for groceries—knowing all the time that they were citizens of the world's finest state. In the country of the almighty GPU, they felt themselves to be the freest of the free.

But the most important part of the system, the Party pyramid, was clearly unsatisfactory. In senior posts there were many disgruntled feudal barons, corrupted by their exorbitant power at the time of the Revolution and sadly cherishing the memory of fallen idols. The incipient rebellion of 1932 had shown how precarious it all was. And the Seventeenth Congress had proved conclusively that in order to tame the country completely he would have to transform the Party.

The necessary machinery had already been created. The successful trials of intellectuals were a splendid dress rehearsal, mounted by the very people with whom he must part company.

Nevertheless, a breathing space was needed before the offensive began. The warm spell continued. Let the enemy enjoy themselves, let them become more brazen still. Ivan the Terrible was always pretending to be at death's door, while his minions listened in to the treasonable talk of boyars who had begun to scent freedom.

Stalin's Third Teacher

In 1933 Hitler became chancellor of the German Reich.

Ever since the beginning of the Bolshevik regime its leaders had, because of Russia's international isolation, concentrated their minds almost entirely on internal policy. But Germany was, to the Bolsheviks, a special country.

Once in power, with the aid of German money, they had conceived a paradoxical plan: they would abandon the "German imperialists" who had funded them and incorporate Germany in a Union of Proletarian Republics. Germany was assigned first place on the map of world revolution. Germany's crushing defeat in World War One made that dream realistic. At the Versailles Conference, where the Germans accepted humiliating peace terms, Lloyd George had circulated a memorandum: "The greatest danger I see in the present situation is that Germany may link its destiny with Bolshevism and put its resources, its brains, and its enormous organizing abilities at the service of revolutionary fanatics who dream of conquering the world for Bolshevism by force of arms." Since then Germany had been, in fact, threatened several times by proletarian revolution.

Later, when the hope of revolution in Germany had faded, the two outcasts of Europe, Bolshevik Russia and defeated Germany, were gradually drawn together by economic interests. Under the Versailles Treaty the Germans had no right to train tank crews and air force personnel on German soil. Hence they set up training establishments in Russia. There, too, secret branches of German arms firms were established, and top-secret experiments leading to the creation of a German chemical weapons industry were carried out. Each side had its own agenda: the Germans wanted to preserve their army, the Bolsheviks to create an army with the aid of the Reichswehr, in order to destroy at some later date imperialism of the German and all other varieties. In high military circles, Tukhachevsky often gave credit to the Reichswehr for teaching the Red army to handle the most modern weaponry. This collaboration went on until Hitler, who had declared himself a relentless enemy of Bolshevism, came to power. He seemed to embody the Bolsheviks' old fear that military intervention by the imperialists was inevitable. Hitler had written that "if Germany needs *lebensraum* in Europe it can be found only in Russia."

The accession of Hitler, as some saw it, was the result of a grave miscalculation on the Boss's part. He who had managed the Comintern as his own fief had forbidden the German Communists to ally themselves with the Social Democrats. The anti-Hitler coalition was split as a result and had lost to Hitler.

In fact Stalin needed Hitler to expedite his next move. If Hitler had not existed Stalin would have had to invent him. The threat of Hitler, the threat of intervention, conferred on him enormous powers, justified the most extreme measures. It also compelled European radicals to support him in spite of everything. He, after all, was the focal point of opposition to fascism, the object of hatred for fascism. Hitler put an end to the international isolation of the USSR. The Entente nations had to seek alliance with the USSR. The Soviet rapprochement with America confirmed this trend. Furthermore, the large number of votes cast against Hitler in the elections to the Reichstag held the promise of future upheavals. The mirage of world revolution reappeared. Old Bolsheviks wrote in a letter to *Pravda* that "Hitler will hold on for a few months, followed by total collapse and revolution." The ironies of history! These two leaders hated each other, yet there were uncanny coincidental resemblances. Like Stalin, Hitler was a third son, and his older siblings too had died. Hitler too was born in poverty, he too was, according to legend, illegitimate, and his father had even earned his living for a time as a shoemaker. Hitler's only love, like Stalin's, had committed suicide, though everyone would think that he had killed her. Their regimes exchanged expressions of hatred, and yet mirrored each other. For that reason, each had useful lessons for the other. After Lenin and Trotsky, Hitler was Stalin's third teacher.

In 1934, as he pondered his next move, he must have taken Hitler's example into account. The way in which Hitler had settled the fate of certain Party comrades, after they had brought him to power, was instructive. They had been a bunch of unruly malcontents, very much like Lenin's Party. Hitler, who had also created a mighty state subservient to its leader, found a drastic solution to the problem. He denounced his comrades of yesterday as traitors, and personally took charge of their extermination. Stalin was able to observe that event in June 1934, while he was still digesting the results of the Seventeenth Congress, held in January and February.

Meanwhile, he encouraged the growing "anti-German hysteria"—as the Germans called it—in the newspapers. What the Russians called "anti-Bolshevik hysteria" was just as actively encouraged by the other side, to the advantage of both leaders.

"Red Russia Is Becoming Pink"

While he planned his murderous change of policy at home, he let the warm spell continue.

An article in *Komsomolskaya Pravda* declared, "Not so long ago any music critic who saw a saxophone, or Utesov, in his dreams would wake up in a cold sweat. . . . But now . . . there's jazz wherever you go—Utesov, Rensky, Berezovsky, English jazz, Czechoslovak jazz, women's jazz, even Lilliputian jazz." *The Days of the Turbins* returned to the stage of the Arts Theater, and Stalin went to see his favorite show again.

"Red Russia Is Becoming Pink," proclaimed a headline in the *Baltimore Sun.*

In 1934, when the warm spell was at its warmest, H. G. Wells arrived in the USSR. With Hitler ruling Germany, Wells, who hated Fascism, wanted very much to like Stalin. For Stalin too the visit had a special importance. Wells had met Lenin in 1920 and enthused over the "Visionary of the Kremlin" in a book. That had been a year of famine, but endless banquets were given in honor of Wells. They were learning already how to bewitch eminent Western friends, though the artist Annenkov quoted a quite unexpected speech heard by Wells at one such banquet: "We've been eating rissoles and cakes, and they have more of an attraction for us than meeting you, believe me. You see us here decently dressed, but not one of the worthy people here present would be prepared to unbutton his waistcoat, because he'd have nothing underneath except a scrap of dirty old rag which, if I remember rightly, once went by the name of 'shirt.' "

Now, in 1934, Wells would not be hearing anything of that sort. The Boss had taught the intelligentsia to behave themselves.

Wells was delighted with all he saw. Or, to be more precise, with all that was shown him. "Something very significant is happening in the USSR," he wrote. "The contrast with 1920 is striking. The capitalists must learn from the USSR. . . . The financial oligarchy has outlived itself. . . . Roosevelt is already intent on a thorough reorganization of society, and the creation of a planned economy."

The Boss received Wells, and succeeded in enchanting him—while making no concessions. He dismissed the possibility of a planned economy in capitalist conditions. He even defended revolutionary violence: "Capitalism is rotten through and through, but the old order will not collapse by itself. It is naive to hope for concessions from the power holders." Wells did not give up completely. As president of the Pen Club, he expressed a wish to discuss with his old friend Gorky the possibility of Soviet writers joining that organization. He told Stalin that the Pen Club insisted on "the right of all to express their opinions, including the opposition, freely. I don't know, however, whether such broad freedom can be permitted here." The Boss answered laughingly, "We Bolsheviks call it self-criticism. It is widely practised in the USSR."

A mere two years later Wells would realize what freedom of expression meant in the USSR. The tragedy of 1937 would leave him stunned, and he would write a novel called *The Wrath of God* about a man who betrays a revolution.

But for the time being Wells had served a purpose. He had confirmed that "Stalin is Lenin today."

Brother Kirov

On June 2, 1934, the State Prosecutor's Office of the USSR adopted an "order concerning the prevention of infringements of legality with special reference to technical experts and managers." The terrible trials seemed to be a thing of the past.

After the Seventeenth Congress it was rumored in the Party that Kirov was to be transferred to Moscow, where, as the Boss's closest friend, a member of the Politburo, and a secretary of the Central Committee, he would shortly occupy the second place in the Party hierarchy.

This raised the hopes of the Party and the intelligentsia, since Kirov was becoming more and more conspicuously the protagonist of the warm spell. He said in a speech in Leningrad that "the old enemy groupings have melted down in the course of the struggle for the Five-Year Plan, and we need no longer reckon with them." (Kirov was referring to the program of intensive industrialization launched in 1929, and known as the Five-Year Plan.)

The Boss loved Kirov and knew that he was loyal. But he had become dangerous. After all the blood spilled, all the slave laborers left dead during the construction of the White Sea–Baltic Canal (his pet project), after his ruthless war on the kulaks, nobody could accuse Kirov of spinelessness. But he had taken the warm spell at face value. It came as no surprise that a maudlin Kalinin, in Leningrad and in Kirov's presence, had interrupted a poet who was singing the praises of the Cheka and said, "We shouldn't be extolling the Cheka, but looking forward to a time when the Cheka need no longer raise its punitive hand." Kirov had applauded him. Kirov was being used more and more frequently by the Boss's enemies. Stalin knew that Bukharin had grown fond of visiting Leningrad. In a letter written shortly before his death (now in the President's Archive), Bukharin said, "When I was in disgrace and fell sick in Leningrad, Kirov came to see me, spent the whole day with me, wrapped me up warmly, put his own railroad carriage at my disposal, and sent me off to Moscow with such tender care." The Boss knew about this "tender care" shown to an enemy of his.

Gorky, too, was putting more pressure on him, pleading for someone or other all the time, and invoking Kirov's name as he did so. Kirov's latest charitable proposal was that Uglanov, one of the rightist leaders, should be allowed to resume an active career. The Boss, however, remembered very well what the penitent Uglanov had written in March 1933. The catalog of treacherous acts was endless: "We acknowledged our mistakes at the November plenum of the Central Committee in 1929. . . . A few months went by . . . in the course of collectivization and the liquidation of the kulaks a number of difficulties arose . . . and again . . . we were in a mood to fight against the Party. . . . At the Sixteenth Congress we acknowledged our mistakes and assured the Party that we would work conscientiously, but in autumn 1933 some of my supporters resumed the struggle. Discussing the situation in the country with them, I came to the conclusion that a leadership headed by Stalin was incapable of overcoming the immense difficulties . . . and that it was necessary to bring Rykov, Bukharin, Tomsky, Zinoviev, and Kamenev back into the leadership of the Party and the country." And this was the man for whom Kirov sought forgiveness! Where would it end? Start forgiving such people and you would have another Seventeenth Congress—Congress of Traitors—on your hands.

Stalin's resolve had ripened. Further delay was pointless. It was time to attack. His enemies were writing Kirov's name on their banner. He would have to sacrifice his loyal brother. They gave him no choice.

Using the sort of logic he favored, he could say that *objectively* they were Kirov's killers. Just as they had been Nadya's killers. The killers of the two people dearest to him. They had earned his hatred and his vengeance.

While the country still basked in the warm spell, preparations for the offensive went on at full speed. On July 10, 1934, the GPU was renamed the NKVD—People's Commissariat of Internal Affairs. This seemed to mean that the secret police was now detached from the Party and from the Politburo. As, of course, it had to be, with the destruction of the Party and of certain members of the Politburo imminent. Faithful Yagoda retained his post, now as People's Commissar. He would lead the offensive. Yagoda had by then compiled a dossier on all those at the top of Lenin's Party. The servants of important bureaucrats had to be approved by Yagoda's department. Housemaids, chauffeurs, and other domestic staff reported several times a month. The amorous exploits of Kremlin boyars helped swell the dossiers. Jan Rudzutak, for instance, a candidate member of the Politburo, had raped the fifteen-year-old daughter of a Moscow Party official, and when in Paris had lavished money belonging to the state on prostitutes. Then there were the escapades of A. Enukidze, secretary of the Central Executive Committee, and of Karakhan, one of the senior officials in the People's Commissariat for Foreign Affairs, among the ballerinas. This bawdy reading matter was sent regularly to the Boss. But what he evidently valued most was information on provocateurs. This must explain the fact that the obliging Yagoda inserted false accusations of collaboration with the tsarist security services in the dossiers of many old Bolsheviks.

A Dangerous House

Early in the thirties the architect B. Jofan designed a new building for high Party officials. It looked out on the Kremlin, across the Moscow River, and became known as the "House on the Embankment." The most fashionable apartments were in Blocks 1 and 12. That was where N. Postyshev, a member of the Politburo, Marshal M. Tukhachevsky, Jan Berzin, head of military intelligence, and a number of other officeholders lived.

Jofan, the architect, took one secret to the grave with him. The building had one unusual entrance. It was shown on all the plans and in all the documentation, but in reality it was nonexistent. Instead, there was a "back stairway," approached from the kitchens of the enormous apartments in fashionable Block 12. You could go down these stairs to an underground passage leading to the Kremlin. This tunnel under the Moscow River, which still exists, was bored in the time of Stalin's favorite tsar, Ivan the Terrible. Yagoda's men could use the backstairs to materialize suddenly in the rooms of high-ranking tenants.

The Soviet military intelligence chief, Jan Berzin, who had become famous under the name of General Grishin during the Spanish Civil War, was lying peacefully in bed one night with his Spanish wife, the beautiful Aurora, beside him. The Boss's emissaries entered his bedroom from the backstairs.

That would be at the end of 1937. But we are still in 1934, and they are all living undisturbed in the house reserved for them. Armed guards kept watch not only at each entrance but on every landing. They were there only to protect tenants, but they noted every step taken, eavesdropped on every conversation.

O. Lepeshinskaya, daughter of one of Lenin's comrades-in-arms, remembered when her family was moved into prestigious Block 1. The apartments had seven rooms, the balconies were two hundred feet long, there were solariums and double walls. That was where the eavesdropping devices stood. *Stood* is the right word: they were animate creatures. Lepeshinskaya recalled how she "once woke up at 3:00 A.M. and heard the silence broken with the words 'that's enough for today, let's go home.' "

All was ready for the offensive. Time to begin. At the end of 1934, he waited only until his birthday celebrations were over, and . . . began.

"Revolutionaries Should Be Sent to Join Their Forefathers at Fifty"

The events of 1935–1938, which led to the total destruction of the Leninist Party, remain the greatest riddle of Stalin's reign. Why did he destroy the Party, now completely subservient to him, with such inordinate cruelty? The most frequent explanation is mental disorder. Stalin, it is said, was a schizophrenic. The story usually told by way of proof is that when in 1927 the great Russian medical scientist Vladimir Mikhailovich Bekhterev was called in to examine Stalin, whose withered arm was troubling him, he diagnosed advanced paranoia and recommended immediate retirement. Shortly afterward, Moscow witnessed the eminent scientist's funeral.

In August 1989, in the days of perestroika, a number of psychiatrists took part in an amusing roundtable discussion in the offices of the *Literary Gazette*. They were looking for an answer to the question: was Stalin mentally ill or not? One of those invited was academician N. Bekhtereva, daughter of the great Bekhterev. She said, among other things, "I myself do *not* know whether Vladimir Bekhterev decided that Stalin was paranoiac, but our family never heard anything to that effect." That puts an end to a very popular legend.

A number of interesting points were made in the course of the discussion. Kornetov, for instance, said that "such an illness is hardly compatible with his skill in manipulating personnel, recruiting supporters, and accurately timing his attacks on opponents." Dr. N. Levin asked, "When were Stalin's ideas out of focus, or abnormally dominant in his consciousness, as is the case with paranoiacs? Stalin was a cruel man, incapable of pity . . . but a pragmatist."

As Stalin contemplated the destruction of the old Party, he must surely have consulted the two men who had influenced him most—Lenin and Trotsky. He could have found in Trotsky's works a complete answer, equally acceptable to Lenin: "Lenin often ridiculed so-called old Bolsheviks, and even said that at fifty revolutionaries should be sent to join their forefathers. This grim joke makes a serious point; at some critical stage every generation of revolutionaries becomes a hindrance to the further development of the idea which they have carried forward."

The Seventeenth Congress had finally convinced Stalin that they would never let him create the country of his dreams—a military camp where unanimity and subservience to the Leader reigned. Only with such a country could the Great Dream be realized. The Great *Secret* Dream.

A tremendous task confronted him. The creation of a Party united in obedience to himself. Ilyich had seen the need for it, but experience showed that he had left the task unfinished. Now Stalin was resolved to complete it.

The bloody purge was also designed to solve another problem. In the system he had created, Party bosses were all-powerful. But these were professional revolutionaries, with little understanding of technology and management. The course of industrialization had demonstrated their incompetence.

In mid-February 1937, his protégé, the young engineer Malenkov, now a secretary of the Central Committee, wrote a report which revealed that seventy percent of oblast Party secretaries had only an elementary education, and that for district secretaries the figure was even higher—eighty percent. In the language of the Boss himself, "a very acute personnel problem has arisen."

Moreover, after twenty years in power, Party functionaries were showing their age, and had accumulated families, in-laws, mistresses. Two expressions used by Molotov in his character sketches of Party functionaries stand out in my mind: they were "beginning to go to pieces" and "manifesting a desire to rest." In these words you hear the mocking voice of the Boss himself.

The destruction of the semiliterate establishment, with its manifest "wish to rest," would make room for a new, educated generation which had grown up under Stalin.

But how was he to get rid of their predecessors, painlessly and without wasting too much time? Retire them? That would mean creating an opposition. His handling of the kulaks supplied the answer. He would do it by the same revolutionary method. He would annihilate them. Too cruel? Well, had they been any less cruel? Weren't *they* always parroting Lenin's murderous words "You can't make a revolution in white gloves"?

In the President's Archive is Stalin's visitors' book, in which the duty officer meticulously noted the arrivals and departures of all the Boss's visitors. "November 28, 1934. Kirov. Arrived 1500 hours, left 17.25." The Boss's "friend and brother" spent over two hours with him in his study. The Boss suggested that Kirov should move to Moscow, where he would become number two in the Party. Kirov left, intending to go Leningrad to wind up his affairs there. On November 29 he was still in Moscow, but was not granted an audience.

Yagoda, however, was a daily visitor.

On the evening of the 29th Bulgakov's wife, Stalin, and Kirov were together at the Arts Theater. The Boss took Kirov to the station, and kissed him on the platform: it is no easy thing to renounce a brother.

He would kiss Kirov once more—as he lay in his coffin.

On December 1, Kirov was walking along a corridor in the Smolny Institute. The onetime headquarters of the October coup had been the seat of the Bolshevik leadership in Leningrad ever since. As he turned into the narrow passage leading to his private office a young man detached himself from the wall. Strangely enough, there were no security guards around. The young man pulled a revolver out of his briefcase and fired. Chudov, a secretary of the Leningrad City Party Committee, ran out of the office and rushed up to Kirov. But Kirov was dead.

This assassination was the beginning of an enormous catastrophe which was to destroy millions of people.

The evening of Kirov's murder, the Boss dictated a decree of the Central Executive Committee of the USSR "on the procedure to be followed in dealing with terrorist acts against officials of the Soviet regime." Investigation of such cases was to be completed in not more than ten days, cases were to be tried without a public prosecutor or counsel, and appeals and petitions for pardon were not allowed. The death sentence must be carried out immediately.

That same night he set off for eternally rebellious Leningrad, together with faithful Molotov and the high executioners Yezhov and Yagoda. Medved, the head of the security police in Leningrad, met them at the station. Without a word Stalin struck him in the face—as much as to say "You should have looked after Kirov properly." He then took over the investigation.

A whole floor of the Smolny and a suite of rooms in the NKVD building were put at his disposal. He conducted the interrogations personally. Certain details began to emerge. According to the deposition of L. Nikolaev, Kirov's assassin, he had been put up to the murder. Asked where he obtained the revolver he pointed to Zaporozhets, the deputy head of the Leningrad branch of the NKVD and said, "Why are you asking me? Ask him."

"Take him away," Stalin commanded. And as soon as the door closed he barked at Yagoda, "That prick!"

That is how the defector Orlov, an ex-general in the NKVD, described the scene.

Stalin banished the Leningrad NKVD chiefs, Medved and Zaporozhets, to the Far East for "negligence." There they would live in comfort until their turn came to play a part in the thriller Stalin was concocting.

The preliminary examination of Kirov's assassin was concluded in twenty-seven days. The findings were signed by the Assistant State Prosecutor, A. Vyshinsky, and L. Sheinin, an investigating officer in especially important cases.

I talked to Lev Romanovich Sheinin in the seventies. Fat Sheinin, who had sent so many people to their deaths in the years of terror, looked like a benevolent Mr. Pickwick. In retirement he had started writing plays, so he was a colleague of sorts. He liked showing off his knowledge of secrets, and was quite delighted when I asked him whether Stalin had ordered Kirov's murder. He smiled, and answered amiably, "Stalin was the Leader, not a thug, my dear fellow."

During Khrushchev's Thaw a commission was set up to decide once and for all whether Stalin really did order Yagoda to kill Kirov. They hoped to find documents—and of course found none. Not because they had been destroyed. I am convinced that they never existed. What Sheinin said was not untrue: Stalin gave Yagoda no direct instructions. He could not do so. True, he personally had asked for "evidence" everyone knew was false to be beaten out of unfortunate engineers and scientists. But that was different. For the good of the Party you could do whatever you liked to "non-Party scum," as intellectuals were often called. Non-Party people were not regarded as human beings; they were the manure on which the society of the future could be grown. But Party members, those who were not criminal oppositionists of some kind, were quite a different matter. Lenin's heir could not call on the head of the NKVD to murder a loyal Leninist. On the contrary—he summoned the head of the NKVD on a number of occasions and asked him to watch over Kirov as carefully as possible. Yagoda's task could not have been simpler: he had only to translate the Boss's wish from "in-depth language,"and then carry it out.

Kirov's assassin, Nikolaev, was a young Party member. He turned out to have a military background. He had gone to the front at the age of sixteen, when Yudenich and the whites were attacking, and had joined the Communist Youth Organization at the front. After working in the GPU he had moved to Murmansk, where he had held some minor post. Since then he had been a disappointed man, haunted by a sense of failure. He dreamed up an imaginary romantic period in the Party's past. He wrote in his diary about the betrayal of former Party traditions, and said that someone must sacrifice himself to draw attention to the deadly dangers of the present situation. He interwove political and personal themes. Unnamed friends informed Nikolaev that his former wife was having an affair with Kirov. Yet another proof of the Party's degeneration!

The really surprising thing is that Nikolaev spoke openly about these fevered imaginings. The ears of Yagoda's establishment missed nothing, and must have heard. Yagoda must have known, too, of Nikolaev's mysterious friends, who aggravated the neurotic young man's delusions. It is difficult not to suspect that someone encouraged the hysterical Nicolaev to make his mad decision. And then enabled him to act on it unhindered. It emerged in the course of the investigation that the Smolny guard had detained Nikolaev on a previous occasion and had found him armed. In spite of this, he was allowed into the Smolny again on the day of the assassination.

The Museum of the Revolution contains the unpublished memoirs of Alex Rybin, a member of Stalin's bodyguard in the thirties. Regarding Kirov's assassination he wrote: "As someone who knows all the fine detail of the security arrangements for members of the Politburo . . . I can see what must have happened. Who could have allowed Nikolaev to sit for some considerable time on a window ledge in the corridor? Why was Kirov not accompanied by a personal aide, waiting to receive orders? Why was Nikolaev released on a previous occasion, although he had a weapon?"

The public asked similar questions. Hence the mischievous ditty "Stalin murdered Comrade Kirov/in his office corridor."

The Boss was in no hurry to answer all the people's questions. His mind was on the long and bloody crime in which millions would take part—and millions would perish. And, as in any good detective story, the questions would all be answered, but only at the very end.

But the drama was only just beginning, and the dramatis personae, marked down by him to die, were eating, drinking, worrying, and pitying the man who had lost a "brother." Maria Svanidze wrote in her diary, "I got back from the dacha at 9:00 P.M. and heard the shocking news. Everyone is terribly sad. Especially for J. [Joseph]. Kirov has been killed by an evil man. . . . It was a staggering blow for me. J. is strong, he bore the pain of losing Nadya heroically. But two such trials in such a short time. . . . A terrorist act of any sort is terrible enough. . . . This White Fascist terrorism is frightening in the hatred it shows."

It was undoubtedly painful to him—two such shocks, two such losses! Now he had neither wife nor friend. They, his enemies, had deprived him of everything. Now he would rid himself of *them.* His faithful brother would serve him still, even in death.

When Yagoda contrived Kirov's death he had not realized that the Leader was thinking on the grand scale. He had envisaged no more than the removal of a single dangerous figure around whom hostile forces were beginning to rally. The Leader had not initiated him into his cosmic plan. As a result, Yagoda hurried to arrest priests, ex-landowners, and so on, intending to lay Kirov's murder at the door of the usual culprits, the class enemy. Even the astute Radek missed the point, and started writing about the hand of the Gestapo killing a loyal Stalinist.

The Boss had to point out to Yagoda precisely where the main blow should fall: among the Zinovievites. Yagoda was too set in his ways and remained unconvinced. The Boss saw that he would never overcome his pious inhibitions when faced with the Leninist old guard. So he harnessed him to a diminutive fellow with a quiet voice, one Nikolai Yezhov, the chairman of the Party Control Commission.

Molotov described Yezhov as "Bolshevik from before the Revolution, worker by origin, never in any of the oppositions, Central Committee Secretary for some years, good reputation."

Secret file 510, in the archive of the former KGB, contains a curriculum vitae of this person of "good reputation": "Yezhov, Nikolai Ivanovich. Born May 1, 1895. Resident in Moscow, Kremlin. Social origin—worker. Education—incomplete primary. . . . In 1919 tried by military tribunal and sentenced to imprisonment for one year."

The Boss had first seen Yezhov during his excursion to Siberia to speed up grain deliveries and had subsequently introduced him into the apparatus of the Central Committee. By the beginning of the thirties Yezhov was already head of its Cadres Department. At the Seventeenth Congress he was elected to the Central Committee and to the vice-chairmanship of the Central Control Commission. In 1935 he became chairman of that body, and a secretary of the Central Committee.

Yezhov was typical of those who rose from nowhere to high positions in this period: semiliterate, obedient, and hardworking. His dubious past made him particularly eager to shine. Most important of all—he had made his career after the overthrow of the October leaders. Yagoda now served Stalin, but until recently had been the servant of the Party. Yezhov had served no one but Stalin. He was the man to implement the second half of Stalin's scheme. For him there were no taboos.

At the height of the Terror Yezhov would be portrayed on thousands of posters as a giant in whose hands enemies of the people writhed and breathed their last. In the Central Asian republics, poets regularly described him as the *batyr* (epic hero). The epic hero was in reality a tiny man, almost a dwarf, with a feeble voice.

This was somehow symbolic.

Like Zhdanov, Malenkov, and others whom the Boss would from now on co-opt to the highest offices, Yezhov was merely a pseudonym for Stalin himself, a pathetic puppet, there simply to carry out orders. All the thinking was done, all the decisions were made, by the Boss himself.

While Yezhov familiarized himself with the way things were going, kept an eye on Yagoda, and gave him a prod when necessary, the Boss was drumming the plot of his thriller into the heads of his closest associates. And that is why afterward Bukharin said, "Two days after the murder Stalin sent for me and announced that the assassin, Nikolaev, was a Zinovievite."

Molotov understood at once the grandiose character of Stalin's scheme. As he wrote, "Until 1937 we lived the whole time with opposition. After that—there were no more opposition groups! Stalin took the whole difficult business upon himself, but we helped. . . . Stalin wanted 1937 to be a continuation of the Revolution . . . in a complicated international situation."

A continuation of the Revolution necessary, it would be said, because the leaders had grown slack, bourgeois, degenerate. It was time to return to the old ideals, and open fire on degenerate cadres. This was made particularly important by Hitler's menaces. For the Party, then, a continuation of the Revolution. And for those outside the Party? The end of the Revolution. The destruction of the Leninist old guard, associated in the minds of the people at large with October and the Red Terror.

The newspapers were whipping up hysteria: new "terrorist outrages" were expected. Stalin returned to Moscow for "Brother Kirov's" funeral. The ceremony took place in the Hall of Columns of the House of Unions. Maria Svanidze recorded in her diary that on December 5, 1934,

> Tverskaya Street was closed, trucks and groups of Red army men stood at the corner, blocking the entrance to it. . . . Redens [head of the NKVD in Moscow, and Anna Alliluyeva's husband] had us escorted to where the family and friends were standing. The hall was brilliantly lit, decorated with a profusion of plush banners and in the middle stood . . . a simple coffin, lined with red calico. . . . His face was a greenish yellow, his nose had become sharper. . . . Between the temple and cheekbone there was a bruise from his fall. His unhappy wife and sisters stood on the right of the coffin. His sisters are village schoolteachers and living out in the wilds they never even knew that their brother had become such a big man. They wrote to him when they saw his picture in the papers but could never get away to visit him . . . now they've seen him. The general public were excluded and admission to the hall was restricted to a small group of people. . . . We all felt the tension, we looked around apprehensively, wondering whether everybody had been properly checked, whether there was anybody who didn't belong there, hoping that it all would go off without incident. J. [Joseph] took his stand by the dead man's head, surrounded by his comrades-in-arms. . . . The floodlights were dimmed, the music stopped. . . . The sentries were ready to screw down the coffin lid. Joseph went up the steps of the catafalque . . . his face was sorrowful. He bent down and kissed the dead man's forehead. . . . It was a heart-rending picture for anyone who knew how close they were. . . . Everyone in the hall was weeping. Through my own sobs I could hear men sobbing loudly. J. is suffering terribly. Pavel was with him at the dacha a day or two after Kirov's death. They were sitting in the dining room together. J. rested his head on his hand (I've never seen him do that) and said "now I'm all alone in the world." Pavel says it was so moving that he jumped up and kissed him. J. told Pavel that Kirov used to look after him like a child. After Nadya's death Kirov had of course been closer to Joseph than anyone, he could approach him with simple affection and give him the warmth he was missing and peace of

> mind. We all feel too shy to drop in just to see him and have a chat. . . . I'm not shy myself, but Alyosha gets suspicious, and brings an element of jealousy into it, says he's afraid he would be intruding, and J. doesn't like women visiting him.

Alyosha Svanidze, who knew his kinsman pretty well, evidently had misgivings and thought it best to keep his distance.

Entries in Stalin's visitors' book recommence after his return to Moscow, on December 3. For a whole month the NKVD chiefs were in and out of his office, all day and every day. Yezhov, the eye of the emperor, was always last to leave, usually in the dead of night.

Nikolaev shortly confessed that he had killed Kirov on the instructions of a Trotskyist-Zinovievite group. He was then shot in a hurry.

Kirov's vile murderers were branded at innumerable public meetings. Zinoviev joined in at a meeting of the board of the Central Council of Cooperative Unions in Moscow, unsparingly abusing the "foul killers." But on December 8 supporters of Zinoviev and Kamenev in Leningrad were arrested and on December 16 Zinoviev and Kamenev themselves were arrested in Moscow.

In the perestroika period a Politburo commission was set up "to further examine materials connected with the repressions which took place between 1930 and 1940 and at the beginning of the fifties." The commission retrieved the hapless Zinoviev's letters from the depths of secret archives.

Within minutes of his arrest Zinoviev wrote a hysterical note to Stalin:

> It is now December 16. At 7:30 this evening Comrade Molchanov and a group of Chekists arrived at my apartment and carried out a search. I tell you, Comrade Stalin, honestly, that from the time of my return from Kustanai by order of the Central Committee, I have not taken a single step, spoken a single word, written a single line, or had a single thought which I need conceal from the Party, the Central Committee, and you personally. . . . I have had only one thought—how to earn the trust of the Central Committee and you personally, how to achieve my aim of being employed by you in the work there is to be done. I swear by all a Bolshevik holds sacred, I swear by Lenin's memory . . . I implore you to believe my word of honor. I am shaken to the depths of my being.

Yagoda sent this letter to Stalin. He did not reply. But I can imagine him reading it with a smile. "Shaken to the depths of my being"! Zinoviev would discover what it was really like to be shaken when he heard of the role assigned to him in Stalin's thriller.

Stalin knew that in starting with Zinoviev and Kamenev he could not possibly lose. He never for a moment doubted they would cave in. Zinoviev's nickname was "Panic," and Kamenev was weak in misfortune, a timid intellectual. They were the best possible candidates for what Stalin had in mind. But Yagoda let him down. He simply could not rid himself of his subconscious respect for former leaders. Yagoda and his interrogators were obviously handling Zinoviev and Kamenev with kid gloves, and the two men refused to admit responsibility for the murder.

The year was drawing to a close. Less than two decades had gone by since the October coup, and some of its leaders could look back on it from their prison cells.

From Maria Svanidze's diary:

> 21.12.34. We celebrated the Boss's birthday. We gathered at the nearer dacha around 9. All the close friends were there (the Molotovs—both of them, Voroshilov—alone, Enukidze, Beria, Lakoba, Kalinin—alone, the Svanidze relatives—the Redens couple—and the Alliluyevs). We were at the table till 1 A.M., then the party got noisy. The Boss got out the gramophone and some records, wound it up himself. . . . We danced. He made the men partner the women and take a few turns. Then the Caucasians sang some doleful songs—the Boss took the lead with his light tenor. . . . Then J. said, "Let's drink to Nadya." My eyes are full of tears again as I write this, just as they were at that moment. Everybody rose and silently went up to J. His face was full of suffering. He has changed greatly after his two heavy losses. He has become gentler, kinder, more human. Till Nadya died he was unapproachable, a marble hero. . . . The Alliluyevs and the Redenses . . . the only one of that quartet you can talk to is Zhenya. She's clever, a live wire, interested in everything. Pavel, Zhenya's husband, is in my opinion deteriorating intellectually, he never reads anything, it's no good trying to talk to him. Nyura [Anna Alliluyeva, Nadya's sister] is obsessively kind, and intellectually null. Her spouse [Redens] is pompous, stupid, conceited, and bogged down in trivial chores. . . . Alyosha has

been promoted—appointed Vice Chairman of the USSR State Bank.

The grief-stricken Marble Hero had become gentler and kinder. He sang in his light tenor. He danced and made merry with them. And all the time he knew what was in store for them.

The New Year had arrived, and still Yagoda had not succeeded in linking Kamenev and Zinoviev with Kirov's murder. The first version of the case for the prosecution is in the President's Archive. It was drawn up on January 13, 1935. It states that Zinoviev and Kamenev had not admitted their guilt. But suddenly, on that very same day, Zinoviev wrote a "statement to the investigators":

> The time allowed for the investigation is running out . . . and I want to disarm myself completely. . . . After the Fifteenth and especially after the Sixteenth Congress I told myself on many occasions that I should leave it at that . . . the Central Committee and Comrade Stalin had been shown to be right about everything . . . but when fresh difficulties arose I started vacillating again: 1932 provides a vivid example—I have described the events of that year in detail in my depositions. . . . Subjectively I had no wish to harm the Party and the working class. But I became in effect the mouthpiece of the forces which sought to disrupt the building of socialism in the USSR. [Objectively he admits that he is an "enemy."] My speech at the Seventeenth Congress was meant sincerely . . . but in reality two souls still lived within me. . . . We proved unable to submit fully to the Party, to merge with it completely . . . we continued to look backward and to live in a stifling atmosphere of our own . . . our whole situation condemned us to . . . duplicity. . . . I asserted under investigation that from 1929 "no center for former Zinovievites" had existed in Moscow. My thought was that you couldn't really call it a center, it was just Zinoviev plus Kamenev plus one or two others, but in actual fact it was a center since Zinoviev's former followers, or what was left of them, refused to merge fully with the Party and looked to that handful of people for leadership. My former adherents always voted for the Party

> line, but among themselves they went on talking in a criminal way that was hostile to the Party and to the state, so whether we wanted it or not, we remained in actual fact one of the centers of struggle against the Party and its great work . . . and the center's role was of course anti-Party and counterrevolutionary. . . . From the first interrogation onward I was outraged to find myself confused with the wretches who had sunk so low as to murder Kirov. . . . But facts are stubborn things, and when I learned (from the newspapers) all the facts set out in the indictment I had to acknowledge the moral and political responsibility of the former Leningrad opposition, and myself personally, for the crime committed. . . . After my return from banishment in 1933 I was criminally negligent in that I did not expose to the Party all the people involved in tentative conspiracies against it. . . . I am full of repentance, the most fervent repentance. . . . I am ready to do all I can to help the investigation. . . . I am naming . . . all those whom I remember as former participants in the anti-Party struggle . . . and I will continue doing so to the end, mindful of the fact that this is my duty. I can only say that if I had the opportunity to do penance before the whole people it would be a great relief to me. . . . Let others learn from my grievous example what deviation from the Party path means, and where it can lead. . . . January 13, 1935.

Kamenev, too, began by denying everything, but the next day, January 14, suddenly admitted that a central Zinovievite directorate had existed and remained active up to and throughout 1932.

Something crucial must have happened to make both former leaders capitulate on the same day. Someone had succeeded where Yagoda and his investigators had failed. It is not hard to guess who that someone was. There are no entries in Stalin's visitors' book from January 11 to 17. He obviously had visitors of a variety best not recorded. *They*—Kamenev and Zinoviev—were brought before him. They spent the whole week bargaining. He could of course show them proofs of their secret meetings with his enemies. And he did what Yagoda had not been clever enough to do. He got them to admit their moral and political responsibility for Kirov's murder, and to betray their supporters. In return he evidently promised to pardon them—soon—but demanded an act of contrition before the whole people. Hence Zinoviev's plea "to do penance before the whole people."

Zinoviev, however, had not yet realized *what* he would have to do public penance for. The plot was only just beginning to unfold and it is doubtful whether anyone could have guessed the fantastic denouement the author had in mind.

On January 16, 1935, Zinoviev was sentenced to ten years' imprisonment, Kamenev to five. The former leaders were now known as the "Moscow Center" of the conspiracy. The members of the Leningrad Zinovievite group were tried simultaneously. One of them was Georgi Safarov, who would say whatever the investigators required against his former friends. He was sentenced to five years' imprisonment in 1935. In 1942, Safarov, one of those mainly responsible for the execution without trial of the imperial family, would be shot without trial himself.

The wave of mass arrests continued over the winter months and throughout the spring of 1935. People outside the Party somewhat humorously described this as the "Kirov stream." Two of Koba's old acquaintances from 1917, the erstwhile young leaders of the Petrograd Bolsheviks, Zalutsky and Shlyapnikov, were among those arrested. Both were shown Safarov's testimony that they had "carried on illegal work against the Party." Shlyapnikov was given five years. But kind Joseph commuted his prison sentence to banishment to Astrakhan. Shlyapnikov still had a part to play: the Boss had thought up a suitable role for him in the thriller.

As spring came to an end Kamenev and Zinoviev looked forward to the customary change in their fortunes. For Kamenev change was in fact not long delayed, but it was not at all the one he had expected.

That carefree Lothario and aficionado of the Bolshoi ballerinas, Avel Enukidze, started grumbling about the arrest of Kamenev and Zinoviev. Avel, secretary of the Presidium of the Central Executive Committee of the USSR, was a close friend of the Boss. But he was also an old Bolshevik, completely tied to the old Party, which now had to disappear. So friend Avel was written into the plot of the thriller. What is more, he was—the Boss had a sense of humor—linked with Kamenev, whom he had tried to defend. In June 1935 Yezhov presented a report to the Central Committee "on the Secretariat of the Central Executive Committee and Comrade A. Enukidze." It appeared that because of Enukidze's criminal negligence several terrorist groups were active within the confines of the Kremlin itself. People were horrified to read the staggering news of plots to assassinate their Leader. Kamenev was declared to be the immediate organizer of an assassination attempt. The conspiracy had allied Trotsky and Zinoviev with monarchists who had wormed their way into the Kremlin thanks to Enukidze's slackness. Certain garrulous witnesses of events surrounding Nadya's death were added to the list of conspirators. Thus, Alekxei Sinelobov, the Kremlin commandant's aide, was shot and his sister was jailed for four years. This was also when the Kremlin cleaner Korchagina was sentenced for "spreading defamatory rumors about government leaders." Neither she nor Sinelobova returned from the camps. Yagoda added to the "terrorist group" Kamenev's brother Nikolai Rozenfeld and his wife, who worked in the Kremlin library. Also, Trotsky's son Sergei Sedov. For the "Kremlin affair" Kamenev was given an additional five years, so he was now Zinoviev's equal, while Rozenfeld and his wife each got ten years, and Sergei Sedov five. Other "terrorists" included Kamenev's wife, Olga Davidovna. She had once lived in the Kremlin and she was Trotsky's sister—ideally suited, in short, for a part in the conspiracy story. Altogether 110 people were sentenced to various terms of imprisonment. Avel Yenukidze, Stalin's friend for many years, and the godfather of his deceased wife, Nadya, was expelled from the Party because of his "political and moral degeneracy," in the words of a Central Committee resolution dated June 7, 1935. The scale of things to come was already foreshadowed in the Kremlin affair.

From Maria Svanidze's diary: "I firmly believe that we are advancing toward a great and radiant future. . . . Avel has received the punishment he deserved. . . . This nest of treachery and filth terrified me. Now all is light again, all the evil has been swept away . . . and everything will get better and better."

He was, indeed, methodically working on that bright future, in which Maria too would meet her end. That same spring, in April 1935, a new law was promulgated: children twelve and older were to pay the same penalties for their crimes as adults. Up to and including the death penalty. So during future trials his victims would have not just themselves but their posterity to think about.

Meanwhile, arrests were becoming less frequent. There were no public trials. People had been expecting something on the scale of the Red Terror, and after the mighty thunderclaps in the press they were rather disappointed. Things were settling down in the same old boring rut. Before long Gorky was making a nuisance of himself with pleas for Kamenev's release. The Boss had fooled them all again. They supposed that the show was over, whereas the curtain had only just risen. The main events in his great work of imagination were all in the future.

That spring was marked by a new entertainment for the people, one which overshadowed the punishment of the old leaders. The Moscow

Metro was opened, another token for all to see of what the future paradise held. Those magnificent underground palaces were intended to show the toilers what sort of homes their children would live in under communism.

From Maria Svanidze's diary: "29.4.35. We started talking about the Metro, Svetlana expressed a wish to take a ride and we all agreed to go with her—myself, Zhenya, the nurse. Suddenly there was a commotion. J. [Joseph] had decided to take a ride with us. They sent for Molotov. Everybody was terribly excited. There was a lot of whispering about the danger of such an outing without proper preparation. Kaganovich was more agitated than anybody. . . . He suggested going at midnight when the Metro would be closed to the public. . . . But J. insisted on going right away. In Okhotny Ryad . . . the public rushed to greet the leaders. . . . They cheered, and ran along behind us. We got separated, and I was almost crushed against one of the columns. The enthusiasm and the ovations reached superhuman dimensions. J. was merry . . . the enthusiastic crowd overturned an iron lamppost. . . . I think that, austere as he is, he was touched by the people's love for their leader. There was nothing contrived or formal about it. He once said of the ovations he received, 'The people need a tsar,' i.e., someone to reverence, someone to live and work for."

He mentioned the need for a tsar on various occasions. N. Chagin, an old Bolshevik, has recorded an episode at a dinner given by Kirov. On this occasion Stalin said: "Bear in mind that in Russia the people were under the tsar for centuries, the Russian people are tsarist, the Russian people are used to having one single individual over them."

Now, as he prepared to destroy the refractory Leninist old guard, his mind was on the monarchy of the future. One émigré aptly remarked after yet another bloody purge that "a lot of blood has to be shed to give birth to a Russian autocrat."

"You'd Have Done Better to Have Become a Priest"

At the end of the year he went at last to see his mother. Throughout the year, as always, he had written to her regularly: "11.6.35. I know that you are not well. You mustn't be afraid of sickness, be strong and it will pass. I'm sending my children to see you. Make them welcome and give them lots of kisses. They are good children. If I can manage it I'll try to come and see you."

It was indeed high time for him to pay her a visit. She was frequently ill, and he had to see her while he could, the sooner the better.

After he'd arranged just what he intended to do, it would be difficult for him to go to Georgia. Difficult and dangerous. He decided to let his mother see her Soso in all his glory now. Before he became anathema.

His mother had been moved to Tiflis some years ago and installed, as befit the mother of a tsar, in the former palace of the Viceroys of Georgia. Grand dukes had once resided there. With all the palace to choose from, his mother had chosen one miserable little room away from the main building, a room quite like the hovel in which they had once lived.

He had provided for Keke generously. Two female hangers-on in black caps waited on her. She lived on a pension, and a special doctor kept an eye on her health: Lavrenti Beria, Party leader in the Caucasus, saw to it personally that Keke wanted nothing.

Molotov recalled meeting the young Beria more than once in Lenin's office. He had joined the Party in 1917, but his rise really began under the Boss. Stalin made the young Chekist Beria a leader, and valued him more and more as time went by. On the Boss's last birthday Beria had been among his guests.

Beria skillfully turned the Boss's meeting with his mother into an occasion of ideological significance. With his shrewd guidance, the newspapers published touching tales of the radiant love between the Great Mother and the Great Leader; the image of the Virgin Mary was clearly discernible in the pages of the press. "Seventy-five-year-old Keke is cordial and lively," *Pravda* reported. "She seems to light up when she talks about the unforgettable moments of their meeting. 'The whole world rejoices when it looks upon my son and our country. What would you expect me, his mother, to feel?' " In fact he was with her only briefly. As their meeting ended she asked him, "Joseph, what exactly are you now?" And he answered, "Do you remember the tsar? Well, I'm something like the tsar."

"You'd have done better to have become a priest," she replied.

During all this time he had not stopped thinking about the wife who had gone. Even after her death he went on quarreling with her passionately. "We got talking about Yasha [his son Yakov]," Maria Svanidze wrote in her diary. "He remembered again his (Yasha's) despicable treatment of dear Nadya, his marriage, all his mistakes, his suicide attempt. Then he said, 'Nadya was so down on Yasha for behaving like that—how could she then go and shoot herself? She did a very bad thing, she crippled me.' [I said,] 'How could she leave two children?' [And he said,] 'Never mind the children. They'd forgotten her a few days later. But she left me crippled for life.' "

After her death, as though to revenge himself upon her, he changed completely the former pattern of his home life.

Agents of the secret police now took charge of the household. Nikolai Vlasik, who commanded his bodyguard, now supervised the upbringing of Stalin's children. Vlasik had emerged from the depths of rural Russia to serve in the ranks of the Cheka, and from there had been seconded to Stalin's bodyguard on Menzhinsky's recommendation. Vlasik was assisted in his task of supervising the children by S. Yefimov, an NKVD officer and commandant of the dacha at Zubalovo, where Vasya and Svetlana spent the summer months.

The effects of this regime on Vasya soon showed themselves. In the President's Archive we find Yefimov's reports to Vlasik, who promptly submitted them to the Boss. "22.9.35. Greetings, Comrade Vlasik. I write to inform you how things are with us. First, Svetlana and Vasya are in good health and feel well. Svetlana is taking her schoolwork seriously, Vasya is neglecting his lessons. . . . He stayed away from school altogether, saying that he had a sore throat, but he would not let the doctor look at it."

From Maria Svanidze's diary: "17.11.35. At dinner we talked about Vasya. He's doing badly at school. J. [Joseph] has given him 2 months to show an improvement, and threatened to turn him out of the house and adopt three able lads instead."

Vasya was afraid of his father, but knew how to defend himself. Yefimov reported to Vlasik that "On 19.10.35 he (Vasya) wrote his name on a sheet of paper, and wrote down below: 'Vasya Stalin, born 1921, died 1935.' This inscription is worrying. Has he got something in mind?"

Vasya evidently knew (had probably overheard) something about his mother and was using this as a weapon to alarm his father. Maria Svanidze wrote in her diary: "J. knows them both [Svetlana and Vasya] inside out. . . . What an analytical mind he has, what an exceptional psychologist he is." For once her enthusiasm may have been justified.

What follows is the Boss's description of Vasily in a letter to Oleg Martyshin, his teacher (published in *Uchitelskaya Gazeta,* Teachers' Newspaper, in 1988):

> To Comrade Martyshin, Schoolteacher. I have received your letter about the misbehavior of Vasily Stalin. I am very late in an-

swering because of an excessive workload. Please forgive me. Vasily is a spoiled youth, of average ability, a little savage (a sort of Scythian), not always truthful, he likes to blackmail weak supervisors, is often insolent, has a weak, or rather disorganized will, has been spoiled by all sorts of "godfathers and godmothers" who sometimes make too much of the fact that he is "Stalin's son." I am glad that in you he has at least one teacher with self-respect, who insists on the impudent boy complying with general school rules. Vasily gets spoiled by headmasters like the one you mention, spineless creatures who do not belong in a school, and if Vasily does not succeed in ruining himself it will be because there are in our country some teachers who will not give way to young master's caprices. My advice is to be stricter with Vasily, and not to fear a spoiled boy's blackmailing threats of suicide. Unfortunately I have no time to spend on Vasily, but I promise to give him a good shaking every now and then—Yours J. Stalin. 8.4.38.

The son about whom he wrote so pitilessly was the one he loved. His other—unloved—son also sprang a surprise on him.

From Maria Svanidze's diary: "17.11.35. Yasha has got married for the second time. To Yulia Isaakovna Bessarb. She is quite pretty, somewhere between thirty and thirty-two, a bit of a flirt, talks nonsense self-confidently, she had made up her mind to leave her husband and make a career . . . and she has done just that. . . . Her things are still at her former husband's place. I don't know how J. will take it! . . . 4.12.35. J. now knows about Yasha's marriage. His attitude is that of a loyal—but ironical—father. After all, Yasha is twenty-seven or twenty-eight!"

Stalin's birthday had come round again. From Maria Svanidze's diary: "26.12.35. Twenty-one of us wrote J. a little letter. (We congratulate dear Joseph on his birthday. There are no words to express all the beautiful things we wish him.) He was in a splendid mood. Everybody was noisy and full of fun at dinner. J. turned to Alyosha and said, 'But for you none of this would be happening. I'd completely forgotten the day.' "

How he enjoyed himself. With those soon to die!

16

"THE PEOPLE OF MY WRATH" DESTROYED

Ah, Assyria, the rod of my anger, the staff of my fury. Against a godless nation I send him and against the people of my wrath I command him.
—Isaiah 10:5–6

I slew your young men with the sword . . . yet you did not return to me, says the Lord.
—Amos 4:10

A Necessary Illusion

It was 1936. He was planning to hold bloody show trials at home, but his foreign policy seemed quite enlightened. He enjoyed moving in opposite directions simultaneously. While he was turning his country into a closed and unassailable fortress, he established diplomatic relations with the United States. He joined the League of Nations and became the main champion of collective security. The constitution then in preparation, with its promises of democratic freedoms, was intended to palliate the coming bloody purge. Against the background of the show trials the constitution served to create the necessary illusion that a democratic state, free of those terrible Leninists, was being created in Russia. He knew that the West would have to further that illusion. Hitler had lived up to his hopes: Germany had rearmed, and the West had fallen behind. They had realized at last that without that dreadful Stalin they would never defeat Hitler. Luck was on his side. During the trials, Hitler would be on the rampage all over Europe, and Franco would raise a rebellion in Spain. In the Spanish general election of 1936, victory went to the parties of the left, and General Franco, supported by Hitler, led a revolt against the government of the Republic. In the cruel Civil War which followed, antifascists all over the world helped the Republican army. Stalin's reaction was instantaneous and, once again, enlightened: Soviet advisers, tanks, and planes were rushed to the aid of democracy in Spain—together with a large number of NKVD agents. All this coincided with a good harvest, and the people were getting their breath back after the years of upheaval. He had chosen a good year for his carefully planned offensive. Its objective was the destruction of the Party.

"Conspiracy"

The NKVD held a conference of its highest officials. They were informed that a gigantic conspiracy had been uncovered, with Trotsky, Kamenev, Zinoviev, and a number of other opposition leaders at its head. It appeared that they had set up terrorist groups in every large town. All those attending the conference were seconded to a secret political department of the NKVD to assist in the investigation. The Leader himself would supervise their work. The Leader would be assisted by Yezhov.

The whole gathering of course realized that there was no conspiracy. But they also knew the "in-depth" language. They had been told that the Party must have a conspiracy. It was essential for success in the struggle with world imperialism and the schismatic Trotsky.

In conclusion, a secret circular from Yagoda was read. The People's Commissar warned them that the use of illegal methods of interrogation such as threats and torture would not be tolerated. In "in-depth language" this meant that such methods were necessary because the accused must be ruthlessly "broken."

Some hundreds of miscellaneous oppositionists were taken from prisons and places of exile and delivered to Moscow. They were required to admit their participation in terrorist acts and to play their parts in a show trial. After the recent trials of intellectuals the public would not be greatly surprised by the bloody theatrical event ahead. The great difference was that those cast as murderers and spies were the old Leninist guard, yesterday's Party leaders. They would lead the way, marching as leaders should at the head of the old Party—leading it to its death.

For the Party's Sake

Meanwhile Zinoviev, who was to play the lead in the forthcoming production, was writing letter after letter to his onetime ally, now the Boss. There is a well-known story that when Zinoviev and Kamenev were brought to Moscow, the Boss himself tricked them into performing at the trials by promising to spare their lives. And that Zinoviev was tortured by deprivation of air and so on. But we need only read Zinoviev's harrowing letters, recently made available.

> April 14 [1936]. In my soul there is one burning desire—to prove to you that I am no longer an enemy. There is no demand with which I would not comply to prove it to you. . . . I have reached the point at which I spend a long time gazing on pictures of you and other members of the Politburo in the newspapers, and thinking, dear friends, look into my soul, surely you can see that I am no longer your enemy, that I belong to you body and soul, that there is no demand with which I would not comply to earn forgiveness, clemency.
>
> May 6. I am treated humanely in prison here. I get medical attention etc. But I am old and badly shaken. In the last few months I have aged twenty years. Help me. Trust me. Do not let me die in prison. Do not let me go mad in solitary confinement.
>
> July 12. My condition is very poor. . . . I fervently beg you to publish the book I wrote in Verkhne-Uraisk. I wrote it with my heart's blood. . . . Also, may I be so bold as to put in a plea for my family, especially my son. You knew him when he was a little boy. He is a talented Marxist with a scholarly bent. Please help him. I am now yours heart and soul.

Once he had lost power, tasted imprisonment, and undergone just a fraction of the torments to which he had doomed others, Zinoviev was a broken man. He was not tortured—on the contrary—"I am being treated humanely, I get medical attention etc." There was no need, then, for further meetings with his onetime ally, the Boss. The old, formidable Zinoviev no longer existed. There was only this unhappy, sick slave yearning to serve his master. And willing to slander himself and others. "There is no demand with which I would not comply." And no humiliation he would not accept: Zinoviev was ready for anything.

In one of my articles I myself repeated the story that Zinoviev and Kamenev were tortured, and also that Stalin sent for them and used persuasion on them. I got one curious response: a letter amusingly signed N-K V.D.:

> You are mistaken, Comrade. No torture was used on Zinoviev. I don't think that Stalin saw Kamenev and Zinoviev while the case against them was in preparation. I do know that his messengers

talked to them. I have heard that Molotov was the one who talked to Zinoviev. He spoke in his usual cold, logical way. "How many times have you lied to the Party? How many times have your lies damaged the Party? You are now asked to calumniate yourself for the good of the Party. At a time when Trotsky is trying to split the workers' movement, and the Germans are preparing to attack us, your lies will undoubtedly be of help to the Party. That is undeniable. So what is there to discuss? If the interests of the Party demand it, it is our duty to sacrifice not only our miserable reputations but our very lives. Although, objectively, you are not being asked to lie. Objectively, everything you did *was* a betrayal of the Party's interests." Zinoviev was, then, treated throughout with the greatest respect. He must have seen in that a possibility of forgiveness. He tried to persuade Kamenev. Kamenev was an intelligent man and he resisted for a while—so they did treat him roughly at times. But there was no torture. The setup was, I repeat, quite different. The prison was more like a clinic. The whole atmosphere suggested that they would surely be pardoned. All they wanted was to be allowed to live. And all those fine words about the Party helped them to preserve, shall we say, their self-respect. They were allowed to stand trial as though they were carrying out a secret Party assignment. Molotov, however, made a mistake. He really believed that they ought to be pardoned. And dared to say so. He very nearly found himself on trial as a result. Especially as all his old friends on the Petrograd Committee, Shlyapnikov and Zalutsky included, were already in jail. We took the point immediately: the official account of the trial of Kamenev, Zinoviev, and the rest of them listed those leaders whom the "Zinovievite assassins" had planned to destroy, including the whole Politburo except Molotov. So when he was sent on vacation before the trial began we were all waiting for something to happen. People were usually picked up en route to somewhere. But Molotov returned after his month off, and was even in time for the opening of the trial. He had learned his lesson. After that, he did occasionally have an opinion of his own. But only when the Boss wanted him to.

Perhaps, with "Stone Arse" away, Stalin had realized how much that indefatigable worker had done for him, and decided to keep him on. At subsequent trials Molotov would be mentioned among other intended victims of the "Trotskyist butchers."

Kamenev was a little harder to handle than Zinoviev. Orlov tells us that his interrogator, Chertok, yelled at him: "You're a coward . . . Lenin himself said so. . . . you were a strikebreaker in October [1917]. You flitted from one opposition group to another. . . . While real Bolsheviks were carrying on the fight underground you were swanning around in Western cafés. . . . Do you imagine that you people are still icons to us, as you used to be? If we let you out the first Komsomol you meet will do you in on the spot. Ask any Young Pioneer who Zinoviev and Kamenev are and he'll say 'enemies of the people.' "

The Young Pioneer in fact needed only to switch on the radio any day of the week to hear the frenzied indignation of the mob. An additional threat was brought to bear: "If you refuse to plead guilty in court a substitute will be found—your son. We have evidence that he monitored the movements of Voroshilov's and Stalin's cars on the highway." When he heard that Zinoviev had agreed to make *any* statement required of him, Kamenev knew that he was doomed, and agreed to play the same role.

The principal actors were now ready to take the stage. A number of other prominent Party members were put on trial with them. Among them were Ivan Smirnov, member of the Party since 1905, who had taken part in the defeat of Kolchak, and the former People's Commissar for Communications, Sergei Mrachkovsky, a worker by origin, an old Bolshevik, and also a hero of the war with Kolchak. They were prepared for trial in the same way, enjoined to confess in the sacred name of the Party. In 1956, during the Khrushchev Thaw, A. Safonova, I. Smirnov's divorced wife, testified that when she was asked to slander her former husband she was told that "it's necessary for the Party's sake."

End of the Old Bear

In the hot summer days of 1936 something also had to be done about Gorky. "The old bear with a ring in his nose," Romain Rolland had sadly called him. But the bear had plainly ceased to be tame. He sought forgiveness for his old friend Kamenev. At the Academia publishing house over which Gorky had presided, Kamenev had been his deputy. The publishing house was, of course, savagely attacked. Gorky again expressed his indignation, and announced his decision to go back to Sorrento for his health. The Boss gave orders that he should not be allowed to leave. Just a little tug on the ring. From then on Gorky's secretary, N. Kryuchkov, became in effect his jailer, openly taking note of all visitors to the house. At the same time Yagoda began an insultingly public affair with Gorky's son's wife. As a prelude to the coming catastrophe the *Maxim Gorky,* the world's largest airplane, built to advertise the country's industrial progress, had ignominiously crashed.

Yagoda delivered to the Boss a letter from Gorky to Louis Aragon in France, in which Gorky begged the famous poet to come and see him immediately. With the scale of the impending trials in mind Stalin was bound to realize how dangerous a rebellious Gorky would be. Gorky repeatedly urged Aragon to visit him. "Gorky had been urging us to go there for the past two months . . . and every summons was more pressing than the last," Aragon wrote later. This must have been when the Boss instructed Yagoda to take good care of Gorky, to do everything possible to prevent enemies from using the writer. Yagoda, of course, did just that . . . by helping him to die.

Yagoda first dealt skillfully with the Communist Aragon and his Russian-born wife, the writer Elsa Triolet. When they arrived to see Gorky they were apparently advised not to be in any hurry to go to him but to stay with Elsa's relatives in Leningrad for a while. Aragon wrote later that they should have hurried on to Moscow. He was right. But they didn't. When they finally arrived in Moscow on June 15, Gorky already lay dying. He died on June 18. The easily persuaded poet had no opportunity to talk to him.

Another visitor turned up at that time—the French writer André Gide, a friend of the USSR. He had been invited to extol the land of the Soviets, but first he intended to visit Gorky. When he arrived in Moscow on June 18 his first question was about Gorky's health. But Gorky had died that very day.

Gorky was given a magnificent funeral. Molotov delivered an address at the memorial service. Gide also spoke: "To this day and in all countries of the world the great writer has almost always been a rebel and a mutineer. . . . In the Soviet Union, for the first time . . . the writer, though a revolutionary, is no longer an oppositionist. On the contrary . . . the Soviet Union has lit new stars in a new heaven." Gide remained in the USSR for a few months, and became the only European radical to write the truth about the terrible land of the "new heaven."

Another incorrigible grumbler died in 1936, the former Commissar for Foreign Affairs Chicherin, a very prominent member of the Party in his day. While so many old Bolsheviks were being shot in the years of terror, others died peaceful but convenient deaths. There existed in the NKVD a splendid toxicological laboratory—the creation of the pharmacist manqué Yagoda.

The Thriller Staged: First Trial of Lenin's Associates

For the trial of Kirov's "murderers" Stalin chose the House of Unions, where not so long ago Kirov had lain in state. Another of history's ironies: the leaders of the land of October were tried in a small hall called the October Room. And, amusingly enough, the premiere of his spectacle on August 19 coincided with the opening of the Moscow theater season.

The stage designers had turned the October Room into a revolutionary court, decorated in different shades of red. The judge's desk was covered with bright red cloth. There were monumental chairs embossed with the arms of the Soviet Union. The defendants were near the right-hand wall, behind a wooden barrier. In back of them stood Red army soldiers with rifles and fixed bayonets. Also behind the defendants was a door, beyond which was, shall we say, the "Wings of His Theater," with a buffet, restrooms for the defendants, and an area for Yagoda and the prosecutor, Vyshinsky, to hold friendly discussions with the accused in the course of the trial, to criticize their performances and give them instructions. There were additional actors in the body of the hall, NKVD agents in mufti acting the part of "the people." If the accused departed from the script as rehearsed, "the people's" job was to drown their voices with cries of indignation.

The charge against the defendants was that acting on Trotsky's instructions they had organized a "center" for the purpose of assassinating the leaders of the Party and the state. They had succeeded in murdering Kirov and created a number of terrorist groups to kill Stalin and his loyal comrades-in-arms.

The state prosecutor, A. Vyshinsky, demanded that these "mad dogs" (the sixteen accused) be executed by shooting. After that the accused, all famous Bolsheviks, eagerly confessed their guilt and declared themselves repentant.

Zinoviev: "My perverted Bolshevism became anti-Bolshevism, and by way of Trotskyism I arrived at fascism. Trotskyism is a variant of fascism." Kamenev: "I stand before a proletarian court for the third time. My life has been spared twice, but there is a limit to the magnanimity of the proletariat." The accused unanimously asked to be shot. Once again, the trial could not have been running more smoothly.

Kamenev: "I should like to say a few words to my children. I have two children, one is an army pilot, the other a Young Pioneer. Whatever my sentence may be, I consider it just. Do not keep looking back, keep going forward. Together with the people, follow where Stalin leads." It was because he knew Koba that Kamenev made this attempt to save his children. It would fail. Koba's plans were much too far-reaching.

Kamenev's son's wife still has the official document which reached her from the NKVD in answer to her inquiry.

> Kamenev, Lev Borisovitch, died 25.8.36, aged 53. Cause of death [deleted].
>
> Place of death—Moscow.
>
> Kamenev, Olga Davidovna, died 11.9.41, aged 58. Cause of death [deleted].
>
> Place of death [deleted].
>
> Kamenev, Alexander Lvovich, died 15.07.39, aged 33. Cause of death [deleted].
>
> Place of death [deleted].

Kamenev's younger son, the "Young Pioneer," would also be shot, at the age of seventeen.

The newspapers were full of deafening curses. But Stalin's main concern was that famous old Bolsheviks still temporarily free should cast stones at their former comrades. The legendary Antonov-Ovseenko (who on the day of the October rising had declared the Provisional Government overthrown) in an *Izvestia* article with the eloquent title "Finish Them Off" spoke of "a special force of fascist saboteurs": the "only way to talk to them," he said, was to shoot them. Inevitably, he went on to praise Comrade Stalin, who with his "eagle eye" saw the prospect ahead, who ensured unity, who had turned the USSR into a "mighty granite cliff."

Antonov-Ovseenko's turn would soon come. Till then, let him make himself useful!

The ex-leaders were sentenced to death by shooting. Their last written words survive in secret files held by the former State Archive of the October Revolution. These are petitions from Zinoviev, Kamenev, I. Smirnov, and other defendants in the case of the united Trotskyist-

Zinovievite center. Kamenev wrote the necessary few lines calmly, in a steady hand. But Zinoviev! Zinoviev wrote in the illegible, childish scrawl of someone crazed by fear.

On the night of August 24–25 visitors entered their cells. Among those in attendance at the execution of the old Leninist leaders were the NKVD chiefs Yagoda and Yezhov, and also the commander of Stalin's personal bodyguard, Pauker. Pauker, once employed as a hairdresser at the Budapest Operetta Theater, had been taken prisoner by the Russians in the First World War. Then came the Revolution and a brilliant career with the GPU. Pauker was still a theater lover, and himself an inimitable clown. Orlov described Pauker's performance of the Boss's favorite turn—an impression of Zinoviev on his way to execution: Pauker's Zinoviev clings helplessly to the GPU men's shoulders, drags his feet, whimpers pitifully, then falls on his knees and howls: "Please, comrade, please, for God's sake call Joseph Vissarionovich." Stalin "laughed uncontrollably."

He laughed all the louder because he knew how the daring raconteur himself would end. Pauker too belonged to the old guard. A similarly comic role awaited the merry fellow in the Boss's thriller. He would be shot, just like Zinoviev, and just like Zinoviev he would beg his murderers for mercy.

Yagoda, who prized historical souvenirs, collected the bullets with which famous revolutionaries had been shot. When Yagoda was shot, his executioner, Yezhov, appropriated the historic bullets. When Yezhov himself was shot later, the bullets were preserved in his case record. The inventory attached to his file lists "revolver bullets, blunted, wrapped in paper, inscribed Zinoviev, Kamenev. . . ."

The bullets were a sort of symbol, a baton zealously passed from one runner to another in a relay race with death at the winning post, while the Boss looked on and laughed.

The One and Only Ryutin

While he was destroying the leftists, Stalin was already getting ready to settle accounts with the rightists, planning a new production with a new cast. On the interrogating officer's insistence Kamenev had testified that Bukharin was also involved in their terrorist plot, but the evidence against him was for future reference, to be used in Act Two of the thriller. Nor, of course, had the Boss forgotten Ryutin. He was brought to Moscow, to the terrible "inner prison" of the NKVD. The only man who really had been brave enough to rebel, Ryutin would play an invaluable part in the coming production—the trial of the rightists.

But here again Ryutin proved unique: he alone refused to play his part, and although—as he himself put it—he was "treated like an animal," he stood his ground. Out of the whole cohort of Party notables one and only one preserved his honor—modest Ryutin. His file contains his last letter, written on November 1, 1936, and made public half a century later, to the Presidium of the Central Executive Committee: "I am not afraid of death, if that is what the investigative apparatus of the NKVD, in glaring contravention of the law, has in mind for me. I declare in advance that I will not plead for a pardon since I cannot confess to things which I have not done, things of which I am completely innocent. But I cannot endure the illegal treatment inflicted on me, and I request protection from it. If I am not so protected I must try again to protect myself by the only means left in such circumstances to a defenseless and innocently persecuted prisoner deprived of all rights, bound hand and foot, cooped up and completely cut off from the outside world." Yezhov passed the letter to Stalin, after which Ryutin was tortured, to no effect, for a further two months. They got nothing out of him. He was shot on January 13, 1937.

Yagoda's Turn

The Boss realized, not for the first time, that Yagoda was not up to the job. He was still "nannying" Party men, just as he always had. Once Stalin had decided to finish with Yagoda he, as was his habit, showered favors on the doomed man. Yagoda was given accommodation in the Kremlin, and told that he "had earned a place in the Politburo." Much would be written later about the Boss's sadism, as seen in the invariable promotion of a victim before liquidation. In fact, he simply wanted his prey to work harder, and to be unaware that the end was near. Above all, he promoted them at the last minute so that people could see how much he loved them, and how they had betrayed his trust.

Happiness made the wily Yagoda stupid. Anticipating further reward, he took steps to speed up construction of the Moscow-Volga Canal. Starving and overworked prisoners died by the thousands. Yagoda hoped that the canal would bear his name. The Boss liked all things "imperial," so Yagoda, eager to please, introduced a splendid dress uniform for the higher ranks of the NKVD: a white tunic with gold facings, pale blue breeches, and a gilded dagger, as worn by officers of the tsar's navy. There was a public changing of the guard outside the NKVD building—like the old ceremony at the tsar's palaces. The luxurious premises of the NKVD club became a replica of the officers' club in one of the tsar's guards regiments. Heads of NKVD departments gave balls. Soviet ladies, the wives of this new aristocracy, flocked to their dressmakers. In September 1936 Slutsky, the head of the Overseas Administration, gave a fancy-dress party. A large, revolving crystal ball suspended from the ceiling created an illusion of falling snow in the darkened room. The men wore tuxedos or uniform; ladies were in long dresses. Masks and theatrical costumes had been borrowed from the Bolshoi for the use of the ladies. But this was a feast in time of plague. The executioners' days were numbered. Their wives would not be wearing their new finery much longer. Slutsky would be poisoned, and nine out of ten dancing in that hall would be shot.

On September 25, 1936, the Boss and his new protégé Zhdanov sent a telegram from Sochi, where they were on vacation, to trusty Molotov and the Politburo: "We consider it essential and a matter of urgency to appoint Comrade Yezhov Commissar for Internal Affairs. Yagoda has shown that he is not up to his task of unmasking the Trotskyist-Zinovievite bloc. The GPU is four years behind in this." Stalin made Yagoda People's Commissar for Communications. But Yagoda knew the Boss and saw now where it would end. The torment of waiting for the denouement had begun.

A Great Army

Yezhov quadrupled NKVD salaries. They were now considerably higher than those in Party and government establishments. The NKVD were given the best apartments, rest homes, and hospitals. Yezhov's people would enjoy these benefits for eighteen months. In 1937, preparing for the final destruction of Lenin's old guard, Stalin converted the NKVD into an enormous army, organized in divisions and numbering hundreds of thousands. NKVD branches were all-powerful at the local level. NKVD "special departments" functioned in all large enterprises and in all educational establishments. A huge network of informers embraced the whole country. Ostensibly, they operated on a voluntary basis, but they received substantial rewards, in particular steady promotion in their professions. Best of all, they could exact a bloody reckoning from those whom they disliked. Their superiors at work trembled before them. At the height of the purges, informers enjoyed a measure of protection, though if their masters fell they might fall with them.

People fought for the right to inform.

Apart from the full-time informers, all citizens were obliged to join enthusiastically in the same activity. And even to inform on themselves. A Party member who learned that someone he knew had been arrested was obliged to report immediately on his relations with that person. Orlov cited an example: Kedrov, the investigator mentioned earlier, was the son of an old Bolshevik, a friend of Lenin. One day he buttonholed Orlov, to consult him on a "delicate matter." It seemed that a certain Ilyin, now under arrest, had been a friend of Kedrov's parents in exile. "What do you think—should my father write and tell the Central Committee that the Ilyins used to drop in to drink tea occasionally?" Kedrov asked, in acute anxiety.

A special department of the NKVD now kept watch on all party bodies, up to and including the Central Committee. Appointments to Party posts were confirmed only with the approval of the NKVD. Within the NKVD, special secret sections were created to keep watch on NKVD personnel themselves. And there was a supersecret special section to keep an eye on the secret special sections. This section too kept files, innumerable dossiers.

When Yezhov was arrested they found in his safe a dossier on Stalin! It included the reminiscences of some Georgian (who had of course vanished in the camps) showing that Stalin had been a provocateur. (So Malenkov, one of Stalin's closest collaborators, told his son.)

The year 1937 had arrived, and the reequipped NKVD under Yezhov set about the total destruction of the old Party. Another batch of Lenin's comrades, identified for this purpose as the "Parallel Trotskyist Center," were tried between January 23 and 30. Those involved included some of the most prominent Kremlin boyars, former supporters of Trotsky who had long ago deserted their idol. That did not help them. The star defendant was Yuri Pyatakov, a member of the Central Committee. Lenin had held him in high esteem, describing him in his Testament as "undoubtedly a person of outstanding strength of purpose and abilities." He had been in the Party since 1905, taken part in the underground struggle, and commanded armies during the Civil War. He had joined opposition groups, had, needless to say, repented, and had been forgiven.

Ordzhonikidze, who was in charge of industry, had made him a vice-commissar, and Pyatakov had become one of the main implementers of the cruel first Five-Year Plan in 1929.

Pyatakov had originally been invited to act as the main accuser at the trial of Zinoviev and Kamenev. He had consented, and got ready to slander his old comrades. It was, he said, a task which showed how great was the Party's trust in him, and he accepted it "with all my heart."

After they saw that Pyatakov was ready to collaborate in any way required, they gave him a more complicated role. In the 1937 trials he joined the defendants, those whom he had meant to blacken. He was arrested, but was at first recalcitrant. Ordzhonikidze in person urged him to accept the role assigned to him in exchange for his life. No one was so well qualified as Pyatakov to destroy Trotsky, his former god and now the Party's worst enemy, in the eyes of the country and the whole world. He finally agreed to do it as a matter of "the highest expediency," and began rehearsals with the interrogators.

Alas, he found at the trial that he had been tricked. As scripted in the thriller, he informed the court that while visiting Berlin on business he had secretly met Trotsky in Norway. The Boss had made an exciting story of it: Pyatakov had flown to Oslo in a German plane to establish contact with Trotsky, Trotsky had told him that he had concerted plans for intervention with the Germans (one of the Boss's favorite themes), etc., etc. Unfortunately, the personnel of the airport at which he was supposed to have landed announced that no foreign planes had touched down at that time.

As might be expected, the Boss also found a star part in the trial for Trotsky's one-time bard Radek. But, in his usual thrifty way he saw to it that the fullest use was made of Radek before his arrest. When Yezhov had asked permission to arrest Karl Berngardovich the Boss replied by telegram from Sochi on August 19, 1936: "I suggest we take Radek's arrest off the agenda and let him write a signed article against Trotsky in *Izvestia.*" That was during Kamenev's trial, and it enabled Radek to trample on Trotsky and other former acquaintances to his heart's content. After which the Author and Producer ordered him to take the stage himself.

Bukharin, Radek's chief at *Izvestia,* was horrified. He wrote to the Boss that "Radek's wife came rushing to tell me that he has been arrested..I have none but positive impressions of Radek. Maybe I am wrong but my inner voices tell me that I must write to you. What a strange business!" Radek realized at once that he would have to play the part assigned to him. But he was clever enough to think of a way of saving his life. He took the investigator's uninspired record of his statements, and instead of signing it said with a laugh, "This is no good. I'll write it myself." He then wrote a "confession," an ingenious tissue of lies, which utterly damned Trotsky. He knew that his literary exercise would be sent to the Boss, and that the Boss would appreciate his servant's cleverness.

In court Radek scintillated. He exposed himself and his comrades unmercifully. It was largely thanks to his inspired performance that the trial was such a success.

The German writer Lion Feuchtwanger, who was present at the trial, wrote that "those who faced the court could not possibly be thought of as tormented and desperate beings. In appearance the accused were well-groomed and well-dressed men with relaxed and unconstrained manners. They drank tea, and there were newspapers sticking out of their pockets. . . . Altogether, it looked more like a debate . . . conducted in conversational tones by educated people. The impression created was that the accused, the prosecutor, and the judges were all inspired by the same single—I almost said sporting—objective, to explain all that had happened with the maximum precision. If a theatrical producer had been called on to stage such a trial he would probably have needed several rehearsals to achieve that sort of teamwork among the accused."

It was simply that the play had such a great producer. And he had found such an excellent actor. The producer thought very highly of him. The trial ended with sentences of death for Lenin's famous comrades-in-arms Pyatakov, Serebryakov, Muralov, etc. Radek got ten years. And Radek "gave the condemned men a guilty smile, as though embarrassed by his luck," wrote Feuchtwanger.

The Boss, however, after showing his gratitude to Radek for the trial, stuck to his original principle: the whole of the old guard must disappear. He needed neither clever Fouchés, nor geniuses like Talleyrand. He needed only faithful servants. Faithful dogs. Radek too would be killed, in the prison camp to which he was sent.

Maria Svanidze wrote in her diary on November 20, 1936: "[They arrested] Radek and others whom I knew, people I used to talk to, and always trusted. . . . But what transpired surpassed all my expectations of human baseness. It was all there, terrorism, intervention, the Gestapo, theft, sabotage, subversion. . . . All out of careerism, greed, and the love of pleasure, the desire to have mistresses, to travel abroad, together with some sort of nebulous prospect of seizing power by a palace revolution. Where was their elementary feeling of patriotism, of love for their motherland? These moral freaks deserved their fate. . . . Poor Kirov was the key that unlocked the door to this den of thieves. How can we have trusted this gang of scoundrels so blindly? It's beyond understanding!"

And in a later entry she wrote: "My soul is ablaze with anger and hatred. Their execution will not satisfy me. I should like to torture them, break them on the wheel, burn them alive for all the vile things they have done."

Beyond understanding indeed! Can she really have believed it all? She, who knew these people? Or . . . ? "Top people were terrified," wrote N. Kotov. "They vied with each other in accusing their former friends. And lied to each other—to friends, to fathers, to mothers, to children, just to demonstrate beyond doubt their loyalty to the mustachioed one. They expected to be arrested from day to day and lied even to themselves, in their diaries, hoping that their lies would be read by the investigators."

Grateful Spectators

The trials, inevitably, met with incredulity in Europe. Trotsky, in exile abroad, helped to reinforce this skepticism.

The Boss knew that the success of a show depends as much on the spectators as on the actors. He needed authoritative spectators, who would approve of his play, and—more important—say so in writing.

He had faith in himself. All those whom he had previously invited to visit the USSR—H. G. Wells, Bernard Shaw, Emil Ludwig, Henri Barbusse, Romain Rolland—had left the country as its friends, full of praise for the Boss. Had they really noticed nothing? Or were they overwhelmed by the technique he had devised of nonstop flattery, dazzling receptions, lavish presents, and fulsome speeches? Was that all there was to it?

Romain Rolland's *Journal,* published many years after his death, shows that one great friend of the USSR understood everything. And saw everything: "I feel pain and indignation welling up within me. I am trying to suppress the need to speak and write about it." But why? Because "rabid enemies in France and throughout the world will use my words as a weapon." Rolland forbade publication of his diaries before 1985. The Communist ideal must not be besmirched. Stalin's cause was more important than Stalin and his myrmidons. An extension of the false argument from expediency in which the Boss had grounded his monstrous trials.

This time things were more serious. What Stalin needed was some eminent European to confirm that the old Party leaders, to a man, had become a gang of murderers and traitors. After long consultations with Comintern the candidate agreed upon was Lion Feuchtwanger, an antifascist and the author of a number of well-known novels, who had been forced to leave Hitler's Germany. He was invited to the USSR, where the Boss in person joined in the game of seducing him. "Comrade Stalin has received the German writer L. Feuchtwanger. They conversed for over three hours," *Pravda* reported.

How It Happened: Karavkina's Reports

The secret archive of VOKS (the All-Union Society for Cultural Relations with Foreign Countries) includes twelve reports, stamped "not to be divulged," written by A. Karavkina, who acted as Feuchtwanger's guide.

I asked a former employee of VOKS to comment on these records. She laughingly told me, "I don't know anything about Karavkina. But in those days any woman interpreter who acted as escort to an eminent foreigner naturally had connections with the NKVD, and was sometimes required to be not just a guide but a 'close friend.' So nothing would escape her notice, by day or by night."

From the Karavkina file:

> 19.12.36. He talked about his visit to Dimitrov [head of the Comintern]. . . . Went specially to talk to him about the Trotskyist trial. Said that Dimitrov was very agitated when talking about this, argued for an hour and a half, but "couldn't convince him." Feuchtwanger informed me that people abroad took a very hostile view of this trial, and that nobody would believe that fifteen high-principled revolutionaries, who had so often risked their lives by participating in conspiracies, would all suddenly and of one accord confess and voluntarily do penance.
>
> 22.12.36. He informed me that he had finished an article on André Gide for *Pravda*. The copy typist will be here tomorrow.
>
> 27.12. Today was a difficult day, as Fekht Vanger *[sic]* couldn't wait to pour out to me his indignation about the article on Gide. It shows, he said, that Gide was right, and that we don't have freedom of opinion, that people cannot say openly what they think, etc. The editors asked him to rewrite certain passages, especially about the "Stalin cult." I explained to him the true nature of Soviet people's attitude to Comrade Stalin, and where it springs from, and told him that it was utterly false to call it a "cult." He went on fuming for some time, saying that he would

> change nothing but . . . finally cooled off, sat down quietly in his study, and made the corrections they'd asked for.
>
> From early this morning Fekht Vanger has been talking interminably about the discomforts of life in the Soviet Union, complaining about service in the hotel, etc. "I should like to see somebody in the USSR print a piece in which I described how uncomfortable your lives here are." He went on to say that however splendid life in the Soviet Union may be, he still prefers to live in Europe.

But what did our author finally have to say about it in his book *Moscow 37?* "To explain the Zinoviev and Radek trials by Stalin's ambition to reign unchallenged and his thirst for vengeance would be simply absurd. When I was there in Moscow, at the trial, when I saw and heard for myself . . . I felt my doubts dissolving like salt in water." And this is what Feuchtwanger wrote about the cult of Stalin's person which he had found so irritating: "It cannot be doubted that the excessive veneration . . . is sincere. People feel the need to show their gratitude, their boundless admiration. . . . The nation is grateful to Stalin for bread, meat, education, and the creation of an army which safeguards its well-being. . . . Add to this that to the people Stalin really is flesh of their flesh. . . . When I remarked on the tastelessly exaggerated veneration shown to him he shrugged and excused his peasants and workers by saying that they were too busy with other matters to develop good taste."

The arrests continued without interruption. Black cars scoured the city every night, picking up Party members and their families and friends. There were no more sensational trials for the present. The victims were picked up quietly, quickly supplied the testimony required, and were quickly put up against the wall. Yezhov's new investigators felt no pious respect for Party members. Moreover, the NKVD had been given a new weapon by the Boss. It was allowed to use torture.

Many works about Gulag, Stalin's system of labor camps, have described the forms of torture used. They were the brainchild of cruel NKVD officers. They were officially authorized. In this twentieth century of ours, torture was given documentary authority. In the President's Archives I read the stenographic record of a Central Committee plenum in 1957, adorned with a number of "top-secret" warnings:

> *Molotov:* The use of physical means was decided upon by the whole Politburo. Everybody signed.

[A voice]: There was no such decision.

Molotov: There was such a decision. It was secret, I don't have a copy.

Khrushchev: Kaganovich said on the eve of the Twentieth Congress that a document exists in which everybody signed his agreement to the beating of a prisoner. . . . We haven't found that document, it has been destroyed.

But it proved impossible to destroy everything. Copies of the following telegram, signed by Stalin, were found in the secret safes of many provincial Party Committees: "The Central Committee of the CPSU . . . wishes to make it clear that the application of physical pressure by the NKVD has been authorized by the Central Committee since 1937. . . . It is well known that all bourgeois agencies use physical pressure on representatives of the proletariat. The question is why should socialist countries have to be more humane with sworn enemies of the working class?" The angry voice dictating that telegram is easily recognized.

The Importance of Fear

He had decided to speed up the process of destroying the Party. That meant speeding up the confession stage. Logic dictated the use of torture. The new generation of Yezhov interrogators quickly mastered the use of the fist and more refined methods. Torture really began before the victims entered the interrogator's office, immediately after their arrest. It began with "cell torture." As one witness described it, "There were sixty people in the cell. It was June, and hot outside. We laid our faces on the cracks in the floor, trying to suck in a little fresh air. And took it in turns to crowd around the door, where a slight draft could be felt through the cracks. Old people succumbed almost immediately." Then came torture by the interrogator: "The first interrogation in the Sukhanov Prison often began with a savage beating, to humiliate the prisoner and break his resistance right from the start. Ordzhonikidze's wife was whipped to death in that place. In the NKVD torture chambers in Leningrad, prisoners were made to sit on the cement floor and covered with a box with nails sticking inward from all four sides. Army commander P. Dybenko, a giant of a man, was covered with a box of this kind one cubic meter in size." Depositions of whatever sort were now signed quickly. Women sometimes put up more resistance than men. The wife of Nestor Lakoba, the deceased dictator of Abkhazia, was taken along for questioning every evening, and dragged back to her cell next morning unconscious and covered with blood. But she answered every demand that she should put her name to "evidence" against her late husband with the same short sentence: "I will not defile my husband's memory." She held out even when they thrashed her son, a sixteen-year-old schoolboy, before her eyes and told her that they would kill him if she did not sign the protocol. She still had not signed when she died in her cell.

Blows and lashes were only the beginning—the entrance to hell. After that the notorious "conveyor belt" was set in motion. Interrogators worked in shifts, while prisoners were kept awake day and night. Kicks, blows, and insults were sustained throughout. The prisoner's mind would be so fogged by sleeplessness that he was ready to sign absolutely anything—usually a version made up by the interrogator himself.

Orlov, an intelligence officer, told this story: "One evening Boris Berman [an NKVD chief] and I were walking along a corridor. We were pulled up short by heart-rending screams coming from the office of an investigator called Kedrov. We opened the door and saw Nelidov sitting on a chair. (He taught chemistry at the Gorky Pedagogical Institute, and was the nephew of the tsar's ambassador in France.) Kedrov was beside himself with rage. He tried to explain. Nelidov, he said, had confessed that he wanted to kill Stalin, and now he had suddenly gone back on it. 'Look!' Kedrov kept yelling hysterically, 'Look at this! Here's what he wrote.' . . . Kedrov was behaving as if he was Nelidov's victim—not the other way round. There was a phosphorescent glow, sparks of madness in his eyes."

The next stage was that of "consolidation." The prisoner was fed, given cigarettes, and told that it was now his turn to think what more he could add to his testimony. He was given paper, and told what direction his thoughts should take. His progress was carefully monitored.

If he had to appear in court—most prisoners were condemned in camera—he would be carefully rehearsed first: "Bear in mind," the investigators would say, "that if you make a mistake in court we shan't just shoot you, we shall torture you, we shall tear you limb from limb." They might also suggest that he not be shot at all, that this was just for the press, that all those condemned were in fact spared. During the trial, the investigators sat under the prisoner's nose. Yet as they were at their cruel work the torturers never stopped talking about the nobler motives for a prisoner to slander himself. It was all for the good of Party and the Motherland. To preserve something of their self-respect, the accused would often join in the game. But, as one victim of Gulag wrote, "Behind all the lofty arguments of an ideological and political character I saw a little imp of fear with a hideous face jigging away."

By then, the country was no longer ruled by the Party, nor even by Stalin. It was ruled by fear. The Roman historian wrote of the age of Nero that "in the city of fear people ceased to exist—nothing but human flesh and bones was left." Ready to do whatever he bade them.

It was now the turn of Trotsky's old friend Alexander Beloborodov, onetime head of the Urals Soviet, who had arranged the execution of the tsar and his family. Terminally ill with cancer of the throat, holding on to his trousers (they had taken his belt from him), the former head of the Red Urals stood before the interrogators and obediently testified against his former friends, the Trotskyists. But he refused to confess to terrorist activities himself. "Stalin to Yezhov. 26 May 37. Isn't it time to put pressure on this gentleman and force him to tell us about his filthy deeds? Where is he supposed to be—in prison or in a hotel?" They "put pressure" on him. They tortured him. They shot him. Did the former boss of the Red Urals ever remember in those terrible days the cellar in the Ipatiev house, where the tsar's wounded son crawled on the floor, while they bayoneted the tsar's daughters?

At last Yagoda himself was arrested. The Boss had not forgotten that back in 1928 Bukharin, talking to Kamenev, numbered Yagoda among his supporters. Later, Yagoda had done a splendid job of betraying Bukharin. And in doing so had inspired a brilliant twist in the Boss's plot. He would unite Bukharin and Yagoda in one and the same conspiracy. A role in the Boss's thriller had been reserved for Yagoda long ago. An unexpected role. And a very useful one.

Yagoda's arrest enabled the Boss to rid himself of the Leninist intake in the NKVD—the old Chekists. They had of course endured in silence the execution of old Party members. They had always carried out orders without a murmur. But they could not have approved. He saw the need for young personnel, with a contempt for all that outworn Party nonsense. People who did their jobs unthinkingly. That was why the old Cheka had to perish together with its creator, the old Party.

Yezhov carried out a general purge of the NKVD with feverish haste. The Boss's sense of humor was at work again: a great number of the Cheka personnel from Lenin's time now had to meet the same fate as the old Party members whom they had so recently written off. Some of them would encounter their recent victims in the camps. The majority would not get that far, but would meet their deaths against the old, familiar Lubyanka wall. The usual itinerary was to the wall to be shot, to the crematorium, then to the bottomless grave number 1 in the Donskoi cemetery, with the ashes of all the other victims. The Boss had another joke up his sleeve: Yagoda had to confess to the innumerable poisonings which he had loyally carried out for the Boss—the murders of Menzhinsky, Gorky, and others.

Yagoda is traditionally supposed to have said in prison, "God does exist after all. From the Boss I deserved nothing but gratitude for loyal service, from God I must have earned the severest possible punishment. Look where I am now, and judge for yourself whether there is a God." He signed everything they put before him. Then he lapsed into a strange state of apathy. Occasionally he wept.

Yagoda's words were reported to the Boss. He laughed. The former seminarist remembered his history, how Attila was called "God's Scourge."

A new constitution was adopted at the end of 1936. Bukharin, traveling abroad that year, took out his fountain pen and solemnly said, "This is the one the Constitution was written with," adding that dear Karl (Radek) had helped him.

It was true. The Boss had entrusted the task to his two most gifted publicists. Their turn to take the stage came only when they had finished this work. The constitution they drafted, proclaiming freedom of speech, universal franchise and the usual civic rights could come into effect only when no one would even think of invoking it. The object of the Terror was to create just such a society. And of course there would be no place in it for those two oppositionists and demagogues.

They had to go. Radek had been first. Now it was Bukharin's turn. Little Bukharin, favorite son of Lenin's Party. Lenin's vanishing Party.

17

THE FALL OF "THE PARTY'S FAVORITE"

All this bloodshed wearies the soul and crushes the heart with grief—I ask one favor of the reader: to permit me not to feel revulsion for these people who so basely allowed themselves to be destroyed.
—Tacitus on Nero's reign of terror

Bukharin Is Trapped

The first warning bell rang on February 10, 1936, when *Pravda* published a harsh critique of Bukharin's views. Yet two weeks later the Boss allowed Bukharin to take his wife abroad, to Paris. He went with a delegation sent to acquire the archives of the German Social Democratic Party, which Hitler had destroyed. They were in the keeping of an émigré Menshevik, B. Nikolaevsky.

In making this move the Boss risked nothing. Letting Bukharin leave the USSR together with his wife obviously made it possible for him to remain abroad. But if he did so, the leader of the rightists would become a "defector," that is, a declared enemy of the USSR, and this would help to justify past and future criminal proceedings against old Leninists. Whereas if he did return, there could be great advantage in that too. Knowing what a peacock Bukharin was, the Boss felt sure that he would not be able to govern his tongue while he was abroad. He would be working with Nikolaevsky, and would not try to avoid meeting other Mensheviks. He and they had too much in common.

It happened just as he had foreseen. Anyone who has lived in the USSR will remember that dangerous sensation of freedom when he finds himself abroad. Bukharin behaved like a free man. There was even an unscheduled meeting with the Menshevik leader F. Dan, during which Bukharin called Stalin "a vicious little man, not a man but a devil." "So how did you come to trust him with your own fate, the fate of the Party, and the fate of the country?" Dan asked him. "It wasn't entrusted to him, but to the man whom the Party trusted. . . . He is a sort of symbol of the Party . . . that's why we all put our heads in his maw knowing that he will surely devour us." "So why are you going back?" "I couldn't live as an émigré, like you do . . . no, whatever happens . . . and perhaps nothing will happen anyway."

Dan made a note of this conversation, and would certainly have told his friends about it. Bukharin prattled endlessly to Nikolaevsky, who recorded it all for future historians. He destroyed his notes after Bukharin's arrest for fear of damaging him, but by then he was certainly not the only one who knew about them. While in Paris, Bukharin secretly met the U.S. ambassador to the USSR, William Bullitt, and told him about the strange, pro-Hitler sentiments which were getting more and more of a hold on Stalin.

Paris was flooded with Stalin's agents: NKVD spies, French Comintern activists, former tsarist officers who had come to believe in the Bolsheviks. Stalin's secret service continued to spirit former tsarist generals out of Paris in broad daylight, and it would be ridiculous to suppose that he would have let Bukharin off the leash without an attendant. He was, of course, watched closely. All in all, Bukharin's trip to Paris supplied a great deal of additional material for his future trial, at which he would be reminded, among other things, of his conversations with Nikolaevsky.

Bukharin returned, and that autumn the Boss sent him on vacation for six whole weeks. While he was enjoying the mountains of Central Asia, his name and those of other rightists began to be heard in the Zinoviev-Kamenev trial. They were accused of complicity in terrorist acts, including Kirov's murder. The state prosecutor, Vyshinsky, announced officially that an investigation was under way. Tomsky interpreted Caesar's command correctly, and on August 22 he committed suicide. *Pravda* announced: "Tomsky, hopelessly entangled in his ties with the Trotskyist-Zinovievite terrorists, has committed suicide at his dacha." Bukharin cut short his vacation and flew back to Moscow immediately.

The Gods Are Athirst

I am sitting in the President's Archive reading letters written by Bukharin shortly before his death. They might be an epistolary novel, written in collaboration by Kafka and Dostoevsky. Everything else that has been written about the Stalinist trials—the most mysterious trials of the century, in which the victims consented to slander themselves in public and glorify their executioner—is no more than myth-mongering, mere guesswork.

In these letters the enigma of the century is unraveled completely.

As soon as he got back Bukharin addressed written statements to the Politburo and to the prosecutor Vyshinsky: "Not only am I not guilty of the crimes attributed to me, I can proudly claim that for the past several years I have defended the Party line and Stalin's leadership with all the passion and sincerity I can command. . . . In this context I have to say that from 1933 I broke off all personal relations with M. Tomsky and A. Rykov, who formerly shared my ideas. This can be confirmed by questioning drivers, analyzing the journeys made by them, questioning sentries, NKVD agents, servants, etc." It was true. Fear had prevented him from meeting old comrades. There had been only one or two meetings with oppositionists, and these he scrupulously listed. "Kamenev—once only . . . I asked him whether he would like to go back to editing the literary pages of *Pravda,* in which case I would speak to Comrade Stalin about it. . . . [But Kamenev said] 'I just want to be forgotten, I don't want Stalin even to remember my name.' (After this philistine declaration I withdrew my suggestion.)" He wrote also about the "Bukharin school": "Stalin personally showed me a number of documents from which it was evident that I could no longer 'keep these people in hand' (as he put it). They had lost confidence in me long ago, and some of them called me a traitor." No links, then, with his devoted pupils either. After this he enthused over the trial. "The trial will have en enormous international significance. . . . So the scoundrels have been shot—excellent: the air has immediately become cleaner."

That is how he spoke of former close associates and friends. But his mind raced feverishly—had he forgotten this or that criminal meeting? He remembered a few more—one of them with a former leader of the Petrograd Bolsheviks. "Some additional facts. I tried as hard as I could to avoid a visit from A. Shlyapnikov, but he managed to catch me. [This was in 1936, shortly before his arrest.] He asked me, in the *Izvestia* office, to pass a letter to Stalin. I told my staff not to let him in again, because 'politically he stinks.' " So much for Shlyapnikov.

He remembered yet another criminal meeting—with the man who had once been number two in the Bolshevik Party. "On one occasion I met Zinoviev in Radek's apartment. . . . He had come to collect a book. . . . We made him drink to Stalin's health. He complained of heart trouble. Zinoviev then sang Stalin's praises (the two-faced rogue!). Let me add that people like Radek and myself sometimes find it difficult to throw out uninvited callers." He was clean. He had betrayed them all, as the Boss required. At the same time, he wrote a hysterical letter to Voroshilov: "As I write I have a feeling of unreality. Is it a dream, a mirage, am I in a lunatic asylum, hallucinating. . . . Poor Tomsky may have got involved in something, I don't know. I don't rule it out, he lived by himself. [He was perfectly ready to regard even his dead friend as a traitor.] I'm terribly glad that those dogs have been shot. The trial means political death for Trotsky, and that will soon become clear. . . . I advise you to read Romain Rolland's play about the French Revolution. I embrace you, for I am clean."

At the end of his letter he couldn't resist an oblique reference to the way in which the Jacobins had exterminated each other. When they picked off Zinoviev and Kamenev, when they gave short shrift to Smirnov, Shlyapnikov, and other former colleagues, he had not been thinking of Rolland's plays. Now it was too late. He himself was a character in a banal revolutionary drama bearing the hoary epigraph "Revolution, like Saturn, kills its children. Beware! The Gods are a-thirst."

The semiliterate Voroshilov, once a metalworker and now a member of the Politburo, had not read Rolland's plays, but he did know the Boss's ways. And just as Bukharin feared the plague-stricken Shlyapnikov and his own pupils, so Voroshilov now feared Bukharin. And was just as eager to throw *him* out. His reply was atrociously rude. Bukharin had branded his own former friends, now Voroshilov branded Bukharin. In the best tradition of the time he promised his onetime friend to "keep as far away from you as I can, irrespective of the outcome of your case" and added that he would henceforth consider Bukharin "a scoundrel." Nevertheless, the "scoundrel" was so terrified that he wrote again: "I got your dreadful letter. My letter ended 'I embrace you,' yours ends with the word 'scoundrel.' Every man has, or rather should have, his own self-esteem. But I should like to remove one political misunderstanding. I wrote a letter of a personal nature (and now regret it) in a state of distress . . . like a beast at bay. . . . I was going out of my mind at the mere thought that someone might genuinely believe in my guilt. . . . I am in an extremely anxious state. That was the reason for my letter. However, I must await the end of the investigation as calmly as I can, since it will, I am sure, prove that I have nothing whatsoever to do with those gangsters." Hunters will recognize the squeal of the hare cornered by dogs and about to die.

The Boss decided that it was too early for the kill. It was as though the second act in the spectacular trial of Pyatakov, Radek, and others was still in rehearsal, and Bukharin's entrance was not due until Act Three. The Boss knew, of course, the reasons for Bukharin's hysterical fear. As soon as he got back to reality, to the USSR, he would have realized how much damage he had done himself abroad. Now he was in agonies at the thought that his friend Koba might know the things he had been saying. The Boss, of course, did know, but he pretended not to. Back from Sochi, he magnanimously and of his own accord halted the investigation, thereby condemning Bukharin to the worst torment of all: waiting for inevitable imprisonment is worse than prison itself. The Boss knew that waiting would crush the spirit of this intellectual. On September 10, 1936, *Pravda* announced that "the investigation has established that there are no grounds for prosecuting Bukharin and Rykov."

Meanwhile, the investigation which was supposed to have been closed was collecting more and more damning evidence against Bukharin and the rightists. "24.9.36. Bukharin to Stalin. I did not ask to be seen before the investigation ended, because I thought it politically awkward. But now I beg you with my whole being not to refuse me. . . . Interrogate me! Turn me inside out! But dot the 'i's so that nobody can put the boot in anymore and generally poison my life." Poor Bukharin even spent one of his sleepless nights writing a "poem about Stalin" which he submitted to his hero for comment. His hero modestly advised against publication.

At a Central Committee meeting in December 1936 Yezhov was allowed to accuse Bukharin outright of counterrevolutionary activity. But the Boss played the part which he had written for himself—that of the Trusting Leader—to the end: "We must not jump to conclusions. The investigation goes on."

This was when Bukharin's life really became hell. Between sessions at the Central Committee, Bukharin and Rykov were confronted with Pyatakov, Radek, and other convicts who had once been comrades of Lenin, brought from their prison cells for the purpose. In the presence of members of the Politburo Bukharin's closest friend, Radek, among others, obediently accused him of complicity in their conspiracy. He hysterically contradicted their statements. But fresh evidence was always obtainable.

"To See Him, Simply to See Him, Made Us All Happy"

Immediately before the new year Stalin managed a great holiday for his people: at the Extraordinary Eighth Congress of the Soviets, he promulgated the constitution drafted by poor Bukharin. The newspapers each devoted a special section to letters from delegates to the Congress. A. Sukov, a worker, wrote: "Amid a storm of enthusiastic applause for the creator of the constitution, the great Stalin, the . . . Congress . . . unanimously resolved . . . to accept the draft as the basis for discussion. It is difficult to describe what happened in the Kremlin hall. Everybody rose and hailed the Leader with prolonged applause. Comrade Stalin, standing on the platform, raised his hand, calling for silence. He invited us several times to be seated. It was no good. We sang the 'Internationale,' and the ovation started all over again. Comrade Stalin turned to those on the platform, no doubt asking them to call us to order. . . . He took out his watch and showed it to us, but we had lost count of time."

These letters had little enough to say about the constitution itself, but a worker named P. Kalinin spoke of the "unforgettable moments when I saw the bright face of our beloved Leader, the genius who has created the constitution." N. Lozhechnikova, a textile worker, hastened "to share with you my immense joy. In the Kremlin palace I saw the man dearest to us of all on earth. I sat as though bewitched, and could not take my eyes off Comrade Stalin's face." Another textile worker, A. Kareva, confided that when "Dusaya and I were told that Comrade Stalin would talk to us next day, I don't know what I looked like, but Dusaya turned bright red, her face lit up, her eyes literally glowed." It wasn't just propaganda, or the ravings of the obtuse crowd. To see *him,* a god on earth, had become a tremendous event, and not just for deluded workers.

This is how the popular children's writer Kornei Chukovsky described Stalin's appearance at a Komsomol Congress: "Something extraordinary had happened to the audience! I looked round . . . every face was full of love and tenderness, inspired. . . . For all of us, to see him, simply to see him, made us all happy. . . . We reacted to every movement of his with reverence, I had never supposed myself capable of such feelings. . . . Pasternak kept whispering rapturous words in my ear. Pasternak and I went home together, both reveling in our own happiness." This was written *in his diary* by one of Russia's cleverest and most highly educated men!

Stalin had by now created a unique image of himself: he was Tsar and God in one. He was the Boss. So what he was about to destroy in 1937 was not Lenin's Party, but all those miserable degenerates who had cherished sacrilegious designs against their Tsar and God. Their Boss.

Living in that deafening medley of panegyrics for the Leader and anathemas for the traitors, in that all-pervading atmosphere of insane idolatry and equally insane fear, the highly strung Bukharin felt that he himself was losing his mind. On the threshold of the new year fresh blows were aimed at him. He wrote at once to his friend Koba: "15.12.36. . . . An article in *Pravda* today [stated] that 'the rightists' . . . 'were hand in glove with Trotskyists, the saboteurs, and the Gestapo.' "

The kindly Boss responded, and angrily rebuked the editor of *Pravda:* "To Comrade Mekhlis. The question of the former rightists (Rykov, Bukharin) has been postponed till the next plenum. Vilification of Bukharin (Rykov) should therefore cease. It does not take great intelligence to understand this elementary truth."

Mekhlis, however, was not only intelligent but familiar with "in-depth language." He knew that what the Boss wrote and what the Boss wanted were not the same thing. So *Pravda* went on baiting Bukharin.

Mourning Dress

The year 1936 was nearing its end. Maria Svanidze recorded in her diary for December 21: "The big event was that we celebrated J.'s [Joseph's] birthday. Lots of guests, all dressed up, noisy, dancing to the radio, went home at 7:00 A.M." He had granted them the happiness of looking upon their god twice. And for the last time. Maria Svanidze: "On the 31st we saw the New Year in at J.'s. Members of the Politburo with wives, and ourselves—relatives. Flat and boring. I was overdressed (long, black frock) and didn't feel quite well. . . . It was all more modest than on the 21st, I thought it would be the other way round." This was their farewell party. They had fun, or tried to, but their god knew their future. For most of his guests, that New Year would be their last. Maria Svanidze's funeral dress was quite appropriate: 1937 was to be the most terrible year in Russia's history.

He sent little Bukharin a New Year's gift: "1 January 37. Bukharin to Stalin. Late in the evening of December 30 I received a whole series of depositions made by Trotskyist-Zinovievite gangsters (Pyatakov, Sokolnikov, Radek, Muralov, etc.)." There follows a long and desperate attempt to defend himself: villains are trying to blacken him because of his devotion to Koba, etc. This time there was no answer. But little Bukharin went on writing: "I am becoming a martyr to myself and making martyrs of all my family. None of us can sleep, we are all so exhausted that we are sick of life. . . . Tell me what to do, send for me!"

He was not sent for. On January 16 Bukharin was dismissed from *Izvestia.* Yet still he went on sending interminable letters to his tormentor: "24.1.37. The whole world has now heard me defamed as a criminal. What am I to do, how can I go on?"

The newspapers stepped up their persecution, and his friend Koba was suddenly helpless, quite unable to stop Mekhlis. Rightists were arrested daily. On the Boss's orders, the "evidence" beaten out of them was sent directly to Bukharin's apartment. He was deluged with accusations against himself. On February 16 he received twenty such statements. And still he wrote and wrote interminable replies, to the Politburo and to friend Koba. When they started evicting little Bukharin from the Kremlin he rang the Boss: "Now they've come to turn me out of the Kremlin." "You tell them to go the Devil," his friend said, and let him stay. For the time being.

Preparations for a plenum of the Central Committee—Bukharin's last—were in hand. The time was drawing near for the friends to part. Bukharin lost his head and said that he would not attend the plenum until the charges of espionage and sabotage were withdrawn, and began a hunger strike in protest shortly afterwards. "7.2.37. I have received the agenda for the plenum of the C.C. Originally it read 'the case of Comrades Rykov and Bukharin.' The word 'Comrades' has been omitted. What does this mean?"

Abraham's Sacrifice: Ordzhonikidze's Secret

The plenum, however, was postponed. Sergo Ordzhonikidze had died.

The noose had been tightening round his neck for some time. Yezhov had arrested his deputy, Pyatakov, and all his immediate entourage, and had ended by arresting Sergo's brother Pavel (Papulya). Ordzhonikidze rang the Boss in a rage, but the only answer he got to his angry shouting was a sigh and "the way that organization is, they might come and search my place." Ordzhonikidze still didn't get the point. He began shouting and raging again. Why had Pyatakov been shot, when he had been promised his life in return for a confession?

What happened on Ordzhonikidze's last day, February 17, has now come to light, thanks to information supplied by his secretary and recently discovered in the Party Archive. Sergo discussed matters with the Boss that morning. They talked for hours, just the two of them, and their meeting seemed to have ended amicably: it would not have been like the Boss to risk a breakdown of relations with one of the main speakers on the eve of the plenum. After that, Ordzhonikidze's workday went smoothly, with no sign of nervous tension. He met Molotov and lunched at home. He left the Commissariat around midnight, after signing a routine telegram expressing his anxiety about a shipment of piping. A man contemplating suicide would hardly get worked up about a few pipes. As soon as he got home he went to lie down. Soon afterward a shot was heard from his bedroom. His wife ran in and found him dead, in his underwear, which was covered with blood. Had he killed himself? Or was the bullet the result of his meeting with the Boss? Had the Boss realized that the ungovernable Ordzhonikidze might spring some unpleasant surprise on him at the plenum? Perhaps Yezhov had taken care of things: perhaps when Ordzhonikidze went to bed his own bodyguard had crept into his apartment through the back entrance.

The Boss, I believe, genuinely grieved for Sergo, just as before he had grieved for Kirov. This was a horrifying trait in his character—he could sincerely grieve for those whom he murdered. (We shall find him grieving again when we come to the story of another of his friends, Kavtaradze.) How indeed could he fail to grieve for loyal Sergo? So many of his memories were associated with Sergo. So many of his best memories. Unfortunately, however, Sergo was part of that Party which had to disappear. Significantly, Sergo had interceded for Pyatakov. The Boss would tell the plenum how Sergo had felt honor-bound not to show his letters from "the vicious oppositionist Lominadze." Could he afford the luxury of such a noble knight, who kept his enemies' secrets? Determined as he was to create a unified society, subject to a single will? For only such a society could carry out the great tasks known to him alone. It was for this great cause that he had to sacrifice his friend. Once again "as Abraham sacrificed his son Isaac."

Maria Svanidze noted in her diary, "I went to see Zina, she has borne her husband's death heroically. . . . She herself took charge of the funeral arrangements, she stood by the coffin throughout." Poor Zina, she was afraid to show her suspicions. But Sergo's relatives showed less restraint, and almost all the Ordzhonikidzes were arrested as a result.

On February 28, 1937, the Boss's relatives were all together in the Kremlin for the last time, at Svetlana's birthday party. Maria Svanidze observed: "Yasha [Stalin's son Yakov] was there with his wife for the first time. She is quite pretty, older than Yasha. He is her fifth husband, not counting other relationships. She trapped him, of course. J. [Joseph] didn't come. Stayed away, on purpose, I think. I'm sorry for J." Maria then detailed a list of "half-wit" and "stupid" relatives of Stalin's late wife Nadya and his own "lazy" and "weak-willed" sons, saying that "the only normal people present" were Alyosha, Maria's husband; Zhenya, Nadya's sister-in-law; and Maria herself. "And Svetochka [Svetlana] who makes up for all the rest." Stalin did not turn up because he was busy at the plenum. The terrible plenum at which he would bid farewell to yet another friend, little Bukharin. Bukharin and Rykov attended the plenum, and were arrested on the spot.

BUKHARIN'S LAST LOVE

Before the plenum Bukharin went on writing Stalin hysterical letters, full of love: "20.2.37. Sergo's death has shaken me to the depths of my soul. I sobbed and howled for hours. I loved that man very much. I wanted to go to Zina, but what if she said, 'No, you are our enemy now.' I really do love you ardently now, though my love is belated. I know that you are suspicious and that you are often wise to be suspicious. I know that events have shown that the level of suspicion should be many times higher than it is." The Boss was not simply torturing him by making him wait for the end. The Boss was being supremely merciful, giving him time to commit suicide. But Bukharin wanted to live. He had a beautiful wife, who had recently borne him a child. Well, the choice was his own.

The plenum opened. Yezhov made a statement on the criminal activity of the rightists. Legend had it that some speakers tried to defend Rykov and Bukharin. This, of course, was untrue. They spoke with one voice, furiously calling for severe punishment. The faithful Molotov was at the fore: "Refusal to confess will prove that you are a fascist hireling. . . . They are the ones who say that our trials are rigged." Mikoyan also invited Bukharin and Rykov to confess at once to activity against the state, and provoked an angry outburst from Bukharin: "I am neither Zinoviev nor Kamenev, and I will not slander myself." (Little Bukharin knew all along, then, that those he had labeled "gangsters" were in fact innocent.)

The most tolerant person present, doing his best to keep the heat down, was of course the Boss. A commission was set up to draft a resolution. Its thirty members included some whom the Boss would allow to live (Khrushchev, Mikoyan, Molotov, Kaganovich, Voroshilov) and others whom he had marked for a speedy end (Yezhov, Gamarnik, Peters, Eikhe, Chubar, Kosarev). These future victims were particularly cruel, particularly violent, in their insistence that Bukharin and Rykov must be shot. Again, it was the Boss who made the most moderate proposal, to "expel them from the Central Committee and the CPSU, but instead of committing them for trial pass the case to the NKVD for investigation." This moderation meant certain but slow death. And torture in the meantime. He had made Lenin's widow, Krupskaya, and sister, Maria Ulyanova, members of the commission: both supported his proposals, and joined in sending Lenin's favorite to Golgotha.

Incidentally, Krupskaya was at the center of a bizarre episode in the course of the plenum. Yezhov declared, "Bukharin writes in his statement to the Central Committee that Ilyich died in his arms. That is rubbish! You're lying! It's utterly false!" "Well, those present when Ilyich died were Maria Ilyinichna, Nadezhda Konstantinovna [Krupskaya], and myself," Bukharin responded. "Is that correct, Nadezhda Konstantinovna?" Neither woman said anything. Bukharin continued: "Did I take Ilyich's dead body in my arms, and kiss his feet?" Both women remained silent, and the audience guffawed at the "liar." Poor Bukharin appealed in vain to the women. Like Bukharin before them, they had lost their voices. Everybody wanted to earn the right to live. It was no time for principles.

In accordance with the plenum's decision, Bukharin and Rykov were arrested. They turned up for one session, and were handing in their overcoats at the cloakroom, when a number of young men surrounded them. The plenum ruled that Bukharin and Rykov had at the very least known about the terrorist activities of the Trotskyist-Zinovievites and that all their letters to the Central Committee were "slanderous." By then they were already in the Lubyanka, undergoing their first interrogation.

At this bloodstained plenum the Boss delivered a famous and terrifying speech, with a typically uninspiring title: "On Defects in Party Work and Measures for the Liquidation of Trotskyists and Other Double-Dealers." It contained in fact his last-minute instructions to the inquisition.

Liquidation: Revolution's Favorite Word

"We must remember that no successes can cancel the fact of capitalist encirclement, that while there is capitalist encirclement there will be sabotage, terrorism, diversions, and spies infiltrated behind Soviet lines. We must smash and jettison the rotten theory that with every advance we make, the class struggle in our country will grow less acute. . . . We lack the will to liquidate our own laxity, our own complacency. . . . Surely we can shake off this ridiculous, this idiotic, malady—we, who have overthrown capitalism, completed the foundations of socialism, and raised high the banner of world communism."

This is from the stenographic record of this plenum and remained hidden in the President's Archive for many years. Throughout the proceedings participants eagerly competed in exposing "wreckers." Fear had now become insanity. One delegate, T. Bogushevsky, exposed a group of saboteurs in the broadcasting service: "On a day of mourning, the anniversary of Lenin's death, they broadcast gypsy love songs, pretending that it was for testing purposes . . . and on January 23, the day when the verdict of guilty against the Trotskyists was broadcast, they played Chopin's Funeral March."

One after another they spoke to the same effect. Yezhov himself spoke of his successes in hunting down human beings and enumerated those arrested in the People's Commissariats. "Those condemned in recent months include 141 from the People's Commissariat for Light Industry, 228 from the People's Commissariat for Education." His audience was indignant that so few Light Industry officials had been arrested. Molotov, called upon to lead the attack, said sarcastically, "Comrade Lyubimov sits there saying nothing. I wonder why."

Yezhov replied: "As far as the Commissariat of Light Industry is concerned we've only just got going. But we have already obtained the conviction of 141 active wreckers and saboteurs. A quite significant number of them have been shot." His audience noisily rejoiced to hear it. Not out of bloodlust—from fear. Fear compelled them to demonstrate their zeal.

R.I. Eikhe boasted: "We have exposed many wreckers in Western Siberia. We exposed wrecking activities earlier than other regions did." The trusty Eikhe had indeed understood the Boss's instructions. But he had not understood their purpose. For Eikhe, who joined with such zeal in exterminating his oppositionist comrades, had been in the Party since 1905 and was doomed to perish with the rest of the old Party. He would do so a little later, in 1940. Two members of the Politburo who spoke, Kosior and Postyshev, were themselves to die shortly. Maria Ulyanova also spoke. They all joined in the general chorus: crucify them!

The Boss could view this contest with satisfaction. And when one speaker mounted the platform and began "angrily" reporting (one couldn't just speak, one had to speak "with uncontrollable anger") progress in the liquidation of enemies, the Boss interrupted him with a joke: "So how are things at your place? Have you driven all our enemies out? Or are there still a few left?" They laughed heartily. With relief. Believing that since he was in such a good mood, perhaps it was all over? They laughed. And the Boss must have laughed with them. For he knew their fate.

The heads of all the branches of the economy reported on their success to date in liquidating enemies, confessed that they had been insufficiently vigilant (this was called "self-criticism"), and fulsomely praised the Boss's speech. After this it was Voroshilov's turn. The People's Commissar for War told them that "happily, we have not as yet discovered many enemies in the army. I say happily in the hope that there are not very many enemies in the Red army. That is how it should be. For the Party sends its best cadres into the army." No, People's Commissar Voroshilov, not a very clever man, had not understood the situation. Molotov, one of the initiated, and leader of the offensive, spoke up sharply: "If we have wreckers in every branch of the economy, can we imagine that in one place alone, the War Department, there are none? It would be absurd to do so." His next words were ominous: "The War Department is a very large affair, and its work will be checked not now but a little later. And it will be examined very rigorously."

". . . Examined Very Rigorously"

After the Party, the army was Stalin's main concern. And his main target. Trotsky had controlled the army for several years. When he had replaced Trotsky with Voroshilov he had ruthlessly dismissed former commanders. He had resumed the process in the early thirties, and 47,000 were dismissed. But there were several who could not be touched: Yakir, Uborevich, Shmidt, Blyukher, Kork. Volumes had been written about them, their names were in history textbooks. Yakir, the youngest of his marshals, son of a Jewish pharmacist, was renowned for his bravery and his obscene language. The bearded giant Uborevich who had, together with Frunze, conquered the supposedly impregnable Crimea, was now in command of the Belorussian military district. Shmidt, the son of a Jewish shoemaker, had taken part in the bloody massacres of the Civil War from the age of fifteen. He was monstrously ugly, but famous for his amorous conquests. Marshal Blyukher had smashed the White armies in the South and the East, was the first to be awarded the Order of the Red Banner, and now commanded the Far Eastern army. Kork, whose head was as bald as a billiard ball, had defended Petrograd together with Trotsky, had completed the destruction of Wrangel in the Crimea, and was head of the Military Academy. They despised him. They remembered what a poor figure Koba had cut in the Polish campaign. Informers let him know what they said about him. Could he rely fully on the army while they and their associates were still around? The biggest worry was that as they saw the Party being destroyed they would unite against him. Out of fear. Could stupid Voroshilov read Tukhachevsky's mind? Time was getting short. He must act. So, in the Boss's thriller, the high command had to form part of a military-political conspiracy. Yagoda and the

NKVD could be thrown in for good measure. Plus his old friend Enukidze, onetime keeper of the Kremlin. The leader of this whole gang was of course Trotsky. And behind them all, needless to say, stood Hitler. The army, the Kremlin, the Party, the NKVD were all accomplices of Hitler and Trotsky. This was as good as anything he had written so far. It was not difficult to find proof of espionage, since the army had previously had close connections with the Reichswehr. To arrest a few senior commanders and force them to supply the necessary testimony was a mere "technicality." So while little Bukharin was in jail the Boss's thriller provided him with new comrades-in-arms—the military chiefs, German spies, and minions of Trotsky.

Extermination of the former commanders had, of course, to begin with the most dangerous of them, Tukhachevsky.

A typical tsarist officer, well groomed and self-possessed, Tukhachevsky had some sort of mysterious power. He was born to command. During the Civil War his appearance on the scene was enough to pacify mutinous units. His thunderous command of "Attention!" brought insubordinate soldiers to their senses. He was as cruel as the bloody times he lived through.

Voroshilov hated Tukhachevsky, who despised him in return. He was fond of telling stories which showed Voroshilov—"our Klim, the Lugansk metalworker, as Kliment Efremovich Voroshilov likes to call himself"—in a ridiculous light. During the First World War Tukhachevsky was for some time in a German POW camp. In the period of military cooperation between the USSR and Germany after the war, and before Hitler came to power, he had often sung the Reichswehr's praises. The impending investigation would have no difficulty in producing compromising material.

At the same time, Hitler's intelligence service, taking advantage of the atmosphere created by the purges, had set out to weaken the Soviet army by forging a letter in which Tukhachevsky announced his intention of carrying out a Napoleonic coup. Whether this occurred to German intelligence spontaneously or was inspired by Stalin's agents is a matter for conjecture. V. Krivitsky, a high official of the NKVD who later defected, claimed that the scheme originated with the Boss himself. The forged letter reached him in January 1937, but by then it was superfluous. V. Primakov, second in command of the Leningrad military district, and V. Putna, Soviet military attaché in the United Kingdom, both arrested in autumn 1936, had already provided the necessary evidence against the "German spy Tukhachevsky."

A. Kork, head of the Military Academy, was arrested first, in May 1937. Tukhachevsky himself was arrested on May 27. By the 29th, as his case record shows, the hero had confessed to all the false charges brought against him. There are reddish-brown marks on some pages of his deposition. Forensic examination has shown that they are bloodstains. When he introduced torture, the Boss had been thinking ahead. Since the military were bound to be a bit tougher than civilians, torture should prove useful. It did.

On May 29 I. Uborevich was arrested at a railway station. Marshal I. Yakir was arrested next.

The arrested officers had to be tried quickly. Marshal Blyukher arrived, and asked Gamarnik, head of the army's Political Administration, to help with the trial. But Gamarnik never got there. Next day when he was expecting Blyukher, NKVD men arrived to seal his safe, and ordered him to stay at home. In "in-depth language" this was an invitation to take a certain action. Gamarnik went into the next room and shot himself. The Boss liked to allow his victims this alternative.

In May 1937, the journalist Mikhail Koltsov, who had fought heroically in Spain, spent three hours with the Boss. When he got home he told his brother, "Stalin stood near me, put his hand on his heart, and bowed. 'What should one call you in Spanish, Mig-u-el?' 'Mig-el, Comrade Stalin.' 'Right then, Don Mig-el. We noble Spaniards heartily thank you for your interesting report. Goodbye for now, Don Mig-el.' " But when he reached the door the Boss called to him and a strange conversation followed:

"Have you a revolver, Comrade Koltsov?"

"Yes, Comrade Stalin."

"But you aren't planning to shoot yourself with it?"

"Of course not."

"Well, that's just fine. Thank you again, Comrade Koltsov, goodbye for now, Don Mig-el."

On December 17, 1938, Koltsov was arrested, and later shot.

The Army Council met in the People's Commissariat of War from June 1 to 4. Stalin arrived with the Politburo. More than a hundred military chiefs had been called in from the provinces because the ranks of the Military Council itself had by then been thinned out catastrophically: a quarter of its members had been arrested as conspirators.

Before the council began work, folders containing documents were distributed to the participants. Their comrades of yesterday, the army's idols—Tukhachevsky, Kork, Uborevich, Yakir, and the rest of them—had confessed that they were spies for Hitler's intelligence service. Voroshilov reported to the council on the discovery of an extensive counterrevolutionary conspiracy by the NKVD: "I am very greatly to blame. I did not detect these base traitors. But I cannot point to a single warning signal from you." His audience realized that they were being accused of complicity. After this, what was left of the council, and all the others in the hall, eagerly denounced their former friends and superiors.

The Boss himself spoke on June 2. He never published this terrible, tense speech, but the stenographic report is in the President's Archive. He spoke of spies, of the skillful way in which German intelligence had "recruited malcontents," who had become "slaves in the hands of the Reichswehr." This speech added one lurid touch to his thriller. "A certain woman" made her appearance, a perfidious beauty by the name of Jozefina Genzi. "She is a beautiful woman. A spy. She recruited people with her woman's wiles. She recruited Karakhan [onetime Vice-Commissar for Foreign Affairs]. She was also the one who recruited Enukidze. She had Rudzutak in her clutches." The names were those of Party members well known for their amorous exploits. Yagoda's dossiers had proved helpful.

Stalin called the unmasked military chiefs "spies," contemptuously denying them the appellation "counterrevolutionary." He explained the distinction: "If, for instance, the suicide Gamarnik had been a committed counterrevolutionary—in his place I would have asked to see Stalin, bumped him off first, and *then* killed myself." The former terrorist could never forget how easy it is to kill people.

A summary trial took place on June 11. Stalin staged his favorite show: friends sent friends to their deaths. Tukhachevsky, Uborevich, Yakir, Primakov, and the others were tried by their army comrades—Dybenko, Blyukher, Belov, Alksnis. The sentence, of course, was death. Stalin knew that the judges who passed sentence ultimately would also perish. All those old commanders were part of the old Party, and must therefore disappear.

The destruction of the old command went on throughout 1937 and 1938. This wholesale massacre left the army weak. That at least is the generally accepted view. But Marshal Konyev, one of the heroes of the Second World War, was of a different opinion. He wrote in his memoirs: "Of the commanders destroyed—Tukhachevsky, Yegorov, Yakir, Kork,

Uborevich, Blyukher, Dybenko—only Tukhachevsky and Uborevich can be regarded as modern military leaders. . . . Most of them were on a level with Voroshilov and Budenny. Those heroes of the Civil War, cavalry army men, living on their past. Blyukher bungled the Khasan operation, Voroshilov would bungle the war with Finland. If they had remained at the top the war would have turned out quite differently." The Boss, indeed, knew that the repressions would weaken the army for the present but strengthen it in the long run. It was another example of his favorite, murderous method of selecting personnel. The mass murder of former officers meant that on the eve of war, command passed to men much more up-to-date in their training and their thinking, men for whom the Civil War was just a heroic myth.

Bukharin, then, while in jail, became one of the leaders of a military-political conspiracy. All that remained was to obtain his consent. For, unlike the soldiers, who were tried in camera, Bukharin was to be granted the favor of a magnificent public trial. There are many legends about the tortures which induced him to take part in this ignominious farce. It is a pity to debunk a good legend, but let Bukharin's letters speak for themselves.

> Night of April 15, 37. Koba! . . . I have been meaning to write to you for several nights now. Simply because I want to write to you, cannot help writing to you, since I now feel you to be someone so close to me (let those who want to laugh up their sleeves). . . . Everything that is most sacred has been turned into a game by me (so it was said at the plenum). In my despair I swore by Ilyich's dying hour. And I was told that I was trading on his name, and even that I was lying when I said that I had been present when he died. . . . I could barely stand on my feet and they accused me of clowning and play-acting. [His thoughts wandered. He seemed now to be remembering his visit to Koba, when Koba said "I'll kill you" and he decided that Koba was jealous of him and Nadezhda.] I want to tell you honestly and openly about my private life. Let me say that I have known only four women intimately. [There follows a minutely detailed account of his excruciating disputes with them.] You were wrong in thinking that I had "ten wives." I never lived with more than one at a time. ["He's lying again," Koba might have told himself. "He's settled down now that he's got a young beauty for a wife. But earlier on. . . ." Every step he took, every one of the "wom-

anizer" Bukharin's women had been accounted for by the NKVD.] All my dreams recently have come down to one thing—to stick closely to the leadership, and to you in particular . . . to work with all my strength, subordinating myself completely to your advice, instructions, and requirements. I have seen the spirit of Ilyich rest upon you. Who else could have resolved upon Comintern's new tactics? The resolute implementation of the Second Five-Year Plan, the arming of the Far East, . . . the organization of reform, the new constitution? No one . . . I had an unusual feeling when I was fortunate enough to be with you. . . . Even fortunate enough to touch you. . . . I began to feel toward you as I felt toward Ilyich—a feeling of close kinship, of tremendous love, unbounded trust, the feeling you have for someone to whom you can say anything, write anything, complain of anything. . . . Is it at all surprising that in recent years I have even forgotten the times when I fought against you, when I was embittered. . . . [I can imagine Stalin reading this and remembering all that Bukharin had so recently said about him abroad. Stalin was too down-to-earth to understand that Bukharin *did* now really love him, with the love of a hysterical intellectual, the love of a victim for the executioner, of weakness for strength. How Russians love these Dostoevskyan perversities!]

I have it in my mind to write a book. I should like to dedicate it to you and to ask you to write a short foreword, to show everyone that I consider myself entirely yours. How horribly contradictory my situation here is. I regard every warder, every Chekist in the prison as one of my own people while he looks upon me as a criminal, though he treats me correctly. I think of the prison as "my own." . . . Sometimes I find myself dreaming, why can't they plant me somewhere outside Moscow, in a little cottage, give me a different passport and two Chekists to watch over me, let me live with my family, make myself useful to society by working on my books, on translations (using a pen name, or anonymously), let me dig the ground so as not to disintegrate physically (never going farther than my own backyard). And then, one fine day, X or Y will confess that he has slandered me. [Poor romantic!]

As it is I am perishing here. The rules are very strict, you can't even talk loudly in your cell, or play checkers or chess,

> when you go out into the corridor you aren't allowed to talk at all, you can't feed the pigeons at your window, can't do anything at all. On the other hand, the warders, even the very junior ones, are always polite, reserved, correct. We are well fed. But the cells are dark. Yet the lights are on day and night. I swab floors, clean my slop pail. Nothing new in that. But it breaks my heart that this is in a Soviet prison. My grief and anguish know no bounds.

With the letter went a request that "no one should read it before J. V. Stalin." But Stalin wrote on it "circulate," and sent it by special messenger to all members of the Politburo. It was as if the benevolent Boss was asking, "Ought we to pardon him in spite of everything?" His henchmen could be under no misapprehension. Heads were falling daily. They did their duty, vied with each other in ruthlessness:

"Read it. In my view written by a con man"—Molotov.

"Con man's spiel"—Chubar.

"I'm not me and the horse isn't mine!"—Kaganovich, Kalinin.

"Undoubtedly a con man's letter"—Chuba.

Once again, the Boss was forced to bow to the collective.

Little Bukharin went on writing to him, forty-three letters, forty-three unanswered declarations of love.

> Greetings, Joseph Vissarionovich! [The familiar "Koba" had vanished.] . . . I have been talking to you for hours in a hallucinatory state—I have spells like that. (You were sitting on my bunk, so close I could touch you.) Unfortunately, it was just my delirium. . . . I wanted to tell you that I would be willing to carry out any demand of yours without the least hesitation or reservations. I have already written (besides an academic book) a large volume of verse. All in all, it is an apotheosis of the USSR. . . . Byron said that to become a poet you either have to fall in love or be a pauper. (Both are true of me.) My first efforts now seem infantile (but I am rewriting them, except for my "Poem on Stalin"). . . . I have seen neither my wife nor my child in the past seven months. I have made several requests, but without success. I have lost my sight twice because of nerve trouble, and have had two or three attacks of hallucinatory delirium . . . J. V.! Give them permission to visit me! Let me see Anyuta and my little boy! Anything may happen! So let me see my dear ones. . . .

> Or if that is impossible at least let Anyushka bring a photograph of herself and our child for me. I know that it may seem ludicrous to you when I say that I love you with all my soul but I can't help that. You must think what you will of me.

So the prison regime was strict, but they were perfectly polite, and the food was good. No, there was no torture. And it seems unlikely that the delicate and hysterical Bukharin would have written so many literary works in the intervals of torture. He tortured himself—with his despair, his fear of being shot, the anguish he felt for his family. His was too delicate an organism for prison life. He was a poet, not a politician. Nervous strain gave him hallucinations and caused him to lose his sight. He knew already that he could not hold out, that he would consent, as Kamenev had, to "lie about himself," even without being tortured. "I wanted to tell you that I would be willing to carry out any demand of yours without the least hesitation or reservation." Almost word for word what that other unfortunate, Zinoviev, had said.

Early in June Bukharin did accept, and put his name to, all the charges made against him. His wife, Anna Larina, was convinced, and later wrote, that in return the Boss promised him his life and then went back on his word. She did not know that there exists a letter in which the hapless Bukharin told the whole story himself.

It is Bukharin's forty-third, and final, letter to Stalin.

> Top Secret, Personal, Please do not read without permission from J. V. Stalin.
>
> 10.12.37. I am writing what may be my last letter before I die. Let me therefore write it without formalities, especially as I am writing to you alone . . . the last page of my drama, and perhaps of my physical life, is about to be turned. ["Perhaps" shows that he still had some hope, remembering that at the previous trial neither Radek nor Sokolnikov had been sentenced to death.] I am trembling all over in agitation, and from a thousand emotions. I can scarcely control myself. But precisely because the end may be near I want to say goodbye to you before it is too late. . . . To avoid all misunderstandings let me tell you right away that for the sake of peace (social peace) (1) I am not going to retract any of the things to which I have signed (2) I do not intend to ask you for anything, to beg you for anything that might throw the whole affair off the rails along which it is

> rolling. I write only for your personal information. I cannot leave this life without writing these last lines to you, because I am a prey to torments of which you should know. I give you my word of honor that I am innocent of the crimes which I acknowledged under interrogation.

Why then did he acknowledge them? As it happens he was the first of all those self-slanderers to explain in detail why.

> I had no recourse except to confirm the accusations and depositions of others: if I had not done so it would have meant that "I was not laying down my arms." I thought over what was happening and reached roughly the following conclusion: that there is some great and bold political idea behind the general purge, that because of (a) the fact that we are in a prewar period and (b) the transition to democracy—the purge embraces (a) the guilty, (b) the suspect, and (c) the potentially suspect. I could not hope to be left out. Some of the above are rendered harmless by one means, others by another, others still by yet another. . . . For heaven's sake do not think that this is a roundabout reproach. I have been out of diapers long enough to recognize, even in my private thoughts, that great plans, great ideas, and great interests overshadow all else. It would be petty of me to put the fortunes of my own person on the same level as those tasks of world-historical importance, which rest above all on your shoulders.

So then, it was all in the name of the higher expediency, of a world-historical task. What had once been the excuse for killing outsiders was now an excuse for killing one another. Now that he had discovered the great idea Bukharin calmed down. It was no longer anything as petty as fear for his life and for his family that had made him betray himself. It was the great idea! In the world of ideas he felt at home. He was no longer a coward, but almost a hero: sacrificing his honor, going to his death for the sake of something great. Enraptured, he soared above the real world. He longed now to do penance.

> I am not a Christian. But I have some peculiar notions . . . and one of them is a belief that I am paying for the years when I re-

ally was fighting against you . . . that is what weighs on me most heavily. When I was with you once in summer 1928 you said to me, "Do you know why I am friends with you? It's because you are incapable of intrigue, aren't you?" I said yes. And that was the very time when I was running to Kamenev. That fact haunts me as original sin haunts an observant Jew. God, how infantile and idiotic I was, and now I'm paying for it with my honor and my life. For that—forgive me, Koba. I weep as I write, I have no more need of anything. When I was hallucinating I saw you several times, and on one occasion Nadezhda Sergeevna. She came up to me and said, "What have they done to you, Nikolai Ivanovich? I've told Joseph to get bail for you." It was so real that I nearly jumped up to write and ask you to get bail for me. I know that N.S. would never believe that I ever meant you any harm, and it's not surprising that my subconscious self produced this hallucination.

He hopes against hope that Koba will forgive him! If only he had known how it would infuriate Koba to see words put into his dead wife's mouth in a letter from her "murderer."

With you I converse for hours on end. Lord—if only there was some instrument with which you could look into my lacerated and tormented soul! If only you could see how *devoted* I am to you . . . but all that is just psychology, forgive me. There is no angel now to deflect Abraham's sword, and what is fated will come to pass. Permit me finally to turn to my last small requests.

(a) To die would be a thousand times easier for me than to go through the coming trial: I simply do not know how I shall manage to control myself. . . . If I could, I would beg you on bended knees, abandoning all shame and pride, not to let it happen, but that is probably now impossible . . . so I should like to ask you to make it possible for me to die before the trial, although I know what a strict view you take on such matters.

(b) If [some words deleted] you have already decided on the death sentence, let me ask you in advance, let me urge you by all that is dear to you to let me, instead of being shot, take poison in my cell (give me morphine so that I can go to sleep and never wake up again). Take pity on me, let me spend my last minutes in my own way. You know me well enough to understand: I sometimes look death in the face with clear eyes. . . . I am capable of brave actions, yet sometimes the same me is so panic-stricken that there is nothing left of me. . . . So if I am condemned to death I ask you to let me have the poisoned cup (like Socrates).

(c) Let me say goodbye to my wife and son before the trial. My reason for this is that if my family see the things I have confessed to, the shock might drive them to suicide. I must somehow prepare them. This would, I think, be a help to the case and its official interpretation.

If my life is to be spared my request is—either send me to America for x years. Arguments in favor: I could mount a publicity campaign about the trials, wage war to the death on Trotsky, win over large sections of the vacillating intelligentsia. I would be in effect an anti-Trotsky, and I would do all this with great energy and enthusiasm. You could send a trained Chekist with me, and as an additional guarantee I would leave my wife here for six months while I show how good I am at bashing Trotsky. Or if there is the slightest doubt about this, banish me, for 25 years if you like, to Pechora or Kolyma, to a camp, where I could start a university, learned institutes, a picture gallery, zoological and photographic museums. Though to tell the truth I have little hope of that.

Joseph Vissarionovich! You have lost in me one of your ablest generals, and one of those really devoted to you. But I am preparing myself spiritually to depart from this vale of tears, and I feel, toward you, toward the Party, toward the cause as a whole nothing but great and boundless love. I embrace you in my thoughts, farewell forever, and think well of your unhappy N. Bukharin.

This letter gives us the final key to the trials. It tells us everything. No, Stalin had not promised to pardon him. Bukharin went on hoping, but the Boss was silent. Bukharin had consented to everything, endlessly professed his love for his torturer, and the Boss had remained silent.

So we see Bukharin, the Party's greatest theoretician, voluntarily inventing a rationale for the trials on Stalin's behalf—"the great and bold" political idea behind a general purge—although he did not know whether there really was such a thing. To have acted simply out of fright would have been too disgraceful. And so he cooperated to the full with his interrogator, although the God Stalin promised nothing. We must try to understand the mentality of this Russian intellectual: the upright liar, the helpless strongman, the noble scoundrel, the bold coward—and at the same time immensely talented even in his humiliation. Incapable of saying, "I simply dread the wrath of these hideously cruel people," he has to invent a "great idea" to justify his behavior. How well I understand and—yes—love him. For I too am a child of fear. My whole conscious life has been lived in that land of fear. Have pity on me. "You, who know me so well, will understand."

Yes, Stalin knew them all so well. Which was why he had devised the trials.

"The Fortunes of Individuals are Transient and Trivial"

The Boss granted none of his prostrate enemy's requests. He allowed Bukharin only to write to his wife immediately before the trial.

> My dear, my precious Annushka, my darling. I am writing to you on the eve of the trial, and I write for a particular purpose, which I underline three times: whatever you read, whatever you hear, however horrible the implications, whatever they say about me, and whatever I say, take it all bravely and calmly. Prepare the family for it, help them, I'm afraid for you and for the others, but above all for you. You must not in any event become embittered, remember always that the great cause of the USSR lives on, that is the main thing, the fortunes of individuals are transient and trivial in comparison with that. A great ordeal awaits you, I beg you, my own, do everything you can, tighten the strings of your soul, but do not let them snap. Don't talk to anyone unnecessarily about anything. You are nearer and dearer to me than anyone. I implore you by all that was good in our life together to brace yourself by a supreme effort so that you can help yourself and the family to live through this terrible phase. I don't think my father and Nadya ought to read the newspapers for those few days: let them pretend to be asleep for a while. . . . If I ask you this believe me that I have arrived at my present state of mind, and this request, through suffering, and that it will all be as great and supreme interests demand that it should be. I am tremendously anxious for you, and if you were allowed

> to write and give me a few reassuring words on what I have just said some of the weight at least would be lifted from my mind. Please try, my dearest. This is no place to carry on about my feelings, but you know, and will read between the lines, how immense, how profound my love for you is.

No one was prepared to pass this letter to his wife. Bukharin's infinitely dear Annushka was already under arrest. Not until she was an old woman, fifty years later, would she be given the letter which her husband had once written to the young and beautiful Anna Larina. For almost half a century her husband's name was an obscene word in the country which he had helped to found. "Great and supreme interests" demanded that it should be.

Then came the trial—in March 1938—the last in the series of trials of famous Bolshevik leaders. The work of exterminating Ilyich's comrades-in-arms was nearing completion. This trial was the climax of the Boss's thriller. As all storytellers should, he drew all the story lines together and left nothing unexplained. It now emerged that Bukharin and Rykov had collaborated simultaneously with the Trotskyist-Zinovievites, with Tukhachevsky and the other German spies in the high command, with the nationalist underground, and with wreckers in the NKVD represented by Yagoda and his associates. The main organizer of the previous trials, Yagoda, thus became one of the stars of the Bukharin trial. "Murdering doctors" who had allegedly helped him to carry out his "perfidious schemes" were tried with him. These were eminent physicians unfortunate enough to have treated Kremlin leaders—Pletnev, Levin, and Kazakov, among others. The Boss exerted himself to answer all the people's questions. One of the accused, for instance, was the former People's Commissar for Agriculture, Chernov, famous for his reign of terror in the countryside during collectivization; the ironical author now invited this enemy of Bukharin's ideas to take part in the trial—side by side with Bukharin. What accounted for the horrors of collectivization? Chernov was contrite and told the court how he had deliberately misinterpreted the correct policy of collectivization on instructions from Bukharin and Rykov! What could account for the unavailability of butter and the continual interruptions in the supply of bread in a country of victorious socialism? This was the cue for Zelensky, head of the Central Council of Cooperatives, to confess: it was all caused by acts of sabotage which he had carried out on the instructions of the rightists.

There is a widely reported story that the Boss watched the trials—

that behind one of the heavily curtained windows overlooking the platform in the hall, one could occasionally see puffs of smoke from his pipe rising behind the cloth. It was of course quite possible. The chief producer ought to see how the show is going. One weakness of previous spectaculars had been the suspicious readiness of the accused to agree with every charge against them, and it was evidently in recognition of this that a few "surprises" were introduced into the Bukharin trial. N. Krestinsky, a member of the Central Committee in Lenin's time, suddenly declared, "I do not plead guilty. . . . I did not commit a single one of the crimes of which I am accused." The audience was stunned. But the author saw to it that the sensation was short-lived. On the very next day Krestinsky said, "I ask the court to record my statement that I acknowledge myself to be completely and utterly guilty. . . . Yesterday, in a moment of false shame caused by finding myself in the dock, I was incapable of telling the truth."

Bukharin also exerted himself at the trial and thoroughly revised a chapter of history. Lenin's favorite told the court how in order to obstruct the Brest treaty, he had been ready to cooperate with the Left SRs in arresting his beloved Lenin. Bukharin not only called himself a despicable fascist but carried out the promise in his letter and stoutly defended the authenticity of the trials against Western critics. But he could not sustain his role. As the trial went on the Boss saw more and more clearly that Bukharin was playing a double game. Admitting everything was his way of admitting nothing in particular. Stalin also appreciated another crafty move of his "most talented general." Bukharin suddenly mentioned that he had an understanding with Nikolaevsky, who had undertaken to organize a public protest if there should be a trial. This was the cunning Bukharin's way of reminding European socialists that he had once organized a campaign in defense of the Left SRs and asking them to repay their debt by organizing a campaign in *his* defense. The Boss realized yet again that some people never learn. Only the grave would teach them.

A campaign in defense of Bukharin was, of course, organized, but times had changed. Some people were suborned by the NKVD, while others believed that Stalin was the last bulwark against Hitler and were afraid of "playing into the hands of the fascists." As Nikolaevsky wrote, "a number of very influential organs of the Western press suddenly became apologists for Stalin's terrorist policies." Romain Rolland, however, did send Stalin a message: "An intellect of the Bukharin type is a treasure for his country. We are all to blame for the death of the chemist of genius Lavoisier, we, the bravest of revolutionaries, who cherish the memory of Robespierre—nonetheless profoundly regret and grieve. I beg you to show clemency." Stalin did not deign to reply.

After sentence of death had been passed, the defendants appealed for a pardon. Rykov confined himself to a few formal lines. Bukharin, of course, went into much greater detail, but ended with the words "On bended knee before my Motherland, my Party, my people and its government, I plead for forgiveness." The interrogators evidently told them that petitions were not enough. They had to work a bit harder. So the next day, March 14 Bukharin wrote another, very long petition: "I have mentally disarmed and have rearmed myself in the new, socialist style. . . . Give this new, this second Bukharin a chance to grow—we'll call him Petrov if you like. This new man will be the complete opposite of the one who has died. He has been born already, give him the chance to do some sort, any sort, of work." He had reverted to his favorite romantic notion. Shoot Bukharin, he must be shot in the name of Great Interests—but let *me* go on living under the name of Petrov.

Yagoda also submitted a petition: "Before the whole people and the Party on bended knees I beg you to forgive me and spare my life." The interesting thing is that the policeman Yagoda and the aesthete Bukharin both use the words "on bended knees." This prayerbook language gives the editor of petitions away.

They came for him. Only then did Bukharin realize that the business of the petitions was merely the final torture—torture by hope. All were executed as sentenced. Friend Koba had not granted Bukharin's request for the poisoned cup. Instead of dying like Socrates, Bukharin died at the hands of "our people." They shot him last. Stalin had not forgiven him for his behavior at the trial. And abroad. Nor for his wife. He let him experience the full torment of waiting for death.

There is an extraordinary feat of proofreading in the President's Archive: Stalin personally prepared the stenographic record of the trial for publication and edited the speeches, deleting words used by the deceased and writing in others. The fastidious author worked away at his thriller to the very end.

Free of the Past

He had been writing to his mother all this time: "I'm told you are well and in good spirits. Is it true? We are obviously a hardy breed. Keep well, and live for many years, Mama dear." He knew that it was not true. His mother was sick. Tiflis was a small city, and she had heard about

Ordzhonikidze and his brothers. There were arrests every night. Old nationalists as well as the old Bolsheviks who had fought them were doomed to die. Horror gripped the city.

In that terrible year his mother fell mortally sick. "Greetings, Mama dear. I'm sending you a shawl and some medicines. Show the medicines to the doctor before you take them. It's for him to decide on the dosage." In the middle of the red hot summer of 1937 he was informed that "on June 4 at 23:05 after a long and grave illness Ekaterina Georgievna Dzhugashvili died at home in her apartment."

This was at the height of the repressions. He knew that Caucasians were skilled in vengeance, and he did not dare go to Georgia for her funeral. This was something else he would never forget: that his enemies had prevented him from saying farewell to his mother.

Stubborn Keke had departed this life without ever forgiving him for her dear Soso, murdered by the revolutionary Koba. I found among his papers a pathetic list of the things left by the mother of the man who ruled half the world. She had lived the life of a solitary pauper. And died poor, and alone. After her death his letters, which she had carefully preserved, were returned to him.

Now he was completely free of the past.

18

Reading this tedious catalog of never-ending arrests and trials, we are bound to imagine that the country's state of mind in that terrible year 1937 was one of deep depression. Not a bit of it! The great majority of the population woke up happily to the relentless blare of loudspeakers, sped eagerly to work, participated enthusiastically in the daily public meetings at which their enemies were anathematized, and read skimpy newspaper reports of the trials which showed how very reliable the secret police were. They knew how hard the lot of workers was in the West. They felt pity for persecuted blacks in the United States and for all whose lot it was not to live in the USSR. Our nearest neighbor, in our communal apartment, was a young professor of biology at Moscow University, sharing a single room with his wife, mother, and daughter. He always hummed happily as he stood perusing the newspaper in the queue for the communal lavatory. During the October Revolution holiday the whole family took part in a "demonstration": they went to Red Square and later told the professor's paralyzed mother how they had seen Stalin. The old lady was deaf, and they shouted so loud that the whole apartment heard them. Were they afraid of the NKVD? The question would have aroused their indignation. They knew that only enemies feared the NKVD. Did they know about the arrests? Of course they did. Many people they knew had been arrested. But they had subsequently turned out to be enemies. Anyway, arrests took place after midnight. Moscow's peculiar night life was not something they knew about. It didn't concern them. At night they slept the sleep of the just. To wake up happily again in the morning, and sing as they stood in line for the lavatory.

The public trials, with their magnificent ritual of retribution, were one of the distractions from everyday life. As a true Caesar should, Stalin arranged many such diversions for his fortunate fellow citizens. Ruby-red stars, for instance, appeared over the Kremlin, and the country exulted—whole families trooped to Red Square to watch them light up at night. Everyday life resounded with the thunder of marching music, for this was the land of victors. Monarchists, Mensheviks, Socialist Revolutionaries, Kadets, the White Guard—all beaten by them in the Civil War. And now they were winning peacetime victories. In the space of two or three Five-Year Plans they had caught up with the rest of the world and would soon leave it behind. Every day the papers reported the victory of some champion worker and the country rejoiced. They had vanquished religion. Nothing was left of Holy Russia except its decapitated churches. And at every political trial the Boss's Chekists were defeating enemies and spies. They had conquered death itself: Ilyich lay incorruptible in his Mausoleum, waiting to receive his fellow citizens. Every day Stalin presented the inhabitants of the world's first socialist state with some new victory. The aviator Chkalov and his crew were driven round the city in open cars; they had been the first in the world to fly nonstop from Moscow to the United States. Then there were the annual military and gymnastic parades on Red Square. And finally the ceremonies in honor of the greatest victors of all—the heroes of labor.

In 1935 when Stalin was launching the "wrecker" trials, he had arranged for the "discovery" of a miner able to produce an enormous quantity of coal; the miner would, moreover, have to dig at a mine where intellectuals engaged in sabotage would inevitably obstruct his heroic labor. This was the Master's script, and it was quickly put into production. The miner was a nice-looking country boy called Stakhanov. A record-breaking shift was organized, and the Stakhanovite movement spread all over the country. Very high output rates were obtained with unmodified equipment. Industrial accidents were put down to wreckers, who had been found at the mine. The records set by Stakhanovites were supposed to spur on others. From time to time, the Boss organized festive congresses of Stakhanovites. The masses, the collective, were everywhere in evidence. He had created a country of collectives. Everything was collective. You worked collectively, lived collectively in a communal apartment, enjoyed your leisure collectively, perhaps on a collective excursion into the countryside. Holidays were collective—Miners' Day, Construction Workers' Day, Metalworkers' Day. Every profession had its own holiday, so that on that one day its collectives could drink and frolic to their hearts' content, and—most important—all together.

Stalin opened Parks of Culture and Rest all over the country. There, under the guidance of specially trained leisure organizers, people could enjoy themselves—as always—collectively. At the height of the Terror, in 1938, there were carnivals for workers' collectives in the Moscow Central Park of Culture and Rest. One hundred thousand happy, carefree people joined in the revels. He was right when he spoke the words afterward quoted on millions of billboards: "Life has become easier, life has become more joyful." In making each park a center for collective amusement, he personally took care that it was furnished with "visual propaganda." Every avenue was lined with quotations from himself and the God Lenin and with current Party slogans. Statues of his new saints and martyrs—Pavlik Morozov, the Young Pioneer murdered by kulaks, and Sergei Kirov, murdered by Trotskyist-Zinovievites—shone white among the foliage. On the central square of each park were statues of the God Lenin and the God Stalin. Along remoter paths were plaster gymnasts with swelling thighs, buttocks, and bosoms. Like Hitler in Germany, the Boss wanted the next generation to grow up strong. On his orders, shooting galleries and parachute towers were set up in the parks for mass target practice and mass parachute jumping. He was already preparing a new generation to make the Great Dream a reality. This constant emphasis on the mass—mass congresses, mass holidays—this dissolution of the individual in the mass produced something which he prized above all else: a collective conscience. Personal responsibility died; there was only collective responsibility: "the Party has ordered it," "the country has ordered it." This collective conscience enabled people to enjoy life unconcernedly when the Terror was at its most cruel. Woe to anyone troubled by a conscience of his own. The writer A. Gaidar found himself in a psychiatric hospital. He wrote to a writer friend, Ruvim Fraerman, "I'm troubled by my thoughts. . . . I no longer know whether I'm telling the truth or not . . . sometimes I come very close to it . . . then sometimes . . . just as the truth is about to slip off my tongue I seem to hear a voice peremptorily warning me—beware! Don't say it! Or you're done for!" He wasn't done for. The psychiatric hospital helped him. The truth stopped "troubling" him so acutely. His private conscience happily fell asleep.

The most popular holiday from everyday life was football. It was, incidentally, the favorite entertainment of the intelligentsia. At a football match, the anger and resentment normally suppressed by fear spilled out in noisy displays of emotion. At the stadium you could find relief from the suppressed terror in your unconscious. The main rivalry in the football world was between the NKVD's club, Dynamo, and the Trades Union team, Spartak. All the intelligentsia were fanatical supporters of Spartak. It was a tolerated form of dissent.

When these two teams met, the head of the NKVD was always in the government box at the stadium. At first it was Yagoda. Yagoda was shot, and Yezhov appeared in the box. When Yezhov was shot, a third

People's Commissar, Beria, would be seen there. They all hated Nikolai Starostin, founder and manager of Spartak.

The whole country knew Starostin. After Lenin's and Stalin's, his was the most popular name. The brothers Starostin were the country's four most famous footballers. When the oldest, Nikolai, gave up playing, he founded Spartak. It was he who started the great Spartak-Dynamo rivalry. His three famous brothers played for his team. Nikolai's inventiveness as an organizer of sport was inexhaustible. When in 1936 the annual gymnasts' parade was due to take place on Red Square, Alexander Kosarev, the head of the Young Communist League and organizer of this ceremony, decided that it should include a demonstration of football skills right there on the square. Spartak was chosen to provide it. Dynamo's devotees were indescribably jealous. In the course of the parade Kosarev gave a signal and a gigantic carpet was thrown over the whole of Red Square: it was meant to represent an emerald-green field with a cinder path around it. Spartak's players raced onto the field and began demonstrating their skills. Kosarev stood next to Stalin, who was clasping a white handkerchief. It had been agreed that if the game was not to the Boss's taste a wave of the handkerchief would put a stop to it immediately. The Boss did not like football: perhaps he was jealous of its popularity as a spectacle. But that day he chose to like it. His comrades-in-arms up on the Mausoleum were insanely enthusiastic. Voroshilov jumped up and down and even shouted.

Below their feet lay the unburied God Lenin.

Stalin, then, did not wave his handkerchief and the footballers interpreted this to mean that they had found favor. They were mistaken. The Boss was simply allowing these pathetic, puny creatures to amuse themselves. For the last time. Kosarev, Chubar, Postyshev, Rudzutak, and most of those who had so childishly enjoyed the football game would vanish together with the old Party.

He exploited his fellow citizens' foolish weakness. The national sensation of 1938 was not the trials: the country had no thought for anything except the visit of the Basque footballers. Yet another holiday for his people: he himself had sent for these famous footballers, at that time the best in the world. The country was overjoyed. The Basques played Dynamo and thrashed the NKVD's team twice. The country was plunged into mourning. The Boss turned nasty, and ordered a win. Yezhov then recommended letting Spartak take the field. His thought was that losing to the Basques would be the end of them.

The Spartak players were driven into Moscow with ceremony, in open Lincolns. On the way tires started bursting: the NKVD had not been asleep on the job. If Spartak arrived late, they were finished. They arrived just in time. As the referee ran onto the field, they changed on the spot, in the cars, watched by delighted fans, and hurried onto the field. For the Basques it was just a game of football, for Spartak it was a matter of life and death. When the match ended, the incredible figures on the scoreboard were Spartak 6, Basques 2.

The country went wild, people kissed each other in the streets, Starostin became the country's idol, and the NKVD gnashed its teeth.

In 1937, 1938, and 1939 Spartak did the impossible: they won both the championship and the cup. They had gone too far.

After shooting Yezhov, Beria began occupying himself with Dynamo in earnest. He had been a footballer himself in his youth, had even played for a major Georgian team, and was fanatically devoted to the game. From that moment Starostin was doomed. But he was too popular, and the Boss at first said no.

It would happen during the war, when football was unimportant. On May 20, 1942, Starostin was awakened by a bright light, a pistol was held to his face, and a harsh voice ordered him to get up. He was taken outside, shoved into a car, and driven to the Lubyanka. There they confronted him with depositions made by Kosarev, who had already been shot. He had been forced to confess that he was planning to liquidate the Party and government leaders at the next athletes' parade, and that for this purpose he had organized a hit squad headed by Nikolai Starostin. The three other Starostin brothers were arrested on the same night. They were all given ten years in the camps—a very lenient sentence by the standards of the time.

19 NIGHT LIFE

From that moment Starostin had entered that other life—the Life after Dark—which everyone tried not to talk about or even think about.

Those black cars used to drive out onto the streets of Moscow after midnight. Everything to do with that other life existed in the dark, and was secret. If someone was arrested in a communal apartment, the neighbors would pretend not to hear, however much noise was made, and would not leave their rooms. Next morning, standing in line for the lavatory, they would avert their eyes from the family of the man who had vanished in the night, and his family would avert their own tearful eyes. They were like plague victims. The whole apartment waited expectantly. They did not have long to wait. As a rule the whole family vanished soon afterward, and a new resident appeared in the communal apartment, humming as happily as the rest as he stood in line for the communal lavatory.

There were no communal apartments in the government House on the Embankment. This was where the new elite—old Bolsheviks, high-ranking officers, Comintern leaders, and not least the Boss's in-laws, the Alliluyevs and Svanidzes—lived in enormous self-contained flats. But fresh blobs of sealing wax now began to appear every morning on the high doors of those magnificent dwellings. The population of the house was dwindling from day to day.

This hectic Night Life went on throughout 1937. Prosecutors signed blank forms, on which NKVD investigators could enter any name they pleased. The prisons were overfull, but the Boss found a solution for the problem. From July 1937 "troikas" began operating in all major NKVD directorates. These three-man boards comprised the head of the local branch of the NKVD, the head of the local Party organization, and either the head of the local Soviet or the district public prosecutor. The troikas had the right to pronounce sentence of death without observing the normal rules of legal procedure. The accused was not present to hear sentence passed. The deadly conveyor belt began its work. A ten-minute trial was followed by execution. The trial of the Boss's friend Enukidze was one of the longest: it lasted fifteen minutes. The Boss urged the troikas on with telegram after telegram: "The established practice is that sentences passed by the three-man boards are final. Stalin." He was always in such a hurry.

Self-Destruction of the Party

The troikas showed such zeal that in 1938–1939 they were ready, to the last man, to share the fate of their victims.

The minutes of the 1957 Central Committee plenum contain the following exchange:

> *Khrushchev:* Every single member of these troikas was shot.
> *Kaganovich:* Not every one.
> *Khrushchev:* The great majority.

In his haste to build a monolithic society Stalin inaugurated a self-service system of elimination: each victim killed his predecessor, and was killed by his successor. Thousands of senior Party officials were members of troikas which passed sentence. But Stalin wanted to involve as many people as possible in the work of destruction. At hundreds of public meetings, millions of citizens welcomed the orgy of arrests and voted for death sentences for "enemies of people." Newspapers printed daily appeals from workers demanding the execution of Trotskyist-Zinovievite-Bukharinite murderers. In 1937 he involved hundreds of thousands of others with the powers of darkness: warrants for the arrest of senior officials now had to be countersigned by the heads of their departments.

The irony of history! In 1937 the Cheka, pioneer of Night Life, celebrated its twentieth anniversary. The Boss turned the occasion into a great national occasion. Poets sang of the people's love for the secret police. The panegyrics went on all through the year, in tandem with the savage destruction of the heroes of the occasion, the old Chekists who had worked with Yagoda. There were mass arrests every night in the luxurious homes of the NKVD. A ring at the door—the occupant is awakened and the man who only yesterday was master of other people's destinies is led out of his apartment. Knowing what their institution was capable of, many did not open up: the nocturnal ring at the door was answered by a shot within. Gorky's friend Pogrebinsky, head of the

NKVD in the city of Gorky, and founder of labor communes for criminals, shot himself, and was followed soon afterward by Kozelsky, a well-known Ukrainian Chekist. Such a listing could be prolonged endlessly. There were innovators in the art of escape. The Moscow Chekist F. Gurov threw himself out of his office window, and jumping was soon all the rage: Chertok, Kamenev's inquisitor, jumped from a twelfth-story balcony as soon as they came for him.

They fell into the street by night, in full view of the occasional dumbfounded passerby. Dying like flies: a pandemic. Many of them must have echoed their chief Yagoda's words: God does exist after all!

The Boss forbade Yezhov to touch Yagoda's prize executioners . . . for the time being. Pending their disappearance, these outstandingly competent executioners were sent, on the Boss's orders, to work for a while in the republics. The Chekist M. Berman (whose brother was in charge of Gulag) had worked for years in Germany, and had tried to organize a revolution there on orders from the Comintern. This Cheka romantic hated Stalin but nonetheless brought back from the West material compromising to Bukharin, whom he loved. Berman was one of the team of investigators who had prepared the case against Zinoviev and Kamenev, and he had played a part in the Ryutin case. Early in 1937 the Boss promoted him to the post of People's Commissar for the Interior in Belorussia. Berman saw danger looming, and exerted himself to "repress" some 85,000 oppositionists, together with their families. But his time had come—"the Moor has done his work"—and the powerful Berman, who possessed all the secrets of the Kremlin trials, went home to the Lyubanka, this time as a prisoner. He had shown particular zeal in destroying rightists. The Boss, whose sense of humor was intact, had Berman shot as a member of a "conspiratorial organization of rightists in the NKVD."

Berman too had discovered that God does exist after all.

It was now the turn of another nocturnal star: the Boss's chief bodyguard, Pauker. Pauker had done a lot to strengthen the Boss's security. Stalin's bodyguard now resembled an army. The route to his nearer dacha was guarded by more than three thousand agents, as well as patrol cars. Whenever his car left the Kremlin the whole twenty-mile route was on a war footing. Pauker sat beside him in the car, ready to take an assassin's bullet in his breast. The Politburo had decided, on Pauker's suggestion, that the Boss should be forbidden even to walk around the Kremlin unguarded. And Stalin, of course, always bowed to Party decisions without a murmur. But the buffoon and lickspittle Pauker was unfortunately a Chekist of the old school. Besides which, crafty Pauker had served all members of the Politburo, including those who had now begun to disappear. He had supplied them with cars, dogs, clothes for their wives, toys for their children, and, unfortunately for him, had become their friend. Pauker, tightly corseted and with the Order of Lenin on his chest, still rode around in his Lincoln, a present from the Boss, but his fate had been decided. He vanished into the darkness quietly and without a trace, following his friends, the mighty Chekists of Dzherzhinsky's day.

The Boss forgot no one, even the legendary organizers of the original Red Terror who had retired from the Cheka: Peters, Latsis, and the famous Latvian riflemen, Lenin's faithful bodyguard, all would be shot.

Into the night went Nikolai Krylenko, the first Bolshevik commander-in-chief, and later the dread state prosecutor who had sent so many to execution—gentlefolk, SRs, and Bolsheviks alike. Krylenko first lost his post as People's Commissar for Justice. But the Boss wanted everyone to know that he was fighting for the life of the faithful commissar who had unflinchingly betrayed so many of his old friends. Stalin therefore telephoned the dacha in which Krylenko was living in fear to say a few kind words. Happy Krylenko slept peacefully, until on one peaceful night he was arrested. Now they could all say God does exist after all.

Krylenko's place as state prosecutor was taken by A. Vyshinsky. This was another of history's jokes. This former enemy of the Bolsheviks, a man who had called for Lenin's arrest in 1917 as a traitor and a German spy, was now accusing the victorious leaders of the Bolshevik Party of betraying Lenin and of spying. This time the charges stuck and all the accused were executed. At the trials Vyshinsky showered insults on the former Bolshevik leaders in a sort of sadistic ecstasy: "stinking heap of human garbage," "wild beasts in human form," "degenerate specimens of the human race," "mad dogs," etc. Vyshinsky's own career to some extent explains his bloodthirsty frenzies and his sinister personality. He had been a Menshevik, but became a Bolshevik in 1920 because only by doing so could an ambitious young man make a career. Orlov (the previously mentioned NKVD general who decided to remain in the West) described in his memoirs his experience of working with Vyshinsky in the public prosecutor's department in the 1920s. Orlov, who hated the man, obviously relished the contempt with which Vyshinsky's old Bolshevik colleagues treated the ex-Menshevik. They despised everything about him, even his "polite manners, recalling those of tsarist officers." Vyshinsky was, however, as Orlov acknowledged, "one of the ablest and best-educated prosecutors."

Throughout the twenties the former Menshevik lived under constant threat of exclusion from the Party. Orlov tells us how Vyshinsky wept in his office on one of several occasions when he was in danger of losing his Party card. Expulsion from the Party would mean the end of his career, and perhaps of his life. We can, then, easily imagine how he hated old Bolsheviks, and what dark passions festered in that ambitious soul. The Boss had, in his own words, "found the man he needed for the job he needed done."

Orlov, in his memoirs, contrasted Lenin's public prosecutor, the honest old Bolshevik N. Krylenko, with Stalin's man, the unprincipled careerist Vyshinsky. The former NKVD general forgot that all the great public trials of the twenties—the wreckers' trials and the trial of the "Industrial Party"—were conducted jointly by Vyshinsky, as presiding judge, and Krylenko as leader for the prosecution. It was from those same old Bolsheviks that Vyshinsky had learned to hold human life cheap.

The dread prosecutor Vyshinsky lived all his life in a torment of fear. He knew that if ever he lost the Boss's favor, his past would be held against him. At every turn he saw reminders of the doom which might be in store for him. Even the dacha in which he lived had belonged to one of those whom the Boss had sent to his death—A. Serebryakov, a member of Lenin's Central Committee. So he served his master slavishly, like a devoted dog.

Stalin gave Vyshinsky the task of formulating new principles of Bolshevik legal procedure. Dzherzhinsky had asked, back in 1918, "What better proof can there be than the accused's confession?" In semiliterate Russia, unaccustomed to the rule of law, the fact that "he admitted it himself" was conclusive. The Boss understood this very well, and all his show trials were based on this "popular principle." Vyshinsky's numerous works are a scholarly exposition of the Boss's ideas: "the confession of the accused is the basis of the case for the prosecution," "the confession of the accused is the empress of proofs." Such were the terms in which Vyshinsky formulated the principles of legal procedure in the "land of socialism."

Throughout 1937 the Boss was busy casting out veterans of the 1905 and 1917 revolutions. M. Spiridonova, B. Kamkov, and other Left SRs, Right SRs, aged survivors of the People's Will Party, anarchists. He brought irreconcilable foes together in the cells: Mensheviks, Bolsheviks, SRs, previously untouched aristocrats. They had fought each other for so many years, only to meet in the same prison. The story is told of a half-mad Kadet who rolled on the floor laughing when he saw this revolutionary Noah's Ark. A bullet in the night would end all their troubles.

He liquidated the famous Society of Former Political Prisoners and Exiles, which was a rallying point for old Bolsheviks. The famous journal *Prison and Exile* was also suppressed. He gave members of the society and the staff of the journal an opportunity to study prison and exile at first hand in the state which he had founded, and to compare them with their tsarist counterparts.

Throughout 1937, the elevator in the House on the Embankment was busy every night, all night. Old Party members arrested included the People's Commissars of Heavy Industry, Finance, Agriculture (two of these), Trade, Communications, War Industry, State Farms and Education, as well as the whole board of the State Bank. Molotov, chairman of the Council of People's Commissars, lost all his vice-chairmen, Kaganovich lost all his railroad chiefs. Nameplates were wrenched off doors in the commissariats, waste paper littered office floors, and younger people were appointed to senior posts.

One of those arrested was Jan Rudzutak, who had tasted all the highest Party offices, including associate membership and full membership of the Politburo. He was tortured, but refused to slander himself and insisted on seeing members of the Politburo. A fascinating feature of the times was that though in the end law counted for nothing, the letter of the law was observed. Since the request had come from a candidate member of the Politburo, the Boss sent Molotov (his usual proxy) to see the battered Rudzutak, fresh from the torture chamber.

In old age, Molotov recalled in an interview that "Rudzutak admitted nothing. He showed strength of character. We—several members of the Politburo—went along to the headquarters of the security services. He complained about the Chekists, said they'd beaten him badly, and thoroughly tormented him."

"Surely you could have spoken up for him—after all, you knew him well," Molotov was asked.

"You couldn't just go by personal impressions. They had proofs. He was one of my deputies. I used to meet him at work, he was pleasant and clever, but at the same time . . . he was always getting mixed up with somebody or other, hell, I mean with women. I couldn't completely vouch for him. He was friends with Antipov and Chubar. We interrogated Chubar—also one of my deputies. . . . He had personal ties with Rykov. Antipov, another of my deputies, and a member of the Central

Committee, testified against him." They would both perish—the denouncer Antipov and Chubar, whom he denounced.

"Was Stalin told?"

"He was." And was, we may be sure, told what he wanted to hear. Men fighting for their lives strained every nerve to condemn their former comrade. That was why Caesar had sent them to him.

Last Days of the Functionaries

Life in the night world was hectic. From dusk to dawn, enemies were flushed out. The following is from a letter written to his wife by E. Shchadenko, a member of the Special Commission for the Liquidation of the Consequences of Sabotage among the Troops of the Kiev Military District: "July 18, 1937. My dear, darling Marusyenka. I am writing to you from the ancient Russian capital, Kiev. I have so much work that I can't away from headquarters before two or three in the morning. The swine have been up to their filthy tricks for years, and we have not only to clear up the results in a matter of weeks, or at most a month, but also to go on from there as quickly as we can." That month Shchadenko personally sent tens of thousands to their deaths.

One doomed Party boss was P. Postyshev, candidate member of the Politburo, who had been so "irresistibly jolly" and "danced (with Molotov!) with such abandon" at the "infinitely kind Joseph's birthday party," as Maria Svanidze noted in her diary. We have recently learned about Postyshev's last days from his son's reminiscences. They enable us to imagine what former Kremlin officials went through on the eve of their destruction.

Postyshev, now fifty years old, had, as leader of the Communist Party of the Ukraine, supported Stalin against all those who had opposed him. But unfortunately for him he had been a member of the Party since 1904 and had connections with all the old Bolsheviks now on the way out. So Postyshev too had to depart into the night. In 1937 in an organized campaign Ukrainian Communists wrote to the Central Committee to inform it of the "unhealthy situation in the Party" and the "conceited" behavior of Postyshev. Postyshev was removed from the Ukraine and sent to run the Kuibyshev province. He did his best, carried out his duties diligently, but to no avail. The old Bolshevik Postyshev failed to realize that no amount of murderous zeal could save him. In fact, when the Boss decided that the time had come, this very zeal would be held against him.

At a plenary meeting of the Central Committee in January 1938

Postyshev's subordinate, the second secretary of the Kuibyshev Provincial Committee, N. Ignatov, was put up to denounce him. His speech gives us an insight into the atmosphere of homicidal madness in the province during those years of terror.

"Comrade Postyshev," said Ignatov, "has acquired a style of his own: he started saying everywhere and anywhere, at the top of his voice, that there are no decent people to be found, that there are enemies everywhere. Postyshev often summoned representatives of district Party committees, picked up a magnifying glass, and began examining schoolchildren's exercise books. The covers were torn off all the exercise books, because Postyshev imagined that he could see a fascist swastika in the ornamental design. All the city and district Party secretaries armed themselves with magnifying glasses. Postyshev dissolved thirty district committees, declaring their members enemies of the people."

Postyshev repented, but was accused by the Boss of "politically damaging and obviously provocative activities." Summing up at the plenary meeting of the Central Committee, the Boss said that "some measures must be taken with regard to Comrade Postyshev. The prevalent opinion is that he should be removed from the panel of candidate members of the Politburo." Postyshev was replaced in the Politburo, and in the Ukraine, by a new protégé of the Boss, Nikita Khrushchev.

There followed days of total isolation. And of waiting. Days during which the unfortunate Postyshev must have realized what his own recent victims had gone through, all those nameless district secretaries, as well as Kamenev, Bukharin, Zinoviev. At this stage, he was evidently summoned by the Party Control Commission and confronted with information about his wife's activities: she had allegedly initiated gatherings of rightists at his apartment. Postyshev was called upon to betray his wife, but he preserved his dignity and defended her. He was expelled from the Party. Then—more waiting. In acknowledgment of his past services the Boss gave him the right to avoid further suffering. "They want me to commit suicide, shoot myself. But I'm not going to be their assistant," Postyshev's younger son recalled being told. The son, a test pilot, had arrived on a visit to his parents on February 21, 1938. "Look," his father went on to say, "this meeting is most probably our last. We shall never see each other again. Your mother and I will be arrested, and there is no coming back. My well-wishers think I've made a mistake, that I shouldn't have tried to save your mother from arrest . . . nor certain others. But a man who sends some other, completely innocent Bolshevik to his death just to save himself should not remain in the ranks of the Party."

Thus spoke Postyshev, who had betrayed so many! That is how the unhappy man wanted his son to remember him. "My mother listened to this long monologue in silence," the son recalled, "then said quietly: 'If they try to make you disown us—disown us, and to hell with them. We won't hold it against you.' Only then did I look into her tear-filled eyes. 'How can you talk like that?' was all I could say."

They were arrested the following night. Postyshev said "I'm ready" and went as he was, in his slippers. He, his wife, and his older son were all shot. His younger son, author of the memoirs, got ten years.

At last it was the legendary P. Dybenko's turn. A member of the first Soviet government, and now an army commander, Dybenko had obeyed the Boss's every order. He had conscientiously betrayed everyone, taken part without demur in the trials of other military leaders who had been his friends, loyally exposed "wreckers," but . . . But now he was accused of being an American spy! The semiliterate army commander tried to defend himself. "I don't know the American language, Comrade Stalin. I beg you to look into it thoroughly," he pleaded in a note to Stalin. But it was all over. This hero of the Revolution, now a craven, heavy-drinking, aging boyar, had not understood the situation. It was not just he who was leaving the scene—the Boss was consigning Dybenko's whole world to oblivion. Marshals Yegorov and Blyukher, who had the misfortune to belong to that same world, were sent into the darkness with him.

Stalin spared only two of them—Voroshilov and Budenny. Budenny, however, encountered serious problems. In July 1937 Yezhov told the Marshal that his wife, the beautiful Mikhailova, a singer at the Bolshoi Theater, faced arrest. The charges against her were typical of that mad time: she was accused of visiting foreign embassies, which put her under suspicion of being a spy. Budenny knew what he had to do. The only way in which he might earn the right to live was by betraying his wife. The intrepid cavalryman, holder of the St. George Cross in the tsar's army, participant in all the wars of the twentieth century, obediently took his wife for questioning to the Lubyanka, from which she was not released. Only after Stalin's death did Budenny write to the public prosecutor's office pleading for his wife's rehabilitation and demonstrating how nonsensical the case against her had been. She returned, and told how she had been the victim of gang rape in the camp. Budenny called her stories crazy.

At the top, the Boss was working tirelessly, looking through endless "lists," with recommended sentences alongside the names of people who had once run the country, or won fame in the world of the arts. I saw these lists when I worked in the President's Archive. Such lists were regularly submitted to the Central Committee for confirmation by Yezhov. The Boss scrupulously observed Party rules. He examined the lists in consultation with his comrades-in-arms. Molotov was his most frequent cosignatory.

He never got tired, reading those thousands of names, and even sometimes added comments of his own. He had a truly diabolical memory. "Comrade Yezhov. Pay attention to pages 9–11. About Vardanyan. He is at present secretary of the Taganrog district Party committee. He is undoubtedly a crypto-Trotskyist." Attention was duly paid, and Vardanyan vanished. He remembered his enemies. Every one of them. But while he mercilessly stepped up the repressions, it was Yezhov who always had to supply proof of the treachery of old Party members. The Boss's role was to resist the evidence, to show surprise that people could sink so low, to call for further inquiry.

One should not make the mistake of taking the Boss seriously, though. In one of his memos, reporting the arrest of yet another batch of Party officials, Yezhov writes that "information on another group of suspects is being checked." This is peremptorily rebuked by the Boss: "You should be arresting, not checking."

Only he, only the Boss, was allowed to play at legality. His servant Yezhov had a job to do: quickly and efficiently destroy the old Party. He was trying his hardest.

On November 12, 1938, Yezhov, writing in haste on scraps of dirty paper (he was short of time—shootings were going on night and day), sent Stalin a list of people arrested on capital charges. It is marked "all 3,167 persons to be shot," and signed by Stalin and Molotov. Occasionally, but not very often, he crossed names off these terrible lists—those of Pasternak and Sholokov, among others. They might still be useful to the Party.

His signature appears on 366 such lists, totaling 44,000 names.

They went meekly to the scaffold, and died fervently praising the Leader. The old Bolshevik Eikhe, who had taken such an enthusiastic part in the repressions himself, accepted all the false accusations leveled at him, and died shouting "Long live Stalin!" Yakir, a Civil War hero denounced as a German spy, wrote in his last letter: "My dear, my own Comrade Stalin! . . . I am dying with words of love for you, the Party, and the country on my lips, and fervently believing in the victory of communism." On this declaration of love, the Boss wrote, "villain and prostitute. Stalin." Afterward he circulated the letter among his associates: "A completely accurate description. Molotov." "For this scum, bastard, and whore there's only one punishment: the death penalty. Kaganovich." (Kaganovich had to show special indignation. Yakir was his friend.)

Madness Born of Blood

At the beginning of 1938 the Bolshoi Theater was making preparations for a state concert. No one slept—the rehearsals went on through the night.

A. Rybin, who had been transferred from Stalin's bodyguard to guard the government box, later wrote that "half of the officers of the government guard were arrested in the theater on the eve of the concert." Rybin lay down for a doze in the course of the nocturnal rehearsal and "woke up to find that more than half of my superior officers were already behind bars. So I became overnight military commandant of the Bolshoi Theater."

In these years of terror, the NKVD went completely mad. Junior officials, seeing their comrades destroyed, decided that their best hope of survival was active involvement. In an excess of zeal they arrested even children as spies. They discovered Trotskyist agents in the most unlikely professions. In Leningrad, for instance, they arrested all the eminent astronomers—almost the whole staff of the Pulkovo Observatory, among them the brilliant young astronomer Nikolai Kozyrev. In the terrible Dmitrov jail, and in the cattle truck that took him to the prison camp, Kozyrev continued his work. He was preoccupied with lunar volcanoes. He was sent to hell—to the camps in the Turukhansk region where "kind Joseph" had once lived in exile. Even in that hell Kozyrev went on thinking and talking about science. One night, in conversation with another prisoner, also an intellectual, he casually remarked that he completely disagreed with Engels's description of Newton as "an inductive ass." Alas, the other intellectual was a stool pigeon, Kozyrev was sent for by the prison authorities, and after a brief ideological debate he was sentenced to death for insulting a classic Marxist. The firing squad was overworked at the time, and he had to take his place in the queue. While he was waiting, Moscow canceled the order to shoot him and contented itself with an extension of his sentence. He continued meditating on lunar volcanoes and after his release became famous for his work on the subject.

Meanwhile, something rather comic but also rather frightening happened to those of the astronomers who were still at liberty. The Boss had finally transformed day into night. He himself did all his work at night, and so the heads of all institutions had to stay awake with him. Late one night the Moscow Planetarium got a telephone call from the Boss's dacha, where the usual midnight junketing was in progress. Comrade Molotov and Comrade Kaganovich had got into an argument. Molotov asserted that the star over the dacha was Orion, Kaganovich identified it as Cassiopeia, and the Boss in his wisdom ordered them to ring the planetarium. Unfortunately, the director, who was keeping vigil, was, unlike his disgraced predecessor, not himself an astronomer, but an NKVD officer. He begged for a little time to ask the astronomers—those of them still left—about the star. To avoid discussing a matter of such moment on the telephone, he sent someone to fetch the eminent astronomer A. Now A. was a friend of the recently arrested Leningrad astronomer Numerov, and while he waited his turn he no longer slept at night. When he heard a car pull up outside he thought the end had come. There was a ring at the door. A terrifying, peremptory ring. A. went to open up—and died of a heart attack in the doorway. The car had to be sent for a second eminent survivor. Astronomer B. heard the car drive up at 2:30 A.M.—the hour at which night life was in full swing. He looked through the window and saw it: the same black car. When they rang the doorbell he had already made up his mind. He was sixty years old, and had no wish to be tortured. He opened the window, and flew toward his beloved stars. Only downward, not upward. It was 5:00 A.M., and they had lost yet another astronomer, when the director discovered the name of the star. He rang the dacha: "Please tell Comrades Molotov and Kaganovich . . ." "There's nobody to tell, they all went to bed long ago," the duty officer said. A writer named Kapler told me this story, laughing heartily. He himself had spent several years in the camps because Stalin's daughter had fallen in love with him.

Many people denounced each other in writing, sometimes simply out of fear, to affirm their loyalty, and not get involved with the night people. Informing became synonymous with good citizenship. Mikoyan, in a speech at a meeting held in the Bolshoi Theater to celebrate the twentieth anniversary of the Cheka, put it like this: "In our country every worker is on the staff of the NKVD."

This was the time when serious consideration was given to the erection on Red Square of a gigantic statue of Pavlik Morozov, the Young Pioneer who had denounced his kulak father. The former seminarist, however, knew the story of Ham, and limited himself to erecting a monument in every park. An enormous number of Pavlik statues were required, and the demand resulted in tragicomedy. The frame used by the sculptor, Viktoria Solomonovich, who specialized in Pavliks, proved unreliable. One of the plaster Morozovs collapsed and killed her with its plaster bugle.

Night Madness

We know of cases in which an enemy hand has skillfully introduced into an ordinary photograph pictures of enemies of the people which are clearly visible if you examine the newspaper or photograph from all angles.
—Bolshevik *magazine, August 1937*

Party secretaries in every oblast armed themselves with magnifying glasses, and many successes were reported. The secretary of the Party committee at the Ivanovo Textile Combine, for instance, took out of production a material it had been making for many years because "with the aid of a magnifying glass he detected a swastika and a Japanese helmet in the design," repeated *Komsomolskaya Pravda* in January 1938.

Wherever he looked, laudable zeal was all that the Boss could see.

Exporting Terror

Stalin was simultaneously cleaning up abroad. The biggest wasp's nest was outside the USSR. At one time he had sent oppositionists abroad, to disqualify them from the political contest; now he wanted them back.

He was compelled, of course, to dismantle the intelligence service, which had such close ties with all those diplomats and Comintern officials. The service had been set up when Zinoviev and Bukharin lorded it over the Comintern, and Yagoda ran the NKVD. Its members must surely fear that their fate would be the same. How could he possibly rely on them? How could he trust them? They must all disappear. He treated them all alike. Summoned to Moscow for promotion, they were suspicious—but they hoped—and went.

Antonov-Ovseenko was recalled from Spain to be appointed People's Commissar of Justice—and was duly appointed, to reassure his colleagues abroad. Lev Karakhan was recalled from Turkey, with an offer of the embassy in Washington. Both were arrested and shot in Moscow. One of Antonov's cellmates remembered that he knew just what was happening when they came to take him for execution: "He said goodbye to us all, took off his jacket and shoes, gave them to us, and went out to be shot half-undressed." Twenty-one years earlier in the Winter Palace—hair down to his shoulders, artist's hat at a rakish angle—he had announced the overthrow of the Provisional Government. Now he was led barefoot to the execution cell.

Karakhan, a former ambassador and Vice-Commissar of Foreign Affairs, was shot in distinguished company, that of Avel Enukidze, former Secretary of the Supreme Central Executive Committee. These two aging Adonises were very fond of the ballet, or, rather, of young ballerinas. Their names were often mentioned together in tales of the court theater's love life. Stalin's arrangement for them to be shot together shows kind Joseph in a playful mood. They were executed on the eve of the Boss's birthday, which had so often been an enjoyable occasion for his friend Enukidze.

The extermination of diplomats and intelligence agents continued throughout 1937. The head of the Soviet intelligence service, Slutsky, was poisoned and given a lavish funeral, so as not to alarm agents in the field. When an agent came home he would be appointed to a different country and would tell colleagues abroad about it. Before taking up his new post he would be sent to some luxurious sanatorium for a well-earned holiday. On his return he would pick up the necessary papers for his new clandestine work, and friends would come to see him off. There would be kisses and farewells. Then, at the very first station into his compartment came visitors. . . .

Rumors of this mass destruction reached agents abroad. They nonetheless went meekly home. Only a handful refused to return. In 1937 two Soviet intelligence officers, Reiss and Krivitsky, defected. Another agent, General Alexander Orlov, shortly followed. His real name was Lev Feldbin. In the second half of the twenties he was a "resident" (spy) in Paris, and in 1933–1935 he operated in Germany, Austria, and Switzerland. In 1936, while the show trials were in progress, Orlov was sent to Spain, where General Franco was fighting, with Hitler's support, against the left-wing Republican government, which was aided by Stalin.

Stalin exploited the Spanish Civil War to the full. Besides supplying Soviet arms to the Republicans, he flooded their army with Soviet "military advisers," genuine or spurious, but in reality mostly NKVD agents. From Spain, Stalin's spies infiltrated other European countries, while in Spain itself they recruited additional agents from among the antifascists. Stalin made Orlov deputy chief military adviser to the Republican army. His official assignment was to organize intelligence and counterintelligence activities and guerrilla warfare behind Franco's lines.

He had a further, unofficial task. Stalin had a secret and extremely important aim in Spain: to eliminate the supporters of Trotsky who had gathered from all over the world to fight for the Spanish revolution. NKVD men, and Comintern agents loyal to Stalin, accused the Trotskyists of espionage and ruthlessly executed them. As the Stalinist spy Sudoplatov said in his memoirs: "When the Spanish Civil War ended there was no room left in the world for Trotsky."

But Orlov's main service was the top-secret assignment which he subsequently described in his book. When General Franco's forces were approaching Madrid, Orlov received an encoded telegram from a certain "Ivan Vasilievich." (Stalin sometimes signed secret telegrams with the Christian name and patronymic of his greatest hero, Ivan the Terrible.) The telegram ordered Orlov to persuade the government of the Spanish Republic to transfer the country's gold reserves to the USSR. His efforts were successful. The gold had been stored in a cave at Cartagena. To the end of his days, Orlov remembered entering the cave and suddenly seeing a mountainous pile of boxes containing six hundred tons of gold. The Boss had insisted in his telegram that there should be no trace of Russian involvement in the export of the gold, and Orlov realized that he had no intention of returning it. Ever thrifty, the Boss obviously regarded the gold as a form of payment by the Republicans for his help in the war. Orlov supervised the export of the gold as "Mr. Blakeston, representative of the National Bank of America."

While all this was happening Orlov carefully read the reports of the Moscow trials in *Pravda*. He realized that they spelled the complete destruction of the old Party. It was not difficult for him, as an old Party member and a GPU officer since 1924, to foresee what his own end might be. So when, in 1938, he was told to return quickly on a Soviet motor vessel, allegedly for secret consultations, he did not hesitate. His hour had come, and, like Reiss and Krivitsky before him, he chose to remain in the West. Knowing how ruthlessly the Boss punished defectors, Orlov wrote to him proposing a deal: if the Boss spared him and his family he undertook to keep secret all that he knew. The Boss did not reply, but acted accordingly, and Orlov survived. He did not publish his book about the secrets of the NKVD, from which I have so frequently quoted, until after Stalin's death.

The Soviet ambassador to Bulgaria, Fyodor Raskolnikov, also refused to return. He later described how, in 1936, he was struck by the extraordinary silence in the Kremlin dining hall: the highly placed functionaries using it were literally afraid to open their mouths, afraid of each other, paralyzed with fear.

Raskolnikov himself, however, also kept very quiet in those days. His wife, M. Kanivez, described in her memoirs how she often woke up in the middle of the night and found her husband sitting hunched over a radio listening to the reports of the trials. He knew very well that the proceedings were a grotesque lie from beginning to end. He knew, for instance, that Pyatakov, who confessed to meeting Trotsky in Norway, had been in Germany at the time in question; Raskolnikov and Pyatakov had, in fact, as Kanivez tells us, been members of the same dinner party. But Raskolnikov said nothing. And suffered torments. Until, in 1937, he found his own *Kronstadt and St. Petersburg in 1917* on the list of forbidden books. Only then did he speak out, in an open letter to Stalin: "Over the main door of the cathedral of Notre Dame there is a statue of St. Denis meekly carrying his own severed head." Refusing to follow St. Denis's example he remained in the West. "You," he wrote, "cultivate power without honesty, and socialism without love for mankind. . . . On various sordid and fraudulent pretenses you have staged trials on charges far more nonsensical than anything in the medieval witch trials of which you know from your seminary textbooks." The Boss must have smiled when he read this letter. Where had "love for mankind" been when sailors, led by the young midshipman Raskolnikov, were killing their officers at Kronstadt? And Stalin's trials were reminiscent not only of "medieval witch trials." There was also, for instance, the trial of the Right Socialist Revolutionaries in 1922, conducted by Raskolnikov's good friend Public Prosecutor Krylenko, at which, on Lenin's insistence, eleven innocent people were sentenced to death.

Like other defectors Raskolnikov was declared an "outlaw." The Boss set up "mobile groups" within the NKVD to carry out sentences on these people. As early as September 1937 Reiss was brutally murdered in Switzerland. Raskolnikov died in Nice in 1939. Officially, the cause of death was pneumonia complicated by meningitis. But it was immediately rumored that he had been poisoned. The Boss could not, after all, leave his insolent letter unanswered.

In February 1941 another defector, Krivitsky, was found in a pool of blood in a Washington hotel room, with a gun beside him. The police announced that he had committed suicide. But Ralph Waldman, Krivitsky's (and also Trotsky's) lawyer, remained convinced that it was murder.

In 1989, working on this book, I kept trying to find one of the former "residents." The Boss seemed to have made a clean sweep. Time went by, and I had found nobody. Then, suddenly, a miracle.

An American Millionaire in a Communal Apartment

One day in 1989 I was being interviewed for a radio program. The conversation got around to Armand Hammer, and I said: "How extraordinary that this American millionaire is the only person mentioned in Lenin's works who is still alive." "You are wrong," the interviewer replied, "there is one other, also, incidentally, a famous old man and also an American millionaire—in the distant past, it's true. I am speaking of Theremin." "Theremin still alive? Impossible! How old can he be?" I remember half-rising from my chair in my excitement. I had already learned a great deal about Theremin.

Soon afterward, I found myself sitting in a Soviet communal apartment on the Lenin Prospect in a room cobwebbed with electrical wiring. Facing me sat a man of ninety-three, perhaps the last of the great men of the twenties still living. In Western encyclopedias the date of his birth is given as 1896, and he is mistakenly said to have died in 1936. That, in fact, was simply the date of his arrest, after which he managed to live on for more than half a century. His ancestors were Huguenots who had fled from France after St. Bartholomew's Day. In the thirties this Russian Frenchman had owned a six-story house in New York—he still remembered the address.

Theremin was just an ordinary genius who had graduated from the Petersburg Conservatoire, from the Military Engineering School, and from the Electro-Technical School. In 1917 he had sided with the Bolsheviks.

As a Bolshevik engineer, Theremin bombarded Lenin with ideas. In the collected works of Lenin there is a letter to Trotsky dated April 4, 1922: "Discuss the possibility of reducing guard duties of Kremlin Kadets by introducing electric signal system. An engineer called Theremin showed us his experiments in the Kremlin." Theremin had invented his electrical "Radio Sentry." It was immediately put on the secret list and installed in the State Bank.

In the twenties he invented the famous "Theremin," an electric musical instrument which sounded like a violin. He exhibited his device at the All-Russia Electrical Congress in 1921 and Lenin once played a tune on it. After a concert attended by Lenin, Theremin's "electromusic" began a triumphant progress round the country. The Theremin was regarded as the instrument of the future. He supplemented the sound with colored lights and a mechanism for reproducing odors. The aged Glazunov and the young Shostakovich both attended his concerts. He went abroad and made successful appearances at the New York Metropolitan Opera House and Carnegie Hall. He performed with the conductor Leopold Stokowski, played duets with Albert Einstein—Theremin on his instrument, Einstein on his famous violin. The Theremin was mass-produced by the thousands, and its inventor became a millionaire.

Only Yagoda knew for whom this strange genius was really working, and why he had gone to America. The GPU had been keeping a watchful eye on him for some time. Yagoda had sent him first, with his Theremin, to an international exhibition in Frankfurt. He was an enormous success. People called him a "second Trotsky" because he threatened to carry out a "world revolution in music" with his instrument. Next, Yagoda dispatched him in the full blaze of his glory to America, where he was to cooperate with the GPU, and regularly pass on interesting information to the embassy. His acquaintances included a number of Jewish physicists, whom he was supposed to sound out as possible collaborators. He got married, and bought a six-story house on 54th Street in New York City. But then he was recalled to Moscow. It was near the end of 1938; not one of his former NKVD acquaintances was still around. Like other "residents" he was accused of being a double agent. But whereas his colleagues had all been shot, he was given what was by the standards of the time a generous sentence—eight years' imprisonment. This was not just a matter of luck. There was no such thing in those days. No, the genius Theremin and his work had remained in the Boss's excellent memory, and he was quickly transferred from a normal prison camp to a *sharashka*. This was one of the Boss's most impressive inventions: a closed research institute in which imprisoned scientists could continue their work. Theremin helped the great Korolev and the famous Tupolev, both prisoners, to develop a radio-controlled, pilotless plane. Then he was taken to another sharashka, where he developed a unique system of remote eavesdropping. This system was called the "Snowstorm," and it earned its incarcerated inventor a Stalin Prize.

Life was like that in Stalin's time: from high honor to prison, from prison to high honor again, back to freedom and daylight. In 1947, thanks to the Boss's clemency, Lev Theremin, Stalin Prize winner, reappeared in Moscow.

As I was leaving his apartment, he said: "I am young. The secret of Dr. Faustus is simple: old age hides when you are working." And he promised to live at least to a hundred.

I did not see him again, but I heard recently that he did not keep his promise. His granddaughter Maria told me about his mysterious end. As his hundredth birthday drew near, perestroika made it possible for him to travel abroad. His triumphal progress took him to Sweden, Holland, and of course France. He visited America. All this time he continued working on new inventions. When he returned in 1993 from one of his excursions, his laboratory had been wrecked, and the archive which he valued more than his life had vanished. The police were powerless. Someone was evidently very interested in the ideas of this strange twentieth-century Dr. Faustus. This was too much for Theremin, and he died, aged ninety-seven, before the year was out.

Purge of the Tower of Babel

In 1937 the Boss felt obliged to destroy Comintern. It was inseparably tied to people whom he had shot as enemies. And here he was playing one of his long chess games. He was contemplating an abrupt change of foreign policy. He had calculated long ago that he needed to ally himself with Hitler. How could he be sure that Comintern, which had fought fascism tooth and nail, would tamely accept an about-face? As he began his bloody purge of Comintern he was already planning to establish an international body in which the very thought of questioning his decisions would seem sacrilegious. Only with a Communist International of that kind would he ever realize his secret objective—the Great Dream. The secret Comintern files give us a glimpse of what happened.

He began the extermination of Comintern at a signal from the head of Comintern itself. In 1937, Dimitrov wrote (or rather found that he had written) a letter to the Central Committee: "The Comintern leadership has screened the whole staff and 100 people altogether have been dismissed as politically insufficiently reliable. . . . Several sections of the Comintern were found to be in the hands of the enemy." The fight against "the enemy" began at once. Comintern became an arena for NKVD operations. An endless series of arrests followed in the first half of 1937—members of the German, Spanish, Yugoslav, Hungarian, Polish, Austrian, Estonian, Latvian, Lithuanian, and other Communist Parties. Bela Kun, the leader of the Hungarian Soviet Republic and a close associate of Zinoviev and Trotsky, was summoned to a meeting of the Comintern's Executive Committee in the spring of 1937. Across the table sat leading Western Communists: Pleck, Togliatti, and representatives of the French Party. The Soviet representative, Manuilsky, stated that according to information supplied by the NKVD, Bela Kun had been recruited by the Romanian intelligence service in 1923. And not one of those present, most of whom had known Kun for years, said that this was insane; not one of them protested or demanded proof. They had passed their exam; they'd won the right to go on living, and to work in the new-style Comintern.

An NKVD car was waiting at the door for Kun. Twelve former commissars of the Hungarian Soviet Republic followed their leader. The Communist Parties of Mexico, Turkey, and Iran also lost their general secretaries without a murmur.

G. Dimitrov now had to prove, from day to day, his own right to live. He served diligently, and succeeded. He authorized the arrest of his own comrades-in-arms in the Bulgarian Communist Party. When some of the Bulgarian leaders protested, his only answer was a helpless gesture and "It's not in my power. It's all in the hands of the NKVD." Yezhov, in his own words, "liquidated Bulgarians like rabbits."

The old Comintern had to vanish completely. Fritz Platten, founder of the Swiss Communist Party, who had organized the return of Lenin, Zinoviev, Radek, and the others to Russia in 1917, was shot. Of the eleven leaders of the Mongolian party only Choibolsan survived. The leaders of the Indian and Korean parties were destroyed. Of the German Communist leadership only Pieck and Ulbricht went unscathed. Yezhov commented in a memorandum that "it would be no exaggeration to say that every German citizen living abroad is a Gestapo agent." A large group of German Communists was handed over to Hitler. Ironically, many of them survived Hitler's camps, while those imprisoned in the land of socialism all perished. Many Italian Communists disappeared into the night. Togliatti's son-in-law was arrested, to keep the Italian leader on his toes. It did.

Leopold Trepper, a Jewish Communist later famous as a Soviet intelligence agent, has described in his memoirs life in Comintern at that time: "In our hostel, where Party activists of all countries lived, no one went to sleep before 3:00 A.M. We waited with our hearts in our mouths. At 3 A.M. precisely, light from automobile headlamps pierced the darkness and swept over the facades of buildings. . . . You were crazy with fear, your guts ached. . . . We stood at the window waiting to see where the NKVD car would stop. . . . When we realized that they were making for the other end of the building we calmed down until the following evening."

Trepper's Jewish Communist friends were also ruthlessly suppressed. The leaders of the Communist Party of Palestine were liquidated one after another. Ephraim Leszinsky, a member of the Central Committee of the Palestine Communist Party, was savagely beaten to make him confess and name his accomplices in espionage. He went mad, and, according to Trepper, banged his head against the wall shouting, "What's that other name I've forgotten? What's that other name?"

Daniel Auerbach, one of organizers of the Communist Party of Palestine, was in the USSR, and in Comintern, in 1937. Trepper writes that "his son and his brother had already perished. But they were a long time coming for Auerbach himself. The agonizing suspense drove him mad. His wife's brother ran about the apartment shouting, 'My God, shall we ever find out what they're arresting us for?' "

Leopold Trepper met Auerbach's wife many years later, in Khrushchev's time. The old woman was hugging a shabby handbag holding the family photographs she had treasured through all her ordeals. She told Trepper that "my husband, my sons, my brother, and my husband's brother were all arrested and killed. I'm the only one who survived. But do you know—in spite of everything I believe in communism."

And in spite of everything, Trepper himself went on working for the USSR. After all that he had gone through, he became a Soviet agent in Germany. He was indignant at the silence of Western Communist leaders. But he had a ready explanation for his own silence. "What could we do? Give up the fight for socialism? We had dedicated our whole lives to it. Protest, try to intervene? We remembered what Dimitrov had said to the poor Bulgarians."

The Boss was familiar with this way of thinking. He had judged them all correctly, and made child's play of destroying the Tower of Babel.

One by one the old Comintern hands disappeared. Stalin left only those who had passed their examination in servility by betraying friends. Another who vanished was M. Gorkic, head of the Yugoslav Communist Party. Josip Tito, future president of Yugoslavia, was his betrayer. In his letter to Dimitrov, Tito said that "nobody in the country knows him, except a few intellectuals. What has happened to him [his arrest] can have no serious consequences for the Party." When Tito visited Moscow in 1938 he found that eight hundred prominent Yugoslav Communists had been arrested. Dimitrov tested his loyalty in long discussions. On this visit Tito had to betray not only his friends but his former wife. She had been arrested as a Gestapo agent, and Tito wrote an explanatory note to the Boss, which is preserved in the Party Archive: "I thought that she was reliable because she was the daughter of a poor working man, and subsequently the wife of a prominent member of the German Communist youth movement, who was sentenced to fifteen years in a German labor camp. . . . I now consider that I was not sufficiently vigilant and this is a big blot on my life. I believe that various people intent on harming our Party may use this against me, and that must be taken into account." Tito need not have worried. By abandoning someone so close to him without demur he had passed his exam, like Kuusinen, Togliatti, Kaganovich, Kalinin, Molotov, and so many others who renounced their nearest and dearest without a murmur. Nothing now stood between Tito and a general secretaryship. And in 1939, when the legendary Yugoslav Communist P. Miletic arrived in Moscow after many years in prison, Stalin showed his preference for Miletic's tried and tested rival. The hero and martyr Miletic disappeared into the cellars of the NKVD.

A new Comintern was born. In 1939 this well-drilled and absolutely docile body would approve the Soviet pact with Hitler, and, a little later, when the Boss found it necessary, it would obediently self-destruct.

20

TENDING TERROR'S SACRED FLAME

The madness of Terror, when the arrest of each "enemy of the people" was followed by the arrests of all his relatives and acquaintances, when people were picked up for a careless word, or a misprint in a newspaper, when textile designs were scrutinized through magnifying glasses—all this, needless to say, served good practical purposes. Every arrest helped to build the magnificent Bonfire of Fear. Every arrest threw a little chip of its own onto the mysterious nocturnal fire which needed to burn forever; only constant fear kept the country and the system stable. (One day the collapse of the Communist empire would confirm this.) The Boss had to tend the sacred fire unremittingly, to keep the flames leaping higher and higher. However fiercely it burned, it stopped short of reducing the country to ashes.

Twentieth-Century Slaves

The Terror, originally directed against the Party, suddenly turned upon the masses. The families of enemies of the people, their acquaintances, acquaintances of their acquaintances—endless chains of people were turned into convicts. In the hands of the army, mass terror consigned thousands of physically strong people to the camps. The Boss now had at his disposal the army of unpaid laborers of which Trotsky once dreamed. Stalin could carry out the most incredible projects at the lowest possible cost. His prisoners built the great White Sea–Baltic and Moscow-Volga Canals, laid roads in impassable places, erected factories beyond the Arctic Circle. In the thirties a considerable proportion of the country's copper, gold, coal, and timber was produced by this secret unpaid labor force. Before any major project was begun, the NKVD received direct instructions about the number of arrests it needed to make. The Boss himself devised the ruthless regime of the camps, and kept a close watch on those whom he had ordered into the night.

The everyday reality of the camps was hideous. In Kolyma, in the northeast corner of Asiatic Russia, a godforsaken region of marshland and permafrost, a wild beast called Garanin was let loose as commandant. He used to parade sick prisoners who were suspected of malingering, walk along the ranks and shoot them point blank, while camp guards followed with a change of pistols. The bodies were stacked by the camp gates, and parties of prisoners on their way to work were told they'd get the same treatment if they tried slacking. I shall not attempt to describe the hell of Gulag. Volumes have been written about its horrors. The banks of Russia's canals are studded with the graves of their nameless constructors. After all these years, communal graves are sometimes waterlogged by the spring floods and human bones rise out of the ground to confront us.

The Boss valued the labor of these slaves of the land of socialism very highly. On August 25, 1938, when the Terror was ebbing, the Presidium of the Supreme Soviet discussed the possibility of early release for prisoners who had distinguished themselves in the camps. But the Boss said, "Can't we find some other way of showing appreciation of their work? From the point of view of the economy it is a bad idea. The best people would be freed, and those left would be the worst." In 1939 he decreed through the Presidium that "a convicted person must serve the full sentence." "The best" were left to die slowly.

"Let Them Eat Cake—but Don't Let Them Out"

The arrest of scientists and technicians was an inspired part of the Boss's plan to provide cheap labor. Molotov touches on this in the book of conversations with him that the poet Chuyev published. Asked why brilliant engineers like Tupolev, Stechkin, and Korolev were arrested, he answered, "People have said all sorts of things. . . . Tupolev belonged to that part of the intelligentsia which the Soviet regime very much needed. But at heart they were very much against us, it was as natural as breathing to them. So a way was found around the problem. The Tupolevs were put behind bars and the Chekists were told to make sure they had the best possible conditions. Let them eat cake, but don't let them out. Let them work, construct things the country needs, things for the army."

I had heard of the Boss's secret plan for scientists and technicians, and had always thought that it was just another myth. But the fundamentals of the plan emerge quite clearly from Molotov's account. Intellectuals were at heart against the Soviet regime. They could therefore easily be drawn into anti-Soviet activity. For that they were liable to be liquidated. Obviously, the best of them should, for their own sake, be isolated. Once isolated, they should be given perfect working conditions: food, books, and even visits from women. Bringing these intellectuals together created a favorable work situation and made it easier to keep them under observation. Most important of all, isolation ensured maximum secrecy. This was very important for military reasons. Determined as he was to realize the Great Dream, he wanted the country's best minds to be working day and night, with no distractions, and under strict control, on its military needs. This was why he had invented the sharashki, scientific institutes staffed by convicts. Most of the country's outstanding technical brains—engineers and scientists—were destined to end up sooner or later in the sharashki. The intelligentsia were gradually rehoused in these prison institutes. The first rehabilitation program (when he decided to release a number of scientists to show that he was trying to combat illegality) and then the war prevented complete realization of the plan. But he would reactivate it after the war.

The Boss had given a great deal of thought to the creative intelligentsia. [Terror was meant to transmute secret hostility with its sacred fire.] He began his 1936 campaign with an abrupt attack on culture. A "restructuring of the cultural front" was proclaimed. Art must henceforward be comprehensible to the toiling millions. The remnants of the avant-garde were smashed. Shostakovich was lambasted. Under the headline "Chaos instead of Music" the January 28 *Pravda* published an annihilating criticism of his opera *Lady Macbeth of Mtsensk*. Everybody understood who was behind this unsigned article. All Party organizations, and indeed the whole country, were required to study it. Shostakovich's name was on everybody's lips. Standing in the shops, or in the Metro, people discussed the noxious composer. Workers met to condemn in the same breath enemies of the people and an opera of which they knew nothing. The bombardment continued all through 1936. Party critics wrote menacing articles against non-Party writers. *Literurnaya Gazeta* advised Pasternak to "ask himself where his present path of parochial arrogance and conceited preciosity is leading him." The rumor in Moscow was that the poet's days of freedom were numbered. A *Pravda* review, "External Brilliance—Spurious Content," demolished Bulgakov's play *Molière*. His wife wrote in her diary: "Misha's lot is clear to me. He will be alone and hunted till the end of his days."

Ideological terror persisted throughout 1936. "We saw the New Year in at home," Bulgakov's wife wrote. "We made a lot of noise smashing cups inscribed '1936.' God grant that 1937 will be happier than the past year."

In 1937 the Boss called a halt. The Party administrators of the arts, the Party critics had done their job. The ideological bombardment had left the artistic intelligentsia scared.

Now the dread accusers were to be destroyed themselves. Under the plan for the destruction of the old Party, all the former leaders of RAPP (the Russian Association of Proletarian Writers), the group that had persecuted Pasternak and Bulgakov, perished one after another in 1937–1938. The old Bolshevik Kerzhentsev, who had been in charge of cultural matters in the Central Committee, was also shot. Two of Bulgakov's old enemies, Lev Bezymensky and A. Afinogenov, were expelled from the Party.

The Party critics disappeared one by one into the night. Bulgakov's wife was in raptures as she listed in her diary each day those who had "got it in the neck": "Article after article in *Pravda,* they go flying head over heels, one after another. It is comforting to think that Nemesis exists after all. . . . The day of reckoning has arrived: very bad things about Kirshon [an important figure in Soviet theater]. . . . As we were walking along the lane Olesha caught up with us. He urged Misha to go to the meeting of Moscow playwrights which begins today. They are going to give Kirshon his deserts. [Bulgakov, however, refused to persecute the persecutors.] . . . Everybody who reads the papers thinks that Misha's position must change for the better." That is how she felt about 1937. And many people in Moscow were glad to think that the Terror, *this* Terror, spelled the end of that hateful and bloody revolution.

A Novel about the Boss

"Misha read his novel about Voland," Bulgakov's wife wrote in her diary on May 15. Bulgakov's novel *The Master and Margarita,* published only after the author's death, would become the favorite novel of the Russian intelligentsia. Its main hero is the Devil, operating under the name Voland. But this is an unusual kind of Devil. The epigraph to the novel is from Goethe's *Faust:*

> Say at last—who art thou?
> That power I serve
> Which wills forever evil
> Yet does forever good.

At large in Soviet Moscow, Voland visits the fullness of his diabolical power on those in authority who act illegally. He also deals with the persecutors of a certain writer whom Bulgakov calls "the Master." Bulgakov wrote his novel under the burning summer sun of 1936 and 1937, during the Moscow show trials, when another devil was destroying the Devil's Party, and Bulgakov's literary enemies were perishing one after another. It is not difficult to see who was the model for Voland.

Bulgakov, like all writers of note, was kept under continuous surveillance by the NKVD and was surrounded by informers. The omniscient Boss must, therefore, have known about the strange novel, parts of which were often read aloud to Bulgakov's guests. But the novelist's fascination with the activities of his strange devil evidently pleased the Boss. Perhaps this was what first gave him the idea of commissioning a play about himself from Mikhail Bulgakov?

A. Bulgakova's record of the horrors of 1937 continues: "June 6. Read *Pravda*. Rushed to wake Misha. . . . They've arrested Arkadiev, the manager of the Moscow Arts Theater. . . . The artist Dmitriev (to whom he had promised a new apartment) was laughing, telling how Knipper, Chekhov's widow, quite speechless, thrust the paper with the piece about Arkadiev under his nose. . . . Misha kept imitating Knipper, in a white peignoir, wringing her hands."

It had become a laughing matter! Only Chekhov's widow, with her nineteenth-century mentality, was still horrified by executions. The new generation of intellectuals preferred to laugh. And in that laughter, from the author of the novel about Voland, there was something diabolical.

Bulgakova's diary goes on describing all-night parties, practical jokes, excursions to the Moscow river, canoeing, while all around her people were disappearing in the "unbearable heat" of that bloody summer.

But however hard they tried to suppress their dread of the interminable vengeance exacted by Voland, however hard they tried to persuade themselves that only "nasty people" were perishing, it was then that the fun-loving Bulgakov became, as his wife wrote in her diary, "afraid again to walk in the streets."

The writers sacrificed that year were mainly the Party hacks who ran RAPP. Bulgakov himself was left alone, as were Shostakovich and Sholokhov. Nor would the Boss authorize Pasternak's arrest. The newspapers at the time were printing an endless series of enthusiastic responses from Soviet writers to the show trials. Pasternak alone dared to refuse to add his signature to a demand for the execution of the "vermin, wreckers, and spies." His pregnant wife implored him to sign, but he was adamant. And yet the Boss permitted him to live. There was plenty of time.

Mandelstam he did not forgive. Mandelstam tried to defend himself, even writing verses extolling the Leader, but the ex-poet who had written such poor verses could neither accept nor forget certain good ones. Stalin was purging the country, and could not leave in it a man who had openly insulted him. Mandelstam was arrested, for the second time, on May Day, when the drunken merrymaking was in full swing.

There are many strange legends about Mandelstam's death. The truth is this: A madman, as poets always have been, an overgrown child in the camp, he quickly turned into a living corpse. He caught typhus, and did not survive it. A fellow prisoner, Yuri Moiseenko, told the story: "He was sick with typhus for four days, lying motionless in bed, his nose (pardon me) was running, and he didn't wipe it, just lay there with his eyes open, not saying anything, his left eyelid kept twitching, he said nothing, but his eye kept winking. Maybe it was from his thoughts, he couldn't go on living without thinking of something." That was how the greatest Russian poet of the century departed: silently, in pain, lying in the filth of a prison camp. Bulgakov's wife had noted Mandelstam's arrest in her diary, without comment. She was happy at the time: Misha had been commissioned to write a play about Stalin.

Hurrah for Terror!

Many Russian émigrés supposed that the Great Terror spelled the end of revolution. They remembered V. Shulgin's prophecy, from his book, *1920:* "Lenin and Trotsky cannot renounce socialism. They must carry that burden to the last. Then someone else will come along. He will be truly Red in strength of will, and truly White in the objectives he pursues. He will be a Bolshevik in energy, and a nationalist by conviction." G. Fedotov wrote in the magazine *Sovremennye Zapiski* (Contemporary Notes) in 1937: "This is a real counterrevolution, carried out from above. . . . The Marxist symbols have not yet been abolished, and they obscure the reality: that Stalin is indeed a Red tsar."

At about this time the eminent writer Kuprin returned from emigration. Prokofiev also opted to return to "Bolshevizia" for good. Shortly after his arrival he composed his ballet *Romeo and Juliet* and *Peter and the Wolf.* But terror soon teaches people how to behave. Before 1937 was over he was writing his *Cantata for the Twentieth Anniversary of October,* on texts from Marx, Lenin, and Stalin. In 1939 Prokofiev met a young girl named Mira Mendelson, and married her after a whirlwind romance. The Boss was reassured. Now Prokofiev was securely hooked.

Apart from ideological considerations, there was one other reason—

simple and terrible—for approving the Terror. Voland, in Bulgakov's novel, looks at the Moscow crowd and says with a sad smile, "Just ordinary people—only—the housing problem has corrupted them."

The population of Moscow huddled together in overcrowded rooms. With every arrest a little extra "living space" became vacant. Happily moving into a new home, people told themselves that the former occupants had deserved what they got. The actress Vera Yureneva remembered moving into an apartment where the kettle was still warm on the stove. The families of those arrested often had no time to collect their belongings before vacating their homes. Where the Boss was sending them, everything was provided by the government.

Relatives of "Enemies of the People"

Stalin was constructing a homogeneous society of "contented" citizens. This meant solving the problem of what to do with the families of "enemies." In the idyllic days of the first trials there was no difficulty: wife and children publicly branded husband and father as an enemy of the people and disowned him. But Stalin had been reared in the Caucasus, where the blood feud was a living tradition, and he was afraid that he might be rearing his own future assassins. As always, he found a revolutionary solution. At Yezhov's (and not, of course, the Boss's) suggestion, the Politburo adopted a secret resolution on July 5, 1937. I have read it in the President's Archive. The wives of convicted enemies of the people were sent to prison camps for a term of five to eight years. Children under the age of fifteen were cared for by the state (that is, they were consigned to a dreadful state orphanage). As for children over fifteen, each case was "decided individually"—they too were sent to the camps.

This was the beginning of a second destruction of the aristocracy: the first was the tsarist aristocracy after 1917; this time it was the Soviet aristocracy. In June 1937 after Gamarnik's suicide his wife and daughter were banished to Astrakhan, together with the families of Tukhachevsky, Uborevich, and the other army commanders. Shortly afterward, their wives were all arrested, and their children sent to the Astrakhan orphanage. Mirra Uborevich, Veta Gamarnik, and Sveta Tukhachevskaya were only little children, and they had been used to quite a different life, with housekeepers and nannies. This was when P. Stukalov, Komsomol secretary in the Kursk oblast, called on the youth movement to expel children of enemies of the people from its ranks, urging his audience to "keep your hatred on the boil, let your hand not tremble." We can easily imagine how these unfortunate children were treated in the orphanage.

Adolescents whom both Lenin and Koba had once petted—the children of Lenin's comrades-in-arms Zinoviev and Kamenev—were arrested, and all perished in prison.

Molotov was once questioned about this period by an interviewer:

> *Q.* Khrushchev said this about you. They brought a list of women sentenced to ten years. Molotov crossed out the sentence next to one name and wrote "highest penalty."
>
> *A.* There was such an occasion.
>
> *Q.* Who was the woman?
>
> *A.* That is unimportant. . . . They had to be isolated to some extent. As it was, they spread all sorts of complaints and unnecessary fuss and demoralization.

We see indeed that the hand did not tremble.

It was high time for the Boss to surrender his own kinsfolk.

Maria Svanidze was still keeping her diary. But with gaps. By now her husband's colleagues in the State Bank had all been imprisoned. Old acquaintances—Budu Mdivani, Orkhelashvili, Eliava—had also been sent out into the night. But Maria was still full of praise for the vigilance of kind Joseph: "27.8.37. No letup in the removal of well-known people. . . . I often walk along the street, look into people's faces, and think 'where are they hiding?' Millions of people whose social position, upbringing, and psychology made it impossible for them to accept the Soviet system, somehow managed to disguise themselves. . . . Now, twenty years after the revolution, these chameleons have been exposed in all their falsity." She had to edit her diary, crossing out the names of vanished acquaintances and noting in the margin "swine lie beneath these crosses." For whom was this intended? For *them*, of course. If she should be arrested she could prove that she had disowned people she once knew. One of her last entries was such a disavowal. The final pages of the diary have been torn out. Perhaps kind Joseph was given the diary after her arrest, and did a little work on it, or perhaps she censored it herself, when she saw that arrest was inevitable. I found traces of the final pages in a little scratch pad she kept with the diary. There, she had ventured to note that on November 21 Alyosha had waited in vain for an audience in the Kremlin, and that on the 22nd he had "been seen," but that it had been "unpleasant." Evidently, kind Joseph had turned him away on the 21st, and on the following day given him the unpleasant news that it was getting more difficult all the time to defend him, when so many of his acquaintances had been arrested. A cryptic note by Maria dated December 7 reads: "evening, Kremlin discussed work." Evidently Alyosha had asked to be transferred, since all his colleagues had been removed. On the 12th she was "in the country with Zhenya [Alliluyeva, Stalin's mistress, his wife Nadyn's sister-in-law]." She believed that Zhenya had some influence on her terrible lover, and of course asked her to "put in a word." The 21st was Joseph's birthday. She went to the hairdresser's—but for the first time she was not invited to the party. After that, we find nothing but blank pages in her diary.

Instead of Kind Joseph's Birthday Party

Kira Alliluyeva-Politkovskaya, the niece of Stalin's wife Nadya, wrote in her memoirs: "In 1937 we moved to another apartment in the House on the Embankment. [So many splendid apartments there were then becoming vacant.] We had a housewarming party. Alyosha Svanidze and his wife, Maria Anisimovna came. Our entrances were next to each other. After the housewarming she put on an overcoat over her velvet dress and they went home. Two or three hours later their son Tolik ran in, white in the face, and said 'Evgenia Alexandrovna, did you know Mama's been arrested? They came and took Mama, and Papa.' . . . The search went on till morning . . . they sealed the apartment, there was nobody there, they'd taken them all to prison. We were shattered, Papa was stunned."

According to records in the President's Archive Alyosha was sentenced to death by shooting on December 4, 1940. The sentence was commuted to fifteen years' imprisonment in January 1941. That was the Boss's decision. But on August 20, 1941, shortly after Hitler invaded, Alyosha Svanidze was shot. Maria Svanidze herself was shot on March 3, 1942.

Why? We shall return to this story later.

The inoffensive Pavel's turn had come. His daughter Alliluyeva-Politkovskaya tells us: "When they started arresting people Papa was very upset, because so many friends, people he had worked with, were jailed. He would speak to Stalin, they would be released. Stalin obviously got tired of this. We have always suspected that Papa was killed . . . I came home from school one day and saw Mama, Grandpa, and all of them in tears. Grandpa put his arms around me and said, 'Kira, we have a great sorrow—your papa has died.' I was petrified. Papa was only forty-four. He had died so suddenly. He had got home the night before from his holiday in Sochi, had drunk coffee and eaten a hardboiled egg the next morning, and—at two o'clock there was a call from his office: 'What did you give your husband to eat? He's feeling sick.' Mama wanted to go to him, but was told not to—'We'll get him to the Kremlyovka [Kremlin Clinic] right away,' and by the time they telephoned to say that she could come Papa was already dead. The doctor said, 'He kept asking why Zhenya didn't come.' They obviously didn't want her there, they were afraid he might tell her something. Mama felt that there was something suspicious about it."

In his private archive the Boss kept a most curious postmortem report on Pavel: "2.11.38. P. Alliluyev's death was caused by paralysis of a diseased heart. According to those around him Comrade Alliluyev felt well when he returned from Sochi on 1.11.38, and was lively and cheerful. On the morning of November 2 he arrived at work in the same good mood. At 1100 hours he suddenly felt ill, vomited, and was in a semiconscious state. At 1300 hours a doctor on the staff of the Kremlin Clinic was called, and she had him taken there. When he was admitted he was unconscious, cyanotic, and apparently dying. The patient did not recover consciousness, and death occurred twenty minutes later." The same "cyanosis" and vomiting would be observed when Nadezhda Krupskaya died just a few months later.

Alliluyeva-Politkovskaya wrote that "Papa was buried with great ceremony. His coffin stood where Nadezhda Sergeevna's [Stalin's wife] had once stood. He was so beautiful. He had just returned from Sochi, and was sunburned. His eyelashes were so long."

The unhappy Zhenya understood the meaning behind her husband's death only too well. That was evidently why she remarried in such a hurry—to escape her frightening admirer. How she must have reproached herself!

Next it was Redens's turn—the husband of Nadya's older sister Anna. He had worked with Yagoda, and had been one of Yezhov's deputies. When those two ceased to exist, he was posted to Kazakhstan, where he was a paragon of ferocity in the hunt for "enemies." His fate, however, had been decided. The Boss intended to pick off this family one at a time. They were too closely connected with the exterminated Party, and with the life of the long-vanished Koba.

Vasily Stalin wrote in a letter to Khrushchev: "When Beria spoke of arresting Redens, Comrade Stalin protested sharply. . . . But Beria was supported by Malenkov. And Comrade Stalin said, 'look into it very carefully . . . I don't believe Redens is an enemy.' " Stalin's son completely missed the point. Beria, like all those around Vasya's father, had only one duty—to understand what the Boss really wanted. If they hadn't understood they would never have dared arrest Redens. But kind Stalin could not consent immediately. Their duty was to persist. They did—playing their part in this theater of the absurd, working hard to convince the Leader that his close relative was a spy!

Redens was shortly recalled to Moscow and arrested. His wife, Anna Alliluyeva, asked kind Joseph to see her. But he told Vasya, who brought the message, "I was mistaken in Redens. I won't see Anna Sergeevna. Don't ask me." And Redens was shot.

21

THE TURN

As 1937 drew to a close Stalin could look back to the beginning, a mere twenty years before, when the Promised Land of Socialism had seemed so near. A few years later it had seemed unattainable. Now he had set foot in that land. He had realized all the dreams of the God Lenin. In the economy, the private sector had been abolished, capitalism was finished forever, the countryside was collectivized. He had manhandled a miserable agrarian country into industrialization. Modern mills and factories had been built. He had concentrated unprecedented productive forces in the hands of the new state. He had a mighty army. A young and united army. An army of unquestionable loyalty. At the head of the state stood the Party, sole ruler and utterly unopposed. In this tamed country, no one would dare challenge its rule. And with all this, he had given his docile people the feeling that they were victors. His society was united as no other had ever been. Now he could concentrate on realizing the Great Dream. If those whom he had liquidated were true Leninists, they would soon have to forgive him for their deaths.

In talking to the makers of the film *Ivan the Terrible,* Stalin said to Eisenstein, "One of Tsar Ivan the Terrible's mistakes was that he did not finish off the five great feudal families." Stalin would not repeat his favorite tsar's mistake. He would kill as many as necessary. But the Keeper of the Sacred Flame of Terror knew that it was time for a pause. The country could stand no more. It might burn itself out.

All this time the NKVD had been cultivating the myth that Stalin knew nothing about Night Life. Innumerable spies who had insinuated themselves into the NKVD concealed the Terror from Stalin. The intelligentsia tried hard to believe this fable, to ease their consciences. They fawned on him and flattered him, but did not want to lose their self-respect. Pasternak, for instance, said to Ehrenburg, "If only somebody would tell Stalin about this," and Meyerhold often said, "They keep all this from Stalin."

A number of similar remarks are on record in the Party

Archive. Here is People's Commissar F. Stebnev: "It looks as if they are deliberately destroying the Party cadres. I'm willing to bet my life Joseph Vissarionovich doesn't know about it."

It was time to buttress the myth with solid "proof." This meant that Yezhov's turn had come. At the end of 1939 A. Zhuralev, head of one of the NKVD's main departments, put it on record that he had frequently reported to Yezhov the suspicious behavior of NKVD personnel who persecuted innocent people, and that Yezhov had ignored him. Zhuralev's statement was immediately discussed by the Politburo. Kind Joseph was, of course, indignant. A Politburo commission was set up, and Yezhov was severely criticized in its report. In the Boss's office his former favorite wrote a contrite letter: "I give my word as a Bolshevik that I will give due attention to my errors." But the inspection of the NKVD was already well under way. Just as Yezhov had once assessed the performance of the doomed Yagoda, so now Lavrenti Beria, summoned for the purpose from Georgia, would look into Yezhov.

Yet Another "Double Agent"

As a humble official in the Baku Soviet, Beria had caught the eye of Bagirov, head of the Cheka in Azerbaijan, who invited him to join that organization. On the Cheka's orders Beria made contact with the intelligence services of the Azerbaijani nationalists. He became a "double agent" and carried out important assignments. Molotov wrote that he saw the young Beria in Lenin's office. Under the Boss, Beria rose rapidly. He became head of the GPU in Georgia, and then, in 1931, First Secretary of the Georgian Central Committee. In December 1938 the Boss appointed him head of the NKVD. But Stalin was in no hurry to declare the Terror at an end. Yezhov was slow-marched to the grave. For some time he remained secretary of the Central Committee and chairman of the Commission of Party Control, while his assistants were arrested one after another. Once the Boss's most publicized comrade-in-arms, he was no longer mentioned in the newspapers. Nowadays Yezhov stole quietly into his office and sat at his desk all day long in a state of prostration. His portrait still hung in every institution, even in the Central Committee building, but no one now entered his office. He was shunned like the plague, one of the living dead. It was his turn now to learn that God does exist.

In March 1939, the Party held its Eighteenth Congress. The kind Boss spoke candidly about "serious mistakes" on the part of the NKVD—more mistakes, he said, than should have been expected. The country rejoiced, celebrating this latest warm spell. Stalin's new aide Zhdanov made the Congress laugh with examples of the insane things done during the Terror: "A doctor was asked for a certificate. 'Because of the state of his health Comrade So-and-so is not to be utilized by any class enemy for his own ends.' " The Congress laughed merrily. Madmen laughing at madness.

At the Congress the new Party paraded for inspection, the Party he had created. The Boss announced the results of the Terror. Half a million new appointments had been made to responsible posts in the state and the Party. In the higher ranks of the Party 293 out of 333 regional Party leaders were new appointments. Ninety percent of leading personnel were under forty years of age. The Boss's new comrades moved up to replace Ilyich's exterminated comrades. Two short, fat men had been elevated: forty-three-year-old Andrei Zhdanov, son of a tsarist inspector of public schools and Kirov's successor in Leningrad, and forty-five-year-old Nikita Khrushchev, who had replaced Postyshev in the Ukraine. But Molotov remained the Boss's most trusted aide.

The new Party broke previous records in homage to their God on earth. "The genius of the modern era," "the wisest man of the epoch," as he was called at the Congress, was henceforward always greeted by an audience on its feet. There was now a prescribed ritual for the Boss's entrances. One stenographic record of the Congress is typical: "All the delegates, standing, greet Comrade Stalin, with a prolonged ovation. Shouts of 'Hurrah,' 'Long live Comrade Stalin,' 'Hurrah for the great Stalin,' 'Hurrah for our beloved Stalin,' etc."

Stalin began openly introducing more of the trappings of the old empire. Those attending a GPU anniversary celebration in the Bolshoi Theater were startled to see a group of Cossack headmen in a box. What astonished the audience was that their uniform was that worn in tsarist times, with gold and silver aiguillettes. The reappearance of the Cossacks, a major symbol of the overthrown empire, was significant. One of the old Party members who had miraculously survived said to his neighbor, "This is their handiwork," and bent his head so that everyone could see the scar made by a Cossack saber.

New history textbooks also appeared, propounding ideas which must have made earlier revolutionaries turn in their graves. All the conquests of the Russian tsars were said to have had a progressive significance and to have been in the best interests of the conquered peoples! For the first time since October 1917, textbooks contained a long list of progressive tsars, princes, and military leaders.

An empire was rising on the grave of the old Party. An atheist empire, without a god, but with a Boss.

Appropriately, Lenin's widow died shortly before the Eighteenth Congress, the new Party's first. During the Eighteenth Congress the Boss need see none but pleasant faces.

Krupskaya may in fact have been helped to die. The Party Archive holds the "history of Comrade Krupskaya's illness," which is now declassified. I read there that on January 13, 1939, "Comrade Krupskaya was examined by Prof. Gautier F. A. and an irregularity of pulse and shortage of breath were noted. . . . Digalen was prescribed, but Krupskaya refused to take it, stating that her bowels were too sensitive."

It is likely that she was afraid by now to take any of their medicine. She had good reason. A little more than a month later Krupskaya was admitted to the Kremlin Clinic with a sudden attack of appendicitis. She died on February 27, 1939. The death certificate is very curious: "The illness began with severe pains throughout the abdomen, accompanied by repeated vomiting, a very fast pulse, and cyanosis of the nose and the extremities . . . cardiac arrest set in and Comrade Krupskaya died."

As in Pavel Alliluyeva's case, the doctors had to account directly to the Boss. He kept their final report in his personal archive: "Death followed a fall in the level of cardiac activity resulting from toxicosis caused by necrosis of part of the blind gut with consequent peritonitis."

Members of the Politburo acted as her pallbearers, led by kind Joseph. Behind the coffin walked the old Bolsheviks. . . . the few members of Lenin's Party whom Stalin had left as exhibits. He did permit himself an occasional weakness. Among the crowd escorting Lenin's widow was Aron Solts, the same Aron Solts with whom Koba had once shared a bed in Petrograd. Some people called Solts the conscience of the Party. During the famine this asthmatic Jew had been responsible for distributing foodstuffs. One day, some workers, driven to despair by their miserable rations, went to his house to inspect his own stocks. All they found was two frozen potatoes. At the height of the purge in 1937 this same Solts had spoken out in public against Vyshinsky. He was dragged from the platform, but the Boss did not touch him. When a woman related to him was imprisoned, Solts wrote a sharp letter. Again the Boss gave orders that he was not to be touched: he was merely put in a psychiatric hospital for a month. Once, on the anniversary of the October Revolution, Solts was called on to give a talk at the Museum of the Revolution. He told his audience that "those were the days when we knew nothing about Stalin." Once again, he was not touched—but those who had invited him were cruelly punished. His old acquaintance Koba allowed him to die his own death. Sick and demented, Solts wrote down endless columns of figures before he died. The writer Trifonov thought that he had been writing something important in underground code. Those pages vanished after his death. The Boss had still not forgotten him.

To go with the new Party, the country was given a new Party history. In 1938 the *Short Course in the History of the Communist Party of the Soviet Union,* Stalin's New Testament, was published in millions of copies. It told the story of the advent of the God Stalin. It was also a thriller, in which the leaders of the vanished party were shown to have been secret traitors and spies: "These midges forgot that the master of the Soviet land is the Soviet people, and that Messrs. Rykov, Zinoviev, Kamenev & Co. were only temporary servants of the state. . . . The despicable lackeys of the fascists forgot that the Soviet government had only to raise its little finger for them to vanish without trace." In this book we hear Stalin's furious voice and feel the terrible energy of his hatred.

THE FIRST REHABILITATIONS

In April 1939 Yezhov disappeared. The rehabilitation of people unjustly condemned had already begun. The kind Boss freed 327,000 people, among them many military men. When Konstantin Rokossovsky, a future marshal, left prison, all his teeth had been knocked out. He, future army General Gorbatov, and a number of others who were to lead the Soviet armies in the Second World War, were the lucky beneficiaries of this "First Rehabilitation," as it was popularly known. The aircraft designers Tupolev and Polikarpov, the microbiologist A. Zilber, and other eminent engineers and scientists were also released.

The kind tsar had pardoned them all, the just tsar who saw and understood everything. He enjoyed that role. Sometimes. In the dangerous days when Koba was a terrorist, his friend Sergei Kavtaradze had risked his own life to help him hide from the security police. In the twenties Kavtaradze had been head of the Georgian government, and had then become a prominent oppositionist. After Kirov's assassination he had been banished to Kazakhstan. From there he wrote a penitent letter to his friend Koba. It was returned to him. As might be expected, Kavtaradze and his wife were arrested in 1936. One of the charges against them was that they had planned to assassinate Comrade Stalin—whose life they had once saved. Kavtaradze was sentenced to be shot. His little daughter Maya, a Young Pioneer, wrote repeatedly to the Father of all Soviet Children, telling him that her father was innocent. More than a year went by, and Kavtaradze was still in the death cell. Suddenly, he was taken to Beria's office. His wife, greatly changed by her spell in a prison camp, was waiting there for him. On the Boss's orders they were both set free. Stalin made Kavtaradze a Vice-Commissar of Foreign Affairs. During the war he would take part in the Yalta and Potsdam conferences.

After the Boss's death Kavtaradze started to tell a remarkable story. One day, after a meeting, Koba took him home to his dacha. It was a stuffy July evening. They strolled around the garden before dinner, with the Boss crooning in his light tenor a favorite Georgian song, "Suliko." "I sought my sweetheart's grave, but could not find it," he sang. Kavtaradze was about to join in and harmonize quietly—the Boss loved that. But suddenly, the Boss broke off in the middle of a verse, and Kavtaradze distinctly heard him say, "Poor, poor Sergo." Then he started singing again—"I sought my sweetheart's grave." And once again Kavtaradze heard him murmur, "Poor, poor Lado." Kavtaradze broke into a sweat, but the Boss went on singing and murmuring . . . "Poor, poor Alyosha. . . ."

Kavtaradze walked behind him, numb with horror; these were the names of their Georgian friends, whom he had destroyed. The Boss gave an extended performance of "Suliko," repeating the verses several times over to include all the names. Then he suddenly turned around and said, "They've gone . . . they've gone . . . not one of them left." There were tears in his eyes. Kavtaradze couldn't contain himself, he too burst into tears and collapsed on Koba's breast. Instantly, Koba's face was flushed with rage; his fleshy nose, his glaring yellow eyes came closer, closer, and he pushed Kavtaradze away, whispering, "They've gone! Not one of them left! You all wanted to kill Koba! But it didn't come off, Koba killed all of you instead, sons of whores." Then he rushed down the path, kicking his bodyguard, who didn't jump out of his way quickly enough.

The Boss never invited his friend to the dacha again, but did not touch him. Kavtaradze died in 1971 at the age of eighty-six.

Case 510: A Portrait of the New Man

Yezhov went to his grave quietly. His arrest was not announced in the press. Where the people's favorite had been, now there was nothing. This gave rise to legends that the Boss had spared his loyal executioner and that he had died a natural death. The truth can be found in Case File 510, which is still there in the KGB Archive.

Yezhov's file contains letters written to him by Stalin's close associates. He carefully preserved the evidence of their ardent love for him. The whole country had been singing the praises of this marvelous Communist for years. We find in his file hymns to the "hero Yezhov" written by the Kazakh poet Dzhambul. A pun heard often in those days was *"Yezhovye rukavitsy"*—literally, "hedgehog's gauntlets" (but also "Yezhov's gauntlets"): to hold someone in hedgehog's gauntlets is "to rule with a rod of iron." Mikoyan urged Party members to "learn from Comrade Yezhov, as he has learned, and learns, from Comrade Stalin." This "heroic figure"—a tiny man with a faint voice—was the holder of many Party offices and distinctions, at once Commissar for State Security, Secretary of the Central Committee, and head of the Party Control Commission, in spite of his "incomplete primary education."

The case file tells us that "Yezhov N. I. was arrested on April 10, 1939, and is held under guard in the Sukhanov Prison" (the most terrible of prisons, in which he had tortured his own victims). The formal indictment against Yezhov, dated February 1, 1940, reads in part: "Yezhov has been detected in treasonable espionage contacts with the Polish and German intelligence services, and with the ruling circles of Poland, Germany, England, and Japan, countries hostile to the USSR, and has headed a conspiracy in the NKVD." The Boss generously bestowed on Yezhov all the standard foreign contacts which he usually wished upon his victims. Nor did he forget the "conspiracy against the Leader," one of Yezhov's favorite weapons: "Yezhov and his confederates were in effect planning a putsch for November 7, 1938," the report continues.

Yezhov had to admit it all. But in court he said, "I was always by nature unable to stand violence against my person. For that reason I wrote all sorts of rubbish. . . . I was subjected to the severest beating." The torturer had been given what he had done to others. But there were points in the indictment which he did not care to deny: "I had sexual relations with men and women, taking advantage of my official position. . . . In October or November 38 I had an intimate liaison with the wife of a subordinate and with her husband with whom I had a pederastic affair." So stated the main guardian of the puritanical Bolshevik regime.

Yezhov's insatiable blood lust had finally unhinged him. He really believed that the enemy was everywhere. He suspected everybody. He tormented his wife beyond endurance with his suspicions, and was on the verge of arresting her. There are letters from her in the file: "Kolya darling, I earnestly beg you to check up on my whole life, everything about me. I cannot reconcile myself to the thought that I am suspected of duplicity." He ended up poisoning her. This was the "firm and modest Party worker" of whom Molotov spoke.

The last item in the file is the record of a closed session on February 3, 1940, of the military panel of the Supreme Court. His feeble, confused mumblings are there preserved: "I purged 14,000 Chekists, but my enormous fault is that I did not purge enough of them. My position was that I would give instructions to this or that department head to conduct the interrogation of a prisoner and all the while I was thinking, 'You've been interrogating him today, but tomorrow I'll arrest you.' There were enemies of the people all around me . . . enemies everywhere. . . . As far as Slutsky is concerned, I had instructions from the directing organs—don't arrest Slutsky, get rid of him some other way. . . . Otherwise our own agents abroad would have run for safety. So Slutsky was poisoned." The "directing organ" issuing orders to the almighty Yezhov is not hard to identify. The Puppet Master was always in control.

Nikolai Yezhov was a product of the society created by the Boss, a perfect example of the Stalinist senior executive.

Reading the poet Chuyev's account of a conversation with Molotov, I remembered my one meeting with him. I could not get over my impression that this dull man, with the intellect of an ordinary bookkeeper, had never in his life made a witty remark or a single profound observation. "File 510: The Yezhov Case" confirms what we already knew: that Molotov, Yezhov, and all the rest of them were faceless slaves, obedient tools, pathetic puppets in the hands of the Puppet Master. Stalin pulled their strings, and when they had played their part he pitilessly removed them from the scene, replacing them with other puppets, equally pathetic. A joke current at the time was very much to the point: "Stalin is a great chemist. He can turn any prominent government figure into a lump of shit, and any lump of shit into a leading government figure."

Yezhov's last request was: "Tell Stalin that I shall die with his name on my lips." A note in the file tells us that "the sentence of death by shooting on Yezhov, Nikolai Ivanovich, has been carried out in the city of Moscow, February 4, 1940."

A Luxurious Office

The Boss now gave the bloody swing a push in the other direction. Whereas earlier the NKVD had destroyed the Party, the new Party founded by Stalin now destroyed the old Yezhov personnel of the NKVD. The Central Committee adopted resolutions on Party control of the NKVD. Party commissions began weeding out NKVD agencies. The heads of yesterday's executioners rolled. The recoil from terror was just as bloody, just as fearful, as the Terror itself.

We are in the office of the Moscow NKVD chief: a molded ceiling, walls with beautiful bas-reliefs, Venetian windows. In the mid-thirties the imposing, gray-haired occupant of this office was Redens. He was shot. His seat was taken by the purple-nosed, mad-eyed inveterate drunkard Zakovsky, who had never heard of any punitive measure other than shooting. He was shot. At the beginning of 1939 the sadist N. Petrovsky moved in, and shot himself three weeks later. He was replaced by Yakubovich, who was arrested the very next day. And shot. P. Karutsky appeared for two days: introduced himself on the first and shot himself on the second. Korovin, appointed next, soon vanished, as did his successor Zhuvralev, who was sent for by Beria and never returned.

You can see slapstick comedians running like that in silent films. They appeared, flickered briefly, vanished. *They* were doing the killing—and *they* were being killed.

Was this reversal of policy genuine? It is true that after Yezhov's removal the NKVD seemed to arrest selected individuals rather than whole categories of people. But what individuals they were! The years 1939–1940 saw the arrest of several men of genius: the producer Meyerhold, the brilliant writer Isaac Babel, the eminent scientist Nikolai Vavilov, the brilliant avant-garde poet Danil Kharms. Was this a random selection of names? With the Boss nothing was ever random. The records of the Babel case have now become available, and they throw some light on the story.

Babel was forced to confess that he was a member of an underground Trotskyist espionage ring, to which he had been recruited by the writer Ilya Ehrenburg. The list of underground terrorists included some of the most eminent people in the world of the arts: L. Leonov, Katayev, Olesha, Eisenstein, Alexandrov, academician Shmidt, Mikhoels, Utesov, and so on. A new spectacular trial was evidently in the making. Plans had been laid in Yezhov's time. But when the Boss decided to get rid of that faithful servant he remembered one of his well-tried schemes: he would include Yezhov in the last act of the thriller. As he had once included Yagoda. He liked linking trials: novels with a sequel appealed to him. What made it more attractive was that Babel knew Yezhov well.

Plans for the trial included the arrest of Vsevolod Meyerhold. On the evening of his arrest in Leningrad, Meyerhold had spent some hours with an artist friend of his called Garin. When Meyerhold went out into one of Leningrad's white nights, Garin looked through the window and saw in the half-light three rats run across his path.

We have the testimony of witnesses present at Meyerhold's interrogations. One of the twentieth century's greatest theatrical producers lay on the floor with a fractured hip and blood streaming down his battered face while an interrogator urinated on him. He was accused of belonging to a Trotskyist organization and of engaging in espionage on behalf of four countries: Japan, England, France, and Lithuania. Pasternak, Shostakovich, Olesha, and Ehrenburg all made their appearance in the stenographic record of Meyerhold's interrogation, the dramatis personae in what was meant to be a unique spectacle.

It had never been his intention to stop at Yezhov.

But as he observed the course of the interrogations, he lost faith in the possibility of getting Babel, Meyerhold, and the others to play their part in the trial as planned. He could no longer rely on these strange people. Babel, for instance, admitted everything, and then, on October 10, 1939, retracted his deposition. The Boss realized that these excitable artists were dangerously unpredictable—they were too quick to agree, and just as quick to go back on their word.

He was disappointed in his cast. Babel, Meyerhold, and Koltsov were all quietly shot, after the required statements had been obtained. The search went on for worthy performers in the last act of the thriller. But it was interrupted by the war.

While Meyerhold was under investigation, his wife, the actress Zinaida Raikh, wrote letters to Stalin and went around Moscow talking about the injustice of it all. This was rebellion, and the Boss reacted accordingly. Assassins broke into her apartment through the balcony door. They murdered her slowly and sadistically, inflicting seventeen knife wounds. She screamed wildly but no one came to her aid. Cries in the night frightened people in those days.

Beria's sixteen-year-old mistress and his chauffeur moved into Meyerhold's flat. A Satanic finale, in the spirit of Voland.

Very soon afterward a miracle happened. Strange rumors were heard—that the famous people supposedly shot were still alive and simply denied the right to correspond. They were secretly held in special and perfectly decent places of detention. The Boss had not permitted the NKVD to extinguish these talents. Mikhail Koltsov's brother, the artist B. Efimov, was visited by people "recently released from the camps," where they had often seen Koltsov alive and flourishing. Babel's wife, A. Pirozhkova, told the same story: she had been informed by a number of different people that Babel was alive. One of Meyerhold's friends had actually had in his hands a postcard from Vsevolod Emilievich. These games ended abruptly after the Boss's death. They were intended in their day to authenticate his favorite image of himself—as the very kind Boss.

Voland Is a Dangerous Playmate

The year 1939 was nearing its end, and Stalin's sixtieth birthday had arrived, the sixtieth birthday of the new tsar. It was quite logical that he should commission a new play, to be produced by the Moscow Arts Theater in honor of his anniversary, from Bulgakov, the bard of the White officer corps. Bulgakov, however, had broken the taboo: he had asked to see documents about the life of Koba. The play was banned.

This decision was more than Bulgakov could bear. He knew, of course, by then that "evil for the sake of good" had destroyed millions, the guilty and the innocent alike. But he had forced himself not to see, to believe in the "Scourge of God." He had so longed for, so passionately hoped for a change in his fortunes. Instead he had been spat upon, slapped in the face. Evil did not need his services. Evil had allowed him to live—and that should be enough. According to her diary, Bulgakov said to his wife, "Do you remember when they banned *Days of the Turbins,* when they took that other play off, when they rejected my *Molière* manuscript . . . I never lost heart, I went on working, but look at me now: I lie here before you full of holes." Shortly afterward he fell fatally ill.

In the novel, Voland helped the Master. In real life, the Devil had killed the Master. It is dangerous to play games with the Devil.

GLORY, GLORY TO OUR RUSSIAN TSAR

In February 1939 the Bolshoi Theater staged the favorite opera of the Romanov tsars—Mikhail Glinka's *A Life for the Tsar.* It had been performed in celebration of Nicholas II's coronation, and to mark the tercentenary of the Romanov dynasty. Now it was performed again on the same stage, though under a different name. It was now called *Ivan Susanin.*

Stalin sat at the back of his box. Music that had not been heard since the Revolution filled the theater. "Glory!" But the famous words which had become the tsarist national anthem had been changed to "Glory, Glory to Thee, My Russia!" Sergei Gorodetsky, a poet of some note before the Revolution, had adapted the text at Stalin's bidding. The Boss himself had checked and edited the new version. He was an opera librettist as well as everything else!

He celebrated his sixtieth birthday to the strains of "Glory to Thee!" He had long been tsar. A lonely Russian tsar. His comrades-in-arms, or rather his servants, lived in mortal fear of him. The writer E. Gabrilovich recounted a story told by Khrushchev, about how he was once the Boss's guest at his dacha near Gagry, in Georgia, where he was on holiday:

> Stalin was sitting in a summer house in the garden. They were drinking tea and chatting. Time passed. It got dark. And Stalin became gloomy. Khrushchev said, "Well, I'd better be going home, Joseph Vissarionovich, my wife must be wondering where I am."
>
> "You won't go anywhere," Stalin said abruptly. "You'll stay here."
>
> "My wife will be expecting me, Joseph Vissarionovich." Stalin looked up at Khrushchev. With that look of his: his yellow eyes full of rage. Khrushchev, of course, stayed. But slept badly. Next morning he dressed and went out into the garden. Stalin was sitting in exactly the same position, in the summer house, sipping tea. Khrushchev asked him about his health.
>
> "Who are you? How did you get here?" Stalin asked peremptorily, between sips.
>
> "I'm . . . Khrushchev, Joseph Vissarionovich."
>
> "I shall have to go and find out who exactly you are," Stalin said. He pushed the tumbler away, and left the summer house.

> Trembling with fear Khrushchev walked along the garden path toward the exit. He was overtaken by one of the guards and prepared himself for the worst.
>
> "Nikita Sergeevich. Comrade Stalin is asking for you. He's been looking everywhere for you." Khrushchev hurried back to the summer house. Stalin was sitting there drinking tea.
>
> "Wherever were you, Nikita Sergeevich?" he asked affectionately. "You shouldn't stay in bed so long, I've been waiting all this time for you."

He liked playing games, the Boss. They were all specks of dust—his mighty bureaucracy. He made them suffer constant, unremitting fear. He sent the wife of Kalinin (then the nominal head of state, as president of the Supreme Soviet) to a camp. There, the president's wife picked the lice from prisoners' underclothes before they were laundered, while Kalinin, a pathetic old man, pleaded for her release in vain. Stalin also sent to the camp the wife of his faithful secretary, Poskrebyshev. Poskrebyshev also importuned the Boss to bring his wife back. And also to no avail. The head of the government, Molotov, was also deprived of his wife. Stalin imprisoned her. Three of the most important people in the Soviet Union had wives behind bars. Just so they wouldn't forget that they were nothing. Blind kittens. He could send them after their wives at any moment. Besides, he had no wife of his own. He was simply evening things up. Now they could serve the Great Dream, without any of silly Khrushchev's family distractions, and forgetting petit bourgeois happiness.

HOME

He was tsar and God. He knew that the divinity of power resides in its mystery. The mysterious darkness with which he surrounded his life, the dread concealed by his subjects' joie de vivre, the mysterious Night Life—the black cars, with their sweeping headlights, the nocturnal police raids of the searchlights over darkened trains carrying people to the camps, the secret shootings of yesterday's lords of creation, the secret graves in cemeteries . . . all part of the mystery. The whole country believed that he lived in the Kremlin. A light was kept burning all night in one particular window of the Kremlin, looking out over the wall. In fact, a number of large Zil automobiles would leave the Borovitsky Gate in the dead of night. They would accelerate to an enormous speed and rush along the government route. The darkened, unbreakable windows of these bulletproof cars made it impossible to see who was inside. They all looked alike, and nobody knew in which of them he was sitting. Only when they were about to enter the grounds of the nearer dacha would his car move to the head of the cortege, with the others following.

The nearer dacha, half an hour's drive from the Kremlin, was his home—and another carefully kept secret. He had moved into this brick villa, built in the thirties, after his wife's death. The grounds were surrounded by a fence fifteen feet high. In 1938 he had a second fence built, with observation slits. Inside the villa there was a foyer and a big dining room, in which he and his Politburo comrades "dined"—his term for the midnight meal which was more like supper and breakfast in one. His nocturnal lifestyle was also secret. The villa was staffed by NKVD officers and maidservants.

One of the maidservants was the youngish Valechka Istomina. She had joined his staff in 1935. She ironed his trousers and his semimilitary tunic. He had no valet. He had never changed his habits, and did most things for himself. Valechka would work there for seventeen years. She made his bed for him, and grew old beside him. "Whether or not she was Stalin's wife is nobody else's business," Molotov told Chuyev.

The maidservant in fact became his secret wife, while the new head of his bodyguard, Nikolai Vlasik, took charge of his children. The compact little villa was his palace, and the setting in which he would spend the rest of his life. This too was where death would overtake him.

ALONE

Before the war, in 1940, he received a present: Beria succeeded in organizing the murder of Trotsky. He had been ruthlessly persecuting Trotsky's relatives all along. He began with the arrest of Trotsky's younger son Sergei, a scientist living quietly in Moscow.

Trotsky's wife, Natalya Sedova, vainly appealed for help to Romain Rolland and Bernard Shaw, among others. The names of many other progressive writers appeared in her open letter. But they all remained silent. Why? In 1933, answering a request from Max Eastman to speak out against the arrest of Trotsky's supporters, Theodore Dreiser wrote as follows: "I have reflected seriously, as if at prayer, on this Trotsky business. I have great sympathy with his supporters, but a problem of choice arises. Whatever the nature of the present dictatorship in Russia, Russia's victory is more important than anything else." The victory of the workers' and peasants' state was more important than mere human lives. The familiar appeal to the higher expediency.

The Boss, then, could be sure of their silence. To madden his enemy, he physically destroyed all his relatives, even the most distant. And even his grandson's nanny!

The Boss's agents stalked Trotsky throughout the thirties. This was yet another form of torture: torture by the constant threat of death. At last, in 1940, one of the Boss's emissaries, R. Mercader, a former lieutenant in the Spanish Republican army, split Trotsky's skull, exposing the brain of which he had been so proud.

Of all the old Bolshevik leaders, beginning with Lenin, he was the sole survivor. The legacy of the Revolution was now his by right. His was the loneliness of a celestial being.

Genghis Khan's gigantic empire had been reerected in Eastern Europe. It was now ready to pounce.

Until 1938, foreign policy remained subservient to domestic policy. But now that he had created a new country he could afford to begin realizing his external aims. Or rather his main aim. The secret one. The Great Dream!

We see that with the accession of Stalin nothing had changed. It was just that the Great Leninist Dream, world revolution, which the activists of Lenin's Party, all those defunct big mouths, had openly shown their eagerness to export, had become a secret. The Boss had relegated it to the underground. So in 1936, in an interview with the American journalist Roy Howard, reproduced in *Pravda,* when asked, "Has the Soviet Union abandoned its plans to carry out world revolution?" Stalin calmly replied, "We never had any such intention."

He was playing his favorite game: quieting the enemy's suspicions. But propaganda at home was preparing his people for something quite different. His tame writers extolled the Great War for the realization of the Great Dream. The poet Pavel Kogan prophesied that his countrymen would "advance to the Ganges" and "die in battles to come" so that the "radiance" of the Soviet Union would shine from England to Japan. Another "poet," Mikhail Kulchitsky, looked forward to a time when "only one Soviet nation, and only the people of a Soviet nation," would exist.

I found traces of these preparations for a major war in the President's Archive. The Red army was rapidly rearming in the thirties—even before the advent of Hitler. As a result Tukhachevsky wrote Stalin an anxious letter: "Dear Comrade Stalin! I fully understand that one has not just to win a war but to preserve one's economic might while doing so. . . . By working along those lines you can most profitably solve the problems posed by a Great War. Communist greetings. Tukhachevsky. Leningrad 19.6.30." There followed a detailed plan for the rearmament of the Red army for a "war of engines"—a Great War. This was where Tukhachevsky clashed with Voroshilov. We need not go into the substance of their disagreement. What is important is that both Voroshilov and Tukhachevsky were preparing for a Great War.

The Great War of the Future also influenced a gigantic construction project put in motion at the beginning of the thirties. While the plans for the Moscow Metro were being drawn up, planes dropped high-explosive bombs on the site. These bombardments helped to determine the depth at which the tunnels for the future underground railway must be bored, to make it invulnerable in an air raid. With the future war in mind, the Boss gave orders that no section of the track should run aboveground. (This information on the building of the Metro was given by the engineer and historian M. Yegorov in the newspaper *Arguments and Facts.*)

In March 1938, Hitler annexed Austria. Clouds gathered over Czechoslovakia. It was as the Boss had expected. Hitler really was drawing Europe into war, and Germany would bring down in ruins the whole capitalist system. It was no longer a mirage, no longer a dream—world revolution was advancing on empire. All that was needed was to egg Hitler on.

These were the favorable circumstances in which the Grand Master began his first major game beyond the frontiers of his own country.

In 1938, while he was engaged in talks on collective security with France and England, the Boss began trying to make contact with his worst enemy, Adolf Hitler. The Soviet ambassador in Berlin, Yakov Surits, a Jew, was recalled, and replaced by Merekalov.

At the same time, negotiations with France and England were pursued with greater urgency. This was a typical Stalin ploy. He knew in advance that the Western democracies would never trust the new Genghis Khan. He inspired in them only fear and revulsion. The talks were meant to gain leverage on Hitler. This gambit worked. Fearing an alliance between Stalin and the Western democracies, Hitler was soon responding to Soviet advances. The customary fulminations against the USSR disappeared from official German statements, and the campaign of mutual insult petered out. A new phase had begun: the irreconcilable foes seemed to have stopped noticing each other.

Meanwhile, Czechoslovakia was about to become Hitler's next victim. The Boss immediately offered to help the Czechs, but only on condition that England and France did the same. This was courageous of him—and quite safe: he knew that Poland and Romania would never agree to let Soviet armies cross their territory. *They* knew that letting Stalin in was easy, but getting him out again would be difficult. And Poland's leaders had shortsightedly swallowed Hitler's bait and grabbed a chunk of dismembered Czechoslovakia. Stalin had behaved nobly in the eyes of the Western European public, with no risk at all. The Politburo demonstratively discussed possible forms of aid while Czechoslovakia's Western allies were washing their hands of the country. Once the Munich Agreement was signed, Chamberlain and Daladier were sure that they had appeased Hitler. The powerful line of Czech fortifications passed into German hands without a shot fired, and the battle-trained Czech divisions ceased to exist. As, very soon, did Czechoslovakia itself, in spite of the British and French guarantees.

Moscow learned about the Munich Agreement on September 29. At an all-night emergency meeting of the Politburo, Litvinov, the People's Commissar for Foreign Affairs, abroad at the time, was assailed as—supposedly—a supporter of alliance with the Western democracies. "Supposedly" is the word. Only one person was behind the Soviet Union's diplomatic moves—the Boss. But he blamed Litvinov for policies which had resulted in the Munich Agreement and exposed the USSR to German aggression: this treachery had made it necessary to seek new ways of preventing a German attack. These statements contained the excuse he had wanted all along for an about-face. The Boss was feeling his way toward an alliance with Hitler—a latter-day version of Lenin's Brest-Litovsk Treaty.

He had no doubt that his scheme would succeed. He sensed that Hitler was like him—insatiable. Czechoslovakia was just the beginning. But to go any farther Hitler needed an alliance with the USSR. He would give Hitler his alliance—to make sure that farther would mean farther away from the Soviet Union.

After Litvinov's dismissal, at a Politburo session on May 3, 1939, Molotov, while remaining head of government, also took over the Commissariat of Foreign Affairs, to emphasize the overriding importance of foreign policy.

Litvinov was given no new post. He took this to mean that he was doomed. While he waited for the end he wrote suppliant letters to the Boss. They went unanswered. Everyone expected that he would shortly be arrested, and everyone was amazed to see that he was not touched. This was one sign that in seeking alliance with Hitler the Boss was thinking several moves ahead. In the game he was playing, Litvinov symbolized alignment with the Western democracies. He might yet be needed. And so it was. When war with Hitler came, Litvinov, prudently preserved, would be appointed Vice-Commissar for Foreign Affairs.

With Hitler poised on the Polish frontier, Chamberlain felt compelled to assure the Poles that Britain would help them in the event of a German attack. Alliance with Stalin now became a matter of urgency for Hitler. The Boss found ways of egging him on. A military delegation led by Voroshilov held talks with England and France. Their only result was to speed up German Ambassador Schulenberg's secret negotiations with Molotov. In Germany, Ribbentrop, long the bugbear of the Soviet press, was ready to leave for Moscow. The fascists were inviting the Bolshevik state to join them in partitioning Europe.

Hitler was now in a hurry to clarify the situation before he attacked Poland, and Ribbentrop showered Schulenberg with ciphered telegrams. Soviet intelligence kept the Boss informed about the Führer's impatience. It was now the middle of August, and Hitler could delay no longer: once the rains set in, the Polish roads would be too muddy. Hitler accepted the Boss's terms without qualification, and telegraphed on August 19 to say that Ribbentrop was on his way.

A New Era

For Stalin, this change of orientation had no ideological implications. Hitler and the Western democracies alike were enemies. Alliance with either side was merely a turn on the tortuous road to the Great Dream. But in shelving his hatred for Hitler, he had sacrificed his claim to be a champion of democracy. He would obviously have to sacrifice Comintern. He knew that he could someday recover all that he had given up, and in the meantime he would gain territory.

Ribbentrop, on arrival in the Kremlin, was greeted with the words "It's been a lovely shoving match, hasn't it?" He and Stalin then spent three hours in perfect harmony, carving up Eastern Europe. The Boss's supplementary proposals were accepted with startling ease. The Non-Aggression Pact and its secret protocol were signed—for the Soviet side not, of course, by the Boss, but by Molotov. The proceedings ended with a state reception—one of those lavish feasts, with lavish toasts, that Stalin enjoyed so much. Molotov, hardened veteran of the Boss's junketings, amazed the German guests with his ability to drink without getting drunk.

Stalin raised his glass to Hitler, and the Reichsminister raised his to Stalin. After this, the German delegation had to drink deep—to the pact and to the new era in Soviet-German relations. The Boss had not, however, lost his sense of humor. He proposed a toast to Kaganovich, who was present, and Ribbentrop found himself drinking to a Jew. Still, Kaganovich himself had to drink Hitler's health. The negotiations were over. The secret protocol specified the price which Hitler was paying him for the pact: freedom to "make territorial and political modifications in the Baltic States" and the right to "assert the Soviet Union's interest in Bessarabia." Stalin also received a piece of Poland. After the signing he gave Hitler a present: the German and Austrian Communists, remnants of the old Comintern, held in Soviet camps were deported to Germany, to the Gestapo.

The next day Voroshilov smilingly told the British and French delegations that "in view of the changed situation there is no point in continuing these discussions."

The Boss personally thought up an explanation of the new alliance for the Soviet people. In army units, a comic drawing was displayed. It showed two triangles. The caption over one of them read "What did Chamberlain want?" At the apex of the triangle was the word "London" and at the two lower corners "Moscow" and "Berlin." Meaning that Chamberlain wanted to bring the USSR and Germany into conflict. The caption over the other triangle was "What did Comrade Stalin do?" Now the word at the apex was "Moscow." Stalin had brought Berlin and London into conflict, leaving the USSR on top.

The country unanimously rejoiced, passing yet another obedience test. It was indeed a new country that he had created.

SECOND WORLD WAR

Hitler invaded Poland, and England and France declared war on Germany. Stalin's tactics had proved correct: Hitler had, as expected, drawn Europe into a world war. The path to the Great Dream lay open. These were the first results of sacrificing his queen, the Comintern.

But the match went on. He went into action himself, taking back parts of the empire of the Romanovs lost after the Revolution. On September 17 his troops entered Poland, which the Germans had already brought to its knees. "Since the Polish state has ceased to exist, Soviet troops have entered Poland to protect the rights of the Belorussian and Ukrainian minorities (against Hitler)." That was how Stalin announced the annexation of Eastern Poland to the country and the world. Hitler had no choice but to accept the new status quo, and, what was more, accept a doctored text of the Soviet-German communiqué. Hitler's bellicose declarations were replaced with ideological phraseology of the sort Stalin favored: "To restore peace and order in Poland . . . suppress disorders caused by the collapse of the Polish state . . . and to give help to the Polish people . . ." In short, Poland had been occupied for Poland's sake. Another example of "in-depth language."

The western Ukraine and western Belorussia, parts of the former

Romanov empire, had returned to the bosom of Stalin's empire. He took the opportunity to bestow a gift on Lithuania—the city of Vilnius. Lithuania rejoiced. But intelligent people were gloomy. "Vilnius belongs to us—but it looks as if we belong to Russia" summed up their feelings.

When Ribbentrop reappeared in Moscow at the end of September, the Boss was now asking for the whole of the Baltic States, including Lithuania, previously in the Reich's sphere of interest. He also asked for, and was given, the Polish oil fields around Borislaw and Drogobycz—which oil-starved Germany sorely needed itself. In return, Stalin promised to sell the Germans oil, and Hitler had to be satisfied with this. He was very much afraid that Stalin might desert him and join the Anglo-French alliance. Once again, there was a banquet in the Kremlin, and once again the Reichsminister had to endure the endless toasts—among other things to friendship between peoples and to peace throughout the world. The Boss never lost his sense of humor.

A Meeting

There were many rumors about a meeting between Stalin and Hitler, which was supposed to have taken place somewhere on the territory annexed from defeated Poland. In 1972, an old railroad man told a story about a train that drew into Lvov in October 1939. The station was closely guarded and no one was allowed into the area around it. Railroad traffic came to a halt. The man even remembered the date—October 16. I recalled this date with something of a shock when I read in the Soviet newspaper *Comsomol Pravda* a document said to have been found in the National Archives in Washington. The newspaper printed a photocopy of the document.

Federal Bureau of Investigation
United States Department of Justice
Washington, D.C
July 19, 1940

PERSONAL AND CONFIDENTIAL
Honorable Adolf A. Berle, Jr.
Assistant Secretary of State, Department of State
Washington, D.C.

Dear Mr. Berle:

Information has just been received from a confidential source to the effect that after the German and Russian invasion

> and partition of Poland, Hitler and Stalin met secretly in Lvov. Poland, on October 17, 1939. It is alleged that foreign governments have not yet become aware of this meeting. During these secret negotiations, Hitler and Stalin reportedly signed a military treaty to replace the previously consummated Non-Aggression Pact. It is reported that on October 28, 1939, Stalin made a report to the Political Bureau of the Communist Party of the Soviet Union, in which he furnished the seven members of the said Bureau, full details concerning his negotiations with Hitler.
> I thought you would be interested in these data.
> Sincerely yours,
> J. Edgar Hoover

Yes, the document was signed by the long-standing chief of the F.B.I. Notes on the document indicate that it had been declassified in 1979.

Even after having been convinced of the document's authenticity, I continued to doubt its accuracy. After all, the report sent to Hoover may have been false. But publication of this document sent me back to the diary in which I had noted the railroad worker's story. And once again, October! I understood that it was unlikely I could verify this. I knew that all documentary records of this meeting, if it had taken place, would have been carefully destroyed by Stalin. So I decided to consult what may seem a surprising source. The President's Archive contains Stalin's visitors' book. I looked up the entries for October 1939. No, Stalin was in his office in Moscow on October 16. And on the 17th there was a long list of visitors. I was about to give up, but took a look at the 18th just in case and found that on the 18th he saw nobody. Stalin was missing from the Kremlin on that day. The 18th fell on a Thursday, an ordinary workday—the workweek then included even Saturday. He was also absent on the 19th until 8:25 P.M., when he returned to his office to receive visitors. I knew about his indefatigable work habits. He was a typical workaholic. His absence from the office in the middle of the week could only occur for one of two reasons: either he was severely ill, or he was absent from Moscow.

The list of visitors on the eve of his absence is also interesting. The People's Commissar for Defense, Voroshilov, and several of the military chiefs—Zhukov, Kulik, Kuznetsov, Isakov—came to see him. But it was the Commissar for Foreign Affairs, Molotov, who spent the most time in his office on that day.

In fact, something very important seems to have happened during his absence. For, according to the visitors' list for October 19, after Stalin turned up in his Kremlin office late that evening, he was closeted for one and a half hours with the second man in the state, Commissar for Foreign Affairs Molotov. In the course of their discussion Zhukov (the commander who was to become the main hero of the Second World War) was summoned to Stalin's office once again, and Kaganovich, third man in the state after Stalin and Molotov, was also called in.

Can the meeting with Hitler really have taken place? It would have been the secret meeting of the century. Who could possibly describe it? They would have sat facing each other, the two Leaders, both Gods on earth. Strange doubles. So alike, and so different. If they did meet, Stalin must have realized all over again how much Hitler needed him. At the end of 1939 he already felt bold enough to spring a surprise on the Führer. He tried to conquer Finland. Hitler accepted that too. Stalin had read him correctly.

Stalin had begun putting pressure on Finland even before concluding his pact with Hitler. K. Meretskov, who commanded the troops of the Leningrad Military District, was called in by the Boss. He described later how he "found in his office an important Comintern official and well-known activist of the world Communist movement, Kuusinen. I was told of the concern caused to our leadership by the anti-Soviet line of the Finnish government. Finland could easily become a bridgehead for anti-Soviet action, by either of the two main imperialist groupings—the German or the Anglo-French. If Finland should strike, various counteractions were open to us. . . . I was made responsible for drawing up a plan to protect the frontier from aggression, and to plan a counterattack against the Finnish armed forces."

An amazing scene! Not one of those present, of course, seriously thought that little Finland would attack the immense empire. Nobody seriously believed that Hitler, with whom they were just concluding successful negotiations, or England and France, to whom they were also talking, would launch an "action against the Soviet Union" from Finland.

The three men in conference all knew that they were really talking about preparations for the annexation of Finland. The "well-known activist of the world Communist movement" Kuusinen, a Finn, would be called upon to form a puppet government. That was how the obligatory "in-depth language" worked: "attack" would always be called "defense," and "aggression" a "response to aggression."

The game was played to the end. The Finns were offered the usual unacceptable exchange of territory: they were asked among other things to cede areas of Karelia through which ran the defensive Mannerheim Line. Negotiations inevitably reached an impasse. Shortly afterward the Soviet government announced: "On November 26 without warning our forces came under artillery fire from the Finnish side . . . as a result of which four men were killed and ten wounded." The Finns tried in vain to prove that the artillery fire had come from the Soviet side and that the Soviet forces had killed their own soldiers. The war had begun.

For its "aggression against the Soviet Union," Finland was expelled from the League of Nations.

Kuusinen immediately formed a "government of the Finnish Democratic Republic" from the pathetic remnants of the Finnish Communist Party which had not vanished without trace during the Terror. Kuusinen himself, "well-known leader of the Communist movement," had been told nothing about the fate of his comrades, or indeed that of his own family. He was just as ill-informed about the future proposed for Finland.

Marshal Konyev noted in his memoirs that when they were beginning the Finnish war the Boss said in the presence of Admiral Isakov and Voroshilov, "We shall have to resettle the Finns. . . . the population of Finland is smaller than that of Leningrad, they can be resettled." Poor Kuusinen may have been slated to vanish with his government and his people. The Boss was good at carrying out such grandiose projects. If God had planted them in the wrong place, the Boss would correct God's mistake.

God's mistake, however, went uncorrected. The USSR expected to win the war by a blitzkrieg. "Our orders were to act on the assumption that the war would last twelve days," wrote Molotov. Instead, crushing defeats followed. It cost the Red army an incredible effort to check the Finnish advance. "Two hundred thousand [Soviet soldiers] lie in snowdrifts staring at our overcast sky with unseeing eyes—and it is no fault of ours," said the Finnish leader Mannerheim. Add to that 300,000 disabled or missing. Little Finland had stood its ground.

The Soviet high command, headed by Voroshilov, had demonstrated its incompetence, much to Hitler's relief. But in spite of its victory, Finland, with its meager resources, had to make peace and to cede territory. The coveted Karelian isthmus and the area around Lake Lagoda went to the USSR. Stalin had drawn his conclusions. He drove Voroshilov out of his Commissariat. The newly appointed People's Commissar for Defense, S. Timoshenko, told the Finnish military attaché that "the Russians have learned a great deal in this hard war."

The Empire Reestablished

Meanwhile Hitler was reaping rewards beyond his dreams all through 1940. Denmark, Norway, Holland, Luxembourg, and finally France fell swiftly. After each act of aggression Stalin unfailingly congratulated Hitler on the Wehrmacht's "brilliant success." But with these congratulations he always called in a bill. One by one, he occupied the Baltic States. This was done, so he claimed, to "put an end to intrigues [in those countries] by which England and France are attempting to sow discord between Germany and the USSR." The great humorist, as we see, had occupied the Baltic States solely in the interests of friendship with Germany. Estonia, Latvia, and Lithuania—needless to say, "at the request of their peoples"—found themselves back in the Russian Empire.

He turned hurriedly toward the Balkans. In summer 1940 he presented Romania with an ultimatum, demanding the return of Bessarabia, annexed by Romania in 1918, and of northern Bukovina. A powerful army group was concentrated on the Romanian frontiers. Romanian oil was feeding the whole German war machine, and Hitler, fearful of a possible military conflict on Romanian soil, was compelled to put pressure on that country's government.

Romania meekly consented to cede the disputed territory.

While grabbing more than had been agreed upon, Stalin still tried to demonstrate his loyalty to Hitler. When the new British ambassador spoke to him of a possible alliance against Germany in the summer of 1940, he immediately sent Hitler the text of his reply: "Stalin has found no desire on the part of Germany to absorb other European countries. . . . He does not consider that Germany's military successes present any danger to the Soviet Union." Whom was he trying to fool? The British? Or Hitler? Or both?

In the occupied territories he worked ruthlessly to create a "morally and politically unified society." The NKVD purged the annexed areas of "alien elements." Train after train carried fresh convicts—the bourgeoisie, intellectuals, well-off peasants. White émigrés, politicians—to swell his labor force in Gulag. They were carried in freight cars—two tiers of plank beds, with a discharge pipe for the sanitary bucket in the middle of the car, tiny barred windows which admitted little air. One such freight car carried into imprisonment a Jew arrested in Lithuania: Menachem Begin, the future prime minister of Israel.

Hitler was efficiently destroying the Old World. Was it time for Stalin to do one more about-face, and set out this time along the road that led straight toward the Great Dream?

This change of direction was connected, in his mind, with the fortunes of Britain. Britain was holding out. Bleeding profusely, but holding out. The iron-willed Churchill, who had replaced Chamberlain, declared: "We shall defend our island whatever the cost. We will fight them on the beaches . . . we will fight them in the fields and on the streets. . . . We will never surrender, even if this island or a large part of it is enslaved and people begin to die of hunger. If that happens, our empire beyond the seas will fight on . . . until, God willing, the New World acts to liberate the Old."

Hitler planned his invasion of England. The British bombed his landing craft and frustrated the operation. Then the unexpected happened. In August 1940, the RAF bombed Berlin for the first time. The Germans had never thought it possible. It was a great shock to them. The war had come to Germany.

Hitler, infuriated, launched air raids of unprecedented ferocity on London. Huge columns of fire rose over the city. But even this did not break the will of the British. Far from it—they were gradually beginning to win the war in the air.

Meanwhile Hitler and Stalin regularly assured each other of their friendship. Molotov was sent to Berlin on a forty-eight-hour visit, to discuss future spheres of influence. The talks took place in an air-raid shelter, amid the din created by yet another British air raid. "England is finished," Ribbentrop said firmly. "So why are we sitting in this place?" was Molotov's curt reply.

Stalin knew well enough that Hitler had not "finished with England."

A Baffling Story

The generally accepted version is that this was when Hitler finally decided to attack his unsuspecting ally. That the mad Führer began preparing for Barbarossa (code name for his invasion of the Soviet Union) precisely at this point. He put his signature to the plan in December 1940. In other words, he had made his final decision some six months before the declaration of war.

Throughout that half-year not only Churchill but the Comintern spies who had voluntarily remained behind in Germany kept warning the Boss that Hitler meant to attack. Richard Sorge gave him the same message. This clandestine member of the German Communist Party, grandson of an associate of Karl Marx, was working in Japan at the time, masquerading as a "Nazi journalist." He regularly supplied Moscow with intelligence reports, and among other things managed to communicate the exact date of the German invasion.

Stalin, however, did not believe Sorge, or any of the others. The sudden invasion took him completely by surprise. His first game in an international tournament ended in a debacle. That, at least, is what people have generally believed.

But this version of events beggars belief.

The wily Boss, a leader whose first rule was "trust no one," whose whole strategy consisted in misleading the enemy, suddenly proves gullible in his dealings with the archenemy, is suddenly himself so easily gulled that he pays not the slightest attention to repeated warnings, but puts implicit trust in the liar Hitler, who has betrayed so many and broken his word so often. . . . It would be believable if we were talking about a different man, and not our Stalin. He had proved conclusively in the sixty years of his life that he was not a bit like that.

What, then, did happen?

As early as March 1941 his intelligence service had supplied him in effect with the full details of Barbarossa. The date set for the German invasion was somewhere between May 15 and June 15. But the Boss was a pragmatist and expected people to behave rationally. Hitler simply could not afford such a risky venture. As a Marxist, Stalin respected economic realities. It seemed incredible to him that Hitler would wage war simultaneously on several countries whose combined resources were incomparably greater than those of Germany. As for Churchill, he made a comic error with one of his predictions. He had warned Stalin of a possible German attack in May 1941, but in that month the Germans attacked the British on the island of Crete instead. The Boss could ask with his quiet smile why British intelligence, which showed such concern for the Soviet Union, was unable to help itself. The answer, as he saw it, was easy: Britain was losing too much blood in an unequal fight, and Churchill wanted to push Stalin into the war at any price. He could not, then, believe Churchill. Nor could he believe his own agent Sorge. Sorge had refused to return to the Soviet Union. How could the Boss believe a defector?

When Hitler began his Balkan campaign early in 1941, Stalin had reason to feel reassured. The Yugoslavs capitulated in April, and Hitler moved against Greece. Hitler's objective now seemed clear to the Boss: once he had seized Greece he would be able to destroy the British in Egypt and take Suez. Churchill, incidentally, was thinking along the same lines when he pleaded with the United States to come into the war: "I beg you, Mr. President," he wrote to Roosevelt, "to weigh carefully the serious consequences of collapse in the Near East. . . . Such a blow could be the end of the British Empire."

There was yet another proof—an amusing one—that Hitler could not possibly attack the Soviet Union in the near future. In May he was in the Balkans, so an attack could not possibly take place before the end of June. Hitler would then have to be prepared for the Russian winter. One sure sign that the Germans intended to attack so late in the year would be the provision of sheepskin coats. Millions of them would be needed. If Hitler really had decided to attack, he should be treating sheepskin coats as a matter of urgency. That would mean a fall in the price of mutton, and a rise in the price of fleece. Nothing of the sort was reported by Soviet intelligence. All in all, Stalin was entitled to conclude that Churchill was determined to draw the United States into the war by supplication, and Russia by false information.

Why did Hitler, in spite of everything, make the most illogical decision of his life at its most critical moment? To understand, we must forget all the generally received versions.

Vladimir Rezun, an officer in the intelligence division of the KGB, chose to remain in the West in order to publish a discovery which had troubled him all his life. In the Military Academy, Rezun had heard in lectures on strategy that if the enemy is planning a sudden assault he must first (a) concentrate his forces near the frontier and (b) locate his airfields as closely as possible to the front line.

In lectures on military history Rezun heard that Stalin, because he had trusted Hitler, was completely unprepared for war. He had committed a number of very serious mistakes. In particular, he had (a) concentrated his best units near the frontier and (b) located his airfields right on the boundary in occupied Poland. Rezun began studying the question, and was astonished to find that trustful Stalin had stepped up arms production with feverish haste after the conclusion of the Molotov-Ribbentrop pact, and that on the eve of war he had deployed more and more divisions on his frontier with Hitler. He was following the strategic rules for a surprise attack. What, Rezun asked himself, was the obvious inference? Was it that Stalin was planning to attack Hitler?

He Was Planning to Attack First

The Boss's pact with Hitler had indeed been intended to spur him on to fresh conquests. And while Hitler, intoxicated with his victories, was destroying capitalist Europe, the Boss was planning his great about-face: his Great War with Hitler. Once he had won that war he would become the liberator of a Europe bled dry. And its lord and master. First there would be an "All-European Union of Soviet Socialist Republics." And later there would exist "only one Soviet nation," as the poet Kulchitsky had promised.

The Boss had appreciated to the full the importance of Hitler's emergence for the triumph of the Great Dream.

Ideological preparations were in high gear. Newspapers and films glorified the army. The main play of the prewar season, *A Lad from Our Town* by Konstantin Simonov, had a military theme. Significantly, the Boss sent both of his sons to army schools. Soldiering became the most prestigious profession. Composers did their socialist duty, and a large number of songs were written about a great war and a speedy victory.

At this time *Pravda* published a speech made by Baidakov, a famous airman: "What happiness and joy will be seen on the countenances of those who, in the Kremlin Palace, receive the last republic into the brotherhood of all countries in the world. I can picture clearly the bombers reducing the enemy's factories, railroad junctions, warehouses, and military positions to ruins, the assault planes launching a hail of fire, the landing craft putting divisions ashore."

On orders from Stalin, work began on plans for the redeployment of the Soviet armed forces immediately after the conclusion of the Non-Aggression Pact. The main concentration of Soviet strength was to be on the western front. In the 1939 "Field Regulations" we read that "the Red army will be the most attack-oriented of all attacking armies ever known." The army was now training airborne troops in unprecedented numbers. By 1941 Stalin had more than a million parachutists. Y. Chadayev, then chief administrative assistant to the Council of People's Commissars, tells us in his unpublished memoirs (deposited in the Archive of the October Revolution—we shall return to them in other contexts) that the Boss asked him in 1941 to "produce a summary of decisions on defense and economic matters during the Civil War . . . [and] kept pestering me, wanting to know how the construction of the new air-raid shelter in the Kremlin was going." Chadayev answered that "work is going on round the clock, it will be ready in two months." To which Stalin said, "Take the necessary steps to get it finished earlier." Hitler, obviously, knew all this. His intelligence service was not idle. Hitler also knew why Stalin had stationed an extremely powerful striking force on the Romanian frontier. He had known all along that Bessarabia was just an excuse. Romania hid Germany's heart's blood, its oil. That was the reason for Barbarossa. Neither of these enemies-and-allies, needless to say, ever trusted the other for a moment. But they both knew for sure that neither of them was fully prepared to take the offensive, and both were reassured by this knowledge. To prove that his intentions were peaceful, Stalin showed the Germans his old front-line fortifications. Hitler, however, knew that Stalin's army was poised on his frontier.

In February 1941 the Boss relocated his command posts. But then in May, as if to ingratiate himself with Hitler, Stalin closed down the embassies of Belgium, Norway, and Greece—countries hostile to Nazi Germany. Yet on May 5, 1941, he said openly, at a graduation banquet for officers at the Red Army Academy, "There will be war, and the enemy will be Germany." In the same speech he announced that the army had been "radically reorganized and greatly expanded." He spoke of "three hundred divisions, one-third of them mechanized." But it is the misfortune of dictators to be told what they want to hear. The Boss did not know that a quarter of the three hundred divisions were not yet up to strength, and that the military schools which he was setting up in such a hurry turned out poorly trained officers.

He explained further in the course of the banquet: "Now that we have reconstructed our army, and more than satisfied its need for the technology of modern warfare, now that we are strong, we must go over from the defensive to the offensive. In conducting the defense of our country we must act by taking the offensive." Chadayev, who heard it, wrote of this speech that "Stalin's remark that 'there is going to be a war' was omitted from the published text. *Pravda* published a very laconic report of the speech. A spurious version was put out via the correspondent of the German Information Bureau. In this, Stalin laid special stress on the Non-Aggression Pact, and emphasized that we did not expect to be attacked by Germany."

Still, in May 1941 a project for the establishment of a Supreme Headquarters was submitted to Stalin. Military training was to be speeded up, and the country put on a war footing under the direction of the General Staff. A Party conference devoted to "defense questions" had been held back in February, and Stalin had proposed a seventeen to eighteen percent increase in industrial capacity. He was thinking of war industry.

"BEGIN IT OURSELVES"

"No, Stalin was not planning an attack on Germany in 1941." That is the view of D. Volkogonov, author of a book on Stalin. A lieutenant general and eminent Russian historian, Volkogonov was the first person to be permitted to work in all the secret archives. He wrote in an article in *Izvestia*: "I have before me several documents addressed to Stalin and Molotov. Marshal S. Timoshenko, People's Commissar for Defense, and G. Zhukov, Chief of the General Staff, submitted an amplified plan, prepared on March 11, 1941, for the deployment of the armed forces of the Soviet Union 'in the West and in the East.' It says in this plan that the existing political situation in Europe compels us to pay exceptional attention to the defense of our western frontiers. The military leaders believe that Germany may strike its main blow southeastward, with the primary object of occupying the Ukraine, with an auxiliary offensive against Dvinsk and Riga. On May 4 Timoshenko and Zhukov sent particularly important directions to the commanders of the Western, Baltic, and Kiev Military Districts. Nowhere is there a single word about a strike against the German forces. All the documents call for defensive measures to be taken." But Volkogonov, a former official of the army's Political Administration, ought to know the importance of ideological words. "Defense" is an ideological word. In "in-depth language," as became clear during the Finnish war, "defense" often signified "attack."

Volkogonov also cited an extraordinary document drawn up by Zhukov, as Chief of the General Staff, for Stalin. The document is dated May 15, 1941: "In view of the fact that Germany at present keeps its army fully mobilized with its rear services deployed, it has the capacity of deploying ahead of us and striking a sudden blow. To prevent this I consider it important not to leave the operational initiative to the German command in any circumstances, but to anticipate the enemy and attack the German army at the moment when it is in the process of deploying and before it has time to organize its front and the coordination of its various arms." Volkogonov pointed out that Zhukov did not sign the document, and concluded that it was not submitted to Stalin.

I see the situation differently.

The document cited by Volkogonov has been preserved in full and is to be found in the Historical Archive and Military-Memorial Center of the General Staff.

The title of the document is "Reflections on a Plan for the Strategic Deployment of the Armed Forces of the Soviet Union in the Event of War with Germany and Her Allies." It is addressed to Stalin.

The authors devote fifteen pages of text to discussing plans for a *surprise attack on Germany.* "At present," they say, "Germany and its allies can field 240 divisions against the USSR." They therefore suggest "forestalling the enemy in deploying our forces and attacking. . . . Our armies would be set the strategic objective of smashing the main forces of the German army . . . and emerging by the thirtieth day of the operation along a front from Ostrolenko to Olomuc. . . . To ensure the realization of the plan set out above it is necessary (1) to carry out a secret mobilization of our forces, representing it as a call-up of reserve officers for training; (2) to carry out the secret concentration of troops nearer to the Western frontier, on pretense of moving them to summer camps; (3) to bring aircraft in secretly from outlying areas and concentrate them on forward airstrips, and to begin establishing rear services for the air force immediately."

The main offensive was to be on the southwestern front in the direction of Cracow and Katowice. Its objective was to cut Germany off from its southern allies—Italy, Hungary, and especially Romania, with its oil—the lifeblood of the German war machine.

The document is furnished with detailed maps and diagrams. It was produced and signed in black ink in his own hand by Major General A. Vasilievsky, Deputy Chief of the General Staff. Corrections to the documents were made by the First Deputy Chief of the General Staff, Lieutenant General N. Vatutin. Space was left for the signatures of the Chief of the General Staff, Zhukov, and the People's Commissar for Defense, Timoshenko. Their signatures are in fact missing. But this does not mean that the document was not submitted to Stalin. What we have here is a typical handwritten rough draft. The master copy was most probably destroyed during one of the routine weedings of the archives: a document containing evidence of plans for a Soviet attack on Germany could obviously not be allowed to survive. But minutely detailed work of this sort on the part of the General Staff could not have been carried out without the Boss's knowledge. It is significant that according to Stalin's official engagement book Zhukov, Timoshenko, and Vasilievsky—all three of them—were in and out of Stalin's office on

May 12, 19, and 24. It was, moreover, on May 15, 1941 that units received a directive from the Main Political Administration intended to stiffen morale: "Many political officers," they were told, "have forgotten Lenin's well-known statement that 'just as soon as we are strong enough to defeat capitalism as a whole, we shall take it by the scruff of its neck.' " The same directive explained that a false distinction is sometimes drawn between "just" and "unjust wars": "If a particular country is the first to attack, its war is considered an unjust one, whereas if a country is the victim of attack and merely defends itself, its war must be considered a just one. The conclusion drawn is that the Red army is supposed to wage only defensive war: this is to forget that any war waged by the Soviet Union will be a just one."

It could not be put more clearly.

The Face of the War God

Hitler too had decided to make the first move. Knowing that Stalin was planning an offensive and that he discounted the possibility of a German attack, Hitler made an insane decision. In fact, he had no alternative. Stalin might attack tomorrow himself. Counting on the weakness of Stalin's army, and on the advantage of surprise, Hitler believed that he would win with lightning speed. For only a successful blitzkrieg could save him.

Stalin, meanwhile, still did not believe that Hitler would make such a mad move. Convinced that time was on his side, he went on calmly making ready for his turnaround—the sudden blow of which his generals had written in their "reflections." But for all his certainty, he grew nervous as the fateful day approached. There were too many reports of German troop movements near the frontier.

He sent up a trial balloon. On July 14 a press release from the official news agency, *Tass,* stated: "the rumors which have appeared in the British and not only the British press that war between the USSR and Germany is imminent are clumsy propaganda put out by forces hostile to the USSR and Germany." He waited, but there was no response from Hitler. Meanwhile, members of the German embassy staff were going home. This was the normal leave period, but they seemed to be departing en masse. Again he reviewed the situation, and again he concluded that Hitler could not attack at that time. Summer would soon be ending, and the German army was not dressed for winter. Stalin saw only one explanation: Hitler is obviously scaremongering. Perhaps he's afraid himself. Perhaps he's looking for guarantees. Good, let's give him some, let's pull back some of our divisions. Then move them up again. His well-drilled high command dared not contradict him. Molotov knew when to argue with the Boss (or rather when he wanted to be argued with). Molotov's job now was the same as that of the Soviet ambassador in Germany, Dekanozov, and all the other lickspittles—to confirm the Boss's own thinking.

On June 18 he was passed reports from agents in Germany about the movement of German fighter planes and the appointment of future heads for the Russian territories that would be occupied. His response: "You can tell your sources to go to . . . !"

It was, however, too much for the Commissar for Defense. Chadayev has quoted Timoshenko as saying in conference that "Germany's preparations obviously mean that war will begin this year, and soon." He was told curtly, "Don't try to frighten us, Hitlerite Germany is simply trying to provoke us."

While all this was happening, the Boss, as usual, took a hand in everything. A scientific expedition was at work on Uzbekistan. Mikhail Gerasimov, an expert in reconstructing human faces to fit skulls, had suggested opening the sepulchre of Tamerlane, and Stalin had agreed. He wanted to see the great conqueror's face.

Tamerlane was entombed in Samarkand, in the Guri Emir Mausoleum. When the expedition first started work, the Boss had been told about a local tradition that "the War God's sleep must not be disturbed." If it was, disaster would follow; Tamerlane would return on the third day, bringing war. So said the old men in the Samarkand bazaar. But after seeing Russian saints tipped out of their coffins, churches blown up, and priests murdered, the Boss must have just smiled. He himself was an Eastern god. What were Tamerlane's bones to him! On the night of June 19–20, 1941, the Guri Emir Mausoleum was floodlit. A news crew was there to film the opening of the tomb. A gigantic marble slab was lifted from it. In the dark recesses of the marble sarcophagus stood a black coffin under a rotting cloth-of-gold baldachin. Tamerlane had died a long way from Samarkand and had been brought back to his burial place in this coffin. An old man who worked in the mausoleum begged them not to open the coffin. They laughed at him. Huge nails were pried from the lid. Gerasimov triumphantly removed Tamerlane's skull and held it up for the cameraman. The film was rushed to Moscow, and the Boss saw the War God's skull staring at humankind.

On June 21 he was informed that, according to a German deserter, a sergeant major, war would begin at dawn the next day. Reason told him that this was a provocation. But reports of German troop movements kept coming in from the frontier throughout the day, and that evening he felt bound to issue a cautious order: "In the course of June 22–23 a German attack in front-line areas is possible. The attack may begin with provocative operations. Our troops must not be taken in by any sort of provocation, but must at the same time be completely ready for action, so that they can withstand a sudden assault by the Germans and their allies. During the night they should surreptitiously occupy weapon emplacements in fortified areas. All aircraft should be dispersed to field airstrips and thoroughly camouflaged. The air force must be on permanent alert." Admiral Kuznetsov, chief of naval forces, was ordered to contact fleet commanders: the navy must be ready for battle.

At 9:30 P.M. Molotov summoned Ambassador Schulenberg to express his government's anxiety. Molotov asked the ambassador, "what is the reason for the mass departure of your embassy staff? Why is Germany dissatisfied—if it is? Why was there no reply to Tass's pacific declaration?" Schulenberg's reply was unintelligible. He was obviously depressed. Molotov must have known just what it meant. But no one must ever think—heaven forbid!—that Molotov had understood what the Leader had failed to understand. He chose not to understand Schulenberg's embarrassment.

The Politburo was in session all day long. After the meeting, the black limousines carried the Boss and his comrades-in-arms to his dacha. He needed distraction. Molotov recalled that "on June 21 we were with Stalin at his dacha until 12:00 P.M. We may even have watched a film." But Stalin's forced cheerfulness was a failure, and he instructed Molotov to send an encoded telegram to the Soviet ambassador in Berlin, telling him to put to Ribbentrop the questions which Schulenberg had been asked.

Molotov drove to the Commissariat for Foreign Affairs and a telegram was sent to Berlin at 12:40 A.M.

At 3:30 A.M. German planes bombed Belorussia. At 4:00 A.M. the Germans were already bombing Kiev and Sevastopol.

At that time the Boss was sleeping peacefully at the nearer dacha. Zhukov tells us in his memoirs:

> The Commissar ordered me to ring Stalin. The man on duty asked me in a sleepy voice, "Who's calling?"
>
> "Zhukov, Chief of Staff. Please connect me with Comrade Stalin, it's urgent."

"What, right now? Comrade Stalin is sleeping."

"Wake him up immediately, the Germans are bombing our cities."

Three minutes later Stalin was on the telephone. Zhukov reported the situation, and was answered by silence.

"Did you understand what I said?" Zhukov asked. Again there was silence. Then, finally, "Where's the Commissar? Bring him down to the Kremlin. Tell Poskrebyshev to summon the whole Politburo."

That was how, on June 22, the war began, three days after the opening of Tamerlane's sarcophagus.

23

THE FIRST DAYS OF WAR

THE WITNESS

The street lamps were still burning when his car drove into the Kremlin. The Germans had attacked on Sunday—attacked a country that took its day of rest seriously. So many hungover citizens were sleeping off Saturday night's revelries. Stalin anxiously awaited news of casualties.

He was the first to arrive at the Kremlin. The other members of the Politburo, awakened by Poskrebyshev, filed into his office shortly afterward.

I am looking again at the entries in Stalin's visitors' book on that terrible day. Or, to be exact, for the first, warm daylight hours.

On June 22 he saw Molotov, then Beria, Timoshenko, Mekhlis, Zhukov, Malenkov, Mikoyan, Kaganovich. . . . Among those who entered his office was one whose name was not recorded, because he was not a visitor.

Y. Chadayev, chief administrative assistant to the Council of People's Commissars, had been chosen to take brief notes at all meetings of the Politburo and of the government held in Stalin's private office. Chadayev mentions several times in his memoirs that he was "the only one whom Stalin allowed to take notes." His recollections of the beginning of the war, in the manuscript of his memoirs (written after Stalin's death), are therefore of the greatest interest. When he himself died, his manuscript seems to have made the rounds of various secret archives before coming to rest in the Secret Fund of the Archive of the October Revolution. That was where I managed, during Gorbachev's perestroika, to read these still unpublished memoirs, to which the author gave the title *In Time of Dread.*

IN TIME OF DREAD

There is a persistent legend that in the first days of the war Stalin, stunned by Hitler's attack, was at his wits' end, incapable of action. He then left the Kremlin for the nearer dacha, where he remained, bewildered and inactive. Knowing Stalin's character as I did, I found this behavior strange. And my knowledge of his biography (the lesson he had learned in the Civil War, when the Bolsheviks lost three-quarters of their territory and still emerged victorious) made it seem doubly strange.

It was only after reading Chadayev's memoirs that I began to understand Stalin's behavior. They, together with the dispassionate visitors' book, give us a quite different picture of those first days after the catastrophe.

Chadayev writes that "at dawn all the members of the Politburo, plus Timoshenko and Zhukov, were assembled. Timoshenko made his report: the German attack must be considered an accomplished fact, the enemy had bombed the main airfields, ports, and major arterial junctions. . . . Then Stalin began speaking. He spoke slowly, choosing his words carefully, occasionally his voice broke down. When he had finished everybody was silent for some time, and so was he. In the end he went up to Molotov and said: 'We must get in touch with Berlin again and ring the embassy.' " He was still clinging to the hope that it was just a "provocation." Chadayev goes on: "Molotov rang the Commissariat for Foreign Affairs from Stalin's office and said to somebody there, with a slight stammer, 'Tell him to come.' He explained that Schulenberg was asking to see him. Stalin just said 'Go!' "

Vatutin, First Deputy Chief of the General Staff, left the office for a few minutes to get the latest news, and announced on his return that German troops were rapidly moving deep into Soviet territory, without meeting any strong resistance.

Molotov went to his own office in the Kremlin, the one looking out on the church of Ivan the Terrible, and Schulenberg was shown in to him. Chadayev continues: "After talking to Schulenberg Molotov returned to Stalin's office, and said: 'The German government has declared war on us.' The Politburo were thrown into confusion." They had believed him, and had gone on hoping that it was all a mere provocation, a trial of strength, and that Molotov's talk with the ambassador would sort it all out.

Chadayev writes: "Stalin said calmly, 'The enemy will be beaten all along the line.' Then, turning to the military leaders: 'What do you recommend?' Zhukov said: 'Order the troops on the frontier to attack along the whole front and halt the enemy—he's gone too far too fast.' Timoshenko: 'Not halt—destroy.' "

It was decided that "our armies will fall upon the enemy with all the forces and all the means at their disposal, and destroy them in areas where they have breached the frontier. Pending further orders the frontier will not be crossed. Our planes will bomb enemy forces including those on occupied territory. On that first day of war everyone was in a quite optimistic mood . . . they believed that this was a short-lived venture which would shortly fail."

There, I think, Chadayev was wrong. Timoshenko and the Politburo were simply playing up to the Boss. They dared not say anything different. He would never forgive them, he would harbor a grudge, and he would make them pay for it later. The Boss was also feigning optimism: he realized, of course, that what had happened was a disaster. Hitler had all the advantages of the aggressor. But what were the dimensions of the disaster? Chadayev writes, "I caught a glimpse of Stalin in the corridor. He looked tired, worn out. His pockmarked face was drawn and haggard. During the first half of the day the Politburo approved an appeal to the Soviet people, and Molotov read it over the radio at noon." He put Molotov on display deliberately: Molotov had signed the pact—let him take the consequences. But he and Molotov—both of them Party journalists, both former editors of *Pravda*—had drafted the appeal together. Molotov said that "Stalin did not want to come forward first . . . he wanted to get the picture, decide what the tone should be and what approach to take."

The country heard the government's appeal on June 22. In many towns and cities, people heard it with bombs crashing around them. Molotov was obviously embarrassed. He spoke with difficulty, stammering slightly, and ended his speech with words written by Stalin: "Our cause is just, the enemy will be smashed, victory will be ours." All through the war this sentence would be endlessly repeated, drummed into people's minds. It would become the Boss's mantra.

Chadayev writes: "At 2:00 P.M. I was called to Molotov's office, and Stalin came along. He said, 'Well, you sounded a bit flustered, but the speech went well.' " Molotov was happy. He knew the Boss: he would start looking for people to blame. But Molotov would obviously not be one of them.

The country was waiting for the omniscient one to speak, but the God was for the moment silent. He was waiting to see what would happen at the front, and selecting his first culprits. Chadayev writes, "That evening Stalin was in a somber mood, and said angrily: 'Pavlov [commander on the western front, who had taken the first blow from the Germans] isn't even in communication with the headquarters of his army groups, he says the order reached him late. Why was it late? And what if we hadn't managed to give an order? With or without orders, surely the army ought to be completely ready for action, surely I shouldn't have to give my watch orders to keep working?' " The first culprit had been identified. Stalin, says Chadayev, went on to say, "We must order them to evacuate the population and the enterprises eastward. Nothing must fall into the hands of the enemy."

This sentence implied the burning of towns, villages, and factories by retreating armies—the "scorched earth" tactic. At that moment of retreat and panic, it was wishful thinking. But it would become reality in the near future.

The day of madness continued. Desperate news arrived from the front. Chadayev writes:

> Timoshenko reported that the attack had exceeded all expectations. In the first hours of war enemy planes had made mass attacks on airfields and troops.
>
> Stalin: "I expect many Soviet planes were destroyed right there on the ground?" He worked himself up into an indescribable state of indignation, pacing up and down the office. "Surely the German air force didn't manage to reach every single airfield?"
>
> "Unfortunately it did."
>
> "How many planes were destroyed?"
>
> "At a preliminary estimate around seven hundred."

In reality it was several times more.

The western front suffered the heaviest losses. Pavlov was anathematized all over again. According to Chadayev, "Stalin said, 'This is a monstrous crime. Those responsible must lose their heads,' and immediately instructed the NKVD to investigate the matter."

The twelve-hour workday ended at 5:00 P.M. Beria was the last to leave the Boss's office, no doubt after the usual parting instruction: shoot those responsible! The culprits, however, were lying dead beside their planes.

Work began again during the night. From 3:30 A.M. to the middle of the following night he received an uninterrupted succession of visitors. In the course of the day an instrument which he had thought of in May was finally created. This was the GHQ of the High Command, now the highest administrative organ for the armed services. He called it "Stavka" (General Headquarters), like its equivalent in the days of the deposed Nicholas II. This was no accident. Nor was it by accident that he shortly brought back the officers' epaulettes which all revolutionaries had loathed. Internationalism and world revolution went at once to the bottom of the agenda. The emphasis was on the nation, the Russian state, the idea of the Fatherland.

While he looked around for a commander for his military, he appointed Timoshenko as chief of GHQ High Command ad interim.

It was now June 24, and Stalin's last visitors, Molotov and Timoshenko, did not leave his office until 6:00 A.M. The mask of impassivity, his favorite, was dropped. Now he could be himself. There was no sign of exhaustion, of helplessness. His constant state was one of rage. He hated everybody and everything—for the error he had committed. Chadayev writes: " 'Although our troops are bravely endeavoring to carry out the orders to counterattack,' Timoshenko reported, 'they have not yet achieved the expected results.' Stalin, when he heard all that Timoshenko had to say, flew into a rage. He blamed the western command for everything. Then he heaped reproaches on Vatutin and Timoshenko. They turned pale, but hid their resentment and asked to be sent to the front. 'The front can wait for you a bit longer,' he said, 'but who's going to clear up the mess we have here at GHQ, who's going to correct the present state of affairs?' " Their request had only fueled his indignation. The People's Commissar for Tank Production, V. Malyshev, was then summoned to the meeting. "Stalin interrupted his report: 'You're a long time getting a move on,' he said, and started asking concrete questions about ways to expand arms production, and how best to organize production of armor plating. It was decided to create a new base for tank production in the Urals and Siberia."

If worst came to worst, if the Germans occupied the whole of European Russia, then the limitless expanses of Siberia, and the Urals, with their great mineral wealth, would still be left. The war could be carried on from there.

Chadayev writes: "In conclusion, he instructed Vasilievsky, Deputy Chief of the General Staff, by telephone to 'convey immediately to the commanding officers on each of the fronts our extreme displeasure that the troops have retreated.' " This "most attack-oriented of armies," trained only to attack, had proved helpless in defensive warfare. The army was in headlong retreat.

Chadayev writes: "G. M. Popov, Secretary of the Moscow City Committee of the Party, and the city district secretaries, who had been sitting in the waiting room, were called in. Stalin stroked his mustache with the telephone receiver and said: 'The Central Committee is receiving a large number of requests from the Soviet people for the creation of a citizens' militia. . . . To meet the wishes of the citizens of Moscow we shall set up a number of volunteer divisions of citizen-soldiers.' " A murderous scheme was taking shape in his mind. He would husband his reserves, hold back and keep fresh the new divisions then being formed in Siberia, a land of hunters, full of young men skilled in fighting. For the present he would plug the holes at the front with cannon fodder—the people's militia, the "four-eyed" intelligentsia, who could hardly be taught to fire a gun, boys fresh from universities and technical colleges, together with the hemorrhaged remnants of the retreating armies.

The patriotic call to the militia was sounded. Joining up was supposedly voluntary. But that was "in-depth language." Those who refused to sign on were showered with contempt and promises of retribution.

Meanwhile the search for scapegoats went on. Chadayev writes: "In Molotov's office Stalin said to Dekanozov, lately ambassador in Germany: 'A duckling knows the water while it's still in the egg, and you've been around a bit. In our private conversations you repeatedly asserted that we need not expect an attack before 1942. . . . How could you. . . . In a word, you have not lived up to our expectations.' . . . He came down heavily on Marshal Kulik, an incompetent soldier, one of those whom he had substituted for the purged marshals. 'That good-for-nothing Kulik needs a kick in the ass.' " Day after day was filled with frantic activity, fits of rage, and tireless drudgery. By now there was no disguising the real dimensions of what had happened. It was a military catastrophe. Chadayev writes: "Timoshenko reported that our forces were regrouping to check the enemy's advance. Stalin: 'You mean you are no longer getting ready, as you were previously, to smash the enemy quickly?' 'No, that can't possibly be done right off, but after we've concentrated our forces we shall undoubtedly smash him.' " He began to lose his temper more and more frequently. This was now his normal condition. "Stalin stood in front of the map, with his comrades-in-arms looking reproachfully at his back. Before they had time to do one thing he was asking them to do something else." He decided that it was time to stop playing games. He must begin cautiously speaking the truth. The others still dared not speak it. "Stalin said, 'We were hoping against hope that the enemy was about to be halted and smashed at any moment, but he continues to edge forward.' He fell silent. He looked tired and worried."

THE BLACK CAPITAL

Chadayev reports: "At 3:00 A.M. on June 24 an air-raid warning sounded. The zonal commander of antiaircraft artillery reported that enemy planes were flying toward Moscow, sirens hooted, the population took refuge in air-raid shelters, antiaircraft guns opened fire." Damaged planes left a fiery trail as they crashed to the ground. (How often we wartime children drew pictures of those blazing planes!) Chadayev continues: "But clarification soon followed. The district commander of antiaircraft telephoned to say: 'Our people have made a bit of a mess of things. It turns out we've been firing on our own planes coming back from a bombing raid.' " He omitted to add "and succeeded in shooting them down."

From the very first days of the war, panic and fear reigned in Moscow. Windows were blacked out. Street lamps were unlit. "A paradise for lovers—they could kiss out in the streets," one poet wrote.

Chadayev says, "On June 25, Poskrebyshev summoned me urgently to Stalin's waiting room. Someone was needed to take minutes. I went straight into the office. There was no one there except Stalin, Timoshenko, and Vatutin. Vatutin was just finishing his report. Stalin said: 'To sum up briefly, the situation is extremely serious on all fronts.' After this Timoshenko asked Stalin whether or not his son Yakov, who was very keen to go, should be sent to the front line. Stalin, trying to contain his anger, said: 'Some—to put it mildly—inordinately zealous officials are always trying too hard to please their superiors. I don't include you in that number but I advise you never to ask me questions like that again.' " What did an unloved son matter? His country was perishing.

As always, Stalin tried to take a hand in everything. Chadayev reports that "he concerned himself, for instance, with the choice of design for a sniper's automatic rifle, and the type of bayonet which could most easily be fixed to it—the knife-blade or the three-edged kind. . . . When I went into Stalin's office I usually found him with Molotov, Beria, and Malenkov. . . . They never asked questions. They sat and listened." But he was now beginning to pay for the universal fear which he had inspired. "Reports coming in from the front as a rule understated our losses and exaggerated those of the enemy. All this helped to convince him that the enemy could not take such losses for long and would shortly suffer defeat." The Germans, however, were advancing rapidly. Minsk was expected to fall at any moment, which meant that Smolensk would also fall, and the way to Moscow would lie open.

Chadayev writes: "Stalin often sent for the heads of People's Commissariats, gave them heavy assignments, and insisted quite unrealistically that they should be carried out in a very short time. People left his office in a state of deep depression." And he was quicker than ever to notice looks exchanged by members of the Politburo behind his back.

Chadayev reports:

> On the morning of the 27th the members of the Politburo assembled as usual in Stalin's office. When the meeting was over, I left the office and saw through the window Stalin, Molotov, and Beria getting into a car. Poskrebyshev hesitated for a moment and then said, "The Germans have obviously taken Minsk." Shortly afterward the government telephone rang, and Poskrebyshev told me that the call was from Vlasik, chief of Stalin's bodyguard, to say that "the Boss," and also Malenkov, Molotov, and Beria, were at the People's Commissariat for Defense. Vatutin told me later that their arrival at the Commissariat had caused great surprise. The staff of the Commissariat seeing Stalin for the first time couldn't make up their minds whether they were really seeing the Leader or were dreaming. He went into Timoshenko's office and said abruptly that they had to acquaint themselves on the spot with the reports coming in from the front, and with progress in planning further measures. . . . Stalin stood by the operations map without saying a word, obviously trying to control his fury. At a sign from Timoshenko, Zhukov and Vatutin remained in the office. Stalin asked, "What's happening at Minsk? Isn't the position stabilized yet?"
>
> Timoshenko: "I am not yet able to report on that."
>
> Stalin: "It is your duty to have the facts clearly before you at all times and to keep us up to date. At present you are simply afraid to tell us the truth."
>
> Zhukov, who had been on edge before Stalin's arrival, flared up. "Comrade Stalin, have we your permission to get on with our work?"
>
> Beria butted in: "Are we perhaps in your way?"
>
> "You know [Zhukov said in exasperation] that the situation on all fronts is critical, the front commanders are awaiting instructions from the Commissariat, and it's better if we do it ourselves, the Commissariat and the General Staff."

> It degenerated into a squabble.
>
> Beria (testily): "We too are capable of giving orders!"
>
> Zhukov: "If you think you can—do it!"
>
> Beria: "If the Party tells us to, we will."
>
> Zhukov (as angrily as before): "So wait till it tells you to. As things are, we've been told to do the job."
>
> There was a pause. Then Zhukov went up to Stalin and said, "Excuse my outspokenness, Comrade Stalin, we shall certainly get it all worked out and then we'll come to the Kremlin and report on the situation."
>
> Stalin looked at Timoshenko, who said: "Comrade Stalin, our first priority must be to think how we can help the armies at the front. After that we can give you the information you want."
>
> Stalin: "You are making a crass mistake in trying to draw a line between yourselves and us. . . . We must all join in thinking how to help the fronts."
>
> Then he looked gloomily at each of the Politburo members in turn and said, "There we are then, let them get it sorted out themselves first. Let's go, comrades."
>
> He was the first out of the office.

He had seen it with his own eyes. The most dreadful thing possible had happened: they were no longer afraid of him. And if they were no longer afraid of him—it could be the end. Chadayev writes: "As he left the Commissariat for Defense he said angrily: 'Lenin founded our state, and we've fucked it up!' " Molotov has also described the visit to the Commissariat: "I went with Stalin to the Commissar for Defense. Stalin spoke rather rudely to Timoshenko and Zhukov, though he rarely lost control of himself. Then we went out to the dacha, where he said, 'We've fucked it up!' The 'we' was meant to include all of us!" Molotov was right. It included everybody and everything.

A Moment of Panic, or a Brilliant Move

Chadayev describes the rest of that day and the next few crucial days at the start of the war:

> In the latter half of June 27 I looked in on Poskrebyshev. The government telephone rang and Posk. answered: "Comrade Stalin is not here, and I don't know when he will be." The Vice-

Commissar for Defense, Mekhlis, came in and asked whether he should ring Stalin at the dacha. Posk. told him to go ahead. Mekhlis dialed the number of the nearer dacha on the hot line and waited half a minute. No answer.

"I don't understand it," Poskrebyshev said.

"Maybe he's on his way here, but if so the guard would have rung me."

We waited a few minutes longer, then decided it wasn't worth waiting and went to see Molotov. . . . While we were there the phone rang and Molotov told somebody that he didn't know when Stalin would be in the Kremlin. . . . Next day, I went to Stalin's outer office, but he hadn't arrived. Nobody had any idea what could have happened. The following day, I went to the outer office again to sign papers, and Poskrebyshev told me at once and categorically, "Comrade Stalin is not here and is unlikely to be here."

"Has he perhaps left for the front?"

"Why do you keep bothering me? I've told you he isn't here and won't be here."

There have been many legends about Stalin's disappearance in those dreadful first days of the war. Now we have Chadayev's eyewitness account:

In the evening I went along to Poskrebyshev again with some papers, and yet again Stalin failed to appear. I had a great pile of papers for signature, and since Voznesensky was First Vice-Chairman of the Council of People's Commissars I asked him to sign. Voznesensky rang Molotov, listened to him for quite a time, then put down the receiver and said: "Molotov asks you to wait one more day, and wants members of the Politburo to meet in his office in two hours' time. So hang on to the documents for a bit."

Voznesensky picked up the hot line phone, waited a minute, and said, "No reply from the dacha." . . . It was a mystery; something must have happened to him at that critical moment.

Chadayev went back to Stalin's outer office that evening.

"The Boss isn't here, and won't be here today," Poskrebyshev said.

"He wasn't here yesterday, either."

"No, he wasn't here yesterday either," Poskrebyshev said, with a trace of sarcasm.

I assumed that Stalin was ill, but didn't like to ask. . . . Stalin usually got to the Kremlin by 2:00 P.M. For half an hour black cars would drive out of the dacha gates one after another, with Stalin in one of them, no one knew which. Stalin's workday went on till 3:00 or 4:00 A.M. All members of the Politburo, the top military men, and People's Commissars had to observe this routine. And suddenly he had failed to turn up. His closest associates were alarmed, to say the least. We all knew that he usually summoned one official after another, with not much of an interval in between. But now the telephones were silent. We knew only that he was at the nearer dacha, but nobody felt bold enough to go and see him. During the days of his seclusion members of the Politburo met in Molotov's office, trying to decide what to do. According to the dacha staff Stalin was alive and well, but had shut himself up, away from everybody, was receiving nobody, and wasn't answering the phone. The members of the Politburo decided unanimously to visit him in a body.

What, then, had really happened? Stalin's great hero was Ivan the Terrible. One curious work in his personal library was A. N. Tolstoy's play *Ivan the Terrible,* published in Moscow in 1942, the most terrible year of the war, and read by Stalin while the Soviet Union was suffering one heavy defeat after another. He read it carefully, amending the style in bold handwriting, and crossing out expressions of grief. His favorite tsar's speech must be like his own, clipped and laconic. The cover of the book, with his pensive doodles, is particularly interesting.

One word written over and over again on the cover is "teacher." Others include "We'll hold out." "We'll hold out"—that was what then filled his thoughts. But let us not forget the word "teacher," which he inscribed on the play about the terrible tsar.

No, the Man of Steel was not behaving like a highly strung person. In the Commissariat for Defense that day he had seen a change in attitude, and drawn his conclusions. He knew that Minsk would fall any day, and that the German avalanche would roll on toward Moscow. If it did, his pathetic slaves might take fright and rebel. So Stalin emulated his teacher: Ivan the Terrible's favorite trick was to pretend that he was dying, watch how the hapless boyars behaved, then rise from his sickbed and cruelly punish them, to discourage all the others. Ivan also made a habit of disappearing from the capital, to show the boyars how helpless they were without their tsar. The Boss was behaving as his teacher had. Poskrebyshev and Beria, the head of the NKVD, were, I am convinced, in on the secret, and took note of what his comrades said in his absence. The experienced courtier Molotov saw through his game immediately, and was wary of signing important papers. *Not* signing was a proof of loyalty. The Boss had chosen his comrades-in-arms well. Without him they were "blind kittens" (as he would one day call them). By leaving them to themselves he made them feel their insignificance and reminded them that, without him, the military would sweep them away. Molotov quickly organized a pilgrimage to the dacha. There the great actor performed a well-known play called "The Retirement Game."

Chadayev records what happened, as described to him by Marshal Bulganin (a Politburo member):

> We were all struck by Stalin's appearance. He was thinner. . . . His sallow, pockmarked face was haggard. He looked gloomy. He said: "The great Lenin is no more. . . . If only he could see us now. See those to whom he entrusted the fate of his country. . . . I am inundated with letters from Soviet people, rightly rebuking us, saying surely you can halt the enemy. Maybe some among you wouldn't mind putting all the blame on me."
>
> Molotov: "Thank you for your frankness, but I tell you here and now that if some idiot tried to turn me against you I'd see him damned. We are asking you to come back to work, and for our part we will do all we can to help you."
>
> "Yes, but think about it: can I live up to people's hopes anymore, can I lead the country to final victory? There may be more deserving candidates."
>
> Voroshilov: "I believe I shall be voicing the unanimous opinion: there is none more worthy." There was an immediate chorus of "right!"

They earnestly pleaded with him. They knew that the less insistent would be doomed. The game was over: now they had begged him yet again to be their Leader, as if they had reinvested him with power.

Consulting the visitors' book, I see that Chadayev's memory has misled him by only a day. On June 28 Stalin was still receiving visitors. But for the 29th and 30th there are no more entries. On those two days

Stalin was indeed absent from the Kremlin. He reappeared there only on July 1.

SOSO'S BRIEF REAPPEARANCE

On July 3 Stalin at last made his long-awaited appeal to the people: "Comrades, citizens! Brothers and sisters! Warriors of the army and the fleet! I call upon you, my friends." That was how he began. Together with the standard revolutionary form of address—"comrades"—the Christian form of address—"brothers and sisters"—had resurfaced from his seminary days. "Brothers and sisters"—they, the people, were the ones who would have to defend their Motherland. In films made at this time church bells were sometimes heard.

He declared the war a Great Patriotic War, a holy war fought by the people against aggressors, like Tsar Alexander I's war against the aggressor Napoleon. As if to support this idea, Hitler had launched his campaign on the anniversary of Napoleon's invasion—June 22. The analogy was bound to inspire hope. In 1812 too the Russians had retreated, and even surrendered Moscow to the enemy, but they had emerged victorious.

The Party, of course, figured in his speech. He called on everyone to "rally round the Party of Lenin *and Stalin,*" and no one saw anything strange in these words, coming from Stalin himself.

During his mysterious retreat the ex-seminarist had decided to involve the aid of the God he had rejected. He had already heard that the Patriarch of Antioch had appealed to all Christians to come to Russia's aid.

A note scribbled in the play *Ivan the Terrible* reads: "Speak to Shaposhin"—Boris Shaposhnikov, then Chief of the General Staff. In his memoirs, Zhukov recalled that "Stalin always called him by his first name and patronymic, and never raised his voice to him. . . . He was the only person allowed to smoke in Stalin's office." Boris Mikhailovich Shaposhnikov was a former colonel in the tsarist army who never disguised his religious beliefs. Another of the senior people on the General Staff, Vasilievsky, was a priest's son. In the early days of the war both of them were very close to the Boss. Presumably from them he heard of an incident that shook the Orthodox world. Ilya, Metropolitan of the Lebanon Mountains, had shut himself up in an underground cell and gone without food or sleep while he knelt in prayer for Russia to the Mother of God. And he had a miraculous vision, which he described in a letter to the leaders of the Orthodox Church in Russia. On the third day the Mother of God had appeared to him in a pillar of fire and given him God's sentence: "The churches and monasteries must be reopened throughout the country. Priests must be brought back from imprisonment, Leningrad must not be surrendered, but the sacred icon of Our Lady of Kazan should be carried around the city boundary, taken on to Moscow, where a service should be held, and thence to Stalingrad [Tsaritsyn]."

These words must have sounded like something from Stalin's forgotten childhood. A little while before he had proclaimed a "Godless Five-Year Plan," by the end of which (in 1943) the last church was to be closed and the last priest destroyed. But now the Boss decided to act on Ilya's vision. This was the beginning of his remarkable, and short-lived, return to God.

Was it that? Had he seen the light? Had fear made him run to his Father? Had the Marxist God-Man simply decided to exploit belief in God? Or was it all of these things at once? Whatever the reason, after his mysterious retreat, he began making his peace with God. Something happened which no historian has yet written about. On his orders many priests were brought back from the camps. In Leningrad, besieged by the Germans and gradually dying of hunger, the inhabitants were astounded, and uplifted, to see the wonder-working icon of Our Lady of Kazan brought out into the streets and borne in procession. From Leningrad the icon went to Moscow, and was then sent to besieged Stalingrad. It was displayed in each of the three great cities which had not surrendered to the enemy. Twenty thousand churches were reopened, including those of the Monastery of the Trinity and St. Sergius, and the Monastery of the Caves in Kiev. He and his generals sent troops into battle with the words "God go with you." On October 17 *Pravda* reported that the head of the Bolshevik Party had met the interim head of the Patriarchate, Metropolitan Sergei—the first occasion of its kind since October 1917. In the course of their meeting, it was said, Stalin had "reacted sympathetically to the proposal to elect a Patriarch, and said that no obstacles would be put in its way by the government."

Once back at work, Stalin was tireless in his efforts to concentrate power in his own hands. On July 1 he created the State Committee for Defense. This was now the supreme authority in the state, and he was its chairman. Ten days later he also appointed himself Chief of Staff and, shortly afterward, Commander-in-Chief, People's Commissar for the Defense, and Chairman of the Council of Ministers. He remained, of course, Leader of the Party.

Now that he held all the levers of power, he resolved to open negotiations with the steadily advancing Hitler. According to information given by Marshal Zhukov to the historian Y. Pavlenko, Stalin instructed Beria to make an attempt via the Bulgarian embassy in Berlin to start peace talks with the Germans. Marshal K. Moskalenko, who heard it from Beria himself, has told the same story.

He was most probably only trying to slow down the lightning German advance and give his armies a breather. The Brest-Litovsk Treaty could serve as a precedent, and an excuse. Hitler, of course, was not interested.

Father and Son

In those days of military disaster he was fated to suffer his cruelest humiliation. On July 19, 1941, he was handed a monitored news flash from Berlin. His older son, Yakov, had been taken prisoner by the Germans. Yakov, it was reported, had in his own words "realized that resistance was pointless and voluntarily come over to the German side."

Stalin kept the following report among his private papers: "A leaflet was dropped by fascist aircraft. . . . It showed a group of German officers talking to Yakov. Yakov was wearing his tunic, without belt. The caption read: 'Stalin's son, Yakov Dzhugashvili, full lieutenant, battery commander, has surrendered. That such an important Soviet officer has surrendered proves beyond doubt that all resistance to the German army is completely pointless. So stop fighting and come over to us.' " On August 7, 1941, he was sent another leaflet. The Germans were showering such leaflets upon his army. One of them included the text of a letter written by Yakov: "Dear Father, I am quite well and shall shortly be sent to one of the camps for officers in Germany. I wish you good health. Greetings to everybody. Yasha." It was his son's handwriting. He was a traitor. There could be no doubt about it.

Stalin's personal archives contain a "Biography of Yakov Dzhugashvili": "His wife—Julia Isakovna Meltser. . . . Until 1935 he lived at his father's expense, and studied. In 1935 he graduated from the Institute of Transport. In 1937 he entered the Artillery Academy." Entering the academy had signified reconciliation with his father, who had always wanted his sons to be soldiers. Yakov had graduated from the academy on May 9, 1941, six weeks before the outbreak of war.

He had left for the front on the first day of the war. His father had no time to see him before he left. Yakov had telephoned from his younger brother Vasily's dacha, where a merry farewell party was in progress. Under interrogation by the Germans Yakov said: "On June 22 my father told me over the phone to 'go and fight.' "

"Go and Fight"

Many soldiers gave themselves up at that stage of the war, or ran home to their villages, where their parents hid them in the cellar. But many were taken prisoner only after heavy fighting, and because they were wounded. Stalin nonetheless decided to treat them all alike. He drafted a decree saying that "all service personnel taken prisoner are declared outside the law and their families are subject to punishment." He further decreed that "men who find themselves surrounded must fight on to the last, try to break out and join their own side, while those who choose to surrender are to be destroyed by any means possible, and the families of Red army men who surrender are to be deprived of state grants and assistance."

That left his soldiers two possibilities: they could either fight and win, or they could die. And while he was contemplating this decree German planes were dropping leaflets telling soldiers that his son had surrendered. He had never loved Yakov, and he concluded that the wolf cub was seeking revenge—for constant humiliation, for his father's neglect and dislike, for the arrest of his mother's relatives the Svanidzes. . . . Stalin now hated everything connected with the traitor, including all the Svanidzes. It was no coincidence that Alyosha Svanidze, the traitor son's uncle, was shot the following month, on August 20, 1941.

Maria Svanidze, Yakov's aunt, also had committed an irreparable mistake. Kira Alliluyeva-Politkovskaya, the daughter of Stalin's mistress (and his wife's sister-in-law) Zhenya, recorded in her memoirs: "Someone who happened to be passing through brought Mama a letter from Maria Anisimovna. She wrote that she was in a camp, that she was having a very hard time there, and that she was dying. When Stalin was in a good mood Mama gave him the letter. He read it and said, 'Zhenya, don't ever do this again.' "

He had read Maria's diary by then, and the thought that the traitor's relative, Maria, had "observed him" with Zhenya, and had taken advantage of her discovery to petition him through Zhenya, infuriated him. Intrigue was forbidden to everyone except himself. As always, he chose a radical solution: the hated Svanidzes must all disappear. Maria and Mariko Svanidze, Alyosha's sister, were shot early in 1942.

So strong was Stalin's belief that his son was a traitor that when the Germans offered through the Red Cross to discuss Yakov's release he simply did not reply.

In the army, rumor had it that the Germans had offered to release Yakov in exchange for a captured field marshal, but Stalin had said, "We don't trade ordinary soldiers for field marshals"—to let everybody know that to Stalin they were all equal, that as far as he was concerned his son was like all other soldiers, and that all soldiers were his sons. At the same time a number of special operations groups were formed to try and snatch Yakov from his place of internment, or to kill him so that the Germans could no longer make use of him. They all perished.

Yakov's wife, Julia Meltser, mother of Stalin's granddaughter, was duly consigned to the Lubyanka. She would be released two years later, when he finally learned that his son was not a traitor. For the time being, Mekhlis invented a story for dissemination in the army: Stalin's son had enjoyed no privileges, and had been wounded before he was taken prisoner. The German leaflets were just lying propaganda.

Documents in Stalin's private archive prove his unfortunate son's innocence. They include, for instance, a letter to Vasily, which was immediately passed on to his father.

> Dear Vasily Iosifovich, I am the colonel who came to your dacha with Yakov Iosifovich on the day he left for the front. On July 12 the regiment was sent into battle with a handful of infantry and without ammunition, and outnumbered ten to one. . . . The divisional commander abandoned them and left the battlefield in a tank. He drove past Yakov Iosifovich showing not the slightest interest in what became of him. . . . [Signed] Ivan Sapegin, Commanding Officer, 303rd Light Artillery Regiment.

The Boss was to learn soon afterward that the story thought up by his propagandists was no more than the truth. His suspicions had been unjustified. His son had been loyal to the end. Zhukov remembered this conversation:

> "Comrade Stalin," I said, "I've been wanting for some time to ask you about your son Yakov. Is there any more news of his fate?" He did not answer my question immediately. He took at least a hundred steps around the room, then said in a strangely muffled voice: "Yakov will never escape. They'll shoot him, murdering

> swine that they are. From what we've been able to learn he is kept isolated from the other prisoners and is under pressure to betray his Motherland." He was silent for a moment, and then added confidently that "Yakov would sooner die than betray his Motherland." . . . He sat at the table for a long time in silence without touching his food.

He would not know the whole story until Hitler was finally defeated. Stalin was then sent the record of Yakov's interrogation, impounded in Germany. What follows is an excerpt from the report of interrogation at Luftwaffe headquarters on July 18, 1941:

> "Did you come over to us voluntarily, or were you captured in battle?"
>
> "I had no choice. We were surrounded. It caused such a panic that everybody started running. I was with the divisional commander at the time. . . . I started running toward my own battery, but a group of Red army men who wanted to break through to the Soviet side called out to me and asked me to take command and lead them in an attack on your forces. I did so, but the soldiers took fright and I found myself alone. . . . If my own ranks had retreated, if I'd seen my own division retreating, I'd have shot myself, but these weren't my men, they were infantry. . . . I was trying to join my own unit. . . . I exchanged clothes with a peasant in some village—gave him my uniform in exchange for civilian clothes. . . . I went into the cottage and the peasant said, 'Go away now or we'll report you.' . . . The woman couldn't stop crying. She said they'd kill her and her children and burn the house down. There was nothing else for it . . . I was surrounded and had nowhere to go. So I came along and said, 'I'm surrendering.' "
>
> "Does the Red government consist mainly of Jews?"
>
> "That's all rubbish, stupid talk. They have no influence at all. On the contrary, I personally don't mind telling you that the Russian people has always hated the Jews. All I can say about them is that they are incapable of work. . . . From their point of view all that matters is trade."
>
> "You know, don't you, that your father's second wife was Jewish? Because Kaganovich is a Jew, isn't he?"
>
> "Nothing of the sort. She was Russian. What are you talk-

ing about? Nothing like that ever happened. His first wife was Georgian and his second was Russian, and that's all there is to it."

"Wasn't his second wife's name Kaganovich?"

"No, no, that's just rumors, nonsense! . . . His wife died . . . Alliluyeva. She was Russian. He's sixty-two now. He was married. Now he isn't."

"About this business of burning all the foodstocks when they're abandoning a place. That's a dreadful disaster for the whole population. . . . Do you think it's right?"

"Frankly, I do."

"Do you know that we've found a letter—from a Russian officer. It says in part, 'I'm doing my exam for second lieutenant in the reserve. I should like to come home this autumn, but I can only manage it if we aren't sent on an outing to Berlin. June 11. Viktor.' "

[The interrogator made a note of his immediate reaction:] He read the letter and said "I'll be damned!"

"Was there really any such intention?"

"No, I don't think so."

In conclusion Yakov said, "I don't know how I could face my father. I'm ashamed to be alive."

Stalin did not make this interrogator's report public. His son was right: it was a disgrace that he was still alive. His son had realized it when the decree on prisoners of war, signed by his father, had reached him. It was an order to him to die. Yakov obeyed his order in the following year.

Stalin would receive information about Yakov's tragic end, a statement made by Gustav Wegner, the officer commanding the SS battalion guarding Yakov's camp. Wegner wrote: "Late in 1943 the prisoners were taking their exercise—Dzhugashvili wouldn't go with them, and asked to see the commandant of the camp. . . . An SS man went to the phone to call the commandant. While he was telephoning the following happened: Dzhugashvili was walking around, and absentmindedly crossed the no-go area and went toward the (electrified) fence. The sentry shouted 'Halt!' Dzhugashvili kept straight on. The sentry shouted 'I'll shoot!' The sentry fired at his head and killed him. . . . As the shot was fired Dzhugashvili simultaneously seized the high-tension wire and immediately collapsed onto the first two rows of barbed wire. He hung there in that position for twenty-four hours, after which his body was taken away to the crematorium."

The dreadful month of July went by, with the Soviet armies rolling back toward Moscow. Marshal Konyev remembered receiving a telephone call at Vyazma from Stalin. To his surprise, it was an impassioned monologue. "Comrade Stalin is not a traitor. Comrade Stalin is not a turncoat. Comrade Stalin is an honorable man . . . he will do everything in his power to correct the present situation." He did just that. He began by re-creating an atmosphere of terror, so that he would never again have to deliver pathetic monologues for the benefit of generals. His decrees on deserters were accompanied by the shooting of soldiers and officers. Then some of the generals were executed. The former High Command of the western front were court-martialed on July 22. The generals asked to be sent to the front as ordinary soldiers, to atone with their blood for the defeat of their armies, but their duty now was to help him restore unquestioning obedience to the new Supreme Commander. He decreed that "army general D. Pavlov, formerly commanding the western front, V. Klimovski, a former chief of staff, A. Grigoriev, former chief of communications, western front . . . being guilty of cowardice, inaction, mismanagement, and deliberate disorganization of the troops . . . are to be shot." This made his generals remember 1937, and who had the power.

In mid-July German troops belonging to the "Center Group" were already outside Kiev, and a mere 150 miles from Moscow. The German front was moving forward along a line from the Baltic to the Black Sea. Outwardly, everything was just as it had been when Poland was attacked: the Germans took many prisoners, whole Russian armies were surrounded, mindless confusion reigned in the retreating units. But right from the start there was a difference. The German General Blumenrit wrote: "The conduct of the Russian troops in retreat was strikingly different from that of the Poles or the Western Allies. Even when they were surrounded they did not leave their positions." Partly, of course, this was because his soldiers were brave, but the terrible decree also had a considerable effect. General Halder's diary is even more interesting: "Russia, a colossus that deliberately prepared for war, was underestimated by us. . . . When the war began we had 200 divisions against us. . . . Now, on August 11, 1941, after the bloody losses they have suffered, we estimate the number of divisions is 360. Even if we smash a dozen of them the Russians will organize another dozen." Stalin could afford to sacrifice millions. There were other millions where they came from. Hitler believed that Stalin would be overthrown by his own people as soon as he suffered a heavy defeat in the field: "One good kick at the door and the whole rotten structure will collapse immediately," Hitler told General Halder.

But the Soviet people did not even dare ask why their Leader had been caught napping by the German invasion, why the army was unready to defend itself and go on to win. Independent thought had evaporated almost completely in the white heat of Terror. He had created a new society, united by an aggressive pagan creed. And by fear, the great engine of despotism. The people dared not doubt the God Stalin. The armies had meekly retreated, dying with the words "For the Motherland! For Stalin!" on their lips. With this war cry, coined by him and his ideologies, the generals led their soldiers into futile attacks. His name was often the last sound men heard before they died.

"If you only had come earlier!" This was how White officers, who had miraculously survived the purges, greeted the Germans. But Hitler was a help. The bestial atrocities of the Germans stiffened resistance and made former White Russians rescind their greeting in a hurry.

At the same time what the Boss had hoped for all along began to happen: Hitler's resources were dwindling. He decided to halt the advance on Moscow temporarily and concentrate his efforts on the Ukraine and the Caucasus. He needed grain and oil to continue the war. Hitler counted on the traditional animosity toward Russia of the Ukraine and the descendants of Cossacks, who had special reasons to hate the Bolsheviks. But the inevitable happened: the fascists made enemies even of those who originally sympathized with them. The brutality and the looting of the occupying armies in the Ukraine gave impetus to the partisan war which the Boss so skillfully organized. Hitler's desire to exterminate the Jews mobilized the most dynamic section of the population against him: yesterday's timid intellectuals became selfless heroes. Throughout the whole period, there was only one serious defection: Lieutenant General Vlasov and his army were surrounded in summer 1942, and went over to the Germans.

Vlasov, second in command on the Volkhovo front, had distinguished himself in the fighting near Moscow. His very modest part in the Civil War, his obscurity in the Trotsky period, and his lack of contacts with old Leninists had enabled him to make a career during the years of terror. Did he go over to Hitler because he saw no hope for himself once he was taken prisoner? Or did he really hate Stalin and dream of a new Russia, as he claimed? But how could Vlasov hope to build a new Russia in alliance with Hitler, who meant to destroy Slavdom?

Vlasov called his units the Russian Liberation Army (ROA). He was joined by White generals well known to Stalin from the battles for Tsaritsyn—Ataman P. Krasnov and General Shkuro.

After his victory he would find Vlasov, Krasnov, and Shkuro, and make them all pay. The NKVD would hunt soldiers who had served in the ROA all over Europe. They would be shot, or more often end on the gallows. The gallows at Gori had remained in his memory from childhood, as a symbol of disgrace. Besides the ROA the Germans created Caucasian, Turkestanian, Georgian, and Armenian legions. These were all small formations, useful mainly for propaganda purposes. Only in the North Caucasus, in the Chechen-Ingush and Kabarda-Balkar "autonomous republics" did Hitler obtain some semblance of collaboration by exploiting the hatred of Moslems for Russians.

The Boss could claim that the empire had stood the test.

Under the Walls of Moscow

At the beginning of October 1941, the offensive against Moscow was resumed. Hitler announced that "the enemy is prostrate. The territory to the rear of our armies is twice as large as that of the German Reich in 1933."

But the Boss knew that there was still plenty of territory ahead of Hitler's troops. And also ahead was the winter, for which the German army was unprepared.

The Germans continued their attack, but it was already getting difficult as the autumn rains washed away nightmarish Russian roads, causing trucks, tanks, and artillery to sink into the mud.

And then—a miracle happened. Metropolitan Ilya had spoken the truth. The Mother of God had not deserted the land. Heavy snowfalls began earlier than anyone remembered—at the beginning of October. In the Moscow area the weather is usually fine and warm at that time of year, but in 1941 the first snow fell on October 7. "There was never a hint that we would be getting winter uniforms," wrote General Blumenrit. On November 3 the temperature dropped to –8 [16°F]. Petrol and lubricating oil began to freeze in the engines of tanks. The Germans lay down on the ice under their tanks and lit fires, and General Guderian begged in vain for winter clothing.

Meanwhile, around Vyazma and Bryansk, five Soviet armies had been surrounded because their commanders had blundered, and were now fighting to the death. They did what he meant them to do, and pinned down the Germans who were gradually destroying them, bleeding them dry. They perished, but the German troops emerged on the road to Moscow drained, exhausted.

By mid-October German units were within twenty miles of Moscow. Hitler was getting ready for a victory parade through the Moscow streets. On October 15 the Boss decided to evacuate the city. Government departments and foreign embassies began withdrawing to Kuibyshev, deep in the rear.

Departure of the Sacred Remains

While all was in collapse, and hundreds of thousands were encircled and doomed to die, Zbarsky, custodian of the Body of Lenin, was summoned to the Kremlin. The presence of Molotov, Kaganovich, Beria, and Mikoyan in the Boss's office underlined the importance of the meeting. Zbarsky was informed of the Politburo's decision to evacuate the precious Body deep into the rear—to distant Tyumen. Zbarsky later recounted the story to the playwright A. Stein, who wrote about it in his memoirs:

> "What will you need?" [they asked Zbarsky.]
>
> "I shall need a coffin."
>
> "What size?"
>
> "We're the same size."
>
> "Take his measurements" [Mikoyan said to his aide.]

While the custodian was reverently measured, he spoke at length on the Body's requirements. There was a lot to be done. They would have to equip a freight car with the mechanism necessary to maintain the optimum microclimate, and with special shock absorbers to prevent jolting. With chaos and panic all around him, the Boss gave orders that the Body was to want for nothing, and shortly afterward a special-purpose train left Moscow in the utmost secrecy. The Body arrived in Tyumen and was secretly housed in a former tsarist modern school. For secrecy's sake all the scientists on the Body's staff lived with it in the school. Sentries, however, were still mounted at the Mausoleum, to conceal the Body's departure. In those October days of praise and evacuation Moscow had to go on believing that "Lenin is with us."

The Boss, too, was due to leave the capital soon afterward. Members of his bodyguard recall how his daughter, Svetlana, helped with the packing. His library had already been transferred to Kuibyshev, along with his personal papers. Maria Svanidze's diary was evacuated with them. The nearer dacha was booby-trapped. A secret train awaited him in a siding. Four planes and his own Douglas aircraft stood ready at the airfield. And then he made a startling decision.

"We Will Not Surrender"

Severe cold had set in. "General Frost" was helping Russia. Field intelligence reported that German tanks were stalling, that men were already dying from frostbite. Meanwhile, Stalin had concentrated a powerful striking force just outside Moscow. A woman who lived in the village of Nikolina Gora recalled how "on the eve of the battle Siberian troops were stationed right there in our woods. Lads with fat, red faces, wearing newish white sheepskin coats. They contrived to sleep, standing up, leaning against trees. The snoring was terrible." Molotov recalled that "at this juncture all the subunits were calling for reinforcements. Operations in the Moscow area were under Zhukov's command. But however hard he begged, Stalin wouldn't give him so much as a battalion. He just told him to hold on at any price. Stalin then had five armies up to full strength and equipped with modern arms [including the new, heavily armored T34 tank]. We thought at the time that Stalin was making a terrible mistake. But when the Germans had lost enough blood he activated these units." His soldiers had already died in the millions wearing the enemy down. He had already appeased the War God's hunger. His strategy was triumphing. As in the wars between ancient empires, he first exhausted the enemy and then prepared to throw in the troops whose strength he had husbanded. And to do it beneath the very walls of the capital.

His son Vasily's family, his son Yakov's daughter, and his daughter, Svetlana, were now moved to Kuibyshev. He himself had a secret bunker ready there. The People's Commissariats and the General Staff were already working in Kuibyshev.

Moscow was being prepared for the arrival of the Germans. Smoke from bonfires hung over the capital—they were burning archives. Prisoners were hastily shot in the cellars of the Lubyanka. On the night of October 15–16 Beria called a meeting of leading Party personnel and ordered them to "evacuate everybody who is unable to help defend Moscow. Foodstuffs in the shops should be distributed to the population so as not to fall into enemy hands." The highway was choked with people leaving the city. Special trains carried women and children to the rear. Thieves were busy in deserted apartments. House managers often told them which were the wealthy ones. Pictures and jewelry were sold dirt cheap.

And then Stalin decided that the time had come. As A. Rybin, one of his guards, reported, after his usual long, long day at headquarters he set off for the nearer dacha, which was already mined. The guards were amazed to see him. There were no lights burning, and they were about to blow the place up. He played the scene to perfection. Why, he wanted to know, were there no lights? He was told why. He shrugged and said simply "Clear the mines at once, and light the stove. I'll get on with some work in the meantime." He informed the astonished guards that he was "not leaving Moscow for anywhere else, and you are staying with me. We will not surrender Moscow." He sat down in the summer house to work. That same night, men in the familiar NKVD uniform appeared in house managers' offices. One house manager in ten was arrested and shot. The following morning they were shooting people trying to loot shops. Everyone realized immediately that the Boss was still in Moscow.

His daughter wrote to him from Kuibyshev on September 19: "Dear, dear Papa, my precious joy, hello, how are you, I've settled down comfortably here. But oh, Papa dear, how I long to come to Moscow, just for one little day! Papa, why do the Germans keep creeping nearer and nearer all the time? When are they going to get it in the neck, as they deserve? After all, we can't go on surrendering all our industrial towns to them. . . . Dear Papa, how I long to see you. I'm hoping for your permission to fly to Moscow if only for two days."

People could be shot for asking some of these questions. But he was confident that he would soon be able to answer her. The battle of Moscow was about to begin. Moscow was a symbol, and he was resolved to save it.

He allowed Svetlana to fly in for two days. The Germans were already scrutinizing the city through their field glasses, and he received her in the recently completed air-raid shelter. She was happy and wanted to talk, but he was irritable and got angry with her for distracting him.

As soon as Svetlana had left he put on his brilliant propaganda show. It was a sort of sequel to his dacha stunt. Hitler had already informed the world of the fall of Moscow. The Boss's reply was to celebrate the approaching anniversary of the October Revolution with the traditional meeting in the Bolshoi Theater. The world, and the country, must see the customary ceremonies in *his* capital. He summoned the senior city officials three days before the anniversary and they discussed it in detail. There was an enormous bomb crater in the Bolshoi Theater, where the gala and the traditional Red Square parade usually took place. They decided to hold it instead underground, at the Mayakovsky Square Metro station, disguised for the occasion as the Bolshoi. They erected a stage like that of the Bolshoi, and brought in the familiar rostrum, seats, and flowers. Two thousand NKVD men acted the part of an audience. Trains standing at the platforms served as dressing rooms and buffet bars.

That night German planes tried for five hours to breach the city's air defenses, but failed. Stalin rose to speak at 7:30. His speech was followed by the traditional concert. Meanwhile, preparations for the parade went on in deep secrecy. It would take place under the open sky, a stone's throw from the enemy. It was timed to begin two hours earlier than usual. A field hospital was set up in GUM, in case the parade was bombed. He gave orders that it should not be canceled even if the bombers broke through. Those taking part in the parade did not know themselves what they were rehearsing for. They thought that these were normal training exercises. The parade was marshaled by Artemiev, the Kremlin commandant, and inspected by Marshal Budenny, a great favorite with the public. Troops taking part were already lined up on Red Square at 5:00 A.M. A cold wind was blowing. But God came to the rescue again. As it got light, a heavy snowfall set in, which camouflaged the troops and made flying impossible. Budenny rode out from the Kremlin gate on his white horse. The marshal had put on weight, but had not forgotten how to ride. He rode gracefully over the slippery cobblestones.

The Boss's famous speech to these troops, addressed "from the Mausoleum," was in fact recorded in a Kremlin studio. On film, the fact that his breath did not steam as it left his mouth was a giveaway. In this speech he recalled the victorious military leaders of the tsarist empire, then sent the troops straight from the parade ground to the front.

The Battle

Zhukov, now Commissar for Defense in place of Timoshenko, was bold and above all ruthless, very like the Boss himself. He would see to it that the troops would "shrink from no sacrifices for the sake of victory."

When Hitler launched his attack on Moscow on December 1 his

soldiers had already come more than five hundred miles: what could a mere twenty more mean to them? Just one final spurt was needed. A German reconnaissance battalion was—with difficulty—forced back from the Khimki Bridge. They were practically in Moscow. The panicky city was haunted by rumors of German motorcyclists breaking through to Sokolniki Park—twenty minutes' drive from the Kremlin.

In reality the German attack was getting nowhere. Zhukov's armies were fighting to the death and the attack had begun to run out of steam. Guderian's tanks were brought to a standstill by the fierce cold. The whole two-hundred-mile-long arc of the attacking German forces came to a halt, paralyzed by the cruel frost. That was when Zhukov brought in his fresh reserves, and the battle for Moscow began in earnest. Carnage on such a scale had never before been seen. More than one hundred divisions were involved in the battle. Fresh units fought beside those hardened by bloody retreat. The Germans could not withstand the shock.

The blitzkrieg was in ruins, and Hitler's army was facing a winter for which it was unprepared. It was the turning point of the war. There were still victories ahead for Hitler, but he would never recover from this blow.

The Supreme Commander

Unlike his comrades-in-arms from the Civil War, Voroshilov and Budenny, Stalin had succeeded in becoming a modern military leader. The price of this knowledge was millions of lives, and he paid it without turning a hair. His office at GHQ was the heart of the army. His marshals have portrayed him at work there. Konyev has written: "His body language was extraordinarily limited, and it was impossible to guess from the look on his face what he was thinking. . . . There was never a superfluous gesture, his carefully contrived manner had become second nature. He maintained his reserve even at times of victory and rejoicing." And Zhukov observed: "Usually calm and reasonable, he lapsed occasionally into extreme exasperation . . . his looks became grim and harsh. I don't know many people who would have been brave enough to stand up to his anger."

He spent whole days, and often nights as well, at headquarters. Zhukov wrote: "In discussion he made a powerful impression. . . . His ability to summarize an idea precisely, his native intelligence, his unusual memory . . . his staggering capacity for work, his ability to grasp the essential point instantly, enabled him to study and digest quantities of material which would have been too much for any ordinary person. . . . I can say without hesitation that he was master of the basic principles of the organization of front-line operations and the deployment of front-line forces. . . . He controlled them completely and had a good understanding of major strategic problems. He was a worthy Supreme Commander."

Stalin and his marshals together went on to devise a new strategy that would win the major battles in that great war. The essence of their strategy was the coordination of timing and objectives for armies operating simultaneously on a number of fronts, all obeying his will alone. The zone in which Soviet armies assumed the offensive was sometimes as much as four hundred miles long. These gigantic operations involved thousands and thousands of tanks, tens of thousands of planes, hundreds of thousands of soldiers on the field of battle, tens of thousands of whom would shortly be in their graves.

The next great milestone in the war was the city that bore his name—Stalingrad. This was the key to the oil and grain of the South. He had once commanded the defense of that city; now the outcome of the war was to be decided there. He turned the city into a wasteland stuffed with scrap iron and corpses, but he would not let it be surrendered. By December 1942 he had prepared a counterattack that defied belief, with a huge number of troops and thousands of tanks and planes. His armies to the north and south clasped the German armies in their embrace and held them while hunger and cold slowly forced them to their knees. Field Marshal Paulus sat helpless, at his wits' end, in the basement of a department store, the command post of his dying army. On February 2, 1943, the German army at Stalingrad ceased to exist.

Stalin provided his fellow Muscovites with a new entertainment. I can still remember the cry heard in my childhood: "They're bringing them!" We war children would rush out to see German prisoners of war led along Gorky Street, ragged, dejected, unshaven, in filthy greatcoats. We were *his* pupils, and we happily threw stones at them. The militiamen lining the street scolded us with a friendly smile. . . . We took that as encouragement, and resumed pelting the prisoners with well-aimed stones.

The Spectral City

Three cities became symbols in that war: Moscow, Stalingrad, and the city named after the first God-Man, Leningrad. There was fierce fighting around the former capital of the tsarist empire. The fascists thought it a good idea to drive captured women, children, and old people before their attacking forces. Soviet soldiers were reluctant to open fire, but a typical Stalin edict was issued immediately: "Hit the Germans and their delegates, whoever these may be, with all you have, mow down your enemies, no matter whether they are voluntary or involuntary enemies." Children, old people, the sanctity of human life, these things had long since ceased to mean anything to him. Nothing mattered except his goal, and victory.

The Germans had already reached the outskirts of Leningrad, and Lake Ladoga, in July 1941. The city was cut off. Only a pathetic little trickle of foodstuffs reached it over the icebound lake. The siege that followed lasted nine hundred days. But Stalin did not surrender the city.

Olga Friedenburg, a scholar of some note who lived through the blockade, wrote in her diary at the time: "People stand in line in the fierce cold waiting for a delivery of horrible bread wet through after ten hours in a biting frost. The electricity was cut off long ago, the streetcars aren't running, apartments, pharmacies, office buildings are all shrouded in darkness. If you go into a shop you have to grope for the end of the line, or wait till you hear a voice. The salespeople work by the light of a stinking candle. . . . There are no matches in the city, the piped water supply came to an end long ago, and toilets cannot be flushed. There is no fuel, and so no electricity. There are air raids every day, night and day, with only short breaks. . . . The noise of bombs exploding round the clock drives people mad." Every day thousands of hungry people collapsed in the streets. "They would go to visit friends for half an hour, sit down, and die. They would leave home on business and die on the way. Thousands of people sat down on the ground for a rest, couldn't get up, and froze to death. The militia immediately stole their ration cards."

These spectral creatures, scarcely able to crawl, had to sign up in citizens' militia units. "They were sent for and invited to volunteer," Friedenburg recalled. "Their fear prevailed over their weakness, they marched and marched, fell down in the ranks, and died. There was no limit to what Soviet man could take, he could be stretched like a thing made of elastic. . . . No suffering inflicted on a living people . . . nothing whatsoever could have made the regime surrender that city. True to the usual law, omnipotence trampled human beings under foot, and spoke of patriotism and the heroism of the besieged."

This monologue of despair was unfair, in that if Stalin had surrendered Leningrad the lives of the besieged would not have been saved. Witness Hitler's directive of September 29, 1941: "The Führer has vowed to wipe St. Petersburg from the face of the earth. The objective is to approach the city as closely as possible and destroy it totally by artillery fire and constant attacks from the air. Requests to be allowed to surrender will be rejected. . . . We have no interest in preserving any part of the population of that large city."

And another question: could the Boss have broken the blockade earlier? The answer seems to be yes. But, for tactical reasons, he used the slavish patriotism of people who died without complaint for ninety days and nights. Perhaps no other nation in the world could have tolerated this—only this people trained by him to be so meekly obedient. Was it really true, then, that only one form of totalitarianism could destroy another? And save humanity?

HIS DAUGHTER'S "TERRIBLE DISCOVERY"

In a letter from Sochi just before the war, Svetlana told Stalin: "I'm not going to write any more 'orders.' I'm no longer a child to amuse myself in that way."

Stalin's daughter was fifteen on the eve of war. She had grown up, and her father knew it. Svetlana describes how furious he was when he saw her with bare knees and arms. He scolded her, gave orders that her skirts should be longer, that she should wear trousers. She did not realize that he was jealous, that he did not want to share her with any other man. After all, Lenin's sister had devoted her whole life to that great leader! But Stalin understood his daughter's temperament. He attached an NKVD watchdog to her. She went everywhere under escort—to school, to concerts, to the theater. He told her that it was for her safety.

Evacuated to Kuibyshev, she pined for Moscow. "I don't like this city. . . . There are such a lot of . . . lame people, blind people, cripples of all sorts. Every fifth person you see in the streets is a cripple." The men who weren't cripples were in his army.

Stalin did not allow his daughter to come home for good until the summer of 1942, when the Germans had been driven back from Moscow. Unknown to him, she was a different Svetlana. In the preceding winter she had, as she later wrote, been overwhelmed by a terrible discovery. Someone had thoughtlessly given her a British magazine to read, and her mother's suicide was mentioned as a generally known fact. She was "stunned." She didn't believe her eyes.

The dacha at Zubalovo, damaged in the war, was rebuilt and Svetlana moved in there. Her brother Vasily was a frequent guest. His wife and child, and Yasha's daughter with her nurse, shared the house with her. Vasily regularly brought friends home—fliers, athletes, actors. They drank recklessly, played music on the phonograph, and danced. "You wouldn't have thought there was a war on," Svetlana wrote.

PRINCE VASYA

After scraping through his lower and middle levels of school, the twenty-year-old Vasya had been sent where all Soviet youngsters dreamed of going in those days—to the Air Force Training School. Stalin preserved letters about Vasya's "exploits" there in his personal file. We read in a report from Beria that "on the way [to Flying School] he told the senior staff members who went to welcome him that 'Papa is supposed to be coming to Sevastopol for a holiday this year, he'll probably look in on me.' " The terrified staff were put on the alert. "Vasya," Beria wrote, "was quartered not in the trainees' hostel but in a house reserved for visitors . . . his meals were prepared separately . . . he went around in a car put at his disposal by the school." His father gave harsh instructions as to how the "crafty little brat" should be treated: "Nobody should show such consideration or concern as to create special conditions of any sort."

Let us try to imagine what it was like to be a dictator's son, for all practical purposes fatherless as well as motherless in adolescence. His mother's suicide, the imprisonment of his relatives, the execution of family friends who had shown him so much affection—these were the horrors he had lived with in childhood.

Stalin kept Vasily's graduation certificate from the Air Force Training School: "An excellent pilot, enjoys flying, promoted to rank of lieutenant." But he knew what such scraps of paper were worth. In March 1941, after Vasily had graduated, his father sent him to summer training camp at Lyubertsy, with what was known as the Palace Garrison. This was an elite air force unit which took part in ceremonial flybys and aerobatic displays in front of the Leader. Only ace pilots were recruited to it.

At the Boss's request, V. Tsukanov, commander of this famous unit, himself became Vasily's instructor. He reported honestly that "Vasya is an able flier, but will always get into difficulties because of his drinking."

Then came the war. After Yasha was taken prisoner, the Boss would not let Vasya fly. He became an air force inspector, sitting in a big office on Pirogov Street, with nothing much to do, except drink. The front line was the place for meteoric rises in careers. But, knowing how insanely ambitious his pipsqueak son was, the Boss saw to it that he didn't fall far behind. Vasya quickly rose to be head of the air force inspectorate.

Fall from Grace

Life at Zubalovo became jollier, and boozier, all the time. Vasya fell in with a fun-loving crowd of filmmakers, among them the scenario writer Alexei Kapler, Moscow's champion lady-killer. One husband, told that his wife was having an affair with this legendary figure, famously observed that "mere husbands shouldn't bear a grudge against Kapler." I knew him well. He was a friend of my father. He was fat and ugly and not a very good writer. His talent lay elsewhere: he was a raconteur of genius. When he spoke, it was like the Siren's song—you were spellbound. Another member of the group was the documentary filmmaker Roman Karmen, an equally famous playboy in his day. Vasya plunged happily into the life of pleasure. When he was drunk he would shoot at chandeliers in restaurants—this was called "the cut-glass chimes." He had endless brief affairs—his famous name gave him an immediate entrée to women's hearts. One of his drinking companions later told this story: "One day I went home and found my wife, L. Tselikovskaya [a Soviet film star of the late thirties], with her friend V. Serova [also a film star] and an air force officer unknown to me. He persuaded us to go out to his dacha. On the way there Serova told me that this was V. Stalin. At the dacha he began making shameless advances to my wife, and tried to drag her off to some secluded spot. I intervened pretty sharply, he apologized, and nothing much happened during the rest of the meal except that after a few drinks Vasya took a cinder from the hearth and decorated the faces of Slutsky, the cameraman, and Karmen while they sat at a table." And they, of course, put up with it.

It was during that time of carousing and conquests that Vasya took Alexei Kapler out to Zubalovo and introduced him to Svetlana.

Like many other writers at the time, Kapler was then working as a war correspondent. He had just come back from an assignment: he had been dropped behind German lines and taken part in sabotage operations with partisans in Belorussia. Now he was getting ready to leave for Stalingrad, where the bloody battle was reaching its critical stage.

Vasya brought him along during the October holidays. Kapler was bewitched as soon as he set eyes on the attractive and intelligent young girl. Half-dead with shyness, a little girl in the low-heeled shoes her father liked her to wear, Svetlana danced a foxtrot with him. It was fatal—once Kapler started talking. After her brother's rambling anecdotage, her father's silences, and the stuffiness of his colleagues, the spellbinder Kapler overwhelmed her. Her loneliness was at an end. She had found someone who understood her. That evening she told him everything—among other things that this was the tenth anniversary of her mother's death, and how horrible it was that no one remembered it.

They began to meet regularly. Those were dangerous meetings. Kapler lent her an unpublished translation of a Hemingway novel, and praised the great disgraced poets—Gumilev, executed in 1921, and the semi-forbidden Akhmatova. In the language of the time, he was "ideologically corrupting" the Leader's daughter. That alone could cost him his life.

She fell in love with him. She did not know what sort of world she was living in, or what sort of man her father was. But Kapler, a man of forty, knew these things only too well. How can he have been so rash? Quite simply—he too was in love. He delighted in her childlike enthusiasms. Nothing else mattered to him. The forty-year-old man waited for the schoolgirl in a doorway opposite her school. They went to the unheated Tretyakov Gallery, they went to hear *The Queen of Spades.* A hangdog NKVD man trailed after them along the blacked-out streets of wartime Moscow—and Kapler occasionally gave him a cigarette to relieve his boredom.

The Boss, of course, was told all about it. But he was completely absorbed in Stalingrad, where he was getting ready for his greatest victory. Nor did he realize how serious the situation was before Kapler left Moscow with all the other correspondents to await the great event at Stalingrad.

And then the Boss read in *Pravda,* his *Pravda,* which he had once edited, a piece by Kapler. This was an account in the form of a "letter from Lieutenant L.," of events in Stalingrad, and also of the author's recent visits with an unnamed sweetheart to the Tretyakov Gallery and their walks around Moscow by night. The obviously insane lover ended with the words "It must be snowing now in Moscow. From your window you can see the crenellated wall of the Kremlin." Just so that there could be no possible doubt as to the identity of his sweetheart!

Stalin's fury is easy to imagine. But he controlled it. For the first time in his life he did not know what to do. Shortly afterward, one of the officers of his bodyguard telephoned Kapler and suggested an assignment to somewhere more remote. Kapler told him to go to hell.

When Stalin was told Kapler's answer, he must have realized how much the war had changed people. Familiarity with death was overcoming fear. Some people had ceased to fear altogether. There would be work to do after the war.

Throughout February Svetlana and Kapler continued their visits to the theater and their nocturnal strolls around Moscow, with the security man plodding behind them. On her seventeenth birthday, they turned up at Vasily's apartment. They embraced in an empty room, trying not to make any noise. The unhappy NKVD man sat in an adjoining room straining his ears. He had to write some sort of report on each meeting.

Kapler was arrested two days later. Her father arrived with a savage glare in his yellow eyes. She had never seen him like that. "I know everything. I've got your telephone calls here," he said, tapping his pocket. "Your Kapler is an English spy, he has been arrested." But she was her mother's daughter. And his. She was not easily frightened. "I love him," she said, and was slapped twice, for the first time in her life. He knew, though, that pain alone would not break her resistance. He had come armed with the most humiliating thing he could think of: "Just look at yourself. Who do you think would want you? He's got women all over the place, you fool!"

She stopped talking to him for several months. But for him it was all over. He felt betrayed for the second time. Her mother's death had been the first.

In fairy tales the tsar often cuts off the heads of those who try to carry off the princess. He had to control himself. He remembered her mother's end. He knew how dangerous it was to reduce those crazy Alliluyevs to despair. The "spy" Kapler was banished to Vorkuta for five years. It could have been worse, but not much.

He was furious with Vasya too. Vasya had produced Kapler—it was at Vasya's brothel of a dacha that they had met. It was about then that Vasya acquired his wound. Not at the front, like others, but as the result of a drunken prank: while stunning fish in a river with aviation shells, Vasya was wounded in the cheek and in one leg.

J. Stalin, People's Commissar for Defense, ordered that "the regiment and its former commander Colonel V. Stalin be informed that he is hereby relieved of his command for drunken and disorderly behavior which tends to damage and corrupt the regiment."

Vasya was sent to the front. But after what had happened to his half-brother he was seldom allowed to take part in aerial combat, and only with heavy cover. This infuriated him: he was brave and eager to show his prowess. The Boss nonetheless saw to it that his son rose in the service. Vasya was never kept in the same place for more than two years. He had begun the war as a twenty-year-old captain. He ended it as a twenty-four-year-old general.

24

THE SECOND FRONT

A great deal has been written about the course of the war, and the opening of a second front by the Western allies. I shall touch on this crucial period only briefly.

After Hitler's attack on Russia, Churchill became Stalin's reluctant ally. The Boss understood his attitude very well: the ideal war for Churchill would be one in which the rival dictators bit through each other's throats. But, as Churchill himself put it, "if Hitler occupies Hell I will ask the House of Commons for aid for the Devil." Late in 1941, the Japanese attack on Pearl Harbor brought the USSR another ally. Now Litvinov came to be useful. The disgraced Jew was appointed ambassador to the United States. To strengthen his arm, Stalin created in February 1942 a Jewish Antifascist Committee. The Yiddish theater in Moscow and the Yiddish poets were all drawn into it. It was headed by the great actor Mikhoels, director of the Yiddish theater. Their immediate task was to attract funds from wealthy American Jews. But a still more important objective was to influence Western public opinion in favor of the second front. Anti-Semitism was forgotten. Litvinov signed an agreement with the United States under which the Soviet Union would get aluminum for aircraft, gasoline, antiaircraft guns, machine guns, and rifles (as well as generous food parcels—I can still remember the taste of American chocolate in frostbound, hungry Moscow).

Stalin desperately wanted the Allies to open a second front in the terrible months of 1941–1942, but Churchill was in no hurry. He preferred to watch the Soviet armies bleed. The Boss understood this way of thinking very well. In his place he would have done the same.

The Allies did not open a second front in 1942 or in 1943. Instead of invading the continent, Churchill flew to Moscow, to that "grim Bolshevik state, which I once tried hard to suffocate at birth and which until the emergence of Hitler I regarded as the worst enemy of civilized freedom."

The Boss greeted Churchill like an old friend. They were alike in some ways. His intelligence service had told him that Churchill knew in advance about the Japanese attack on Pearl Harbor, but had kept it from his American friends to make sure of drawing them into the war. There, too, he would have done the same himself. Churchill went to the Bolshoi, was entertained by the Boss at home, was introduced to Svetlana, and told her that the hair which had vanished from his head had been as red as her own. But he refused to open a second front, saying that the Allies were not ready.

Churchill had in a way done Stalin a favor in leaving him to fight alone. With support from the Allies in weapons and food supplies his army acquired fantastic strength as it fought. Hitler's generals and Europe's strongest army were its teachers. By the end of 1943 Stalin had the greatest military machine that had ever existed, and Hitler's fate was sealed. The Boss had already made plans for the mighty blows that would carry the war beyond Russia's frontiers into Europe. The Great Dream was reborn. Stalin chose that time—spring 1943—to dissolve Comintern, in order, he told a Reuters correspondent, "to refute Hitler's lie that Moscow intends to interfere in the lives of other states and to Bolshevize them." In "in-depth language" this meant: Moscow will interfere in the lives of other states and will Bolshevize them. The personnel of the dissolved Comintern would become the rulers of Eastern Europe.

The dissolution of Comintern, the restoration of the Patriarchate in Russia, the reintroduction of tsarist ranks in the army—all these things seemed to signify the end of Bolshevism. Stalin assiduously cultivated this notion in the minds of his allies, in preparation for the decisive assault on Europe.

HONEYMOON

In 1943 the Big Three met in conference at Teheran. The Western Allies were now themselves in a hurry to open a second front, before Stalin arrived in Europe. He had not grown out of Koba's youthful habit: he arrived a day late. Let them wait. He was the Boss now.

At Teheran he met Roosevelt for the first time. Roosevelt, whom Stalin saw as an idealist, and Churchill were comically incongruous partners. Which of them did he like better? Asked this by Molotov, he replied, "They're both imperialists," the appropriate answer to a person of Stone Arse's limited understanding. The fact was that they were both very much to his liking. He saw at once how he could cause a collision between Roosevelt, with his avowed aversion to under-the-table deals, and Churchill, who felt sure that without such deals they stood no chance against the dread Uncle Joe. "If I had to pick a negotiating team, Stalin would be my first choice," said Anthony Eden, the British Foreign Secretary.

During the Teheran honeymoon they exchanged protestations of eternal love. Churchill presented the Boss with the Stalingrad Sword. "Marshal Stalin," he said, "can take his place beside the major figures in Russian history, and deserves to be known as 'Stalin the Great.' " The Boss modestly replied that "it is easy to be a hero when you are dealing with people like the Russians." The main subject of discussion was the second front. But Churchill couldn't resist asking about territorial claims once the war was won. Stalin answered that "there's no need to talk about that at present: when the time comes we shall have our say."

He knew even then that Churchill would suggest a tradeoff. In 1944 the Western Allies landed in Normandy, while Stalin's armies crossed the Soviet frontier and began rapidly overrunning Poland, Hungary, Romania, Yugoslavia, Czechoslovakia. Bulgaria and Finland withdrew from the war. The Balkans were at Russia's mercy. The Communist-dominated National Liberation Army took control of the whole of mainland Greece. A partisan army led by the Communist Tito, helped by Soviet forces, was victorious in Yugoslavia.

Churchill made haste. On October 9, 1944, he and Eden were in Moscow, and that night they met Stalin in the Kremlin, without the Americans. Bargaining went on throughout the night. Churchill wrote on a scrap of paper that the Boss had a 90 percent "interest" in Romania, Britain a 90 percent "interest" in Greece, both Russia and Britain a 50 percent interest in Yugoslavia. When they got to Italy the Boss ceded that country to Churchill. The crucial questions arose when the Ministers of Foreign Affairs discussed "percentages" in Eastern Europe. Molotov's proposals were that Russia should have a 75 percent interest in Hungary, 75 percent in Bulgaria, and 60 percent in Yugoslavia. This was the Boss's price for ceding Italy and Greece. Eden tried to haggle: Hungary 75/25, Bulgaria 80/20, but Yugoslavia 50/50. After lengthy bargaining they settled on an 80/20 division of interest between Russia and Britain in Bulgaria and Hungary, and a 50/50 division in Yugoslavia. U.S. Ambassador Harriman was informed only after the bargain was struck. This gentleman's agreement was sealed with a handshake.

The percentages—the idea that the Boss would accept anything less than one hundred percent authority—were a comic fiction.

Churchill knew very well that Stalin could not be trusted, and he tried to act in the way they both favored. But the Boss was unconcerned. He knew that Roosevelt would not countenance any breach of faith, however compelling the arguments in favor of it. When Churchill tried to enter into secret negotiations with Germany, the Boss immediately informed Roosevelt. Roosevelt indignantly protested and the talks were broken off. (When Roosevelt died on April 12, 1945, too soon to see Uncle Joe's new Europe, the Boss wrote to Churchill that "for my part I feel particularly the grievous loss of that great man, our common friend.")

Hitler, in any case, had succeeded in consolidating the alliance of the Big Three by the end of 1944. The Germans made a sudden attack on the Allies in the Ardennes and inflicted heavy losses. Stalin nobly came to the rescue, and distracted the Germans by launching a premature offensive. The help he gave them was to be credited to his account when the time came to divide Europe.

The Third Reich was within months of its end when the Allied powers met at Yalta. Roosevelt and Churchill were Stalin's guests in the Livadia Palace, the favorite home of the Last Tsar and his family. The Conference adopted high-sounding decisions on the peaceful Europe of the future, on the establishment of the UN, on the demilitarization of Germany. But its main business was to complete the partition of Europe, and help to give substance to the Great Dream. This time Stalin was able to include Poland in his maneuvers.

The monstrous Katyn affair caused complications. After the collapse of Poland more than twenty thousand captured Polish officers had been quartered in prison camps near the Soviet frontier. When Stalin was getting ready to attack Germany, the thought of keeping so many potential enemies within the Soviet Union alarmed him. He remembered the mutiny of the Czechoslovak prisoners of war in 1918. As usual, he found a quick and drastic solution: the prisoners were "liquidated." When General Anders began forming the Polish army in the West, Stalin released some two thousand Poles from the camps. But Poles abroad asked where so many thousands of officers had disappeared to. The answer given was that they had run away from the camps at the beginning of the war. The Polish government in exile was not satisfied, and persisted in asking about the missing officers.

A little play-acting was called for. In the presence of the Polish representative Stalin telephoned Molotov and Beria to ask whether all Poles had been released from Soviet jails. They both said yes. But when the Germans occupied Smolensk they had found in the nearby Katyn forest a gruesome burial ground containing row upon row of corpses with bullet holes in the backs of the neck, the remains of the Polish officers. Stalin of course accused Hitler of a grotesque provocation. He changed his story: the Poles had not run away, but had been transferred to the Smolensk area to work on building sites. There the Germans had captured them, shot them, and blamed the USSR for it. A special Soviet commission was set up, with the Boss's own writers, academics, and clergy as members. The commission, of course, confirmed his story. Roosevelt and Churchill had to take their ally's word. The monstrous scale of the tragedy has only recently become known. A. Krayushkin, head of one of the directorates of the Federal Security Service (as the former KGB is now called), at a press conference in Smolensk in April 1995, informed the Russian and Polish journalists present that the number of Polish prisoners killed in various camps was 21,857.

The documents concerning those shot were destroyed, with Khrushchev's consent, in 1959. What remains is a letter from A. Shelepin, then head of the KGB, informing Khrushchev that "in all, 21,857 people were shot on orders from the KGB, including 4,421 in the Katyn forest, 6,311 in the Ostashkovo camp (Kaliningrad oblast), and 3,820 in the Starobel camp near Kharkov."

Shelepin's letter then asks Khrushchev for permission to destroy the records of those shot, since they have "neither operational nor historical importance."

On the site of the terrible mass grave in the Katyn forest there now stands a dacha built by one of the "new Russians"—a rich businessman.

August 1944 was the month of the Warsaw rising, organized by the Polish government in exile. Stalin's armies had halted in sight of Warsaw, but he ordered them not to advance, and they stood there watching while the Germans destroyed the city. His main objective now was to get rid of the émigré Polish government. Repeated Allied attempts to talk to good old Uncle Joe about a democratic Poland were met with a sharp "no." The logic of his position was simple. He had won the war in order to have good next-door neighbors. He would allow the Western Allies to surrender Poland by easy stages: Roosevelt, he knew, had to think of the Polish vote at home. But that was as far as he would go. He had, then, in the final stages of the war erected the framework of a future Communist Eastern Europe.

He also had plans for Asia. At Yalta they had discussed the part Russia might yet play in the war against Japan. Stalin had of course consented to join in. It would enable his armies to move into China and onward, toward realization of the Great Dream.

At the very end of 1944 yet another ally arrived in Moscow—General de Gaulle, now Prime Minister of liberated France. The French visitors' rooms were bugged, and the Boss was kept informed of their regular conversations about the bloodthirsty Stalin.

At the Kremlin banquet lanky de Gaulle and the diminutive Boss made a comic duo. Stalin proposed a toast to Kaganovich—"a brave man. He knows that if the trains do not arrive on time"—he paused, and then concluded affectionately—"we shall shoot him." Then he proposed a toast to Air Marshal Novikov—"a good marshal, let's drink to him. And if he doesn't do his job properly"—with a kindly smile—"we shall hang him." The French no longer found him such a comic figure. He finished his teasing by saying laughingly, "People call me a monster, but as you see I make a joke of it. Maybe I'm not so horrible after all."

On the train de Gaulle said incredulously, "And these are the people we shall be dealing with for the next hundred years!" The French visitors, however, also carried away another impression. "In his behavior you caught a glimpse of something resembling the despair of a man who has reached such heights of power that he has nowhere else to go," one of them wrote. On that same occasion in the Kremlin, Hitler's conqueror had suddenly remarked to de Gaulle that "in the long run death is the only victor." It was December, and his sixty-fifth birthday was drawing near.

Preparing the Country for Victory

Stalin had every right to call himself a "monster."

De Gaulle can have had no idea what was then happening in the jocular dictator's country. For that matter, the monster's own soldiers, who were finalizing their victory, did not know all that had happened deep in the rear, in many cases to their own families.

Terror had almost vanished from the land by 1944. On the threshold of victory, Stalin began reviving it. What troubled him most were reawakened nationalist aspirations. At the beginning of the war his commissars could speak of a Ukrainian, a Georgian, a Moldavian, an Armenian, an Azerbaijani "fatherland." While the country stood on the brink of the abyss he had encouraged such talk, to stiffen the morale of the non-Russians. Now he needed to eradicate these ideas, to burn them out of people's minds. He had always known that nationalism was dynamite. (Dynamite indeed. Half a century later it would blow his empire to bits.)

Late in 1943, when the war was at its most critical stage, Stalin had convened the Politburo to lecture them for over an hour on a screenplay written by Dozchenko.

Dozchenko, a great filmmaker, was also a Ukrainian. His *Earth* was at the time one of the most famous films ever made. Before the war the Boss had condescended to take a stroll with him after a conference. They walked along the Arbat, which was deserted except for security men and NKVD cars parked along the sides of the street. Dozchenko talked incessantly, as artists will, while his companion listened. That evening told the Boss all that he needed to know. From then on he watched Dozchenko closely. One day he was told that the director had written a new screenplay and had read it to Khrushchev, then in charge of the Ukraine. Khrushchev, who was relaxing at his dacha, no doubt with the help of a few drinks, liked the script. The Boss asked to see it, and realized immediately that he had been right about Dozchenko. The cunning director had used a device to which writers would often resort in the post-Stalin period. His most challenging ideas, those he prized most, had all been put into the mouths of negative characters. A German officer, for instance, was made to say, "Your nation has a fatal Achilles' heel: people are incapable of forgiving each other for their differences of opinion. They have been living for twenty-five years with negative slogans—rejection of God, property, the family, friendship. The word *nation* no longer exists except in the adjectival form." And so on. Such sallies of course met with the orthodox answers, but how feeble the answers looked compared with those insidious criticisms. Stalin noted in particular Dozchenko's central idea: "Whichever front we fight on, it's the Ukraine we are fighting for. For a people forty million strong which has never found itself. For a people lacerated and fragmented." He quoted this passage to the Politburo, in a meeting to which Dozchenko was invited, and commented that "there is no separate Ukraine! It does not exist! In fighting for the USSR you are fighting for the Ukraine also." He had shot hundreds of thousands to teach them this lesson so that they would never forget it. And here he was again. The Boss savaged Dozchenko unmercifully: "He is trying to criticize our Party. . . . If we were to publish this story Soviet people would give him such a going-over there'd be nothing left but a damp patch on the ground." Dozchenko sat there pale and helpless.

The Boss gave Khrushchev a chance to correct his own mistake. He set to work with a will. Dozchenko was lambasted at innumerable meetings and was driven out of the Kiev Film Studio. As he wrote in his diary, he was "hacked to pieces, and the bloody remains were distributed for desecration wherever an ugly mob could be gathered."

As soon as he glimpsed victory in 1944, the Boss decided to hit nationalism hard, hard enough to draw blood. They must never forget that they belonged to the Union of Soviet Socialist Republics. Beria took the hint and quickly provided the country with an object lesson. During their occupation of the Caucasus the Germans had promised independence to the Chechens, the Ingush, the Balkars, and the Kalmyks. Members of these ethnic groups did sometimes collaborate with the Germans. The same was true of the Crimean Tartars. Beria knew the rules: the Boss could not be seen as the initiator of reprisals. He himself had to seek the Leader's permission.

I saw one of Stalin's top-secret "special files," a file that bore witness to a bloodbath of which the army, the country, and the world at large knew nothing. I saw a note from Beria to Stalin: "The Balkars gave a friendly welcome to the German occupation of the Caucasus. As they retreated before the blows of the Red army, the Germans organized Balkar detachments." Nationalism leads to treason—that was the ideological lesson to be learned. And if these people had betrayed, how could they possibly deserve to go on living in the Caucasus, that earthly paradise? The birthplace of the Living God of communism? Stalin had his solution ready. On March 11, 1944, Beria reported that "37,103 Balkars have been loaded onto special trains and dispatched to their new areas of settlement in the Kazakh and Kirghiz republics. There were no incidents requiring attention during the operation."

He continued punishing errant ethnic groups and rooting out nationalism throughout the spring and summer of 1944, that year of victories.

While the Allies were singing his praises and discovering a new Stalin unlike their old picture of him, thousands of soldiers wearing NKVD uniforms arrived in the mountainous regions of the Caucasus, with the February snows falling. The local inhabitants were summoned to a meeting—it was the anniversary of the foundation of the Red army. They arrived, and found their hosts ready for them. Beria reported: "On February 23 there was a heavy snowfall, which caused difficulties in transporting people, especially in mountainous regions." But by February 25, in spite of frost and snow, settlements in which people had lived for thousands of years were deserted. The inhabitants had been driven out under escort. Cattle trucks were waiting down in the valley. They were crammed full of people and sent off to Siberia.

On the same day, Beria reported that "the eviction of the Chechens and Ingush is proceeding normally: 342,647 people were loaded onto special trains on February 25 and by [February 29] the number had risen to 478,479 of whom 91,250 were Ingush and 387,229 Chechens. . . . The operation proceeded in an organized fashion, with no serious instances of resistance, or other incidents. There were only isolated cases of attempted flight."

There were of course "no incidents" in a report meant for Stalin, but in reality the NKVD had found it hard work. Ruslan G., a bank manager, recalled how "they combed the huts to make sure there was no one left behind. It was cold, and the floor was coated with hoarfrost. The soldier who came into the house didn't want to bend down. He raked the hut with a burst from his tommy gun. Blood trickled out from under the bench where a child was hiding. The mother screamed and hurled herself at the soldier. He shot her too. There was not enough rolling stock. Those left behind were shot. The bodies were covered with earth or sand, carelessly. The shooting had also been careless, and people started wriggling out of the sand like worms. The NKVD men spent the whole night shooting them all over again."

"Incidents" there were. But no resistance—there Beria had spoken the truth. The country had not altogether forgotten its earlier lessons. Fear was rapidly returning. One ethnic group after another was driven out of the Caucasus. "The operation to resettle persons of Kalmyk nationality in eastern regions (the Altai, the Krasnoyarsk Krai, the Amur, Novosibirsk, and Omsk oblasts) proceeded successfully. In all 93,139 people were entrained. The operation was conducted without excesses—People's Commissar Beria."

Beria had also exerted himself in the Crimea: "To Comrade Stalin. In compliance with our decree an operation to cleanse the Crimea of anti-Soviet elements was carried out in the period April–June, and Crimeans, Tartars, Bulgars, Greeks, Armenians, and persons of foreign nationality have been deported to the eastern regions of the USSR. Altogether 225,009 persons have been evacuated. . . . 23,000 officers and other ranks of the NKVD took part in the operation. The NKVD hereby applies for the award of medals to those who have distinguished themselves."

Jewish nationalism also had to be dealt with.

By the end of the war, Stalin was getting ready to play the Jewish card. Almost all of the well-known Jews in the Soviet Union were on the Jewish Antifascist Committee which he had set up. As well as Mikhoels, its members included the poets Fefer and Markish, and the academician Lina Stern, director of the Institute of Physiology. Stalin appointed Lozovsky, the head of the Soviet Information Bureau, to the committee as, to all intents and purposes, its political commissar. He also found a use for Molotov's wife, Polina Zhemchuzina, a fanatical Communist, as patroness of the committee.

In 1944 the committee wrote to Stalin on behalf of all Soviet Jews, recommending the establishment of a Jewish Socialist Republic in the Crimea, on vacant land from which the Tartars had been evicted. The letter was, of course, written by Lozovsky, but a man of his experience would never have risked writing such a thing without the Boss's agreement. One of the initiators of the letter was Zhemchuzina. But would Molotov's wife have gone so far without consulting the Boss? He was obviously somewhere in the wings. "A California in the Crimea"—just the thing to win the hearts of American Jews and, of course, untie their purse strings. Besides, the rumor that good old Uncle Joe was going to give the Crimea to the Jews would help divert attention from the fate of the deported peoples.

The Crimean Jewish Republic was, however, just another Trojan horse. The members of the Antifascist Committee did not realize what a dangerous position they had strayed, or rather been inveigled, into. The enticer had their future mapped out. The long game was always his preference.

VICTORY

His armies met those of the Allies on the Elbe. They fraternized, they got drunk together . . . this boozy display of brotherly love might have gone on forever, had the Boss not known his history. The Russian officers who defeated Napoleon had brought back from Europe the spirit of freedom, and founded secret societies. Stalin was particularly annoyed with Zhukov. The marshal was busy giving interviews to foreign news agencies, more often than not forgetting the obligatory refrain about "the greatest war leader of all times, Comrade Stalin."

Victory had arrived. Stalin allowed Zhukov the supreme privilege of formally accepting Germany's unconditional surrender. Zhukov was also allowed to inspect the victory parade. Such honors bestowed by the Boss were dangerous. If Zhukov's head had not been turned by victory, the shades of vanished marshals might have told him so.

During the victory parade, on a rainy day when "even the skies wept for the fallen," as his poets wrote, Stalin's mind was on tomorrow, on the day after victory.

His cities lay in ruins. The face of the country was pitted with the graves of his soldiers. Half of Europe was seeded with their bodies. When he got around to it he would think of a number which was not too frightening—around seven million. After his death the numbers would grow from year to year. At an international conference held in the Russian Academy of Sciences in 1994 the majority of experts present agreed on the following figures: the army had lost around 8,668,000 men, and the civilian population 18 million: 26 million in all.

For the present—let the soldiers who had survived this cruelest of all wars march over Red Square and fling the banners of Hitler's defeated army at the foot of the Mausoleum. At *his* feet. But he must soon give some thought to the future, after demobilization of these soldiers who had learned to kill skillfully and without compunction. He was well aware that criminal gangs had sprung up in the capital. As his daughter wrote to him early in 1945: "It's getting so that even in the central districts people are afraid to go out after dark."

While they were fighting, they had forgotten how to work, and how to be afraid. Or rather, they had forgotten what work was because they had forgotten what fear was.

"I heard today," his daughter wrote, "a rumor that Stalin had returned to Moscow and decreed that gangsterism and thieving are to be liquidated by New Year. People are always crediting you with something good." He lived up to expectations, and gave his favorite order: shoot them all. Not just the looters, but those who could not put a stop to the looting.

The gangs were swollen by hundreds of homeless and destitute people. Many of them were war cripples, men who had lost arms or legs or been disfigured and were afraid or reluctant to return to their families. Those who did return often found that their wives had received a "burial chit" and had married again. So these men would join one of the tribes of beggars or gangsters.

The NKVD reports are still in his files: "A large number of professional beggars have turned up in Arzamas region. The largest concentration of beggars is round the 'Dawn' refinery. The refinery disposes of its waste products to the local population as animal feed. The beggar element now uses these waste products as food. Up to 20,000 people so far have visited the territory of the refinery.—L. Beria." The beggars helped to reinforce the camp population.

The country desperately needed a dose of terror. The counterespionage service zealously intercepted letters from the front, Beria regularly reported their contents, and the Boss saw that the worst had happened: together with a sense of personal responsibility, the war had reawakened independent thought. A relentless struggle with independent thinking would soon follow.

Vengeance

He also solved the problem of prisoners of war liberated from German camps. They had to pay for disobeying his orders to die on the battlefield. They had dared to survive as prisoners. And of course he had in mind the dangerous ideas they would have "picked up" (a favorite phrase in his propaganda) in multinational camps.

Their fate, then, was decided in advance. These unfortunates, who had survived years of nightmare as prisoners, and lived to see their country victorious, were to be sent straight from German to Soviet prison camps.

Marshal Zhukov told a plenary meeting of the Central Committee in 1957 that "126,000 officers who returned from captivity were stripped of their rank and sent to the camps."

A sad fate also awaited civilians forcibly deported to Germany by the Germans. In Stalin's logic anyone in contact with foreigners was infected with an incurable disease. These plague victims had to be segregated from healthy people. They too were destined to swell the population of his camps.

Many of those due to return were in areas occupied by the Allies. They knew that, according to the Boss, only "traitors to their homeland let themselves be taken prisoner" and begged not to be dispatched to the USSR. But the Boss, as always, had provided for this. At the Yalta conference he had concluded an agreement with Roosevelt and Churchill under which all Soviet citizens taken prisoner or interned by the enemy during the war must be returned to the USSR.

The Allies relentlessly carried out this agreement. In his book *Victims of Yalta,* Count Nikolai Tolstoy-Miloslavsky, great-nephew of Lev Tolstoy, presents evidence collected from eyewitnesses and from participants in the tragedy. Sergeant D. Lawrence (one of the British military escort for motor vehicles carrying Soviet citizens to be handed over to

Soviet representatives) told the following story: "When the former prisoners arrived at Graz (Austria), where the Soviet reception point was located, a woman rushed to the parapet of the viaduct over the River Mur . . . threw her child into the water and then jumped in herself. . . . Men and women were herded together into a huge concentration camp fenced with barbed wire. . . . That nightmare will remain with me for as long as I live."

But these were citizens of the USSR. And as the Boss's favorite hero, Ivan the Terrible, wrote about his subjects: "The tsar is free to reward them and free to punish them [put them to death] also."

The Boss also succeeded in claiming another set of victims. Thousands of his former enemies, who had fought in the White armies during the Civil War and then fled from Russia, found themselves in countries now occupied by his armies: Czechoslovakia, Yugoslavia, Bulgaria, Romania, and Hungary. His secret police sought them out and deported them to the USSR, to the camps.

Some of his former foes, however, were in areas of the defeated German Reich occupied by the Western Allies. But although only "those who had been Soviet citizens before being deported to Germany or taken prisoner" were supposed to be repatriated, he obtained from his allies what should have been impossible: the Cossack General Krasnov, General Shkuro (awarded the British Order of the Bath for his feats of valor against the Bolsheviks in the Civil War), General Solomatin, and General Sultan-Girei were handed over by the British.

In vain did Sultan-Girei don the uniform of a tsarist general, in vain did General Kuchuk-Ulugai flourish his Albanian passport before a British officer's eyes. They were handed over by the British to officers of the NKVD. The Boss had compelled his allies to do his bidding.

When they heard what had happened, thousands of Cossack émigrés in Austria fled to the mountains. But British patrols hunted down the refugees and handed them over to the Soviet authorities.

The Boss's old enemies, the Civil War heroes Andrei Shkuro (now sixty) and Peter Krasnov (now seventy-eight) were put on trial, anathematized by the press, condemned, and hanged.

The church also received his attention. By now he had forgotten his appeal to God. Soso's youthful fears seemed ridiculous to Stalin. It was he—the God Stalin—who had won the war, the greatest war in history. It was he who had liberated the peoples.

When he reinstated the Patriarchate he had arranged for close supervision of the church. The Council on Church Affairs watched its every move. Formally, the council was answerable to the Council of People's Commissars (from 1946, the Council of Ministers). In practice, he put a very different body—the NKVD—in charge of the Council for Church Affairs and installed an NKVD colonel, G. Karpov, at its head. Karpov was also head of the Fifth Department of the NKVD, whose assignment was to combat the "counterrevolutionary clergy." In the NKVD Karpov's duty was to fight the church, in the council to assist it.

But he also wished to show his gratitude. In 1947 he invited Metropolitan Ilya to the Soviet Union, and awarded him a Stalin Prize. The prelate would not accept it. He explained to the ex-seminarist that a monk did not need money, and donated $200,000, supplementing the Stalin Prize with money of his own, to a fund for the relief of war orphans.

In July 1945 Stalin traveled by train to Potsdam for the peace conference. Seventeen thousand NKVD men were on duty along the route, six to fifteen security men for every kilometer of the line. Eight NKVD armored trains stood by. All this was a demonstration of the might of the God Stalin. The sacred train sped over the ruined land, filling his subjects with dread.

MOLOTOV AND "DRUZHKOV"

Stalin's fellow honeymooners were missing from the conference. Roosevelt was in his grave and Churchill flew from Potsdam to take part in a general election and did not return—the Labour Party, led by Attlee, had won. The Boss commented that Western democracy must be a wretched system if it could exchange a great man like Churchill for Attlee.

The Western Allies, then, were represented by Truman and Attlee. Stalin had succeeded in outsmarting two Titans; what hope had these two against him?

The partition of postwar Europe went on, at Potsdam and afterward, all through 1945. In the course of the negotiations the Western Allies were greatly impressed by Molotov. This was when the enigmatic Foreign Minister acquired a sort of charisma. The westerners were fascinated by his extraordinary taciturnity, his steely inflexibility, his cunning gamesmanship. Molotov mesmerized them with his slow responses, and at times perplexed them by refusing to say either "yes" or "no" to the simplest of questions. How did Molotov suddenly become a great diplomat? Documents in the President's Archive gave me the answer to this riddle.

It turns out that throughout 1945 Molotov received minutely detailed instructions from a certain "Druzhkov" in Moscow. These telegrams have not been published to this day. It is not difficult to work out who was hiding behind the pseudonym "Druzhkov." Who would be giving orders to Molotov, the second man in the state? It was, of course, Stalin. By signing himself "Druzhkov" (which in Russian suggests "friendliness") the Boss was evidently demonstrating his affection for Molotov. In these coded messages the Boss dictated literally every diplomatic move Molotov made, just as he had dictated his policies at home. Molotov the Soviet Metternich did not exist. There was only Molotov the transmitter of the Boss's wishes, who dared not make a single decision independently. Hence his awe-inspiring leisureliness, his enigmatic ambiguity in the simplest of matters.

In the last days of Hitler's Germany, while the Allies-and-rivals were engaged in their headlong race for Berlin, the future of Poland was also being decided. Truman and Churchill in a joint démarche had stood firm for a democratic Poland. Druzhkov ordered Molotov not to give ground, however, and even told him exactly what to say. "The joint message from President Truman and Churchill is mild in tone, but in content shows no improvement. If they question the general principles of the Polish program you may reply that these principles are set out in Stalin's message, and that unless they are accepted you see no possibility of reaching an agreed decision. Druzhkov."

Before the conference, Harriman informed Truman that Stalin attached importance to aid from the Allies, that he needed to rebuild his ruined country, and that consequently pressure could be brought to bear on him at Potsdam. The Western Allies, and Truman in particular, who arrived as the Americans were about to carry out a successful test of the A-bomb, braced themselves to defend Poland and as much of Eastern Europe as possible.

But the moment Truman began asking Stalin to make concessions he was met, to his amazement, with a peremptory and unconditional "nyet." "Nyet" because his armies had occupied Eastern Europe; "nyet" because he had purchased that "nyet" with the lives of millions of Soviet soldiers. "Nyet," Molotov echoed, and went on repeating relentlessly, until Stalin had installed his protégé Bierut in Poland.

On August 9 Stalin joined in the war against Japan. His timing was perfect. Soviet troops shattered the Japanese army in Kwantung. They annexed the Kuriles and southern Sakhalin, avenging tsarist Russia's defeat by Japan in 1905. What was more, the defeat of Japan and the occupation of Manchuria made it possible for Stalin to support Mao Tsetung openly. Soviet experts and Soviet weapons helped Mao seize control of Northern and Central China. China, with its enormous reserves of manpower, was about to join in realizing the Great Dream.

Haggling over the future of Europe continued at the London session of the Council of Foreign Ministers. On September 12 Druzhkov instructed Molotov that "it is essential that you stand firm. No concessions with regard to Romania." Molotov consulted Druzhkov at every step. "Molotov to Druzhkov. In cipher. 15.9.45. Invited by Attlee this evening to dinner at the Prime Minister's residence. Attlee and Bevin (Foreign Secretary) were present with their wives. Dinner and after-dinner conversation passed off in a relatively relaxed atmosphere. Attlee, and more particularly Bevin, suggested expanding unofficial contacts between Russian and English peoples. He recommended sending Soviet football teams, and an opera and ballet group to London. It would be good if I could give them more definite answers on both of these matters." Without instructions from Druzhkov the minister could give no "definite answer" even in the matter of the ballet dancers. He could only maintain his enigmatic silence.

Druzhkov was assiduous in his fine-tuning. "Should the Allies show signs of intransigence in regard to Romania, Bulgaria, etc., convey to [U.S. Secretary of State James F.] Byrnes and Bevin that the government of the USSR will have difficulty in agreeing to the conclusion of the peace treaty with Italy."

Toward the end of the conference of foreign ministers Druzhkov ordered his minister to launch a determined attack: "It would be better to let the Council of Foreign Ministers collapse rather than make substantial concessions to Byrnes. I think we can now tear off the veil of amity, some semblance of which the Americans are so eager to preserve."

Honeymoon Over

Molotov, however, still did not fully understand how his master's mind was working. He knew as well as Harriman that the USSR needed aid from its allies. He continued reporting Western proposals and mentioning possible compromises. And the answer was always an ear-splitting "no." "27.9.45. The Allies are putting pressure on you to break your will, force you into making concessions—obviously you must be absolutely inflexible. The conference may end in complete failure. Even if it does we need shed no tears."

Molotov finally began to understand. It was desperately important for him to anticipate the Boss's secret wishes. His very life depended on it. Druzhkov *wanted* the foreign ministers' conference to end in failure. He did not intend to cooperate with the Allies any longer. The honeymoon with the capitalists was over. Molotov immediately became icily arrogant. Harriman was mistaken: in 1945 Stalin not only did not want help from the Allies, he was eager to part company with them. But why?

There were several reasons. One was that he wanted to hold on to occupied Eastern Europe and the Balkans, and to forget his promises about "percentages of influence." He intended to create a powerful, integrated socialist camp opposing the West. Molotov changed his tune. He quarreled openly, and often, with the other foreign ministers and repulsed every attempt to moderate his demands.

After the Americans dropped the atomic bomb, victory went to their heads. Since they were obviously about to lose China, they concentrated on the future of Japan. The Boss resented what he saw as an attempt to sideline him, and he let loose one of his famous "raucous no's": "26.9.45. To Molotov. In cipher. I consider it the height of impudence on the part of the Americans and the British, who regard themselves as our allies, that they have refused to give us a proper hearing on the question of the Control Commission in Japan." His recommended remedy (one of his favorites) was blackmail: "We have information that the Americans have laid hands on gold reserves in Japan estimated at 1–2 billion dollars, and have made the British their accomplices. You must drop a hint that we see this as the reason why the Americans and British are opposed to the organization of a Control Commission, and are unwilling to allow us any part in matters Japanese." Shortly after this telegram, Harriman presented Molotov with a note on the Control Commission: "30.9.45. An Allied Military Council will be established under the presidency of the Supreme Commander of the Allied Powers. The members of the Council will be the USSR, China, and the British Commonwealth." Stalin had won again, in spite of the bomb.

The Bomb

The Potsdam conference had been timed to coincide with the first test of the twentieth century's superweapon, the nuclear bomb. At the conference, Truman was delighted to hear that "the baby has been born." The hegemony of Stalin's war machine was no more. Truman's great moment had arrived: he triumphantly informed Stalin that the superweapon had been tested. But Stalin was remarkably unperturbed by Truman's announcement. The president could only suppose that the aged generalissimo had failed to understand how powerful the new weapon was.

If the Boss appeared unmoved by Truman's announcement it was because he had been kept informed about the "baby's" progress long before its birth. How this grand old man of the theater must have smiled to himself when Truman moved in to stun him with the news. In fact, the damnable new weapon had troubled him all along. It meant life or death to the Great Dream. He had been frantically trying to catch up in the nuclear race for some time. He had started very late, but, as always, he was determined to catch up with a single bound.

In the Gorbachev period, the Archive of the October Revolution took over from the KGB "Comrade Beria's Special Files." These files included position papers and reports, stamped "Top Secret," meant for the eyes of the almighty head of the NKVD. One of these files, for 1946, contained an inspector's progress report on construction projects No. 817 (Kurchatov's) and No. 813 (Kikoin's). Isaac Kikoin and Igor Kurchatov were Soviet physicists engaged in developing a nuclear bomb.

In 1946, Stalin divided Beria's all-powerful NKVD department into two ministries—State Security and Internal Affairs. Beria, as a Vice-Chairman of the Council of Ministers, continued to have overall responsibility for both top-secret departments. His loyal henchman Merkulov was in charge of State Security at first. But the Boss did not like this arrangement, and he replaced Merkulov with someone unconnected with Beria, Viktor Abakumov, the former head of Smersh (the army's security organization). Smersh had not confined itself to counterespionage, but had kept a sharp lookout for political unreliability, had intervened in the appointment of commanders, and had earned notoriety with its ruthless executions at the front.

It was to Beria and his secret departments that the Boss had thought it best to entrust the creation of the bomb. In this context Beria was like Molotov in his diplomatic activity—merely a workhorse driven by the Boss.

When he joined the nuclear race, his scientists were far behind. Well before the war, physicists such as Y. Zeldovich, Y. Khariton, G. Flerov, and A. Rusinov had made advances in nuclear research. But neither Stalin nor any other member of the leadership had realized the importance of this work. They were preoccupied with the weaponry of the coming war—tanks, airplanes, big guns. The oscillating needles of laboratory apparatus which so thrilled physicists left them unmoved. When Zeldovich and Khariton worked out the conditions necessary for a nuclear explosion, and estimated its potential force, Stalin was not even informed.

But then Soviet intelligence relayed from London an item of news which startled him. It came from a theoretical physicist named Klaus Fuchs, a Communist émigré from Germany working in Britain with a team which was trying to develop an atomic bomb. When Fuchs learned that this work was kept secret from the USSR, he began passing information to the Soviet embassy in London. Soviet intelligence contacted him, and this was when the Boss at last appreciated the potential of the new weapon. He decided that the quickest way to close a dangerous gap was to put Beria in charge of a Soviet nuclear program. Beria's spies would obtain the necessary information. Moreover, Beria's department had unlimited resources. Many brilliant scientists were held in the sharashki, the prisons which were also scientific research establishments. The total secrecy of everything to do with Beria's department guaranteed the secrecy of the nuclear program.

This was when the disbanded Comintern became useful. Stalin's spies appealed to those whose friends and comrades had perished in his torture chambers with a formula which he himself had authorized: "Stalins come and go, but the first socialist state in the world remains."

Some of his helpers—the Rosenbergs, Fuchs—were exposed, but many more escaped exposure. I have already written about Lieutenant General Sudoplatov's memoirs. This is a work of disinformation, intended to distract us from the real secrets. And I often recall another intelligence officer, General Vasily Sitnikov. When I first met him he was Vice-Chairman of VAAP (the All-Union Copyright Agency). This office was traditionally reserved for KGB generals no longer on the active list. In VAAP Sitnikov posed as a liberal. He even helped me when I was, not for the first time, refused an exit visa for the United States to attend a premiere of my play. He was Andropov's man, and had high expectations of Gorbachev's perestroika. As it happened, he was one of its first victims—summarily pensioned off when one of the new KGB people needed his job. He cherished wild ideas of revenge. Shortly after his dismissal I met him in the streets, and we got talking. "This," he said, brandishing the back number of *Foreign Literature* he was carrying, "includes a documentary play about the Oppenheimer affair. . . . The interesting thing about it wasn't Oppenheimer himself. . . ." He smiled that familiar know-all smile, the smile I had once seen on the face of the investigator Sheinin. He was silent for a while, then went on: "Beria often said, 'Comrade Stalin teaches us that no public figure in the bourgeois world is incorruptible. You only have to know what sort of bribe to offer. For most of them it's money. And if one of these resists temptation it's because you have been too miserly. Where money won't do the trick, a woman may. And where a woman won't, Marx will.' The best people worked for us for idealistic reasons. If I were to write down all I know about these things . . . I just might do that . . ." Soon after our conversation, I heard that he had died.

After the Boss's return from Potsdam, Beria relayed this message to the physicists: "Comrade Stalin has said that the atomic bomb must be made in a very short time whatever the cost." He promised the scientists a spell in the camps in the event of failure.

Between 1943 and 1946 intelligence reports from the United States had included large quantities of scientific information needed for the creation of a nuclear weapon. When Kurchatov, who was in charge of the Soviet project, learned that a bomb had been successfully tested in the United States, he decided to copy the procedures which had proved successful there. He had ideas of his own, but dared not continue with them once the Boss had demanded completion "in a very short time." Instead, he would re-create the American bomb.

The first Soviet bomb was tested successfully on August 29, 1949. Stalin had gotten what he wanted. The USSR had caught up with the USA, and "in a very short time" at that. After the explosion the Boss lavished awards and distinctions on his scientists, and said: "If we had been a year and a half late it would probably have been tried out on us."

The situation was transformed. Once again, Stalin had the most powerful army in the world. He now gave his scientists their heads, and they did not disappoint him. By 1951 they had created an atomic bomb of their own, more than twice as powerful as the first one and half as heavy. This was important, as he was already contemplating delivery. For, in 1951, he was already preparing to involve his country and mankind at large in the realization of his grandiose and bloody scheme. Apocalypse was drawing nearer.

Map of the Empire in Its New Borders

Stalin liked to repeat that "Russians have always been good at making war, but never good at winning the peace." He, however, had been good at both. Molotov tells us that "when the war was over, a map of the USSR within its new borders was brought out to Stalin at his dacha. He pinned it to the wall with drawing pins, and said: 'Let's see what we've got, then: in the north everything's all right, Finland greatly wronged us, so we've moved her frontier farther from Leningrad. The Baltic States, which were Russian territory from ancient times, are ours again, all the Belorussians are ours now, the Ukrainians also, and the Moldavians are also back with us. So to the west of us everything is normal. [He then turned to the eastern frontiers.] What have we got here? The Kurile Islands are ours, and the whole of Sakhalin . . . and look, isn't it great: Port Arthur is also ours!' He ran the stem of his pipe over China. 'China, Mongolia, all as it should be.' "

The extended borders of the empire were now surrounded with docile satellite countries. Finland, it was true, was still independent.

She had "greatly wronged us" by fighting on the German side. His agents now more or less openly hunted down Russian émigrés who had taken refuge in Finland after the Revolution, and delivered them to Moscow. The Finns had to turn a blind eye.

"Now this frontier I don't like at all," he told Molotov, pointing south of the Caucasus. "The Dardanelles. . . . We also have claims to Turkish territory, and to Libya." His minister turned cold at this. The Boss was speaking of another partition of the world. Molotov's fears were for himself, though, not for mankind at large. He remembered 1937, when the Boss had initiated the Great Terror in preparation for the war they had just fought. Did this talk of another war mean that another great bloodletting lay ahead?

26

THE SOCIALIST WAR CAMP

The Boss needed an open quarrel with the West. As always, he needed enemies. With a new threat to the land of the Soviets, he could stop playing at democracy in Eastern Europe and tighten the screws at home.

Churchill came to his aid with his famous Fulton speech. Both Truman and Attlee deprecated Churchill's outspokenness, but it was too late: Stalin could proclaim that the USSR was threatened with aggression again. The war of mutual anathemas, the cold war which he so much wanted, had begun. The Soviet public was deluged with radio programs about the menace of imperialism and the incendiarist warmongers.

His hands were untied. Between 1946 and 1948 he abandoned all pretense and unceremoniously fashioned his "mighty camp of socialism" from Czechoslovakia, Hungary, Romania, Poland, East Germany, Bulgaria, and Yugoslavia, installing Communist rulers everywhere.

Cominform (the Communist Information Bureau), the legitimate heir to Comintern, was his control lever. Under his direction this body coordinated policy in Eastern Europe and channeled funds and instructions to Western Communist parties. Nothing happened within the camp unless he gave the order. No independent action was possible. The Boss had eyes for everything, and punished mercilessly any attempt to decide things without him.

There were, of course, unpleasant surprises. Stalin learned that Tito, loyal Tito, was engaged in intrigue. First, Tito had tried to annex Albania without consulting the Boss. Then Tito and Dimitrov, the Boss's slave and satrap in Bulgaria, had concluded a mutual security pact without informing him. Tito had gone so far as to suggest that Yugoslavia and Bulgaria should form a confederation. Worse still, he was trying to associate Poland, Czechoslovakia, and even Greece with it. The Boss reacted sharply to this wild stallion who threatened to lead his herd astray. His wrath was awesome. Menacing articles appeared in *Pravda.* He summoned Dimitrov and Tito to Moscow. Remembering the fate of the old Comintern hands, Tito sent some of his comrades instead.

The Boss received both delegations in the Kremlin in the cold February of 1948. He yelled at Dimitrov: "You're kicking up your heels like some young Komsomol. . . . You and the Yugoslavs never report on what you're doing."

The Yugoslav Kardelj, trying to smooth over the situation, told him that "there are no disagreements between us."

This brought a furious outburst from Stalin: "Nonsense! There are disagreements, and very profound ones. You never consult us at all. You do this on principle—you don't just make mistakes."

They resolved to consult each other regularly in the future. But the Boss had made up his mind to rid himself of Tito. He knew that "one bad sheep can spoil the flock." Tito would now be more useful to him as an enemy—as Trotsky had once been. He needed Tito as he had once needed Trotsky, to punish those who associated with him. By anathematizing Tito he would tighten the bonds of obedience within the camp, and he would gradually bring back fear. The other members of Cominform unanimously fell upon Tito, and Yugoslavia was expelled from the camp.

Great China more than made up for little Yugoslavia. In October 1949 Mao Tse-tung's forces occupied Beijing. With the help of China's army, a Communist regime was quickly installed in North Korea. The Boss had a firm footing in Asia. The socialist camp he had created possessed enormous human resources by the middle of the century. The Great Dream was so near to fulfillment. . . . But first he had to reintroduce terror into his own country.

Molotov was not mistaken. The Boss was preparing the country for an unprecedented ordeal. During the war the generals had been a cause of concern. They had become used to having their own way, and they had tasted glory. Even before the German army was driven from the USSR, he was planning to chasten them. V. Abakumov, then head of Smersh, was ordered in 1943 to monitor the future telephone conversations of marshals and generals. Files containing Smersh transcripts have been found in the KGB's archives. Monitoring became even more intensive after the war.

What follows is an excerpt from a conversation recorded eighteen months after the war. The speakers were Colonel General V. Gordov (a hero of the Soviet Union, he commanded the Stalingrad front in the summer of 1942 and was appointed commander of the

Volga Military District in 1946) and Major General Rybalchenko, his chief of staff.

December 28, 1946. The following conversation between Gordov and Rybalchenko was monitored and recorded.
R: The way things are now you might as well lie down and die. . . . Everybody is fed up with his life, people say so quite openly—on the trains—in the Metro, everywhere, they come straight out with it.
G: Everything depends on bribery and bootlicking nowadays. I've been passed over twice because I've never gone in for licking boots.
R: Yes, well. Zhukov's resigned himself to it, he just keeps soldiering on. [Zhukov, the conqueror of Germany, had recently taken the salute at the victory parade and had been relegated by the Boss to a provincial command.]
G: On the face of it he's soldiering on, but in his heart he doesn't like it.

December 31, 1946. The following conversation between Gordov and his wife Tatyana was monitored and recorded.
G: Why do I have to go to Stalin—why do I have to beg and demean myself, crawl to that [obscene and derogatory expressions about Comrade Stalin]?
T: I feel sure he won't last more than a year now. . . .
G: I can't bear to look at him, I can't breathe the same air, yet you keep urging me to go and see Stalin. It's just like the Inquisition, people are just dying. If you knew the half of it. . . . You think I'm the only one, but I'm not, not by a long shot.
T: At one time people with minds of their own could go underground and do something about it. But now there's nothing you can do. They've broken even Zhukov's spirit.
G: They'll keep Zhukov for a year or two, and then he's finished.

Conversations such as these confirmed for Stalin that his fears weren't all idle fantasy. Gordov, his wife, and Rybalchenko were arrested in January 1947 and subsequently shot. But the Boss must have remembered Gordov's words: "You think I'm the only one, but I'm not, not by a long shot."

A number of other military "big mouths" were also shot, among them G. Kulik, a former marshal demoted to the rank of general.

In all this seditious talk among army officers, Georgi Zhukov's name was invariably mentioned. The Boss knew that as long as Zhukov was at liberty the clandestine military opposition would have a center. But an outsize bait would be needed to catch such a shark. He ordered his lackeys to find it. One April night in 1946, Marshal of Aviation Novikov, commander of the Soviet air force, found a reception party waiting outside his home. He was bundled into a car and, as he later described it, delivered to "some sort of room where they stripped off my marshal's uniform and gave me a ragged pair of trousers and a shirt." The joke which de Gaulle had heard was no joke after all. All the top people in the aircraft industry were arrested simultaneously. Abakumov conducted the investigation skillfully, and soon had yesterday's war heroes slandering themselves. They confirmed that they had approved for service planes which they knew to be defective, with the result that a number of fliers had lost their lives. More important, they testified against Zhukov.

On September 18, 1948, Lieutenant General Vladimir Kryukov and his wife, the popular singer Lidia Ruslanova, were arrested. The investigating officer's record has survived. "Can you repeat hostile remarks made by Zhukov about the Party and the government? . . . Can you give further examples of hostile and provocative statements made by Zhukov?" The general obliged. But Zhukov's words were insufficient: criminal acts were required. According to his case file, General Kryukov had brought back from conquered Germany antique carpets, Gobelin tapestries, several antique dinner services, furniture, furs, pictures—all loaded onto four (looted) motor vehicles. In the first flush of victory the Boss had encouraged that sort of thing . . . with an eye to the future. That future had arrived:

> *Investigating Officer:* In the end you sank so low that you turned into a looter and a robber. Can we say that Zhukov, who accepted presents from you knowing their origin, was just as much of a looter and a robber as you were?
>
> *Kryukov:* I sent Zhukov valuable lengths of cloth, carpets, crockery, and many other things. Just as I did to several other generals.
>
> *Investigating Officer:* In what circumstances did Ruslanova pre-

sent Zhukov's wife with a diamond brooch she had appropriated in Germany?
Kryukov: The day after the victory parade in June 1945 Zhukov gave a banquet at his dacha outside Moscow. . . . Ruslanova proposed a toast "to faithful wives," sang Zhukov's wife's praises, and presented her with the brooch saying: "It never occurred to the government to give medals to valiant wives."
Investigating Officer [indignantly]: You both toadied to Zhukov, knowing full well how much he loved flattery. You were the one who started calling him "Georgi, Bringer of Victory" [St. George is so called by the Russian Orthodox Church].

For a short time after the war, Stalin abolished the death sentence. General Kryukov, therefore, got "only" twenty-five years in the camps, and Ruslanova, the country's favorite entertainer, ten years. A drastic purge of the army was meant to be the final stage of his operation, as it had been in the thirties. As long as the generals were a united group, it was too early to arrest Zhukov. Terror had first to be reinstated.

Stalin began, as he had in the thirties, with the intelligentsia, using once again the tactics which had proved effective in the days of the Great Terror. The intellectuals had returned from the war with "private thoughts." As one poet wrote:

Smoke of the Fatherland—Thou art strange to us,
Comrades—it is not as we thought.

Rashly, the intelligentsia looked for changes. The war, the proximity of death, the brief interval of friendship with the Allies had encouraged a derisive attitude to doctrinaire ideology. In 1946, Stalin resumed his ideological bombardment.

Stalin asked for Eisenstein's *Ivan the Terrible, Part II,* recently finished, to be brought to him. Part I he had pronounced a masterpiece and awarded a Stalin Prize.

Eisenstein was in the hospital at the time, and the Boss watched the film about his favorite hero in the company of Bolshakov, Minister of Cinematography. An eyewitness recalls that "when Bolshakov returned he was unrecognizable: his right eye was half-closed, there were red spots on his face and after what he had gone through he was incapable of saying anything for the rest of the day." The Boss had called the film a "nightmare." And his parting words to Bolshakov were: "We could never quite get around to you during the war, but now we'll give you the full treatment."

Shortly afterward came the famous decree "On the Magazines *Zvezda* and *Leningrad*." The two celebrities chosen for demolition were Anna Akhmatova, a poet already famous in tsarist times, and the satirist Mikhail Zoshchenko. The Boss had been watching Zoshchenko closely for some time. Stalin's daughter, Svetlana recalled that "he used to read Zoshchenko to us and sometimes he'd say 'this must be where Comrade Zoshchenko remembered the GPU and changed the ending.' " Konstantin Simonov said that "Zoshchenko and Akhmatova were chosen because their public appearances in Leningrad had been so demonstratively applauded. Their audience had consisted of openly disaffected intellectuals."

The Leningrad intelligentsia were summoned to hear Stalin's henchman Andrei Zhdanov, a pudgy little man with a silly mustache, call the great Akhmatova a whore and vilify Zoshchenko. In the course of his speech, he asked a question which sent a shudder through the hall: "Why are they still free to stroll through the parks and gardens of this city sacred to Lenin?" The Boss, however, decided not to touch them, for the present. Pavlenko told my father that "Stalin personally ordered that Akhmatova should not be touched. The poet Soso had once been fond of her verses." That was a story put about by his secret police. It was Stalin's practice to show clemency while getting ready for a great bloodletting.

All the arts were systematically savaged: literature, the theater, the cinema. Soon it was music's turn. The West's favorites, Prokofiev and Shostakovich, were the two composers most lambasted in a Central Committee edict of February 1947. As soon as the edict was published, Prokofiev wrote a penitential letter. It was published and read out at a general meeting of Moscow composers and musicologists, who all "joined with the Soviet people in warmly welcoming the Central Committee's decision." Prokofiev and Shostakovich waited in dread to see what would come next. Out at his dacha Prokofiev locked himself in his study and burned the works of his favorite author, Nabokov, and a complete set of the magazine *America*.

The Boss did not lay a finger on them either, for the present. He did, however, give them a warning. Prokofiev was then living at his dacha with his young second wife. His Italian ex-wife, Lina, a singer, lived in Moscow with their two sons. At the end of February both sons arrived at the dacha. Prokofiev realized at once what had happened. He went outside to talk to them, and they told him that Lina had been arrested. It was enough to frighten him once and for all.

Prokofiev's son Svyatoslav said that "after all that, my father suffered from exhausting headaches and chronic hypertomia. He was a different man, he always looked sad and hopeless. His ex-wife, the Italian singer, was already in a prison camp, hauling slop buckets on a handcart. The writer Evgenia Taratuta, who was in the camp with her, remembered that she 'sometimes stopped pulling the handcart and stood beside the slop buckets ecstatically telling us about Paris.'" Lina would outlive both Stalin and Prokofiev—she returned from the camp and died in 1991.

Shostakovich, too, tried to make the best of it. He wrote incidental music for propaganda films such as *Meeting on the Elbe, The Fall of Berlin* and *Unforgettable 1919*. He also wrote a symphony called *1905* and another called *1917*. Stalin was already dead when Shostakovich addressed this statement to the party: "Recently I have felt more strongly than ever how much I need to be in the ranks of the Communist Party. In my creative work I have always been guided by the Party's inspiring instructions." So wrote the greatest composer of the century. He too had been frightened once and for all.

The Central Committee's successive edicts on the arts were issued in pamphlet form, and the whole country studied them in "political education groups." The intelligentsia trembled and were silent.

Against this background of ideological pogroms, arrests were already being made. The victims were relatives of the great ones of this world—chosen so that everyone would learn what was happening and be afraid.

Peter Shirshov, People's Commissar for the Merchant Marine, had many titles. He was an academician, had won fame as a member of expeditions to the North Pole, and was a hero of the Soviet Union. He was married to a beautiful thirty-year-old actress, Zhenya Garkusha. They were madly in love with each other. In 1946 she was arrested, and he was not even told why. His daughter Marina has preserved Peter Shirshov's diary.

> In spite of everything I am writing because I can no longer bear the horror of it. Another Saturday has gone by, and at 4 A.M. I simply can't find myself anything more to do in the Commissariat. I go home reluctantly, knowing that I shan't be able to sleep anyway. It is a struggle to keep going, 13–14 hours at

work—and then what? What can I do with myself when I'm alone, what can I do to get away from myself? . . .

Zhenya, my poor Zhenya. . . . It was Sunday, like now, and you whispered to me "Shirsh, we shall have another little Marina soon, but let's hope for a boy this time!" Then you talked about the marvelous time we would have together in the South. . . . It was quite dark when we got up to leave the balcony, and as we went in you snuggled up to me and said "Shirsh! if only you knew how happy I am with you!" That was how our last day passed. Next morning there was the usual mad rush at work—telephones ringing, papers to sign, coded messages, telegrams. Then at 7 P.M. they sent for me and I was told Zhenya had been arrested. They were waiting for her on the riverbank. She was happy and laughing, and she was just as happy and full of life when she got in the car, with nothing over her light summer frock. Among strange, hostile people. . . . Once, in a tent on an ice floe, cut off from the world by a blizzard and the polar night, I listened to the wind howling and dreamt of a great love. I always believed in it and was always waiting for it to happen. And finally I'd got what I'd dreamt of—when I was a gray-headed idiot, still as naive as a little boy in my forties. Listen, that's the wind whistling through the prison bars. How it howls over the roof of the crowded hut they've locked your poor Zhenya in. . . . It will soon be morning. For three months . . . I kept waiting for something to happen, for a miracle, I didn't admit it even to myself, but I was expecting Zhenya to return. Time and time again the telephone has rung, my heart has missed a beat, I had a presentiment that it was Zhenya ringing from home—they'd released her! How often have I come home at night and gone into the bedroom quietly in case the miracle had happened—maybe she's at home, maybe they just haven't told me. For three months I've been trying my hardest to get them to tell me about her, tell me what's happened to her, and every time I come up against a wall of silence. Nobody tells me anything, and they obviously don't intend to. Why am I writing all this? I don't know. I've got more than enough time ahead of me. I'm trying to hold out! . . . I must go on living for your mama's sake, and yours, little Marina. But I hope you will never know what torment it can be to resist taking the easy way out. . . . I hope you'll never know how hard it can be to wrench your hand away from a pistol that has gotten hot in your coat pocket.

Zhenya Garkusha was sent to the gold mines to pan for gold, work so dangerous to human health that women were not normally made to do it. She was thirty-three when she died in the camp. Shirshov remained at his place of work, and held his tongue, as any good Communist should, or any slave. He never found out why she had been arrested. He died of cancer in 1953.

The Boss did not overlook what was left of the Alliluyev family. He had stopped seeing them long ago. They belonged to a forgotten life. Now they would help him reinstate Terror. Beria informed him that Zhenya Alliluyeva, of whom he once had been so fond, was spreading the rumor that her husband had been poisoned. He had never forgiven her for spurning his advances, and for remarrying in a hurry. Beria went to work and in a little while a counterrumor crept around: Pavel had indeed been poisoned, but by his wife! Zhenya had been living with another man and wanted to get rid of her husband, the story went.

Svetlana wrote to her father on December 1: "Papa dearest, about Zhenya. I think your doubts about her arose because she remarried too quickly. She herself has told me more or less why it happened like that. . . . I shall certainly tell you when you get here . . . remember that people have said all sorts of things about me too!" Papa dearest, however, was already taking action.

Zhenya's daughter, Kira Alliluyeva-Politkovskaya, recalled: "It happened on December 10, 1947. . . . I had just graduated from drama school, and life was beautiful. Then came that ring at the door. I opened it. There were two of them standing there: 'Can we see Evgenia Alexandrovna?' I shouted, 'Mama, two citizens want to see you,' and went back to my room. A little later I heard Mama walk along the corridor and say loudly, 'Prison and poverty can't be kept waiting.' When I heard that I dashed out. She gave me a quick kiss on the cheek and left the apartment. When she came back from the camp I asked why she'd walked out so quickly. She said: 'I realized it was the end, and meant to throw myself down the stairwell from the eighth floor, so that they couldn't torture me when they got me there.' [She knew kind Joseph only too well.] But they grabbed her and took her away. Some time later the bell rang in the night. Two men in uniform came in and said, 'Get dressed and take some warm clothes and 25 rubles, just in case.' " That was only a month after her mother's arrest.

He pinned a charge of conspiring against Stalin on Anna Sergeevna, his wife Nadya's older sister, and had her jailed. When she returned she was mentally ill and suffered from auditory hallucinations. In 1948 he banished Dzhonik Svanidze, the son of the friends he had executed. The explanation he gave Svetlana was laconic but honest: "They knew too much and chattered too much. And that helps our enemies."

All Moscow was horrified by these arrests, wondering whether 1937 was about to begin all over again.

1937 Redux

He had already opened fire on his headquarters staff. The destruction of his henchmen had begun.

Who were these henchmen of his? "The all-powerful favorite" Zhdanov was in reality a hopeless drunkard, a lackey on whom the Boss regularly vented his bad temper. Cunning Beria? It doesn't say much for his cunning that a hundred days after Stalin's death he failed to spot the very first conspiracy directed against himself. If he can be called cunning at all it is for his skill in divining the Boss's wishes, and creating the spurious conspiracies which Stalin wanted to see. Beria, like all of them, was a willing workhorse, and no more. Malenkov, that "fat, flabby, cruel toad," as one of his colleagues called him, was left high and dry when his Leader died. They all had a paranoid fear of the Boss, and observed his first commandment: no thinking for yourself. We need only look at Stalin's "special files." Beria reported absolutely everything that happened in the capital, even the discussion of a play in the Maly Theater or the visit of a foreign delegation to a high-rise building—it was all reported to him, read by him, double-checked by him—by the Boss in person. The slightest sign of independence could be fatal. When in 1951 Khrushchev took the initiative in proposing the amalgamation of collective farms into larger units, a bellow of rage followed immediately. Khrushchev had to write a schoolboy letter of apology: "Dear Comrade Stalin—you have perfectly correctly pointed out the mistakes I have made. . . . I ask you, Comrade Stalin, to help me correct my gross mistake and to minimize the damage done to the Party by my erroneous statement." Shortly afterward, an attempt to act without authorization destroyed Voznesensky.

No, the Boss's henchmen were nothing without him. They were handpicked nonentities—chosen because they could not be a danger to him. The idea that they could engage in intrigues of their own is laughable. It was he who organized them in rival groupings and egged them on to destroy each other. One man and one man only stood behind each and every one of the Kremlin cliques: the Boss.

So he began his purge of the country by striking first at his lieutenants. He had grown tired of them. They had got on his nerves. They were overburdened with secrets, and too old. He needed new, obedient young cadres to carry out his will, to realize the Great Dream. The deafening crash of toppled leaders would signal the return of Terror.

As soon as the war was over he had begun harping on his age. His lieutenants, of course, were expected to deny that he was getting old. K. Popovich, one of the Yugoslav leaders who visited Stalin, described how he "took us out to the nearer dacha in the night. A woman served supper on silver dishes without saying a word. Supper, and toasting each other, took a whole hour. Then Stalin started putting gramophone records on and jigging to the music, while Molotov and the others kept calling out 'Comrade Stalin, how fit you are!' But his mood suddenly changed and he said: 'No, I haven't got long to live now.' His comrades shouted 'You'll live a long time yet. We need you!' But Stalin shook his head: 'The laws of physiology are irreversible.' Then he looked at Molotov and said: 'But Vyacheslav Mikhailovich will still be around.' " Molotov must have broken into a sweat.

He evidently said this on other occasions. Molotov told Chuyev, the poet, that "after the war Stalin thought of retiring and once said at table: 'Let Vyacheslav do some of the work now. He's a bit younger than me.' " Molotov did not say what his answer was. But we can imagine how passionately he protested. He must surely have been terrified, and thought: It won't be long now! Nor, indeed, did the Boss keep his lieutenants waiting.

He began by setting a trap. In the President's Archive I read this telegram from the Boss to Molotov, who was in New York. "14.9.46. The academicians ask you not to object to your election to honorary membership in the Academy of Sciences. Please do agree. Druzhkov."

Molotov sent a courteous telegram to the Academy expressing his profound gratitude and signing himself "Yours, Molotov." An angry riposte in cipher followed immediately: "I was astounded by your telegram. Are you really in ecstasies over your election to honorary membership? What did you mean by signing yourself 'Yours, Molotov'? It seems to me that you, as a statesman of the highest category, ought to show more concern for your dignity."

Molotov knew then that it had begun. He hastened to do penance. "I can see that I have acted stupidly. Thank you for your telegram." He knew the Boss's habits. This was just a beginning. When the time came to destroy him, any excuse would be good enough. "Molotov's proposed amendments to the draft constitution for Germany must be regarded as incorrect and damaging." Stone Arse's seat was getting wobblier all the time. But for the moment, as he undermined Molotov, the Boss was regularly promoting Voznesensky. Mikoyan recalled that "at Lake Ritsa in 1948 Stalin said that he had aged and was thinking about successors. He mentioned N. A. Voznesensky as a possible Chairman of the Council of Ministers and A. Kuznetsov as a possible Secretary General of the Central Committee." Molotov, with all his experience, must have heaved a sigh of relief when he heard this: the bell had tolled for others. The Boss had fresher quarry in his sights.

The young Politburo member Voznesensky had come to the fore in the war years. An able economist, he was now First Vice-Chairman of the Council of Ministers, and Stalin's deputy in that body. Another young man, A. Kuznetsov, one of the Secretaries of the Central Committee, acted more and more frequently in alliance with Voznesensky. In some respects Kuznetsov resembled Kirov: he had great charm, he was honest, and he was a hard worker. And, like Kirov, he had previously led the Leningrad Communists. The Boss had brought him to Moscow as a secretary of the Central Committee, making him in effect second man in the Party hierarchy, and had entrusted him with supervision of Beria's two ministries, State Security and Internal Affairs. Unlike Stalin's other henchmen, Kuznetsov and Voznesensky were substantial figures, capable of making independent decisions. Such men had been needed during the war. But the war was now over—and they seemed incapable of understanding that fact.

The Voznesensky-Kuznetsov partnership had obviously arrogated too much power. Stalin would aim his first murderous blow at them. Beria and Malenkov at once sensed what the Boss had in mind. Beria, in particular, resented Kuznetsov's supervising role and could not wait to assail him. The dogs were straining at the leash.

When Stalin made V. Abakumov Minster of State Security, Kuznetsov welcomed his appointment in an enthusiastic speech. He did not know that, on the Boss's orders, he himself was under investigation by the ministry which he nominally supervised. Abakumov would subsequently state that "the case against Voznesensky and Kuznetsov was dictated by the highest authority," that is, by the Boss.

It began with a nonsensical quibble. The Leningrader Kuznetsov was, so it was said, spoken of as the city's "chief," and Leningrad Party members also called Voznesensky "chief." The two of them decided, without informing the Boss, to organize an all-Russian trade fair in Leningrad. The fair itself was unimportant; it was the principle that mattered. From January 10 to 20, 1949, Leningrad hosted the trade fair. Malenkov promptly charged Kuznetsov, and certain senior officials in the city, of pandering to Leningrad's self-importance and of organizing the fair without informing the Central Committee or the Council of Ministers. The Politburo immediately ruled that Kuznetsov had made a "demagogic bid for popularity" with the Leningrad organization, shown disrespect for the Central Committee, and attempted to "alienate the city from the Central Committee." This nonsense was enough to deprive the previously all-powerful secretary of all his offices, while Voznesensky was reprimanded.

For thousands of Party functionaries the nonsense had an ominous ring. In "in-depth language" it meant: "Get ready!" Get ready for a repetition of the days they remembered so well—when the Zinovievite organization was destroyed. They braced themselves, and they were not disappointed in their expectations. The Boss was on the warpath.

While the case against Voznesensky and Kuznetsov was cobbled together, Stalin went on undermining Molotov, who might be thought by some to symbolize the previous foreign policy of the USSR and friendship with the West. His demise was meant to emphasize that friendship with the West was at an end. And someone had to answer for the alliance with Hitler!

A New Pogrom

Moreover, Molotov's wife was Jewish. In the Boss's new plan, a leading role was reserved for the Jews.

He began with the "cosmopolitans," and the Jewish Antifascist Committee (JAC), a symbol of close relations with the United States. As far back as October 1946 the Ministry of State Security had produced a secret memorandum on "nationalist manifestations among JAC personnel": "The JAC makes international contacts with bourgeois public figures without observing the proper class approach . . . and exaggerates the Jewish contribution to the achievements of the USSR, which is a manifestation of nationalism." The Boss gave orders to whip up a case against the JAC, but the great Mikhoels stood in his way; since the war he had become far too famous for the Boss's liking.

Mikhoels's death was surrounded by legends. In 1953, Beria would hasten to dissociate himself from his late master's misdeeds by disclosing "breaches of legality." The relevant documents, however, remained inaccessible for forty years. What follows is an extract from a letter written by Beria to the Presidium (the Politburo was so renamed in 1952) of the Central Committee:

> A review of the documentation in the Mikhoels case has shown that . . . by order of the Minister of State Security, V. Abakumov, an illegal operation for the physical liquidation of Mikhoels was carried out in Minsk in February 1948. In this connection V. Abakumov was interrogated in the Ministry of Internal Affairs of the USSR. . . . Abakumov testified that "in 1948 Stalin instructed me to organize the liquidation of Mikhoels as a matter of urgency, assigning special people to the case. We knew that Mikhoels, and a friend of his whose name I do not remember, had arrived in Minsk. When this was reported to Stalin he gave instructions that the liquidation was to be carried out there and then, in Minsk. When Stalin was informed that Mikhoels had been liquidated he expressed his appreciation and ordered that medals should be awarded, which was done. Various plans for the removal of Mikhoels had been suggested. The one adopted was to invite him, via the secret police, to a social gathering at night, send a car to his hotel, take him to the grounds of an out-of-town dacha belonging to L. F. Tsanava, Minister of State Security of the Belorussian Republic, liquidate him there, then take him to an unfrequented backstreet in the city, lay his body on the road leading to his hotel, and run over it with a truck. This was done. To ensure secrecy Golubov, the agent of the Ministry of State Security who took Mikhoels to the 'party,' was also liquidated."

In January 1948, Stalin limited himself to Mikhoels, and postponed the demolition of the Jewish Antifascist Committee. This was because the Boss was simultaneously watching with close interest the establishment of the state of Israel. Many émigrés from Russia had a hand in its creation, including several former Comintern activists. Disillusioned with the Arab nationalists (who had looked either to the fascist regimes or to Britain for support), the Boss decided to place his bet elsewhere. Already in May 1947 the USSR's United Nations representative, Gromyko, had announced to the UN General Assembly that the creation of an independent Jewish state in Palestine had the full support of the USSR. The Boss's plan was to use an Israeli state under Soviet influence in opposition to Britain, and to bar the way to the Americans. Israel was meant to be his advanced post in the Near East. So the Jewish Antifascist Committee lived on, though without Mikhoels. Mikhoels himself was buried with full honors.

The first ambassador of the new state of Israel, Golda Meir, arrived in the USSR with due ceremony on September 3, 1948. The Minister of State Security, under Abakumov, monitored Jewish reactions to this event, and amassed material for future use. Meir arrived on the day on which the Boss's faithful henchman Andrei Zhdanov was buried. Golda was struck by the millions who went to pay their last respects to him. She did not yet know that grief, like everything else in Stalin's country, was organized.

Meir was warmly welcomed, but Ilya Ehrenburg was commissioned to write an article telling Soviet Jews that Israel had nothing to do with them since anti-Semitism and the "Jewish problem," did not exist in the Soviet Union. In the USSR there was no "Jewish people," only a "Soviet people." Israel was needed only by the Jews in capitalist countries, where anti-Semitism flourished. Soviet Jews, however, did not understand that this was a warning and a threat. They knew only that the great Stalin had supported the creation of Israel, and that Molotov had received "our Golda." The heady spirit of freedom had not yet evaporated. An unprecedented crowd, some fifty thousand strong, gathered outside the synagogue which Golda Meir attended on the Jewish New Year. There were soldiers and officers of the Red army, old people and youngsters. Babes were held up by their parents to see her. She wrote in her memoirs that "people were calling out 'Our Golda!,' 'Shalom, Goldele!,' 'Long life and good health!,' 'Happy New Year!' Such an ocean of love overwhelmed me that I could hardly breathe. I came close to fainting." Her words to the crowd were, "Thank you for still being Jews." A dangerous thing to say in Stalin's kingdom.

At a reception given by the Ministry of Foreign Affairs Meir was approached by Molotov's wife, Polina, who addressed her in Yiddish. "You're Jewish?" Meir asked in surprise. "I'm a daughter of the Jewish people," Polina answered in Yiddish. This was probably just part of the effort to seduce Meir. As always, the Boss had distributed the parts: Ehrenburg could write an article for the general public, but someone had to think about friendship with Israel.

It did not take Stalin long, however, to realize that ungrateful Israel was obviously leaning toward America. He need no longer hesitate to carry out his long-cherished plan.

THE JEWISH CARD

Early in 1949 Stalin launched a massive campaign against "homeless cosmopolitans." That was the name now given to those accused of "kowtowing to things foreign." It was announced that excessive praise of things foreign was an insidious form of propaganda for the bourgeois way of life.

The campaign quickly degenerated into lunacy. Stalinist historians "revealed" that the discoveries of Russian scientists had been pirated wholesale by rascally foreigners. It now appeared that the steam engine was invented not by Watt but by a Siberian skilled workman called Polzunov, the electric lightbulb by the Russian Yablochkov, the radio by Popov, not Marconi. . . . The first successful test flight was made by the Russian engineer Mozhaisky, not the Wright brothers, and Petrov, a schoolteacher, had discovered the electric arc. Whatever later Russians had not invented had already been discovered by Mikhail Lomonosov in the eighteenth century.

Filmmakers, writers, and musicians were in permanent conference, exposing instances of "kowtowing to the West," while unmasked "cosmopolitans" did public penance. The great majority of the unmasked "cosmopolitans" were Jews.

There should be no doubt about the anti-Semitic thrust of the campaign. Stalin combined it with the destruction of the Jewish Antifascist Committee.

Moscow was fed terrible rumors that the late great Mikhoels had been found to be a spy and an agent of the Jewish nationalists. Malenkov summoned the new chairman of the Jewish Antifascist Committee, Lozovsky, who was also head of the Soviet Information Bureau, and roundly abused him. The accusations against him were simple: Meir's reception had shown that thousands of Jews were potential spies whose hearts were in a hostile state. Zionist organizations had made the Antifascist Committee their agent—witness the fact that the committee, with American backing, had planned to create a Jewish outpost in the Crimea. Lozovsky was an old enough hand to know that any attempt to excuse himself by mentioning Stalin's involvement in that scheme would mean a slow and painful death. All he could do was to confess and hope for clemency. But clemency was not to be had. The Boss was planning too far ahead. Lozovsky and the other members of the committee were shortly arrested. They would all be shot (except for academician Lina Stern) later, in the summer of 1952. In 1949 the arrested members of the Antifascist Committee were needed alive, for the big-game hunt in which Molotov was the quarry.

The disbandment of the Antifascist Committee made possible the arrest of Molotov's wife, Polina Zhemchuzina. Molotov told the poet Chuyev that "when Stalin read out at a Politburo meeting the information about Polina given to him by the Chekists my knees were knocking. She was accused of links with Zionist organizations and with the Israeli Ambassador Golda Meir, in connection with their wish to make the Crimea a Jewish republic. She had been on good terms with Mikhoels. . . . She ought, of course, to have chosen her friends more carefully. She was dismissed from her post, but not arrested for some time afterward. . . . Then Stalin said, 'You'll have to divorce your wife.' " A more accurate version of this would read: "Before having her arrested Stalin said 'you'll have to divorce your wife.' " Molotov said of his spouse, "She said, 'If that's what the Party needs, I'll get a divorce.' We parted at the end of 1948. In 1949 she was arrested." Yet again, Molotov has failed to tell the whole story. I found the necessary supplement in the President's Archive.

It turned out that when the Central Committee voted to expel his completely innocent wife from the Party, Molotov heroically abstained. But shortly afterward he wrote the following note: "January 20, 1949. Top Secret. To Comrade Stalin. When the Central Committee voted on the proposal to expel P. S. Zhemchuzina from the Party, I abstained, which I acknowledge to be politically incorrect. I hereby declare that after thinking the matter over I now vote in favor of the Central Committee's decision, which is in accordance with the interests of the Party and the state, and which teaches us the true meaning of Communist Party membership. Furthermore, I acknowledge that I was gravely at fault in not restraining in time a person near to me from taking false steps and from dealings with such anti-Soviet nationalists as Mikhoels." Betraying his wife was the price of liberty. As always, he observed the rules.

Meanwhile his wife was being broken down by the investigators. Three files containing the records of her interrogation and of confrontations with witnesses are to be found in the archives of the former KGB.

She was accused of long-standing connections with Jewish nationalists. Molotov's own name cropped up occasionally in this connection.

She denied everything. She even denied that she had ever visited the synagogue. The following is an excerpt from the record of Zhemchuzina's confrontation with Slutsky, head of the NKVD's overseas administration:

> *Slutsky:* I am a member of the board of twenty responsible for the operation of the Moscow synagogue.
> *Interrogator:* Did you make a statement that Zhemchuzina was present during prayers at the synagogue on March 14, 1945?
> *Slutsky:* Yes, I made such a statement and I now confirm it. . . . The rule in our synagogue is that the men are down below in the hall and the women in the gallery. We made an exception for her, and gave her a particularly honorable place in the hall.
> *Zhemchuzina:* I was not in the synagogue, all that is untrue.

She also denied witnesses' statements that she had taken an active interest in the scheme for a "California in the Crimea." She denied everything. Why? Because the truth was something which she had no right to tell the interrogator. I believe that she was always the right wife for her husband. Attending the synagogue and being a "good Jewish daughter" were for her merely a Party assignment. Her husband knew all about it, and that means that the Boss also knew. She dared not say so; flat denial was all that was left to her.

Stalin contented himself with banishing her. He had a further use for her in the near future. She was exiled in the distant Kustanai oblast, where she was known as "Object Number 12." Female stoolies regularly reported her conversations to the center. But Polina preserved her self-control and was guilty of no treasonable utterances.

In the same year, 1949, Molotov lost his post as Minister of Foreign Affairs. The Boss stopped inviting him to the dacha. Molotov knew from experience that his time was nearly up.

The Boss, meanwhile, was tying up the loose ends of the Kuznetsov-Voznesensky affair. Malenkov was sent to Leningrad in February 1949, and quickly extracted from Party officials under arrest the required confession that a secret anti-Party group had existed in the city. Kapustin, Secretary of the city's Party Committee, confessed to being a British spy.

Stalin staged a revival of his 1937 production not because he lacked imagination, but because old accusations automatically produced the old reflex response: mindless Terror.

For Voznesensky the end had come. The accusations against yesterday's "outstanding economist" were that he had "deliberately set low output targets" in the Five-Year Plan, and that his members "were not honest with the government." In March 1949 he was dismissed from all his posts. The man who had once been Stalin's deputy in the Council of Ministers now sat at home in his dacha working on a book about "the political economy of communism" and waiting for the end.

When he least expected it, he was summoned to the nearer dacha. The Boss embraced him, and sat him down to eat and drink with his former friends in the Politburo. The Boss even drank a toast to him. He went home happy—and was arrested at once. The Boss had liked Voznesensky, and had given a farewell banquet in his honor, but personal feelings were unimportant. The old machinery of government had to be replaced.

The repeat performance of 1937 was now well under way. Two thousand Party officials had been arrested in Leningrad. Voznesensky, Kuznetsov, and a number of others were tried in that city in September. They confessed to all sorts of unlikely crimes, and were sentenced to death. The finale in the courtroom was fantastic. After sentence had been passed, secret policemen draped white shrouds around the condemned men, and carried them like so many sacks right across the courtroom to the exit. They were shot in a single batch one hour later. Trials arising from the "Leningrad case" continued throughout 1951 and 1952.

A Suitable Place

Meanwhile a special prison for Party members was being built in a hurry on Matrosskaya Tishina Street in Moscow. Kuznetsov and Voznesensky were among its first prisoners. A great future was planned for it. After Malenkov's fall, in the late 1950s, documents taken from his aide Sukhanov included lists of the questions to be put to certain important future prisoners, together with the answers which they would be giving. The prisoners-elect were still at large, but their statements were already on file. The Great Storyteller had thought of everything. This special prison was meant to hold forty to fifty people, the elite of the ruling group. Specially selected interrogators had a direct line to the Boss. Stalin intended to supervise the staging of this next grandiose spectacle in person.

He warned Malenkov at the start that Beria was to have no authority over this prison. In other words, Beria too was finished.

All the top Kremlin personnel were under close observation. The results of the NKVD's eavesdropping on Marshals Budenny, Timoshenko, Zhukov, Voroshilov, and other prospective inmates of the special prison run to fifty-eight volumes. They were taken from Malenkov's private safe after his fall. At a plenary Central Committee meeting in 1957 Malenkov tried to excuse himself. "My conversations were also listened to—it was the general practice." An amusing argument—a scene from the theater of the absurd—ensued:

> *Khrushchev:* Comrade Malenkov, you were not bugged. You and I lived in the same building. You were on the fourth floor, I was on the fifth. . . . The eavesdropping device was under my apartment.
> *Malenkov:* No. Both Budenny and I were overheard via my apartment. Remember when you and I were going to arrest Beria—you came to my place, but we were afraid to talk there because we were all of us bugged.

Malenkov in fact was right. They were all being monitored. He had sentenced all of them to end their lives in the new prison. Malenkov had simply been chosen to play Yezhov's former role, and to leave the stage in the same way.

By 1949 the shape of the impending supertrial was clearly discernible. The Jewish connection brought Molotov into it, as an American and Zionist agent. Molotov's testimony would involve the other members of the Politburo. Finally, as in earlier purges, the military would be included as a bonus.

The unified society, forged in the white heat of the purge, annealed once more by Terror, he would lead forward to the third and final world war. To the Great Dream—the worldwide Soviet republic.

THE SUN OF OUR PLANET

As always, an apparent relaxation of his ideological campaign prefaced Stalin's next decisive step. Throughout 1949 he focused the country's attention on the celebration of the day he had chosen as his seventieth birthday. On the eve of the anniversary, Beria diverted him with a letter from another emperor—Henry Pu-Yi, the last emperor of Manchuria, who had been taken prisoner by the Red army. It is still there in his special file:

> It is the highest of honors for me to be writing the present letter to you. . . . I am treated with consideration and generosity by the authorities and by the personnel of the camp. While here I have begun reading Soviet books and newspapers for the first time. For the first time in the forty years of my life I have got to know *Questions of Leninism* and the *Short Course in the History of the Communist Party of the Soviet Union.* I have learned that the USSR is the most democratic and progressive country in the world, the guiding star of small and oppressed peoples. . . . I have asked to remain in the USSR, but so far have received no answer. My interests are identical with those of the Soviet people, I want to work and to toil as Soviet people do, to show my gratitude for your beneficence.

Such was the letter to the God Stalin from a common emperor. We can see in every line how eager poor Pu-Yi was to earn his freedom. But the Boss had other plans. Since Pu-Yi's state was now part of Communist China, he dispatched the dethroned emperor to his brother Communist Mao Tse-tung. The hapless emperor was transferred from captivity in Soviet hands to captivity in China. To be reeducated all over again.

By 1949 Stalin had created his own personal school of literature. Its main object was glorification of the "Leader and Teacher," the "Coryphaeus of Science and Technology," the "Greatest Genius of All Times and All Nations"—appellations now regularly bestowed on him. There were others, even more curious, such as "the Sun of Our Planet." This was Dozchenko's invention—he had learned his lesson.

But what looked like a crass "personality cult," mere madness, had in fact a very serious purpose. One of Stalin's favorite writers was Peter Pavlenko. The Boss had bestowed the highest literary award—the Stalin Prize, First Class—on him four times. Pavlenko, fortune's favorite, was in fact the unhappiest of men. He had joined the Party in 1920, had ties with many victims of the purges, lived in perpetual fear of his own past, and spent his life trying to atone for that past. Since the war he had written the screenplay for two films officially declared "masterpieces of Soviet art": *The Vow* (1946) and *The Fall of Berlin* (1947).

He had in fact only been coauthor of these films. "The vow" of the title was that made by Stalin over Lenin's coffin. Pavlenko showed the manuscript of his scenario to my father. It was lavishly adorned with marginal notes made by the hero himself. Stalin the leader had corrected the portrayal of Stalin the character in the script. Pavlenko told my father that "when Beria handed over the annotated scenario to Chiureli, the director, he told him that *The Vow* must be a 'sublime' film in which Lenin is John the Baptist and Stalin the Messiah." This seminarist's language betrayed the authorship of this observation. Thus *The Vow* became a film about the God-Man. *The Fall of Berlin* further developed the theme. The film ends with an apotheosis: Stalin arrives in the center of conquered Berlin not on a humdrum train, but by plane. Dressed in a dazzling white uniform (of course, the white attire of an angel descending from heaven) he reveals himself to the expectant humans. They represent the rejoicing peoples of the earth. They glorify the Messiah in all tongues. "A mighty 'Hurrah!' is raised." Foreigners hail Stalin, each in his own tongue. A rousing song rings out:

> We follow you to wondrous times,
> We tread the path of victory . . .

The God-Man . . . Konstantin Simonov, one of the most famous writers of the Stalin era, was made a member of the Stalin Prize Committee. In his memoirs, he described Stalin's behavior at a meeting of the committee called to consider works of literature recommended for one of the prizes bearing his name. He walked about inaudibly behind the backs of members of the Committee. This was his usual practice, so that they could not see the God's face. This raised the tension as they struggled to divine and to do his will. . . . He paced the room, sucking his pipe. The Secretary of the Commission called out "the writer S. Zlobin, candidate for a Stalin Prize for his novel *Stepan Razin.* Malenkov unexpectedly intervened: 'Comrade Stalin, Zlobin was in a German POW camp and behaved badly.' There was an astonished silence. Everybody knew that candidates were carefully screened beforehand. Was this meant to test the members of the commission? Stalin's quiet voice broke the silence. 'Should we forgive him, or shouldn't we?' They were all silent. They were afraid. He slowly circled the table, smoking his pipe, and asked again: 'Should we forgive him, or shouldn't we?' Again, a deathly silence was the only answer: the accusation made against Zlobin was a terrible one! He should be losing his head, not winning a Stalin Prize! Now he was making his third round of the table. Again he asked: 'Should we or shouldn't we forgive him?' But this time he answered his own question: 'He is forgiven.' " So instead of being sent to a prison camp Zlobin became a Stalin laureate—raised in the twinkling of an eye to the summit of wealth and fame! Yes, *he* and *he* alone was the arbiter of destinies. It was given to him, the God-Man, to pardon any crime. This was his way of teaching them.

His comrades-in-arms, by now half-mad with fear, racked their brains trying to decide how to celebrate his jubilee. In 1945, for the victory (Stalin's victory) over Germany, they had already bestowed on him the title of "Generalissimus." Marshal Konyev remembered how Stalin had grumbled at the time, "What need has Comrade Stalin of that? Some title you've thought up! Chiang Kai-shek is a generalissimo. Franco is a generalissimo—fine company I find myself in!" But he became "Generalissimus" nonetheless, accepting promotion to what had been the highest military rank in tsarist times. He was portrayed more and more frequently in marshal's uniform, with red stripes on his trousers. These were one of the distinguishing features of the uniform worn by high officers in the tsarist armies.

He had not only renamed the People's Commissariats "ministries"—another throwback to Tsarist times—but reintroduced uniforms for bureaucrats. His henchmen, of course, understood the Boss's aspirations. Obviously they had to think up something very special for his jubilee, a title, equivalent to that of "tsar." But it had to be a revolutionary title. The anniversary was getting nearer and nearer, the tension was growing, and still they couldn't think of anything. I found traces of their agonized lucubrations in the archives. "Secret. December 16, 1949. Project for the introduction of an 'Order of Stalin and a Jubilee Medal' . . . 'Medal for Laureates of the International Stalin Prize.' " They just couldn't think of anything new. He realized yet again how indolent his henchmen had become. He, of course, would not hear of an Order of Stalin, "which would rank below the Order of Lenin," in the words of the planned citation.

They misunderstood him. He was not afflicted with senile vainglory. The realization of the Great Dream was imminent, when he would lead his peoples in their assault on the enemy's stronghold. The image of the god—the God Stalin—would lead them into that last, decisive, and truly bloody battle. That was the whole purpose of the Stalin cult. That was why his newspapers and his radio had to exalt his name day and night. . . . The earth was filled with the thunder of his name. As a contemporary wrote in her diary: "Stalin here, Stalin there, Stalin, Stalin everywhere. You can't go out to the kitchen, or sit on the toilet, or eat without Stalin following you. . . . He creeps into your guts and your very soul, creeps into your brain, stops up all holes, treads on a person's heels, rings you up in your innermost self, gets into bed with you under the blanket, haunts your memories and your dreams."

The Sins of the Father

At the end of his life he said, laughingly, about his henchmen, "They're all great men! All geniuses! But there's nobody to have tea with." At the summit of his power he was utterly alone. His henchmen—soon to die—exasperated him. His daughter had become a stranger. In 1944 she decided to marry a Moscow University student named Grigori Morozov. She had known him for a long time—they had attended the same exclusive school. He was the handsome son of a well-off intellectual family; his father was deputy director of a scientific research institute. But Grigori was Jewish. Svetlana went to the nearer dacha to tell her father the news. "It was May," she wrote in her memoirs, "and everything was in flower." "So you want to get married?" her father said. Then he was silent for a long time, looking at the trees. "Yes, it's spring," he said suddenly, and then added, "Do what the hell you like." But he would not allow her to bring Grigori home. She gave birth to a boy, strangely like Stalin, and gave the child his name. But shortly afterward she got a divorce. Stalin had not pushed her into it; it was her own idea. She then married the son of the deceased Zhdanov. He was pleased with this marriage, but father and daughter still saw little of each other. One day he mentioned her mother to her—for the first time in her life. It happened during the November celebrations—on November 9. This, the anniversary of the October Revolution, was the country's most important official holiday, and also the day on which Nadezhda had died.

"It poisoned the holiday for him," Svetlana wrote in her memoirs, "and he preferred to spend it in the South." On this occasion she had gone there to join him. They were alone together, when he suddenly said angrily: "It was such a wretched little pistol." (He showed her how small it was.) "It was Pavel who brought it! What a present to give her." Then he was silent. They never spoke of it again. His daughter left, and once again there was a long interval before their next meeting. Although he often thought of her and remembered when she was "mistress of the house." For many years now Valechka Istomina, a maidservant at the nearer dacha, had been the woman at his side. She was never "mistress of the house." Just a humble servant. But devoted to him—and that was what mattered.

He was getting old. And, like any aging Georgian, he had become fond of his son. That was why Vasily had risen so rapidly since the war.

At twenty-seven he commanded the air arm of the Moscow Military District. The Boss's son organized those famous aerial displays. The Boss and the whole Politburo drove out to the airfield at Tushino to see them. Together they watched daring aerobatics, and mock air battles, while the whole country sat listening to radio commentaries on the display. The announcer's voice had a steely ring when he spoke of the plane piloted by Vasily. According to Marshal Savitsky, "It is a myth that Vasya led the aerial displays over Red Square or at Tushino. He sat in the right-hand seat, the bomber's—in other words he just sat there while the flight commander was at the controls and actually flying the plane."

People were afraid for Vasya, who was drinking more than ever. After divorcing his wife, he left the House on the Embankment and went to live in a detached house on Gogol Boulevard, taking both children with him. Their mother had no right of access, but visited them secretly. It was *Anna Karenina:* the children's nurse could not bear a mother's grief, and surreptitiously arranged for her to see her children. Vasya, meanwhile, married the famous swimmer Kapitolina Vasilieva. He showed his love as Caesar's son should, and built for her a whole sports complex, which still adorns the Leningrad Prospect. The first 50-meter covered swimming pool in the country is a monument to their love. But this marriage was also short-lived.

Vasily was arrested after Stalin's death and charged with "systematic misappropriation of state property." The records of the criminal proceedings against him are in the President's Archive. The files give a detailed account of his way of life. What follows is from the testimony of his adjutant, Polyansky: "Vasily drank heavily almost every day, did not turn up at work for weeks on end, and could not leave the women alone. . . . He had so many affairs that if I were asked how many I wouldn't know what to say. . . . Using air force funds he established a 55-hectare [135-acre] reserve for hunting in the Pereyaslav-Zalessky area, where three villas were built, linked by a narrow-gauge railroad. . . . Fifty spotted deer, a number of willow grouse, and other game were delivered to the estate." And from the testimony of B. Voitekhov, a writer: "At the end of 1949 I arrived at the apartment of my second wife, the actress Maria Pastukhova, and found her in a state of extreme distress. She said that Vasily had just visited her, and tried to force her to become his mistress. I went to his apartment and found him drinking with other fliers. . . . Vasily knelt down, called himself a heel and a scum, and said that he was sleeping with my wife. In 1951 we made peace with each other. I had money troubles and he gave me a job on his staff, as a consultant. I did no work but received the same wage as an air force sportsman."

And his chauffeur A. Brot recalled: "He had a big garage at headquarters. As far as he was concerned, traffic regulations did not exist. He would be sitting beside me in the passenger seat after a few drinks and put his foot down on the accelerator. He always made me drive fast, often on the same side as the oncoming traffic."

In spite of all this, the drunken Vasya's dream was to be like his father. He longed to make everyone fear him. Major A. Kapelkin testified that "one night, just before the November holiday, he summoned me to his apartment and said: 'We have to interrogate a terrorist.' He said that Colonel Golovanov, the head of the counterespionage service, had 'arrested a group of terrorists' who allegedly intended to carry out a terrorist act against J. V. Stalin. Vasily announced that he himself would be questioning one of them—Major Kashin, formerly of the Personnel Department. He ordered one of his subordinates to take off his shoes and kneel on a chair. He then started beating the soles of the man's feet with a thin rod, trying out the instrument of torture. . . . When Kashin was brought in, Vasily felled him with a blow. After this prelude Kashin was interrogated and denied the charges against him. He was made to kneel on the chair, but the rod broke after the first stroke on the soles of his feet. We tried to beat a confession out of him. Whenever he fell down we kicked him. Then we all started drinking."

Brot, his driver, recalled that "Vasily soon got married for the third time, to a daughter of the war hero Marshal Timoshenko. She was very strict, and could be cruel. She did not like Vasily's children. The cook and I used to give them extra food on the sly. His adjutant told me one day that a trunkload of presents from the High Command was on its way from conquered Germany. It arrived, and the adjutant collected a few things for Vasily, mainly desk sets. He gave orders for the rest to be sent to Vasily's wife, Ekaterina, out at the dacha. It included golden ornaments with diamonds and emeralds, dozens of carpets, a lot of lady's lingerie, a huge number of men's suits, overcoats, fur coats, fur wraps, astrakhan. . . . Her house was bursting with gold, German carpets, and cut glass ever since the war anyway. She asked me to sell it all in commission shops. I was carting stuff there for a whole month, and handing the money over to Ekaterina."

His father had hoped that the Timoshenkos, sensible, thrifty people, might perhaps bring Vasily to his senses. They didn't. One scandalous situation followed another. Trying to deal with them distracted the Boss from the Great Dream.

The Prince and the Sportsmen

Vasily's great passion was sport, and the Air Force Sports Society. Above all, he loved soccer and hockey. In a very few years he had created the famous VVS (air force) hockey team. Living accommodations in the USSR were not bought privately, but were allocated by the state. The star players in Caesar's son's team received the richest of rewards—apartments of their own—besides special rations and other benefits. In a very short time all the great stars were playing for the VVS team. And the elite of Soviet hockey perished to a man after one of Vasily's escapades.

The team was traveling by air to play at Chelyabinsk. A blizzard made it impossible for the plane to land at the Chelyabinsk airfield, and it had to touch down at Kazan. The players got restless and telephoned Moscow. Vasya Stalin, exercising his authority as commander of the Moscow Military District's air arm, ordered the pilot to continue the flight. The plane crashed while attempting to land in the blizzard, and all eleven star players were killed. The plane itself was one which was supposed to take only Politburo members as passengers.

His father was informed immediately. He gave orders that the disaster should be given no publicity. Disasters did not happen in his country! The public knew only that the country's finest hockey players had disappeared. No one dared ask where or why.

What Vasily, and the country at large, loved best was football. His bounty had also created an all-star football team. In the early fifties, only Dynamo, Beria's team, could rival the VVS squad. But although Vasya had recruited brilliant players, the VVS team was a disappointment at first. It lacked an effective trainer—until Vasya remembered that Spartak's famous trainer, Nikolai Starostin, was still serving his sentence in a camp somewhere in the Far East.

Starostin himself has described what followed. One night in 1948 he was awakened and taken by car to the camp commandant's office. Over the secret government telephone line he heard a voice saying, "Hello, Nikolai. This is Vasily Stalin." The personal plane of the commander of the VVS landed on the nearest military airfield shortly afterward. Starostin was flown to Moscow and taken to the detached house on Gogol Boulevard. A decanter holding vodka stood on a table in the middle of an enormous room. Vasya drank to their meeting. A little later Starostin was at home, in the eight square yards which was all they had left of their own enormous apartment, with his wife and daughter beside him weeping for joy. But before he could begin training the VVS team, Beria, the Dynamo fan, struck back. Two uniformed men turned up and told Starostin, "You know very well that you have come here illegally, and you must go back within twenty-four hours."

Vasya was furious. How dare they! He quickly made up his mind. "You'll live with me in my house. Nobody will touch you there." After that the Boss's prisoner and the Boss's son were inseparable. They went together to headquarters, to training sessions, to Vasily's dacha. They even slept in the same extrawide bed.

Vasily went to bed with a revolver under his pillow. He forbade Starostin to leave the house alone. But Starostin missed his family, and one day, when Vasily had drunk himself to sleep, he climbed through a window into the garden and went home. Next morning he was awakened by a ring at the door. Two colonels came in. Starostin was put on a train out of Moscow. But at the very first stop the head of Vasily's counterespionage department boarded the coach and told Starostin, "I've caught up with you by plane. The Boss [Vasya loved to be called that] has ordered me to get you to Moscow by whatever means are necessary." Once Starostin was safely delivered, Vasily grabbed the telephone, rang the Ministry of the Interior, asked for one of Beria's deputies, and said "Two hours ago you told me that you didn't know where Starostin was. . . . He is now sitting here with me. Your people had abducted him. Just remember that in our family we never forgive an insult." In the end his father had to intervene. Order had to prevail. Starostin was sent back.

All this time, Vasily was drinking heavily. Disaster struck in 1952. S. Rudenko, commander of long-distance aircraft, and P. Zhigarev, commander-in-chief of air forces relieved the drunkard of responsibility for the Tushino air display. The display was a brilliant success, and Stalin broadcast his thanks to all those who had taken part. Afterward Vasily, scarcely able to stand on his feet, turned up at a reception attended by his father, his father's henchmen, and high-ranking officers. "What do you mean by this?" his father asked. "I'm on holiday." "Do you often spend your holidays like this?" There was silence. Then Zhigarev said, "Yes, he does." Vasily cursed Zhigarev.

The silence was terrifying. Then Stalin said curtly, "Get out of here." Vasily was relieved of all his posts, and enrolled as a student in the Aviation Faculty of the Military Academy.

But the Boss remembered how his henchmen and the service chiefs—braggarts whose egos had become inflated during the war—had gloated over his son's humiliation, and hadn't even tried to hide it. He knew, of course, why Vasya drank and misbehaved. His poor weak son was mortally afraid of what would happen to him when his aged father was no more. He tried to drown his fear with drink, to deaden it with womanizing. They—Stalin's old henchmen—would rid themselves of Vasily immediately. His son knew far too much about them.

He Becomes a Mystery Even to His Henchmen

It was 1950. His life followed the routine which he had long ago established: the same nocturnal banquets, sometimes prolonged till dawn. After a long day's work in the Kremlin his henchmen still had to drive out with him to the dacha for the torment of a sleepless night's drinking. But to be invited was happiness enough: it meant that he was not yet ready to destroy them. Forty years later his ancient former bodyguards would tell me about the secret life of this lonely man in the hermetically sealed nearer dacha.

When he banqueted with his henchmen, clean plates, cutlery, and wineglasses stood near a luxurious buffet. It was self-service, so that there would be no servants to overhear their conversation. From time to time he would call for a clean tablecloth. The servants would appear, take the festive tablecloth by its four corners, and make a bundle of it—crockery, uneaten food, and all. All would then hear the sound of fine cut glass breaking. Every dish was accompanied by a certificate: "No poisonous substances found." A doctor retained for this purpose periodically tested the air. I. Orlov, commandant of the dacha, said that "portraits of the Politburo hung in the room where they gathered. He liked each of them to sit under his own portrait." The portraits of Voznesensky and Kuznetsov had by then been removed. Molotov was no longer invited, but, knowing that staying close to the Boss meant survival, turned up anyway looking dejected, like a faithful dog. The Boss now openly sneered at the former head of government, calling him an "American spy." He knew that several of the portraits would shortly vanish.

They whiled away the small hours by telling dirty jokes. Among his henchmen he liked using obscene language. He made his guests drink too much. They dared not refuse: to do so meant that they had something to hide and were afraid that drink would loosen their tongue. They would play practical jokes of the sort his daughter Svetlana describes—put a tomato on someone's chair as he stood up to propose a toast, sprinkle salt in a neighbor's wineglass. Or push someone into the shallow pond on the grounds. They were happy: as long as he was making fun of them it meant that he was not angry. He sucked his pipe and watched the humiliation of the living dead. The feasting would end at 4:00 A.M. After that he allowed the exhausted buffoons to go home to bed. His own lonely night was not yet over.

After they had gone he would work in his study, or in the garden. He liked cutting flowers at night, using pruning shears by lamplight. His guards would pick up the severed heads. But his hands were not what they had been. They trembled, and he often cut himself. When a paramedic was called in to dress the cuts, *his* hands trembled too with fear. Stalin would laugh and bandage his finger himself. Toward morning he slept a little—sometimes, in the summer, on a trestle bed under the stairs to the second floor, covering his face with his cap so that the early morning sun would not disturb him. In winter he liked tobogganing on the grounds. But he did this less often. His rheumatism was getting worse, his legs hurt, and he had become very irritable.

Of the many rooms in the dacha he chose one and practically lived there. The servant Valechka made up his bed on the sofa, and he took his meals at his desk, clearing a little space among the clutter of books and papers. A portrait of Lenin hung on the wall. The ex-seminarist kept a lamp burning beneath it day and night: the eternal flame illuminating the God Lenin's face.

When the Politburo clowns were not around, he liked talking to his guards. These semiliterate people were now his best friends: he discussed things with them, and told stories about his years in exile, exaggerating as old men do. He lived more and more in the past. "He was lonely, I felt sorry for him, he showed his age," one former member of his guard told me.

This pathetic old man was in fact the beast of prey he always had been. The aged leopard was resting, preparing to spring. The great purge he had planned was already under way, throughout the country.

As in 1937, members of his own bodyguard began disappearing. "The old fellow couldn't prove his innocence," he would say sadly. He really was sorry for them. But that was the way it had to be. All the old hands had to disappear. Vlasik would shortly have to go, like Pauker before him. The man who had commanded his guard for many years and was burdened with so many secrets would be arrested in 1952.

The year 1950, however, was a quiet one of secret murders. One August night, on Stalin's orders, dozens of high officers, including Gordov and Rybalchenko, were shot. They were followed in autumn by a large number of people arrested in connection with the Leningrad affair. The crematorium near the Donskoi Monastery worked overtime, and the ashes of fresh victims were regularly tipped into the bottomless grave number 1.

Storm Clouds

Meanwhile preparations for the next big show had already begun.

A number of doctors employed in the clinic of the Stalin Automobile Works (ZIS), the largest in the country, were arrested, together with some senior ZIS executives, a few bureaucrats, and even a woman journalist who had written about ZIS. The names of those arrested told their own story: Aron Finkelstein, David Smorodinsky, Miriam Eisenstadt, Edward Lifshits. They were all Jews.

All the accused were shot in November 1950.

He was warming up, in preparation for the "Kremlin doctors" event. It would give the interrogators a little practice. The "ZIS case," as some called it, attracted no publicity whatsoever.

In his last years he published two pamphlets, one concerned with Marxism and linguistics, the other with the economics of socialism.

It had been a long time since he had treated the country and the Party to one of his excursions into Marxist theory. The war had prevented it. But Leninist tradition demanded that the Leader should be a great theorist.

Did he write these two pamphlets himself? No. In both cases the original idea was his, but he graciously permitted his academicians to do some of the work for him. He was, however, far from idle. He rewrote them both, from start to finish, and also added certain previously undisclosed ideas of his own.

In *Economic Problems of Socialism,* for instance, he had a great deal to say about the struggle for peace. He called on a favorite ploy of his: as he prepared for war, he praised the "peace partisans," who were active in several countries under the tutelage of Soviet secret agents, secretly implying that they were meant to become a fifth column in the rear of his future enemy. "In some countries," he wrote, "the struggle for peace will develop into a struggle for socialism." In "in-depth language" this meant: "through the peace movement we shall promote rebellion and revolution."

He dealt also with the likelihood of war, arguing in particular that war between capitalist countries was inevitable. In "in-depth language" this meant: "we shall set them on each other as we did in Hitler's day." At the same time he tried, as had Lenin, to reassure the Western "deaf-mutes." He declared that "war between capitalist countries is more likely than war between the socialist and capitalist camps," but went on to say that war was not inevitable once imperialism was destroyed. Only when the Great Dream prevailed would the miseries of the human race come to an end.

As soon as these works were published, they were extravagantly praised. Eminent philologists and economists wrote innumerable articles on the renascence of their disciplines. Dissertations and multivolume studies were planned.

The campaign expanded, and shortly all branches of scholarship were reporting that Stalin's pamphlets had marked a major turning point. The God on earth had vouchsafed his worshipers a revelation. He had done so not only to gratify his vanity. Like the *Short Course in the History of the Communist Party,* which had appeared after the Great Terror, these works were intended to mark the beginning of a new era. He was writing for the future, for those who would survive the great bloodletting.

The destruction of his top people was about to begin. In 1952 he convened the Nineteenth Party Congress after an interval of thirteen years. He himself spoke only at the end of the Congress. Everyone knew that he was feeling ill. Khrushchev recalled that "he spoke for five to seven minutes and said to us afterward: 'There you are—I can still do it!' We looked at our watches: he'd spoken for five to seven minutes. If that was all he could manage, we came to the conclusion that he was physically very weak."

He had deceived his wretched associates yet again. A plenary meeting of the Central Committee took place immediately after the Congress, and there the "physically weak" Stalin made a long and passionate speech. The writer Konstantin Simonov, who was present, described the occasion in his memoirs. Many years later he still remembered it with horror:

> October 16, 1952. Kremlin. The Sverdlov Hall. He entered from the rear door, accompanied by the other members of the Politburo, and looking grimly purposeful. People began applauding, but he raised his hand to stop them. Malenkov presided, and called on Stalin to speak. His manner was stern and humorless. He spoke without notes.
>
> He fixed his audience with an unwavering gaze. The tone and content of his speech left them numb and dazed. The meeting went on for two hours, and Stalin's speech took up three-quarters of that time. His main theme was that he was old and that the time was approaching when others would have to carry on his work. "But for the present the job has been entrusted to me, and I'm doing it," he said bluntly, almost savagely. He called for courage and firmness, the Leninist firmness of 1918. He recalled how Lenin had "thundered away in an incredibly difficult situation, he thundered on, fearing nothing, he just thundered away." He repeated the word "thundered" three times. He mentioned Lenin—he said—because of the conduct of "certain comrades."

The "certain comrades" shortly acquired names:

> He pitched into Molotov, accusing him of cowardice and defeatism. He spoke of Molotov at length and unsparingly, citing examples of his behavior which have escaped my mind. . . . I realized that Stalin's white-hot anger made these accusations a direct threat. . . . Then he turned on Mikoyan, and his words became angrier and ruder still. There was a terrible silence in the hall. The faces of all the Politburo members were rigid, petrified. They were wondering whom he would attack next. Molo-

> tov and Mikoyan were deathly pale. Having demolished Molotov, Stalin mentioned his age again, and said that he could no longer cope with the task entrusted to him. He asked therefore to be relieved of his post as Secretary General, while remaining Chairman of the Council of Ministers. As he said it he stared at the audience. I saw a look of dread on Malenkov's face—that of a man who realizes that he is in deadly danger. His face, his gestures, his eloquently raised hands beseeched those present to reject Comrade Stalin's request. And voices behind Stalin's back hastily called out "No! Please stay!" At once the whole hall was abuzz with calls of "Please, please, stay!"

I remember a play by Brecht in which as people are killed their faces are daubed with white paint, and they stand motionless on the stage until the end of the act. Molotov's ghastly white face . . . Malenkov's sudden pallor . . . Simonov is right: if they had granted the Boss's request, Malenkov would have been the first to answer with his head. But it is difficult to imagine what it would have cost the rest of the audience. He needed a repetition of the Seventeenth Congress. He needed traitors, so that he could destroy them wholesale. They dared not oblige. He had trained them too well. But they were doomed just the same.

Then came the elections. In preparation for the massacre, he enlarged the Politburo and changed its name to Presidium. It was, in fact, a facade for a small inner group which now performed the functions of the former Politburo. Neither Molotov nor Mikoyan was admitted to it. Everyone considered them as good as dead.

Crosses and Question Marks

After Stalin's death Sharapov, an employee of the Party Archive, was sent to sort out the Boss's library. In one room he found a thick, black-bound volume containing the stenographic record of the next to last Congress, the Eighteenth, in 1939. On the eve of the Nineteenth Congress in 1952 Stalin had looked through the list of those elected to membership or candidate membership of the Central Committee in 1939. He had put crosses against the names of those who, at his own wish, had since ceased to live. He had also generously distributed question marks among the survivors. The first wave of those soon to be purged.

He had acquired an amusing habit. When he destroyed one of his henchmen he gave the victim's dacha to the next in line. Thus, Beria now had Chubar's dacha, Molotov had Yagoda's, Vyshinsky had Serebryakov's. They all would soon be handing over their dachas to new occupants.

We are now entering the last four and a half months of his reign, the terrible months of preparation for Apocalypse.

At the beginning of the fifties the Boss had authorized Abakumov, the Minister of State Security, to arrest a large number of Georgians from Beria's native province, Mingrelia, people whom Beria had planted in important posts. When he began the operation the Boss had told Abakumov in so many words to "look for the big Mingrel in the plot." But progress was slow. Abakumov was obviously afraid to collect evidence against his overlord. The Boss saw how frightened he was, and Abakumov was doomed.

Abakumov was working at the time on the "case of the Kremlin doctors." Back in 1948 Lidia Timashuk, senior electrocardiographer at the Kremlin Clinic, had reported that Zhdanov was not receiving the appropriate treatment. The Author of the 1936–1937 thriller had remembered her letter, and now saw how it could help his story line. Professor Vovsi, for instance, one of the Kremlin doctors, was related to Mikhoels. This prompted the idea of a proliferating Jewish conspiracy utilizing the world's most humane profession. Stalin had vivid memories of the anti-Semitic tracts devoured by the mob in his youth—*Protocols of the Elders of Zion,* the outpourings of the Union of the Russian People. With his mind always on the Great Dream he knew that there were two emotions which could unite society: fear, and hatred of the Jews. His "anticosmopolitan" campaign had been instructive. The results had surpassed his expectations. The public had joined wholeheartedly in vilifying Jews, deliberately distorting the names of their victims. He remembered particularly the enthusiasm of the workers in that factory at the time of the ZIS affair. As one Russian writer put it: "Anti-Semitism makes your vodka stronger and your bread more appetizing." Before leading his people to the Apocalypse he would bestow on them a great claim to superiority: the most downtrodden of Russians would rejoice in the fact that he was not a Jew.

His Last Thriller

He had, then, composed his last thriller. The country would shortly learn its contents.

The storyline Stalin concocted went as follows: the sinister Jewish organization Joint was bent on destroying the Russian people. It had probably begun operations in the days of Trotsky, Zinoviev, and Kamenev. Later, its agents, Mikhoels and other loyal instruments of American imperialism, had infiltrated everywhere. Acting on instructions from Joint, the ubiquitous cosmopolitans were poisoning the country's ideology. But that was the least of it. Traitorous doctors were killing statesmen. (The "murdering doctor" theme had been given an airing at the Bukharin trials. But that was all to the good: it conditioned the public to associate Jews and Terror.)

Zionists had infiltrated even the highest levels of the political elite. This was where Zhemchuzina came in. He had spared her, as he had once spared Zinoviev and Kamenev, for use in a public trial. She was the intermediary through whom Molotov had been recruited as an enemy agent. The Boss could go on from there to write group after group of conspirators into his story. In the early stages they would be destroyed by the Great Mingrel.

But he now had the "socialist camp" to think of, not just the Soviet Union. He therefore broadened the scene of action to embrace the "fraternal countries." He could not forgive Dimitrov for his alliance with Tito. The Bulgarian leader, who had served him so well, was now dying, and the Boss could easily write his close associates into the thriller. One of them, Traicho Kostov, who was also one of the Cominform leaders, was shot. The charge against him was, of course, espionage.

The thriller also took on the required anti-Semitic complexion in the fraternal countries. In Czechoslovakia Slansky, the First Secretary of the Communist Party, was put on trial, and several other senior officials were tried with him. They had one thing in common: all of them were Jews. Slansky was shot as an agent of international Zionism.

Meanwhile the Boss was completing the recruitment of those who were to implement his terrorist scheme.

Abakumov's hesitancy in dealing with Beria called for a decision. Abakumov, the cruel torturer who looked like a gallant guardsman, was consigned to oblivion. Bobkov, the Vice-Chairman of the KGB (the Committee of State Security, which superseded the Ministry in 1953), later remembered "members of the staff wandering round the corridors stunned. They had heard news of Abakumov's arrest and pored over the Central Committee's edict." The Boss, with his unfailing sense of humor, had removed the ruthless executioner for being insufficiently ruthless. The decree stated that "Chekists have lost their vigilance, they are working in white gloves." That was enough. In the drive against the "white-gloved" brigade, many heads of departments and branches in the Ministry of the Interior were arrested. Abakumov's, and so also Beria's, protégés were routed. Ministry of State Security personnel were urged to "apply ruthless pressure to those under arrest." Everyone finally realized that this was indeed 1937 all over again. The Boss appointed Ignatiev, a Party official unconnected with Beria, to the Ministry of State Security.

By then a large group of eminent Jewish doctors—Kogan, Feldman, Ettinger, Vovsi, Grinstein, Ginzburg, and others—had been arrested in readiness for the coming trial. Stalin's story line, however, demanded that the conspiracy should be against himself. There was only one thing to do: he generously added his own doctor, Professor V. Vinogradov, to the list.

In January 1953 a team of secret police brought "Object Number 12"—Polina Zhemchuzina—from her place of banishment to a Moscow jail. A statement made by the "Object" is preserved in the case file: "What the government has decided upon is what must happen." By then Vinogradov, Kogan, and Vovsi had made the required depositions, which also incriminated Zhemchuzina. The "Object" was taken to the Lubyanka for interrogation. Molotov's future was no longer in doubt.

The Molotovs, husband and wife, survived only because of the Leader's death. Yet they both went on praising him for the rest of their days. According to Molotov, his wife "not only never spoke ill of Stalin, she couldn't bear to hear anyone else speak ill of him."

After parting with his doctor, Stalin dispatched another old favorite of his to jail—Vlasik. Semiliterate Vlasik had succeeded the semiliterate Pauker as commander of the Boss's bodyguard, and had inherited his inordinate influence. In 1947 the Boss had made him head of the Chief Administration of Security, whose job it was to appoint the bodyguards of the Boss's henchmen. In practice, he planted informers on them. But he had begun to slip up. Sarkisov, who had been planted on Beria, kept Vlasik informed on "Beria's debauchery." But Vlasik failed to sense the Boss's current wishes. He not only did not pass on this information but rebuked Sarkisov for submitting it. The Boss, who double-checked everything, found out about this, and saw that the old dog's nose was not so keen as it used to be. His drinking bouts and his incessant womanizing made him even less reliable. The obvious solution was to write him into the thriller. On December 15, 1952, Vlasik was arrested.

A verbose petition for pardon, and his testimony before the court, survive. Vlasik, like Yezhov, draws a striking picture.

Vlasik's Trial

He was tried on February 17, 1955, when Stalin and Beria were both dead. This is an excerpt from the interrogation of Vlasik by the presiding judge:

> "When did you meet the artist Stenberg?"
>
> "About 1934 or 1935. He was involved in preparing Red Square for ceremonial occasions."
>
> "How did you and Stenberg become friends?"
>
> "We obviously became friends because of drinking together and because of the women we knew."
>
> "Defendant Vlasik, you revealed the names of Ministry of State Security agents to Stenberg. Stenberg has testified that 'I learned from Vlasik that my woman friend Kirova was an agent of the organs, and that his mistress Ryazantseva also cooperated with them.' "

Vlasik admitted this, but went on to claim that

> "Where my duties were concerned I was always in order. . . . Meetings with women were on account of my health and in my spare time. I admit that I had a lot of women."
>
> "The head of government warned you that such behavior was unacceptable."
>
> "Yes, he said to me in 1949 that I was abusing my relations with women."
>
> "You have testified that Sarkisov reported Beria's debauchery to you, and you said: 'We mustn't interfere with Beria's private life, we have to protect it.' "
>
> "Yes, I kept out of it, because I didn't think it was my business to interfere, as it was connected with Beria's name."

> "How could you permit the enormous overexpenditure of state funds by your department?"
>
> "My literacy is very poor, my whole education consists of three classes in a parish school."

Stenberg testified that "I have to say that Vlasik is a moral degenerate, he cohabited with many women, in particular with [the list includes more than twenty names] and others whose names I do not remember. Vlasik used to get me and my wife drunk and then had sex with her, as he himself cynically told me."

One other activity of his was the subject of questions.

> "Defendant Vlasik, tell the court what captured enemy property you obtained illegally, without payment."
>
> "As far as I remember an upright piano, a grand piano, three or four carpets . . ."
>
> "What about the fourteen cameras? . . . And where did you get cut glass vases, wineglasses, and porcelain tableware in such quantities?"

There was much more of the same.

In the earliest days of revolution they had promised in their anthem to "build a world of our own, to build the world anew." They had built it. So much blood, so many lies, betrayals, and murders had gone to produce them—the Vlasiks, the Yezhovs, Vasya Stalins—people of the new world created by the God Lenin and the God Stalin. The triumph of "loutishness," gloomily predicted in early-twentieth-century Russian literature, was now a reality. Dostoevsky's Devils had conquered.

Stalin's death saved Vlasik. In 1955, Vlasik wrote a petition for a pardon, which contains something extremely interesting. Vlasik tells us that he was originally interrogated by Beria in person. He was astonished to find that Beria knew details of private conversations between himself and the "head of government" (Stalin) which he could have obtained only by "eavesdropping." "Beria," Vlasik wrote, "must have known about the head of government's expressions of dissatisfaction with Beria after the war."

The Boss had, for the first time in his life, been in too much of a hurry. By arresting Vlasik he had deprived himself of an experienced watchdog with no other to take its place.

Like all previous victims, Beria was required to complete the work entrusted to him before his removal. He was more immediately relevant to the Great Dream than anyone else.

The new, more powerful nuclear bomb had been tested under Beria's supervision in 1951. Now, in 1953, his scientists had created a new weapon of unprecedented power. The transportable hydrogen bomb was shortly to be tested. Its yield was expected to be twenty times that of the bomb dropped on Hiroshima. There was nothing else like it in the world. The Boss alone possessed such a weapon. (The bomb would not be tested till August 1953, some months after his death.)

Before this new weapon became available, Stalin had ordered Beria to complete Moscow's rocket defenses. It had been decided at the end of the forties to surround Moscow with special formations armed with enough ballistic missiles to shoot down any plane flying toward the city. Two gigantic concrete rings were built, with antiaircraft rocket installations at intervals around them. The Boss insisted that this work should be carried out in feverish haste. The work was done by the experienced construction workers available to Beria's department. There were six hundred rockets to each emplacement. Twenty rockets could be launched simultaneously. Radar stations tracked the targets, rockets soared . . . but coordination was unsatisfactory. The Boss told Beria to hurry up. The engineers were housed in barracks. Beria summoned the chief designer and told him that the system must be made to work—"or else."

It began to work. By early 1953 the Boss knew that Moscow would soon be looking at the West from behind a picket fence of rockets.

Everything was ready: the superweapon and the most powerful army in the world, which had not yet forgotten the art of killing. It had not been idle talk when Stalin said to Molotov soon after the war: "The First World War delivered one country from capitalist slavery, the Second has created the socialist system, and the Third will finish imperialism for ever." In "in-depth language" this meant: "We shall start a war and we shall finish it." The Great Dream, bequeathed to him by the God Lenin, would come true.

Lighting the Fuse

Ignatiev was told to get everything ready for the trial of the "Kremlin doctors" in the shortest possible time—and was promised that "if they don't confess you'll be where they are."

On January 13, 1953 the country read a Tass communiqué on the "discovery of a terrorist group of poisoning doctors." In an accompanying article, *Pravda* recalled the Leader's words in 1937: "Our successes lead not to the damping down but to the exacerbation of the class struggle. The more insistent our advance, the fiercer the struggle of the enemies of the people will become." *Pravda* was dispelling all doubts: it was 1937 all over again. But the incipient horror had one quite new and decisive ingredient: anti-Semitism. The incitement of a fanatical mob meant that Terror would range more widely than anyone would have thought possible.

All day long loudspeakers barked menacing messages. Their burden was always the same: "Soviet people angrily condemn this criminal gang of murderers and their foreign masters." This was accompanied by a promise that struck a chill into all who understood "in-depth language": "as for those who *inspire* these hirelings, they must be sure that retribution will soon find its way to them."

The "inspirers" were the doctors' "foreign master"—"American imperialism." And retribution, in the shape of war, was already trying to find a way to them. My family spent that winter at a dacha near Mamontovka Station outside Moscow, where several of the "Kremlin doctors" had dachas. Their dachas were deserted. None of them came out there to ski that winter.

The campaign was escalating. *Pravda* published a selection of reports "on the arrest of spies in various towns." In Moscow the black limousines drove around by night, arresting prominent Jews. Sheinin, once Vyshinsky's deputy, was among them. The sacred mummy failed to protect its Jewish custodian, Zbarsky. His role would obviously be that of "the Jew who desecrated the Sacred Body."

Zbarsky was released in 1954, well after Stalin's death. For him it should have been an anniversary: thirty years without a break beside the Body. Later he described his role as Custodian of the Body: "I was connected with the Mausoleum by phone twenty-four hours a day. I instructed my collaborators to call me even if a fly settled on him, and strictly forbade any attempt to remove it in my absence. All my life I used to dream about the telephone ringing and somebody saying 'Boris Ilyich, we're sending a car, there's a fly in the sarcophagus,' and I would jump up and rush off like a madman." Zbarsky died that same year, in 1954. The Body endured.

One Step Nearer Apocalypse

He was now more often than not completely alone at the nearer dacha. His daughter had long been an infrequent visitor. She communicated with him mainly by letter. "26.10.52. Dear Papa, I very much want to see you. Just to see you—I have no 'business,' no 'problems' to discuss. With your permission, and if it would not be a burden to you, I should like to spend two days of the November holiday, November 8–9, with you at the nearer dacha." She was getting divorced again. "10.2.53. I very much want to see you, to tell you face to face what's happening in my life at present. As far as Yuri Andreevich Zhdanov is concerned, we decided to part for good just before the New Year. . . . I'm sorry but I've had enough of that dessicated professor, that unfeeling polymath, let him bury himself in his books, he doesn't really need a wife and family. I have enough money at present—the money you sent me—so it isn't just that." On her rare visits she was alarmed to see strange pictures on the walls. He had taken to cutting out illustrations from magazines and pinning them up. Pictures of children—a little girl giving milk to an elk calf, a boy on skis, children under a cherry tree. The pictures were substitutes for grandchildren.

That terrible year, 1952, was, as Khrushchev wrote in his memoirs, the first year in which he did not go away on holiday. He had no time for holidays, or for children. The world was on the threshold of the Great Dream. He no longer invited Molotov, Mikoyan, Kaganovich, Voroshilov, and others under sentence of death. Only four Politburo members were now entertained at the dacha: Malenkov, Beria, and two recent additions to the inner leadership—Khrushchev and Bulganin. This quartet would be required to act first against the disgraced elders, then against each other, after which they would be replaced by new robots. The Party jail was now quite ready for its new inmates.

The intended victims, like Roman senators in the days of Nero, meekly awaited their fate. Fear, total fear, had paralyzed them. The atmosphere was growing hotter. Women in shops abused and threatened Jewish women standing in line. From one day to the next people expected something terrible to happen.

An ominous signal was given in February.

A Published Confession

Endless accusations of anti-Semitism were heard in the West, and the Cultural Committee's propagandists counterattacked with a collective letter from representatives of the Jewish community, persons eminent in science and the arts. They angrily condemned the "murderers in white gowns," and declared that anti-Semitism did not and could not exist in the USSR, the land of workers and peasants, but that well-deserved punishment awaited a miserable handful of bourgeois nationalists, agents of international Zionism.

There were, subsequently, all sorts of rumors about those who had signed this letter and those who had refused to do so. One of the signatories (I will not mention his name; he punished himself to the end of his days for signing) told me: "Yes, we signed that grotesque letter out of animal fear—for ourselves and our children. At the same time I told myself that the doctors could not be saved, and that we had to save all the others. To put a stop to the anti-Semitic campaign we had to distance ourselves, to separate other Jews from the unfortunate doomed doctors."

The letter was supposed to appear at the very beginning of February, but something unexpected happened. On February 2 bewilderment reigned in the editorial offices of *Pravda:* the newspaper was forbidden to print the painstakingly prepared letter. Everybody realized that only the Boss could have suppressed a letter drafted on instructions from the Secretariat of the Central Committee. The well-known writer and literary critic A. Borshchagovsky, one of the main targets of the anti-Semitic campaign of 1949–1953, wrote in his book *Blood Condemned* that "the peremptory veto came right from the very top. Stalin did not want to divide the Jews into good and bad. He did not want the Jews to purchase immunity by sacrificing a handful of bourgeois nationalists."

Those who knew about this affair were terrified. They knew that if he refused to accept the "handful of bourgeois nationalists" as ransom for the rest, he probably intended to punish all Jews. On February 8 *Pravda* stepped up the campaign against the Jews by substituting for the letter from the Jewish penitents an angry anti-Semitic article entitled "Simpletons and Scoundrels." The article listed the Jewish names of the many "swindlers," "saboteurs," and "scoundrels" to whom the "simpletons"—Russians who had relaxed their vigilance—had given employment.

A new wave of anti-Semitic hysteria followed. Jews were sacked,

Jews were beaten up in the streets. At the end of February rumors went around Moscow that the Jews were to be deported to Siberia. People knew that any rumor of which the Boss disapproved was quickly silenced—and those who disseminated it promptly jailed. But this rumor was more insistent, more widely believed, and more alarming from day to day. As in the days of Nazism many Jews tried to reassure themselves. The man in the next apartment to ours asked my father whether he realized how many freight cars would be needed and said, "No, he simply can't do it!"

They were lying to themselves. They knew very well that he *could* do it. Just as he had been able even at the height of the war to transfer hundreds of thousands of people from the Caucasus to Siberia.

I still remember my mother coming home from work one day and telling my father in a whisper (so that I wouldn't hear) that "the house management committees are drawing up lists of Jews. They know the date already." My father feebly replied, "It's just rumors."

After Stalin's death the whole world would hear of the deportation planned by Stalin. Professor B. Goldberg noted in his book *The Jewish Problem in the Soviet Union* that "Stalin's plan to send the Jews to Siberia reached the West after his death." And in *The Jews of the Soviet Union* Benjamin Pinkus, professor of Jewish history at Ben-Gurion University, wrote that "Stalin saw in the trial [of the doctors] a way to prepare the ground for exiling the Jewish population from the center of the Soviet Union." "Only Stalin's death saved the Jews from this fate." (*The Little Jewish Encyclopedia*, Vol. 1, "Anti-Semitism.") In Siberia and Kazakhstan people still point out the remains of the flimsy wooden huts, without heating, in which hundreds of thousands of Jews were meant to live, or rather to die.

The Apocalypse Interrupted

What did it all mean? What was the purpose of the anti-Semitic campaign, the planned deportation of the Jews, the impending purge of the leadership, and the rising tide of terror?

It is simplistic to explain this (or for that matter the Terror of 1937) by Stalin's paranoia or his brutish anti-Semitism.

The Boss was a cold pragmatist who, throughout the twenty-five years in which he held absolute power, always had precise reasons for his monstrous actions.

My father often repeated a remark made by someone else about Stalin: "Woe betide the victim of such slow jaws."

Stalin, of course, disliked Jews, but he never acted simply to gratify his likes and dislikes. Some of his most trusted associates were Jews, amongst them Kaganovich, third man in the state, and Mekhlis, who had been his secretary and during the war was put in charge of the Political Administration of the Soviet army.

What then was the point of it all?

Could someone as cunning as Stalin fail to understand that his official anti-Semitism would create a wave of revulsion against the USSR in the West, and above all in the United States? That the deportation of Jews could exacerbate American hostility to a dangerous degree?

A strange question. The fact is that for some reason he wanted this confrontation, wanted to fall out with the West once and for all!

Then again—why was he planning a new wave of terror? The Great Terror in the thirties was intended to create a unified society, implicitly obeying the Boss. The terror planned in 1953 had the same aims. It was meant to reestablish the discipline which had been impaired by the war, to bring back the fear which was gradually disappearing, so as to establish once again a unified society implicitly obedient to the Boss.

But, as Molotov correctly explained to Chuyev, the ultimate aim of the Terror in the thirties was to prepare the country for war.

It was the same in the fifties—the Boss needed the terror which he planned in order to . . .

Yes, in order to begin the Great War. War with the West. The last war, which would finally destroy capitalism. A holy war, whose battle cries would be those so dear to the hearts of his deluded people: crush the universal evil of capitalism, crush its agent, international Jewry!

The Boss's propaganda insistently proclaimed that America, "Uncle Sam," was the incarnation of this evil. This was why he sought to provoke a confrontation with the United States. The aged Dictator had resolved to realize the Great Dream with the aid of the Jews.

This was the moment at which he had everything necessary to the achievement of his objective. His troops were stationed in Eastern Europe and in Germany, his battle-hardened army was the most powerful in the world, his capital was protected by a ring of rocket sites, he was expecting from day to day the results of tests on the most powerful weapon in the world (he knew that the Americans were lagging behind), a third of mankind was under his banners, and hundreds of thousands of others sympathized with the conqueror of Hitler.

But all these advantages were temporary. For the time being he was ahead. Tomorrow his half-ruined, half-starved country would inevitably start falling behind.

How could the great predator, who already felt his strength waning and the end approaching, fail to take advantage of this last chance to realize the Great Dream?

In Russia Everything Is a Secret, and Nothing Is a Mystery

I knew very well that there could be no relevant documents. The screening of Stalin's archives began on March 5, 1953, the day of his death. "Malenkov G. M., Khrushchev N. S., and Beria L. P." were instructed "to take steps to ensure that the documents and papers of Comrade Stalin, both current and archival, are put in proper order." (This secret clause in a decision made at a joint meeting of the Central Committee of the CPSU, the Council of Ministers, and the Presidium of the Supreme Soviet on March 5, 1953, was first published in 1994, forty-one years later, in the journal *Istochnik.*)

"Steps" were of course taken, "proper order" was established—and this trio would hardly leave behind evidence of the USSR's intention to launch a world war. But there exists in the USSR, a country where documents were either periodically destroyed or were full of falsifications, an intriguing historical source—the oral testimony of contemporaries. For, as Mme. de Staël, whom we have previously cited, put it: "In Russia everything is a secret, and nothing is a mystery."

A. Borshchagovsky, who is still among us, told me about a remarkable statement supposedly made by Stalin at a meeting of the Bureau of the Presidium of the Party's Central Committee in February 1953. Borshchagovsky had heard it from close acquaintances of his (since, alas, deceased) who were present at the meeting: the writer V. Yakovlev, author of several books about Lenin and speechwriter for a number of Party functionaries, and Colonel General D. Dragunsky, a member of the Central Revision Commission of the Central Committee.

In the course of the meeting, Vyshinsky (who had ceased to be public prosecutor in 1940 and had served as Deputy Minister of Foreign Affairs from 1940 to 1949 and as Minister from 1949 to 1953) told Stalin about the "enormous" reaction in the West to the impending trial of the doctors. Vyshinsky was openly supported by some members of the Presidium. In reply Stalin savaged Vyshinsky, describing his statement as "Menshevik," and berated his comrades-in-arms, calling them "blind kittens." He concluded with this ominous sentence: "We are afraid of no one, and if the imperialist gentlemen feel like going to war there is no more favorable moment for us than the present."

After which Stalin went off to his dacha, never again to leave it alive.

I have heard various other accounts of Stalin's departure for his dacha in February 1953. The most interesting of them I heard by chance in the Union of Soviet Writers at the end of the seventies. The story was told by Yuri Zhukov (one of *Pravda*'s most influential and most "conservative" political commentators and, incidentally, like Dragunsky, a member of the Revision Commission of the Central Committee of the CPSU). Zhukov's story was as follows: In February 1953 Vyshinsky was present when the Boss received some ambassador or other. The ambassador raised the subject of the anti-Semitic campaign in the USSR, and after he left Vyshinsky complained that the "doctors' affair" had made difficulties for Soviet diplomacy. Stalin did not reply. But when Vyshinsky had gone, and some of Stalin's comrades-in-arms came into the office, he suddenly launched into an attack on Vyshinsky, calling his remark "provocative" and mentioning his Menshevik past. Then he turned to his silent comrades and said: "How easy it is for the imperialist gentlemen to intimidate you! We shall obviously have to make it a question of 'either-or.' Either we shall liquidate them, or after my death they will liquidate you like blind kittens." Those present of course began saying that "Comrade Stalin will live many years yet." He dismissed them with foul language and left for the nearer dacha. This was his last appearance in his office. But—in Zhukov's words—"a rather anti-Semitic article was sent to *Pravda* from on high."

All these stories must obviously have some basis in reality. I did, however, find Borshchagovsky's assertion that some of Stalin's associates spoke out against him improbable. To the day he died they never dared contradict the Boss. The second story, therefore, seemed more plausible than the first.

But I saw no way whatsoever of checking these stories against actual events. No record of proceedings at meetings of the Bureau of the Presidium were kept at that time. All that happened was that particular members of the Bureau went into Stalin's office to deal with particular problems—and any such meeting might count as a meeting of the Bureau. Apart from which, as I have already said, no document concerning possible Soviet aggression would have been allowed to survive. It was not until July 1995 that a simple solution occurred to me: I would use once more an objective source which had already proved its value—the visitors' book from Stalin's office—to see what had happened in his office in the last February of his life.

It turned out that February 17 was the last day Stalin spent in his office. After that, he never appeared in the Kremlin again. One person whom he did receive that day was the Indian ambassador, Kumar Menon. But Vyshinsky was not present at their meeting. After the ambassador left, Beria, Malenkov, and Bulganin (newly promoted by the Boss) arrived in the office.

We find, however, that on February 7, from 6:00 to 6:45 P.M. the Argentinian ambassador, Bravo, was received in his office, and that Vyshinsky was present. When Vyshinsky left, Stalin's next visitors were his four closest aides—Malenkov, Beria, Khrushchev, and Bulganin. And the anti-Semitic article previously mentioned—"Simpletons and Scoundrels"—actually appeared in *Pravda* on the following day. February 7, then, was probably the day on which it all happened. The story, as I see it, is as follows.

It may very well be that the Argentinian ambassador raised the subject of the anti-Semitic campaign and that this was where Vyshinsky made his mistake: once he was alone with the Boss he probably complained that the doctors' trial created difficulties for Soviet diplomats. The Boss, more likely than not, made no reply. But when his associates arrived, he attacked Vyshinsky and alarmed them by saying: "If the imperialist gentlemen feel like going to war there is no more suitable moment for us than this."

He probably repeated this thought on subsequent occasions. Then, on February 17, Menon's visit reminded him of Vyshinsky, and he renewed his attack. This time he also vented his anger on his comrades-in-arms. This was possibly when the words "liquidate the imperialists" were first heard.

After February 17 no visitors to Stalin's office are recorded. In fact, he never returned to Moscow after that date. Someone has drawn a red line in the margins of the register, as though closing the account.

Visitors would, however, enter his office on March 2. In his absence.

CAESAR! BEWARE THE IDES OF MARCH!

March was drawing near.

According to rumor March 5 was the day on which the Jews would be loaded onto trucks. And Beria, needless to say, would realize that on March 5, the war which the Boss had in mind would almost be upon them. The second part of the program devised by the Boss would follow at once: the Terror, the great purge, in preparation for war. And that would be the end for all of them.

If Beria wanted to save himself he would have to hurry.

February was drawing to an end, and a sunny March was promised, like that March long ago when the Revolution had just begun, and he had stepped out onto the platform in Petrograd, full of hope . . . a sunny March. But he would not see it.

March 5 was the day on which he intended to lead the world into the Apocalypse, and to destroy the chosen people. But March 5 was the day on which he would close his eyes forever. It was his turn at last to discover that God does exist.

"And I will deliver my people out of your hands, and you shall know that I am the Lord."

28

I still remember that day in March. I remember the voice of Levitan, Moscow Radio's chief announcer, a menacing voice which people had come to associate with the Boss himself, reading the official bulletin on his illness. The country listened, numb with horror, to news of his white blood-cell count. So he had white blood cells just like the rest of us! Did this mean that death would dare to snatch him from us? People bombarded the newspapers with fantastic suggestions, even offering to give their own lives—what mattered was that he should live.

There is no end to the legends about his death. Even K. Simonov, the writer who was also a member of the establishment, knew nothing for certain. In 1979 he wrote, "A quarter of a century after the event I am still tormented by curiosity as to how he really died."

Yet even in the Khrushchev period people passed on in whispers the following story: The Boss did not die in the Kremlin, as stated in the official announcement, but at the nearer dacha. On the night of February 28–March 1 Stalin's guards summoned Beria to the nearer dacha by telephone. They said that "the Boss had not left his rooms for a suspiciously long time." Beria telephoned Khrushchev and Malenkov, and they went out there. They went into his room together and found him lying unconscious on the floor. But suddenly he stirred—and Khrushchev rushed up to him and began strangling him. The others joined in, and together they choked the tyrant. Beria had all Stalin's guards shot that same night. When the country was informed that Stalin was ill, he had in fact been dead for some time.

His life began with one mystery, and ended with another.

Witnesses Come Forward

The first testimony from genuine witnesses of Stalin's death was published in 1989, in D. Volkogonov's book. On the strength of a conversation with A. Rybin, one of Stalin's guards, Volkogonov confirms that Stalin died at the nearer dacha. Another member of his bodyguard, Starostin, found Stalin lying on the floor after a stroke.

I knew even then, however, that Volkogonov was wrong about Starostin. I had read Rybin's unpublished memoirs in the Museum of the Revolution. His manuscript contains some startling pages.

The Boss's Incredible Order

Rybin himself had not served in Stalin's guard since 1935, but on March 5, 1977, the anniversary of Stalin's death, he organized a little gathering. Those present included several members of the guard who had been at the nearer dacha around the time when Stalin died. He wrote down whatever these "officers for special missions attached to Stalin" (to give the watchdogs their official title) could tell him about the event. He first recorded matters on which they all agreed:

> On the night of February 28–March 1, members of the Politburo watched a film at the Kremlin. After this they were driven to the nearer dacha. Those who joined Stalin there were Beria, Khrushchev, Malenkov, and Bulganin, all of whom remained there until 4:00 A.M. The duty officers on guard that day were M. Starostin and his assistant Tukov. Orlov, the commandant of the dacha, was off duty, and his assistant, Peter Lozgachev, was deputizing for him.

M. Butusova, who looked after the Boss's linen, was also in the dacha. After the guests had left, Stalin went to bed. He never left his rooms again.

After this introductory note Rybin recorded separately the testimony of Starostin, Tukov, and Lozgachev. Starostin's statement was the briefest. "At 19:00 the silence in Stalin's suite began to alarm us. We (Starostin and Tukov) were both afraid to go in without being called." So they got Lozgachev to go in, and it was he who found Stalin lying on the floor near the table. But it was the recorded statements of Tukov and Lozgachev themselves that startled me. Starostin, it appeared, had omitted a surprising detail. Before going to bed Stalin had given his guards an incredible order. In Tukov's words: "When the guests left, Stalin told the servants and the commandants *'I'm going to bed, I shan't be wanting you, you can go to bed too.'* . . . Stalin had never given an order like that before."

So then the Boss, with his obsessive concern for his own security, suddenly *for the first time* orders his guards to go to bed. In effect, leaving his own suite unguarded. And that very night he suffers a stroke.

The main witness, Lozgachev, who was the first to see him lying on the floor after his stroke, bears out Tukov's statement. "Stalin said, 'I'm going to bed, you go to bed as well.' . . . I don't remember Stalin ever giving such an order—'everybody go to bed'—before."

I made up my mind to interview Peter Vasilievich Lozgachev.

THE MAIN WITNESS

He proved elusive. I rang him dozens of times. He kept changing his mind and putting off our meeting. He was afraid—they will all be afraid as long as they live. The "secret object" to which they were "attached" (they called themselves "the attached") had not lost its power over them. But my persistence was rewarded. Lozgachev finally agreed.

At his suggestion we met at a Metro station. Lozgachev was a short, broad-shouldered man, still robust in spite of his age. We sat on a bench with passengers bustling around us. I repeated what I had told him so often before: that his testimony was of great historical importance, that all his colleagues were now dead. . . . He listened attentively to the familiar words, thought a while, heaved a sigh, and then took me to a small apartment in a new building. I wrote down his statement in the tiny kitchen.

After typing up my text I visited him again and asked him to sign it. This time he was remarkably ready to oblige, put on his thick-lensed glasses, spent a long time reading the text, then signed at the bottom of the pages with a trembling hand.

Before getting around to that last day, Lozgachev told me a great deal about life at the nearer dacha. One episode seemed to me particularly interesting:

> Shortly before he died the Boss asked me: "What do you think—will America attack us or not?" I said, "I think they'd be afraid to." He flared up and said, "Clear out—what are you doing here anyway, I didn't call you." The guys said to me afterward: "What did you do to make him so angry today?" . . . Suddenly there was a call: go to the house. I went over, and his tone had changed completely: "Forget that I shouted at you," he said, "but just remember this: they *will* attack us, they're imperialists, and they

> certainly will attack us. If we let them. That's the answer you should give."

He was getting ready for the Apocalypse.

Lozgachev finally got around to that last night.

> I was on duty at the dacha. Orlov, the commandant, had just returned from leave, and was off duty. Those on duty in Stalin's quarters were the senior "special attachment," Starostin, his assistant Tukov, I myself, and Matryona Butusova. "The guests," as the Boss called members of the Politburo, were expected. As usual on such occasions we helped the Boss work out the menu. That night it included three bottles, I think it was, of Madzhari—that's a young Georgian wine, but the Boss called it "the juice" because of its low alcoholic content. . . . In the night the Boss called me in and said, "Give us another two bottles of the juice each." . . . Who was there that night? His usual guests —Beria, Malenkov, Khrushchev, and the other one with the beard, Bulganin. Some time later he called me in again: "Bring some more juice." We took it in and served it. Everything was quiet. There were no complaints. Then at 4:00 A.M. . . . or a bit later—we brought the guests' cars around. When the Boss saw his guests off, an "attachment" always saw them off with him, and closed the doors behind them. The "attachment" Khrustalev, when Ivan Vasilievich was closing the doors, saw the Boss, and the Boss said, "Go to bed, all of you, I don't need anything. I'm going to bed myself. I shan't need you today." Khrustalev came and told us, happily: "Well, guys, here's an order we've never been given before," and he repeated the Boss's words. It was true, in all the time I worked there that was the only occasion when Stalin said "go to bed." He usually said, "Want to go to bed?" and looked daggers at you. As if we'd dare! So of course, we were very glad when we got this order, and went off to bed without thinking twice.

"Wait a bit," I said. "Where does Khrustalev come into it? You didn't say that this Khrustalev was also at the dacha." Lozgachev replied, " 'Attachment' Khrustalev was at the dacha only till 10:00 A.M., then he went home to rest. He was relieved by Starostin, Mikhail Gavrilovich." We see now why Starostin did not tell Rybin about the Boss's strange order: he simply didn't know about it.

So then—that night at the nearer dacha only light wine was drunk, no cognac, no particularly strong drink likely to make him ill. The Boss, according to Lozgachev, was "amiable," whereas, Lozgachev also tells us, when he felt ill "his mood would change, and it was best not to go near him." But none of that matters much. The important thing is the surprising sentence that Lozgachev heard from the Boss for the first time ever—"go to bed, all of you."

To be precise, he heard it *not from the Boss but from the attachment Khrustalev. It was Khrustalev who passed on the order,* and left the dacha next morning. The order came as a surprise to Lozgachev and the other guard, Tukov, because the Boss insisted on strict observance of standing regulations. Those alleged words of his were a breach of his sacrosanct routine: they authorized the attachments *not* to guard his rooms. And not to keep an eye on each other.

Lozgachev said, "Next day was Sunday. At 10:00 A.M. we were all in the kitchen as usual, planning the day's work."

Lozgachev, then, obeyed the order, and conscientiously slept through to 10:00 A.M. He obviously could not know what his comrades were doing during the night. What, for instance, was Khrustalev doing, between transmitting the Boss's improbable order and leaving for home next morning? Lozgachev continued his account:

> At 10:00 A.M. there was "no movement" in his rooms—that was the expression we always used when he was sleeping. 11:00 A.M. came, 12:00—still no movement. It began to seem strange. He usually got up between 11 and 12, but he was sometimes awake as early as 10.
>
> 1:00 P.M. came, and there was still no movement. We began to be alarmed. 3:00 P.M., 4:00 P.M.—no movement. People may have been trying to ring him, but when he wanted to sleep his calls were usually put through to other rooms. I was sitting there with Starostin, and he said: there's something wrong, what shall we do? We wondered whether to go in there. But he had given the strictest possible orders that if there was "no movement" no one should enter his rooms. He would punish severely anyone who did. So we sat there in our staff quarters—which were connected with his rooms by a corridor twenty-five yards long, entered through a separate door—for six hours, wondering what to

do. Suddenly there was a ring from the sentry out in the street. "I see the light's gone on in the little dining room." Thank God, we thought, everything's all right. We were all at our posts, all ready for action . . . and still nothing happened! 8:00 P.M.—still nothing. We didn't know what to do. 9:00 P.M.—"no movement." 10:00 P.M.—still none. I said to Starostin—"You go, you're in charge of the guard, you ought to be getting worried." He said "I'm afraid." I said: "You're afraid—what do you think I am, a hero?" About then they brought the mail—a packet from the Central Committee. It was usually our job to take the mail straight to him. Or rather mine, the mail was my responsibility. Oh well, I said, I'll go, if anything happens, guys, don't let me down. I had to go. As a rule we were careful not to creep up on him, in fact you sometimes knocked on the door specially loudly, so that he'd hear you coming. He reacted very badly if you went into his rooms quietly. You had to walk with a firm step. You didn't have to look embarrassed, and you didn't have to stand at attention. If you did he'd say, "Why are you standing at attention like the good soldier Schweik?" Well then, I opened the door, and walked noisily along the corridor, and there's a room where we put the documents, just before you get to the little dining room, and I went into that room, and looked through the open door to the little dining room, and there was the Boss lying on the floor holding up his right hand like this [here Lozgachev showed me—crooking his arm and raising it slightly]. I was petrified. My hands and legs wouldn't obey me. He had probably not yet lost consciousness but he couldn't speak. He had good hearing, he'd obviously heard me coming, and probably raised his hand slightly to call me in to help him. I hurried up to him and said: "Comrade Stalin, what's wrong?" He'd—you know—wet himself while he was lying there, and was trying to straighten something with his left hand. I said, "Shall I call the doctor, maybe?" He made some incoherent noise—like "Dz—dz . . . ," all he could do was keep on "dz"-ing. His pocketwatch and a copy of *Pravda* were lying on the floor. When I picked the watch up the time it showed was 6:30, so 6:30 was when it must have happened to him. I remember there was a bottle of Narzan mineral water on the table, he'd obviously been going to get it when the light in his room went on. While I was questioning him, maybe for two or three minutes, he suddenly gave a little

> snore, like a man snoring in his sleep. I raised the receiver of the house phone. I was trembling, I broke into a sweat, I rang Starostin: "Come over quick, I'm in the house." Starostin came, he was dumbstruck, too. The Boss was unconscious. I said, "Let's put him on the sofa, it's uncomfortable for him on the floor." Tukov and Motya Butusova arrived after Starostin. We all helped to lift him onto the sofa. I said to Starostin: "Go and ring them all up—without exception." He went to ring. I didn't leave the Boss's side. He was lying motionless, just snoring. Starostin rang Ignatiev at the Ministry of State Security first, but Ignatiev was frightened and referred him to Beria and Malenkov. While he was ringing, we talked it over and decided to move him onto the large sofa in the big dining room. . . . We moved him because there was more air in there. We all helped put him on the sofa, and covered him with a rug, we could see he'd got very cold, lying there since 7:00 P.M. Butusova rolled his shirtsleeves down—he must have felt cold like that. In the meantime Starostin had put in a call through to Malenkov. Roughly half an hour later Malenkov rang us and said: "I haven't found Beria yet." Another half an hour went by, and Beria rang to say: "Don't tell anybody about Comrade Stalin's illness."

So an hour had passed, and still no one was hurrying to the dying (former) Boss. Only the attachments sat at his bedside, waiting.

Khrushchev's Version

Only one of Stalin's comrades-in-arms has described that nocturnal tragedy—Nikita Khrushchev. And a very strange story he tells.

> I suddenly got a call from Malenkov. "The Chekists" (he mentioned a name) "have rung from Stalin's place. They're very worried, they say something's happened to Stalin. We'd better get out there. I've already phoned Beria and Bulganin. Go straight out to Stalin's place, I'll be on my way, and so will the others." I called for a car immediately. . . . We agreed not to go straight up to the dacha, but to call at the duty room first.

So, according to Khrushchev, all four of last night's guests set off immediately.

> We looked in at the duty room and asked, "What's wrong?" They explained that Stalin always rang at about 11 in the evening, and asked for tea. . . . This time he hadn't. The Chekists said they'd sent Matryona Petrovna [Butusova] to reconnoiter—she waited at table, a person of very limited intelligence, but honest and devoted to Stalin. She came back and said that Comrade Stalin was lying on the floor, and that the floor under him was wet, he'd wet himself. The Chekists had picked Stalin up and put him on the couch in the little dining room. When they told us what had happened, and that he was now asleep, we thought that it would be rather embarrassing if we turned up there while he was in such an unseemly state. So we went back home.

According to Khrushchev, then, they went out there immediately, but tactfully withdrew, all four of them, when they were told about the Boss's "unseemly state."

Lozgachev told me otherwise: "At 3:00 A.M. I heard a car drive up." Nearly four hours had passed since that first telephone call. Lozgachev recounted:

> Beria and Malenkov had arrived. [And there was no Khrushchev!] Malenkov's shoes creaked, and I remember him taking them off and tucking them under his arm. They came in: "What's wrong with the Boss?" He was just lying there, snoring. . . . Beria swore at me, and said, "What d'you mean by it, starting a panic? The Boss is obviously sleeping peacefully. Let's go, Malenkov." I told them the whole story, how he was lying on the floor, and I asked him a question, and he could only make inarticulate noises. Beria said to me: "Don't cause a panic, don't bother us. And don't disturb Comrade Stalin." Then they left.

So, then—after declaring that a seventy-four-year-old man, who had been lying for 4 hours (or possibly longer) in a pool of his own urine, was "sleeping peacefully," his comrades-in-arms drove off, leaving the Boss still without help.

"I TOOK HIM OUT"

Lozgachev: "I was on my own again, I thought I'd better call Starostin and tell him to get them all up again. I said, 'Otherwise he'll die, and it'll be curtains for you and me. Ring and tell them to come.' "

N. Khrushchev: "After a short time there was another ring. Malenkov was on the line. He said, 'The boys have rung again from Comrade Stalin's place. They say there really is something wrong with Comrade Stalin. Matryona Petrovna did say, when we sent her in, that he was sleeping peacefully, but it isn't an ordinary sleep.' We shall have to go again. We agreed that the doctors would have to be called in."

Lozgachev: "Around 8:00 A.M. Khrushchev put in an appearance. [This then was his first appearance.] Khrushchev said, 'How's the Boss?' I said, 'Very poor, something's happened to him,' and told him the whole story. Khrushchev said, 'The doctors will be here right away.' I thought, 'Thank God!' The doctors arrived between 8:30 and 9:00 A.M.

He had been lying there, without help, for thirteen hours.

We will never know for sure what happened that night in the Boss's locked rooms. But there are only two possible versions. Either the Boss suddenly lost his mind, ordered everybody to bed, and then had a stroke in the night, or Khrustalev was ordered by *somebody* to send his subordinates to bed so that he, or someone unknown to us, could be alone with the Boss.

After Vlasik's arrest, Beria had of course recruited support for himself among Stalin's guard, which was no longer under proper supervision. The Boss had always thought he could count on Beria because he was a man of straw. He had miscalculated. Beria had seized his last chance of survival. Was it Khrustalev himself who ventured into the Boss's room? Or someone else? Perhaps they gave the Boss, who was fast asleep after his Madzhari, an injection? Perhaps the injection caused his stroke? Perhaps the Boss managed to wake up when he felt ill and tried to save himself? But the injection took effect before he got any farther than the table? If that is how it all happened we can easily understand why his henchmen so bravely refrained from rushing to his aid. It looks as though they *knew exactly what had happened,* and that the Boss was no longer dangerous.

Even if we prefer the first variant, the four of them calmly and *deliberately* denied Stalin help and left him to die.

In either case, then, they killed him. Killed him like the cowards they had always been. Beria had every right to say to Molotov—as Molotov later told Chuyev—"I took him out."

TIMETABLE OF A DEATH

Lozgachev explained: "Well, the doctors were all terrified. . . . They kept looking at him. . . . They were all trembling, like us. They had to examine him, but their hands were shaking. A dentist came to take out his false teeth, and they slipped out of his hands, he was so frightened. Then professor Lukomsky said: "We'll have to take his shirt off, to measure his blood pressure." I ripped open the shirt. They started measuring. Then they all took a good look and asked us who was there when he fell. We thought, This is it then, they'll put us in a car and it's goodbye—we're done for! But the doctors, thank God, came to the conclusion that he'd had a hemorrhage. Then a lot of people started arriving, and from that moment we were really out of it all. I stood in the doorway. There were crowds of people behind me, people who'd just come. I remember that Ignatiev, the minister, was afraid for some time to come in. I said, 'Come on in, there's no need to be shy.' "

On March 2 Svetlana was brought in, as she recalled: "They called Vasily in as well, but he was drunk and hurried off looking for the guards. I heard him out there in the staff quarters shouting that they'd killed Father. . . . Then he went off home. They applied leeches, and x-rayed his lungs. The whole Academy of Medical Sciences met to try and decide what else they could try. An artificial respirator was brought in. The clumsy machine stood there unused, while the young technicians looked goggle-eyed at what was going on around them."

He died in the atmosphere he had created, surrounded by fear and false pretenses.

His comrades-in-arms left him dying and drove to Moscow. Straight to his office.

The Boss's office had continued to function while he was dying. On March 2 at 10:40 A.M., according to an entry in Stalin's visitors' book, the trio who returned from the dacha—Beria, Malenkov, and Khrushchev—assembled there. The four who had fallen out of favor—Molotov, Mikoyan, Voroshilov, and Kaganovich—together with the other members of the Presidium, officeholders of the second rank, joined them. They began dividing his power among themselves, there in his office. After which Beria and Malenkov, together with the newly confident Voroshilov and Mikoyan, set out again for the dacha to keep an eye on the dying man.

At 8:30 P.M., according to the visitors' book, they reassembled in Stalin's office and continued discussing the division of power.

The following morning they returned to the dacha.

That was now their daily routine.

The eminent physician A. L. Myasnikov was one of the experts assembled to determine the cause of Stalin's death. He recalled that "Stalin lay there in a heap. He turned out to be short and rather fat. His face was contorted. . . . The diagnosis seemed clear—a hemorrhage in the left cerebral hemisphere resulting from hypertonia and sclerosis. . . . The consultants had to answer Malenkov's question: What is the prognosis? There could be only one answer: 'Death is inevitable.' "

He was helpless, scarcely breathing, close to death, but they still had need of him. Myasnikov recalled: "Malenkov gave us to understand that he hoped that medical measures would succeed in prolonging the patient's life 'for a sufficient period.' We all realized that he had in mind the time necessary for the organization of the new government and the preparation of public opinion. Stalin groaned from time to time. For just one short minute he seemed to be looking at those around him and recognizing them. Voroshilov said: 'Comrade Stalin, we are here—your loyal friends and comrades. How do you feel, dear friend?' But by then there was no expression on his face. On March 5 we spent the whole day giving injections and writing bulletins. Members of the Politburo approached the dying man's bedside. Those of lower rank looked in through the door. I remember that Khrushchev also kept to the doorway. The order of precedence was strictly observed. Malenkov and Beria were in front. Then came Voroshilov, Kaganovich, Bulganin, and Mikoyan. Molotov was unwell, but looked in briefly two or three times."

Molotov recollected: "I was called to the dacha. His eyes were closed, and whenever he opened them and tried to speak Beria rushed over and kissed his hand. After the funeral Beria said, 'The Coryphaeus of Sciences, eh?' and roared with laughter."

March Fifth

Svetlana described his last moments: "Father's death was slow and difficult. . . . His face was discolored and different . . . his features were becoming unrecognizable. . . . The death agony was terrible. It choked him slowly as we watched. At the last minute he opened his eyes. It was a terrible look—either mad or angry and full of the fear of death. . . . Suddenly he raised his left hand and seemed either to be pointing upward somewhere or threatening us all . . . then, the next moment, his spirit after one last effort tore itself from his body."

Each of those present had a different interpretation of that last gesture. The resuscitator G. Chesnokova said that, "the rhythm of his breathing changed abruptly, and signs of agitation appeared. His left hand rose as if in greeting. That was the death agony. Breathing ceased."

Lozgachev told me, "They say that when he died he raised his hand, as he had that other time, by the table, begging for help. . . . But who could help him!"

Myasnikov noted, "Death took place at 21:50."

Comrade Stalin Continues to Fight against Death

Svetlana wrote, "Beria was the first to rush out into the corridor, and in the quiet of the room where we were standing in silence we heard him say in a loud, undisguisedly triumphant voice: 'Khrustalev—the car!' . . . Valechka Istomina, with her round face and snub nose, rested her head on the deceased's breast and wept out loud." This note of Svetlana's has preserved for us Beria's triumphant voice—and the fact that he addressed himself to Khrustalev! Of all the attachments he singled out Khrustalev.

Beria was in a hurry. But the other comrades-in-arms stayed behind. To Beria, Stalin was just the Boss. To some of the others—Molotov, Kaganovich, Voroshilov—he meant their youth, the friends they had betrayed for him, their hopes, their very lives.

But they stayed only a little while before dashing to the Kremlin after Beria, to assume power. The Central Committee of the Party, the Council of Ministers, and the Supreme Soviet held a joint meeting in the Kremlin to legalize what *they* had already agreed on.

The writer Konstantin Simonov, although he was a member of the Supreme Soviet, believed, like the rest of the country, that Stalin was still alive:

> I arrived in the hall forty minutes early, but everybody was already there. We all believed that Stalin was lying somewhere nearby in the Kremlin, unable to recover consciousness. We all sat in complete silence. . . . I would never have believed that three hundred people sitting so closely together could remain so silent for forty whole minutes. I shall never forget that silence. They emerged from a door at the rear of the hall—the Bureau

> of the Presidium of the Central Committee, plus Molotov and Mikoyan. Malenkov made the introductory speech. The gist of it was that Stalin continued to struggle against death, but that even if he won the fight his condition would be so grave that. . . . The country could not be left without leadership. It was therefore necessary to form a new government.

They did as they were told. There was then no point in prolonging the farce. After the meeting Simonov went off to the *Pravda* offices. The editor's phone rang, and as he hung up he told Simonov that Stalin was dead. Lozgachev recalled: "They told us that they'd be taking him to the hospital right away to embalm him. Nobody called us in to say goodbye to the dead man, we went in without being asked. Svetlana was there briefly. Vasya was there too. I wouldn't say he was drunk, but he was overexcited. . . . Then a car came with a stretcher, they put him on it and carried him out, with me watching. And that was it. . . . There was nobody else there—only ourselves standing and watching." I asked Lozgachev whether it was correct that, as some people said, there was a bruise on the Boss's body, as if someone had pushed him. He said "There was no bruise, and there could be no bruise. . . . Nobody pushed him. *Khrustalev was there when they embalmed him*, and told us they'd found something like a cinder in his lungs. Maybe something had got in when they were piping oxygen in. Otherwise there was nothing." What, I asked, became of the attachments afterward? "Afterward they were all sent to different places. . . . One or another would be called in and sent out of Moscow—'leave the city immediately and take your family with you.' " But Starostin, Orlov, and Tukov decided to go and see Beria and ask him not to send them away. When they got to him he said: "If you don't want to be there—you'll be there (pointing at the ground)." So off they went.

What about Khrustalev? I asked Lozgachev. He replied, *"Khrustalev fell ill and died soon after.* Orlov and Starostin were posted to Vladimir, and I remained at the 'object'—the 'object' was vacant, and I was in charge of it. It was handed over to the Ministry of Health. . . . That was the end of the nearer dacha. . . . Valechka Istomina . . . was thirty-eight at the time, she used to look after him, see to his shirts and socks and linen, I don't know what else there may have been between them. She was a clever one, talkative, a chatterbox, I've seen her a few times since, she was sent away somewhere at first. Now she's in Moscow, married, with grandchildren."

Stalin lay in state in the Hall of Columns, and thousands of mourners took to the streets. Trainloads of people arrived from every town, to say goodbye to the God. His fellow citizens, who idolized him, and of whom he had destroyed more than all Russia's wars put together, trampled each other in the struggle to catch one last glimpse of him, to say farewell.

I remember that sunny day, I remember the girl standing in front of me. The crowd was crushing us. The militia were hemming us in, and we were suffocating. I remembered that girl's fear-crazed eyes. Suddenly something gave, and people began falling down. I found myself carried away, pinned between two sets of shoulders, stumbling over bodies, right out of the crowd, where I was flung onto the roadway. The skirt of my overcoat was torn, but I was alive. Thousands were carried off to mortuaries that day. He had refused to depart without a blood sacrifice. . . . The crushed mourners joined the millions he had destroyed in his lifetime.

On the day of Stalin's death, March 5, 1953, another death passed quite unnoticed—that of Sergei Prokofiev. His widow tried to get flowers, flowers of any sort, for his coffin. But everything was closed, nothing was being sold. Her neighbor took cuttings from all the indoor plants so that there would be something at least to lay on the great composer's coffin. Prokofiev's favorite pianist, Svyatoslav Richter, was flying from Tiflis at the time, to play beside the Leader's coffin in the Hall of Columns. It was a special plane, and it was crammed full of flowers. Richter was almost suffocated by their scent.

The Burial Commission was in permanent session, doing its utmost to immortalize the Leader: "The Commission deems it expedient to carry out the long-term embalmment of Comrade Stalin's body in the special laboratory of the Lenin Mausoleum. Comrade Stalin's body must be laid in the coffin in military uniform, with the medals of Hero of the Soviet Union and Hero of Socialist Labor, and also ribbons of his other decorations and medals, attached to his tunic. . . . A decree on the construction of a Pantheon should be drafted." Instructions to the embalmers specified that his shoulder boards, the buttons on his uniform, and his "hero's stars" must be of gold.

The sarcophagus containing the mummy of the second Bolshevik God stood outside the Mausoleum. On the Mausoleum stood the loyal comrades-in-arms who had killed him: Malenkov in a cap with ear flaps, Khrushchev in a squashed fur hat, Beria in a felt hat with the broad brim pulled down over his pince-nez, looking like a Hollywood mafioso. They joined in glorifying the murdered God.

After the funeral the Boss's comrades arranged for his son's apartment to be permanently bugged. The records of his conversations are in the President's Archive. We have Vasily talking to his chauffeur, Fevralev, about the funeral: "All those people crushed—it's terrible! I had a row with Khrushchev about it. . . . Something terrible happened in the House of the Unions. An old woman with a walking stick came in, Malenkov, Beria, and Molotov were standing in the guard of honor . . . and suddenly the old woman says, 'You killed him, you swine, now you can be happy! May you be damned!' " Three weeks after his father's death Lieutenant General of Aviation Vasily Stalin was discharged from the Soviet regular army without the right to wear military uniform. A month after that he was arrested. The once too-powerful general finally came out of prison only in the spring of 1961. He was banished to Kazan, where he died on March 19, 1962. Perhaps, following the tradition established by his father, someone helped him to die?

Beria, who had jailed Vasily, shortly followed him inside. A description of his execution has survived. "They tied his hands behind his back and attached him to a hook driven into a wooden board. Beria said, 'Permit me to say . . .' but the Procurator General said, 'Gag his mouth with a towel.' One protruding eye glared at them wildly over the blindfold. The officer pulled the trigger and the bullet struck him in the middle of the forehead." Malenkov, Molotov, Kaganovich—they all fell in turn. And last of all, Khrushchev.

While his henchmen were destroying each other, people in dirty padded jackets drifted over the expanses of Stalin's empire. The great deliverance from the camps was under way. Alexei Kapler, whom his daughter once loved, was one of those freed. Many years later he told me about it. "I went into a little park and stared stupidly at the children playing. One little boy ran past me, laughing—I saw his skinny, defenseless childish legs. And something happened to me. I burst into tears. I sobbed and sobbed shamelessly—enjoying it, like I used to in my childhood. I wept and wept . . . forgiving them . . . forgiving everybody."

Stalin himself, even after Khrushchev's denunciation, still lay in the Mausoleum. I remember when I first saw him: beside Lenin's doll-like head, his face was that of a living person. Stubble had grown on his cheeks.

Eight years went by before they could bring themselves to remove him. F. Konyev, Commander of the Kremlin Regiment, remembered the occasion.

October 31, 1961. Militia squads cleared Red Square and closed off all the entrances. When it was completely dark they finally got around to digging a grave by the Kremlin wall. . . . They transferred Stalin's body from the sarcophagus to a coffin lined with red cloth. He looked as if he was alive; the Mausoleum staff wept as they switched off the installation. They replaced the golden buttons with brass ones, and also removed his golden shoulder boards. Then they covered the body with a dark veil, leaving only his lifelike face uncovered. At 22:00 the Reburial Commission arrived. No relatives were present. . . . After a minute's silence we lowered him into the grave. We had orders to cover him with two concrete slabs [as if they feared that he might return from the grave]. But we just shoveled earth onto him.

End of an Age

Perestroika arrived, Gorbachev came to power, people began reviewing what they had lived through. I received a letter:

> My name is Yuri Nikolaevich Pepelyaev. I have long been curious about my family. Can you possibly give me detailed information about my relatives, and in particular:
>
> —Pepelyaev, N. M. Major General in the tsar's army, killed 1916, in the First World War.
>
> —Pepelyaev, V. N. President of the Council of Ministers in Kolchak's government, shot in 1920 at Irkutsk.
>
> —Pepelyaev, A. N. Lieutenant General, commanded Kolchak's First Siberian Army, then fought in the Far East, was forced to surrender. Sentenced to death and shot in 1938.
>
> —Pepelyaev, L. N. White officer, killed during the Civil War.
>
> —Pepelyaev, M. N. Staff Captain in the tsar's army, convicted in 1933, died in prison camp.
>
> —Pepelyaev, A. N. Surgeon in Kolchak's army, tried and convicted 1942, died in Siblag [a prison camp] in 1946.
>
> —Pepelyaev, A. I. Member of the Socialist Revolutionary Party, shot by the Cheka at Perm in 1918.
>
> —Pepelyaev, M. E. My grandfather, resident at Blisk, tried and convicted in the thirties.
>
> —Pepelyaev, M. I. Resident at Blisk, killed in the great Patriotic War [World War II].

Pepelyaev's letter is a concise history of Russia in the twentieth century.

Two of the Boss's faithful comrades-in-arms, Molotov and Kaganovich, lived on. They walked about the streets like ghosts. In his last years Molotov began to forget things. At times he imagined that he was Chairman of the Council of Ministers again, called for his suit and a tie, and sat waiting for Gorbachev's ministers to report to him. Not until 1986 did this man who had been born under Alexander III, lived under Nicholas II, worked with Lenin and Stalin, finally seek rest in the traditional Bolshevik red-lined coffin.

Kaganovich dragged on into the nineties. A relative of his told me: "He died in July 1991. The television was broadcasting the latest news of perestroika, showing Gorbachev and Yeltsin. The maid heard him say, 'It's a catastrophe.' When she looked around he was sitting in front of the television set dead."

Three weeks later, in August 1991, the crowd smashed statues of the God Lenin and broke windows in the sacred building of his Party's Central Committee. The USSR, the greatest of empires, built by the Boss to endure through the ages, was crumbling with bewildering rapidity.

The Tower of Babel and the Great Dream were no more.

Alas! alas! thou great city, thou mighty city, Babylon! In one hour has thy judgment come!

—Revelation 18:10

AFTERWORD

I thought that my book was complete, but something needs to be added.

In 1995 the new Russia celebrated the fiftieth anniversary of its victory over Germany. There was a victory parade, as in the past. But this time the man standing on the Lenin Mausoleum, where once the Boss had stood, was President Yeltsin. And a little green curtain hid the inscription "Lenin" on the Mausoleum. Western leaders, among them President Clinton and Prime Minister Major, stood in a group at the base of the Mausoleum. Standing there beside the Sacred Body they watched the veterans march past—the remnants of the great army which had defeated fascism, and which had, in its creator's mind, been destined to conquer the whole world.

Another procession coincided with the victory parade: a demonstration fifty thousand strong. Loudly singing songs from the Stalin era, they proceeded from the Belorussian Station, through the main streets of Moscow, to Mayakovsky Square.

For the first time since his death, dozens of portraits of Stalin floated by, held aloft over the heads of the demonstrators.

Yelling raucous slogans, Communists, monarchists, and Russian fascists marched side by side, at one in their devotion to the Boss.

And rightly so. Was he not a greater national-socialist than Hitler? Had he not created the greatest of monarchist cults and enlarged the empire of the Romanovs? And had he not served the Great Dream—a world in which Bolshevism reigned supreme?

Stalin had bided his time underground for over forty years. While those of his victims who had survived the horrors of his reign of terror died off one by one, and while their children grew old. . . . But now that the Great Amnesia had come upon the land, the Boss had risen from the grave.

People streamed past, with pictures of the Boss bobbing overhead, some of them bearing such eloquent inscriptions as "Jews Beware! Stalin Will Soon Return!"

The Russian religious philosopher Georgi Fedotov, writing at the end of the twenties, foretold with dread a time when "the obsessive malice at present concentrated on the construction of a godless Leninist International is directed instead to the creation of a nationalist and Orthodox Russia. . . . And the hand which today kills kulaks and the bourgeois will kill Jews and non-Russians. And man's black soul will remain as it was, or rather it will become blacker."

Those walking in the procession included priests in cassocks—also under portraits of Stalin.

Was Holy Russia preparing to rise again under a portrait of the Devil?

Fedotov's article, however, has an epigraph: "And Satan exults and mocks you, because you were called Christ's."

Yes, they are ready now to restore his empire, the bloody Babylon of yesterday. Surely it cannot happen again! The suffering and the bloodshed! Surely this unhappy land will have to learn yet again the truth of those words: "Woe, woe unto thee, thou mighty city Babylon, thou strong city!"

"I am the First and the Last, and besides me there is no other God."

SELECTED BIBLIOGRAPHY

ARCHIVAL SOURCES

ARCHIVE OF THE PRESIDENT OF THE RUSSIAN FEDERATION
Documents on security of party documents. F3 O22 D76,78,9.

STALIN'S PERSONAL ARCHIVE
Letters to his mother, E. G. Dzhugashvili. F45 O1 D1549.

Correspondence with his wife Nadezhda. F45 O1 D1550.

Letters from Nadezhda Alliluyeva to Maria Svanidze. F 44 O1 D1.

Letters from Nadezhda Alliluyeva to E. G. Dzhugashvili. F45 O1 D1549.

Letters from Svetlana to her father. F45 O1 D1551–1553.

Prosecution of Vasily Stalin. F45 O1 D1557–1558.

Record of interrogation of Yakov Dzhugashvili at HQ of Commander Aviation, Fourth Army [Translation from the German made for Stalin]. F45 O1 D1554.

Report from NKVD to I. V. Stalin on details of death of Yakov Dzhugashvili. F45 O1 D1555.

Letter from I. V. Sapegin to Vasily Stalin about Yakov Dzhugashvili. F45 O1 D1553.

V. Butochnikov's recollections of Yakov Dzhugashvili. F45 O1 D1554.

Report to Stalin from head of Kremlin Clinic on causes of death of Pavel Alliluyev. F45. O1 D1497.

Medical History ("History of Illness") of N. S. Alliluyeva. F45 O1 D155.

Medical History (History of Illness) of I. V. Stalin. F45 O1 D1482.

Diary of Maria Svanidze. F45 O1 D1.

Letter from Stalin to Politburo, March 21, 1923, on Krupskaya's request for potassium cyanide. F3 O22 D307.

Letter from Tukhachevsky to Stalin and his note on the reconstruction of the Red Army. F45 O1 D447–451.

I. V. Stalin's speech at session of the Military Council of the People's Commissariat of Defense, June 2, 1937. F45 O1 D1120.

Letter from Bukharin to Stalin on Mandelstam. F45 L1 D709.

Letters from Bukharin to Stalin immediately before and after his arrest. F3 O24 DD 236, 262, 270, 291, 301, 427.

Correspondence of I. V. Stalin with V. M. Molotov. F45 01 DD768, 769, 771. (Also *Kommunist,* No. 11/1990; *Izvestia,* Ts.K.KPSS Nos. 7, 9/1991. F45 O1 DD678, 769, 771.)

Letter from the teacher Martyshin to I. V. Stalin. F45 O1 D1552.

"Stalin's Visitors' Book" Nov.–Dec. 1934. F45 O1 D411. October 1939. F45 O1 D412.

Plenum of Central Committee of All-Union Communist Party (Bolsheviks). February 23–March 5, 1937. Stenographic report.

Plenum of Central Committee of Communist Party of Soviet Union. June 22–27, 1957. Stenographic report.

RUSSIAN CENTER FOR THE PRESERVATION AND STUDY OF DOCUMENTS RELATING TO MODERN HISTORY (FORMERLY CENTRAL PARTY ARCHIVE)

Documents on the birth of I. V. Dzhugashvili. F558 O1 D1–2.

P. Kapanadze's reminiscences: Stalin's childhood and adolescence. F558 O4 D669.

Materials on childhood and adolescence of Stalin. F7 O10 D213.

Recollections of various persons of meetings with Stalin during his time at the church school and the seminary. F558 O4 D665.

S. Y. Alliluyeva's manuscript: "In the Fire of Revolution." F558 O4 D668.

Recollections of S. Y. And A. S. Alliluyev on meetings with Stalin before the February Revolution. F558 O4 D659.

Memoirs of Fyodor Alliluyev, 1938–1946. F558 O4 D663.

Notification of death of Ekaterina Svanidze. F558 O4 D97.

Recollections of various persons of Stalin's period in exile at Turukhansk. F558 O4 D662.

Proceedings of the Executive Committee of Comintern: On Work Underground. F495 O3 D23–26.

Documents of the Commission of the Executive Committee of Comintern on Work Underground. F495 O27 D2.

N. Krupskaya: "The Last Year and a Half of Lenin's Life." F16 O3 D13.

Letter from Krupskaya to I. Armand on Lenin's illness. F12 O2 D254.

"Medical History of Comrade Krupskaya, N. K." F12 O1 D47.

Note of Maria Ulyanova on Lenin's attitude to Stalin. F14 O1 D398.

History of Stalin's illness in 1921. F558 O4 D675.

Memorandum on Comrade Dr. Julius Hammer and his son Armand Hammer. F2 O1 D24800.

Uglanov's testimony. F589 O3 D9354.

Letter from Stalin to L. Kamenev. F558 O2 D17.

Stalin's last letter to Lenin, March 7, 1923. F2 O1 D26004.

Fotieva's letter to Kamenev on Lenin's "Letter to the Congress." F5 O1 D276.

Letter from G. Dimitrov, Secretary General of Executive Committee of Comintern, and D. Manuilsky, Secretary of Executive Committee of Comintern, to Central Committee of All-Union Communist Party, October 10, 1937. F17 O120 D259.

Materials on Ordzhonikidze. F85 O1 D143.

BOOKS FROM I. V. STALIN'S PRIVATE LIBRARY WITH HIS ANNOTATIONS

Proof copy of *Short Biography of Stalin*, read and corrected by Stalin, 8.1.1947. F71 O10 D261.

Trotsky, L. D.: *Terrorism and Communism.* F558 O3 D364.

Kautsky, K.: *Terrorism and Communism.* F558 O3 D90.

Tolstoy, A.: *Ivan Grozny.* F558 O3 D350.

Stalin I. V.: "On Shortcomings in Party Work and Measures to Liquidate Trotskyists and Other Double-Dealers." F558 O3 D338.

STATE ARCHIVE OF THE RUSSIAN FEDERATION (FORMERLY CENTRAL STATE ARCHIVE OF THE OCTOBER REVOLUTION)

Report of Agent Fikus to the Police Department. F102.00 for 1910, 1911, 1912. D5 pt. 6, 1913. D5 pt. 7.

Secret instruction of Police Department on organization and conduct of internal surveillance by agents. F102.00 O308 D236.

Documents on Stalin's arrests and escapes. F102.00: 1898: D5–52/152–153; 1906: D145/2; 1906: D150; 1910: D5; 1911: D5–7 9b/50. [Also "Krasny Arkhiv," 1941, vol. 2, pp.12–13, and V. Nevsky, Materyaly dlya biograficheskogo slovarya sotsial-demokratov, no. 1. Petrograd and Moscow, 1923, p. 239.]

Collection of newspaper clippings on Bolshevik links with the Germans in 1917. F130-s O1 D1-a.

Instruction to the guard on V. I. Lenin's Kremlin office, January 22, 1918. F130 O2 D347, 347/18.

Zinoviev and Kamenev: pleas for clemency. F3316 O2 D1842.

Bukharin's pleas for clemency. F7253 O66 D58.

A. G. Korchagina's appeal for clemency to M. I Kalinin with her account of the circumstances of N. Alliluyeva's death. F3316 O2 D2016.

Y. E. Chadayev: V groznoye vremya. Ms. In State Archive collection.

M. S. Vlasik's plea for clemency. F7523 O107.

Comrade Stalin's personal files. F9401-a. O2. DD64, 66, 67, 97, 236, 269, 428.

On formation and work of Commission in connection with seventieth birthday of I. V. Stalin. F7523-S O65-c.

MUSEUM OF THE REVOLUTION (ARCHIVES)
A. T. Rybin: "Zhelezny soldat" (Iron Soldier). Ms. Vs 8920/12.

PUBLISHED PRIMARY SOURCES

Letters of Zinoviev and Bukharin to Stalin 1922–1923. *Izvestia Ts.K.KPSS*, no. 4, 1991.

"On Stalin's Meeting with His Mother." *Pravda* 23 & 27, October 1935.

"Stalin's Letter to Menzhinsky on Testimony of Ramzin, Kondratiev, and Chayanov. *Kommunist*, no. 11, 1990.

"Memoirs of N. S. Khrushchev." *Ogonyok*, nos. 27–37, 1988.

"Reabilitatsiya (Rehabilitation): Political trials of the 1930s–1950s," Moscow 1991. (In the book *Documents of the Politburo Commission on the Further Study of Materials Concerning the Repressions Which Took Place in the 1920s, 1940s, and Early 1950s: Letters of Zinoviev to Stalin at the Time of, and after His Arrest . . .*)

E. Polyanovsky: "Death of Osip Mandelstam." *Izvestia*, May 29, 1992.

E. Maksimova: "They Eavesdropped and Shot." *Izvestia*, June 16, 1992.

"E. Hoover's Letter on the Alleged Meeting of Hitler with Stalin." *Argumenty i Fakty* 11, 9, 1990.

"From the Unpublished Memoirs of Professor A. L. Myasnikov on Stalin's Death." *Literaturnaya Gazeta*, March 1, 1989.

"A. Brot's Recollections of Vasily Stalin." *Argumenty i Fakty*, April 14, 1991.

Proceedings of Joint Session of Central Committee, Council of Ministers and Presidium of Supreme Soviet, March 5, 1953. *Istochnik*, 1/1994.

Perespiska predstavitelei Soveta Ministrov SSSR s Prezidentami S.Sh.A i. Prem'er-Ministrami Velikobritanii (Correspondence of Representatives of Council of Ministers of USSR with Presidents of the USA and Prime Ministers of Great Britain). Moscow, 1976.

Arkhiv russkoy revolyutsii. Vols. 1–12. Moscow, 1991.

Istochnikovedenie istorii Velikogo Oktyabrya. Moscow, 1977.

Podgotovka i pobeda Oktyabryskoy revolyutsii v Moskve: Dokumenty i materialy. Moscow, 1967.

Protsess anti-sovetskogo Trotskistskogo tsentra. Moscow, 1937.

Sudebny otchet po delu anti-sovetskogo pravo-Trotskistskogo bloka. Moscow, 1938.

Protokoly Ts.K RSDRP, Avgust 1917–Fevral 1918. Moscow, 1958.

Shestoy S'ezd RSDRP(b): Protokoly. Moscow, 1958.

7 *Aprel'skaya Konferentsiya RSDRP(b)*. Moscow, 1958.

7 *S'ezd Rossiiskoy Kommunisticheskoy Partii (Bolshevikov): Stenograficheskii Otchet*. Moscow-Petrograd, 1923.

12 S'ezd Rossiiskoy Kommunisticheskoy Partii (Bolshevikov): Stenograficheskii Otchet. Moscow-Leningrad, 1926.

14 Konferentsiya Rossiiskoy Kommunisticheskoy Partii (Bolshevikov): Stenograficheskii Otchet. Moscow-Leningrad, 1925.

14 S'ezd VKP(b): Stenograficheskii Otchet. Moscow-Leningrad, 1926.

15 Konferentsiya Vsesoyuznoy Kommunisticheskoy Partii (Bolshevikov): Stenograficheskii Otchet. Moscow-Leningrad, 1927.

15 Konferentsiya Vsesoyuznoy Kommunisticheskoy Partii (Bolshevikov): Stenograficheskii Otchet. Moscow-Leningrad, 1928.

17 Konferentsiya Vsesoyuznoy Kommunisticheskoy Partii (Bolshevikov): Stenograficheskii Otchet. Moscow, 1934.

KRSS v Rezolyutslyakh i Resheniyakh S'ezdov, Konferentsii i Plenumov Ts.K. (1898–1971). 2nd ed. Vols. 1–7. Moscow, 1976.

Pervy Vserossiiskii S'ezd Sovetov. Moscow-Leningrad, 1932.

Tegeran, Yalta, Potsdam: Sbornik Dokumentov. Moscow, 1970.

Ezhenedel'nik Ch.K. 1918, 1–3.

Istoria Velikoy Otechestvennoy Voyny (1941–1945). Vols. 1–6. Moscow, 1960–1965.

Istoria Vtoroy Mirovoy Voyny (1939–1945). Vols. 1–12. Moscow, 1960–1965.

Vtoraya Mirovaya Voyna: Kratkaya Istoriya M. 1984.

Dokumenty po Istorii Grazhdanskoy Voyny. Vol. 1 M. 1940.

"Perelistyvaya Dokumenty Ts.K": Shornik Dokumentov. Volgograd, 1987.

Kratkaya Evreiskaya Entsiklopedia. Vol. 1. Jerusalem, 1975.

Istochnik [Journal], 1993–1995.

"Konets Veka." *Nezavisimy Almanakh* 4/1992.

"Skol'ko Zhiznei Unesla Voyna." *Argumenty i Fakty* 18–19/1995.

M. Egorov: *Kak Stroilos' Moskovskoye Metro. Nezavisimaya Gazeta*, May 13, 1995.

Fedotov G. P.: *Sud'ba i Grekhi Rossii*. Vol. 2. Moscow, 1992.

SECONDARY SOURCES

Abramov, A. *Nachalo revolyutsionnoy deyatelnosti Stalina 1894–1902*. Leningrad, 1939.

Akoyan, G. S. *Shaumyan: Zhizni'i deyatelnost'*. Moscow, 1973.

Aleksandrov, G. V. *Epokha i kino*. Moscow, 1976.

Alliluyev, S. *Proydenny put'*. Moscow, 1946.

Alliluyeva, A. S. *Vospominaniya*. Moscow, 1946.

Alliluyeva, S. *Tol'ko odin god*. Princeton, 1968.

Alliluyeva, S. I. *Dvadtsat' pisem k drugu*. Moscow, 1989.

Annenkov, Yu. P. *Vospominaniya o Lenine. Novy Zhurnal*, no. 65, 1961.

Armand, I. E. *Stat'i, Rechi, Pis'ma.* Moscow, 1975.

Arsenidze, R. "Iz vospomonanii o Staline." *Novy Zhurnal*, no. 72, 1963.

Avdeenko, A. O. *Nakazanie bez prestupleniya.* Moscow, 1991.

Avrekh, A. Ya. *Masony i revolyutsia.* Moscow, 1990.

Bagirov, M. *Iz istorii bolshevistskikh organizatsii Baku i Azerbaidzhana.* Baku, 1952.

Barbusse, A. *Stalin.* Moscow, 1936.

Batumskaya demonstratsiya 1902. Moscow, 1937.

Bazhanov, B. *Vospominaniya byvshego sekretarya Stalina.* Paris, 1990.

Berdayev, N. A. *Istoki smysl Russkogo kommunizma.* Paris, 1955.

———.*Russkaya religioznaya psikhologiya i kommunisticheskii ateizm.* Paris, 1931.

Berezhkov, V. M. *Kak ya stal perevodchikom Stalina.* Moscow, 1993.

Bol'sheviki: Dokumenty po istorii bol'shevizma byvshego Moskovskogo okhrannogo otdelenia. Telex. New York, 1990.

Bonch-Bruyevich, V. D. *Moi vospominaniya.* Leningrad, 1933.

Bukharin, N. I. *Izbrannye proizvedeniya.* Moscow, 1988.

———.*Zapiski ekonomista. Pravda*, September 30, 1930.

Bunin, I. A. *Okayannye dni.* Moscow, 1990.

Burlatskii, F. M. *Mao-Tze Dun.* Moscow, 1976.

Buyanov, N. I. *Lenin, Stalin i psikhiatriya.* Moscow, 1993.

Chalidze, V. *Pobeditel' Kommunizma.* Paris, 1981.

Chudakova, M. O. *Zhizneopisanie Mikhaila Bulgakova.* Moscow, 1988.

Chuyev, F. I. *Sto sorok besed s Molotovym.* Moscow, 1988.

David, I. *Istoria Evreev na Kavkaze.* Vols. 1–2. Tel Aviv.

Deich, G. M. *Evreiskie predki Lenina.* Moscow, 1991.

Deti o Staline. Moscow, 1939.

Dzhilas, M. *Litso Totalitarizma.* Moscow, 1992.

Erenfeld, B. K. "Delo Malinovskogo." *Voprosy Istorii* 7, 1965.

Ezhevskii [Jerzewski], L. *Katyn.* Telex. New York, 1985.

Ezhov, N. I. *Rech'na sobranii izbiratelei.* Moscow, 1990.

Fadeev, A. *Vstrecha s tovarishchem Stalinym.* Moscow, 1939.

Fel'tishinski, Yu. *Razgovory s Bukharinym.* New York, 1991.

Feuchtwanger, L. *Moskva 1937.* Moscow, 1937.

Gippius, Z. *Peterburgskie dnevniki.* Telex, 1982.

Gorky, M. *Nesvoevremennye mysli.* Moscow, 1990.

Gorodetskii, E. I. *Is istorii oktyabr'skogo vooruzhennogo vosstaniya i 2-ogo s'ezda sovetov. Voprosy Istorii* 10, 1957.

Gronsky, I. M. *Iz proshlogo*. Moscow, 1991.

Iosif Vissarionovich Stalin: Kratkaya biografiya. Moscow, 1939. 2nd ed. Moscow, 1947.

Istoriki otvechayut na voprosy: sbornik. Vypuski pervy-vtoroy. Moscow, 1988–1990.

Ivanitskii, V. *Klassovaya bor'ba v derevne i likvidatsiya kulachestva kak klassa*. Moscow, 1972.

Ivanov, V. *Marshal Tukhachevskii*. Moscow, 1985.

I. V. Stalin v tsarskoy ssylke na severe. Arkhangel, 1936.

I. V. Stalin v sibirskoy ssylke. Krasnoyarsk, 1942.

Kanal Imeni Stalina. Moscow, 1934.

Karabinova, S. *Istoricheskie mesta Tbilisi, Svazannye s zhizn'yu i deyatelnost'yu I. V. Stalina*. Tbilisi, 1944.

Khlebnyuk, O. V. *Stalin, NKVD i Sovetskoye Obshchestvo*. Moscow, 1992.

Khrushchev o Stalin. New York, 1989.

Kolesnik, A. *Khronika zhizni sem'i Stalina*. Moscow, 1990.

Kommunisticheskaya oppozitsiya, 1923–1927. Vols. 1–4. Chalidze Publications, 1988.

Korolenko, V. G. *Pis'ma k Lunacharskomu*. Paris, 1922.

Koznov, A. P. *Bor'ba bolshevikov s podryvnymi aktsiyami tsarskoy okhranki. Voprosy Istorii,* Kpss 9, 1988.

Krasnaya, *Kniga V.Ch.K*. Vols. 1–2. Moscow, 1922.

Krasny, A. *Tainy okhranki*. Moscow, 1917.

Krasny terror v Rossii. New York, 1991.

Krupskaya, N. *Vospominaniya o Lenine*. Moscow, 1989.

Lapshin, V. P. *Khudozhestvennaya zhizn' Petrograda i Moskvy v 1917 godu*. Moscow, 1983.

Larina (Bukharina), A. *Nezabyvaemoe*. Moscow, 1989.

Lenin v pervye mesyatsy sovetskoy vlasti. Moscow, 1933.

Lenin v 1917. Moscow, 1967.

Lunacharskii, A. V. *O Vladmire Ilyiche*. Moscow, 1983.

———.*Siluety*. Moscow, 1991.

Lutskii, E. A. *Zasedanie Ts.K. RSDRP(b) noch'yu 24–25 Oktabrya. Voprosy Istorii,* KRSS 11, 1986.

Makharadze, F. *K 30-letiyu Tiflisskoy organizatsii*. Tiflis, 1925.

Mandelstam, N. Ya. *Vospominaniya*. Moscow, 1989.

Maryamov, G. *Kremlevskii tsenzor*. Moscow, 1992.

Matskevich [Mackiewicz], J. *Katyn*. London, 1988.

Medvedev, R. *Oni okruzhali Stalina*. Paris, 1984.

Melgunov, S. P. *Zolotoy nemetskii klyuch bol'shevikov.* New York, 1989.
"Men'sheviki." Paris, 1988.
Meretskov, K. A. *Na sluzhbe narodu.* Moscow, 1968.
Merezhkovskii, D. *Gryadushchii kham.* Petersburg, 1914.
Mikoyan, A. I. *Istoria velikogo Oktyabrya.* Vols. 1–3. Moscow, 1968.
"Minuvshe": Istoricheskii Al'manakh. Nos. 1–11. Paris, 1988–1991.
Mondich, M. "Smersh." Paris, 1984.
Moskalev, M. *Russkoye byuro Tsk.RSDRP(b).* Moscow, 1947.
Neizvestnaya Rossiya, 20 vek. Moscow, 1992.
Oktyabr'skoye Vooruzhennoye Vosstanie v Petrograde. Leningrad, 1956.
Orlov, A. [L.L. Fel'dbin]. *Tainaya istoriya stalinskikh prestuplenii.* Moscow, 1991.
Pavlov, P. *Provokatory, zhandarmy, palachi.* Petrograd, 1922.
Peregudov, Z. *Metody bor'by departamenta politsii.* "Fakel"-Al'manakh, 1990.
Radek, K. B. *Iz vospominanii. Krasnaya,* November 10, 1926.
———.*Portrety i pamflety.* Moscow, 1933.
"Raketnaya izgorod' vokrug Moskvy." *Moskovskii Komsomolets,* May 28, 1993.
Rapoport Ya. L. *Na rubezhe dvukh epokh: delo vrachei 1953.* Moscow, 1988.
Raskol'nikov F. F. *Kronstadt i Piter v 1917 godu.* Moscow-Leningrad, 1925.
———.*Na boevykh postakh.* Moscow, 1964.
Rasskazy starykh rabochikh zakavkaz'ya o velikom Staline. Moscow, 1937.
Reisner, L. *Izbrannye proizvedeniya.* Moscow, 1956.
Rokossovskii, K. K. *Soldatskii dolg.* Moscow, 1968.
Rossiya pered vtorym prishestviem. Svyato-Troitskaya Lavra, 1993.
Rozanov, G. A. *Stalin, Gitler.* Moscow, 1991.
Rybin, A. T. *Ryadom so Stalinym.* Moscow, 1992.
Ryutin, M. N. *Na koleni ne vstanu.* Moscow, 1991.
Savinkov, B. *Izbrannoye.* Moscow, 1990.
Serebryakov, A. G. "Vospominaniya." *Rodina* 6, 1990.
Shaposhnik, V. *Severno-Kavkazskii voenny okrug.v 1918 godu.* Rostov-on-Don, 1990.
K shestidesyatiletiyu so dnya rozhdeniya I. V. Stalina. Moscow, 1940.
Shitts, I. I. *Dnevnik velikogo pereloma.* Paris, 1991.
Shlyapnikova, G. *Kanun 17-ogo Goda.* Vols 1–2. Moscow, 1923.
Shok ot pakta mezhdu Gitlerom i Stalinym: vospominaniya sovremennikov. Paris, 1989.
Shtein, A. P. *I ne tol'ko o nem.* Moscow, 1990.
Shtemenko, S. M. *Generalny Shtab v gody voyny.* Moscow, 1968.
Shveitser, V. *Stalin v turukhanskoy ssylke.* Moscow, 1940.

Simonov, K. M. *Glazami cheloveka moego pokoleniya.* Moscow, 1990.
Slasser, R. *Stalin v 1917.* Moscow, 1989.
Somov, K. A. *Pis'ma, dnevnik.* Moscow, 1979.
Spiridovich, A. I. *Zapiski, zhandarma.* Moscow, 1991.
Spirkin, A. *Voprosy yazyka i myshleniya v svete rabot t. Stalina.* Moscow, 1931.
SSSR-Germaniya 1939–1941. New York, 1989.
Stakhanov, A. *Rasskaz o moei zhizni.* Moscow, 1938.
Stalin, I. V. SOCHINENIYA. Vols. 1–13. Moscow, 1946–1951.
———.*Beseda s angliiskim pisatelem G. Uellsom.* Moscow, 1934.
———.*Ekonomicheskie problemy sotsializma v SSSR.* Moscow, 1952.
———.*Marksizm i voprosy yazykoznaniya.* Moscow, 1953.
———.*O Lenine.* Moscow, 1921.
———.*O trekh osobennostyakh krasnoy armii.* Moscow, 1949.
———.*O velikoy otechestvennoy voyne.* Moscow, 1950.
Starostin. *Futbol skvoz' gody.* Moscow, 1989.
Sukhanov, N. N. *Zapiski o revolyutsii.* Vols. 1–7. Berlin, 1922–1923.
Suvorov, V. *Ledokol.* Moscow, 1992.
Takker, R. *Stalin-put' k vlasti.* Progress, 1990.
Trepper, L. *Bol'shaya igra.* New York, 1989.
Trifonov, Yu. *Sobranie sochinenii.* Vol. 4, p. 144.
Trotsky, L. *Dnevniki i Pis'ma.* New York, 1986.
———.*K Istorii Oktyabrskoy Revolyutsi.* New York, n.d.
———.*Moya Zhizn'.* Moscow, 1991.
———.*O Lenine.* Moscow, 1924.
———.*Stalin.* Vols. 1–2. Chalidze Publications, n.d.
———.*Stalinskay Shkola Fal'sifikatsii.* Berlin, 1932.
———.*Uroki Oktyabrya.* Moscow, 1925.
Valentinov, N. V. *Nasledniki Lenina.* Chalidze Publications, 1990.
———.*Nep i krizis partii.* New York, 1991.
———.*O Lenine.* New York, 1991.
V.CH.K-G.P.U. Chalidze Publications, 1989.
Viktorov, V. V. *Bez grifa sekretno: zapiski voennogo prokurora.* Moscow, 1990.
Vishnyak, M. *Dan' proshlomu.* Paris, 1954.
Volkogonov, D. A. *Lenin.* Moscow, 1994.
———.*Stalin.* Moscow, 1989.
Volkov, A. *Petrogradskoe okhrannoe otdelenie.* Petrograd, 1917.
Voroshilov, K. E. *Stalin i krasnaya armia.* Moscow, 1937.

Vozhd' Lenin, kotorogo my ne znali. Saratov, 1992.

Vozvrashchennye imena. Bks. 1–2. Moscow, 1984.

Yaroslavskii, E. *O tovarishche Staline*. Moscow, 1939.

Zbarskii, B. I. *Mavzolei Lenina*. Moscow, 1994.

Zhordaniya, N. *Moya zhizn*. Paris, 1968.

Zhukhrai, V. *Tainy tsarskoy okhranki*. Moscow, 1991.

Zhukov, G. K. *Vospominaniya i razmyshleniya*. Moscow, 1969.

Zinoviev, G. *Leninizm*. Leningrad, 1925.

BOOKS IN ENGLISH

Balabanoff, A. *Impressions of Lenin*. Ann Arbor, 1964.

Conquest, R. *The Great Terror.* New York, 1968.

———.*Stalin*. London, 1991.

Deutscher, I. *Stalin: A Political Biography.* New York, 1967.

Fischer, L. *The Life of Lenin*. New York, 1964.

Goldberg, B. *The Jewish Problem in the Soviet Union*. New York, 1961.

Laqueur, W. *Russia and Germany.* Washington, D. C., 1991.

Leonhard, W. *Child of the Revolution*. London, 1957.

Meir, G. *My Life*. London, 1975.

Pinkus, B. *The Jews of the Soviet Union*. Cambridge, 1988.

Piper, R. *Russia Under the Bolshevik Regime*. New York, 1994.

Schapiro, L. *The Communist Party of the Soviet Union*. New York, 1960.

Shirer, W. *The Rise and Fall of the Third Reich*. New York, 1959.

Smith, E. *The Young Stalin*. New York, 1967.

Souvarine, B. *Stalin*. New York, 1939.

Tucker, R. C. *Stalin as Revolutionary: A Study in History and Personality.* New York, 1973.

Ulam, A. B. *Stalin: The Man and His Era*. New York, 1973.

INDEX

o a potential second Holocaust. Radzinsky also takes an intimate look at Stalin's private life, marked by his turbulent relationship with his wife Nadezhda, and re-creates the circumstances that led to her suicide. Finally Radzinsky discovers one of Stalin's elite bodyguards, who breaks forty years of silence to give the strongest evidence yet of the conspiracy behind Stalin's death.

As he did in the *The Last Tsar*, Radzinsky thrillingly brings the past to life. The Kremlin intrigues, the ceaseless round of double-dealing and back-stabbing, the private worlds of the Soviet Empire's ruling class—all become, in Radzinsky's hands, as gripping and powerful as the great Russian sagas. And the riddle of that most cold-blooded of leaders, a man for whom nothing was sacred in his pursuit of absolute might—and perhaps the greatest mass murderer in Western history—is solved.

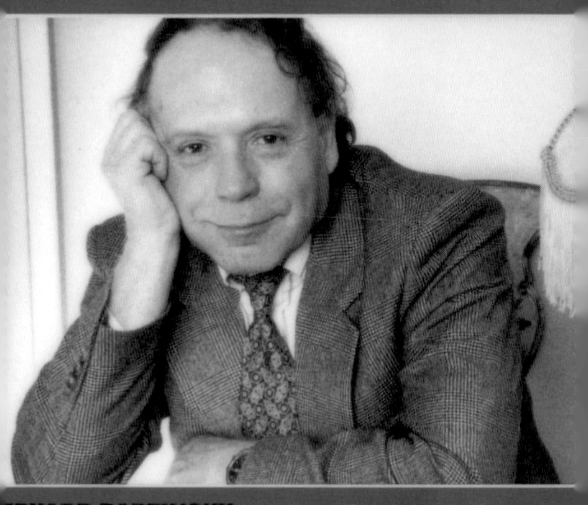

EDVARD RADZINSKY is, after Chekhov, Russia's most frequently staged playwright, and his plays have won him international acclaim. A trained historian, Radzinsky labored for twenty-five years to produce the international bestseller *The Last Tsar*. He is also known in Russia as a popular television personality.